FORT WORTH LIBRARY
P9-BZU-914

The Deliciously Keto Cookbook

Molly Pearl and Kelly Roehl, MS, RD, LDN, CNSC

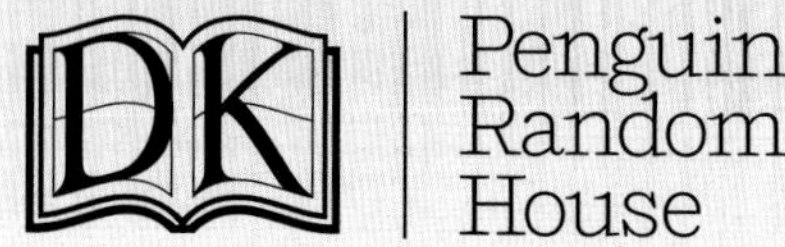

Publisher: Mike Sanders
Associate Publisher: Billy Fields
Senior Acquisitions Editor: Brook Farling
Development Editor: Kayla Dugger
Cover and Book Designer: William Thomas
Photographer: Molly Pearl
Food Stylist: Jason Peters
Illustrator: Clint Ford
Prepress Technician: Brian Massey
Proofreader: Cate Schwenk
Indexer: Celia McCoy

First American Edition, 2016
Published in the United States by DK Publishing
6081 E. 82nd Street, Indianapolis, Indiana 46250

Copyright © 2016 Dorling Kindersley Limited

A Penguin Random House Company

16 17 18 19 10 9 8 7 6 5 4 3 2 1

001–295790–November/2016

All rights reserved.

Without limiting the rights under the copyright reserved above, no part of this publication may be reproduced, stored in or introduced into a retrieval system, or transmitted, in any form, or by any means (electronic, mechanical, photocopying, recording, or otherwise), without the prior written permission of the copyright owner.

Published in the United States by Dorling Kindersley Limited.

ISBN: 978-1-46545-439-3

Library of Congress Catalog Card Number: 2016938282

Note: This publication contains the opinions and ideas of its authors. It is intended to provide helpful and informative material on the subject matter covered. It is sold with the understanding that the authors and publisher are not engaged in rendering professional services in the book. If the reader requires personal assistance or advice, a competent professional should be consulted. The authors and publisher specifically disclaim any responsibility for any liability, loss, or risk, personal or otherwise, which is incurred as a consequence, directly or indirectly, of the use and application of any of the contents of this book.

Trademarks: All terms mentioned in this book that are known to be or are suspected of being trademarks or service marks have been appropriately capitalized. Alpha Books, DK, and Penguin Random House LLC cannot attest to the accuracy of this information. Use of a term in this book should not be regarded as affecting the validity of any trademark or service mark.

DK books are available at special discounts when purchased in bulk for sales promotions, premiums, fund-raising, or educational use. For details, contact: DK Publishing Special Markets, 345 Hudson Street, New York, New York 10014 or SpecialSales@dk.com.

Printed and bound in China

www.dk.com

Contents

Introduction

We live in a toxic food environment in which making healthy choices feels nearly impossible. It's all about convenience, speed, and more. This has led to rising rates of obesity and chronic disease.

What This Book Covers

While most of us are familiar with the old food guide pyramids and the newer plate renditions released by health and government institutions, many have become frustrated with lack of improvement in health despite following these guidelines. This is largely due to the food environment in which we live, as well as a general lack of knowledge of what food is and how to actually prepare it. It's easier and more convenient for us to hit the drive-thru or microwave a prepared meal than to start from scratch, which is what influences those rises in obesity and chronic disease. However, the message to eat less processed food is not enough to promote change—we need a diet that dramatically alters the inflammation and damage caused by a diet of excess sugar and processed fat.

What if I told you there is such a diet, and that by following it, you may actually see improvements in your health? What's more, the diet doesn't limit fat—it actually encourages it? If you're looking to lose weight, lower your blood glucose, impact your neurological health, or just overall feel better, the ketogenic diet (also known as the *keto diet*) is sure to help!

The keto diet has been one of the hottest areas of research within the nutrition, health, and medical community. While many have understood the benefits of the keto diet for years, these benefits are just beginning to be recognized by the medical community—and the health-conscious public is beginning to take notice!

The keto diet is a low-carbohydrate, high-fat, moderate-protein diet that helps transition your body from using sugar or glucose for energy to becoming a fat-burning machine. As you remove high-carbohydrate foods from your diet, your blood sugar will dramatically decline and your body will begin to break down fat for energy, producing ketones that can be used by nearly every cell in the body. This process causes weight loss, decreased cravings and bloating, and improved mental clarity.

This book offers a how-to guide to help you get started on a keto diet, as well as a collection of delicious recipes that were developed with keto philosophies in mind and analyzed by a registered dietitian nutritionist so you can be confident in your keto choices. It's time to embrace not only a diet, but a new and healthy way of life!

Special Thanks to the Technical Reviewer

The Deliciously Keto Cookbook was reviewed by an expert who double-checked the accuracy of what's presented here to help us ensure learning about the keto diet is as easy as it gets. Special thanks are extended to Carolyn Doyle.

Disclaimer

When starting this diet, you should first discuss your plans with your doctor—particularly if you're pregnant or breastfeeding, have kidney disease, or are taking insulin for diabetes. Your doctor and a registered dietition can also help you understand how the diet affects certain baseline risk factors, such as cholesterol levels, diabetes risk, waist circumference, weight, and body mass index.

Getting Started

A ketogenic diet allows you to lose weight, enhance your mental clarity, and improve your overall health without feeling deprived. But how does it work? The first section of this book explains the keto diet, including the benefits of following it; the role of protein, fat, and carbohydrates in your meals; common misconceptions associated with the diet; and ways to achieve success. Once you have a good understanding of how it all works, you'll be able to confidently dive in and enjoy eating the keto way.

What Is a Ketogenic Diet?

Ketogenic diets—often referred to as *keto diets*—are composed of foods low in carbohydrates, high in fat, and adequate in protein to help you maintain a healthy body.

The Nature of the Ancient Human Diet

Historically, humans haven't always had a constant source of food (think hunter-gatherer days). This caused our bodies to become more efficient at conserving energy for use during a time when food was scarce–hence the reason we pack excess calories, or energy, away as fat when we eat more than we need. Although we have evolved to become a highly productive species with ample food availability, our bodies remain physiologically nearly identical to those of our hunter-gather ancestors.

While the diet of our ancestors isn't 100 percent certain, we do know it was a combination of foods that were easy to hunt and gather–such as animals, leafy plants, and nuts–that likely required little time or work to prepare and eat. These were primarily fat, protein, and fiber-rich plants. On the other hand, high-carbohydrate foods like grains, root vegetables, and seasonal fruits were likely a small part of the diet of our hunter-gatherer ancestors due to the need for heat to be edible.

This lack of carbohydrates caused human bodies to become hard-wired to seek carbohydrates and store them for use during a time of need–in other words, a period of days or longer where food is scarce and we're forced to rely on our stored energy, or fat. The only problem is, most humans today rarely go without food for 12 hours, let alone days or weeks. In the current food environment, many of us have access to endless amounts of calories in an easy-to-consume form–and we typically eat too many.

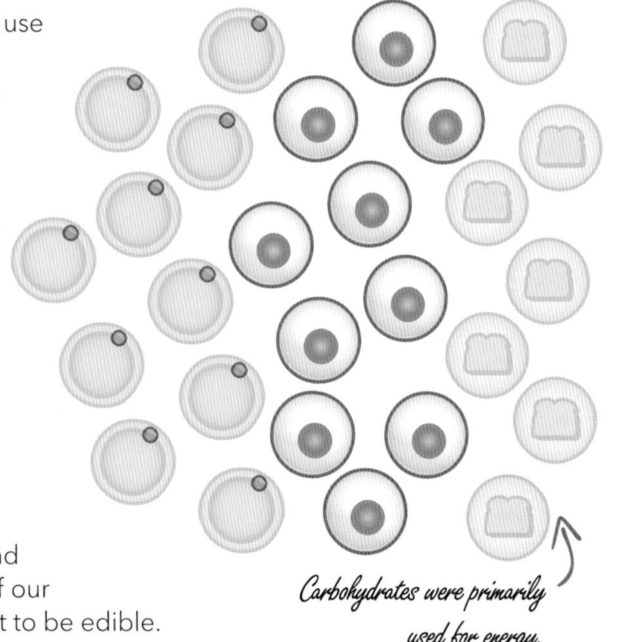

HOW THE BODY USED MACRONUTRIENTS ON AN ANCIENT HUMAN DIET

Because carbohydrates were rare in prehistoric times, bodies became hard-wired to use carbohydrates for energy and store fat. That way, when food was scarce, the body could feed off the stores of fat.

Fat (30%)
Protein (15%)
Carbohydrates (55%)

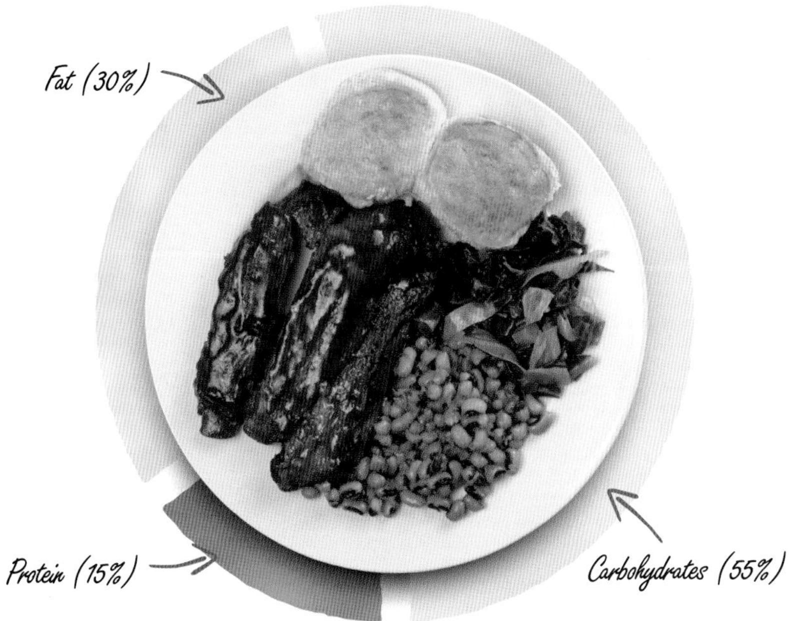

A MODERN WESTERN PLATE
In the modern diet, carbs make up more of the macronutrient intake than fat and protein combined.

Protein (20%)
Carbohydrates
(5)%)
Fat (75%)

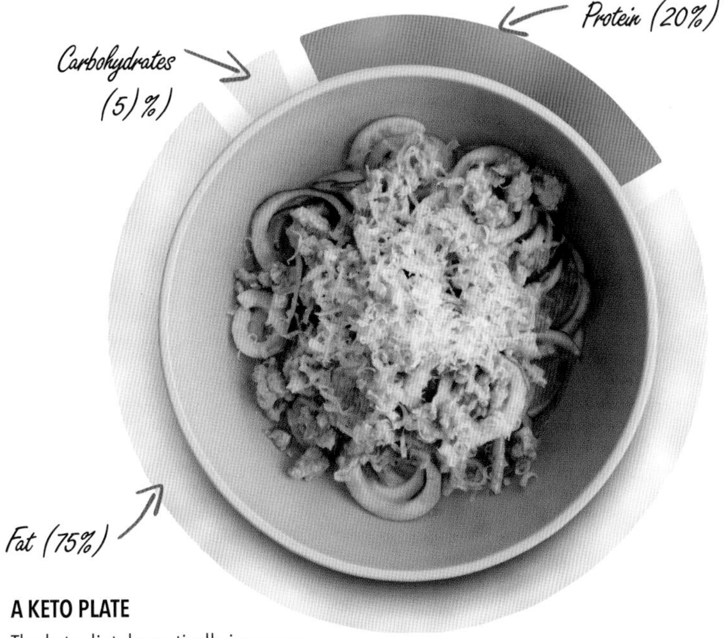

A KETO PLATE
The keto diet dramatically increases fat intake and significantly decreases carbohydrate intake.

How Is a Keto Diet Different?

While carbohydrates, proteins, and fats—also known as *macronutrients*—provide benefits to the human body in certain settings, the right amount of each type of macronutrient in terms of calories remains up for debate. In the modern Western diet, carbohydrates make up about as much of the calories as proteins and fats combined. However, in a keto diet, fats make up a very large portion of the calories, with proteins and carbohydrates incorporated in significantly smaller amounts. This makeup encourages your body to rely on your stored fat rather than glucose (sugar) from carbohydrates for energy, potentially preventing excessive weight gain and promoting overall improvements in health.

The focus of the keto diet is to eat just enough protein to meet your body's needs; limit carbohydrates to those that are rich in vitamins, minerals, color, and fiber to help maintain a healthy gastrointestinal (GI) tract; and incorporate higher amounts of fat into your diet to meet your energy needs. This will cause your body to use fat instead of sugar for energy in the form of ketones—hence the name of the diet.

Benefits of a Keto Diet

Whether you're looking to lose weight, gain more energy, improve your neurological health or sleep, or just feel better overall, the keto diet is a powerful tool that can have a significant impact on your life!

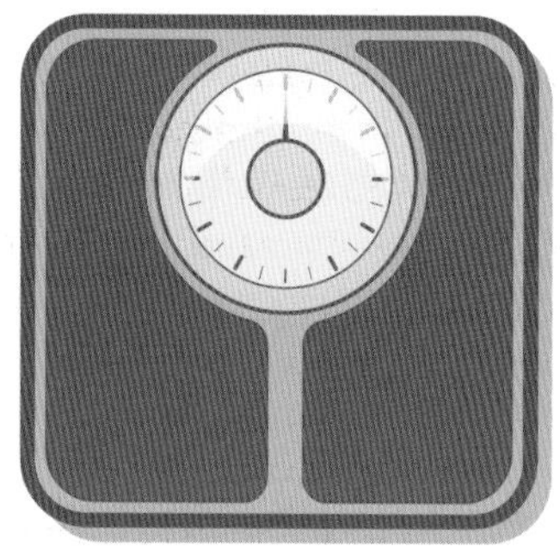

Weight Loss

When you eat a high-carbohydrate diet, your blood glucose is elevated, leading to the release of insulin. This process sends a signal to your body to store energy as glycogen, which is then converted to fat. This can lead to abdominal obesity, a condition in which fat is stored in your stomach area—a risk factor for diabetes and heart disease. A keto diet prevents your body from releasing too much insulin, and instead encourages your body to burn fat for energy. This fat burning helps shrink your waistline and avoid many of those health risk factors—a win-win!

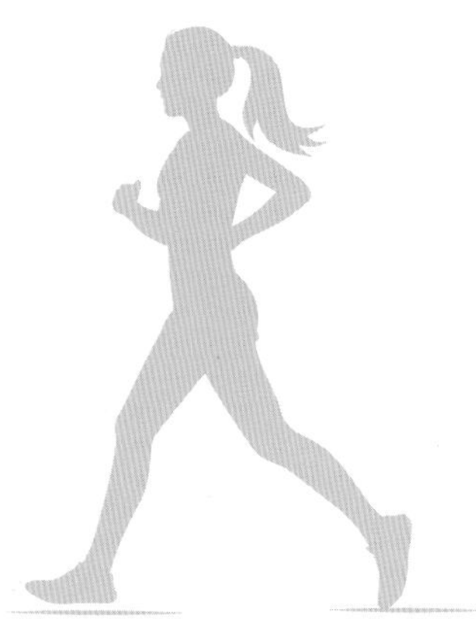

Steady Energy

As you learned earlier, unlike glucose (which is more concentrated in the liver and muscle and is generally limited to less than 1,000 calories total or converted to body fat for use later), ketones are utilized by many different parts of the body for energy. This gives your body a steady source of energy rather than the up-and-down energy you get from eating a high-carbohydrate diet.

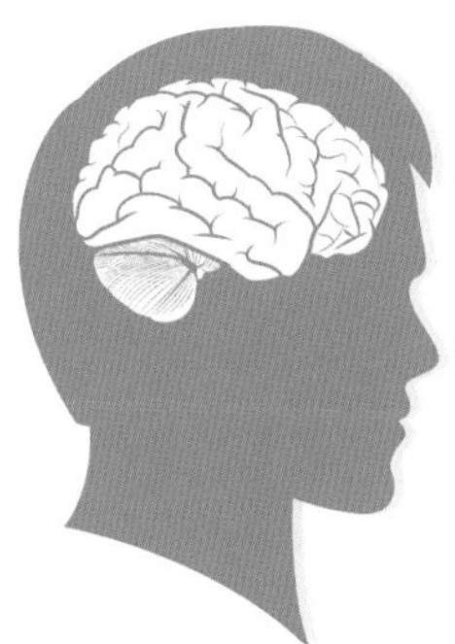

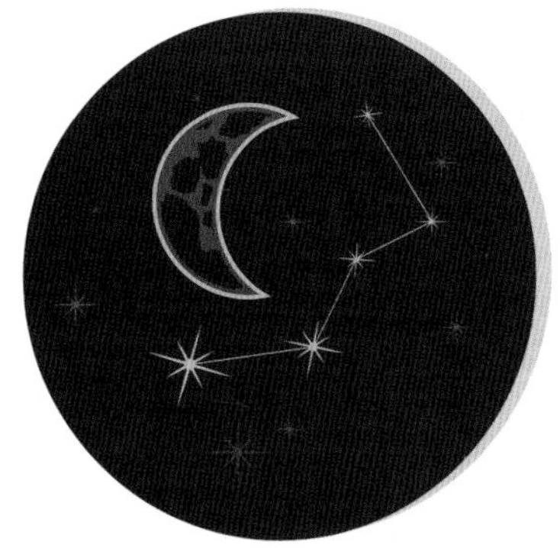

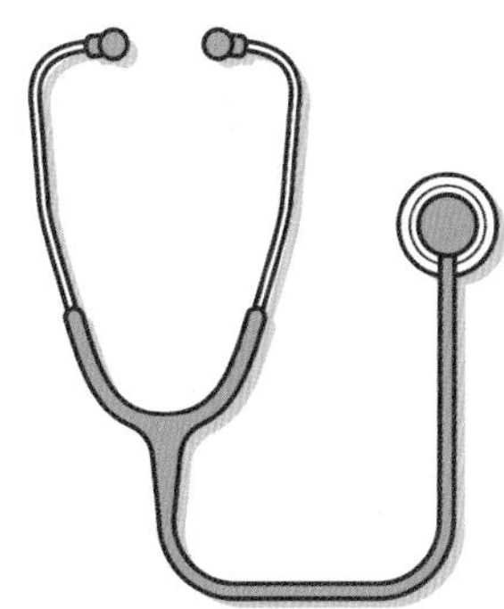

Better Mental Clarity and Focus

Have you ever felt like your thinking was a bit sluggish after you ate? A common problem associated with an improper, high-carbohydrate diet is "brain fog," or lack of focus. This can make concentrating on your daily tasks that much more difficult. A keto diet, on the other hand, helps create a steady fuel source for your brain in the form of ketones. This allows you to begin thinking more clearly and is more likely to sustain that over a longer period of time.

More Restful Sleep

Emerging research suggests that impaired glucose metabolism may interfere with your body's ability to achieve a restful sleep. This may make you feel like you're constantly tired and impact your energy during the day. By eating a high-fat, low-carbohydrate keto diet, you'll find that you begin to experience a more restful sleep. And forget that sleepy feeling you get in the middle of the day–with a more restful sleep and better eating habits, you'll be able to power through your day without the desire to nap.

A Decline in Risk Factors for Chronic Disease

A diet comprised heavily of processed fats and sugar can cause chronic inflammation. This is believed to be the primary reason for the development of many chronic diseases, including heart disease and diabetes. By eliminating or reducing processed carbohydrates, sugar, and trans fats and incorporating healthy fats and vegetables via a keto diet, you may reduce the risk of chronic inflammation, leading to better health over the long term.

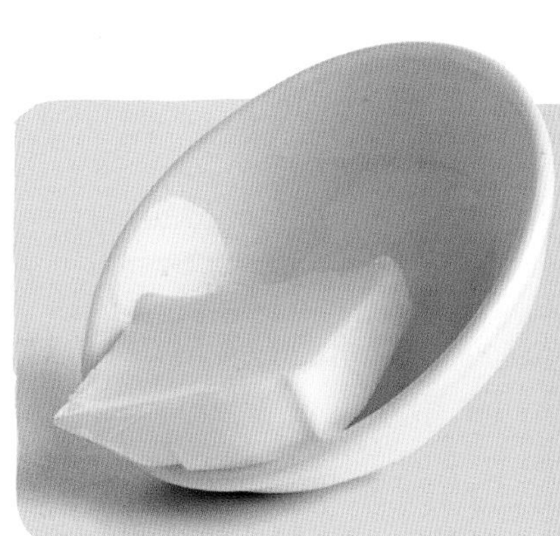

NO SKIMPING ON HEALTH–OR TASTE

Following a keto diet will help you focus on eating more fresh, real whole foods—which provide your body with nourishment in the form of vitamins, minerals, fiber, antioxidants, and color variety—and fewer processed foods that may be harmful to your health. Also, many of the foods typically not allowed on other diets—such as bacon, butter, and cream—are not only allowed, but encouraged on a keto diet!

Ketosis and the Keto Body

How your body produces energy on a keto diet is very different from how it's produced on a higher-carbohydrate diet due to the type of fuel used by each.

Energy from Glucose (Carbohydrates)

Diets rich in carbohydrates cause your body to rely on glucose as the primary source of energy. What isn't used right away is stored in adipose (fat) tissue, causing fluctuations in energy levels and weight gain.

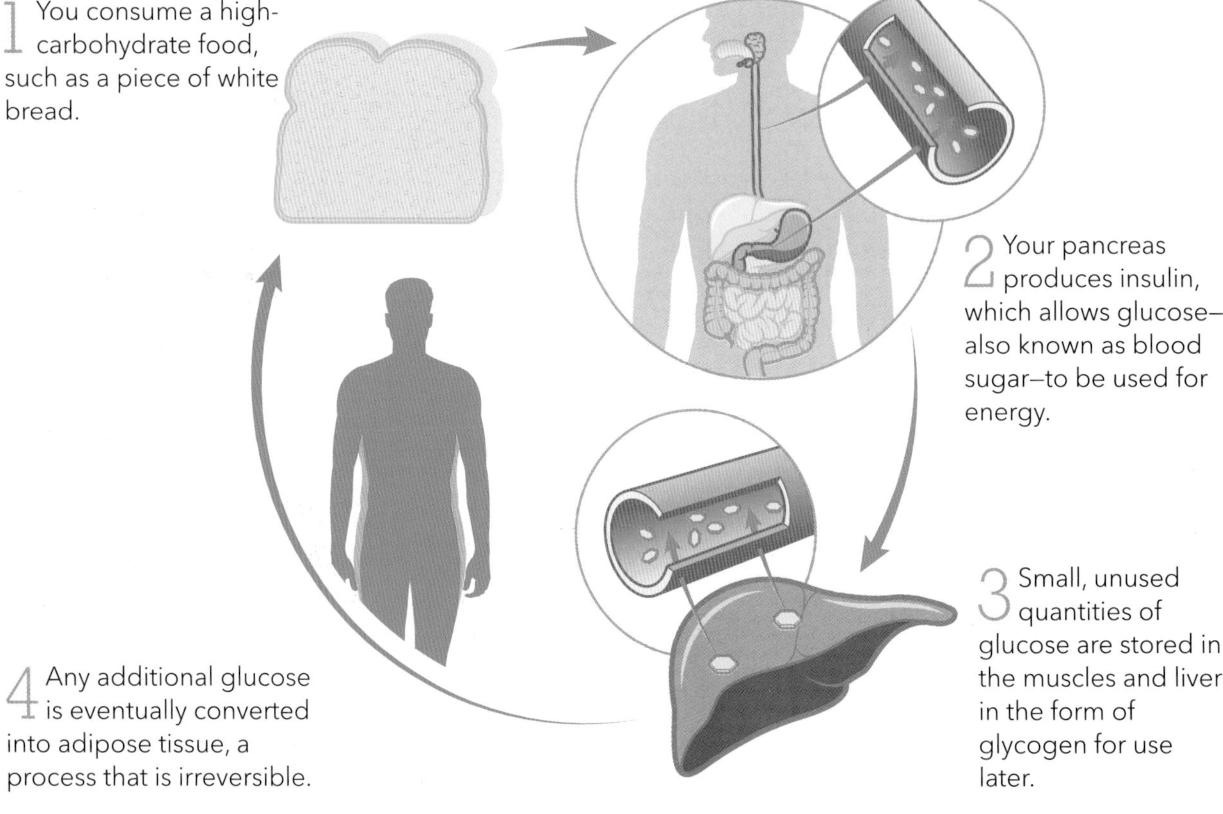

What Is Ketosis?

Ketosis refers to the state in which fat is broken down into ketones and used by the body for energy. When your body no longer has adequate glucose or glycogen stores to convert into energy, your body will begin breaking down fat stored in your fat cells and in the foods you eat. This leads to the production of ketones—fatty-acid molecules that are your body's natural defense against starvation. These ketones are then used by your body for energy. For healthy people who don't have diabetes, ketosis kicks in after about 3 or 4 days of eating less than 50g of carbohydrates. Over a longer period of time, this lowered intake of carbohydrates leads you to become keto adapted, meaning your body becomes very efficient at using fat and ketones for energy throughout its entirety.

Energy from Ketones (Fat)

A high-fat keto diet forces your body to use a process known as *ketosis*. Nearly every cell uses ketones more efficiently than glucose, leading to steadier energy levels and a greater chance of weight loss.

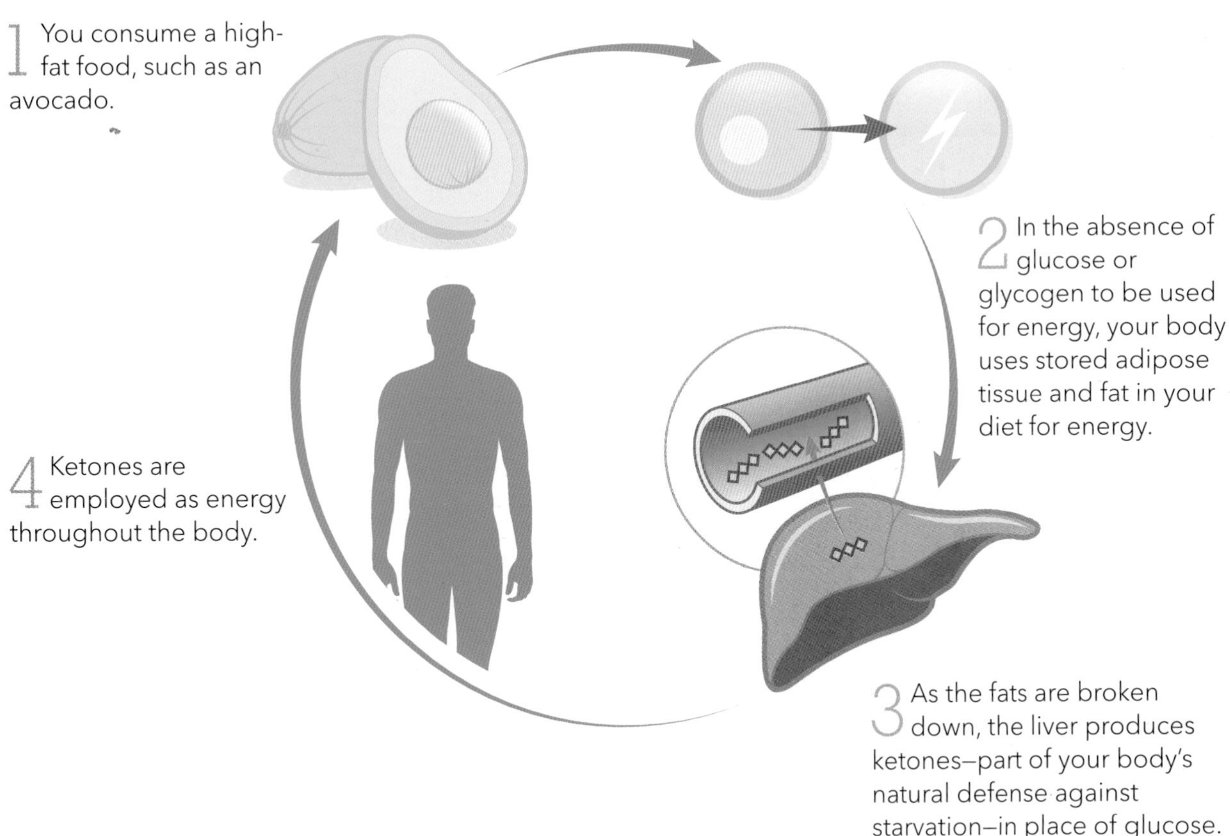

Keto Q&A

Now that you know how the keto diet works, you may wonder just what goes into implementing it. The following address some common questions about the keto lifestyle.

Q Isn't all this fat bad for my health?

A Even with low-fat and fat-free eating quickly falling by the wayside, there's still a stigma around fat in a diet. While it's a widespread belief that saturated fat causes heart disease, there's actually little evidence that saturated or total fat intake increases the risk of cardiovascular disease. Instead, it may be more about overall eating patterns. Although the exact mechanism for this is beyond the scope of this book, by incorporating a good blend of fat from saturated, monounsaturated, and omega-3 polyunsaturated sources, you may actually see improvements in you lipid profile when eating a diet high in fat!

Q Do I need to fast before starting the diet?

A While fasting can certainly help you achieve ketosis faster, it comes at the cost of fatigue, headaches, and potential gastrointestinal (GI) side effects, lovingly referred to as *keto flu*. Instead, focus on adequate hydration and electrolyte and fat consumption starting on the first day of your keto diet. You should then begin to see progress in terms of ketones within 2 to 5 days.

Q Will this diet cause me to gain weight?

A Eating fat doesn't contribute to weight gain on its own; instead, a major factor in weight gain is your calorie intake. When consuming more calories than necessary (especially in the form of carbohydrates), your body releases insulin, which tells it to package up excess calories as triglycerides to be stored away in your adipose (fat) tissue. On a keto diet, the food (carbohydrates) that causes the release of insulin is dramatically reduced, making it challenging for your body to store fat. So you use the fat you eat and that's stored in your adipose tissue for energy, which in turn leads to weight loss.

Q Can I drink alcohol on a keto diet?

A Alcohol can be consumed in moderation on the keto diet—no more than 1 drink per day for women or 2 drinks per day for men. Still, while drinking alcohol itself won't dramatically interrupt your ketosis, certain alcohols are higher in carbohydrates and should be limited.

UNSWEETENED LIQUOR	0g net carb per ounce (25ml)
WINE	Approximately 1g net carb per ounce (25ml)
LIGHT BEER	Approximately 2 to 5g net carb per 12 ounces (350ml)
CRAFT BEER	Approximately 15 to 25g net carb per 12 ounces (350ml)

Q Do I need to take any vitamins while following this diet?

A During the induction phase of a keto diet, some experts recommend taking a high-quality multivitamin or mineral supplement to prevent any deficiencies due to large dietary changes. Also, while not essential, consider asking your doctor to check your vitamin D status. If you're asked to start supplementing, it'll likely be about 1,000 to 2,000 international units (IUs) of vitamin D_3 (the form used by the body) daily. However, vitamin, mineral, and herbal supplements in the United States aren't regulated consistently, so it's best to avoid vitamins beyond those situations.

Q Do I need to count calories?

A One of the best things about a keto diet is that there's no real need to count calories. Because carbohydrate and protein requirements—and therefore intake—should remain static on a keto diet, the best way to determine if you're eating too many calories (too much fat) will be your weight. If you aren't losing weight, eat less fat; if you're losing too much weight or want to maintain your weight, eat enough fat to provide weight stability and satiety. That's all there is to it!

Q Is it sustainable to follow a keto diet?

A While initially it can be challenging to adhere to a keto diet with social obligations and temptations, a keto-adapted individual generally has little desire to break ketosis due to the satisfying effect of initial weight loss, overwhelming improvements in mental clarity, and endless energy associated with following the diet. There's also the satiety achieved through high fat intake, which ultimately can be felt as reduced cravings on the diet. If you view the keto diet simply as a way to quickly cut weight, it's unlikely this way of life will be sustainable. Having the mind-set that keto is your way of life is essential to making it sustainable.

The Role of Fat in a Keto Diet

Fats are organic compounds in foods that provide a concentrated source of energy and vitamins. On the keto diet, fats make up 75 to 80 percent of your total calories.

Fat Is Essential!

Because you're limiting carbohydrate foods, fats will provide the majority of your energy. While the exact breakdown of which fats to incorporate and in which proportions remains unknown, research suggests that the type of fat the body prefers to use on a keto diet is similar in composition to what it stores.

So what type of fat does the body store? Mostly saturated fats (similar in composition to butter and virgin coconut oil) and monounsaturated fats (such as extra-virgin olive oil and nuts and seeds). Therefore, the majority of fat you consume on a keto diet should come from saturated and monounsaturated sources, with a small portion of your diet comprised of polyunsaturated fats (such as salmon and walnuts).

ADDING FATS AND OILS TO YOUR DIET

Choose fats and oils with minimal processing techniques, exposure to light, and/or hydrogenation. Examples of high-quality fats include extra-virgin olive oil from a light-protected bottle or tin, cold-pressed coconut oil, and grass-fed butter or cream.

Generally, fats can be deemed healthy or unhealthy based on the level of heat processing, as well as the exposure to light and hydrogen they receive. For instance, oils that come in light-protected containers are more likely to be extracted via the low-heat cold-pressed technique and to retain more of their green hue, a good indication they contain higher concentrations of antioxidants and anti-inflammatory components.

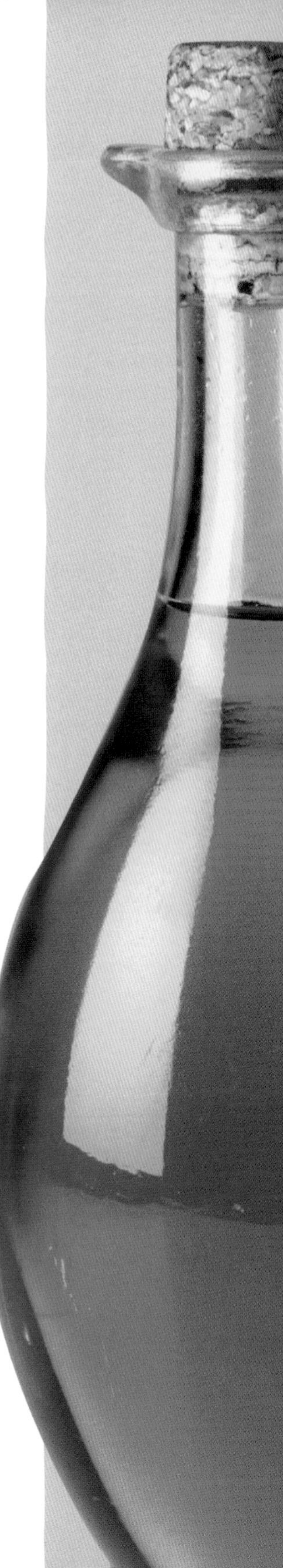

Fats to Eat

Fats can be classified as plant based or animal based. When figuring out the right types of fat to eat, look to natural plant and animal sources for your regular intake, aiming for a good blend of the two for your best overall health.

Plant-Based Fats

Fats and oils found in plant-based foods are generally beneficial for your health if they have been minimally processed (for instance, extracting oil from olives using a more natural cold-pressed process versus extracting oil from soybeans using a chemical process).

- Coconut, olive, MCT, and palm kernel oils
- Mayonnaise made with olive oil
- Unsweetened cocoa powder or cacao nibs
- Unsweetened coconut flakes
- Seeds, such as hemp, sesame, pumpkin, and sunflower seeds
- Avocados

Animal-Based Fats

While animal-based fats have received a bad reputation for being high in saturated fat, the latest research suggests that not all saturated fats are created equal. These fats are packed with flavor and offer many culinary options.

- Butter or ghee
- Heavy cream
- Sour cream
- Fatty fish, such as tuna, mackerel, or sardines
- Bacon or duck fat

ADDING MCTS TO YOUR DIET

Medium-chain triglycerides (MCTs)—found in oils such as coconut and MCT oil—are of particular interest to many keto dieters due to their ketone-boosting potential. Because they require minimal if any digestion before being absorbed and are shuttled right to the liver for ketone production, using MCT-based oils may enhance your level of ketosis.

Fats to Avoid

Not all fats are created equal. Certain fats–including trans fats in processed foods with high sugar and saturated fats created by hydrogenating oils–can have a negative impact on your health.

- Stick margarine
- Vegetable shortening
- Hydrogenated fat and oils of any type
- Low-fat or fat-free salad dressings
- Low-fat spreads
- Salad dressings with added sugars

The Role of Protein in a Keto Diet

Proteins are compounds in foods that provide the building blocks of who you are. On the keto diet, proteins make up around 15 percent of your total calories.

Finding the Right Balance of Protein

Variations of the low-carbohydrate diets—such as the Atkins, South Beach, and Paleo diets—often leave dieters with the impression that all low-carbohydrate diets are ketogenic. While many have the potential to produce ketones, one thing that differentiates a true keto diet from many of the other diets is the protein content. On true keto diets, protein intake is generally limited to an "adequate" level—just enough to keep your cells healthy and your tissues operating appropriately. While the amount of protein your body needs each day varies, you generally need about .8 to 1g per kg of lean mass. For most, this works out to be between 60 and 110g of total protein per day.

> Consuming more protein than your body needs to maintain healthy tissue can actually have an anti-keto effect.

When you limit carbohydrates, you may feel protein should be the bulk of the food you eat at a meal; however, consuming more protein than your body needs to maintain healthy tissue can actually have an anti-keto effect. Therefore, it's important to not eat protein just to fill yourself up. Before you begin the diet, track your baseline protein intake using food-tracking software to gain an understanding of which foods you eat contain the most and least amounts of protein.

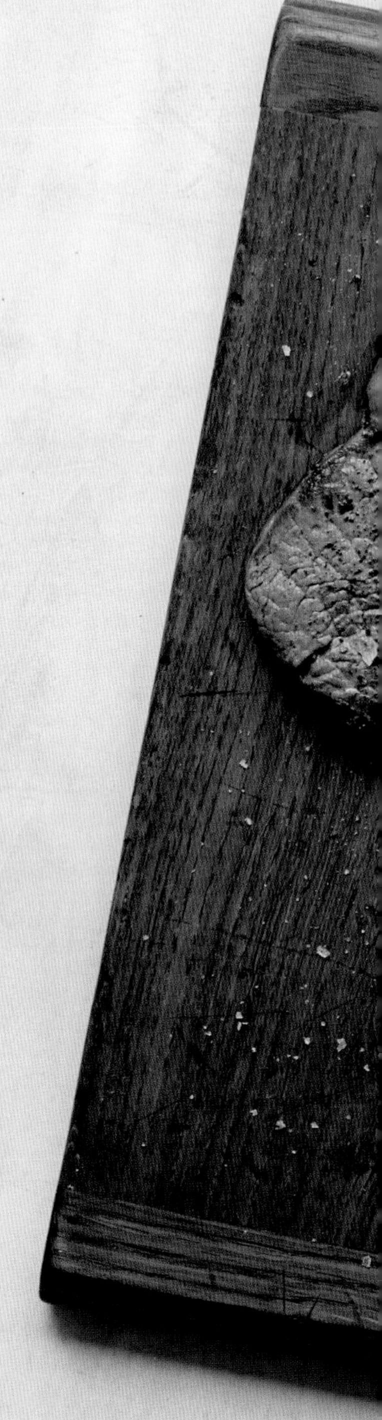

PAIRING PROTEIN WITH FAT

A juicy, protein-rich steak with a fatty sauce will help you feel satisifed and maintain a steady level of energy.

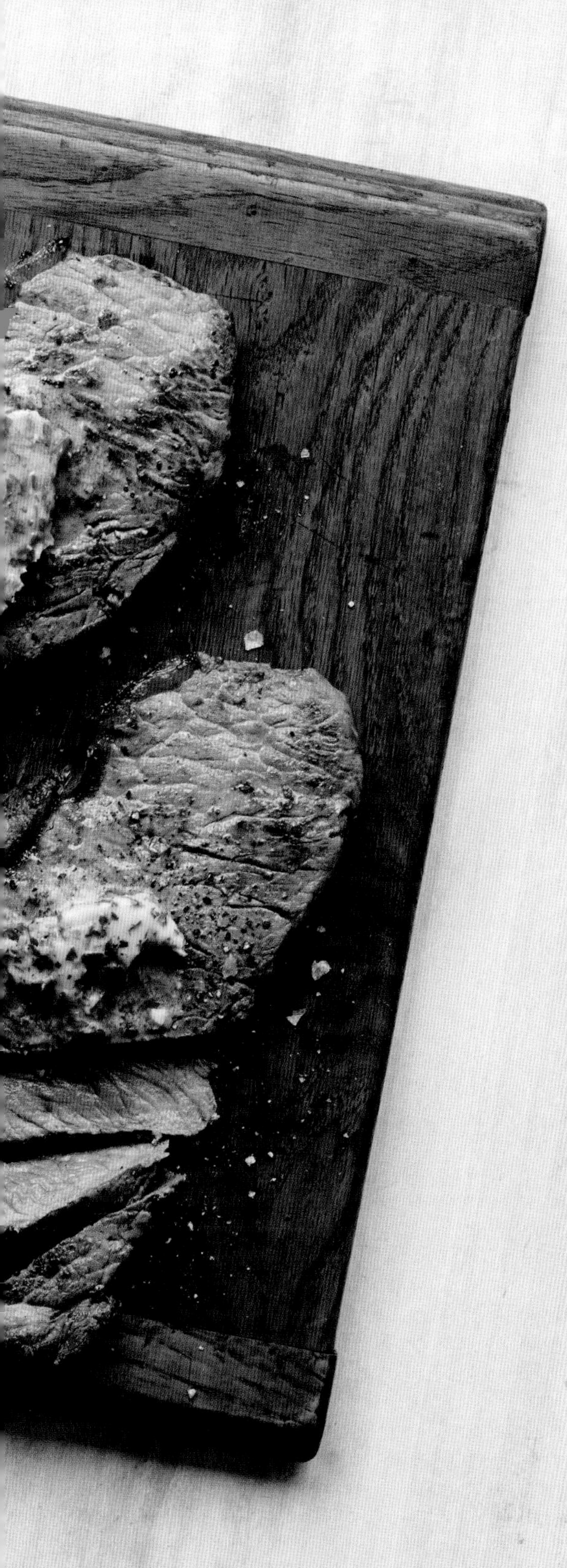

Proteins to Eat

Fresh proteins contain little to no carbohydrates, which means you can consume protein without upping your carb intake.

- Poultry, such as chicken, turkey, and duck
- Meat, such as beef and pork
- Seafood, such as shrimp, scallops, and crab
- Eggs
- Cheese
- Nuts and seeds, such as walnuts, pecans, chia seeds, and flaxseeds

Proteins to Limit

When choosing proteins, it's important to watch out for ones with additives and preservatives, as they may contain high levels of carbohydrates.

- Highly processed lunch meats, such as those flavored with maple or honey
- Any protein breaded with wheat, corn, or breadcrumbs
- Store-bought, deep-fried proteins
- Most beans and legumes (due to high carbohydrate content)

Q Should You Drink Protein Shakes?

A It's probably best to avoid protein shakes while following the keto diet. Researchers have reported that individuals following a keto diet maintain higher levels of specific amino acids in the bloodstream following vigorous exercise, meaning they likely don't break down as many protein stores. Also, many protein powders are laden with carbohydrates or greatly exceed your protein requirements. If you're looking to incorporate protein after a workout, a natural food source (such as cheese or nuts) will do the trick!

The Role of Carbohydrates in a Keto Diet

Carbohydrates are compounds in foods that, once fully digested and absorbed by the body, are broken down into sugars and used for energy or stored as fat. On the keto diet, carbohydrates make up only 5 percent of your total calories.

Keeping Carb Consumption Low

A common misconception is that keto diets are carbohydrate free, when in fact certain carbohydrate foods are essential for health. However, in order for your body to begin producing ketones, carbohydrate foods must be limited. If you eat too many carbohydrates at one meal or throughout the day, it can have an anti-keto effect.

Your carbohydrate intake on the diet will consist of foods that provide the most nutritional value with the fewest grams of net carbohydrate.

Net Carbohydrate

Foods with minimal starch or natural sugars and high fiber content are considered low in net carbohydrate. On the keto diet, your net carbohydrate should be limited to 20 to 60g per day.

COLORFUL CARBS

Foods with the lowest net carbohydrate content include leafy green vegetables, nuts and seeds, and berries.

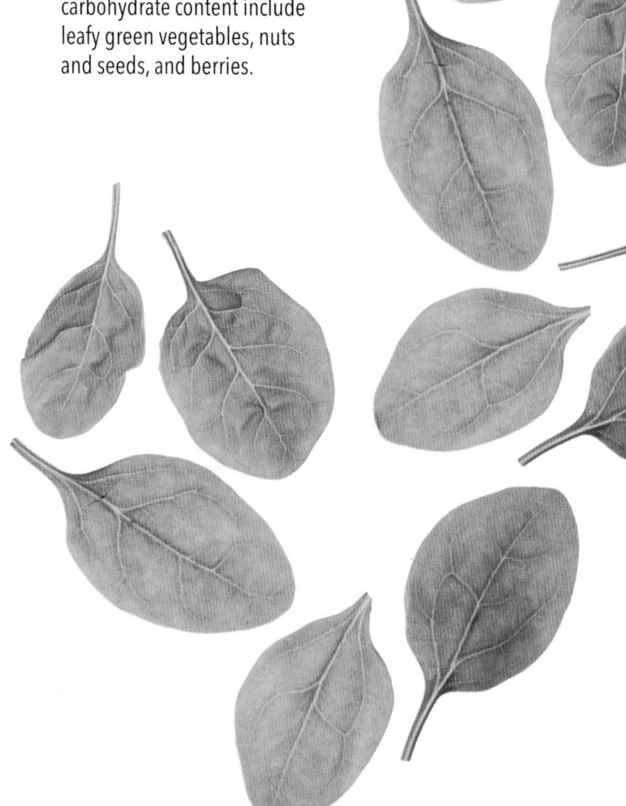

CALCULATING NET CARBOHYDRATE

You can find out the net carbohydrate of a food with this formula:

Net carbohydrate = grams total carbohydrate - grams fiber

Let's use a nutrition label for baby spinach to try it out.

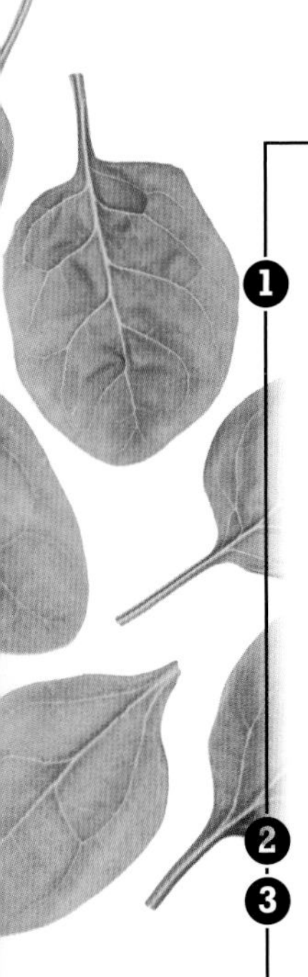

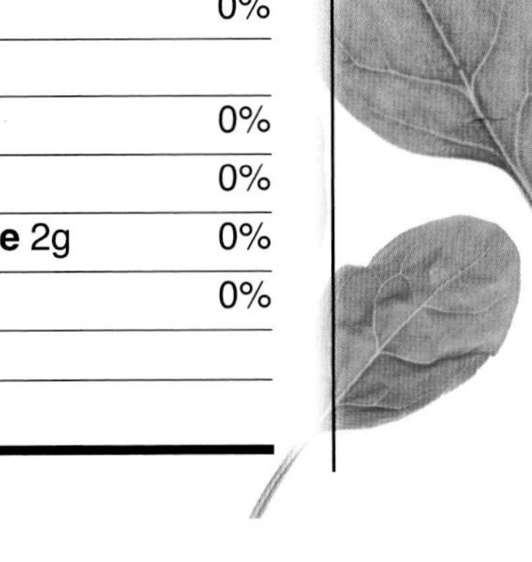

NUTRITION FACTS

❶ Serving Size 1 cup (57g)
Servings Per Container 8

Amount Per Serving	
Calories 15	**Calories from Fat** 0
	% Daily Value
Total Fat 0g	0%
Saturated Fat 0g	0%
Trans Fat 0g	
Cholesterol 0mg	0%
Sodium 45mg	0%
❷ **Total Carbohydrate** 2g	0%
❸ Dietary Fiber 1g	0%
Sugars 0g	
Protein 1g	

1 Take a look at the serving size—1 cup, in this example. All of the numbers on the label will be for 1 cup of baby spinach.

2 Look for total carbohydrate. This food has 2g total carbohydrate in a 1-cup serving.

3 Find fiber, which is often listed as dietary fiber, soluble fiber, or insoluble fiber. A 1-cup serving of baby spinach has 1g fiber.

4 Subtract grams total fiber from grams total carbohydrate. In this case, 2g total carbohydrate minus 1g fiber leaves 1g net carbohydrate.

Carbs to Eat

When choosing carbohydrates to eat, you're looking for ones packed with vitamins, minerals, and antioxidants that are low in net carbohydrate and high in fiber.

- Nonstarchy vegetables, such as green leafy vegetables, zucchini, and eggplant
- Nuts, such as walnuts, almonds, pecans, pistachios, and nut flours
- Seeds, such as sunflower, hemp, sesame, and pumpkin seeds
- Small portions of high-fiber fruit, such as berries

Carbs to Avoid

Certain foods have a net carbohydrate that will likely exceed your needs in one serving.

- Grains, such as wheat, rye, barley, rice, quinoa, oats, cereals, bread, and pasta
- Starchy vegetables, such as potatoes, corn, peas, and winter squash
- Large quantities of fruit
- Fruit juices
- Sugar and honey

Keto Phase 1: Induction

Induction is the initial phase of any keto diet, during which time you'll closely monitor carbohydrate and protein intake. Induction generally lasts for 1 to 3 months; however, it can be followed for however long you need to achieve your goals.

Calorie Intake

While counting calories is generally not necessary on a keto diet, consuming more energy (calories) than you need puts unnecessary stress on your body's metabolism. In most cases, your level of hunger will dictate your energy needs and how much you should eat. Most individuals will find they are most satisfied with 1,500 to 1,800 calories a day.

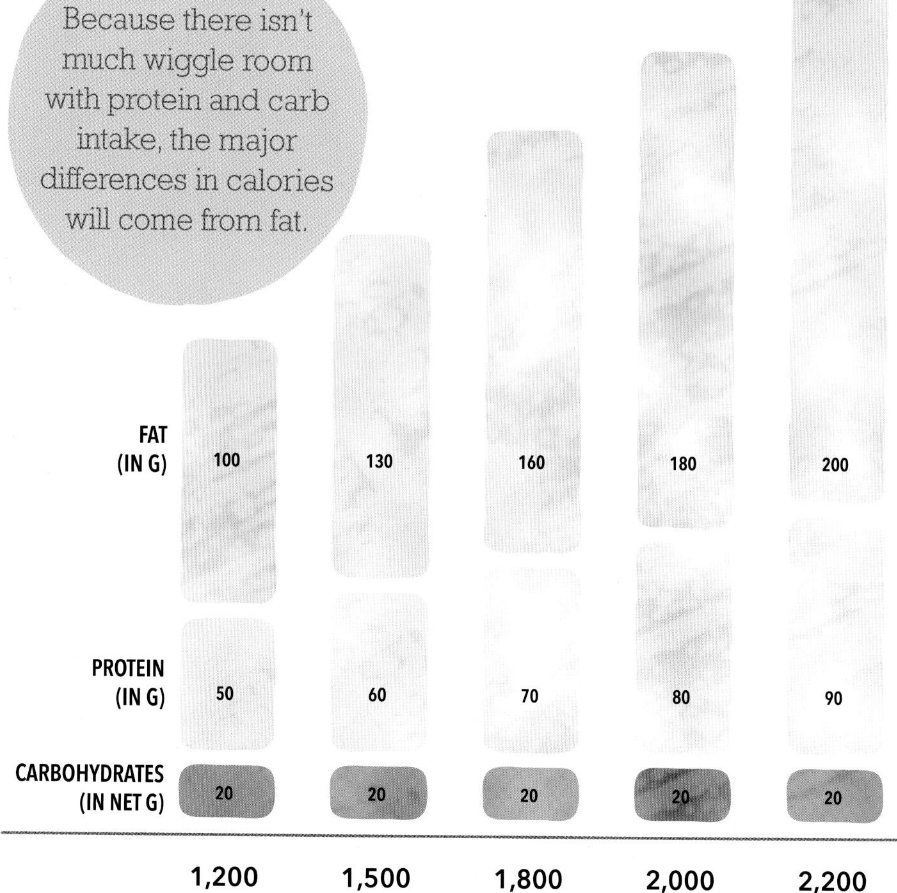

INDUCTION PHASE INTAKE

This table shows you the amount of protein, fat, and carbohydrates you can eat per day based on different calorie levels.

Cutting Carbs

The overall principle for the induction phase is to limit your net carbohydrates to approximately 20g a day in order to achieve a steady state of ketosis and to help your tissues efficiently use fat as the primary fuel. To ensure you consume a variety of essential vitamins and minerals in those 20g, focus primarily on vegetables, nuts, and seeds for your carbohydrate sources.

NUTS AND SEEDS (SUCH AS ALMONDS AND CHIA SEEDS)
5 to 10g
FRUITS (SUCH AS BERRIES)
0 to 5g
VEGETABLES (SUCH AS ZUCCHINI AND CAULIFLOWER)
15 to 20g
PROTEIN FOODS (SUCH AS EGGS AND UNPROCESSED MEATS)
0 to 10g
MISCELLANEOUS (SUCH AS HEAVY CREAM AND UNSWEETENED, MINIMALLY PROCESSED YOGURT)
0 to 5g

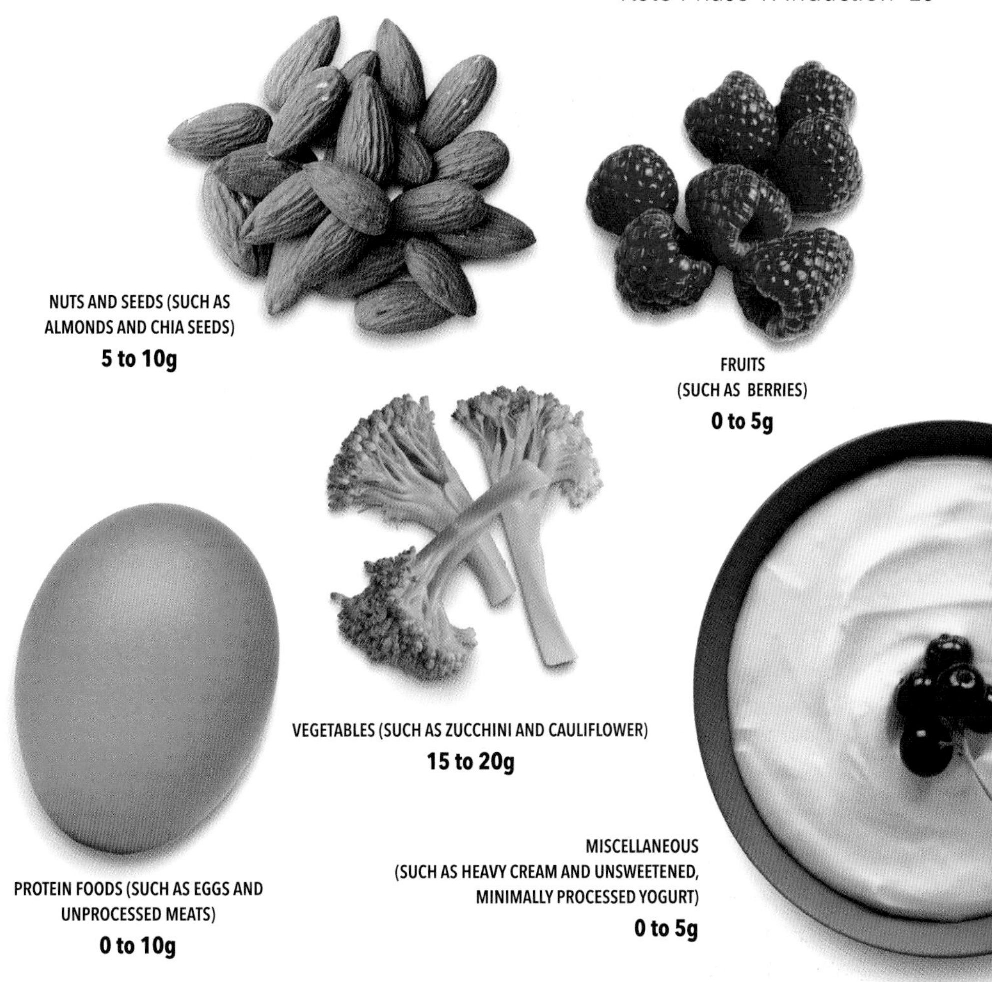

Increasing the Fat

As you begin to limit your carbohydrate intake, it is essential for you to also dramatically increase the amount of fat you consume. Based on your calorie intake, this should be anywhere from 100 to 200g per day. Most of the recommended fats on the keto diet are rarely eaten on their own, so it's pretty difficult to have too many. For those high-fat foods that can be eaten individually, such as nuts and seeds, be careful not to have too many, as they also contain carbohydrates. Suggestions for increasing fat in your diet include adding olive oil to salads and vegetables and creating fat-based sauces using cream or butter.

Finding the Right Balance of Protein

When it comes to protein, finding the right balance is key. Aim for about a deck-of-cards size portion of protein at most meals. You want to get enough to maintain good health, but you don't want to eat enough to kick you out of ketosis. Generally, adults require no more than 60 to 90g of protein per day. If you find that adhering to protein recommendations is challenging and you have a considerable amount of weight to lose, try slowly increasing protein intake (in 7 to 10g increments) until you're satisfied with a maximum protein intake of 90g a day.

Monitoring Ketosis

The purpose of a keto diet is to cause a metabolic shift in your body so fat and ketones are used as the primary fuel source. The best way to determine if you're implementing the diet correctly is to measure your level of ketosis.

Ways to Measure Ketones

One way ketones can be measured is in the blood (as beta-hydroxybutyrate); this method measures ketones available to be used for energy by the body. Other ways to measure them is through your breath (as acetone) or in your urine (as acetoacetate); these methods measure ketones that were produced but are being excreted because they exceed the needs of your body.

While measuring blood ketones is a highly accurate method of testing, it's generally quite expensive (and painful!). Testing ketones on the breath is a less expensive and painless method; however, it is a relatively new method that may not be as accurate as the others. Most keto dieters monitor their level of ketosis in their urine via urine ketone test strips (available at any pharmacy or online) due to the ease of testing and inexpensive cost.

Whichever method you choose, the goal is to achieve positive ketones, generally labeled as small to moderate. Ketones will be highest during the time of day when your metabolism is highest—generally in the afternoon or evening.

URINE KETONE LEVEL	WHAT THIS MEANS
Negative	Your body isn't producing enough ketones to spill into the urine.
Trace	Your body is producing ketones; however, it's probably inconsistent.
Small to moderate	Your body is producing adequate ketones to ensure your brain has an adequate fuel source.
Large	Caution—your body is producing high levels of ketones, which may increase your risk for dehydration.

URINE KETONE LEVELS

Using urine test strips, you can check your ketone levels every 24 hours. Eating too many carbs or protein can have an anti-keto effect, as can starving your body of fat. To boost ketosis, limit net carb intake to 20g per day, keep protein counts in check, and increase fat intake.

Keto Phase 2: Maintenance

Once you've achieved the goals you set out to hit on the diet, you may choose to follow a more liberal version of the diet, referred to as *maintenance.* This phase can be followed for as long as you choose to maintain a keto lifestyle.

Calorie Intake

The maintenance phase allows you to maintain your keto lifestyle while slowing or halting weight loss by eating the just the right amount of calories that your body needs.

Increasing Carbs

During the maintenance phase, you will consume up to 60g net carbohydrate per day. You can continue to use the same recipes as during the induction phase with some carbohydrates added. This can be done by increasing the vegetable content of the recipe, adding a side salad, eating keto-friendly snacks (such as nuts and seeds), or even enjoying more keto-friendly desserts!

Decreasing Fat

Although fat intake may be slightly less on the maintenance phase of your keto diet, it still makes up the majority of your calorie intake. If you find you start to gain weight on the maintenance phase and aren't overeating carbs or protein, try cutting back on fat by 1 o 2 tablespoons per day.

Keeping Protein Stable

Remember that keto diets are not high-protein diets. Protein intake should remain similar to that on the induction phase. If you remember, eating more protein than you need means your body can convert excess protein into glucose, which can disrupt ketosis!

CALORIES	CARBOHYDRATES (IN NET G)	PROTEIN (IN G)	FAT (IN G)
1,200 calories	50	50	90
1,500 calories	50	60	120
1,800 calories	50	70	150
2,000 calories	50	80	170
2,200 calories	50	90	180

MAINTENANCE PHASE INTAKE

This table shows you the amount of protein, fat, and carbohydrates you can eat per day based on different calorie levels.

The Keto Kitchen

The first step in making sure you follow a keto diet is filling your pantry and refrigerator with plenty of keto-friendly items. The following are what we recommend you have on hand for the diet.

Must-Have Pantry Items

The key to any successful keto diet is adding flavor and spice. Filling your pantry with plenty of keto-friendly items will not only enhance your success, but also help you cook up some delicious dishes.

GHEE

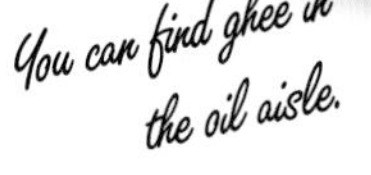

You can find ghee in the oil aisle.

COLD-PRESSED OR VIRGIN COCONUT OIL

Avoid refined or bleached varieties.

SALT, HERBS, AND SPICES
Kosher salt, black pepper, garlic powder, onion powder, crushed red pepper flakes, cayenne pepper, paprika, chili powder, thyme, oregano, basil, bay leaves, and mustard powder

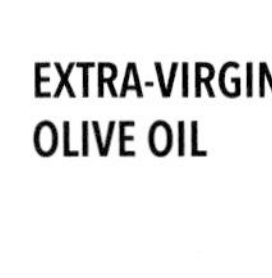

EXTRA-VIRGIN OLIVE OIL

Look for ones in light-protected, green-glass bottles.

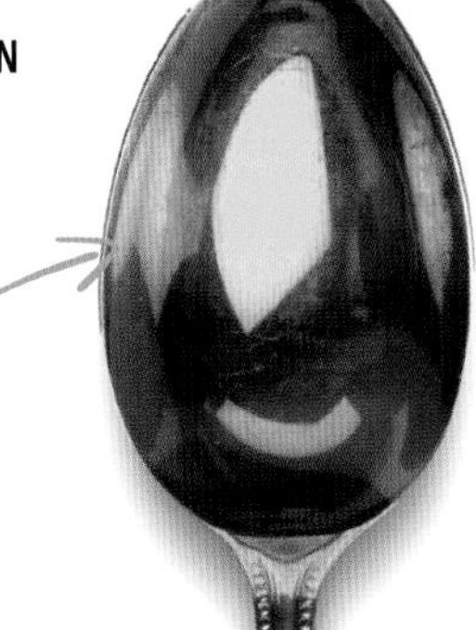

LOW-CALORIE SWEETENERS
Such as stevia

Must-Have Perishable Items

When purchasing perishable items for your keto kitchen, be sure to choose those that are naturally low in net carbohydrates and high in fat. Aim for full-fat dairy products, skin-on poultry, and meats with plenty of marbling.

FRESH VEGETABLES

Spinach, kale, chard, collard greens, carrots, zucchini, eggplant, mushrooms, broccoli, small amounts of peppers, mustard greens, cauliflower, cabbage, and tomatoes

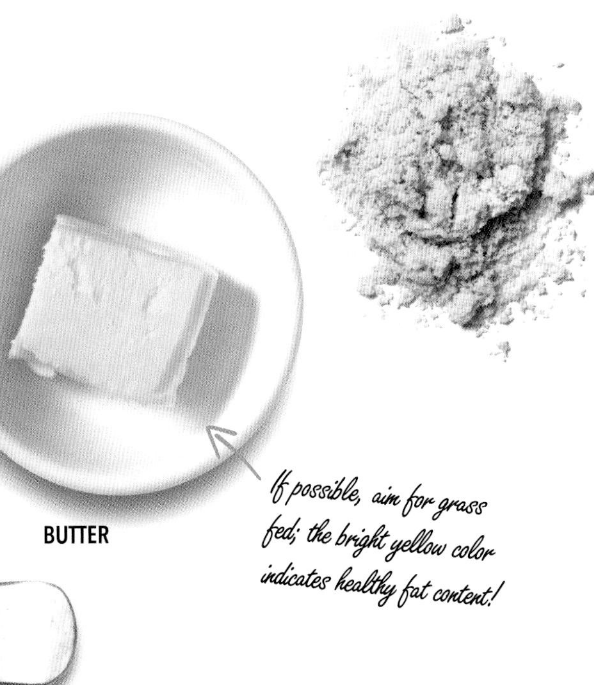

WHOLE NUTS, SEEDS, AND NUT OR SEED FLOURS

Walnuts, almonds, chia seeds, pumpkin seeds, sunflower seeds, almond flour and meal, ground flaxseeds, coconut flour, and unsweetened flaked coconut

CHEESE

Full-fat Parmesan, mozzarella, cheddar, ricotta, and specialty cheeses

BUTTER

If possible, aim for grass fed; the bright yellow color indicates healthy fat content!

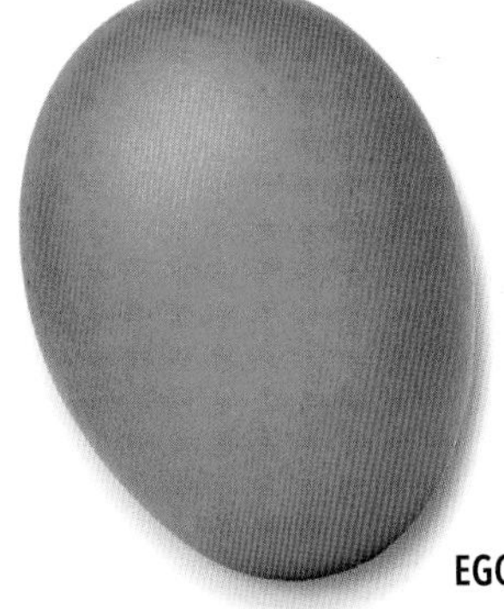

EGGS

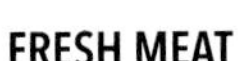

FRESH POULTRY

Skin-on chicken or turkey thighs, wings, drums, or breasts; duck; ground chicken; and ground turkey

FRESH MEAT

Steak, pork chops, tenderloin, ground beef, and certain processed products like sausage without a lot of fillers

FRESH SEAFOOD

Salmon, tuna, trout, sardines, shrimp, scallops, and crab

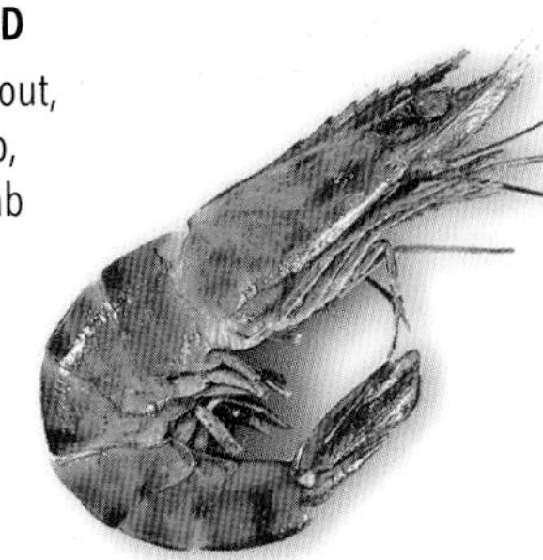

Eating the Keto Way

You've shopped for the ingredients; now it's time to put them together into some delicious meals. In order to construct a keto meal, break it down by the percentages of protein, carbohydrates, and fat you'll have as your total calories.

1. Start with Protein (20 Percent)

Use a deck-of-cards size piece (about 3 ounces [85g]) of protein as the base for your meal. This could be beef, pork, chicken, turkey, fish, seafood, or eggs, for instance. Just remember to be mindful of carbohydrate counts on processed meats, as they may contain preservatives added for flavor and to extend shelf life. Also, don't eat more than you need; otherwise, your body may convert the protein to carbohydrates, which will impact your body's ability to produce ketones.

Generally, you want to keep your protein at an adequate level without going overboard like on a typical Western diet.

ADDING THE RIGHT AMOUNT OF PROTEIN TO YOUR DIET

- Focus on eating protein paired with liberal amounts of fat, such as in a sauce or dip.
- Choose proteins with higher natural fat content to avoid adding fat during cooking.
- Count the proteins in nontraditional protein foods that you eat during the day, such as cheese.

The size of an average deck of playing cards.

2. Make the Carbohydrates Count (5 Percent)

Once you've decided on your protein, choose carbohydrates high in fiber, vitamins, and minerals. Your carbohydrates should be low in net carbohydrate—less than 5g per serving. Examples that fit these stipulations include leafy green vegetables, broccoli, cauliflower, green beans, celery, mushrooms, almonds, walnuts, pecans, and so on. For the vegetables in particular, try to include them in your meals at least twice a day to gain the most benefit.

Because you're trying to limit your intake of carbohydrates, you may wonder how to best fit in these foods. The options on the right illustrate how you can add the largest volume of food for the smallest amount of carbohydrates.

Nuts can be used as snacks and added to salads and sauces.
Include seasonings while being mindful of their carbohydrate content.
Aim for at least one type of vegetable, such as carrots, at lunch and dinner.

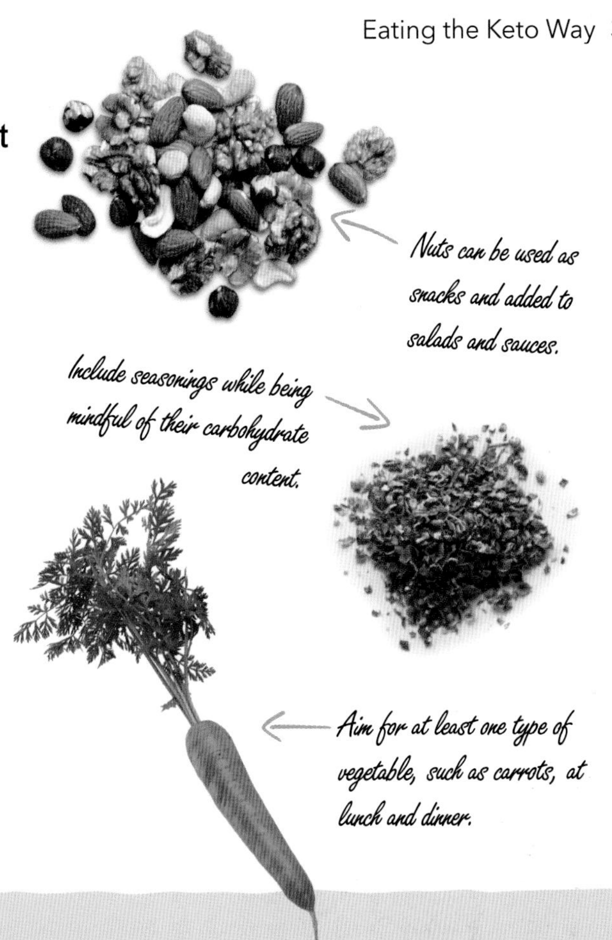

SOURCING YOUR PROTEINS

Antibiotics

Choosing animal products grown without the use of antibiotics may reduce your risk of developing an antibiotic-resistant infection. When shopping for antibiotic-free products, look for key terms such as the following:

- Animal welfare approved
- Certified humane
- No antibiotics used/raised without antibiotics

Hormones

A variety of hormones are given to animals to maximize growth and reproduction. Understandably, there has been much concern about how these factors impact human health. To avoid dairy products that contain hormones, choose ones certified organic or not produced from milk treated with recombinant bovine growth hormone (rbGH).

Grass Fed

Although not essential on a keto diet, the type of fat you get from consuming grass-fed beef is more favorable than that produced by consuming grains. In addition to higher anti-inflammatory omega-3 fats, grass-fed beef has been found to contain higher levels of vitamins and antioxidants, potentially influencing your cardiovascular risk factors.

Cage Free, Free Range, and Certified Humane

The access a bird has to the outdoors is labeled from cage free (simply uncaged), to free range (some outdoor access), to certified humane free range or pasture raised (outdoors for at least 6 hours a day with ample space per bird). The more access to the outdoors, the more likely a bird is to consume a more natural diet. This has been found to produce more omega-3s and vitamins, and less overall fat and cholesterol than grain-fed birds.

3. Finish with Fat (75 Percent)

When it comes to fat, you want to eat about 2 to 3 tablespoons per meal. Butter, coconut oil, extra-virgin olive oil, heavy whipping cream, and mayonnaise are just some of the keto-friendly fats that can be added to your meals.

The nice thing about adding fat is how easy it is to do. For instance, you can work it into sauces, dressings, or spreads to bring out the natural flavors in your foods. However, because fat intake has been discouraged over the past half-century, you may initially struggle with this idea. Check out the sidebar for some different ways you can increase your fat intake.

Five Ways to Increase Your Daily Intake of Fat to Keto Diet Levels

- Sauté cooked proteins and raw vegetables in butter or oil.
- Create herbed butters and oils and use them for sautéing or spreads.
- Add oils or cream to sauces served with your meals.
- Add heavy cream, unsalted butter, or coconut oil to low-carbohydrate beverages, such as coffee or tea.
- Dip each bite of protein (such as beef) into melted butter, ghee, oil, or mayonnaise.

A NOTE ON CARDIOVASCULAR HEALTH AND CHOLESTEROL

High cholesterol is not a contraindication to following a keto diet—in fact, your lipid profile may improve! However, for a small number of people, certain foods high in saturated fat and cholesterol may need to be limited. Consult your doctor and know your risks for developing chronic disease prior to starting this diet.

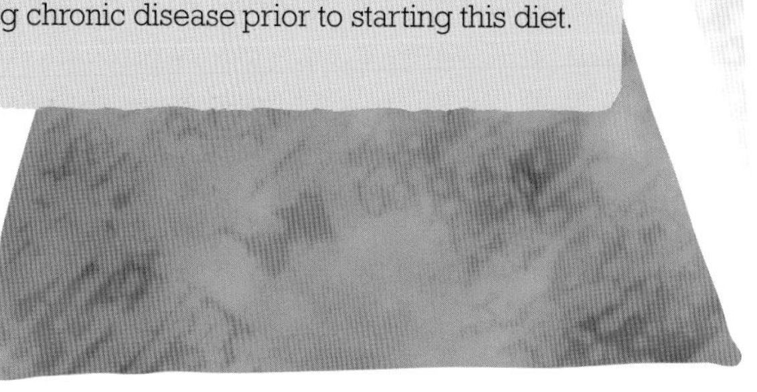

A Sample Keto Day

This sample meal plan—broken down by proteins, carbs, and fats—can provide you with a point of reference.

Breakfast – Baked Eggs with Ham and Gruyère

Fat 76% Protein 21% Net Carb 3% Ratio 1.4:1

Recipe found in **Breakfasts** section.
Serving Size: 1 baked egg

Start your day off right with a delicious egg bake. The fat in this meal will carry you through lunchtime and beyond.

Lunch – Keto Cobb Salad

Fat 75% Protein 20% Net Carb 5% Ratio 1.3:1

Recipe found in **Salads** section.
Serving Size: 1 salad

This salad offers the perfect ratio of fat, protein, and carbs. You may increase or decrease the portion size or share it with a friend if you're still satisfied from breakfast.

Snack – Dilly Dip

Fat 91% Protein 2% Net Carb 7% Ratio 4.3:1

Recipe found in **Snacks** section.
Serving Size: ¼ cup

This dip offers you a way to increase the fat in your day with minimal carbs and protein, making it a perfect snack.

Dinner – Bacon Brie Burger

Fat 73% Protein 24% Net Carb 3% Ratio 1.2:1

Recipe found in **Beef Mains** section.
Serving Size: 1 burger

This burger provides a large portion of your daily protein intake and is sure to keep you satisfied until breakfast the next day.

Daily Total

Net Carbohydrate: 20g Protein: 98g Fat: 164g Calories: 1,948 calories

Achieving Keto Success

Once you've decided to follow the keto way of life, you may wonder how you can maintain it over time. While there's no "perfect" way to stick to the diet, we've provided some pointers to help keep you on the path to success.

Make a Plan

The most important way you can help yourself achieve your keto diet goals is to make a plan. While it can take a few weeks to really understand what a well-balanced keto diet looks like, take time to review recipes and create a menu for the first week of your diet. Also, put some steps into place to minimize the risk for deviation. For instance, experiment with you own breakfast bakes, salads, and protein-veggie dishes. This ensures you seamlessly transition into the keto way of life.

Introduce Variety in Foods

Although eating generous amounts of bacon, steak, butter, and cream while improving your health sounds amazing, after a few weeks, you may hear the pizza or cookies calling your name. No matter how much better you feel on the diet, being bored with your food is a surefire way to fall off the wagon. Keep up your enthusiasm by branching out from what you typically eat. You can also pair your favorite keto-friendly foods with herbs, seasonings, and flavor-enhancing fats to create new sensations for your taste buds.

Choose Healthy Alternatives

Following a keto diet doesn't mean you have to give up your favorite foods. Many of the recipes in this book offer low-carbohydrate, keto-friendly alternatives to your starchy faves. However, if you still get those carbohydrate cravings and need some ideas beyond the recipes, the following are some low-carbohydrate substitutions you can try.

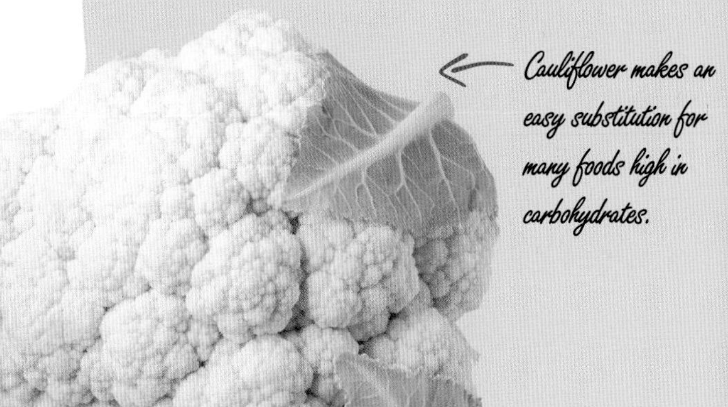

Cauliflower makes an easy substitution for many foods high in carbohydrates.

Be Smart When Dining Out

While you may find that preparing your own meals at home will offer control over portion size and ingredients used, it's hard to avoid eating out. Familiarizing yourself with available menu options will make the choice easier once you're ready to order.

The biggest ketosis-breaking culprits you'll find in restaurants outside of the obvious starches are sauces, gravies, and dressings, as they often contain added sugars. So when ordering, ask for them on the side. You'll also typically find meals on menus that contain a lot of protein and are inadequate in fat. Don't be afraid to box up half of the meal and ask for a fatty side. For instance, if you're having a burger, remove the bun; box half of the meat; and order some cheese, bacon, avocado, and a side of mayonnaise for the half you have.

QUICK TIPS WHEN DINING OUT:

- Be cautious of gravies, dressings, and sauces that may have added sugars.
- To avoid added carbs, choose broiled, roasted, or grilled chicken over battered or breaded.
- Pick sandwiches wrapped in lettuce or take off the bun and eat it with a fork.
- Look at nutrition information before you arrive, so you can make a better decision.

CARBOHYDRATE FOOD	LOW-CARBOHYDRATE SUBSTITUTES
Pasta and noodles	Spiralized zucchini, spaghetti squash (in small quantities), and kelp noodles
Rice	Riced cauliflower and grated zucchini
Mashed potatoes	Mashed cauliflower or celery root
Flour and breading	Almond flour, ground flaxseeds, coconut flower, and crushed pork rinds
Bread	Lettuce wraps, portobello mushroom caps, and sliced and fried eggplant
Chips	Cheese crisps, kale chips, and dried seaweed
Cereal	Homemade nut- and seed-based granola, hemp, and unsweetened coconut flakes
Pizza	Cauliflower- or sausage-based crust and pepperoni and cheese bites
Milk	Unsweetened almond or coconut oil and heavy cream mixed with water

Track Your Success

Research has shown that those who track their diets—whether on paper or in apps—are more successful in achieving their goals. Consider using a diet-tracking program or app to monitor your macronutrient intake. This can help you pay close attention to any spices, sweeteners, sauces, dressings, or gravies added to your foods or drinks, as these often have hidden carbs that wreak havoc on your keto diet.

When tracking your progress, you may want to pay particular attention to foods that contain less than 1g of carbohydrate per serving, as this information is not required to be listed on a label. Examples include eggs (.5g carb per egg), heavy whipping cream (.5g carb per tablespoon), and flax and chia seeds (.5g net carb per tablespoon).

Managing Risks and Side Effects

While there are a few undesirable side effects that can occur when starting the keto diet, most can be easily prevented or quickly remedied. Let's take a look at some of the most common, along with how to prevent or treat them.

Dehydration and Electrolyte Loss

When you're starting out on the keto diet, you may feel fatigue, headaches, dizziness, and muscle cramps. These are symptoms of "keto flu"–side effects that result from dehydration and the loss of electrolytes. This happens because ketosis causes your kidneys to excrete more water and certain electrolytes (such as sodium, potassium, and magnesium) as your body adjusts to the changes in your diet.

To help ward off these undesirable side effects, make sure you consume enough water and electrolytes. In terms of hydration, drink at least 8 to 10 8-ounce (235ml) glasses of fluid (ideally water) a day. If you're properly hydrated, your urine will be a very light yellow color. And while you should avoid taking electrolytes in supplement form, a few good dietary sources can provide what you need.

ELECTROLYTE DIETARY SOURCES

The following are some foods you can consume to replenish certain electrolytes that may be lost when following a keto diet.

- **Sodium:** Broth, pickles, olives, cheese, and salt
- **Potassium:** Avocados, tomatoes, artichokes, brussels sprouts, spinach and other leafy green vegetables, pumpkins, mushrooms, eggplant, green beans, lemons, and limes
- **Magnesium:** Leafy green vegetables, nuts, seeds, and meats

Risk for Kidney Stones

While kidney stones are uncommon, they can be a side effect of high fat intake, particularly in children or in those with a personal or family history of kidney stones. To minimize this, drink plenty of fluids and speak with your doctor to determine your risk.

SYMPTOMS OF KETOACIDOSIS

Ketoacidosis may manifest in different ways. Watch out for these symptoms.

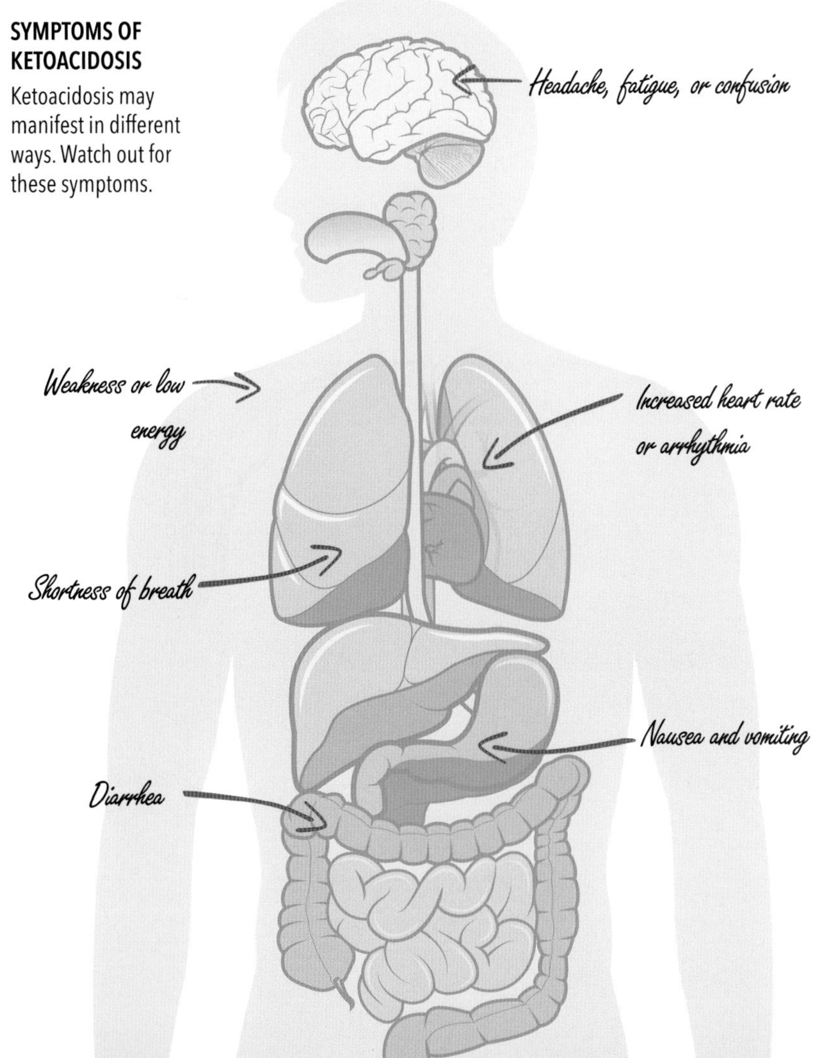

Constipation

Following the keto diet can lead to constipation. However, eating foods high in fiber and maintaining adequate hydration will help you prevent this. Some high-fiber foods you can eat daily to help with constipation include nonstarchy vegetables, nuts and seeds, avocados, and coconut or MCT oils. For a beverage alternative, consider drinking a tea that helps regulate your bowel movements.

Ketoacidosis

Following a well-constructed keto diet with less than 50 g net carbohydrates a day, just enough protein to meet your needs, and sufficient fat helps you enter a state of ketosis referred to as *nutritional ketosis*. In this state, blood ketones generally reach levels of 1 to 8 millimoles per liter (mmol/l) and rarely result alterations in blood pH.

Although unlikely to occur among adults on a keto diet, if blood ketones reach levels greater than 8 mmol/l, it can result in a dangerous condition called *ketoacidosis*. To lower your ketone levels, start by consuming 1 ounce (25ml) of juice and recheck your ketones in 30 minutes, repeating every 30 minutes until they're in the large range or below (see "Monitoring Ketosis"). Once your symptoms have resolved, drink plenty of fluids and eat a keto-friendly meal in the next several hours.

Breakfasts

The word *breakfast* literally means to break the fast from your overnight slumber. So a good breakfast is a way to replenish and prepare yourself for a productive day. From a simple and sweet parfait to savory and filling steak and eggs, these delicious low-carbohydrate, high-fat recipes offer a broad range of keto-friendly foods that generate ample keto fuel to burn fat and help you power through your mornings.

Creamy oven-baked eggs are smothered in bubbling golden Gruyère and sprinkled with fresh thyme.

Baked Eggs with Ham and Gruyère

Prep Time: **10 mins** Cook Time: **7 mins** Yield: **2 baked eggs** Serving Size: **1 baked egg**

Ingredients

- 2 oz. (55g) uncured ham, thinly sliced (about 2 slices)
- 2 TB. unsalted butter, cut into small pieces
- 1 tsp. fresh thyme
- 2 TB. heavy cream
- 2 large eggs
- 2 oz. (55g) Gruyère, grated
- Freshly ground black pepper

1. Preheat the oven to 450°F (230°C). Place uncured ham in the bottom of 2 small oven-proof crocks or ceramic bakers. (Alternately, you can use 2 4-inch (10cm) cast iron skillets.)
2. Add 1 tablespoon unsalted butter, ½ teaspoon thyme, and 1 tablespoon heavy cream to each crock.
3. Carefully break 1 egg into each crock. Sprinkle each with 1 ounce Gruyère and black pepper to taste.
4. Place crocks on a sturdy baking sheet. Bake for 5 minutes, or until eggs are mostly set.
5. Turn the broiler on high and move crocks to the top oven rack, just beneath the broiler. Broil for 1 to 2 minutes, or until cheese is bubbly and golden brown.
6. Remove crocks from the oven and let sit for 5 minutes before serving.

If you can't find Gruyère, use Baby Swiss or another mild cheese that won't overpower the subtle flavors of this dish.

Nutrition per Serving

Fat **76%** Net Carb **3%**
Protein **21%** Ratio **1.4:1**

Calories	Fat	Protein	Total Carbohydrate	Dietary Fiber	Net Carbohydrate
393	33g	21g	3g	0g	3g

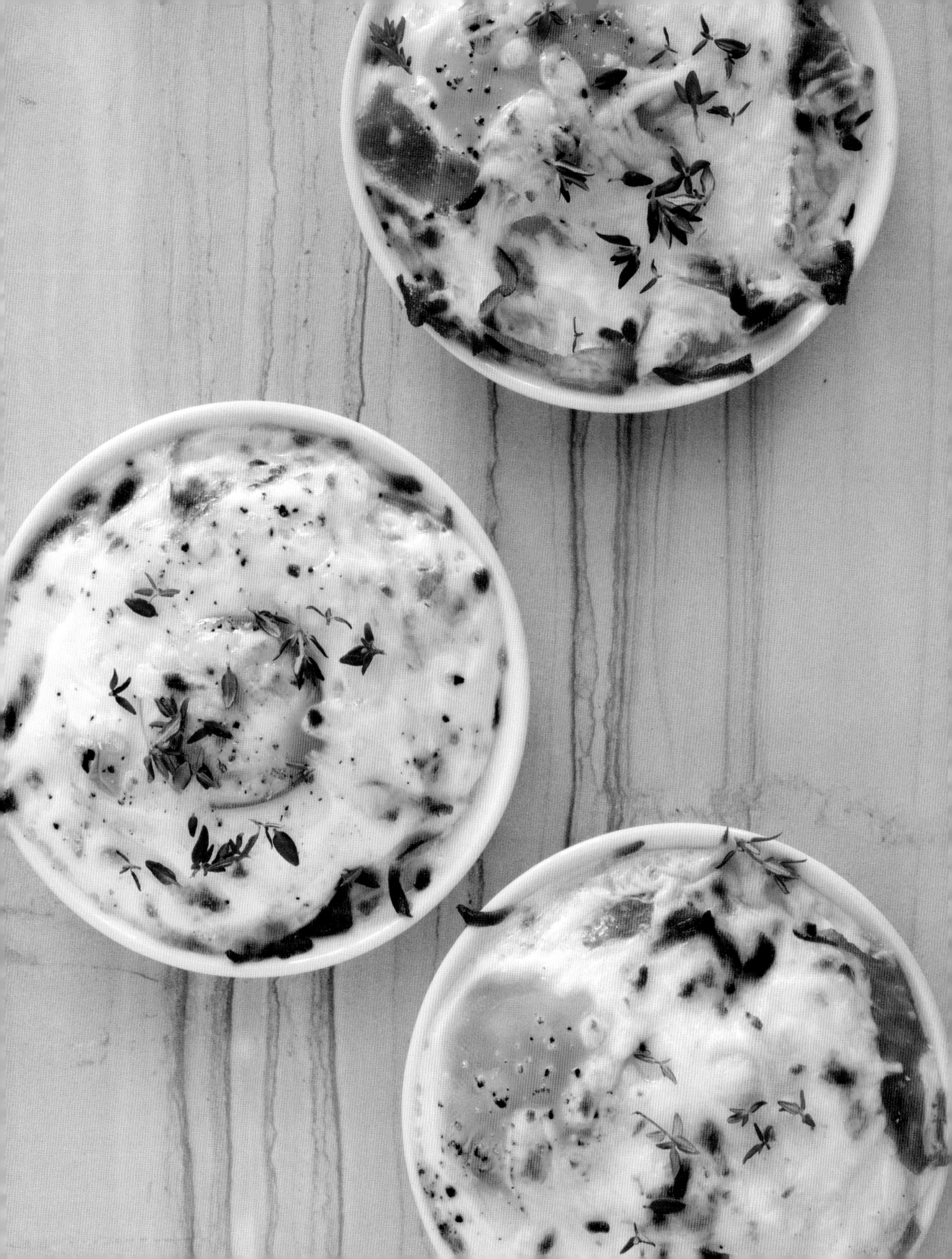

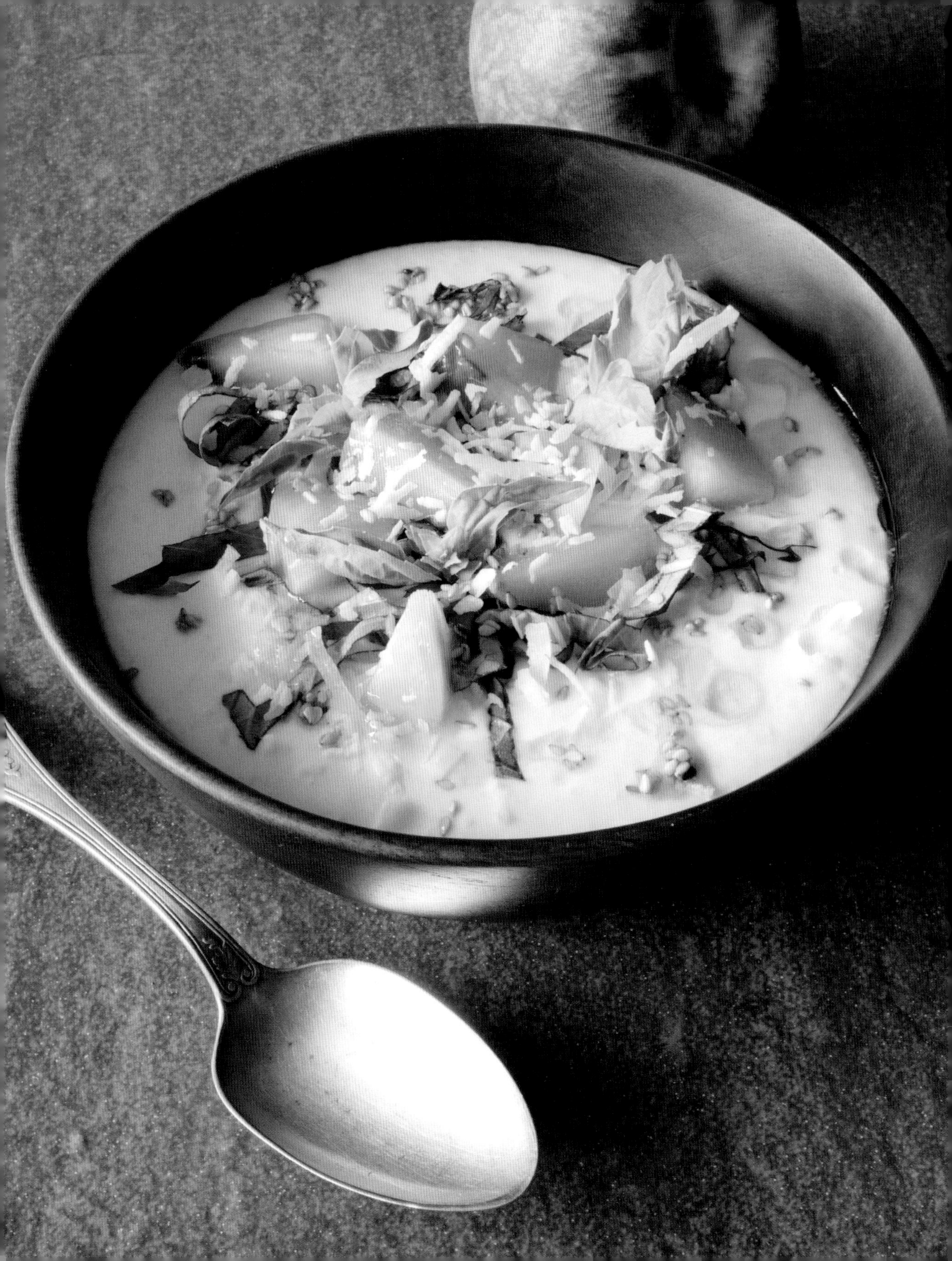

This peach and coconut cream smoothie is topped with fragrant sesame oil, fresh basil, and toasted sesame seeds.

Peaches and Cream Smoothie Bowl

Prep Time: **10 mins** | Cook Time: **none** | Yield: **3 cups** | Serving Size: **1½ cups**

Ingredients

- 1 (14-fl.-oz.; 400ml) can full-fat coconut cream
- ½ cup canned coconut milk
- 2 TB. unsweetened, shredded coconut
- ½ medium peach, sliced (or ½ cup frozen sliced peaches, thawed)
- 2 tsp. toasted sesame seeds
- 2 TB. toasted sesame oil
- 5 basil leaves, thinly sliced

1. Place coconut cream, coconut milk, shredded coconut, and peach into a blender.
2. Pulse for 30 seconds to 1 minute, or until blended to your desired consistency.
3. Pour mixture into 2 small bowls. Garnish with toasted sesame seeds, toasted sesame oil, and basil to serve.

Variation: To make a **Strawberries and Cream Smoothie Bowl,** replace peaches with ½ cup thawed frozen strawberries, and use 2 tablespoons chopped fresh mint instead of basil. Replace toasted sesame oil with almond oil, and use 2 tablespoons chia seeds instead of toasted sesame seeds.

If you're in the maintenance phase, you may be able to increase the peaches for an extra-satisfying smoothie.

Nutrition per Serving

Fat 87% | Net Carb 8% | Protein 5% | Ratio 3.0:1

Calories	Fat	Protein	Total Carbohydrate	Dietary Fiber	Net Carbohydrate
753	73g	8g	18g	2g	16g

Fresh dill and diced avocado complement delicious cold-smoked salmon, peppery arugula, and buttery eggs.

Smoked Salmon Scrambled Eggs with Dill

Prep Time: **5 mins** | Cook Time: **5 mins** | Yield: **2 cups** | Serving Size: **1 cup**

Ingredients

- 4 large eggs
- ¼ tsp. sea salt
- ⅛ tsp. freshly ground black pepper
- 2 TB. heavy cream
- 3 TB. unsalted butter
- 2 oz. (55g) cold-smoked salmon, thinly sliced
- 1 cup baby arugula
- 1 avocado, diced
- 1 TB. fresh dill, finely chopped

1. In a medium bowl, whisk eggs, sea salt, black pepper, and heavy cream. Set aside.

2. Heat a medium skillet or nonstick pan over medium heat. Add unsalted butter to the skillet.

3. When butter is completely melted, pour egg mixture into the skillet. Add cold-smoked salmon and baby arugula.

4. Stirring constantly, cook for 2 to 3 minutes, or until eggs coagulate. Remove the skillet from heat immediately.

5. Divide scramble onto 2 plates. Top with avocado and sprinkle with dill to serve.

Variation: This quick scramble can easily be modified for variety. Replace smoked salmon with 2 ounces (55g) diced hard salami, and use 1 tablespoon fresh chives instead of dill to make **Salami Scrambled Eggs with Chives.**

Nutrition per Serving

Fat **80%** Net Carb **1%**
Protein **19%** Ratio **1.7:1**

Calories	Fat	Protein	Total Carbohydrate	Dietary Fiber	Net Carbohydrate
531	47g	26g	9g	8g	1g

This frothy "latte," loaded with creamy butter and a splash of vanilla extract, is the perfect ketogenic start to the day.

Buttery Vanilla Latte

Prep Time: **5 mins** | Cook Time: **2 mins** | Yield: **2 cups** | Serving Size: **1 cup**

Ingredients

- 16 fl. oz. (475ml) freshly brewed coffee
- 6 TB. unsalted butter
- 1 tsp. pure vanilla extract

1 Place coffee, unsalted butter, and vanilla extract in a blender.

2 Blend on high for 2 minutes, or until a creamy, frothy consistency forms. Divide into 2 mugs and drink warm.

Variation: To make a **Hazelnut Mocha,** substitute hazelnut extract for vanilla extract and add 1 tablespoon unsweetened cocoa powder.

While true lattes use espresso, this high-fat version is a great cheat if you don't have a home espresso machine.

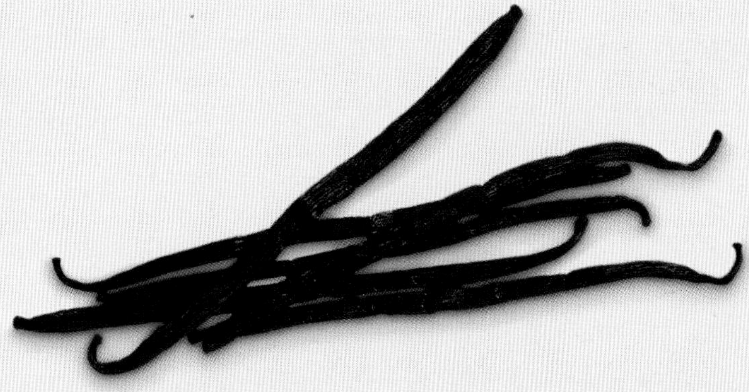

Nutrition per Serving

Fat 99% Net Carb 0%
Protein 1% Ratio 35:1

Calories	Fat	Protein	Total Carbohydrate	Dietary Fiber	Net Carbohydrate
319	35g	1g	0g	0g	0g

Spicy chorizo sausage is baked into a tasty egg and cheese muffin, and topped with sour cream and sprouts.

Chorizo Breakfast Muffins

Prep Time: **10 mins**
Cook Time: **20 mins**
Yield: **12 muffins**
Serving Size: **2 muffins**

Ingredients

2 TB. coconut oil

¾ lb. (340g) fresh chorizo (with no added fillers)

8 large eggs

¼ cup heavy cream

¼ tsp. freshly ground black pepper

1 cup grated cheddar cheese

¼ cup sour cream

½ cup radish or alfalfa sprouts

Nutrition per Serving

Fat **77%**
Net Carb **2%**
Protein **21%**
Ratio **1.5:1**

Calories **516**
Fat **44g**
Protein **27g**
Total Carbohydrate **3g**
Dietary Fiber **0g**
Net Carbohydrate **3g**

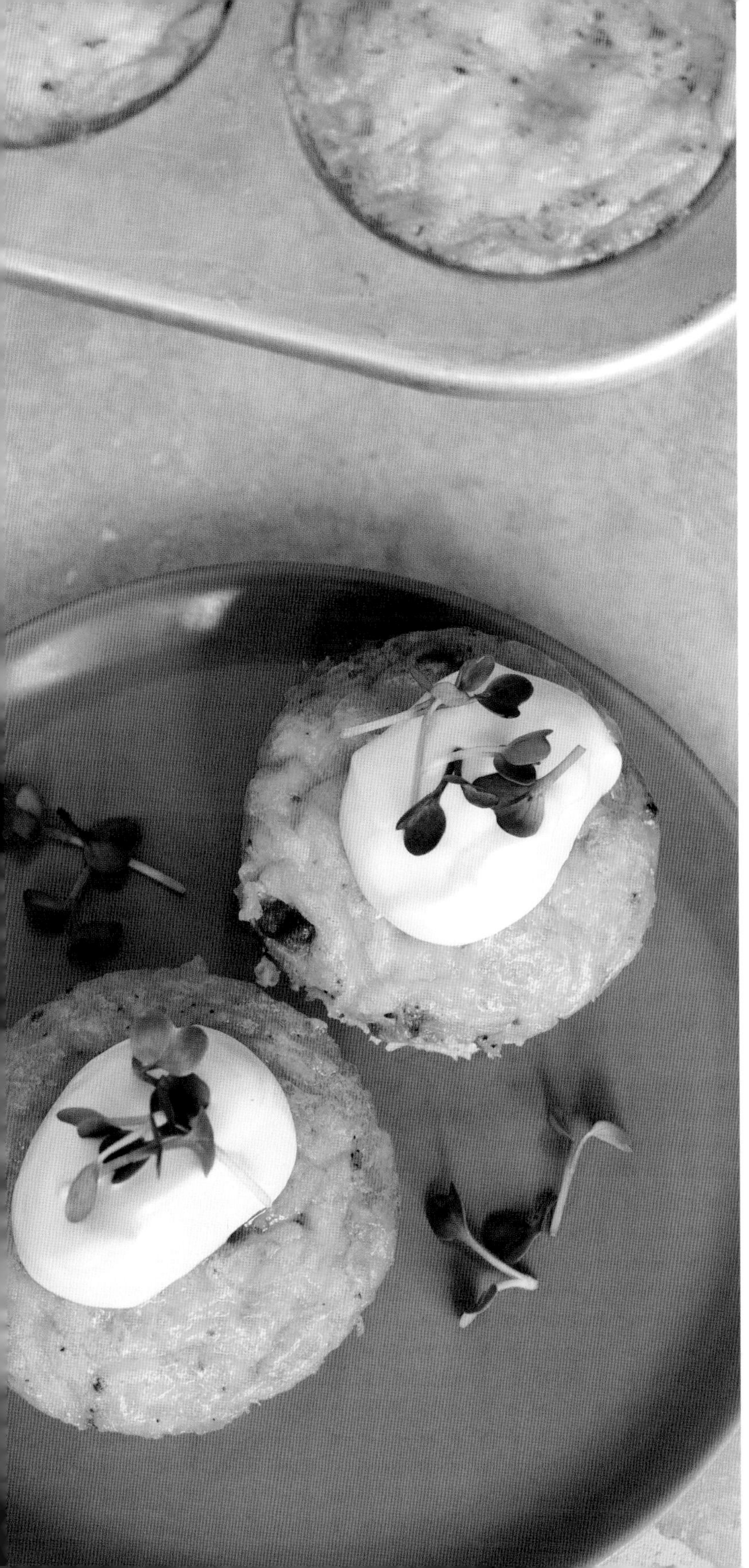

1 Preheat the oven to 350°F (180°C). Place a medium skillet over medium-high heat. Add 1 tablespoon coconut oil and wait for 30 seconds.

2 Add chorizo to hot skillet and cook, stirring frequently, for 4 to 5 minutes, or until browned. Remove from heat and set aside.

3 In a medium bowl, whisk eggs, heavy cream, and black pepper.

4 Use remaining 1 tablespoon coconut oil to generously grease a 12-muffin baking pan.

5 Evenly distribute chorizo into each muffin cup. Pour egg mixture over top and sprinkle with cheddar cheese.

6 Place muffin pan in the oven and bake for 13 to 15 minutes, or until a toothpick inserted into the center of a muffin comes out clean.

7 Remove muffins from oven and allow to cool for 5 minutes. Top with sour cream and sprouts to serve.

Variation: To make a less spicy version, replace chorizo with ground breakfast sausage, and use grated Havarti instead of cheddar cheese for **Sausage and Havarti Breakfast Muffins.** Top with crème fraîche and a hearty sprinkle of fresh dill.

Golden-crisp fritters, loaded with grated Parmesan, are served alongside a fresh basil mayonnaise.

Parmesan Zucchini Fritters with Basil Mayo

Prep Time: **7 mins** | Cook Time: **10 mins** | Yield: **4 fritters** | Serving Size: **2 fritters**

Ingredients

- ¼ tsp. sea salt
- ½ lb. (225g) zucchini, grated
- ⅓ cup mayonnaise
- ¼ cup fresh basil, chopped
- ½ tsp. fresh lemon juice
- ¼ tsp. freshly ground black pepper
- 1 large egg, beaten
- ½ cup Parmesan cheese, grated
- 2 TB. almond flour
- 4 TB. unsalted butter, cut into 1-TB. slices

Nutrition per Serving

Fat 87% | Net Carb 2%
Protein 11% | Ratio 2.8:1

Calories 677
Fat 65g
Protein 19g
Total Carbohydrate 6g
Dietary Fiber 2g
Net Carbohydrate 4g

1 In a medium bowl (or using a colander over the sink), sprinkle sea salt over zucchini. Gently massage zucchini for 1 minute to be sure salt covers completely. Set aside for 5 minutes.

2 Meanwhile, in a small bowl, combine mayonnaise, basil, lemon juice, and black pepper. Set aside for dipping sauce.

3 After 5 minutes, gently squeeze zucchini to release any extra water. Discard water and place zucchini in a dry, medium bowl.

4 Add egg, Parmesan cheese, and almond flour and stir to combine.

5 Heat a nonstick griddle over medium-low heat. When the griddle is hot, scoop unsalted butter slices onto it.

6 Divide mixture in quarters. Spoon zucchini onto melted butter and flatten into 4 thin disks. (The griddle should be hot enough to sizzle slightly.)

7 Cook fritters for 4 to 5 minutes per side, or until deep golden brown and cooked through. Remove from the griddle and place on a paper towel.

8 Serve fritters with basil mayo dipping sauce.

Variation: To make **Cheddar Cauliflower Fritters with Chive Mayo,** replace zucchini with 2 cups grated cauliflower florets and use a pungent sharp white cheddar cheese instead of Parmesan. As a variation on the basil mayo, use finely chopped chives instead of fresh basil.

Juicy rib-eye steaks are smothered in a savory jalapeño-cilantro butter and topped with cheddar scrambled eggs.

Steak with Cheddar Eggs

Prep Time: **15 mins** | Cook Time: **10 mins** | Yield: **1 steak, 2 eggs** | Serving Size: **½ steak, 1 egg**

Ingredients

- 4 TB. salted butter, at room temperature
- 1 small jalapeño, seeded and minced
- 2 TB. fresh cilantro, chopped
- ¼ tsp. freshly ground black pepper
- 2 large eggs
- 2 TB. heavy cream
- 4 oz. (110g) rib-eye steak, about ½ inch (1.25cm) thick
- ¼ tsp. sea salt
- ¼ cup grated sharp cheddar cheese

1. In a small bowl, combine 3 tablespoons salted butter, jalapeño, cilantro, and black pepper until smooth. Set aside.
2. In a separate small bowl, whisk eggs with heavy cream. Set aside.
3. Slice rib-eye steak into 2 equal pieces. Sprinkle both sides of each half with sea salt.
4. Heat a medium skillet over medium-high heat. When the skillet is hot, add remaining 1 tablespoon salted butter.
5. Add steaks to the skillet. (They should sizzle.) For medium doneness, cook for 3 to 4 minutes, turn steaks, and cook for an additional 1 to 2 minutes.
6. Remove steaks from the skillet and spread jalapeño-cilantro butter over top. Let rest for 5 minutes.
7. Reheat the skillet over medium heat. When the skillet is hot, add egg mixture.
8. Cook for 2 to 3 minutes, stirring constantly, until eggs coagulate. Sprinkle with sharp cheddar cheese and remove from heat.
9. Serve cheddar eggs alongside steaks.

Current USDA guidelines indicate fresh beef should be cooked to 145°F (65°C). If you prefer medium-rare steak, cook for 2 to 3 minutes on the first side, and an additional 1 minute after turning.

Nutrition per Serving

Fat **81%** | Net Carb **2%**
Protein **17%** | Ratio **1.9:1**

Calories **435**
Fat **39g**
Protein **19g**
Total Carbohydrate **2g**
Dietary Fiber **0g**
Net Carbohydrate **2g**

Granola clusters are baked with cinnamon and nutmeg, and layered with soft yogurt cream and plump blackberries.

Granola Parfait

Prep Time: **35 mins** | Cook Time: **20 mins** | Yield: **8 parfaits** | Serving Size: **1 parfait**

Ingredients

- ¾ cup raw pecans
- ¾ cup raw walnuts, chopped
- ½ cup slivered almonds
- ¼ cup raw shelled pumpkin seeds
- 2 cups raw hemp seeds
- ¼ cup salted butter, melted
- 2 TB. raw honey
- 1 tsp. ground cinnamon
- ½ tsp. ground nutmeg
- 1 tsp. pure vanilla extract
- 1 cup full-fat plain yogurt
- ½ cup heavy whipping cream
- 6 oz. (170g) fresh blackberries

1. Preheat the oven to 300°F (150°C). In a large bowl, combine pecans, walnuts, almonds, pumpkin seeds, and hemp seeds.
2. In a medium bowl, combine melted salted butter, honey, cinnamon, nutmeg, and vanilla extract. Pour over nut mixture and stir to combine.
3. Spread mixture evenly on a rimmed baking sheet. Bake for 10 minutes.
4. Remove granola from the oven and stir. Return to the oven and bake for an additional 8 to 10 minutes, or until deep golden brown and fragrant. Remove from the oven to cool completely.
5. While granola bakes, whisk full-fat yogurt and heavy whipping cream together until smooth.
6. To serve, layer granola and yogurt cream in parfait glasses or Mason jars, and top with blackberries.

For a quick cold breakfast, skip the fresh berries and use ¾ cup whole milk or heavy cream per ¾ cup granola.

Nutrition per Serving

Fat **79%** Net Carb **7%**
Protein **14%** Ratio **1.6:1**

Calories	Fat	Protein	Total Carbohydrate	Dietary Fiber	Net Carbohydrate
561	49g	20g	17g	7g	10g

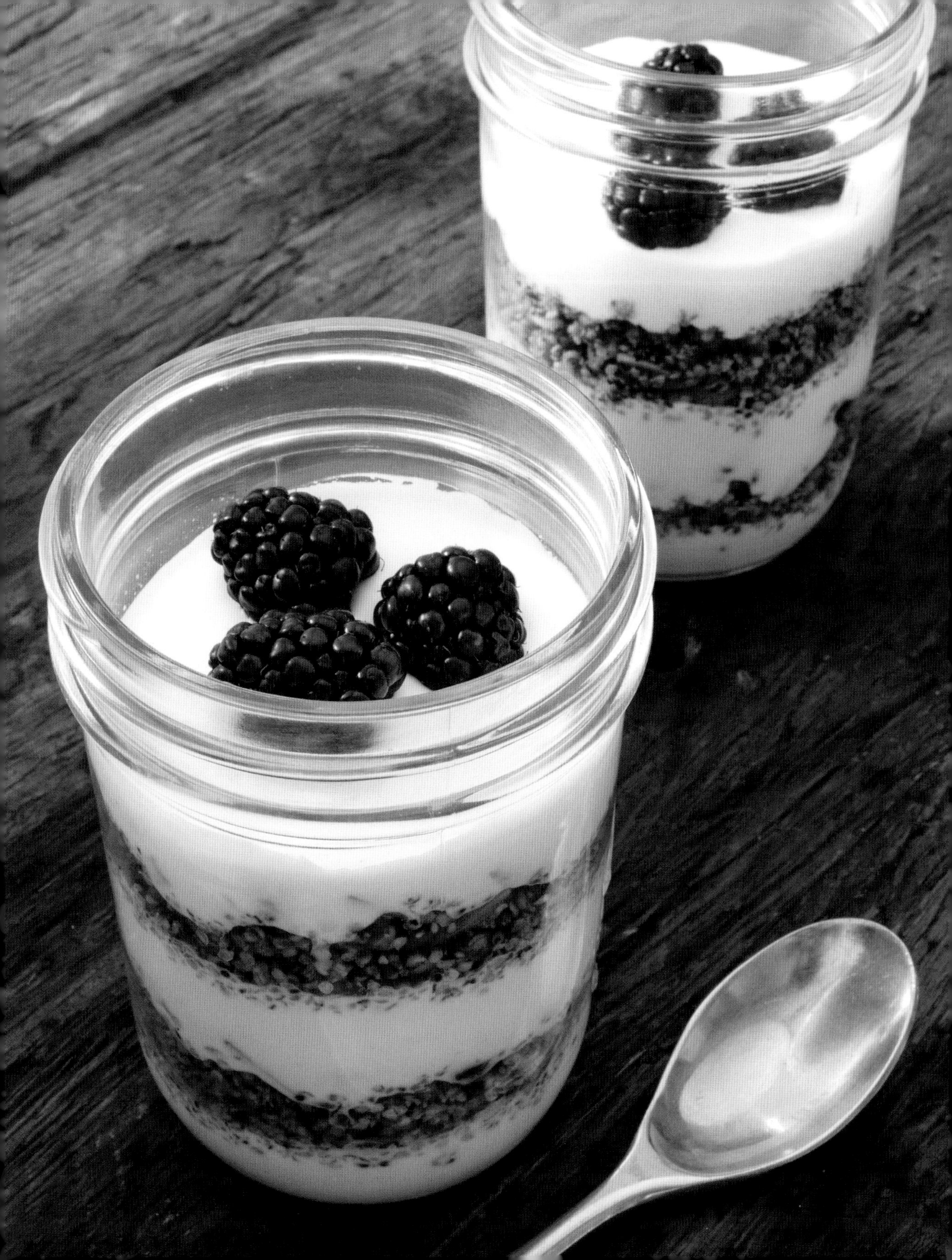

Salty bacon is pan-fried with fragrant garlic in this fluffy omelet, packed with baby spinach and piquant Pepper jack.

Bacon and Pepper Jack Omelet

Prep Time: **5 mins** | Cook Time: **15 mins** | Yield: **1 omelet** | Serving Size: **1 omelet**

Ingredients

- 2 large eggs
- 1 TB. heavy cream
- ¼ tsp. freshly ground black pepper
- 2 oz. (55g) uncured bacon, diced
- 1 garlic clove, minced
- 1 TB. unsalted butter
- ½ cup grated Pepper jack cheese (about 2 oz.; 55g)
- 1 cup baby spinach

Nutrition per Serving

Fat **74%** | Net Carb **4%**
Protein **22%** | Ratio **1.3:1**

Calories **567**
Fat **47g**
Protein **31g**
Total Carbohydrate **7g**
Dietary Fiber **2g**
Net Carbohydrate **5g**

1. In a medium bowl, whisk eggs, heavy cream, and black pepper for about 30 seconds, or until fully combined and slightly foamy. Set aside.

2. Place a medium nonstick skillet over medium heat. Add bacon to the skillet and cook, stirring frequently, for 3 minutes.

3. Add garlic and continue to cook for an additional 1 to 3 minutes, or until garlic and bacon are lightly browned.

4. Immediately remove bacon and garlic. Pour off bacon fat and return 1 tablespoon of bacon fat to the skillet.

5. Reheat the skillet over medium heat and add unsalted butter.

6. When the skillet is hot, pour in egg mixture. Shake the skillet vigorously to spread egg evenly along the bottom.

7. As egg begins to cook and coagulate, use a rubber scraper or spatula to carefully lift cooked edges from the sides of the skillet. Tilt the skillet to allow raw egg to run down lifted edges toward the bottom of the skillet to cook, about 2 minutes.

8. When egg is coagulated but still moist, place cooked bacon and garlic, Pepper jack, and baby spinach on one half.

9. Using a wide plastic spatula, flip empty half of egg over top of vegetables. Cook for 1 minute, and slide onto a plate. Serve immediately.

Variation: To make a **Sausage and Swiss Omelet,** simply replace bacon slices with ¼ pound (115g) ground sausage, and use grated Baby Swiss instead of Pepper jack. You may also need to add an additional tablespoon of butter to make up for the missing bacon drippings.

Smoked chipotle and cumin flavor this cheese-free omelet, loaded with avocado, black olives, and red onion.

Mexican Omelet

Prep Time: **5 mins** | Cook Time: **15 mins** | Yield: **1 omelet** | Serving Size: **1 omelet**

Ingredients

- 2 large eggs, beaten
- 3 TB. heavy cream
- ¼ tsp. ground cumin
- ½ tsp. ground chipotle
- 2 TB. unsalted butter
- ½ medium avocado, diced
- 5 black olives, sliced or chopped
- 1 TB. red onion, finely diced
- ¼ cup fresh cilantro, chopped
- 1 TB. sour cream

1. In a medium bowl, whisk eggs, heavy cream, cumin, and chipotle for about 30 seconds, or until fully combined and slightly foamy. Set aside.

2. Place a medium nonstick skillet over medium heat. Add unsalted butter.

3. When the skillet is hot, pour egg mixture into the skillet. Shake the skillet vigorously to spread egg evenly along the bottom.

4. As egg begins to cook and coagulate, use a rubber scraper or spatula to carefully lift cooked edges from the sides of the skillet. Tilt the skillet to allow raw egg to run down lifted edges toward the bottom of the skillet to cook, about 2 minutes.

5. When egg is coagulated but still moist, place avocado, black olives, and red onion on half.

6. Using a wide plastic spatula, flip empty half of egg over top of vegetables. Cook for 1 minute, and slide onto a plate.

7. Top omelet with fresh cilantro and sour cream to serve.

If you can't find ground chipotle, you can substitute smoked paprika or any red chili powder instead.

Nutrition per Serving

Fat 88% Net Carb 2%
Protein 10% Ratio 3.4:1

Calories	Fat	Protein	Total Carbohydrate	Dietary Fiber	Net Carbohydrate
683	67g	17g	12g	9g	3g

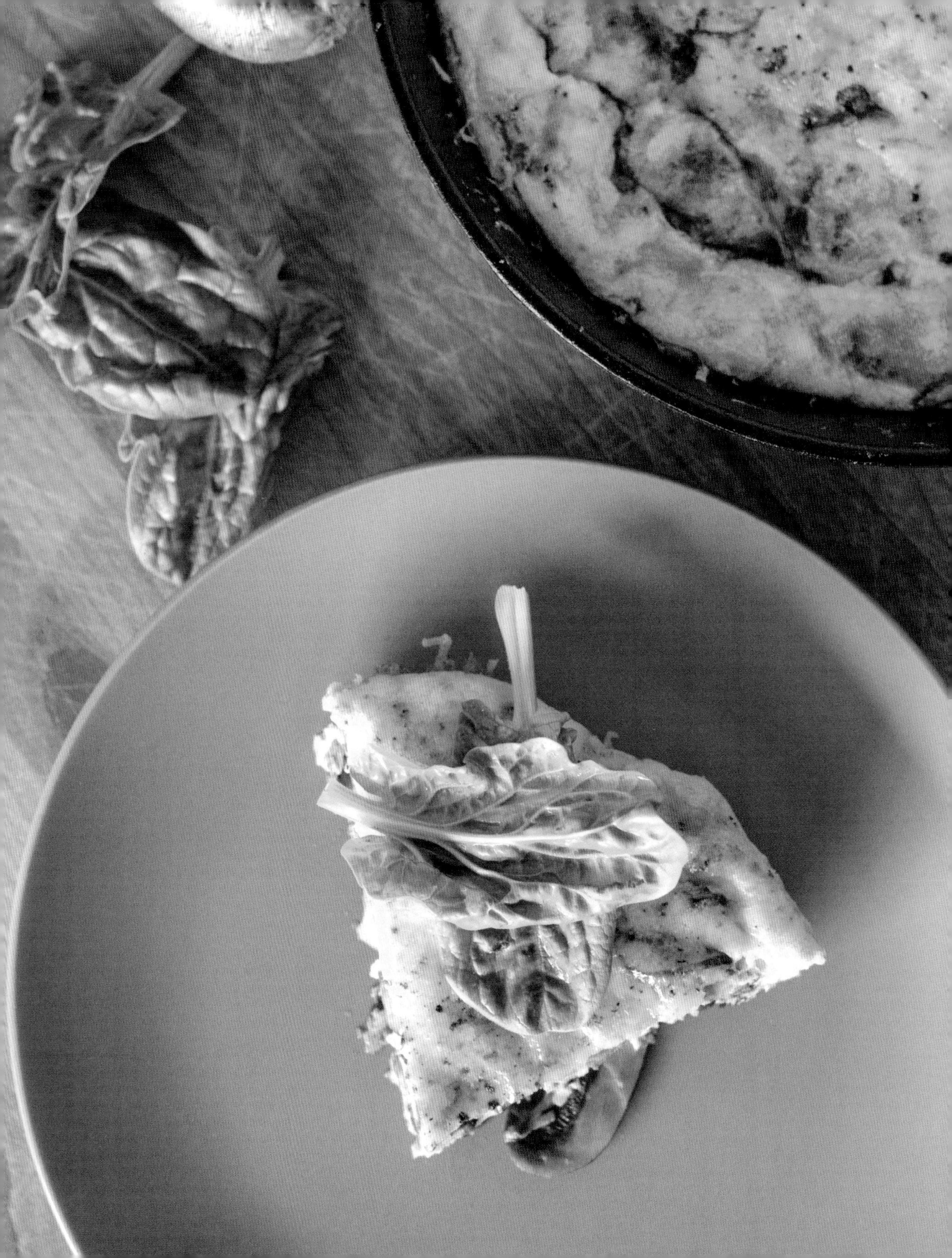

Earthy mushrooms are sautéed with fragrant garlic and fresh spinach, and then sprinkled with mellow Baby Swiss.

Mushroom and Swiss Frittata

Prep Time: **5 mins** | Cook Time: **20 mins** | Yield: **1 frittata** | Serving Size: **½ frittata**

Ingredients

- 4 large eggs, beaten
- ¼ cup heavy cream
- ¼ tsp. freshly ground black pepper
- 3 TB. extra-virgin olive oil
- ¼ lb. (115g) fresh mushrooms, sliced
- 1 garlic clove, minced
- 3 cups baby spinach
- 2 oz. (55g) Baby Swiss cheese, grated

1 Adjust the top oven rack to be in the second shelf from the top position. (Make sure there's enough room above to fit the cast-iron skillet.) Preheat the oven to 350°F (180°C).

2 In a medium bowl, whisk eggs, heavy cream, and black pepper. Set aside.

3 Heat an 8-inch (20cm) cast-iron or ovenproof skillet over medium-high heat. When the skillet is hot, add extra-virgin olive oil and wait for 15 seconds.

4 Add mushrooms to the skillet and sauté, stirring frequently, for 2 to 3 minutes, or until softened.

5 Add garlic and baby spinach and continue to sauté for 1 to 2 minutes, or until spinach is wilted and garlic is fragrant. Remove from heat.

6 Pour egg mixture evenly over top and sprinkle with Baby Swiss cheese.

7 Place the skillet on the top rack of the oven. Bake for 12 to 15 minutes, or until egg is set in the middle and a toothpick inserted in the center comes out clean. Serve hot right out of the pan.

While this recipe is great with white button or cremini mushrooms, it's even better with in-season morels or chanterelles.

Nutrition per Serving

Fat 76% Net Carb 4%
Protein 20% Ratio 1.4:1

Calories	Fat	Protein	Total Carbohydrate	Dietary Fiber	Net Carbohydrate
472	40g	24g	7g	3g	4g

Snacks

Snacks are the glue that holds any diet together, as they can prevent the temptation to reach into the cookie jar. It's therefore critical to have snack recipes on hand that are easy to put together and—most important—taste good. From veggies and dip to pizza bites, these delicious, keto-approved snacks satisfy your between-meal cravings while keeping you on track for meeting your diet goals.

Ruby radishes are accented with velvety butter and adorned with large flakes of pure sea salt in this filling snack.

Buttered Radishes

Prep Time: **5 mins** Cook Time: **none** Yield: **16 halves** Serving Size: **4 halves**

Ingredients

8 medium radishes

8 tsp. unsalted butter, at room temperature

¼ tsp. coarse sea salt

1 Using a small paring knife, trim green tops from radishes and discard. Slice each radish bulb in half, from stem to root.

2 In a small bowl, gently whip unsalted butter with a fork until soft and spreadable.

3 Spread ½ teaspoon butter on each radish half and sprinkle with coarse sea salt before serving.

These radishes rely on the flavor of high-quality butter. Look for a golden yellow variety made from grass-fed or pasture-grazed cow's milk. If you can't find a high-quality butter, use a luxurious triple-cream Brie.

Nutrition per Serving

Fat 100% Net Carb 0%
Protein 0% Ratio 8:0

Calories	Fat	Protein	Total Carbohydrate	Dietary Fiber	Net Carbohydrate
72	8g	0g	0g	0g	0g

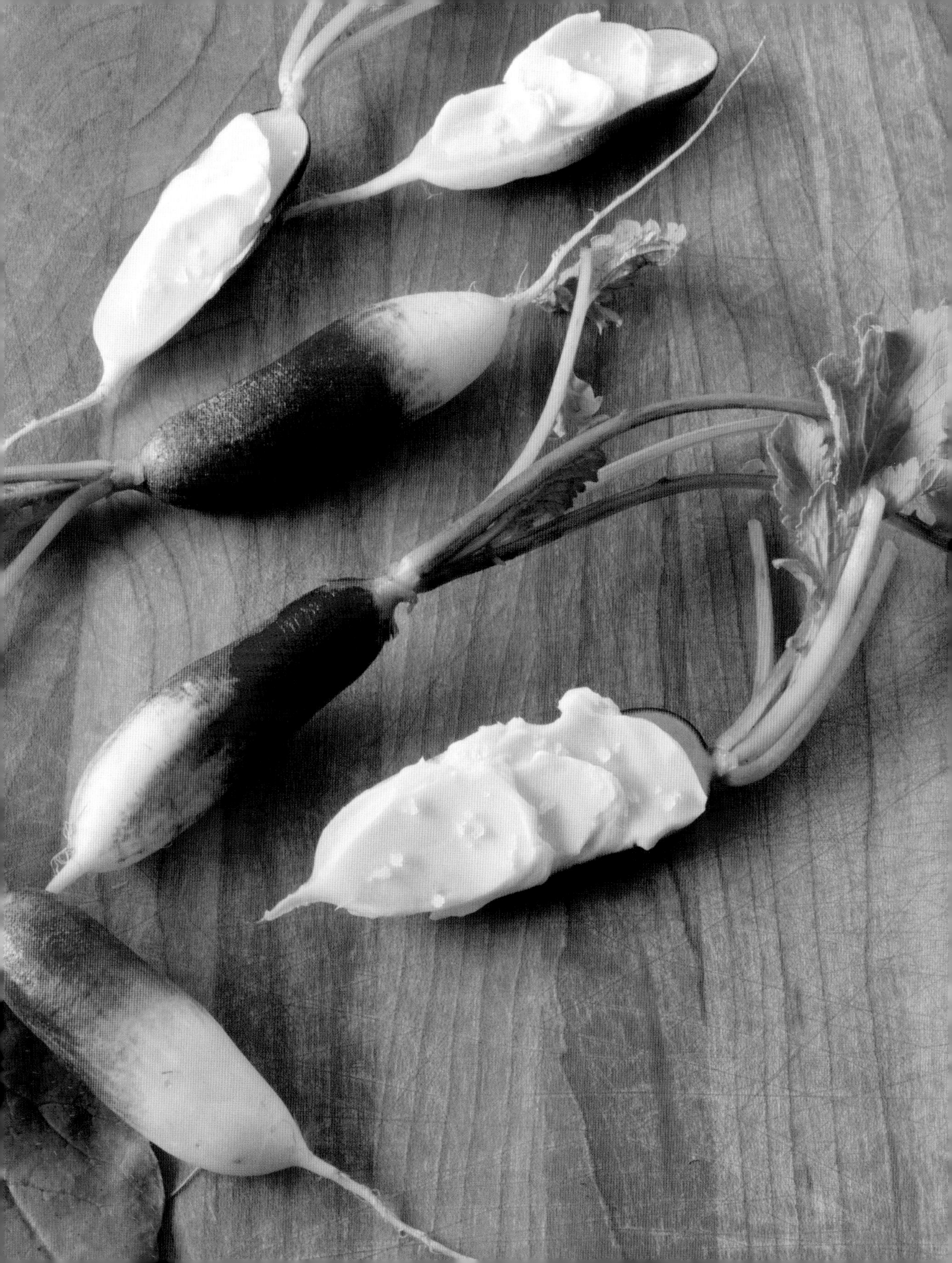

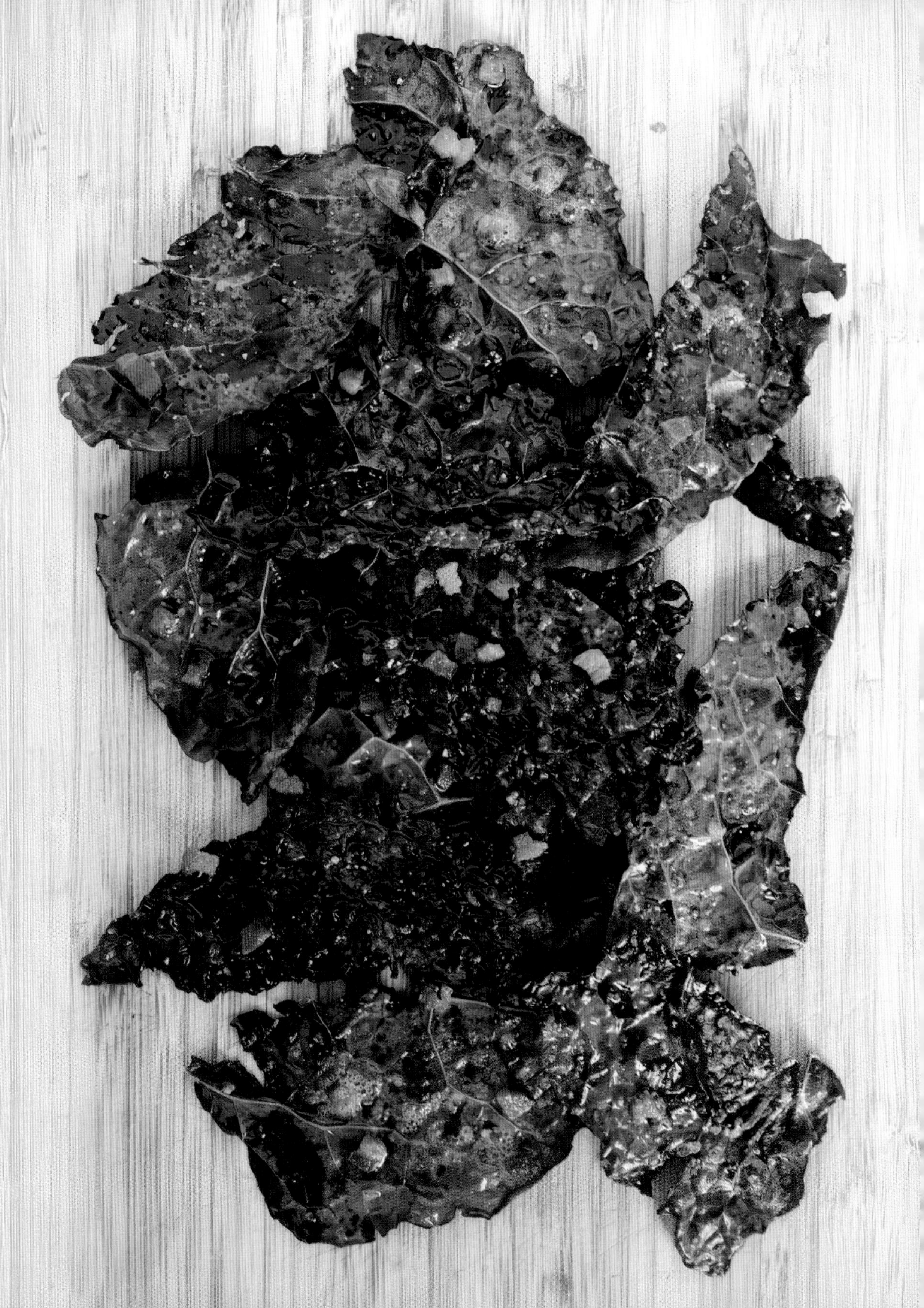

Deep green-blue lacinato kale is oven-crisped with olive oil and covered in salty, bacon-y goodness.

Kale Chips with Bacon

Prep Time: **10 mins** | Cook Time: **15 mins** | Yield: **32 chips** | Serving Size: **8 chips**

Ingredients

- 8 lacinato kale leaves
- 4 TB. extra-virgin olive oil
- 1 tsp. sea salt
- ½ tsp. freshly ground black pepper
- 1 oz. (25g) uncured bacon, minced

1 Preheat the oven to 350°F (180°C). Remove and discard woody stems from lacinato kale leaves. Cut leaves in half lengthwise. (If kale has any residual water from rinsing, use a salad spinner or paper towel to dry before proceeding.)

2 Rub both sides of leaves with extra-virgin olive oil. Spread leaves evenly on a metal baking sheet. Sprinkle with sea salt and black pepper. Bake for 10 minutes.

3 While kale is baking, heat a small skillet over medium heat. When the skillet is hot, add minced bacon and cook, stirring frequently, for 3 to 5 minutes, or until a light golden brown. Remove from heat.

4 Remove kale from the oven. Carefully pour bacon and residual bacon fat evenly over kale chips.

5 Return the baking sheet to the oven and finish cooking for 3 to 5 minutes, or until edges of kale are browned and crisp. Serve straight from the oven or allow to cool to room temperature.

If you have trouble finding lacinato kale, feel free to use curly green or beautiful Red Russian varieties instead.

Nutrition per Serving

Fat **84%** Net Carb **11%**
Protein **5%** Ratio **2.3:1**

Calories **150**
Fat **14g**
Protein **2g**
Total Carbohydrate **5g**
Dietary Fiber **1g**
Net Carbohydrate **4g**

These snappy crackers are made of baked Gouda, with an extra pop from a sprinkling of chia seeds.

Cheesy Crisps

Prep Time: **40 mins** | Cook Time: **7 mins** | Yield: **24 crisps** | Serving Size: **4 crisps**

Ingredients

- 12 oz. (340g) Gouda, grated
- 2 TB. extra-virgin olive oil
- 3 TB. chia seeds
- ½ tsp. freshly ground black pepper

1. Preheat the oven to 350°F (180°C). Cut a piece of parchment paper to line a rimmed metal baking sheet. (Alternately, use a silicone baking mat.) Repeat with a second baking sheet.
2. Using a teaspoon, scoop small mounds of Gouda and place onto the parchment, spacing cheese at least 4 inches (10cm) apart.
3. Drizzle extra-virgin olive oil evenly over cheese. Sprinkle with chia seeds and black pepper.
4. Place the baking sheets in the oven and bake for 5 to 7 minutes, or until edges are a deep golden brown.
5. Remove the baking sheets from the oven and let cool completely. Using a spatula, gently remove crisps from the parchment.
6. Serve at room temperature, or store leftovers in an airtight container for up to 1 week.

Variation: To make **Cheesy Ranch Crisps,** make a mixture of 1 teaspoon dried parsley, ½ teaspoon granulated garlic, ½ teaspoon onion powder, and ¼ teaspoon dried thyme. Sprinkle mixture on the crisps in addition to olive oil, chia seeds, and black pepper.

These crisps are excellent for dipping. You can also crumble a few up for a crunchy and flavorful salad topping.

Nutrition per Serving

Fat **74%** Net Carb **3%**
Protein **23%** Ratio **1.3:1**

Calories	266
Fat	22g
Protein	15g
Total Carbohydrate	4g
Dietary Fiber	2g
Net Carbohydrate	2g

This creamy dip, with a dash of smoked paprika, is an effortless snack served alongside crunchy cucumber slices.

Tuna Dip

Prep Time: **10 mins** | Cook Time: **none** | Yield: **1 cup** | Serving Size: **1⁄4 cup**

Ingredients

- 1 (4-oz.; 110g) can albacore tuna in olive oil, drained
- ¾ cup olive oil mayonnaise
- ½ tsp. sea salt, or to taste
- ½ tsp. freshly ground black pepper
- 1 tsp. smoked paprika
- 2 medium cucumbers, sliced

1. In a food processor, combine albacore tuna, olive oil mayonnaise, sea salt, and black pepper.
2. Pulse for 15 to 25 seconds, or until a rough paste forms. Transfer dip to a serving bowl.
3. Sprinkle dip with smoked paprika and serve alongside cucumber slices.

Make sure to look for albacore tuna that has been canned in olive oil to ensure you avoid bad omega-6 fats.

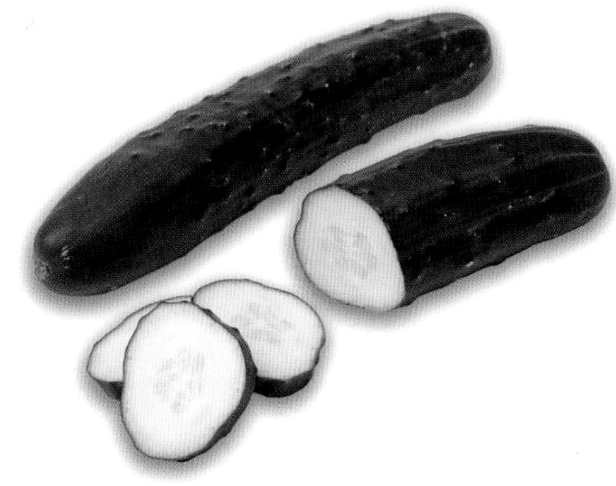

Nutrition per Serving

Fat **83%** Net Carb **6%**
Protein **11%** Ratio **2.2:1**

Calories	Fat	Protein	Total Carbohydrate	Dietary Fiber	Net Carbohydrate
357	33g	10g	6g	1g	5g

Rich, bone-building sardines are accented with fresh dill and a splash of lemon juice, and served on crisp Belgian endive.

Sardines with Endive and Lemon

Prep Time: **5 mins** Cook Time: **none** Yield: **8 leaves** Serving Size: **2 leaves**

Ingredients

- 1 small head Belgian endive
- 1 (3.75-oz.; 106g) can sardines in olive oil
- 2 TB. fresh dill, chopped
- 1 tsp. grated lemon zest
- ½ tsp. sea salt
- 2 TB. extra-virgin olive oil

1. Trim woody end off Belgian endive and separate leaves.
2. Drain sardines, discarding olive oil. Break sardines into large pieces.
3. Place 2 to 3 sardine pieces on each endive leaf. Sprinkle with dill, lemon zest, and sea salt.
4. Drizzle sardine pieces with extra-virgin olive oil before serving.

Brimming with omega-3 fatty acids, vitamin B_{12}, and vitamin D, sardines are also a highly sustainable seafood.

Nutrition per Serving

Fat **72%** Net Carb **3%**
Protein **25%** Ratio **1.1:1**

Calories	Fat	Protein	Total Carbohydrate	Dietary Fiber	Net Carbohydrate
126	10g	8g	5g	4g	1g

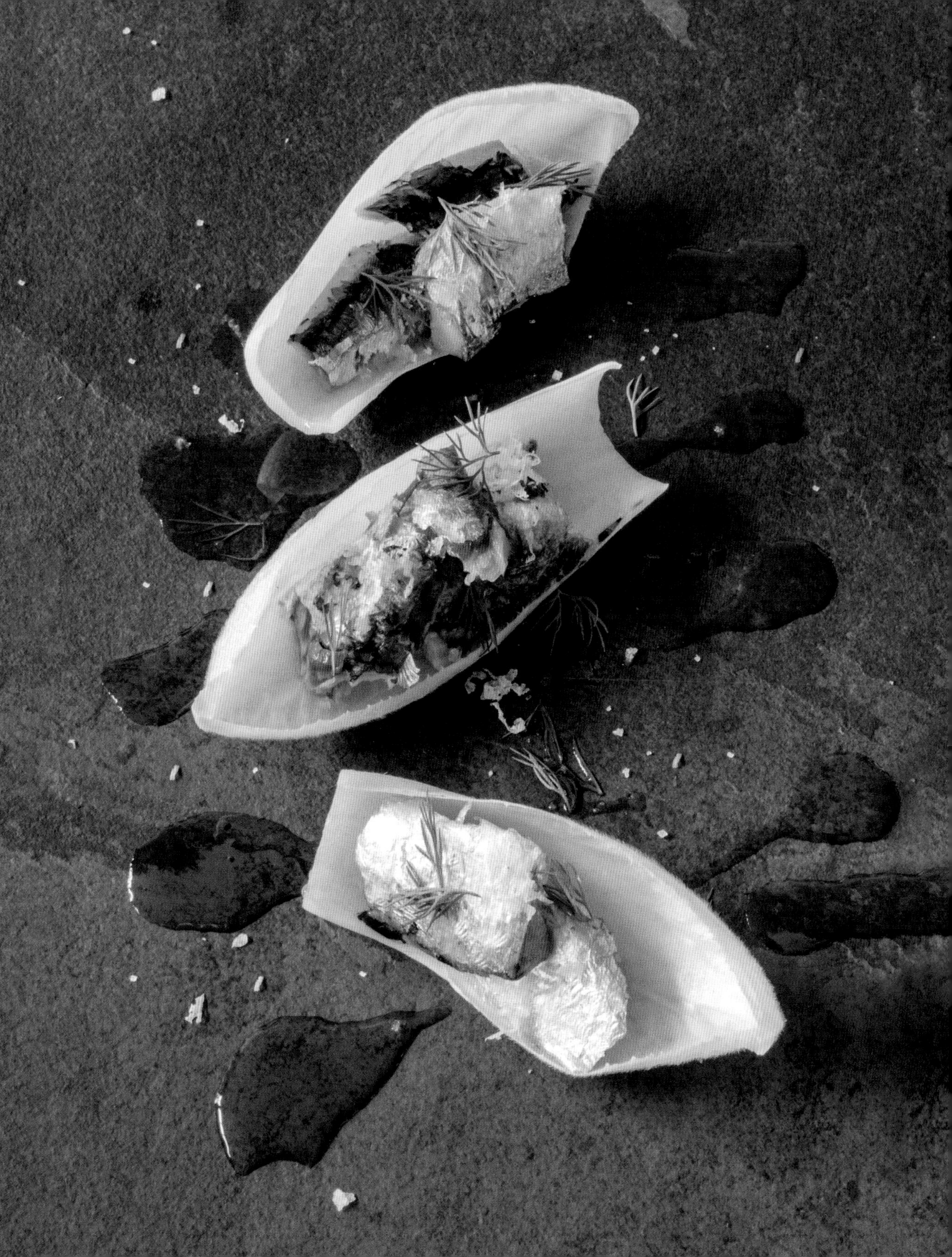

Luscious Brie cheese is steeped in fragrant garlic and aromatic, rosemary-infused olive oil.

Rosemary and Black Pepper–Marinated Brie

Prep Time: **3 days, 1 hr** | Cook Time: **4 mins** | Yield: **20 to 30 pieces** | Serving Size: **2 to 3 pieces**

Ingredients

- 1 cup extra-virgin olive oil
- 3 garlic cloves, sliced
- 1 tsp. whole black peppercorns
- 2 sprigs fresh rosemary
- 8 oz. (225g) double- or triple-cream Brie, chilled

1 Heat a small saucepan over medium heat. Add extra-virgin olive oil and garlic and cook for 3 to 4 minutes, or until garlic is fragrant and just beginning to color. Remove from heat. Add black peppercorns and rosemary and let stand for 1 hour, or until completely cool.

2 Meanwhile, cut Brie (rind included) into small bite-size pieces. Place pieces in a 1-quart (1l) Mason jar with a tight-fitting lid. Keep refrigerated until oil cools.

3 Pour cooled oil, garlic, black peppercorns, and rosemary over Brie. Add additional olive oil, if needed, to cover Brie completely.

4 Refrigerate for 1 to 3 days. Flavors will increase the longer Brie marinates. Serve chilled.

Variation: To make **Lemon Thyme–Marinated Brie,** replace black peppercorns and rosemary with 1 teaspoon grated fresh lemon zest, 1/4 teaspoon crushed red pepper flakes, and 6 fresh thyme sprigs.

Double- and triple-cream Brie have added cream versus normal Brie, so they contain a higher percentage of butterfat.

Nutrition per Serving

Fat **96%** Net Carb **0%**
Protein **4%** Ratio **10.3:1**

Calories **291**
Fat **31g**
Protein **3g**
Total Carbohydrate **0g**
Dietary Fiber **0g**
Net Carbohydrate **0g**

Loaded with fresh dill, a hint of shallot, and a dash of celery salt, this creamy dip is a light and easy ketogenic snack.

Dilly Dip

Prep Time: **10 mins** | Cook Time: **none** | Yield: **2 cups** | Serving Size: **¼ cup**

Ingredients

- 1½ cups sour cream
- ½ cup mayonnaise
- 1 TB. minced shallot
- 2 TB. chopped fresh dill
- 1 tsp. celery salt
- ¼ tsp. freshly ground black pepper
- 1 small cucumber, thinly sliced

1. In a small bowl, whisk sour cream and mayonnaise together until fully combined.
2. Add shallot, dill, celery salt, and black pepper and stir to combine.
3. Serve dip alongside thin cucumber slices. (Alternately, serve with celery sticks or endive leaves.)

This dip is perfect served with any low-carb veggie. Just don't serve it with higher-carb options, such as carrot sticks.

Variation: To make a **Garlic Herb Dip,** replace fresh dill with 1 tablespoon chopped fresh chives and 1 tablespoon chopped fresh parsley, and use ½ teaspoon granulated garlic in place of shallot.

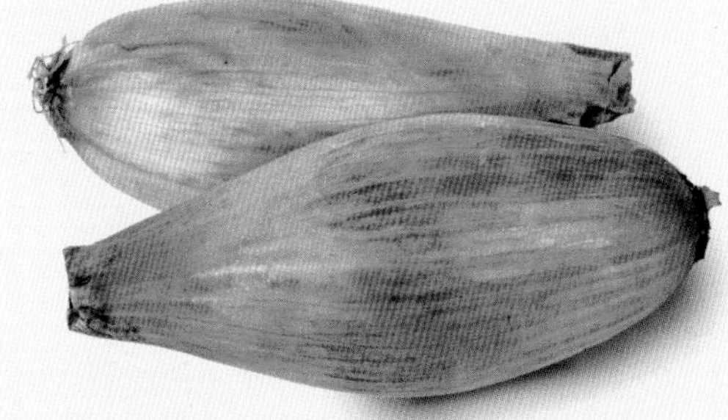

Nutrition per Serving

Fat 91% Net Carb 7%
Protein 2% Ratio 4.3:1

Calories	Fat	Protein	Total Carbohydrate	Dietary Fiber	Net Carbohydrate
169	17g	1g	3g	0g	3g

Silky avocado, laced with lime and ground cumin, is piped into hard-cooked eggs in this savory snack.

Guacamole Deviled Eggs

Prep Time: **15 mins**
Cook Time: **15 mins**
Yield: **24 halves**
Serving Size: **2 halves**

Ingredients

- 12 large eggs
- ½ cup mayonnaise
- ½ medium avocado
- 1 TB. fresh cilantro, chopped
- 1 TB. fresh lime juice
- 1 tsp. ground cumin
- ½ tsp. sea salt
- 1 tsp. chili powder

Nutrition per Serving

Fat **81%** Net Carb **0%**
Protein **19%** Ratio **1.9:1**

Calories **145**
Fat **13g**
Protein **7g**
Total Carbohydrate **1g**
Dietary Fiber **1g**
Net Carbohydrate **0g**

Food safety is a concern when serving deviled eggs. Always be sure to keep filled eggs covered and refrigerated, and serve them on a chilled platter resting on ice, if necessary.

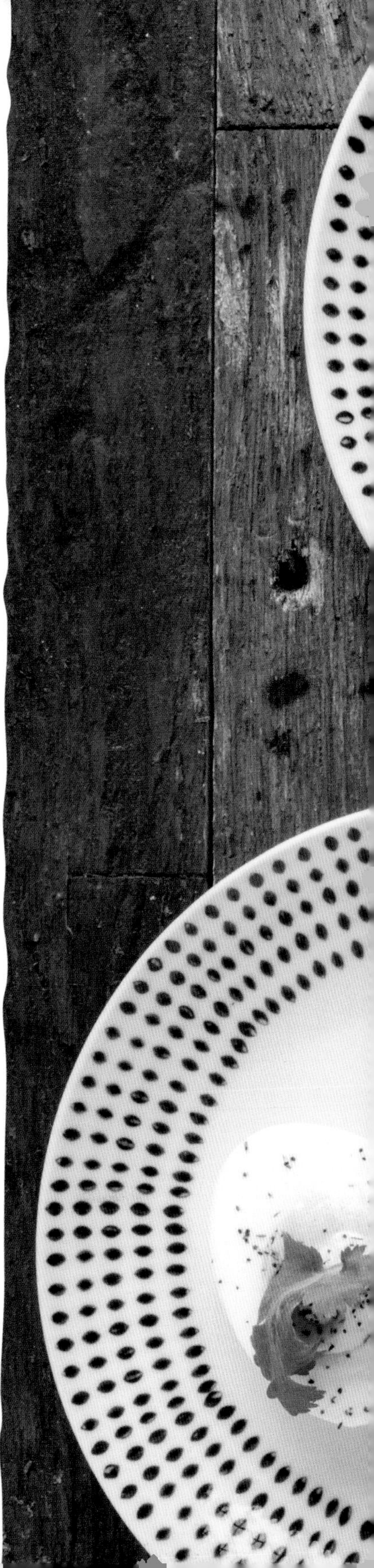

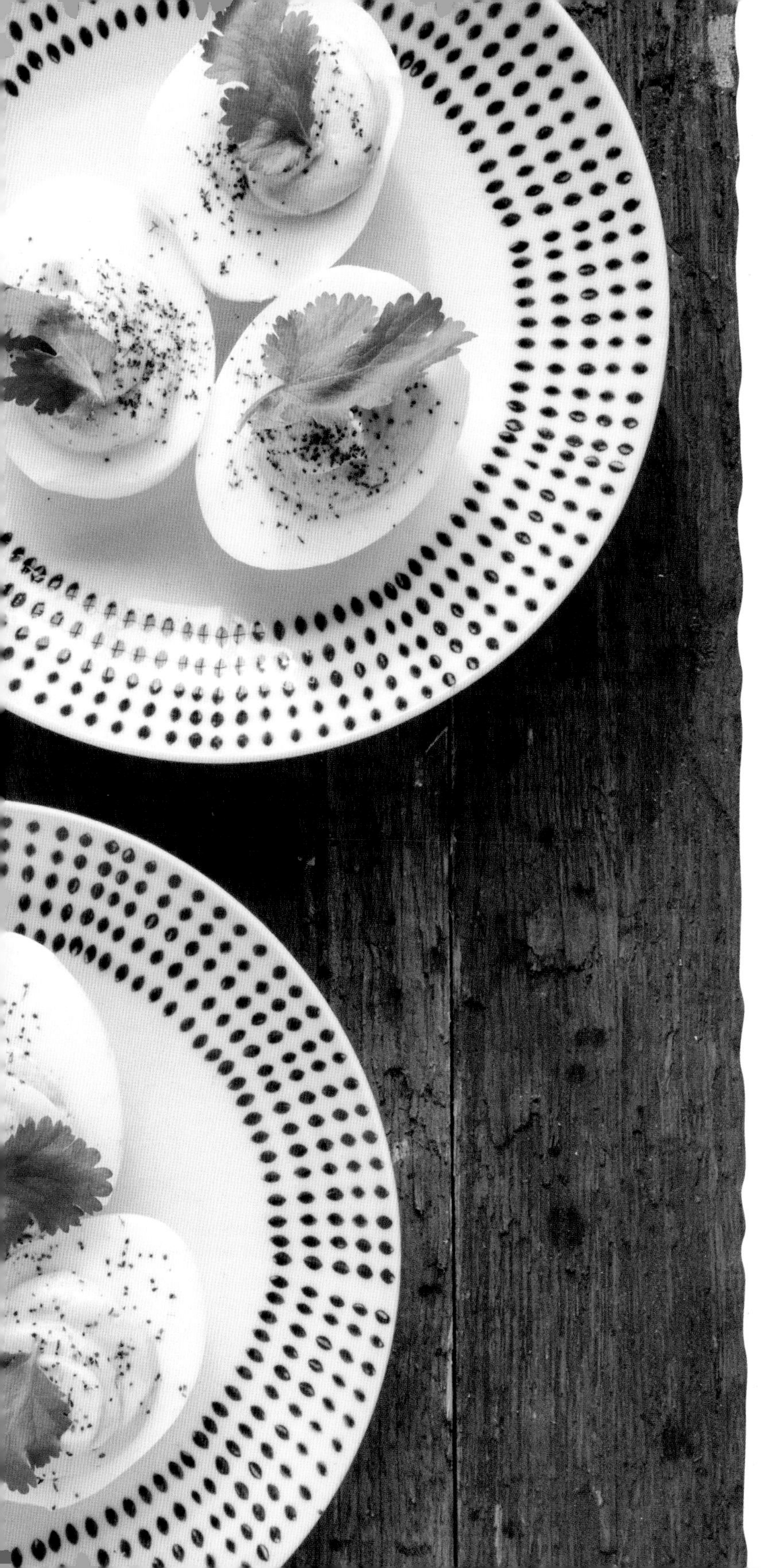

1. Place whole eggs in a 2-quart (2l) saucepan. Fill the pan with cold water to cover eggs. Place the pan, uncovered, over high heat until simmering, about 5 to 10 minutes.

2. Remove the pan from heat, cover, and wait for 13 minutes.

3. While eggs cook, combine mayonnaise, avocado, cilantro, lime juice, cumin, and sea salt in a food processor. Pulse until a smooth paste forms.

4. Drain cooked eggs and plunge under cold water until cool enough to handle. Remove and discard shells immediately, and slice eggs in half lengthwise.

5. Scoop firm yolks out of eggs and add to avocado mixture. Pulse until mixture is fully combined and smooth.

6. Carefully spoon filling into egg halves. (Alternately, use a pastry bag with a decorative tip to pipe filling into eggs.)

7. Dust with chili powder before serving.

Variation: To make **Classic Deviled Eggs,** fill egg halves with a mix of ⅔ cup mayonnaise, 1 tablespoon Dijon mustard, 12 cooked egg yolks, and ½ teaspoon sea salt. Sprinkle with smoked paprika to serve.

Succulent bites of seared rib-eye steak are dunked in a copious amount of lavish horseradish cream.

Steak Bites with Horseradish Cream

Prep Time: **5 mins** | Cook Time: **10 mins** | Yield: **about 20 bites** | Serving Size: **about 5 bites**

Ingredients

- 6-oz. (170g) boneless rib-eye steak, cut into ½-in. (1.25cm) cubes
- ½ tsp. sea salt
- 2 TB. ghee or tallow
- 1 cup crème fraîche
- 2 TB. prepared horseradish
- 1 tsp. lemon juice
- ¼ tsp. freshly ground black pepper
- 1 tsp. fresh chives, chopped

1. Season boneless rib-eye steak bites with sea salt.
2. Heat a medium skillet over medium-high heat. When the skillet is hot, add ghee and wait for 30 seconds.
3. Add rib-eye to hot ghee and cook for 1 minute. Turn each cube and brown opposite side for an additional 1 to 2 minutes. Remove from heat.
4. In a small bowl, combine crème fraîche, horseradish, lemon juice, and black pepper. Sprinkle with chives.
5. To serve, dip rib-eye bites in Horseradish Cream.

There's enough fat in the horseradish cream to support a leaner cut of steak, such as bavette, hanger, or flap steak.

Nutrition per Serving

Fat **86%** Net Carb **4%**
Protein **10%** Ratio **2.8:1**

Calories	Fat	Protein	Total Carbohydrate	Dietary Fiber	Net Carbohydrate
407	39g	10g	4g	0g	4g

These perfect personal-sized pizzas include gooey mozzarella, sliced black olives, and earthy mushrooms.

Pepperoni and Black Olive Pizza Bites

Prep Time: **5 mins** | Cook Time: **15 mins** | Yield: **8 pizza bites** | Serving Size: **2 pizza bites**

Ingredients

- 32 1- to 1.5-oz. (25 to 40g) slices pepperoni
- 1 cup grated whole-milk mozzarella cheese
- ½ cup sliced black olives
- 3 medium white button mushrooms, finely chopped

Nutrition per Serving

Fat **73%** Net Carb **5%**
Protein **22%** Ratio **1.3:1**

Calories **192**
Fat **16g**
Protein **10g**
Total Carbohydrate **2g**
Dietary Fiber **0g**
Net Carbohydrate **2g**

1. Preheat the oven to 400°F (200°C). On an ungreased baking sheet, overlap 4 pepperoni slices to make a larger circle. Repeat with remaining pepperoni to make 8 larger circles.

2. Top larger pepperoni circles with whole-milk mozzarella cheese, black olives, and white button mushrooms.

3. Place the baking sheet in the oven and bake for 10 to 15 minutes, or until cheese is golden brown and bubbly.

4. Using a spatula, remove pizza bites from the sheet and let cool slightly before serving.

Variation: To make **Anchovy and Pepperoncini Pizza Bites,** replace pepperoni with thin-sliced salami. Combine 12 chopped anchovies with 1 tablespoon extra-virgin olive oil. Top mozzarella with anchovy mixture and ¼ cup sliced pepperoncini peppers instead of olives and mushrooms. Just be sure not to add higher-carb toppings such as red bell peppers, onions, or tomatoes without additional fat.

These addictive snacks are loaded with bacon and cheese, and covered in a savory "everything bagel" topping mixture.

Everything Mini-Cheeseballs

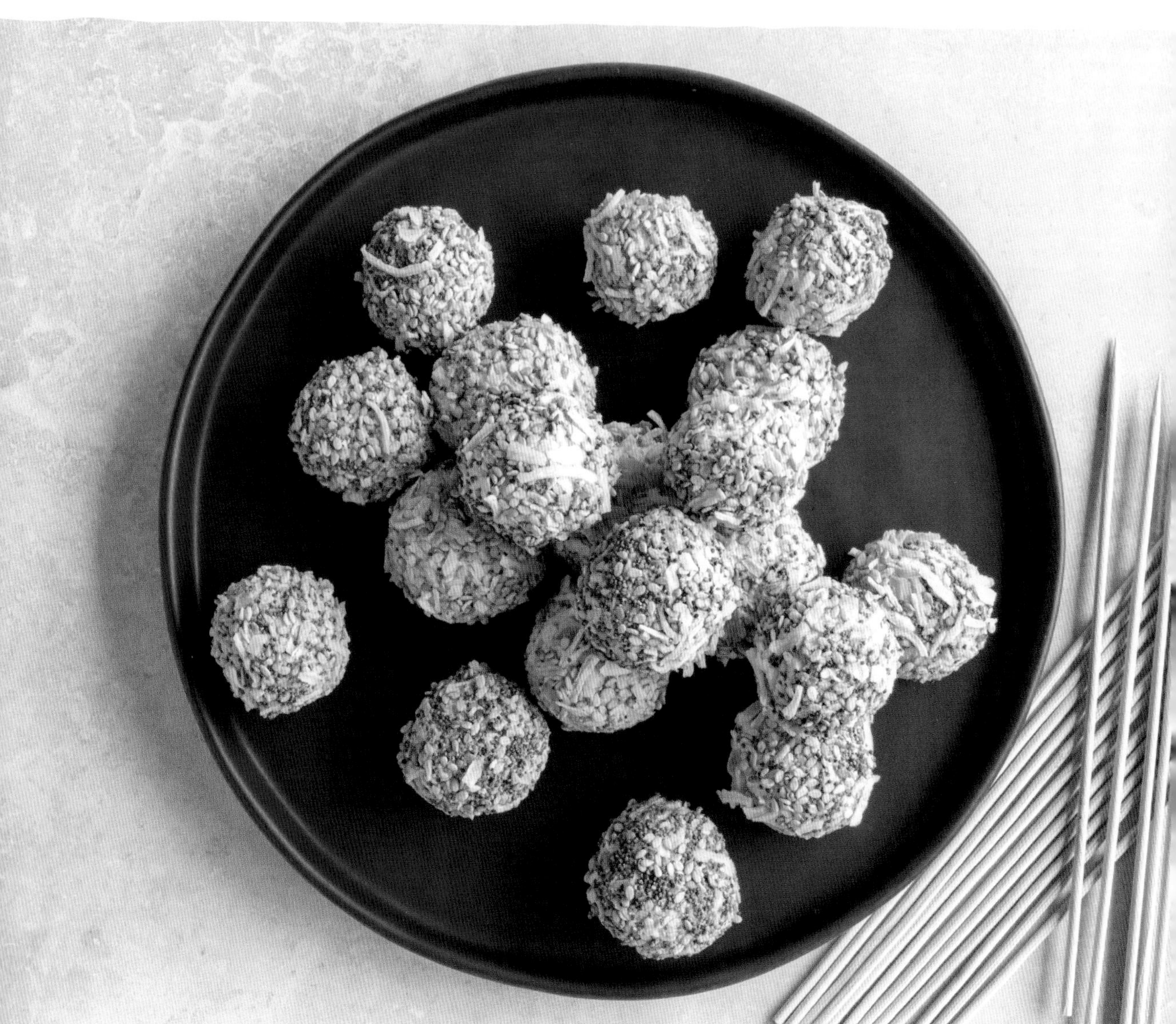

Prep Time: **3 hrs, 15 mins** Cook Time: **6 mins** Yield: **24 cheeseballs** Serving Size: **4 cheeseballs**

Ingredients

2 oz. (55g) uncured bacon, minced

1½ cups grated sharp cheddar cheese

8 oz. (225g) full-fat cream cheese, at room temperature

4 TB. unsalted butter, at room temperature

2 tsp. Worcestershire sauce

2 tsp. dried chives

1 tsp. granulated garlic

1 tsp. freshly ground black pepper

2 TB. poppy seeds

¼ cup toasted sesame seeds

¼ cup dehydrated onions

Nutrition per Serving

Fat **85%** Net Carb **4%**
Protein **11%** Ratio **2.5:1**

Calories **371**
Fat **35g**
Protein **10g**
Total Carbohydrate **5g**
Dietary Fiber **1g**
Net Carbohydrate **4g**

1 Heat a small skillet over medium heat. When the skillet is hot, add bacon. Cook for 4 to 6 minutes, stirring occasionally, until bacon is crisped. Remove bacon bits and place on a paper towel to drain.

2 In a food processor, combine sharp cheddar cheese, full-fat cream cheese, unsalted butter, Worcestershire sauce, dried chives, granulated garlic, and black pepper. Pulse for 30 seconds to 1 minute, or until a smooth paste forms.

3 Add bacon and pulse for 15 seconds to combine. Transfer mixture to a 24×12-inch (61×30.5cm) piece of parchment paper or plastic wrap.

4 Gently fold the long edges of the parchment around mixture and roll into a log about 1 inch (2.5cm) in diameter. Twist parchment ends to close. Refrigerate log until firm, about 3 hours.

5 While cheese log chills, combine poppy seeds, toasted sesame seeds, and dehydrated onions. Keep in an airtight container or Mason jar until ready to use.

6 When chilled, unwrap cheese log and slice into 24 1-inch (2.5cm) sections.

7 Using clean hands, gently roll each section into a small ball and roll in poppy seed mixture. Serve chilled or at room temperature.

Variation: To make **Jalapeño Bacon Mini-Cheeseballs,** replace dried chives with 1 small jalapeño (seeded and minced) and coat cheeseballs with 3 tablespoons dried chives instead of poppy seed mixture.

Appetizers

Whether you're looking to impress guests with your culinary skills or just priming your palate for a main course, appetizers are a great way to start your meals off right. In fact, you may be tempted to make them a meal of their own! From crab cakes to meatballs, the scrumptious recipes in this chapter are both keto compliant and absolutely delicious.

It's hard to stop eating these delightful appetizers, filled with herbed cream cheese and wrapped in crispy bacon.

Bacon-Wrapped Stuffed Mushrooms

Prep Time: 15 mins
Cook Time: 35 mins
Yield: 32 mushrooms
Serving Size: 4 mushrooms

Ingredients

32 medium white button mushrooms

6 TB. unsalted butter, at room temperature

1 garlic clove, minced

2 TB. shallot, minced

8 oz. (225g) cream cheese, at room temperature

2 TB. fresh parsley, chopped

½ tsp. dried thyme

¼ tsp. freshly ground black pepper

16 thin bacon slices, cut in half lengthwise (about 8 oz.; 225g)

Nutrition per Serving

Fat 83% Net Carb 7%
Protein 10% Ratio 2.2:1

Calories 238
Fat 22g
Protein 6g
Total Carbohydrate 4g
Dietary Fiber 0g
Net Carbohydrate 4g

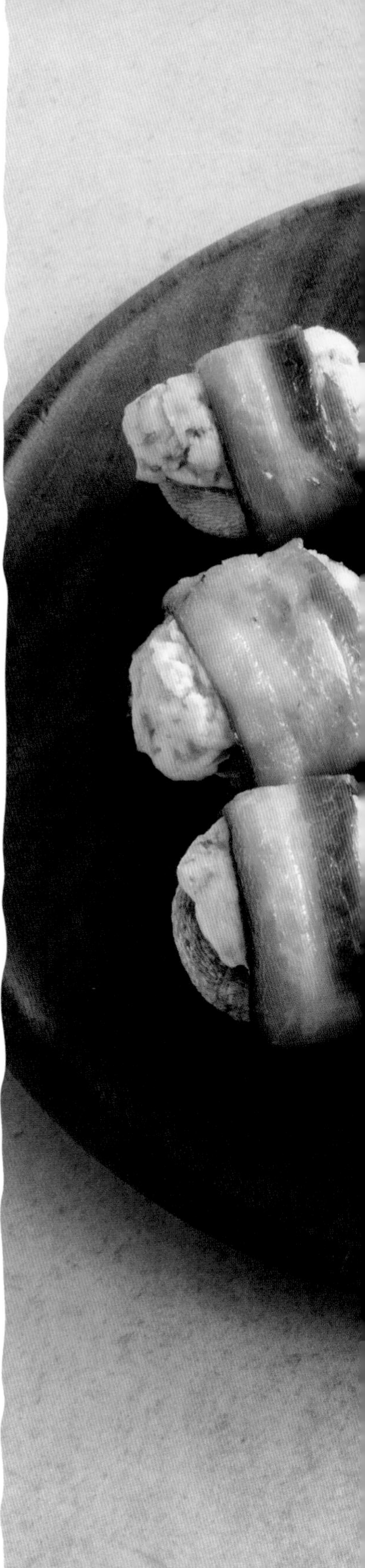

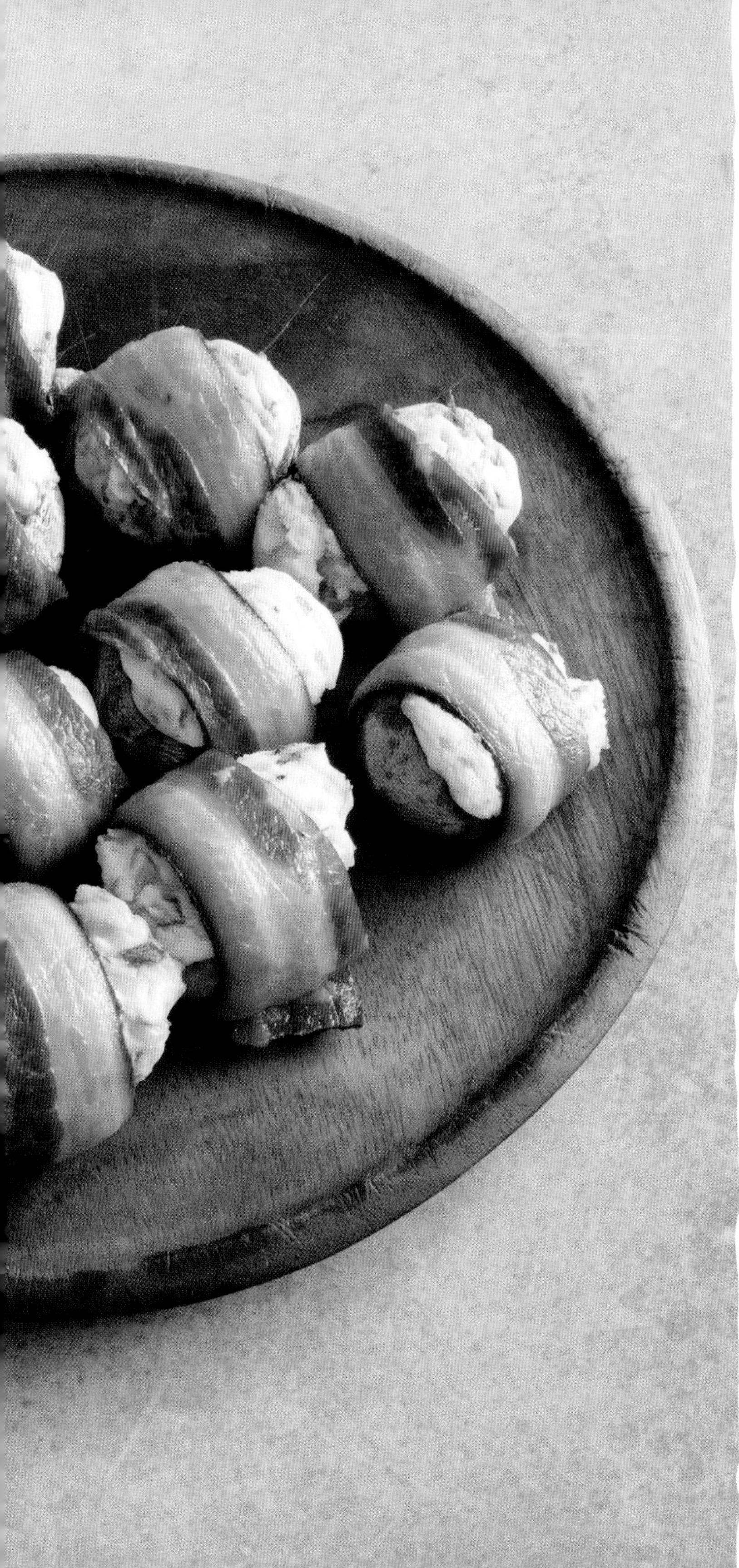

1 Preheat the oven to 350°F (180°C).

2 Remove stems from white button mushroom caps. Set caps aside and finely chop stems.

3 Heat a medium skillet over medium-high heat. When the skillet is hot, add 2 tablespoons unsalted butter.

4 Add garlic, shallot, and mushroom stems to the hot skillet. Sauté, stirring occasionally, for 4 to 5 minutes, or until fragrant and softened. Remove from heat and cool for 5 minutes.

5 In a small bowl, blend remaining 4 tablespoons unsalted butter, cream cheese, parsley, thyme, and black pepper.

6 Stir mushroom stem mixture into cream cheese mixture until fully combined.

7 Spoon filling into mushroom caps. Wrap each mushroom cap with ½ bacon slice so it overlaps on bottom side of cap. Place caps on an ungreased rimmed metal baking sheet with overlap sides down to secure.

8 Bake for 25 to 30 minutes, or until bacon is browned and crisp. Let cool slightly before serving.

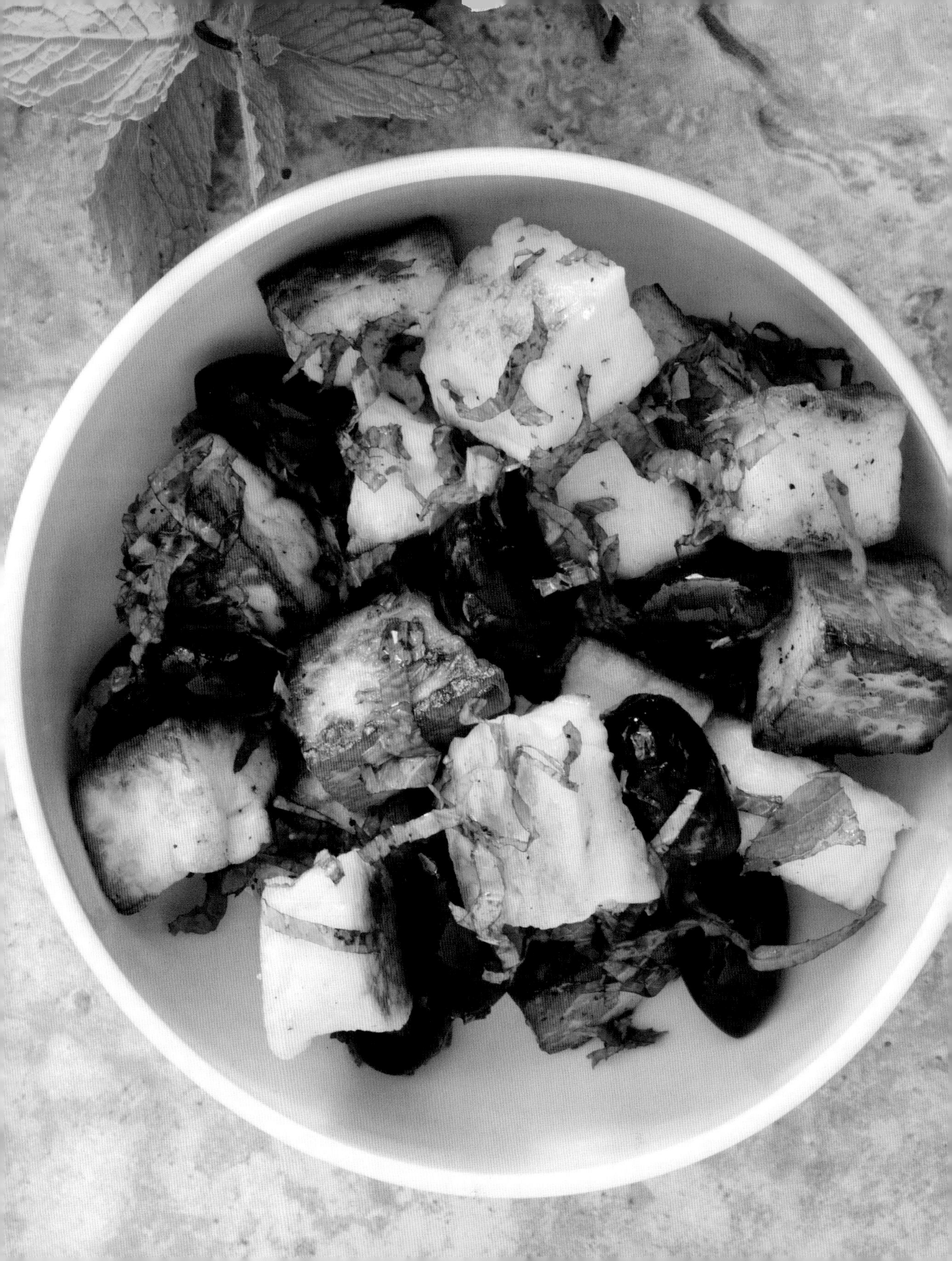

Salty, golden-fried Halloumi cheese is tossed with brined Kalamatas and softened with fresh mint.

Fried Halloumi with Kalamatas and Mint

Prep Time: **5 mins** Cook Time: **5 mins** Yield: **2 cups** Serving Size: **½ cup**

Ingredients

- 8 oz. (225g) Halloumi
- 1 TB. avocado oil
- 1 TB. extra-virgin olive oil
- 12 large Kalamata olives
- ¼ tsp. freshly ground black pepper
- 2 TB. fresh mint, chopped
- 1 tsp. fresh lemon juice

Nutrition per Serving

Fat 79%	Net Carb 2%
Protein 19%	Ratio 1.7:1

Calories 250
Fat 22g
Protein 12g
Total Carbohydrate 1g
Dietary Fiber 0g
Net Carbohydrate 1g

1. Slice Halloumi into ¾-inch (2cm) cubes. Pat cubes dry with a paper towel.
2. Heat a medium skillet over medium-high heat. When the skillet is hot, add avocado oil. Wait for 15 seconds.
3. Place Halloumi cubes in hot oil. Cook for 30 to 45 seconds, or until a deep, golden-brown crust forms. Use a spatula to turn cubes and brown opposite side.
4. Transfer cubes to a small serving dish. Drizzle with remaining avocado oil from the skillet.
5. Add extra-virgin olive oil, Kalamata olives, black pepper, mint, and lemon juice, and gently toss to combine. Serve warm or at room temperature.

Variation: To make **Spicy Halloumi and Castelvetranos,** replace Kalamata olives with buttery Castelvetrano olives and use ¼ teaspoon crushed red pepper flakes instead of mint.

Because Halloumi is heated early in its production, it won't melt when fried like other cheeses.

Whipped lard is combined with butter, fresh orange zest, and rosemary for an unexpectedly delicious ketogenic dip.

Whipped Lardo

Prep Time: **10 mins** | Cook Time: **none** | Yield: **1½ cups** | Serving Size: **2½ TB.**

Ingredients

- ¾ cup salted butter, at room temperature
- ¾ cup pure lard, at room temperature
- ½ tsp. sea salt (or more, to taste)
- ¼ tsp. freshly ground black pepper
- ¼ tsp. granulated garlic
- ½ tsp. fresh orange zest
- ½ tsp. fresh rosemary, finely chopped
- 4 oz. (110g) hard salami, cut into ⅛-in. (3mm) slices
- 2 medium carrots, cut into ⅛-in. (3mm) slices
- 4 large radishes, cut into ⅛-in. (3mm) slices

1. Place salted butter in a stand mixer. Using the whisk attachment, beat butter for 2 minutes.
2. Add lard and continue to whip for an additional 2 minutes, or until light and fluffy.
3. Add sea salt, black pepper, granulated garlic, orange zest, and rosemary and mix until fully combined.
4. Transfer dip to a serving bowl and serve with salami, carrot, and radish slices.

Store leftover whipped lardo in the refrigerator, covered, for up to 1 month. The flavors will increase over time.

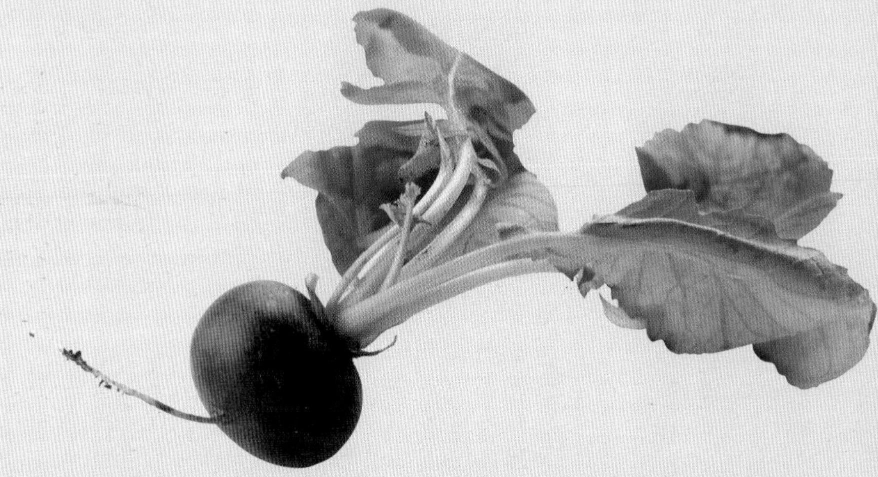

Nutrition per Serving

Fat 93% | Net Carb 2% | Protein 5% | Ratio 6.0:1

Calories	Fat	Protein	Total Carbohydrate	Dietary Fiber	Net Carbohydrate
348	36g	4g	2g	0g	2g

This silky ham spread is livened up with shallots and pepperoncinis and served with crisp bell pepper scoops.

Deviled Ham Dip

Prep Time: **10 mins** | Cook Time: **none** | Yield: **2 cups** | Serving Size: **⅓ cup**

Ingredients

- 8 oz. (225g) thick-cut uncured ham, cubed
- 1 cup mayonnaise
- 1 tsp. Dijon mustard
- 1 TB. shallot, minced
- 3 pepperoncinis, stemmed and minced
- ½ tsp. freshly ground black pepper
- 3 medium green bell peppers, seeded and thickly sliced lengthwise

1 Add uncured ham, mayonnaise, and Dijon mustard to a food processor. Pulse for 60 seconds, or until a smooth paste forms. Add more mayonnaise, if needed.

2 Add shallot, pepperonicinis, and black pepper and pulse a few more times to combine.

3 Transfer dip to a serving bowl and serve with green bell pepper slices.

Don't use cheap sliced deli ham, as it's loaded with sugar and added nitrates. Look for uncured ham from a reputable brand.

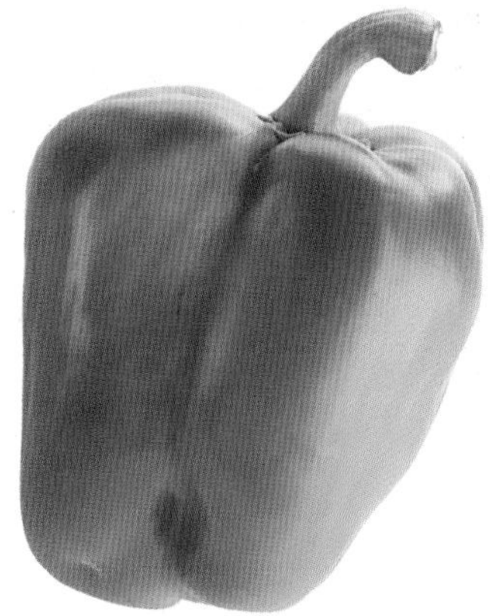

Nutrition per Serving

Fat **84%** Net Carb **5%**
Protein **11%** Ratio **2.3:1**

Calories	Fat	Protein	Total Carbohydrate	Dietary Fiber	Net Carbohydrate
322	30g	9g	5g	1g	4g

Prep Time: **10 mins** | Cook Time: **50 mins** | Yield: **16 to 20 wings** | Serving Size: **4 to 5 wings**

Ingredients

- 2 lb. (1kg) chicken wings and drummettes
- 4 oz. (110g) blue cheese, crumbled
- ¾ cup mayonnaise
- ¼ cup heavy cream
- ¼ cup sour cream
- 1 TB. lemon juice
- ¼ tsp. freshly ground black pepper
- 1 tsp. sea salt
- 6 TB. unsalted butter, cut into cubes
- ¼ cup hot pepper sauce
- 4 celery stalks, cut into sticks

1. Preheat the oven to 400°F (200°C). Cut a piece of parchment paper just large enough to line a rimmed baking sheet.

2. Spread chicken wings, skin side up, evenly over parchment on baking sheet. Bake for 45 to 50 minutes, or until wings are cooked through and skin is crisp.

3. While wings cook, combine blue cheese, mayonnaise, heavy cream, sour cream, lemon juice, black pepper, and ½ teaspoon sea salt in a small bowl. Refrigerate dressing for later use.

4. Heat a small saucepan over low heat. Add unsalted butter. When butter melts, whisk in hot pepper sauce and remaining ½ teaspoon sea salt. Remove sauce from heat.

5. When wings are done, transfer to a large bowl along with sauce and toss to coat.

6. Serve wings alongside blue cheese dressing and celery sticks.

Variation: To make **Five-Alarm Spicy Wings,** whisk ½ teaspoon cayenne pepper and 1 teaspoon habanero hot sauce into the wing sauce. You may want to make extra blue cheese dipping sauce to balance out these fiery wings!

Nutrition per Serving

Fat **82%** Net Carb **1%**
Protein **17%** Ratio **2.0:1**

Calories	Fat	Protein	Total Carbohydrate	Dietary Fiber	Net Carbohydrate
990	90g	43g	4g	1g	3g

Crispy chicken wings are covered in a hot buffalo sauce and served with crunchy celery and a blue cheese dressing.

Buffalo Wings

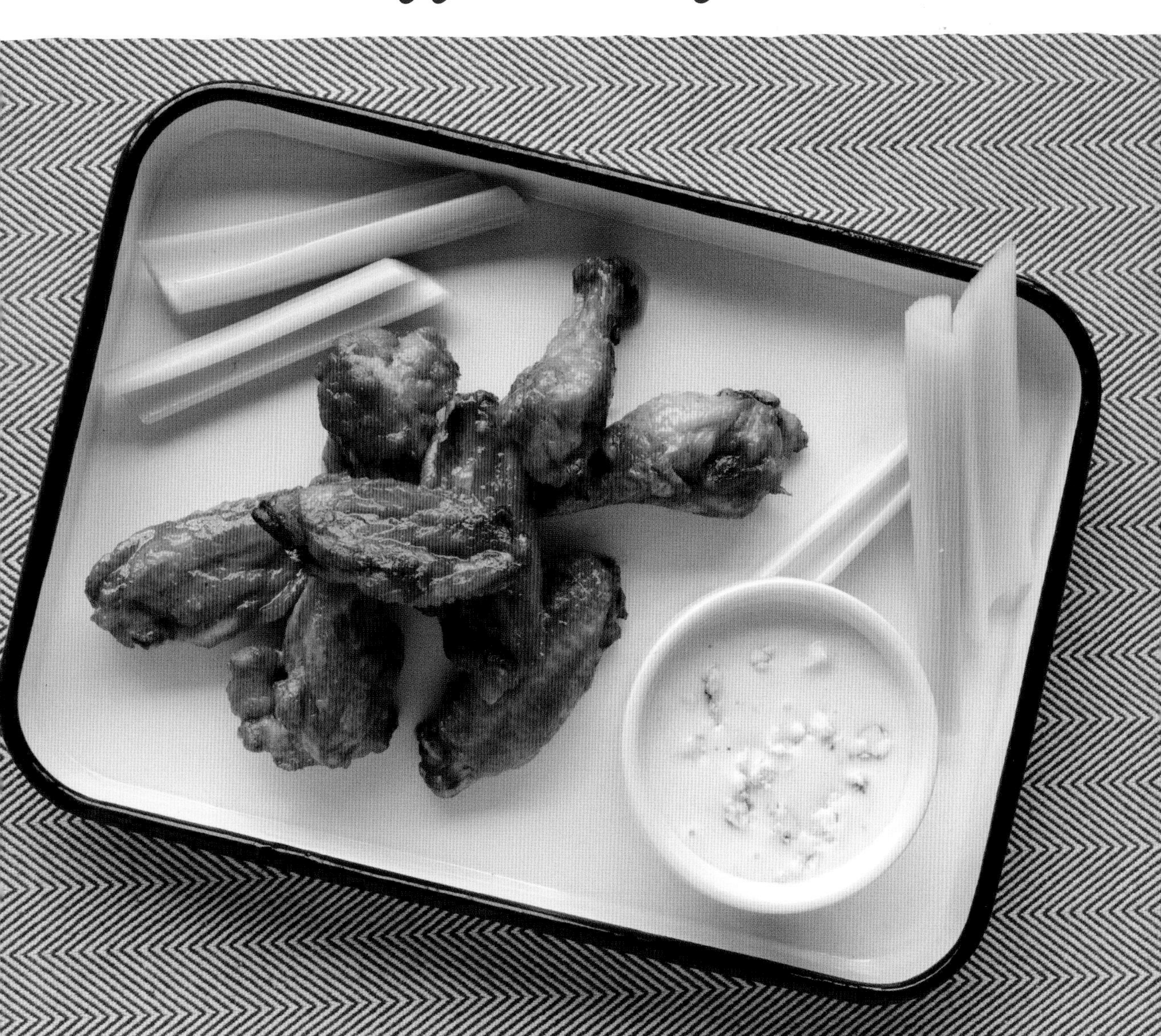

Spicy jalapeño halves are filled to the brim with smooth cream cheese and bubbly Monterey Jack cheese.

Jalapeño Poppers

Prep Time: **10 mins** | Cook Time: **28 mins** | Yield: **20 poppers** | Serving Size: **2 poppers**

Ingredients

- ½ lb. (225g) ground mild Italian sausage
- 8 oz. (225g) full-fat cream cheese, softened
- ¼ tsp. freshly ground black pepper
- 10 large jalapeño peppers, halved and seeded
- 4 oz. (110g) Monterey Jack cheese, grated

1 Preheat the oven to 425°F (220°C). Heat a medium skillet over medium heat. Add Italian sausage and cook, stirring occasionally, for 5 to 8 minutes, or until browned. Remove from heat.

2 Meanwhile, in a medium bowl, combine cream cheese, black pepper, and cooked Italian sausage.

3 Place jalapeño halves, hollow side up, on a rimmed baking sheet.

4 Fill hollowed jalapeño halves with cream cheese and sausage mixture. Sprinkle with Monterey Jack cheese.

5 Place the baking sheet in the oven and bake for 15 to 20 minutes, or until cheese is a deep golden brown and bubbly.

6 Remove the baking sheet from the oven and allow poppers to cool for 5 minutes before serving.

For an extra treat, wrap stuffed jalapeño halves with a thin slice of bacon, secure with a toothpick, and bake as directed.

Nutrition per Serving

Fat 82% Net Carb 2%
Protein 16% Ratio 2.0:1

Calories	Fat	Protein	Total Carbohydrate	Dietary Fiber	Net Carbohydrate
176	16g	7g	2g	1g	1g

Tangy blue cheese and zippy lemon zest make a tasty filling for green olives in this simple yet classy hors d'oeuvre.

Blue Cheese–Stuffed Olives

Prep Time: **10 mins** Cook Time: **none** Yield: **48 olives** Serving Size: **6 olives**

Ingredients

- 8 oz. (225g) blue cheese, crumbled
- 1 tsp. fresh lemon zest
- ½ tsp. freshly ground black pepper
- 4 TB. heavy cream
- 48 large green olives, pitted

1. In a small mixing bowl, combine blue cheese, lemon zest, black pepper, and heavy cream.
2. Use a fork to vigorously mix until a creamy consistency forms.
3. Transfer mixture to a pastry bag fitted with a medium tip. (Alternately, you can cut a small corner out of a small plastic bag and use it as a pastry bag.)
4. Pipe filling into green olives. Serve on toothpicks or in a small serving bowl.

Olives with blue cheese can make for a salty combo. To avoid this, soak olives in cold water for 30 minutes before filling.

Variation: Replace blue cheese filling with a whole Marcona almond to make **Marcona Almond–Stuffed Olives.**

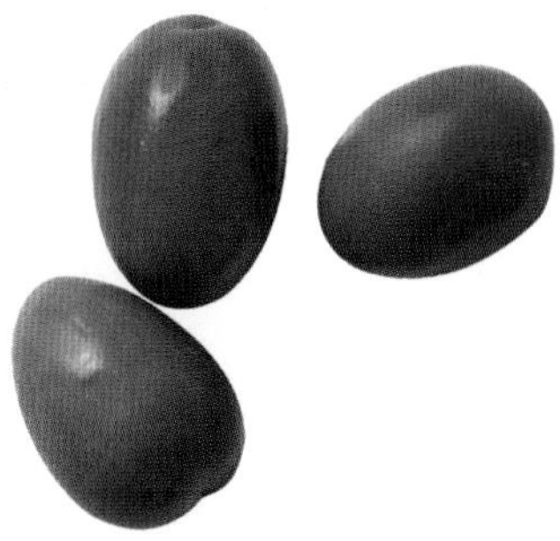

Nutrition per Serving

Fat 80% Net Carb 5%
Protein 15% Ratio 1.8:1

Calories	Fat	Protein	Total Carbohydrate	Dietary Fiber	Net Carbohydrate
158	14g	6g	3g	1g	2g

These little fried cakes, packed full of fresh lump crab meat, are served with a spicy remoulade dipping sauce.

Crab Cakes with Easy Remoulade

Prep Time: **10 mins**
Cook Time: **20 mins**

Yield: **6 crab cakes**
Serving Size: **1 crab cake**

Ingredients

- 1 cup cauliflower florets
- ½ cup plus 2 TB. mayonnaise
- 1 tsp. capers
- 1 tsp. lemon juice
- 1 TB. plus 1 tsp. Dijon mustard
- 1 tsp. Worcestershire sauce
- ¾ tsp. sea salt
- ½ tsp. paprika
- 1 TB. coconut flour
- ⅔ cup almond meal
- 1 large egg, beaten
- 1 green onion, thinly sliced
- 1 lb. (450g) cooked lump crab
- ¼ cup ghee

Nutrition per Serving

Fat **80%** Net Carb **3%**
Protein **17%** Ratio **1.8:1**

Calories **549**
Fat **49g**
Protein **23g**
Total Carbohydrate **6g**
Dietary Fiber **2g**
Net Carbohydrate **4g**

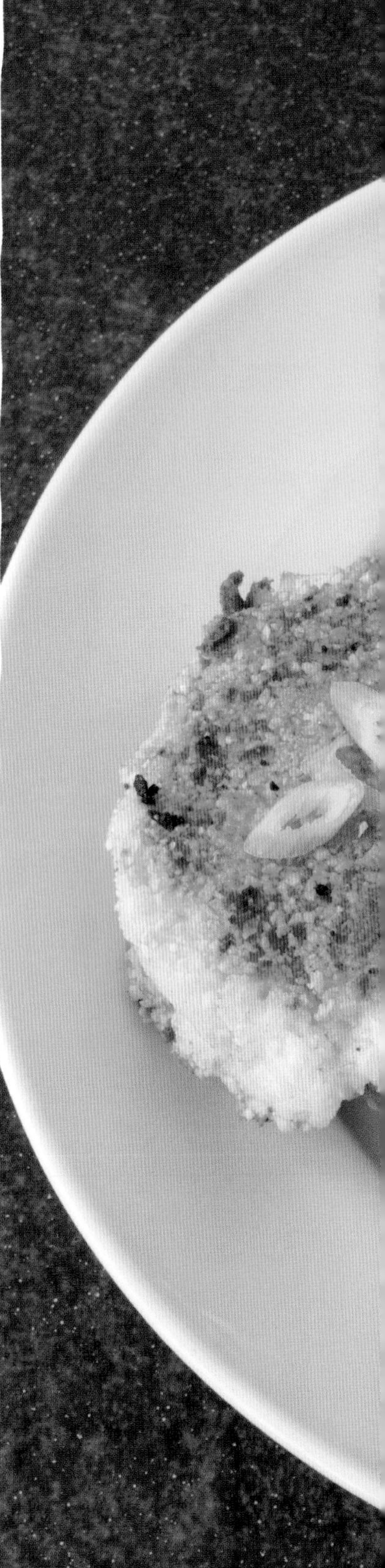

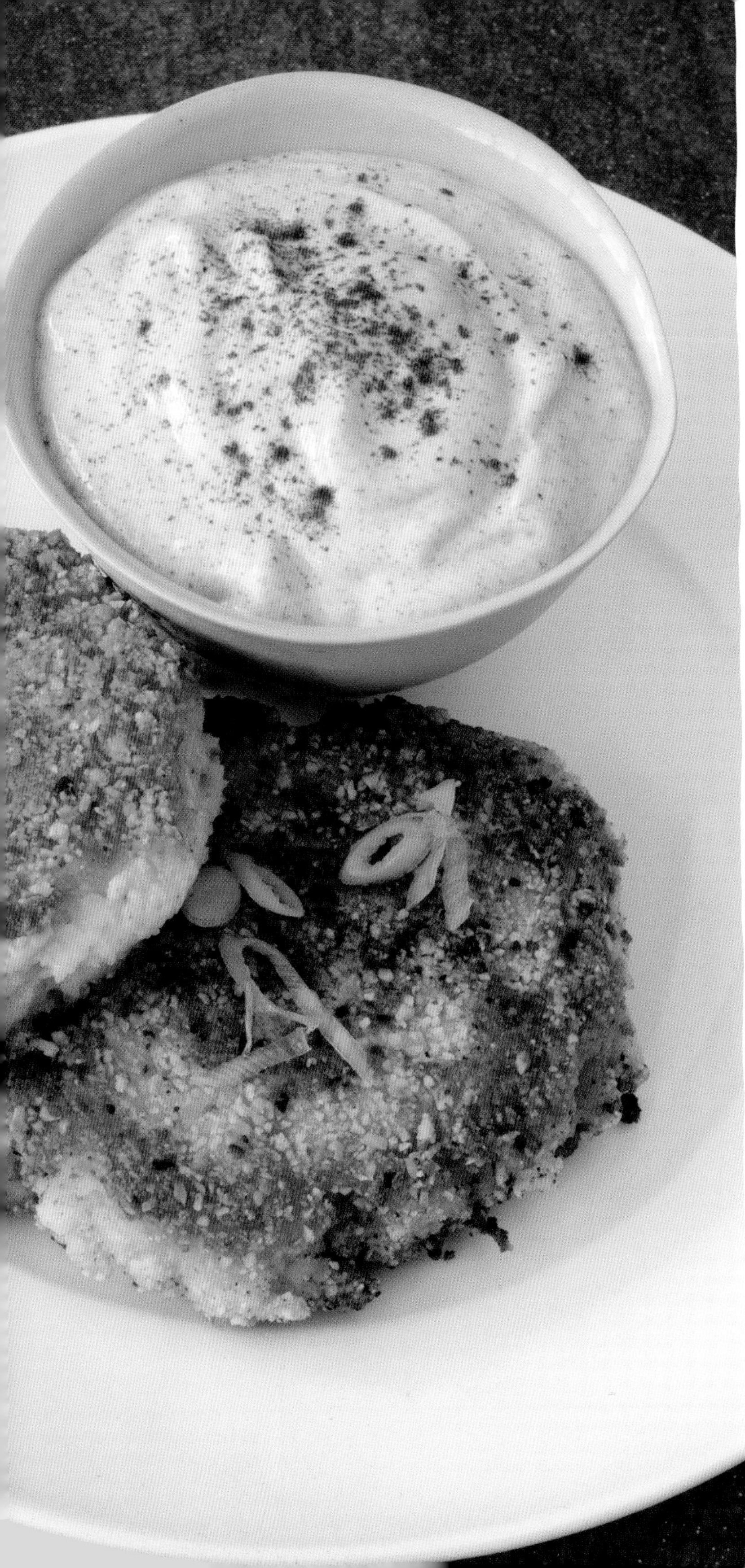

1. Place cauliflower in a microwave-safe bowl with ½ inch (1.25cm) water. Cover and microwave on high for 5 to 10 minutes, or until soft to the touch. Drain and set aside.

2. Whisk ½ cup mayonnaise, capers, lemon juice, 1 tablespoon Dijon mustard, Worcestershire sauce, ¼ teaspoon sea salt, and paprika in a small bowl. Set aside.

3. Use a fork to mash cauliflower into a paste. Stir in coconut flour, remaining 1 teaspoon Dijon mustard, remaining 2 tablespoons mayonnaise, ⅓ cup almond meal, egg, green onion, and remaining ½ teaspoon sea salt. Stir well to combine.

4. Add crab and gently mix. Form into 6 equal-size patties.

5. Place remaining ⅓ cup almond meal onto a plate or shallow dish. Press both flat sides of each crab cake into almond meal to coat.

6. Heat a large nonstick skillet over medium heat. Add ghee and wait for 30 seconds.

7. Place crab cakes in hot ghee. Cook for 2 to 4 minutes, or until deeply browned. Turn and cook for 2 to 4 minutes on the other side until browned and cooked through.

8. Serve warm crab cakes with remoulade.

Bite-size mozzarella and plump grape tomatoes pair with fragrant basil in this spin on the classic Insalata Caprese.

Caprese Sticks

Prep Time: **10 mins** Cook Time: **none** Yield: **16 sticks** Serving Size: **4 sticks**

Ingredients

- 16 long toothpicks or cocktail sticks
- 32 small fresh mozzarella Ciliegine
- 8 grape tomatoes, halved
- 8 fresh basil leaves, finely chopped
- ¼ cup extra-virgin olive oil
- ¼ tsp. sea salt
- ⅛ tsp. freshly ground black pepper

1 Thread 1 mozzarella ball onto a long toothpick or cocktail stick. Thread 1 half grape tomato followed by another mozzarella ball. Repeat for all toothpicks.

2 Place sticks on a small serving platter. Sprinkle with basil.

3 Drizzle with extra-virgin olive oil and sprinkle with sea salt and black pepper before serving.

Ciliegine are bite-size balls of mozzarella. If you can only find larger Bocconcini or Ovolini, cut them into small chunks.

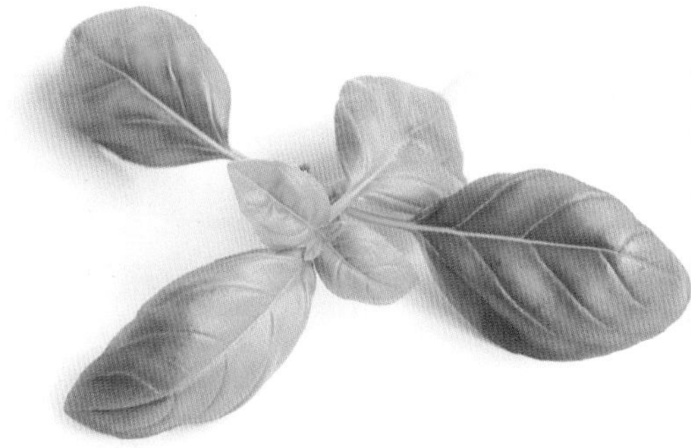

Nutrition per Serving

Fat 88% Net Carb 2%
Protein 10% Ratio 2.4:1

Calories	Fat	Protein	Total Carbohydrate	Dietary Fiber	Net Carbohydrate
331	31g	12g	1g	0g	1g

This decadent dip, loaded with creamy cheeses and savory artichoke hearts, is served with crunchy Belgian endive.

Artichoke Dip

Prep Time: **15 mins** | Cook Time: **40 mins** | Yield: **4 cups** | Serving Size: **½ cup**

Ingredients

- 2 TB. unsalted butter, at room temperature
- 8 oz. (225g) cream cheese, at room temperature
- ½ cup mayonnaise
- ½ cup sour cream
- 1 cup canned artichoke hearts, drained
- 1 cup shredded provolone
- ¼ tsp. granulated garlic
- ¼ tsp. crushed red pepper flakes (optional)
- ⅛ tsp. freshly ground black pepper
- ¼ cup grated Parmesan
- 2 to 3 heads Belgian endive

1 Preheat the oven to 350°F (180°C). Using a hand mixer, beat unsalted butter and cream cheese until well blended.

2 Mix in mayonnaise, sour cream, artichoke hearts, provolone, granulated garlic, crushed red pepper flakes (if using), and black pepper.

3 Transfer mixture to a small oven-proof pan or baking dish.

4 Sprinkle Parmesan over top. Bake for 30 to 40 minutes, or until cheese is golden brown and bubbly. Let cool for 5 minutes.

5 Trim ends off Belgian endive heads and separate into leaves. Serve leaves alongside hot dip.

Variation: To make **Artichoke and Crab Dip,** add 1 cup cooked crab meat to mixture instead of shredded provolone, and use ½ teaspoon paprika instead of crushed red pepper flakes.

Look for unmarinated artichoke hearts. A marinade will add extra sugar and unwelcome spice to this dip.

Nutrition per Serving

Fat **81%** Net Carb **6%**
Protein **13%** Ratio **1.9:1**

Calories	Fat	Protein	Total Carbohydrate	Dietary Fiber	Net Carbohydrate
343	31g	11g	11g	6g	5g

These delectable little meatballs float in a sea of tangy crème fraîche and are topped with a smattering of fresh dill.

Meatballs with Crème Fraîche

Prep Time: **15 mins** | Cook Time: **30 mins** | Yield: **36 meatballs** | Serving Size: **3 meatballs**

Ingredients

- 1 TB. extra-virgin olive oil
- 6 medium white button mushrooms, sliced
- 1 medium shallot, minced
- ½ cup almond flour
- 1 large egg
- 1 tsp. sea salt
- 1 lb. (450g) ground pork
- ½ lb. (225g) ground beef
- 1 cup crème fraîche
- ¼ cup fresh lemon juice
- 2 TB. fresh dill, chopped
- ½ tsp. freshly ground black pepper

1. Preheat the oven to 350°F (180°C). Heat a medium skillet over medium-high heat. When the skillet is hot, add extra-virgin olive oil. Wait for 15 seconds.

2. Add white button mushrooms and shallot and sauté, stirring occasionally, for 3 to 4 minutes, or until softened. Set aside to cool for 10 minutes.

3. Transfer mushroom-shallot mixture to a food processor. Add almond flour, egg, sea salt, pork, and beef and pulse until fully combined.

4. Form mixture into 1-inch (2.5cm) meatballs and place on a rimmed metal baking sheet.

5. Bake meatballs for 20 to 25 minutes, or until meatballs are cooked through.

6. In a medium mixing bowl, combine crème fraîche, and lemon juice and whip until smooth.

7. Transfer hot meatballs to the mixing bowl with crème fraîche mixture and stir to combine. Sprinkle with dill and black pepper to serve.

If you have a hard time finding crème fraîche, feel free to substitute full-fat sour cream, though it may need to be thinned with milk.

Nutrition per Serving

Fat **79%** Net Carb **3%**
Protein **18%** Ratio **1.6:1**

Calories	Fat	Protein	Total Carbohydrate	Dietary Fiber	Net Carbohydrate
263	23g	12g	3g	1g	2g

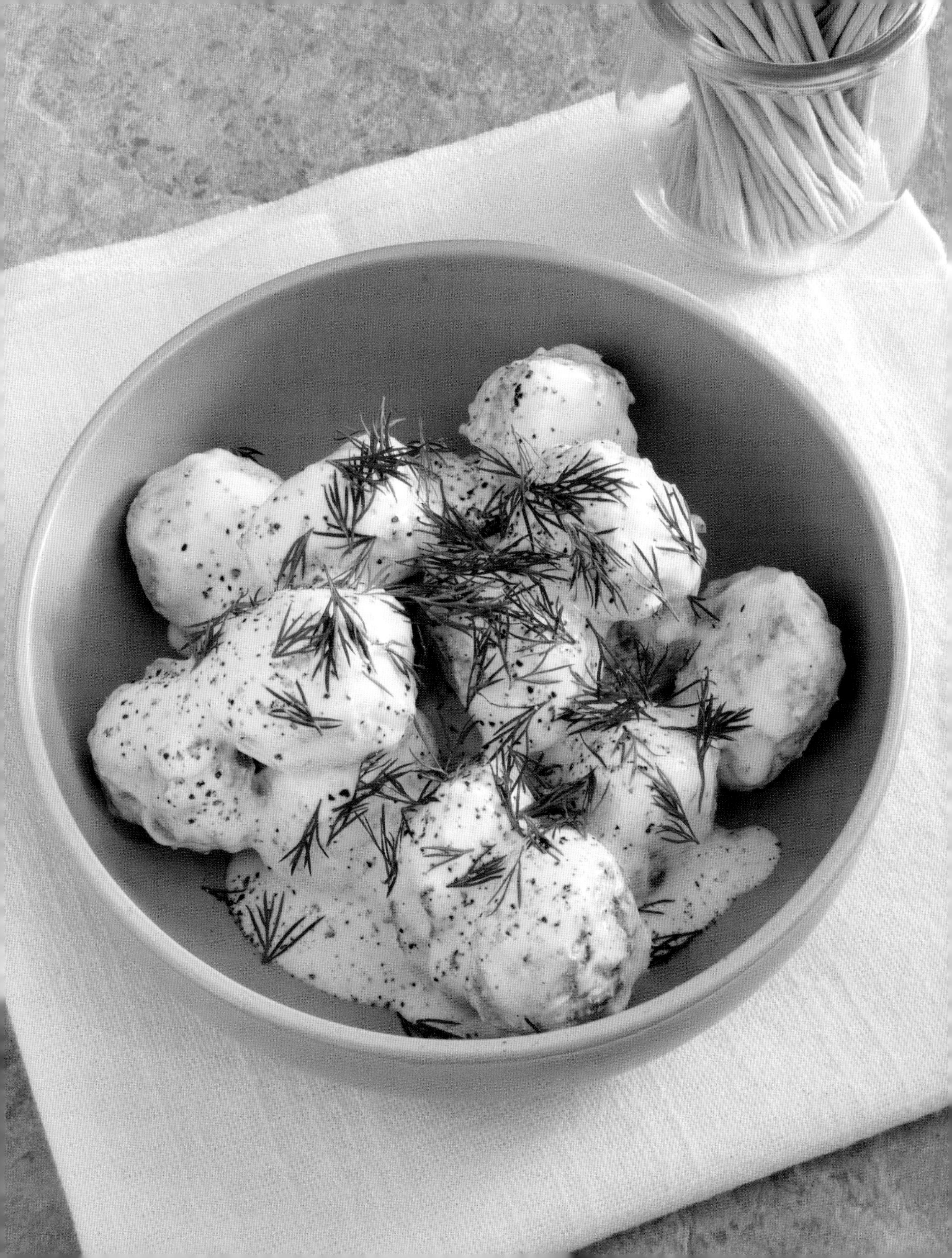

Salads

Salads are easily the fastest—as well as the most nutritious—meal to make when you're eating the keto way. In addition to adding colorful, nutrient-rich antioxidants to your diet, salads are an excellent source of fiber, which is one of your secret weapons when following the keto diet. From a keto-friendly Cobb salad to a delicious kale and Parmesan salad, these fresh recipes can be served as an accompaniment to any main dish, but are also satisfying enough to be eaten on their own.

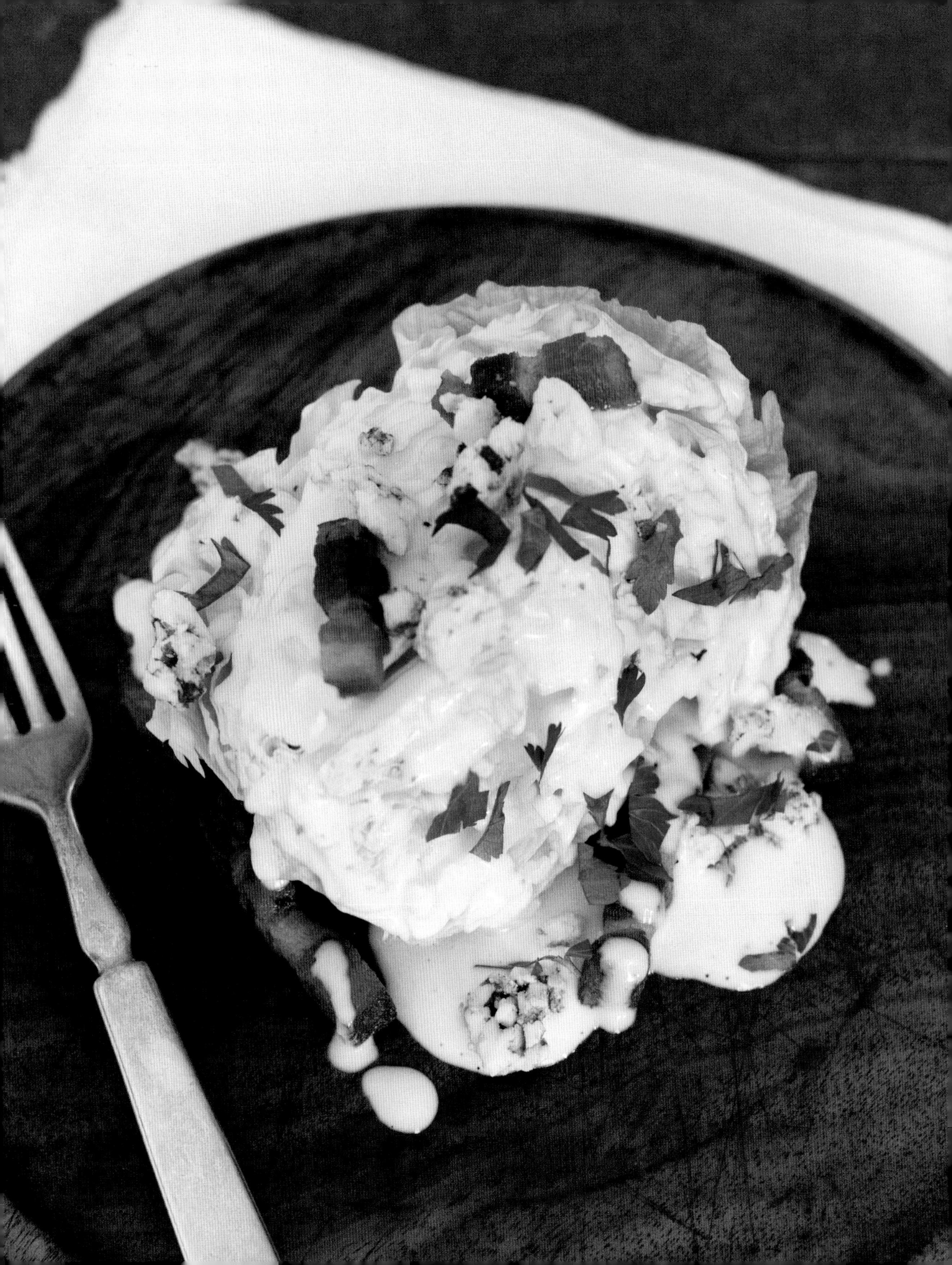

Crisp iceberg lettuce wedges are coated with a tangy blue cheese dressing and sprinkled with crunchy bacon pieces.

Wedge Salad with Bacon and Blue Cheese

Prep Time: **10 mins** Cook Time: **5 mins** Yield: **4 wedges** Serving Size: **1 wedge**

Ingredients

- 4 oz. (110g) thick-sliced bacon (about ¼ in.; .5cm thick)
- 4 oz. (110g) blue cheese, crumbled
- ¾ cup mayonnaise
- ¼ cup heavy cream
- ¼ cup sour cream
- 1 TB. lemon juice
- ½ tsp. sea salt
- ¼ tsp. freshly ground black pepper
- 1 head iceberg lettuce, quartered
- ¼ cup fresh parsley, chopped

1. Slice bacon into ½-inch (1.25cm) squares. Heat a medium skillet over medium heat.
2. Add bacon in an even layer on the bottom of the skillet. Cook for 4 to 5 minutes, turning as needed, until all sides are crisp. Remove bacon from the skillet and place on a paper towel. Discard any bacon drippings left in the skillet.
3. In a small bowl, combine blue cheese, mayonnaise, heavy cream, sour cream, lemon juice, sea salt, and black pepper until well blended.
4. Cut woody core off each lettuce wedge. Place wedges on 4 salad plates.
5. Drizzle with blue cheese dressing and top with crisp bacon and parsley to serve.

Many butcher shops will cut a thick slice of bacon if asked, or you can simply substitute the thickest cut you can find.

Nutrition per Serving

Fat **87%** Net Carb **3%**
Protein **10%** Ratio **2.9:1**

Calories	Fat	Protein	Total Carbohydrate	Dietary Fiber	Net Carbohydrate
624	60g	16g	7g	2g	5g

Verdant broccoli florets are tossed with sweet dried currants, crisped bacon pieces, and sharp white cheddar cheese.

Broccoli Bacon Salad

Prep Time: **15 mins** Cook Time: **8 mins** Yield: **6 cups** Serving Size: **1½ cups**

Ingredients

- ½ lb. (225g) uncured bacon, diced
- ¾ cup mayonnaise
- 1 TB. apple cider vinegar
- 1 TB. red onion, grated
- ¼ tsp. sea salt
- ¼ tsp. freshly ground black pepper
- 4 cups broccoli florets, cut into bite-size pieces
- 2 oz. (55g) sharp white cheddar cheese, cut into small cubes
- 2 TB. dried currants
- ¼ cup raw sunflower seeds

1. Heat a large skillet over medium heat. Place uncured bacon in the skillet. Cook, stirring occasionally, for 6 to 8 minutes, or until crisp. Remove bacon and place on a paper towel. Reserve bacon drippings.

2. In a small bowl, whisk mayonnaise, apple cider vinegar, red onion, sea salt, and black pepper to make a dressing.

3. Place broccoli florets in a large salad bowl. Drizzle with 1 tablespoon reserved bacon drippings.

4. Add sharp white cheddar cheese, currants, and raw sunflower seeds. Drizzle with dressing and toss to combine. Serve at room temperature or chill before serving.

If you're trying to cut down on dairy, you can replace the sharp white cheddar cheese with extra sunflower seeds.

Nutrition per Serving

Fat **77%** Net Carb **3%**
Protein **20%** Ratio **1.5:1**

Calories	Fat	Protein	Total Carbohydrate	Dietary Fiber	Net Carbohydrate
691	59g	34g	9g	3g	6g

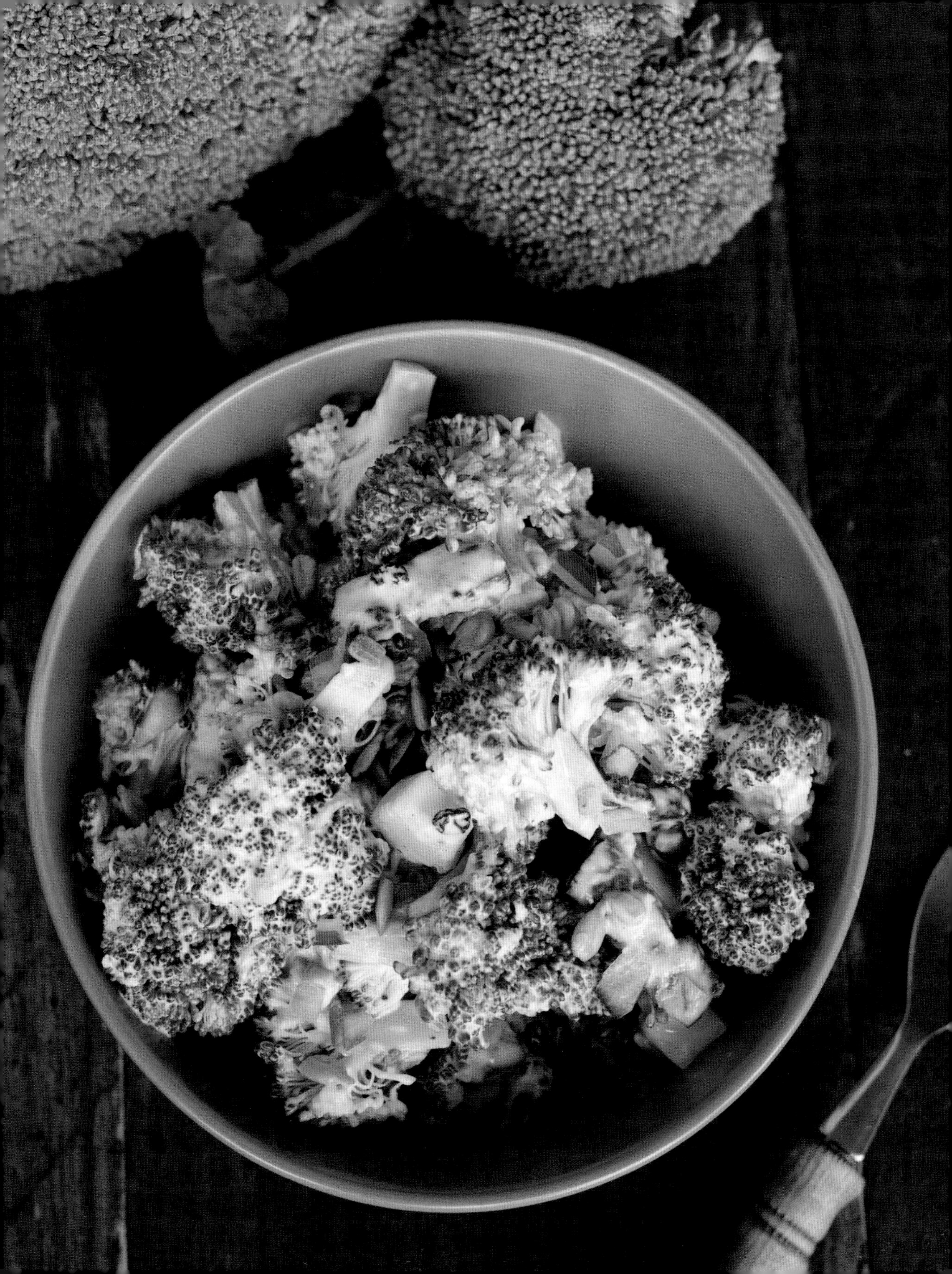

Thin strips of rib-eye steak sit atop fresh baby spinach smothered in a tangy buttermilk-peppercorn dressing.

Steak Salad with Buttermilk-Peppercorn Ranch

Prep Time: **10 mins** Cook Time: **7 mins** Yield: **2 salads** Serving Size: **1 salad**

Ingredients

- 6 oz. (170g) boneless rib-eye steak
- ½ tsp. sea salt
- 1 TB. coconut oil or tallow
- ¼ cup mayonnaise
- ¼ cup sour cream
- 2 TB. buttermilk
- 1 small garlic clove, finely minced
- ¼ tsp. dried parsley
- ¼ tsp. dried chives
- ¼ tsp. freshly ground black pepper
- 6 cups baby spinach
- 2 TB. raw sunflower seeds

1. Season both sides of rib-eye with ¼ teaspoon sea salt. Heat a medium skillet over medium heat. When the skillet is hot, add coconut oil.

2. Place rib-eye in the hot oil. Cook for 3 to 4 minutes. Turn rib-eye and cook for an additional 2 to 3 minutes. Transfer rib-eye to a cutting board and let rest for 5 minutes.

3. While rib-eye rests, in a large salad bowl, combine mayonnaise, sour cream, buttermilk, garlic, dried parsley, dried chives, black pepper, and remaining ¼ teaspoon sea salt.

4. Add baby spinach and raw sunflower seeds and toss with dressing. Divide into 2 bowls.

5. Thinly slice rib-eye. Top each salad with rib-eye slices to serve.

This dressing is so versatile, you may wish to make a double batch and keep it in the refrigerator for easy side salads.

Nutrition per Serving

Fat 82% Net Carb 3%
Protein 15% Ratio 2.0:1

Calories	Fat	Protein	Total Carbohydrate	Dietary Fiber	Net Carbohydrate
585	53g	22g	10g	5g	5g

Creamy blue cheese dressing coats crunchy romaine and the Cobb classics: bacon, eggs, chicken, and avocado.

Keto Cobb Salad

Prep Time: **10 mins** Cook Time: **15 mins** Yield: **2 salads** Serving Size: **1 salad**

Ingredients

- 2 uncured bacon slices (about 2 oz.; 55g), diced
- 4 oz. (110g) skinless, boneless chicken thighs, diced
- ¼ cup extra-virgin olive oil
- 1 tsp. Dijon mustard
- 2 TB. red wine vinegar
- 1 TB. lemon juice
- ½ tsp. granulated garlic
- ¼ tsp. sea salt
- ¼ tsp. freshly ground black pepper
- 1 head romaine lettuce, thinly sliced (about 6 cups)
- 2 oz. (55g) blue cheese, crumbled
- 2 hard-cooked eggs, diced
- 4 cherry tomatoes, thinly sliced
- 1 medium avocado, diced
- 6 fresh chives, thinly sliced

1 Heat a medium skillet over medium heat. Add uncured bacon to the skillet and cook, stirring occasionally, for 4 to 5 minutes, or until crisp. Remove bacon from the skillet and place on a paper towel.

2 Reheat the skillet with bacon drippings over medium-high heat. Add chicken to the skillet and cook, stirring occasionally, for 5 to 7 minutes, or until browned and cooked through. Remove from heat and set aside.

3 In a small bowl, combine extra-virgin olive oil, Dijon mustard, red wine vinegar, lemon juice, granulated garlic, sea salt, and black pepper to make dressing.

4 To assemble salad, toss romaine lettuce with cooked chicken and residual oil. Add dressing and toss.

5 Divide salad onto 2 plates. Top each with equal portions of bacon, blue cheese, hard-cooked eggs, cherry tomatoes, and avocado. Sprinkle with chives and serve immediately.

When you're ready to add more carbohydrates into your diet, you can double the cherry tomatoes in this salad.

Nutrition per Serving

Fat 75% Net Carb 5%
Protein 20% Ratio 1.3:1

Calories	Fat	Protein	Total Carbohydrate	Dietary Fiber	Net Carbohydrate
685	57g	34g	24g	15g	9g

In this classic salad, romaine leaves are slathered in creamy dressing and sprinkled with Parmesan and pine nuts.

Caesar Salad

Prep Time: **15 mins**
Cook Time: **none**

Yield: **4 salads**
Serving Size: **1 salad**

Ingredients

- 2 romaine hearts
- 1 to 2 small garlic cloves
- ½ tsp. sea salt, or to taste
- 6 whole anchovies, coarsely chopped
- 1 large egg yolk
- 2 TB. lemon juice
- ½ tsp. Dijon mustard
- ½ cup extra-virgin olive oil
- ¼ tsp. freshly ground black pepper
- 4 oz. (110g) Parmesan, shaved
- ¼ cup toasted pine nuts

Nutrition per Serving

Fat **88%** Net Carb **3%**
Protein **9%** Ratio **3.3:1**

Calories **266**
Fat **26g**
Protein **6g**
Total Carbohydrate **2g**
Dietary Fiber **0g**
Net Carbohydrate **2g**

Variation: The protein in this recipe is relatively low. If you need more, you can add 8 ounces (225g) cooked boneless, skinless chicken thighs to make **Chicken Caesar Salad.**

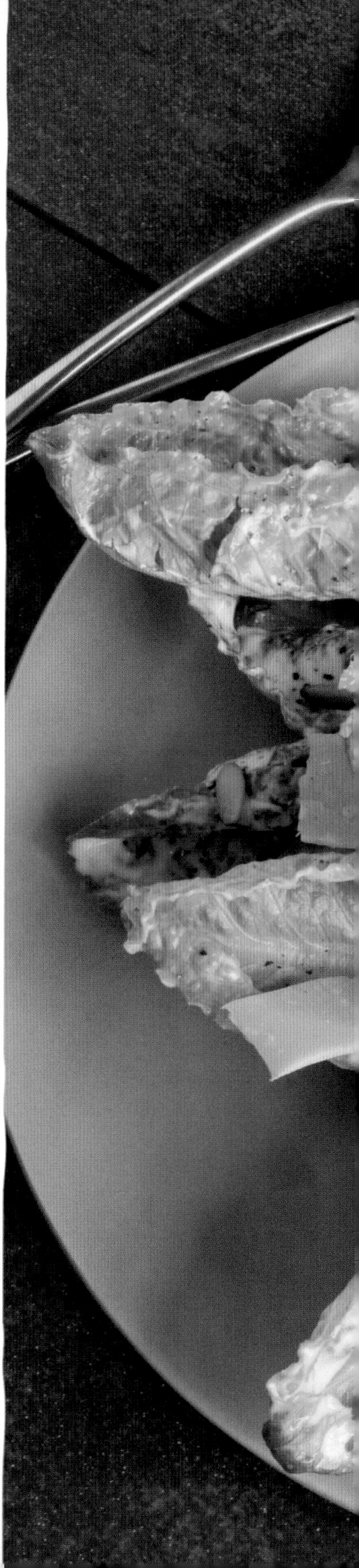

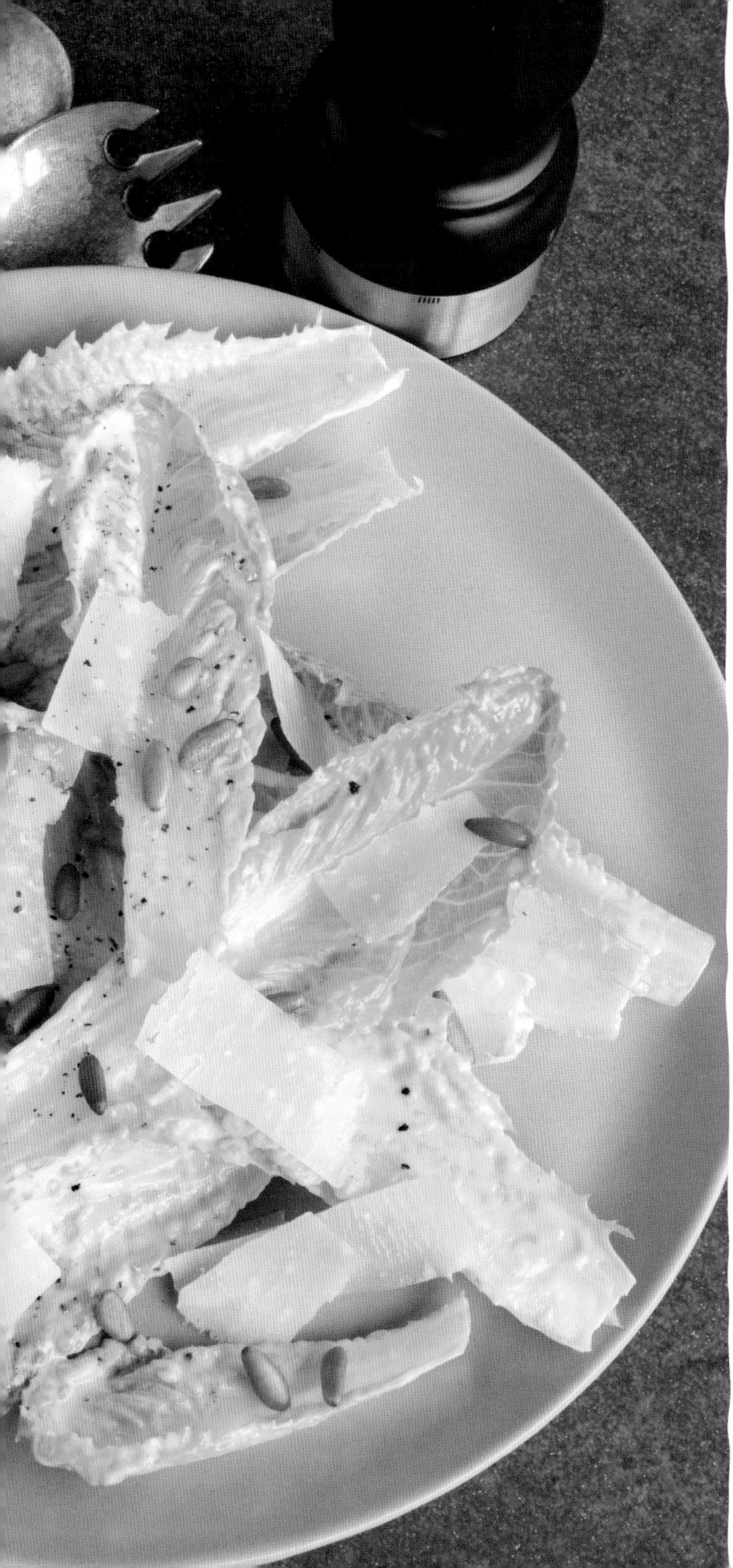

1. Cut off root end of romaine hearts. Gently pull leaves apart and place in a large mixing bowl.

2. Crush and finely mince garlic clove. Sprinkle with sea salt. Using the side of a chef's knife, crush garlic into a smooth paste.

3. In a wide-mouth 1-pint (.5l) Mason jar, place garlic paste, anchovies, egg yolk, lemon juice, and Dijon mustard.

4. Place the head of an immersion blender at the bottom of the jar. Pulse for 15 seconds, or until puréed.

5. Add 2 drops extra-virgin olive oil. Blend for 30 seconds. Add 2 additional drops olive oil and blend for another 30 seconds. Continue adding olive oil ½ teaspoon at a time, blending for 30 seconds in between, 6 times.

6. Slowly drizzle remaining olive oil into the jar, about 2 tablespoons at a time, blending for 30 seconds before adding more. When olive oil is fully incorporated, dressing should be thick and glossy.

7. Taste dressing and season with additional sea salt or lemon juice, if desired.

8. Toss romaine leaves with dressing. Divide onto 4 plates and top with black pepper, Parmesan, and toasted pine nuts to serve.

This salad features thick flakes of albacore tuna, pungent capers, and a dash of fresh dill, wrapped in crunchy lettuce.

Albacore Tuna Salad

Prep Time: 10 mins | Cook Time: none | Yield: 3 cups | Serving Size: 1½ cups

Ingredients

- 1 (6-oz.; 170g) can albacore tuna in olive oil, drained
- ½ cup mayonnaise
- 1 tsp. Dijon mustard
- 1 tsp. lemon juice
- ½ tsp. granulated garlic
- ¼ tsp. freshly ground black pepper
- 1 celery stalk, minced
- 1 TB. red onion, minced
- 1 TB. capers, rinsed
- 1 TB. fresh dill
- 6 to 8 small butter lettuce leaves

1. In a medium bowl, combine albacore tuna, mayonnaise, Dijon mustard, lemon juice, granulated garlic, and black pepper. Mix thoroughly.
2. Add celery, red onion, capers, and dill and mix until incorporated.
3. To serve, scoop tuna salad on butter lettuce leaves.

Variation: To make **Spicy Tuna Salad,** add 1 jalapeño, seeded and minced, and replace fresh dill with ½ teaspoon crushed red pepper flakes.

The ratios in this salad are low enough that you can use up to an 8-oz. (225g) can of tuna, depending on what you can find.

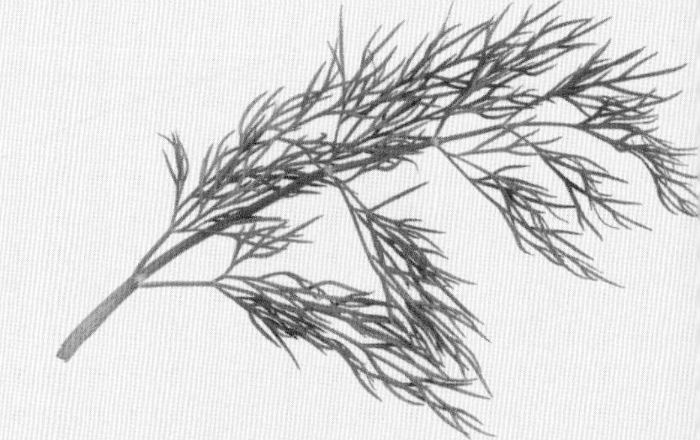

Nutrition per Serving

Fat 79% | Net Carb 2% | Protein 19% | Ratio 1.7:1

Calories	Fat	Protein	Total Carbohydrate	Dietary Fiber	Net Carbohydrate
522	46g	25g	3g	1g	2g

Crisp romaine and snappy celery are tossed with tangy blue cheese dressing and zesty buffalo chicken thighs.

Buffalo Chicken Salad

Prep Time: **10 mins** | Cook Time: **10 mins** | Yield: **4 cups** | Serving Size: **2 cups**

Ingredients

- 2 oz. (55g) blue cheese, crumbled
- ¼ cup mayonnaise
- 2 TB. heavy cream
- 2 TB. sour cream
- 1 tsp. lemon juice
- ¼ tsp. sea salt
- ¼ tsp. freshly ground black pepper
- 1 TB. extra-virgin olive oil
- 4 oz. (110g) boneless, skinless chicken thighs, sliced
- 2 TB. salted butter
- 5 tsp. hot pepper sauce
- 1 romaine heart, chopped
- 4 large celery stalks, thinly sliced
- 2 TB. sliced almonds

1. In a small bowl, whisk blue cheese, mayonnaise, heavy cream, sour cream, lemon juice, sea salt, and black pepper to make dressing. Set aside.
2. Heat a small skillet over medium-high heat. When the skillet is hot, add extra-virgin olive oil.
3. Add chicken thighs and cook for 2 to 4 minutes, or until browned and cooked through.
4. Add salted butter to the hot skillet with chicken. When butter melts and sizzles, add hot pepper sauce and stir. Remove from heat.
5. In a large salad bowl, toss romaine and celery with dressing. Divide into 2 bowls. Top with buffalo chicken and sliced almonds to serve.

If you don't care for blue cheese dressing, you can use ranch to dress the vegetables instead.

Nutrition per Serving

Fat **84%** Net Carb **3%**
Protein **13%** Ratio **2.3:1**

Calories	Fat	Protein	Total Carbohydrate	Dietary Fiber	Net Carbohydrate
644	60g	21g	8g	3g	5g

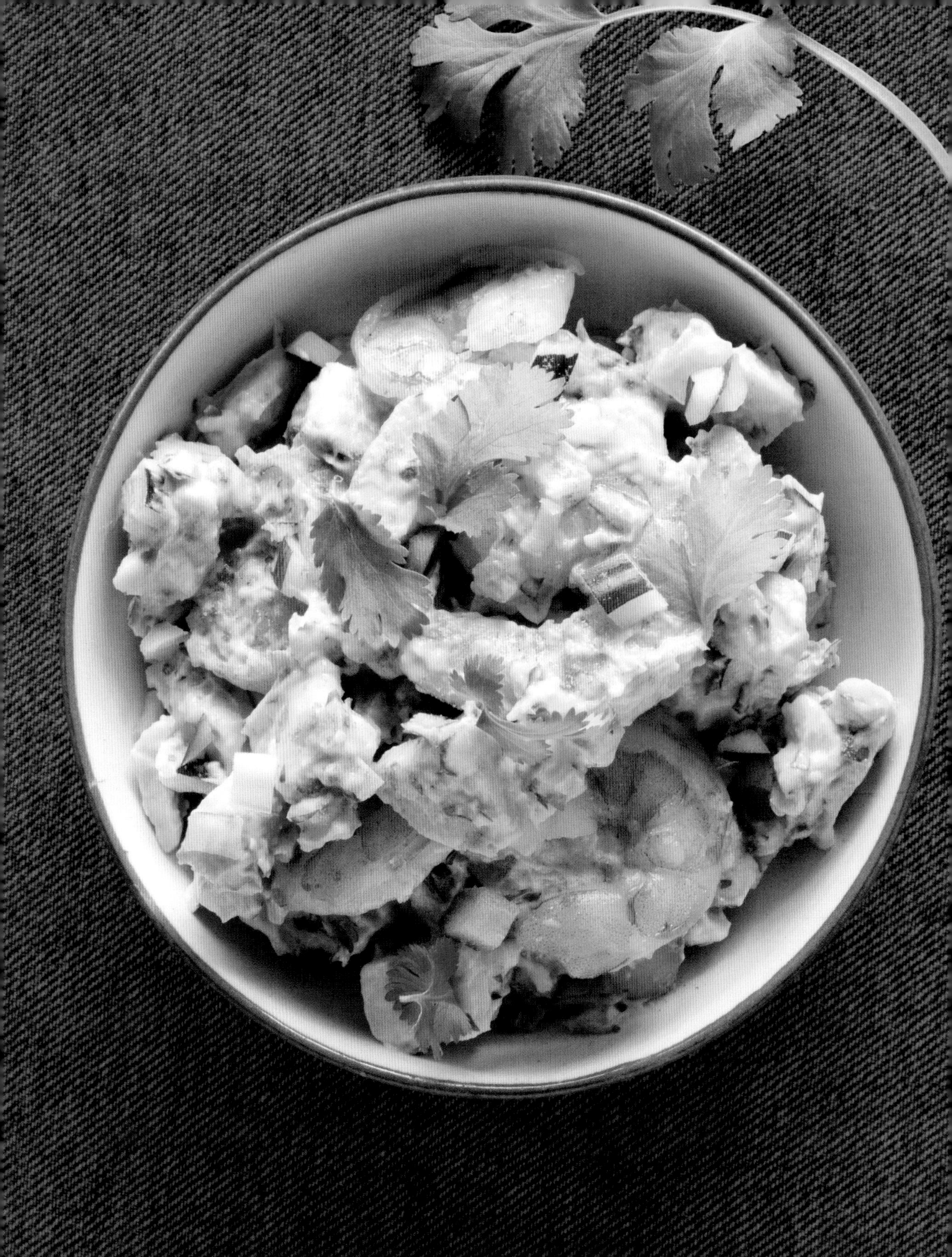

Sweet cocktail shrimp are decadently dressed in creamy avocado with a hint of red onion and a spritz of fresh lime.

Shrimp and Avocado Salad

Prep Time: **10 mins** Cook Time: **none** Yield: **2 cups** Serving Size: **1 cup**

Ingredients

- 1 large avocado
- ¼ cup mayonnaise
- 2 tsp. fresh lime juice
- ¼ tsp. sea salt
- ¼ tsp. freshly ground black pepper
- ¼ tsp. ground cumin (optional)
- ½ lb. (225g) cooked cocktail shrimp, peeled
- 2 TB. red onion, minced
- 2 TB. fresh cilantro, chopped

1 Divide avocado in half and remove pit. Dice one avocado half and set aside.

2 In a medium bowl, mash remaining avocado half into a smooth paste. Add mayonnaise, lime juice, sea salt, black pepper, and cumin (if using), and stir until well blended.

3 Add cocktail shrimp, red onion, cilantro, and diced avocado. Stir gently to combine. Serve immediately.

Variation: To make **Creamy Shrimp and Celery Salad,** replace cilantro with 2 tablespoons chopped dill, use 2 teaspoons fresh lemon juice instead of lime juice, and add 1 large celery stalk, thinly sliced.

Feel free to use frozen cooked shrimp for this recipe. Just be sure to thaw the shrimp in the refrigerator beforehand.

Nutrition per Serving

Fat **70%** Net Carb **4%**
Protein **26%** Ratio **1.1:1**

Calories	Fat	Protein	Total Carbohydrate	Dietary Fiber	Net Carbohydrate
460	36g	30g	11g	7g	4g

This salad is piled high with antipasto ingredients, lightened with fresh basil and parsley, and drizzled with fruity olive oil.

Antipasto Salad

Prep Time: **10 mins** | Cook Time: **none** | Yield: **2 salads** | Serving Size: **1 salad**

Ingredients

- 2 small Persian cucumbers, diced
- ½ cup pitted Kalamata olives
- ½ cup pitted green olives
- 2 thin (2mm) slices red onion
- 6 pepperoncinis, stemmed and sliced
- 3 oz. (85g) hard salami, peeled (if needed) and diced
- 4 oz. (110g) fresh mozzarella, diced
- ¼ cup fresh basil leaves, thinly sliced
- ½ cup Italian flat-leaf parsley
- ¼ cup pine nuts
- 2 TB. extra-virgin olive oil
- ½ tsp. freshly ground black pepper

1. In a large bowl, combine Persian cucumbers, Kalamata olives, green olives, red onion, pepperoncinis, hard salami, mozzarella, basil, Italian flat-leaf parsley, and pine nuts.

2. Drizzle with extra-virgin olive oil and season with black pepper. Toss to combine. Serve immediately, or refrigerate for up to 12 hours.

> While you can use any salami, look for a high-quality one comprised of only pork or beef, salt, garlic, and spices—no fillers.

Nutrition per Serving

Fat **76%** Net Carb **7%**
Protein **17%** Ratio **1.4:1**

Calories	Fat	Protein	Total Carbohydrate	Dietary Fiber	Net Carbohydrate
660	56g	28g	18g	7g	11g

For this unique salad, radicchio is pan-fried in bacon fat and tossed with basil, dill, toasted pine nuts, and Parmesan.

Radicchio and Fresh Herb Salad

Prep Time: **10 mins** Cook Time: **12 mins** Yield: **2 salads** Serving Size: **1 salad**

Ingredients

- ½ cup pine nuts
- 3 TB. extra-virgin olive oil
- ¼ tsp. sea salt
- 2 uncured bacon slices, diced
- 1 medium head radicchio, quartered
- ¼ cup chopped fresh basil
- ¼ cup chopped fresh dill
- ¼ tsp. freshly ground black pepper
- 2 oz. (55g) Parmesan, grated or shaved

1 Heat a medium skillet over low heat. Add pine nuts, 1 tablespoon extra-virgin olive oil, and sea salt. Cook for 4 to 5 minutes, stirring constantly, or until nuts are golden brown and fragrant. Remove nuts and transfer to a large bowl.

2 Reheat the skillet over medium heat. Add uncured bacon and cook, stirring occasionally, for 4 to 5 minutes, or until bacon is browned. Remove bacon from the skillet and transfer to the large bowl with the toasted pine nuts.

3 Reheat the skillet (including remaining drippings) over high heat. When the skillet is hot, carefully place radicchio quarters in the hot bacon fat. Cook for 1 minute.

4 Using long-handled tongs, turn radicchio quarters over. Cook for an additional 1 minute. Transfer to the large bowl.

5 Add basil, dill, black pepper, remaining 2 tablespoons extra-virgin olive oil, and Parmesan to the large bowl. Toss to combine. Divide into 2 salad bowls and serve warm.

You can also grill the radicchio. To keep the ratios the same, simply add the bacon fat to the salad before tossing.

Nutrition per Serving

Fat 86% Net Carb 2%
Protein 12% Ratio 2.8:1

Calories	Fat	Protein	Total Carbohydrate	Dietary Fiber	Net Carbohydrate
584	56g	18g	5g	3g	2g

Delicate kale ribbons are covered with a lemon and pepper vinaigrette and tossed with Parmesan and bacon bits.

Kale and Parmesan Salad

Prep Time: **10 mins** | Cook Time: **6 mins** | Yield: **2 salads** | Serving Size: **1 salad**

Ingredients

- 12 lacinato or dinosaur kale leaves
- ¼ tsp. sea salt
- 4 oz. (110g) uncured bacon (about 4 slices), minced
- 2 TB. extra-virgin olive oil
- 2 tsp. fresh lemon juice
- ½ tsp. freshly ground black pepper
- ¼ cup grated or shaved Parmesan

1 Remove woody stems from lacinato kale. Roll leaves together to form a loose bundle. Carefully slice kale crosswise into very thin slices or ribbons.

2 Place kale in a colander or strainer over the sink. Sprinkle with sea salt and gently massage to coat kale. Let sit for 5 minutes.

3 Meanwhile, heat a medium skillet over medium heat. Add bacon and cook for 4 to 6 minutes, stirring occasionally, until bacon is crisp. Remove bacon from the skillet and place on a paper towel. Reserve bacon drippings.

4 In a small mixing bowl, whisk extra-virgin olive oil with bacon drippings. Add lemon juice and black pepper and whisk together to make dressing.

5 Squeeze any water out of kale. Place kale in a large salad bowl and toss with dressing to coat. Top with bacon pieces and Parmesan to serve.

Variation: To mix it up a bit, replace kale with 3 cups thinly sliced red chicory or radicchio, and use blue cheese instead of Parmesan for a delicious **Radicchio and Blue Cheese Salad.**

The chopping technique used for the kale in this salad is called *chiffonade*. The thin ribbons soften the rigid kale texture.

Nutrition per Serving

Fat 63% Net Carb 8%
Protein 29% Ratio 0.8:1

Calories	Fat	Protein	Total Carbohydrate	Dietary Fiber	Net Carbohydrate
516	36g	37g	14g	3g	11g

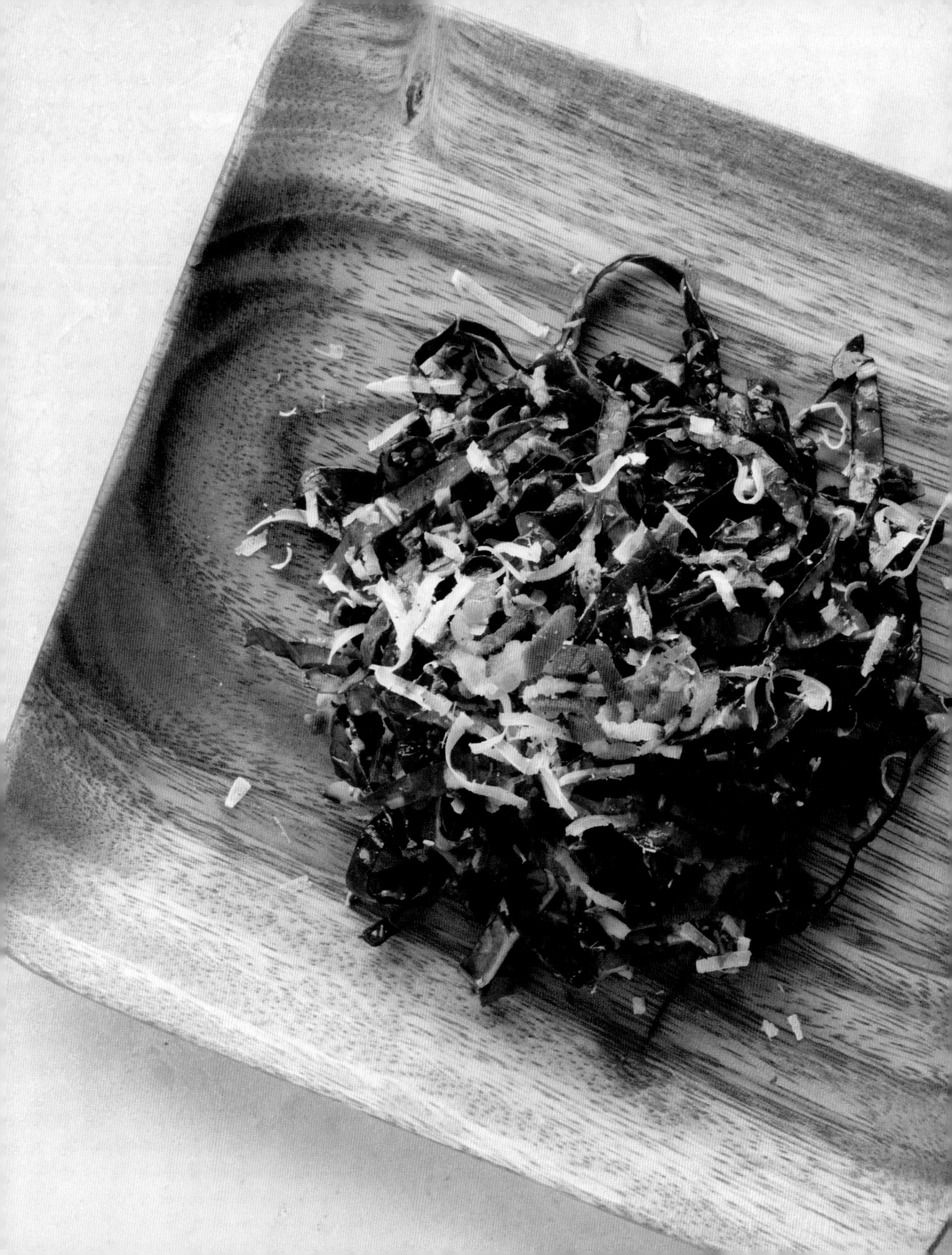

Soups and Stews

What's more comforting than a hot bowl of soup or stew during the cold winter months? Soup and keto go hand in hand due to their perfect blends of fat and salt. From cheddar broccoli soup to chicken stew, these deliciously simple recipes offer ample variety without skimping on flavor. And because they make great leftovers and reheat well, you always can make double batches and freeze them for later.

This foolproof chicken stock is chock-full of fat and collagen, making it a great base for keto soups and stews.

Keto Chicken Stock

Prep Time: **1 hr** Cook Time: **6 hrs** Yield: **2 qt. (2l)** Serving Size: **2 cups**

Ingredients

- ¼ cup extra-virgin olive oil
- 2 lb. (1kg) chicken wings, necks, and backs
- 1 yellow onion, quartered (with peel on)
- 4 qt. (4l) cold water
- 1 lb. (450g) chicken feet (optional; use 1 lb. [450g] additional chicken wings otherwise)
- 1 TB. apple cider vinegar
- 1 bay leaf
- 1 tsp. whole black peppercorns
- 2 tsp. sea salt

1 Heat a large stockpot or Dutch oven over medium-high heat. Add extra-virgin olive oil.

2 When the pot is hot and oil is shimmering, add chicken wings, necks, and backs, as well as yellow onion. Cook, stirring occasionally, until well browned, about 5 to 7 minutes.

3 Add cold water and stir, scraping up any browned bits from the bottom of the pot.

4 Add chicken feet (if using), apple cider vinegar, bay leaf, black peppercorns, and sea salt. Stir and reduce heat to medium-low.

5 Simmer for 4 to 5 hours, occasionally skimming any white scum that comes to surface of stock.

6 To finish stock, remove from heat and let stand for 1 hour. Strain stock to render a clear liquid.

7 Refrigerate or freeze stock immediately in 2- to 4-cup portions for later use.

For a slow cooker: add ingredients, reduce the water to 2 qt. (2l), cover, and cook on low 8 to 12 hours. Cool, strain, and store.

Nutrition per Serving

Fat **67%** Net Carb **3%**
Protein **30%** Ratio **0.9:1**

Calories	Fat	Protein	Total Carbohydrate	Dietary Fiber	Net Carbohydrate
458	34g	35g	4g	1g	3g

This gorgeous dark-colored stock uses roasted bones to create a substantial and deeply flavored base.

Keto Pork Stock

Prep Time: **1 hr** | Cook Time: **6 hrs** | Yield: **2 qt. (2l)** | Serving Size: **2 cups**

Ingredients

- 2 lb. (1kg) pork marrow bones
- 1 lb. (450g) pork trotters
- ¼ cup extra-virgin olive oil
- 1 yellow onion, quartered (with peel on)
- 1 large carrot, quartered
- 1 large celery stalk, quartered
- 4 qt. (4l) cold water
- 1 TB. apple cider vinegar
- 1 bay leaf
- 2 dried shiitake mushrooms (optional)
- 2 tsp. sea salt

1 Preheat the oven to 350°F (180°C). Place pork marrow bones and trotters on a rimmed metal baking sheet. Bake for 20 to 30 minutes, or until browned.

2 Heat a large stockpot or Dutch oven over medium-high heat. Add extra-virgin olive oil. When the pot is hot and oil is shimmering, add yellow onion, carrot, and celery.

3 Sauté, stirring occasionally, until browned, about 4 to 5 minutes. Add cold water and stir, scraping up any browned bits from the bottom of the pot.

4 Add browned bones and trotters, along with any residual drippings from the baking sheet. Add apple cider vinegar, bay leaf, dried shiitake mushrooms (if using), and sea salt. Stir and reduce heat to medium-low.

5 Simmer for 4 to 5 hours, occasionally skimming any white scum that comes to surface of stock.

6 To finish stock, remove from heat and let stand for 1 hour. Strain stock to render a clear liquid.

7 Refrigerate or freeze stock immediately in 2- to 4-cup portions for later use.

Variation: To make **Keto Beef Stock,** replace pork marrow bones with 2 pounds (1kg) beef knuckle bones, and use 1 pound (450g) oxtails or beef short ribs instead of pork trotters.

Nutrition per Serving

Fat **72%** Net Carb **5%**
Protein **23%** Ratio **1.2:1**

Calories	Fat	Protein	Total Carbohydrate	Dietary Fiber	Net Carbohydrate
628	44g	32g	7g	1g	6g

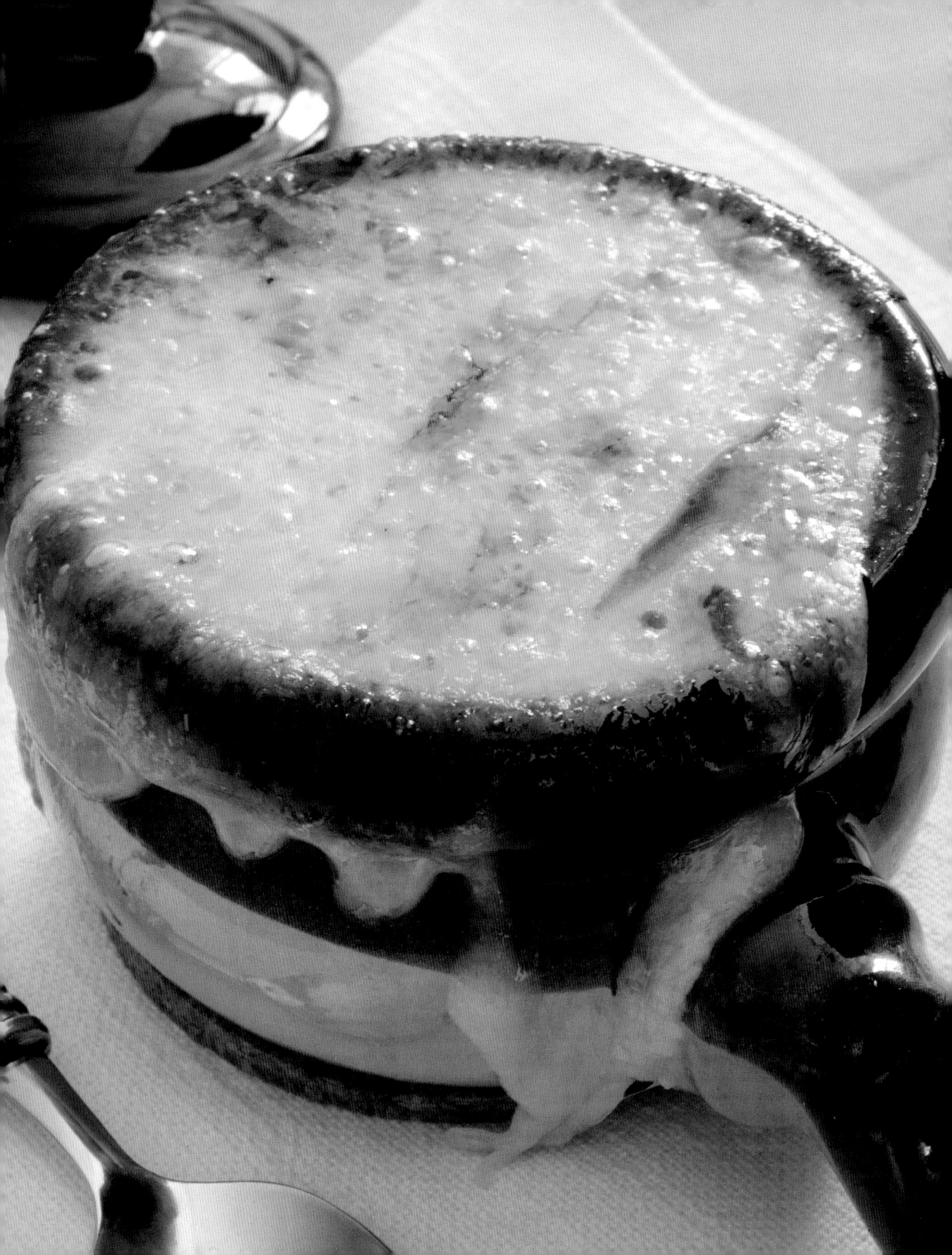

You'll never miss the baguette in this rich beef and onion broth covered with a gooey layer of golden-brown cheeses.

French Onion Soup

Prep Time: **10 mins** | Cook Time: **1 hr** | Yield: **6 cups** | Serving Size: **1½ cups**

Ingredients

- ¾ cup salted butter
- 2 large yellow onions, sliced into thin rings
- 6 cups beef broth
- ½ cup dry white wine
- 1 bay leaf
- 1 tsp. dried thyme
- ½ tsp. sea salt
- ¼ tsp. freshly ground black pepper
- 4 oz. (110g) Gruyère, sliced
- 4 oz. (110g) Parmigiano-Reggiano, grated

1 Heat a medium soup pot over medium-low heat. Add salted butter.

2 When butter melts, add yellow onions. Cook, stirring occasionally, for 20 to 30 minutes, or until a deep caramel brown.

3 Add beef broth, dry white wine, bay leaf, dried thyme, sea salt, and black pepper. Stir, cover, and simmer for 20 minutes. Remove and discard bay leaf.

4 Preheat the broiler to high and place a rack on the highest shelf.

5 Place 4 ovenproof crocks or metal bowls on a rimmed metal baking sheet.

6 Divide soup into the 4 crocks. Cover with Gruyère and Parmigiano-Reggiano.

7 Place the crocks on the top shelf of the oven and broil for 2 to 4 minutes, or until cheese is bubbly and golden brown. Let cool for 2 minutes before serving.

Real Parmigiano-Reggiano can't be beat quality-wise. But if you wish, you may use a different hard cheese, such as pecorino.

Nutrition per Serving

Fat **79%** Net Carb **6%**
Protein **15%** Ratio **1.7:1**

Calories	Fat	Protein	Total Carbohydrate	Dietary Fiber	Net Carbohydrate
601	53g	23g	9g	1g	8g

This full-flavored stew is teeming with zesty Italian sausage, robust kielbasa, sturdy vegetables, and lively seasonings.

Hearty Italian Stew

Prep Time: **10 mins** Cook Time: **45 mins** Yield: **8 cups** Serving Size: **2 cups**

Ingredients

- ¼ cup extra-virgin olive oil
- ½ cup yellow onion, diced
- ½ cup carrot, diced
- 1 garlic clove, minced
- 1 lb. (450g) ground mild Italian sausage
- ½ medium green bell pepper, seeded and diced
- 1 TB. tomato paste
- 4 cups chicken stock
- 8 curly green kale leaves, woody stems removed
- ⅓ lb. (170g) kielbasa, sliced
- 1 tsp. Italian seasoning
- ¼ tsp. crushed red pepper flakes
- Sea salt (optional)
- ¼ cup fresh basil, chopped

1 Heat a large soup pot or Dutch oven over medium heat. When the pot is hot, add extra-virgin olive oil and wait for 30 seconds.

2 Add yellow onion and carrot and cook, stirring occasionally, for 3 to 5 minutes, or until onion begins to soften. Add garlic and cook for an additional 1 minute.

3 Add mild Italian sausage, and use a wooden spoon to break apart in the bottom of the pot. Cook for 5 minutes, or until sausage begins to brown.

4 Add green bell pepper and tomato paste and cook for an additional 2 minutes.

5 Pour chicken stock into the pot, scraping up any browned bits off the bottom of the pot. Add kale, kielbasa, Italian seasoning, and crushed red pepper flakes. Cover, reduce heat to medium-low, and simmer for 30 minutes.

6 Taste soup and season with sea salt to taste, if necessary. Ladle soup into bowls and sprinkle with basil to serve.

Nutrition per Serving

Fat **77%** Net Carb **6%**
Protein **17%** Ratio **1.5:1**

Calories	Fat	Protein	Total Carbohydrate	Dietary Fiber	Net Carbohydrate
525	45g	22g	12g	4g	8g

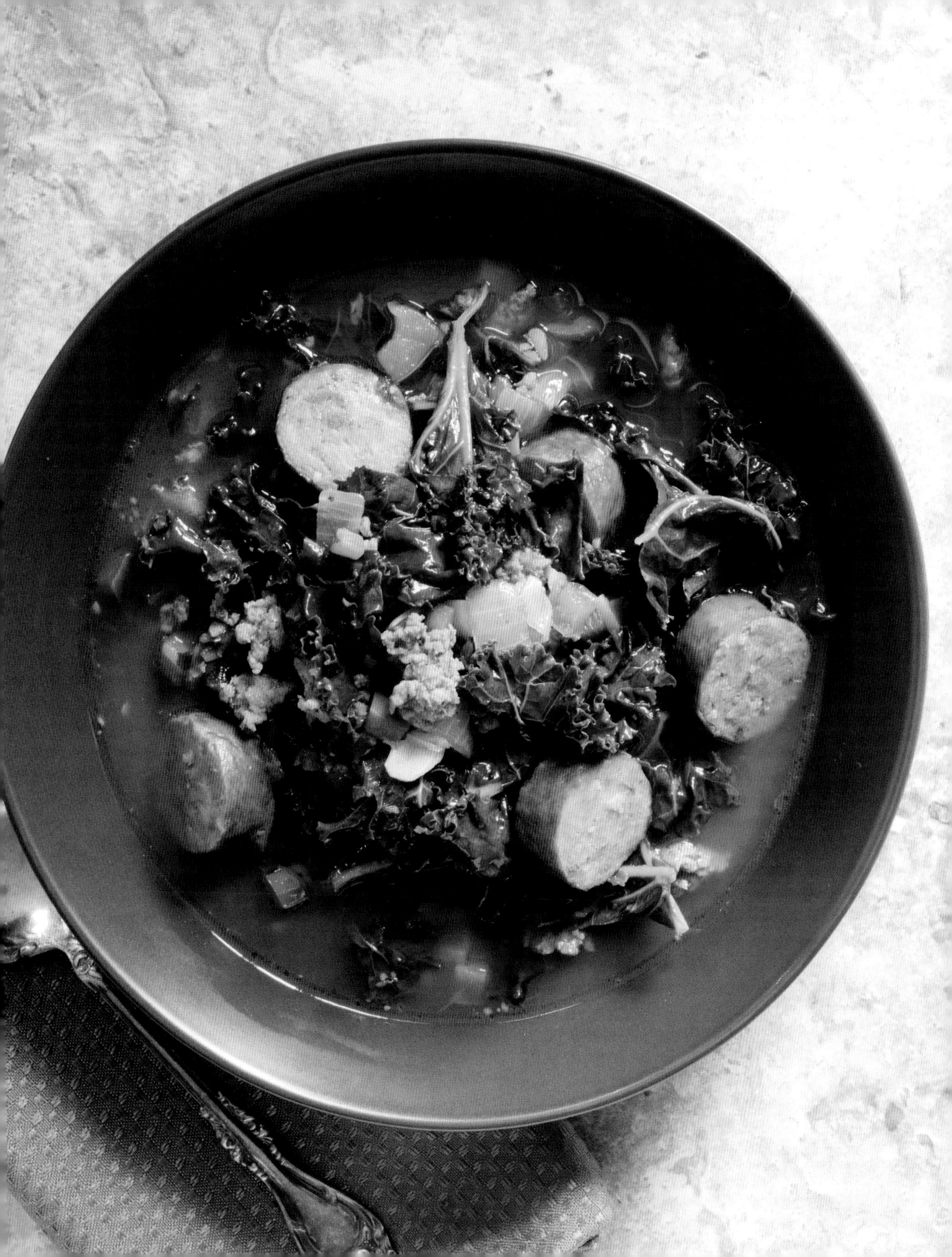

Chewy Manila clams, chunks of salmon, sweet bay scallops, and plump shrimp abound in this flavorful chowder.

Seafood Chowder

Prep Time: **10 mins** Cook Time: **35 mins** Yield: **8 cups** Serving Size: **2 cups**

Ingredients

- ¼ cup unsalted butter
- ¼ cup shallots, diced
- ¼ cup carrots, diced
- ¼ cup celery, diced
- ½ tsp. dried thyme
- 2 cups vegetable broth
- ¼ cup dry white wine
- ¼ lb. (115g) celery root, peeled and diced
- ½ tsp. sea salt
- ¼ tsp. freshly ground black pepper
- 2 cups heavy cream
- ¼ lb. (115g) live Manila clams, cleaned
- ¼ lb. (115g) fresh salmon, cut into 1-in. (2.5cm) cubes
- ¼ lb. (115g) raw bay scallops (out of shell)
- ¼ lb. (115g) raw shrimp, peeled and deveined

1. Heat a large soup pot or Dutch oven over medium-high heat. Add unsalted butter.
2. When butter melts, add shallots, carrots, celery, and thyme. Sauté, stirring occasionally, for 4 to 6 minutes, or until shallots have softened.
3. Pour in vegetable broth and stir, scraping up any browned bits from the bottom of the pot.
4. Add dry white wine, celery root, sea salt, and black pepper. Reduce heat to medium-low and simmer for 15 to 20 minutes, or until celery root is tender.
5. Stir in heavy cream and bring back to a light simmer. Add Manila clams and simmer for 2 minutes.
6. Add salmon, bay scallops, and shrimp and simmer for an additional 1 to 2 minutes, or until seafood is cooked through and clams have opened.
7. Discard any clams that don't open. Serve immediately.

Feel free to vary the seafood you use. Just be sure you don't use more than 1 lb. (450g) to keep an optimal keto balance.

Nutrition per Serving

Fat **81%** Net Carb **7%**
Protein **12%** Ratio **1.9:1**

Calories	Fat	Protein	Total Carbohydrate	Dietary Fiber	Net Carbohydrate
655	59g	20g	12g	1g	11g

Earthy mushrooms and sweet leek flavor this smooth and creamy soup, seasoned with a hint of thyme.

Cream of Mushroom Soup

Prep Time: **10 mins** Cook Time: **30 mins** Yield: **8 cups** Serving Size: **2 cups**

Ingredients

- ¼ lb. (115g) unsalted butter, cut into cubes
- 3 TB. extra-virgin olive oil
- 1 leek, chopped
- 1 garlic clove, minced
- ¾ lb. (340g) cremini mushrooms, quartered
- 4 cups mushroom stock or vegetables stock
- ½ cup dry white wine
- 1 tsp. dried thyme
- ½ tsp. sea salt
- ¼ tsp. freshly ground black pepper
- 2 TB. cornstarch
- 2 TB. cold water
- 2 cups heavy cream

1 Heat a small soup pot over medium-high heat. When the pot is hot, add unsalted butter and extra-virgin olive oil. Wait for 30 seconds.

2 Add leek, garlic, and mushrooms and sauté, stirring occasionally, for 4 to 6 minutes, or until browned. Add mushroom stock, dry white wine, thyme, sea salt, and black pepper. Reduce heat to medium-low, cover, and simmer for 20 minutes. (If desired, remove the pot from heat afterward and use an immersion blender to purée soup before returning to the stove over medium-high heat.)

3 Meanwhile, in a small bowl, combine cornstarch with cold water and whisk until all lumps dissolve. Set aside.

4 Whisk heavy cream into soup. Slowly drizzle in cornstarch mixture and whisk for 1 minute, or until a creamy texture forms. Portion soup into bowls and serve warm.

Variation: To make **Cream of Asparagus Soup,** replace cremini mushrooms with ¾ pound (340g) sliced asparagus spears and simmer for 5 to 7 minutes before adding heavy cream.

This soup will lose its creaminess if frozen and thawed, so be sure to make it fresh for the best consistency.

Nutrition per Serving

Fat 91% Net Carb 6%
Protein 3% Ratio 4.3:1

Calories	Fat	Protein	Total Carbohydrate	Dietary Fiber	Net Carbohydrate
774	78g	5g	14g	1g	13g

Fork-tender chunks of beef shoulder are slow-cooked with piquant ground chorizo in this meaty Texas-style chili.

Texas Chili

Prep Time: **20 mins** | Cook Time: **2 hrs** | Yield: **12 cups** | Serving Size: **1½ cups**

Ingredients

- 2 TB. chili powder
- 2 tsp. ground cumin
- 1 TB. granulated garlic
- 1½ lb. (680g) boneless beef chuck, cut into 1-in. (2.5cm) cubes
- 4 oz. (110g) thick-sliced, uncured bacon, diced
- ½ cup extra-virgin olive oil or lard
- 1 large yellow onion, diced
- 2 garlic cloves, minced
- 4 cups beef broth
- 1 lb. (450g) fresh pork chorizo
- 1 tsp. dried oregano
- 1 TB. red wine vinegar
- 1½ cups grated cheddar cheese
- 1½ cups sour cream
- 1 cup fresh cilantro, chopped

1 In a medium bowl, combine chili powder, cumin, and granulated garlic. Toss beef cubes in spice mixture. Set aside.

2 Heat a large soup pot over medium-low heat. Add uncured bacon and cook for 5 to 7 minutes, or until bacon is crisp. Remove bacon from the pot and place on a paper towel.

3 Add 3 tablespoons extra-virgin olive oil to residual bacon fat in the pot. Reheat the pot over medium-high heat.

4 When oil is hot, place half of beef cubes into the bottom of the pot. Cook for 1 to 2 minutes, or until browned. Turn beef cubes and brown on all sides. Remove beef from the pot.

5 Reheat the pot and add 3 tablespoons olive oil. Repeat Step 4 with remaining beef.

6 Reheat the pot and add remaining 2 tablespoons olive oil. Add onion and sauté, stirring occasionally, for 3 to 5 minutes. Add remaining spice mixture and cook for 1 minute.

7 Pour broth into the pot and scrape up any browned bits. Add 2 cups water, browned beef, pork chorizo, oregano, and red wine vinegar. Reduce heat to medium-low. Cook for 1 hour, 30 minutes, or until beef is tender.

8 To serve, top bowls of chili with cheddar cheese, sour cream, bacon, and cilantro.

Variation: To make **Colorado Green Chili,** replace chorizo with 1 pound (450g) ground pork, beef chuck with 1½ pounds (680g) pork shoulder, and onion with 2 diced poblano peppers; eliminate chili powder.

Nutrition per Serving

Fat **81%** Net Carb **2%**
Protein **17%** Ratio **1.9:1**

Calories	Fat	Protein	Total Carbohydrate	Dietary Fiber	Net Carbohydrate
690	62g	29g	6g	2g	4g

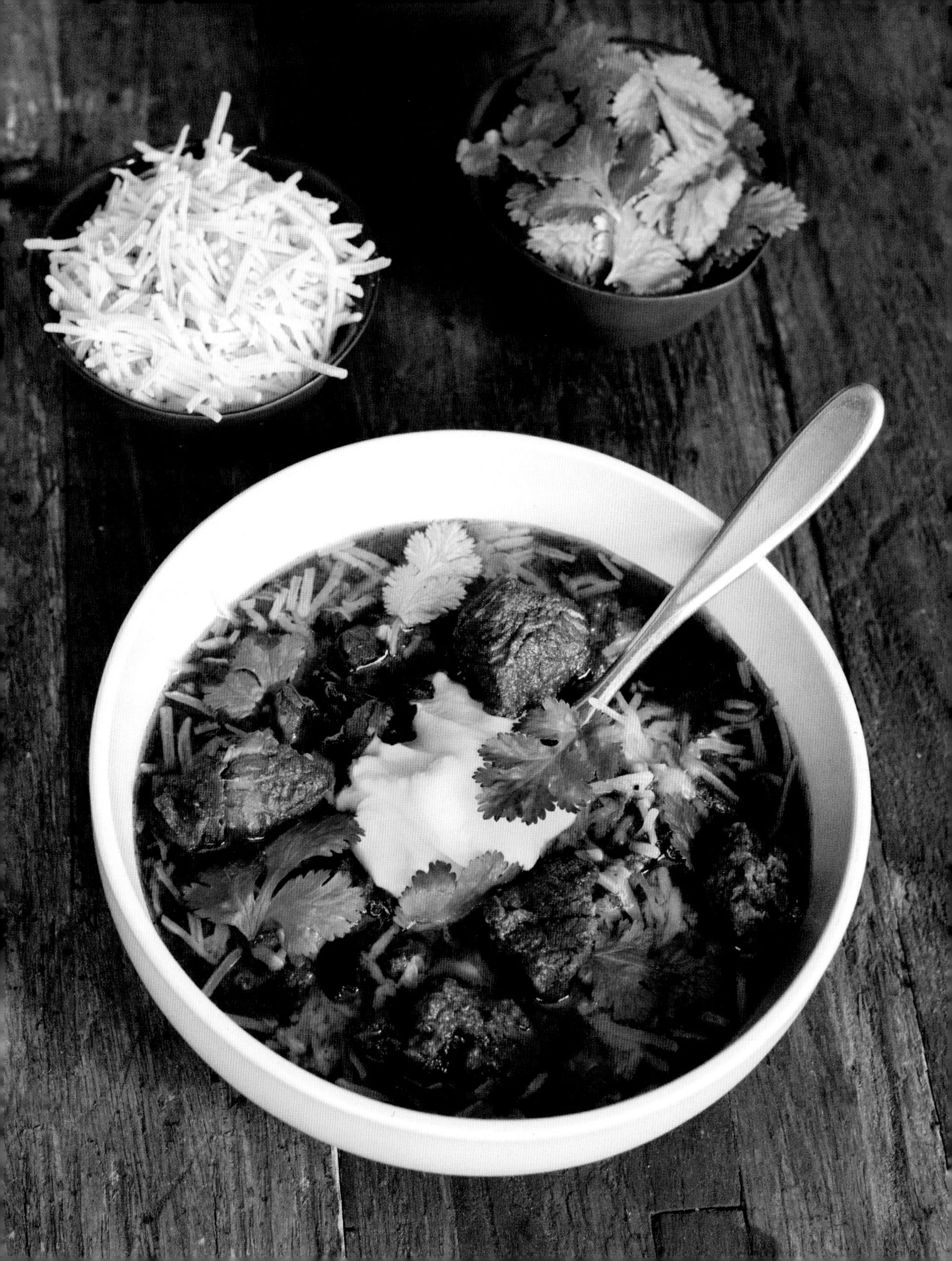

This stew is brimming with shredded chicken, celery root, mushrooms, and fragrant rosemary in a rich, creamy broth.

Rosemary Chicken Stew

Prep Time: **15 mins** Cook Time: **45 mins** Yield: **8 cups** Serving Size: **2 cups**

Ingredients

- ¼ cup extra-virgin olive oil
- 1 TB. fresh rosemary, chopped
- 4 cloves garlic, minced
- 8 medium white button mushrooms, quartered
- 4 cups chicken broth
- 2 cups water
- 1 medium carrot, trimmed and sliced
- ¾ lb. (340g) celery root, peeled and diced
- 1 lb. (450g) skinless, boneless chicken thighs
- ½ tsp. sea salt
- ½ tsp. freshly ground black pepper
- 1 tsp. lemon zest
- 1 cup heavy cream
- 2 TB. arrowroot powder
- ¼ cup cold water

1 Heat a large soup pot over medium heat. When the pot is hot, add extra-virgin olive oil and wait for 15 seconds.

2 Add rosemary, garlic, and white button mushrooms. Cook, stirring occasionally, for 4 to 6 minutes, or until mushrooms are browned.

3 Pour chicken broth into the pot. Stir, scraping up any browned bits from the bottom of the pot.

4 Add water, carrot, celery root, chicken thighs, sea salt, and black pepper. Reduce heat to low, and simmer uncovered for 30 minutes, or until chicken is cooked through and vegetables are firm but tender.

5 Remove chicken thighs from soup. Using 2 forks, pull thighs apart into shredded pieces. Return chicken to soup. Add lemon zest and heavy cream and stir.

6 Mix arrowroot powder with cold water. Pour mixture into soup and stir to combine. Simmer for 3 to 5 minutes, or until creamy. Serve warm.

Celery root—a low-carb alterative to potatoes—turns brown quickly after peeling, so keep it in water with lemon juice.

Nutrition per Serving

Fat 73% Net Carb 10%
Protein 17% Ratio 1.2:1

Calories	Fat	Protein	Total Carbohydrate	Dietary Fiber	Net Carbohydrate
553	45g	24g	15g	2g	13g

Bright broccoli florets float in a rich cheddar cream sauce in this silky soup, topped with crunchy bacon crumbles.

Broccoli Cheese Soup

Prep Time: **5 mins** | Cook Time: **25 mins** | Yield: **9 cups** | Serving Size: **1½ cups**

Ingredients

- 4 TB. unsalted butter
- ¼ cup yellow onion, diced
- ¼ cup carrots, diced
- 1 garlic clove, minced
- 2 cups vegetable broth
- 2 cups heavy cream
- 1 lb. (450g) broccoli florets
- ½ tsp. sea salt
- ¼ tsp. freshly ground black pepper
- 2½ cups grated cheddar cheese
- 4 bacon slices, cooked and crumbled (about 4 oz.; 110g)

1 Heat a large soup pot or Dutch oven over medium-high heat. Add unsalted butter.

2 When butter melts, add yellow onion, carrots, and garlic. Sauté, stirring occasionally, for 4 to 5 minutes, or until vegetables have softened.

3 Pour in vegetable broth and stir, scraping up any browned bits from the bottom of the pot.

4 Add heavy cream, broccoli florets, sea salt, and black pepper. Reduce heat to medium-low and simmer for 15 to 20 minutes, or until broccoli is tender.

5 Using a wooden spoon, stir in cheddar cheese and continue stirring until smooth. Top with bacon crumbles to serve.

If you want a creamier texture, use an immersion blender to purée the soup before topping with bacon crumbles.

Variation: You can add ½ pound (225g) skinless, boneless chicken thighs, cut into thin slices, to make **Cheesy Broccoli Chicken Soup.** Simply add chicken along with the broccoli florets and simmer until cooked through. (Don't purée this variation.)

Nutrition per Serving

Fat **82%** Net Carb **4%**
Protein **14%** Ratio **2.0:1**

Calories	Fat	Protein	Total Carbohydrate	Dietary Fiber	Net Carbohydrate
673	61g	23g	11g	3g	8g

Layers of umami flavor this slow-cooked broth, loaded with low-carb kelp noodles and all the traditional ramen toppings.

Low-Carb Ramen

Prep Time: **15 mins** | Cook Time: **3 hrs, 35 mins** | Yield: **8 cups** | Serving Size: **2 cups**

Ingredients

- ¼ cup sesame oil
- 1 lb. (450g) pork spare ribs
- 6 chicken wings
- 3 pieces kombu
- 12 scallions, thinly sliced
- ½ cup bonito flakes
- 4 garlic cloves, crushed
- 1 3-in. (7.5cm) piece fresh ginger root, peeled and halved
- 1 tsp. sea salt
- 1 oz. (25g) dried shiitake mushrooms
- 3 TB. tamari or coconut aminos
- 1 TB. rice wine vinegar
- ½ lb. (225g) thick-sliced bacon (about ¼-in.; .5cm thick), cut into 4 or 8 equal pieces
- 1 24-oz. (680g) pkg. kelp noodles
- 4 nori sheets, cut in half
- 2 TB. toasted sesame seeds
- 2 large eggs, hard-cooked, peeled, and halved

1. Heat a large soup pot over medium-high heat. When hot, add 2 tablespoons sesame oil.

2. Add spare ribs and chicken wings to hot oil and brown on all sides, about 3 to 5 minutes.

3. Add 4 quarts (4l) water to the pot, scraping up any browned bits from the bottom. Cover pot and increase heat to high.

4. When water boils, add kombu. Boil for 10 minutes. Remove and discard kombu.

5. Add 10 scallions, bonito flakes, garlic, ginger root, and sea salt. Reduce heat to medium-low and simmer, uncovered, for 3 hours, or until spare ribs fall off the bone.

6. Strain broth. Remove large pieces of pork and chop. Return pork to the pot.

7. Return broth to the pot and place over medium heat. Add shiitake mushrooms, tamari, and rice wine vinegar and cook for 8 to 10 minutes, or until mushrooms are tender.

8. Meanwhile, heat a small skillet over medium heat. When the skillet is hot, add remaining 2 tablespoons sesame oil. Place thick-sliced bacon in hot oil and cook until browned and crisp, about 3 to 5 minutes per side. Remove bacon and reserve oil.

9. Rinse kelp noodles under cool water. Add noodles to hot broth and cook for 2 to 3 minutes, or until softened.

10. Ladle soup and noodles into 4 bowls. Top each bowl with 1 nori sheet, 2 scallions, toasted sesame seeds, 1 hard-cooked egg half, and bacon. Drizzle with remaining oil from the bacon pan and serve.

Nutrition per Serving

Fat **72%** Net Carb **4%**
Protein **24%** Ratio **1.1:1**

Calories	Fat	Protein	Total Carbohydrate	Dietary Fiber	Net Carbohydrate
1,078	86g	65g	16g	5g	11g

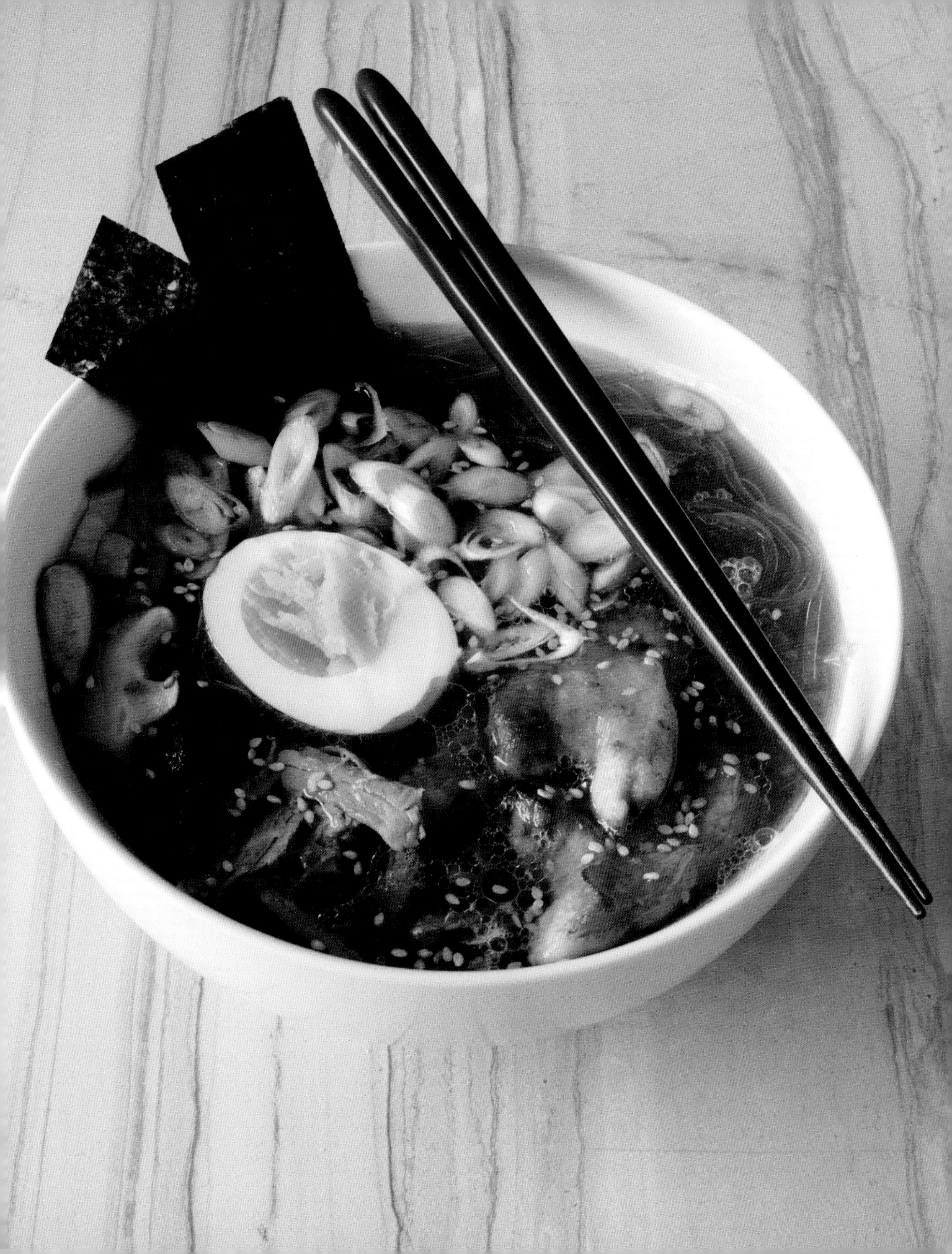

Silky ribbons of egg float in golden chicken broth in this simple soup, finished with a drizzle of toasted sesame oil.

Egg Drop Soup

Prep Time: **5 mins** | Cook Time: **15 mins** | Yield: **4 cups** | Serving Size: **2 cups**

Ingredients

- 4 cups chicken broth
- 1 tsp. fish sauce
- 2 large eggs, slightly beaten
- 2 TB. toasted sesame oil
- 1 green onion, thinly sliced

1 In a small soup pot over medium heat, bring chicken broth to a simmer, about 5 to 10 minutes. When broth is simmering, stir in fish sauce.

2 While continuously whisking broth with one hand, slowly drizzle in eggs with the other. Eggs will immediately coagulate into ribbons. Remove from heat.

3 Ladle soup into 2 bowls. Drizzle with toasted sesame oil and sprinkle with green onion to serve.

Nutrition per Serving

Fat **77%** Net Carb **5%**
Protein **18%** Ratio **1.5:1**

Calories **223**
Fat **19g**
Protein **10g**
Total Carbohydrate **3g**
Dietary Fiber **0g**
Net Carbohydrate **3g**

Many American versions of this soup add cornstarch for a thicker broth. As you are able to increase carbs, you may wish to whisk in 2 TB. arrowroot powder mixed with 2 TB. cold water and let simmer for 2 minutes before whisking in the egg.

Meaty beef oxtails are simmered alongside rich aromatics and a hearty selection of diced root vegetables in this stew.

Oxtail and Root Vegetable Stew

Prep Time: **10 mins** Cook Time: **3 hrs, 10 mins** Yield: **6 cups** Serving Size: **1½ cups**

Ingredients

- 1 lb. (450g) beef oxtails
- ½ tsp. sea salt
- ¼ tsp. freshly ground black pepper
- 8 TB. extra-virgin olive oil
- 2 TB. diced shallots
- 2 garlic cloves, minced
- ½ tsp. ground allspice
- ½ cup dry red wine
- 2 cups beef broth
- 2 cups cold water
- 2 bay leaves
- 1 sprig rosemary
- 1 medium carrot, trimmed and sliced
- ½ lb. (225g) turnips, peeled and diced
- ¾ lb. (340g) celery root, peeled and diced

1 Heat a large soup pot or Dutch oven over medium-high heat.

2 Season beef oxtails on all sides with sea salt and black pepper.

3 When the pot is hot, add 3 tablespoons extra-virgin olive oil and heat until shimmering.

4 Add enough oxtails to cover the bottom of the pot (don't overcrowd). Cook for 3 to 5 minutes on all sides, until deeply browned. Remove from the pot and repeat with 3 tablespoons olive oil and remaining oxtails.

5 Reheat remaining olive oil in the pot over medium heat. Add remaining 2 tablespoons olive oil, shallots, garlic, and allspice. Cook for 2 to 3 minutes, or until shallots are browned and garlic is fragrant.

6 Add dry red wine and stir, scraping up any browned bits from the bottom of the pot. Cook for 1 minute.

7 Pour in beef broth and cold water. Add bay leaves, rosemary, and browned oxtails. Cover and reduce heat to low. Simmer, stirring occasionally, for 2 hours.

8 Add carrot, turnips, and celery root. Replace cover and simmer for an additional 1 hour, or until vegetables and oxtails are tender.

9 Remove and discard bay leaves and rosemary sprig before serving.

Nutrition per Serving

Fat 63% Net Carb 12%
Protein 25% Ratio 0.8:1

Calories	Fat	Protein	Total Carbohydrate	Dietary Fiber	Net Carbohydrate
615	43g	38g	22g	3g	19g

This Cajun-style stew of okra pods, shrimp, and Andouille sausage is served with low-carb cauliflower "rice."

Gumbo

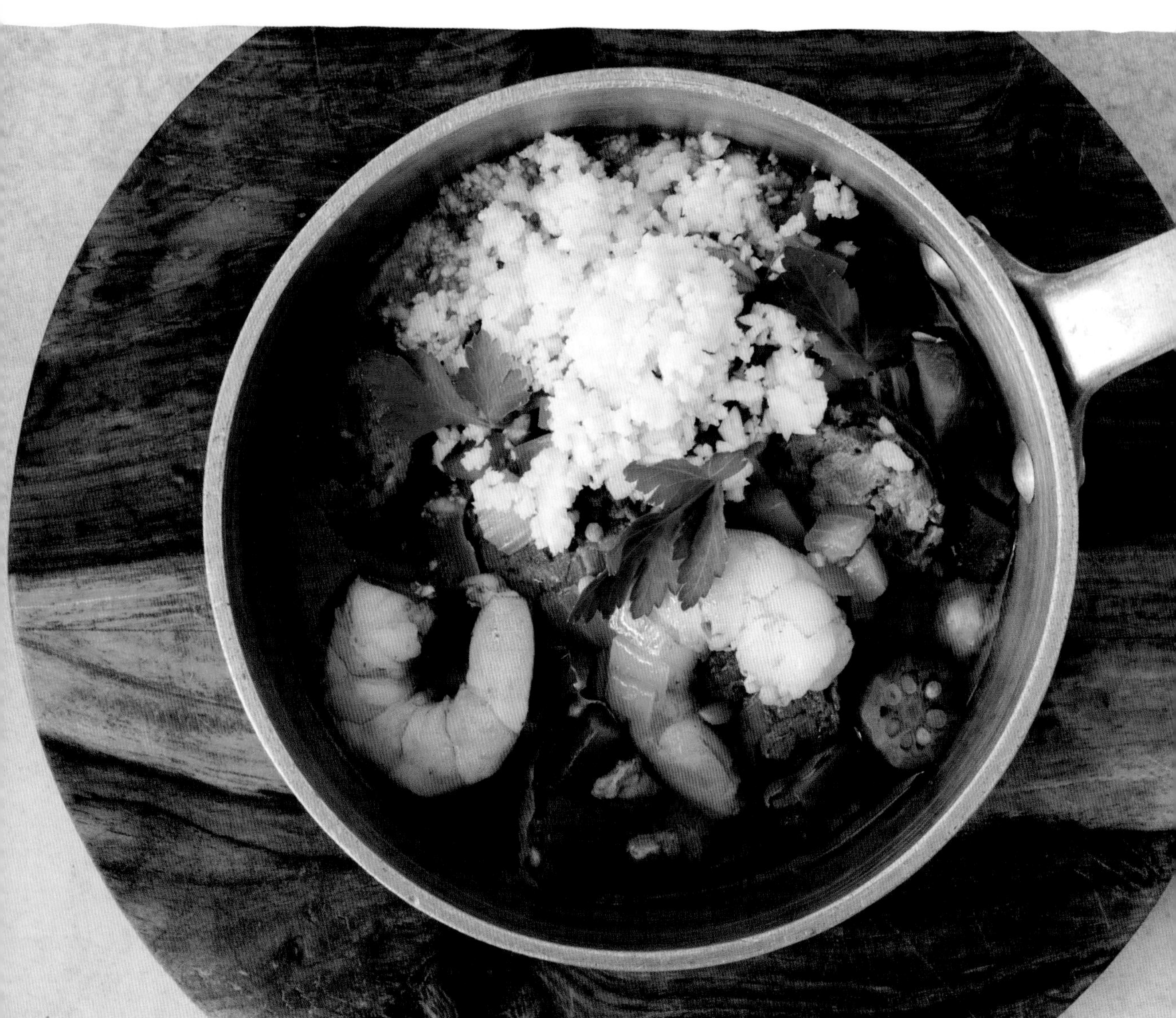

Prep Time: **10 mins** | Cook Time: **30 mins** | Yield: **12 cups** | Serving Size: **2 cups**

Ingredients

2 TB. extra-virgin olive oil

6 oz. (170g) skinless, boneless chicken thighs, diced

8 TB. unsalted butter

½ large yellow onion, diced

2 garlic cloves, minced

1 cup celery, diced

½ medium green bell pepper, diced

2 TB. tomato paste

2 TB. Worcestershire sauce

4 cups chicken broth

2 tsp. Cajun spice blend

10 oz. (285g) package frozen sliced okra, thawed

3 cups cauliflower florets

1 lb. (450g) Andouille sausage, sliced

½ lb. (225g) raw shrimp, peeled

½ cup chopped fresh parsley

½ tsp. sea salt

1 Heat a large soup pot or Dutch oven over medium-high heat. When the pot is hot, add extra-virgin olive oil and wait for 30 seconds.

2 Add chicken thighs and brown for 2 to 3 minutes per side. Remove from the pot and set aside.

3 Add 2 tablespoons unsalted butter to the hot pot. When melted, add yellow onion, garlic, and celery. Sauté, stirring occasionally, for 4 to 5 minutes, or until softened and fragrant.

4 Add remaining 6 tablespoons unsalted butter, green bell pepper, tomato paste, and Worcestershire sauce. Stir to combine.

5 Pour chicken broth into the pot. Stir, scraping up any browned bits from the bottom.

6 Add browned chicken, Cajun spice blend, and okra. Reduce heat to medium-low and simmer, uncovered, for 20 minutes.

7 While soup simmers, place cauliflower florets into a food processor. Pulse for 30 seconds, or until a ricelike consistency forms. Set aside.

8 Add Andouille sausage, shrimp, and parsley to soup. Cook for an additional 1 to 2 minutes, or until sausage is warmed through and shrimp are bright pink. Season with sea salt (if using).

9 To serve, ladle gumbo into bowls and place ½ cup cauliflower "rice" on top of each bowl.

To make your own flavorful Cajun spice blend, combine 1 tsp. cayenne, 1 tsp. freshly ground black pepper, ½ tsp. white pepper, ½ tsp. ground cumin, and ½ tsp. granulated garlic.

Nutrition per Serving

Fat **66%** Net Carb **8%**
Protein **26%** Ratio **0.9:1**

Calories	Fat	Protein	Total Carbohydrate	Dietary Fiber	Net Carbohydrate
436	32g	28g	12g	3g	9g

Poultry Mains

When it comes to poultry, you may think you're limited to the same boring boneless, skinless chicken breast recipes that are so common to other diets. However, the keto diet allows you to eat a variety of poultry—even beyond the chicken and duck options listed in this chapter. From chicken alfredo to duck confit, these recipes allow you enjoy indulgent poultry-based meals without any guilt.

Prep Time: **10 mins** | Cook Time: **40 mins** | Yield: **9 cups** | Serving Size: **1½ cups**

Ingredients

- 1 lb. (450g) broccoli florets, cut into small florets
- ¼ cup unsalted butter
- 1 lb. (450g) boneless, skinless chicken thighs, diced
- ½ tsp. sea salt
- ¼ tsp. freshly ground black pepper
- 10 medium white button mushrooms, sliced
- 2 garlic cloves
- 1½ cups heavy cream
- 2½ cups sharp cheddar cheese, grated

1. Preheat the oven to 400°F (200°C). Evenly spread broccoli florets on the bottom of 9-inch (23cm) square baking dish.

2. Heat a large skillet over medium-high heat. When the skillet is hot, add 1 tablespoon unsalted butter and chicken thighs. Sprinkle with sea salt and black pepper. Cook, stirring occasionally, for 3 to 4 minutes, or until chicken is browned. Remove from the skillet and place on a plate.

3. Reheat the skillet and add 2 tablespoons unsalted butter. Add white button mushrooms and sauté, stirring frequently, for 3 to 4 minutes, or until mushrooms are lightly browned. Add garlic and sauté for an additional 1 minute. Transfer vegetables to the plate with chicken.

4. Reheat the skillet over medium-high heat. Add remaining 1 tablespoon unsalted butter and wait until melted.

5. Add heavy cream in a slow stream and whisk constantly, scraping up any browned bits from the bottom of the skillet. Simmer for 2 minutes.

6. Add 1½ cups sharp cheddar cheese and continue to whisk until mixture thickens, or about 1 to 2 minutes. Pour mixture evenly into the baking dish over broccoli.

7. Transfer chicken and mushrooms and spread evenly over broccoli and cheese sauce.

8. Sprinkle remaining 1 cup sharp cheddar cheese over top and bake for 15 to 20 minutes, or until chicken is cooked through and cheese is browned and bubbly. Let sit for 5 minutes before serving.

> Add black olives, sliced kielbasa, or even a dash of hot pepper sauce to this versatile casserole to mix it up.

Nutrition per Serving

Fat **74%** Net Carb **5%**
Protein **21%** Ratio **1.2:1**

Calories **392**
Fat **32g**
Protein **21g**
Total Carbohydrate **7g**
Dietary Fiber **2g**
Net Carbohydrate **5g**

This classic—chock-full of broccoli, mushrooms, and a rich sharp cheddar cheese sauce—gets a ketogenic makeover.

Cheesy Chicken Broccoli Casserole

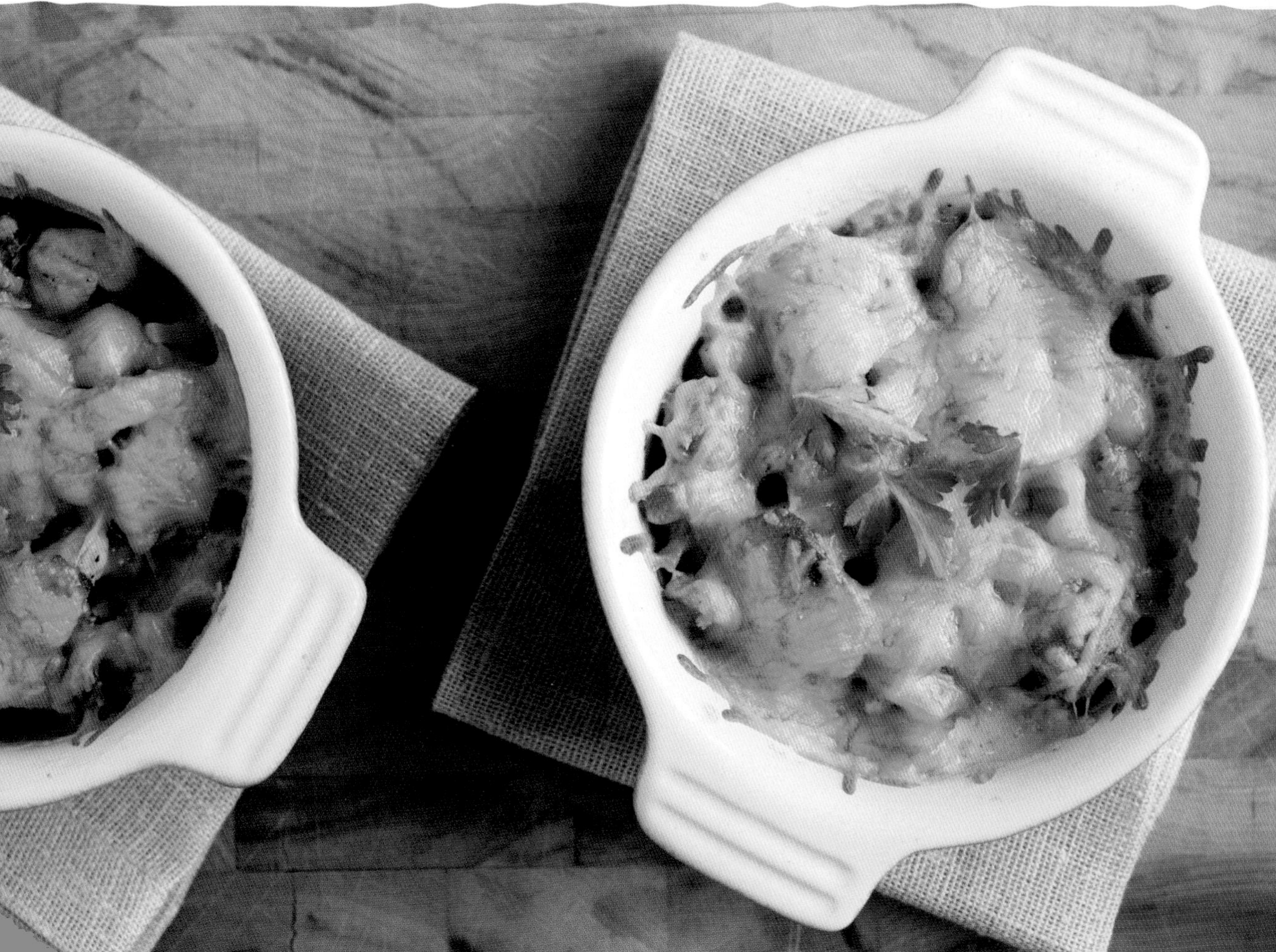

Duck breast is pan-roasted to perfection and drizzled in a golden brown butter sauce with sage.

Duck Breast with Brown Butter and Sage

Prep Time: 5 mins
Cook Time: 20 mins

Yield: 1 breast
Serving Size: ½ breast

Ingredients

1 (6-oz.; 170g) skin-on duck breast

¼ tsp. sea salt, or to taste

⅛ tsp. freshly ground black pepper

1 small head radicchio (about 4 oz.; 110g), core removed

¼ cup unsalted butter

6 fresh sage leaves, finely sliced

Nutrition per Serving

Fat 76% | Net Carb 2%
Protein 22% | Ratio 1.4:1

Calories 393
Fat 33g
Protein 22g
Total Carbohydrate 3g
Dietary Fiber 1g
Net Carbohydrate 2g

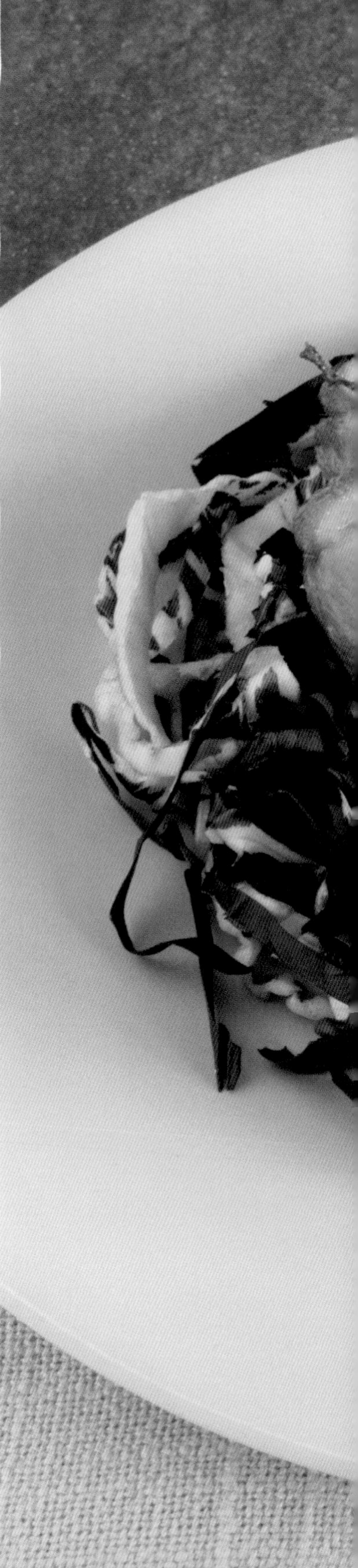

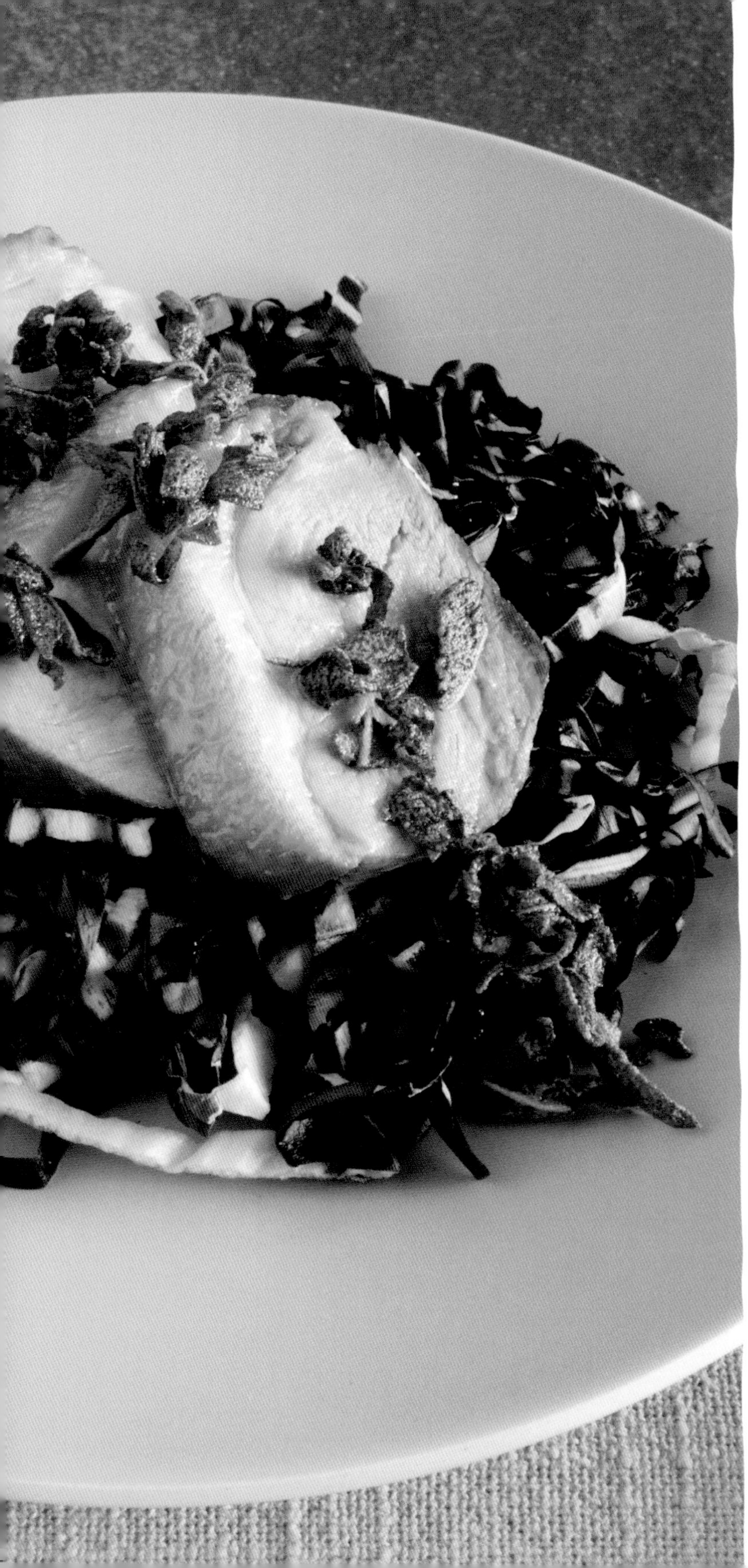

1. Preheat the oven to 400°F (200°C). Pat duck breast skin dry with a paper towel. Season both sides of duck breast with sea salt and black pepper.

2. Heat an ovenproof skillet over high heat. When hot, place duck breast in the skillet, fat side down. Sear for 3 to 4 minutes, or until fat turns deep brown.

3. Turn duck breast over and place the skillet in the oven. Roast, uncovered, for 9 to 11 minutes, or until desired internal temperature is reached.

4. While duck breast cooks, cut radicchio in half. Remove and discard woody white core and thinly slice leaves. Set aside.

5. Remove the skillet from the oven. Transfer duck breast, fat side up, to a cutting board to rest for 5 minutes.

6. Reheat the skillet over medium heat. Add unsalted butter and sage, and cook, stirring constantly, for 3 to 4 minutes, or until butter is a deep golden brown. Remove from heat.

7. After duck has finished resting, cut into 6 equal slices.

8. Divide radicchio onto 2 plates. Top with slices of duck breast and drizzle with browned butter and sage sauce to serve.

Velvety alfredo sauce, accentuated with a pinch of nutmeg, smothers pan-fried chicken thighs and bright broccolini.

Chicken Alfredo with Broccolini

Prep Time: **5 mins** Cook Time: **25 mins** Yield: **3 cups** Serving Size: **1½ cups**

Ingredients

- ½ lb. (225g) broccolini, ends trimmed
- 3 TB. unsalted butter
- 6 oz. (170g) boneless, skinless chicken thighs
- 1 cup heavy cream
- ¼ tsp. freshly ground black pepper
- ⅛ tsp. nutmeg
- ¾ cup grated Parmesan

1 Bring a medium saucepan of water to a boil over high heat. Add broccolini and boil for 2 minutes, or until bright green and fork tender. Immediately plunge broccolini into cold water to stop cooking. Set aside.

2 Heat a medium skillet over medium-high heat. When the skillet is hot, add 1 teaspoon unsalted butter.

3 Add chicken thighs to the hot skillet and cook for 4 to 5 minutes per side, or until browned and cooked through. Transfer chicken to a cutting board and cut into ½-inch (1.25cm) slices. Set aside.

4 Reheat the saucepan over medium heat. Add remaining 2 tablespoons and 2 teaspoons butter. When butter melts, whisk in heavy cream, black pepper, and nutmeg. Bring to a light simmer and cook for 2 minutes.

5 Whisk Parmesan into cream to thicken. Add sliced chicken and broccolini, and toss in the warm pan to fully coat. Serve immediately.

Broccolini is similar to broccoli, but has longer, thinner stalks and a milder flavor. But if you can't find it, use broccoli florets.

Nutrition per Serving

Fat **80%** Net Carb **5%**
Protein **15%** Ratio **1.8:1**

Calories **834**
Fat **74g**
Protein **32g**
Total Carbohydrate **14g**
Dietary Fiber **4g**
Net Carbohydrate **10g**

Crispy almond-crusted chicken breast rolls are filled with a delicious lemon, garlic, and tarragon butter.

Chicken Kiev

Prep Time: **3 hrs, 15 mins** Cook Time: **45 mins** Yield: **2 breasts** Serving Size: **½ breast**

Ingredients

- 8 TB. unsalted butter, at room temperature
- ½ tsp. sea salt
- ¼ tsp. freshly ground black pepper
- ½ tsp. granulated garlic
- 2 TB. fresh tarragon, chopped
- 1 tsp. fresh lemon zest
- 2 boneless, skinless chicken breasts
- 1 large egg, beaten
- 1 cup almond flour
- ¼ cup sunflower oil

1. In a small bowl, combine unsalted butter, sea salt, black pepper, granulated garlic, tarragon, and lemon zest.
2. Using a meat tenderizer, gently flatten both chicken breasts to ¼ inch (.5cm) thickness. (You may want to lay plastic wrap above and below chicken breasts before pounding.)
3. Spread butter mixture over one side of each chicken breast. Gently roll chicken into a tight log. Slice each log in half, and secure ends with toothpicks. Refrigerate for 3 hours.
4. Preheat the oven to 425°F (220°C). Dip rolled chicken in egg, and then cover in almond flour.
5. Heat a medium oven-proof skillet over medium-high heat. Add sunflower oil.
6. When oil is hot and shimmering, place chicken in the skillet. Brown for 3 to 4 minutes on each side.
7. Remove toothpicks and bake for 30 to 35 minutes, or until chicken is cooked through. Serve immediately.

Fresh tarragon has an unmistakable licorice-like flavor. If you don't care for black licorice, use chopped fresh parsley instead.

Nutrition per Serving

Fat **83%** Net Carb **3%**
Protein **14%** Ratio **2.2:1**

Calories **586**
Fat **54g**
Protein **21g**
Total Carbohydrate **7g**
Dietary Fiber **3g**
Net Carbohydrate **4g**

Yogurt and spice–marinated chicken thighs are blackened and simmered in a vibrant tomato and cream curry.

Chicken Tikka Masala

Prep Time: **1 day, 15 mins**
Cook Time: **50 mins**
Yield: **8 cups**
Serving Size: **2 cups**

Ingredients

- 4 garlic cloves, minced
- 2 TB. fresh ginger root, grated
- ⅓ cup plain whole-milk yogurt
- 3 TB. Curry Spice Mixture
- 1 lb. (450g) skinless, boneless chicken thighs, cut into large pieces
- 5 TB. unsalted butter
- 2 TB. minced shallot
- 2 TB. tomato paste
- 2 serrano peppers, seeded and minced
- 1 cup canned diced tomatoes, with juice
- 2 cups heavy cream
- 1 cup chicken broth
- 1 tsp. sea salt
- 3 cups cauliflower florets
- ½ cup fresh cilantro, chopped

Nutrition per Serving

Fat **75%** Net Carb **8%**
Protein **17%** Ratio **1.3:1**

Calories **768**
Fat **64g**
Protein **33g**
Total Carbohydrate **20g**
Dietary Fiber **5g**
Net Carbohydrate **15g**

To make Curry Spice Mixture, combine 4 tsp. garam masala, 2 tsp. turmeric, 1 tsp. ground coriander, 1 tsp. ground cumin, and 1 tsp. ground cardamom.

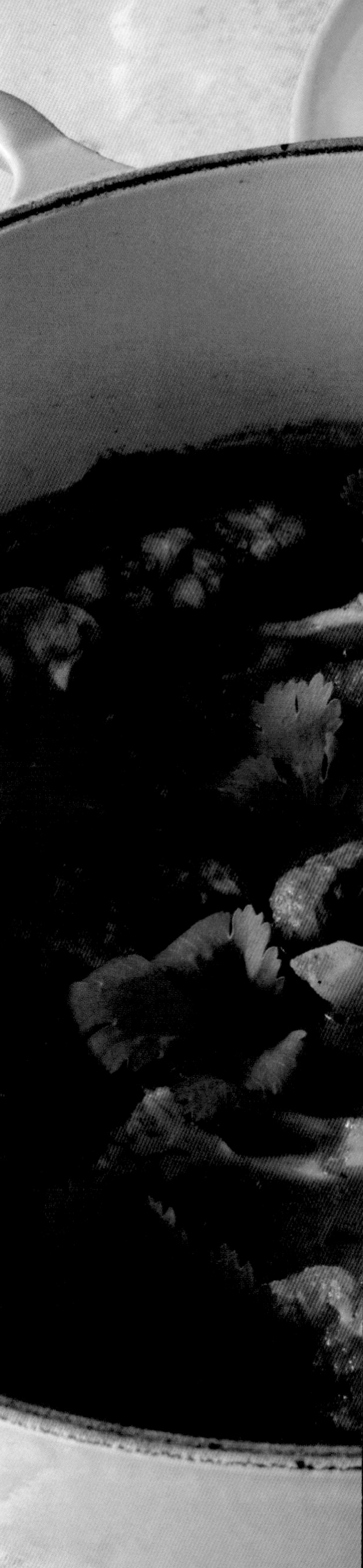

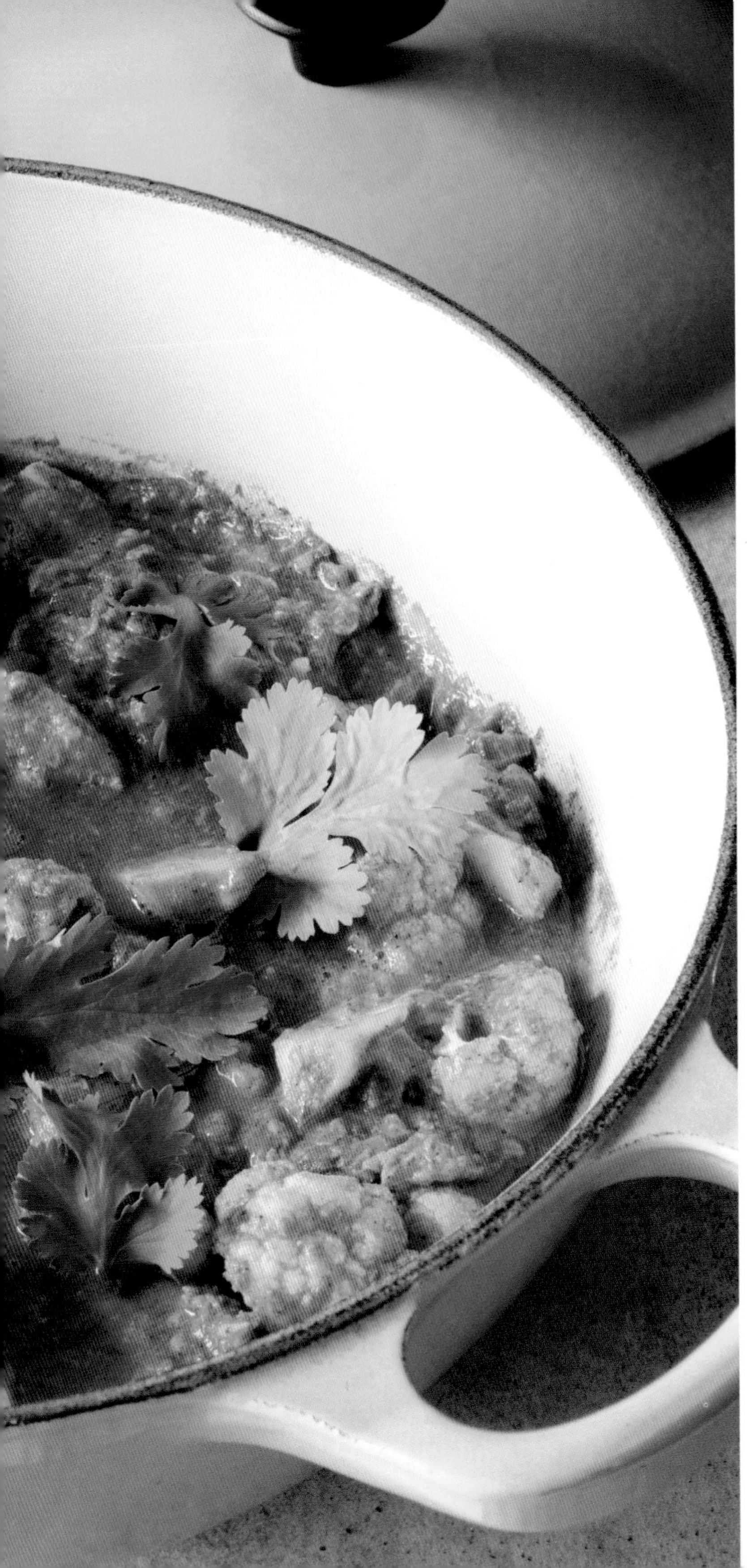

1. Combine 2 garlic cloves, 1 tablespoon ginger root, yogurt, and 1½ tablespoons Curry Spice Mixture in a resealable plastic bag. Add chicken, seal the bag, and gently massage contents to mix. Refrigerate for 12 to 24 hours.

2. Heat a Dutch oven over medium heat. Add unsalted butter and stir until melted.

3. Add remaining 2 garlic cloves, shallot, remaining 1 tablespoon ginger root, tomato paste, and serrano peppers. Cook, stirring frequently, for 3 to 5 minutes, or until shallot softens. Add remaining 1½ tablespoons Curry Spice Mixture and cook for 1 minute, or until fragrant.

4. Add tomatoes, scraping up any browned bits from the bottom. Add heavy cream, chicken broth, and sea salt and bring to a simmer. Cover and simmer for 15 minutes.

5. Meanwhile, arrange the oven rack to the highest position. Preheat the broiler on high.

6. Scrape yogurt mixture off chicken pieces and discard mixture. Arrange chicken on a wire rack over a rimmed baking sheet. Broil for 8 to 12 minutes, or until lightly blackened on top.

7. Add chicken and cauliflower florets to sauce. Cover and simmer for 10 to 15 minutes, or until chicken is cooked and cauliflower is tender. Sprinkle with fresh cilantro to serve.

Duck quarters are marinated in garlic, bay leaves, and orange zest, and slow cooked in fat until crisped and tender.

Duck Confit

Prep Time: 1 day, 15 mins | Cook Time: 3 hrs | Yield: 2 legs | Serving Size: ½ leg

Ingredients

- 2 whole duck legs, cut into thighs and drumsticks (about 1 lb.; 450g)
- 2 bay leaves
- 2 garlic cloves, halved
- 1 tsp. fresh orange zest
- ½ tsp. freshly ground black pepper
- ½ cup extra-virgin olive oil
- 1 tsp. sea salt
- 6 cups chopped frisée
- 2 TB. balsamic vinegar

1 Place duck legs and thighs in a small baking dish. Make sure the dish is as small as possible to fit duck in one layer, tightly packed in the bottom.

2 Tuck bay leaves and garlic clove halves around duck. Sprinkle with orange zest and black pepper, and drizzle with extra-virgin olive oil. Cover and refrigerate for 1 day.

3 Preheat the oven to 350°F (180°C). Sprinkle duck with sea salt. Bake for 3 hours, basting every 30 minutes, until duck is cooked through and tender.

4 Remove finished duck from the baking dish and set aside. Carefully pour hot fat into a heatproof container and reserve.

5 In a medium bowl, toss frisée with balsamic vinegar and ¼ cup of reserved fat. Serve alongside duck quarters.

Traditional duck confit is a laborious task using all parts of the duck. This modified version requires much less hands-on prep.

Nutrition per Serving

Fat 83% | Net Carb 2%
Protein 15% | Ratio 2.1:1

Calories	Fat	Protein	Total Carbohydrate	Dietary Fiber	Net Carbohydrate
348	32g	13g	5g	3g	2g

Chicken, sour cream, and green chilies sit atop roasted leeks, and are covered in enchilada sauce and cheese.

Chicken Enchilada Casserole

Prep Time: **20 mins** | Cook Time: **50 mins** | Yield: **1 casserole** | Serving Size: **⅛ casserole**

Ingredients

- 2 large leeks, trimmed to 6-in. (15.25cm) stalks
- 2 TB. extra-virgin olive oil
- 1 lb. (450g) skinless, boneless chicken thighs
- 4 TB. unsalted butter
- 2 TB. chili powder
- 1 tsp. ground cumin
- 1 tsp. granulated garlic
- 1 tsp. dried oregano
- 1 tsp. sea salt
- 1 cup chicken broth
- 1 TB. arrowroot powder, mixed with 2 TB. cold water
- 1½ cups sour cream
- 1 (4-oz.; 110g) can diced green chilies, drained (optional)
- 1 (8-oz.; 225g) can sliced black olives, drained
- 2 cups grated Monterey Jack cheese
- ½ cup fresh cilantro, chopped

1. Preheat the oven to 425°F (220°C). Cut leeks in half lengthwise. Rinse halves under cold water to remove any dirt.

2. Place leeks in a layer at the bottom of a 9×13-inch (23×33cm) casserole pan. Drizzle with extra-virgin olive oil and rub to coat. Place chicken thighs on top of leeks and bake for 15 to 20 minutes, or until cooked through.

3. Heat a medium saucepan over medium-high heat. Add butter. When butter melts, whisk in chili powder, cumin, garlic, oregano, and sea salt until fragrant. Whisk in chicken stock and bring to a simmer.

4. Drizzle in arrowroot mixture while whisking stock. Simmer for 1 minute, or until thickened. Remove from heat.

5. When chicken thighs are fully cooked, remove from the pan and shred using 2 forks.

6. Combine shredded chicken with sour cream and green chilies (if using) and mix well.

7. Spread shredded chicken mixture evenly over roasted leeks. Cover with black olives. Pour sauce over casserole and sprinkle with Monterey Jack cheese.

8. Reduce the oven temperature to 350°F (180°C) and bake casserole for 20 to 25 minutes, or until cheese is brown and bubbly.

9. Let casserole sit for 10 minutes before slicing and scooping into bowls. Sprinkle with cilantro to serve.

Nutrition per Serving

Fat **71%** Net Carb **9%**
Protein **20%** Ratio **1.1:1**

Calories	Fat	Protein	Total Carbohydrate	Dietary Fiber	Net Carbohydrate
391	31g	19g	11g	2g	9g

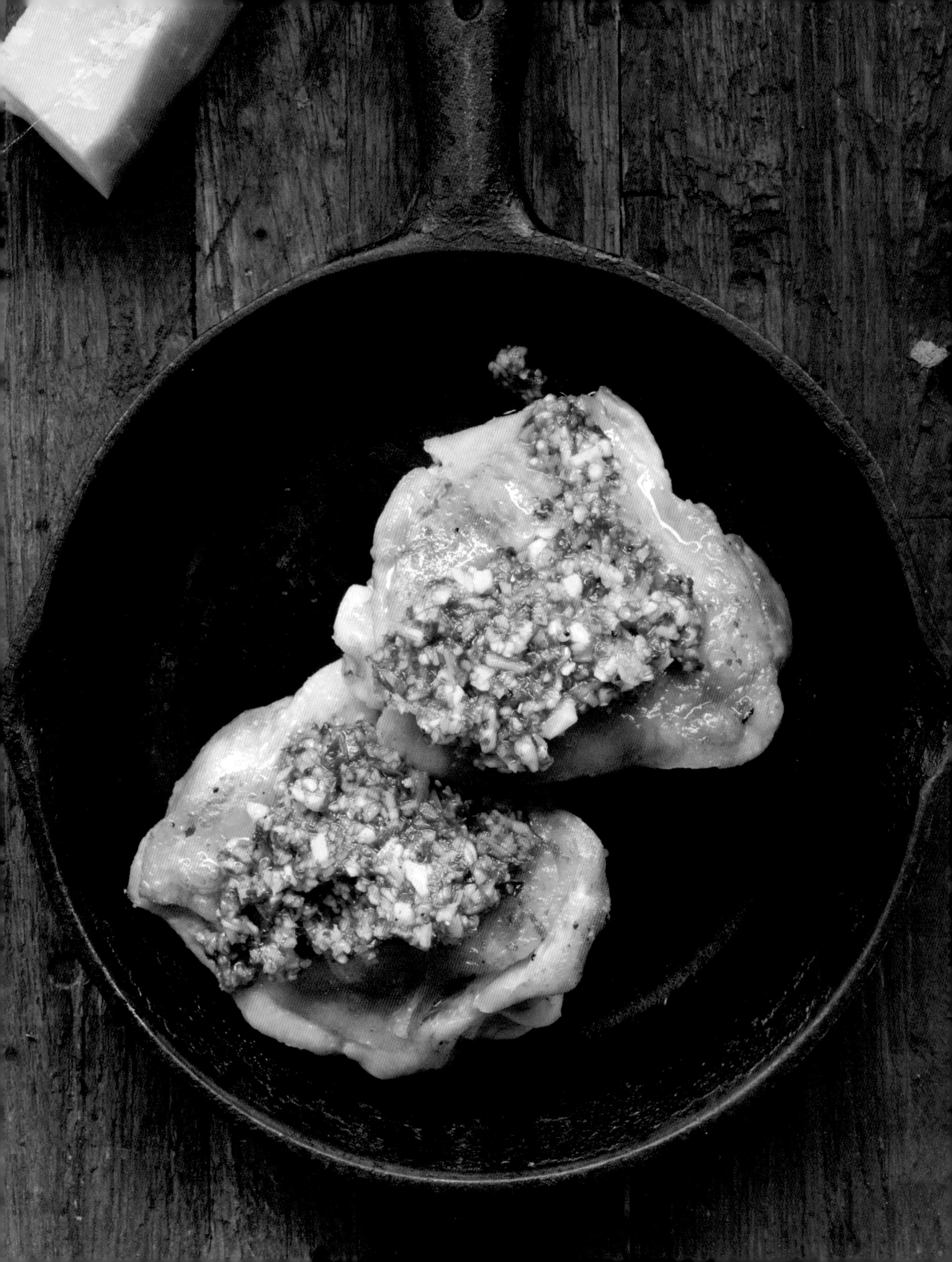

Whole chicken thighs are perfectly roasted until the skin is crisp and golden, and then coated in a tasty pesto sauce.

Roasted Chicken Thighs with Pesto

Prep Time: **10 mins** | Cook Time: **35 mins** | Yield: **4 thighs** | Serving Size: **1 thigh**

Ingredients

- 4 (4 oz.; 110g each) skin-on, bone-in chicken thighs
- ½ cup plus 1 TB. extra-virgin olive oil
- ½ tsp. sea salt
- ¼ tsp. freshly ground black pepper
- 1½ cups fresh basil leaves
- 2 garlic cloves
- 1 TB. lemon juice
- ¼ cup pine nuts
- ¼ cup grated Parmesan

1 Preheat the oven to 375°F (190°C). Coat chicken thighs with 1 tablespoon extra-virgin olive oil and sprinkle with sea salt and black pepper.

2 Place chicken thighs, skin side down, on a rimmed metal baking sheet (or use a large cast-iron pan). Bake for 20 minutes.

3 While chicken bakes, place basil, garlic, lemon juice, pine nuts, Parmesan, and remaining ½ cup extra-virgin olive oil in a food processor. Pulse for 1 to 2 minutes, or until a smooth paste forms. Add additional olive oil, if needed. Taste and season with additional sea salt or lemon juice, if desired.

4 After 20 minutes, remove chicken from the oven. Turn chicken and bake for an additional 10 to 15 minutes, or until chicken is cooked through and skin is crisp. Top with pesto and serve.

> Marinate chicken in ¼ cup olive oil, 1 tsp. oregano, 1 tsp. lemon zest, and 1 minced garlic for up to one day for extra flavor.

Nutrition per Serving

Fat **83%** Net Carb **1%**
Protein **16%** Ratio **2.2:1**

Calories	Fat	Protein	Total Carbohydrate	Dietary Fiber	Net Carbohydrate
445	41g	18g	2g	1g	1g

Beef Mains

Because saturated fat has been demonized for years, red meat—with its high saturated fat content—has received a lot of negative attention. The truth is, saturated fats are important for maintaining proper bone density, a healthy immune system, and normal testosterone levels. So from burgers to stroganoff, you can savor the rich, flavorful recipes in this chapter while also benefitting your health.

Prep Time: **10 mins** | Cook Time: **25 mins** | Yield: **8 oz. (225g)** | Serving Size: **4 oz. (110g)**

Ingredients

- 2 TB. whole black peppercorns
- 8 oz. (225g) boneless rib-eye steak, cut in half lengthwise
- 2 tsp. sunflower oil
- 2 TB. unsalted butter
- 1 small shallot, minced
- ¼ cup cognac or brandy
- ½ cup beef broth
- ½ tsp. sea salt
- 1 tsp. fresh thyme
- ½ cup heavy cream

Nutrition per Serving

Fat **83%** Net Carb **3%**
Protein **14%** Ratio **2.1:1**

Calories **65**
Fat **60g**
Protein **23g**
Total Carbohydrate **7g**
Dietary Fiber **2g**
Net Carbohydrate **5g**

1 Place whole peppercorns in a resealable plastic bag. Close the bag and place on a sturdy cutting board. Use a meat tenderizer or the back of a heavy metal spoon to crack peppercorns into coarse pieces.

2 Transfer cracked peppercorns to a plate. Press rib-eye halves into peppercorns to fully coat. Turn over rib-eyes and repeat to coat both sides.

3 Heat a medium cast-iron pan over medium-high heat. When the pan is hot, add sunflower oil and wait for 15 seconds.

4 Add rib-eyes to the pan. Cook for 3 to 6 minutes, or until a browned crust has formed. Turn over rib-eyes and cook for an additional 2 to 4 minutes, or until cooked as desired. Remove rib-eyes to a cutting board to rest.

5 Reheat the pan over medium-high heat. Add unsalted butter and shallot and cook for 2 to 3 minutes, or until lightly browned.

6 Carefully pour cognac into the pan to deglaze, scraping up any browned bits from the bottom.

7 Add beef broth, sea salt, thyme, and heavy cream and bring to a simmer. Stirring constantly, simmer for 7 to 10 minutes, or until reduced by half.

8 Remove from heat and season with more sea salt, if desired. Pour sauce over steaks to serve.

Variation: To dress this recipe up a bit more, you can add 2 ounces (55g) blue cheese crumbles along with heavy cream, and replace thyme with 1 tablespoon chopped fresh dill to make **Steak with Cognac Blue Cheese Sauce.**

Take care when adding any alcoholic beverage to a pan at higher heat. The alcohol could ignite and quickly burn out.

Mouthwatering rib-eye steaks are covered with an indulgent creamy cognac and black pepper sauce.

Steak Au Poivre

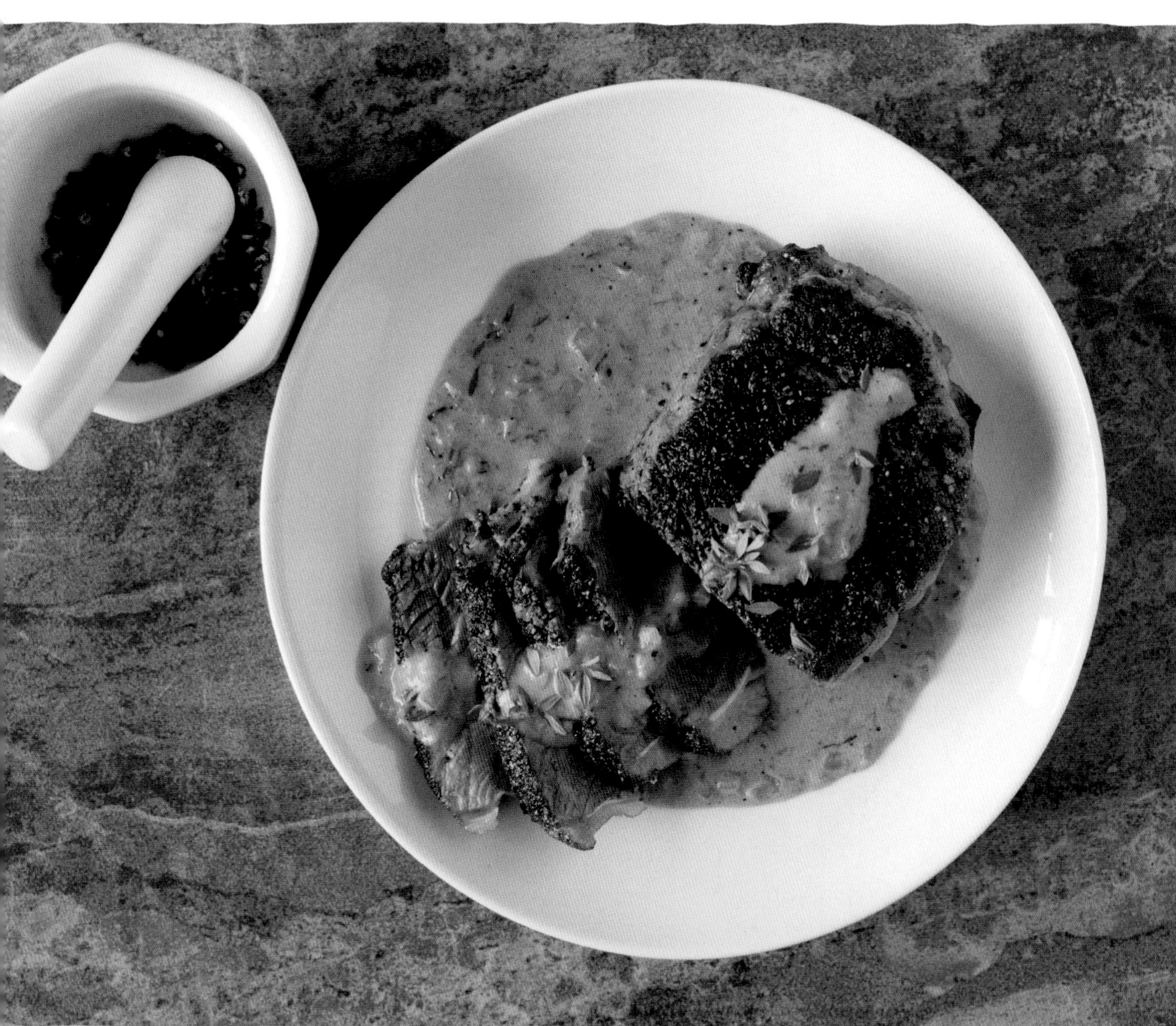

Beef patties—piled high with creamy Brie, crisp bacon, and fresh arugula—are sandwiched between portobello caps.

Bacon Brie Burger

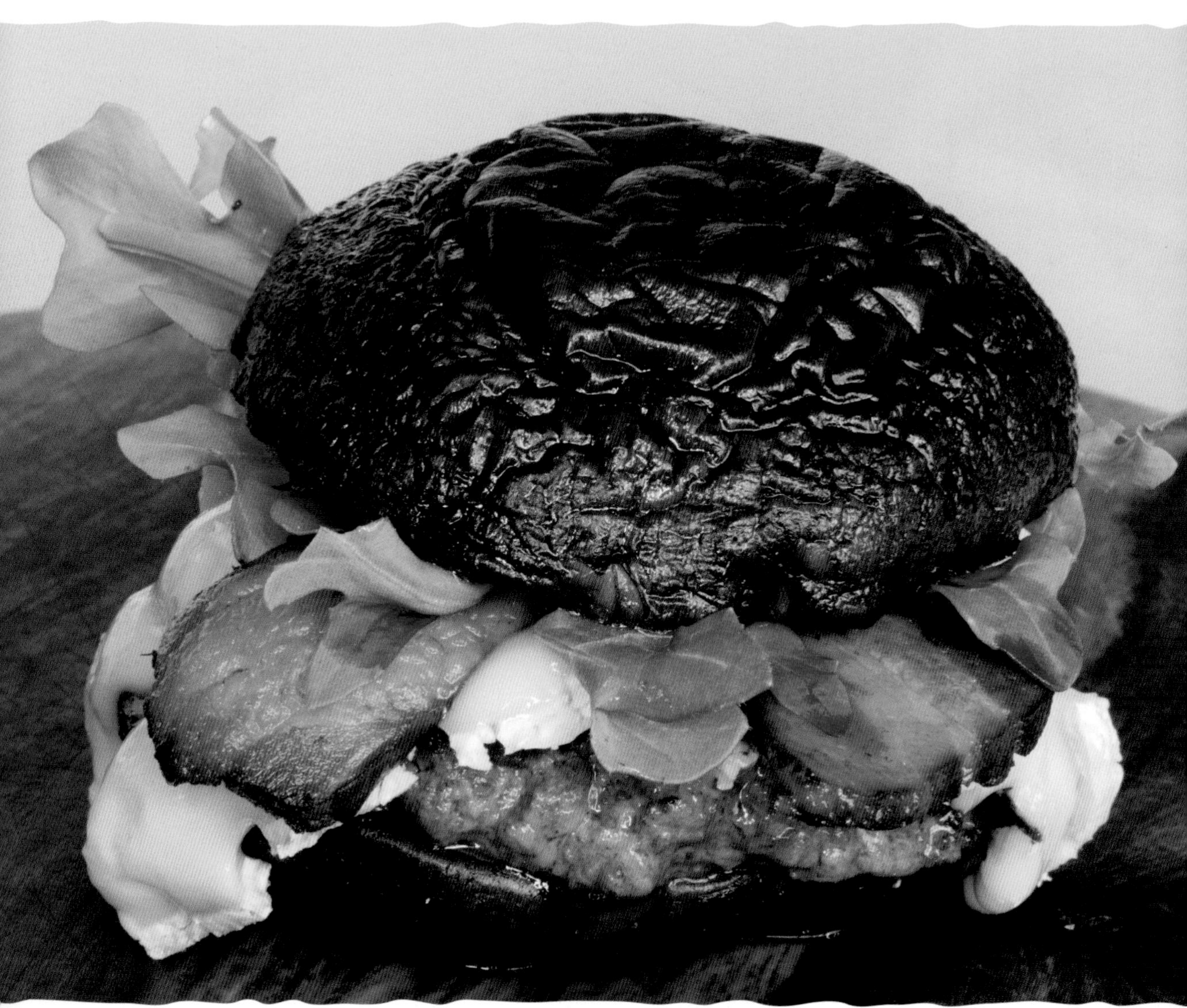

Prep Time: **5 mins** | Cook Time: **20 mins** | Yield: **2 burgers** | Serving Size: **1 burger**

Ingredients

⅓ lb. (170g) ground beef

2 oz. (55g) uncured bacon slices, cut in half lengthwise

¼ cup extra-virgin olive oil

4 large portobello mushroom caps, stems and gills removed

2 oz. (55g) double- or triple-cream Brie, cut into 4 slices

1 cup baby arugula

1 Form beef into 2 equal-size patties that are as thin as possible. Set aside.

2 Heat a medium skillet over medium heat. Add uncured bacon to the skillet and cook, turning occasionally, for 4 to 6 minutes or until bacon is crisp. Remove bacon from the skillet and place on a paper towel.

3 Reheat the skillet over medium-high heat. Add extra-virgin olive oil to residual bacon fat. Wait for 30 seconds.

4 Place portobello mushroom caps, smooth side down, in the skillet. Cook for 2 to 3 minutes, or until lightly browned. Turn caps, and cook for an additional 2 to 3 minutes, occasionally spooning fat over top. Remove from the skillet and place on a paper towel smooth side up.

5 Reheat the skillet over medium-high heat. Place beef patties in the skillet and cook for 3 to 4 minutes, or until browned. Turn patties and place 2 Brie slices on top. Cook for an additional 2 to 3 minutes, or until patties are cooked through.

6 To assemble burgers, place 1 portobello cap on each plate smooth side down. Stack cap with burger patty and bacon slices. Top with arugula and remaining portobello cap smooth side up. Serve immediately.

Variation: To make an **American Bacon Cheeseburger,** replace Brie with 3 ounces (85g) sharp cheddar cheese slices, and use 1 cup thinly sliced iceberg lettuce instead of arugula.

Nutrition per Serving

Fat **73%** Net Carb **3%**
Protein **24%** Ratio **1.2:1**

Calories	Fat	Protein	Total Carbohydrate	Dietary Fiber	Net Carbohydrate
701	57g	42g	7g	2g	5g

Tender ribeye steaks are pan-fried in clarified butter and drizzled with a creamy gravy made from pan drippings.

Chicken Fried Steak with Pan Gravy

Prep Time: 20 mins | Cook Time: 15 mins | Yield: 6 oz. (170g) | Serving Size: 3 oz. (85g)

Ingredients

- 6 oz. (170g) rib-eye steak
- ¼ tsp. sea salt
- ¼ tsp. freshly ground black pepper
- 3 TB. almond meal
- 1 TB. tapioca flour
- 1 large egg, beaten
- 5 TB. ghee
- ¾ cup heavy cream
- 1 TB. cornstarch, mixed with 2 TB. cold water

Nutrition per Serving

Fat	84%	Net Carb	5%
Protein	11%	Ratio	2.3:1

Calories 979
Fat 91g
Protein 28g
Total Carbohydrate 14g
Dietary Fiber 2g
Net Carbohydrate 12g

1 Place steak on a sturdy work surface. Using a meat tenderizer, pound steak to ½-inch (1.25cm) thickness.

2 Cut rib-eye steak in half. Season all sides of steak halves with sea salt and black pepper.

3 In a shallow bowl or pie pan, combine almond meal and tapioca flour.

4 Pour egg into a second shallow bowl or pie pan.

5 Dip steak halves into egg, and then coat in almond meal mixture. Set aside.

6 Heat a medium cast-iron pan over medium heat. When the pan is hot, add 2 tablespoons ghee.

7 Place steaks in hot ghee. Cook until deeply browned, about 3 minutes. Turn and repeat on opposite side. Remove steaks from the pan and place on a wire rack to rest for 5 minutes.

8 Meanwhile, reheat the pan over medium-high heat. Add remaining 3 tablespoons ghee and stir, scraping up any browned bits from the bottom of the pan.

9 Add heavy cream and bring to a light simmer. Reduce heat to low.

10 Whisk in cornstarch and water mixture and simmer for an additional 1 minute, or until thickened. Drizzle steaks with pan gravy to serve.

Fall-off-the-bone beef short ribs are slow cooked with red wine, a fragrant herb bundle, pearl onions, and mushrooms.

Short Rib Beef Burgundy

Prep Time: **10 mins** Cook Time: **3 hrs** Yield: **16 short ribs** Serving Size: **2 short ribs**

Ingredients

- 6 oz. (170g) thick-cut uncured bacon (about ½ in.; 1.25cm thick), diced
- ½ cup ghee or extra-virgin olive oil
- 2 lb. (1kg) beef short ribs
- 1 tsp. sea salt
- ½ tsp. freshly ground black pepper
- 2 medium carrots, peeled and sliced
- ½ cup diced celery
- 3 garlic cloves, minced
- 2 whole cloves
- 1 cup dry red wine
- 2 cups beef broth
- ½ lb. (225g) pearl onions, peeled, halved, and root ends cut off
- 1 lb. (450g) white button mushrooms, quartered
- 2 bay leaves
- 4 sprigs thyme
- 4 sprigs parsley

1 Preheat the oven to 350°F (180°C). Heat a Dutch oven or covered braising pan over medium-high heat. Add bacon and cook for 4 to 6 minutes, or until crisp. Remove bacon from the Dutch oven and set on a paper towel.

2 Reheat residual bacon fat and 4 tablespoons ghee over medium-high heat.

3 Season short ribs with sea salt and black pepper. Place 4 pieces in the hot Dutch oven and brown on all sides. Remove from the Dutch oven and set aside. Repeat with remaining beef.

4 Reheat the Dutch oven and add remaining 4 tablespoons ghee, carrots, celery, garlic, and cloves. Sauté, stirring occasionally, for 4 to 5 minutes, or until fragrant.

5 Pour dry red wine into the Dutch oven and stir, scraping up any browned bits from the bottom of the Dutch oven.

6 Pour beef broth into the Dutch oven. Add browned short ribs, bacon, pearl onions, and white button mushrooms, and stir gently to evenly distribute in the Dutch oven.

7 Using undyed cooking twine, tie bay leaves, thyme, and parsley together. Tuck into cooking liquid.

8 Cover and bake for 2 hours to 2 hours, 30 minutes, or until beef is tender. Remove herb bundle and cloves before serving.

Nutrition per Serving

Fat **75%** Net Carb **5%**
Protein **20%** Ratio **1.3:1**

Calories	Fat	Protein	Total Carbohydrate	Dietary Fiber	Net Carbohydrate
567	47g	29g	8g	1g	7g

Fall-off-the-bone beef short ribs are braised with fiery Thai chilies, fresh ginger, and luscious coconut cream.

Thai-Style Braised Beef Short Ribs

Prep Time: **15 mins**
Cook Time: **3 hrs, 30 mins**

Yield: **8 cups**
Serving Size: **1⅓ cups**

Ingredients

- 6 TB. peanut or sesame oil
- 2½ lb. (1.1kg) bone-in beef short ribs
- 1 medium yellow onion, diced
- 4 small Thai red chilies, stemmed and halved lengthwise
- 2 cloves garlic, minced
- 1 TB. fresh ginger, minced
- 1 small lime, zested and juiced
- 4 cups beef broth
- 2 TB. high-quality fish sauce
- 1 TB. unseasoned rice wine vinegar
- 1 (14-fl.-oz.; 400ml) can full-fat coconut cream
- 20 fresh green beans, trimmed and sliced (about 2 cups)
- 2 cups cauliflower florets
- ¼ cup fresh basil, chopped

Nutrition per Serving

Fat **75%** Net Carb **8%**
Protein **17%** Ratio **1.3:1**

Calories **602**
Fat **50g**
Protein **26g**
Total Carbohydrate **14g**
Dietary Fiber **2g**
Net Carbohydrate **12g**

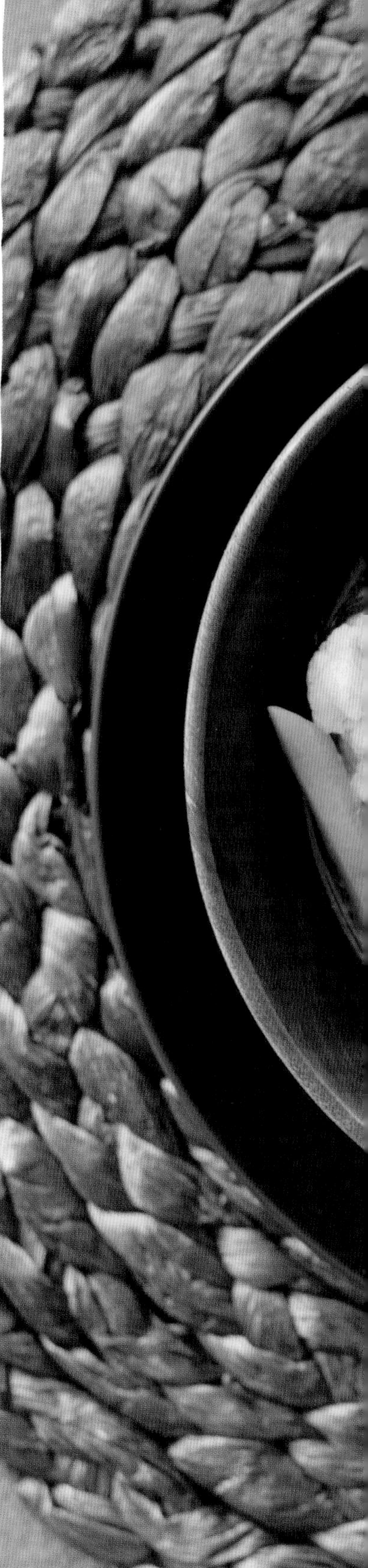

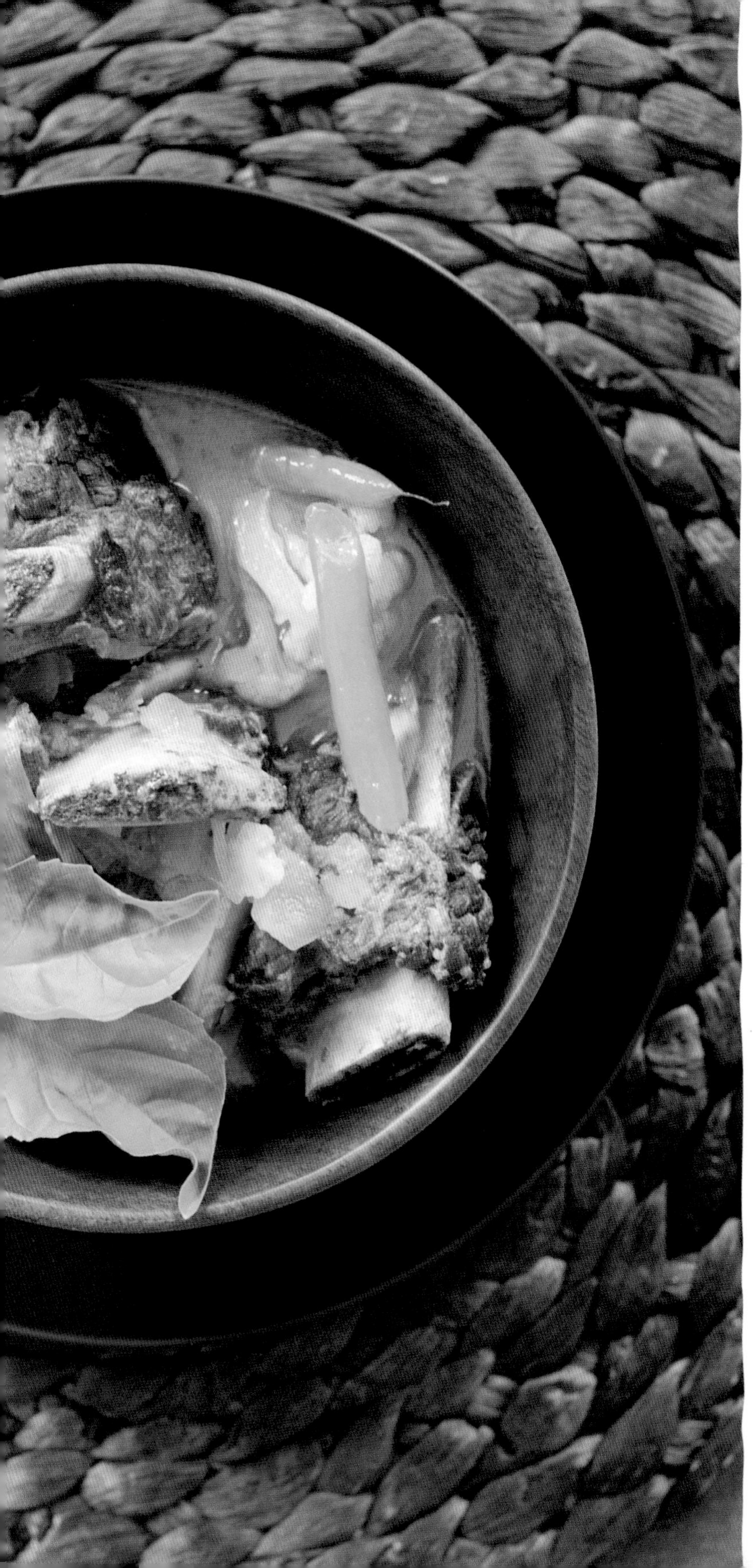

1. Preheat the oven to 350°F (180°C). Heat a large Dutch oven over medium-high heat. Add 2 tablespoons peanut oil and wait for 30 seconds.

2. Cover the bottom of the Dutch oven with half of short ribs and cook for 2 minutes, or until deeply browned. Turn and repeat on the other side. Remove short ribs and set on a plate.

3. Reheat the Dutch oven and add 2 tablespoons peanut oil. Wait for 30 seconds and repeat Step 2 with remaining short ribs.

4. Reheat the Dutch oven and add remaining 2 tablespoons peanut oil. Add yellow onion, Thai red chilies, garlic, ginger, and lime zest. Stirring frequently, cook for 2 to 4 minutes.

5. Pour in beef broth and scrape up any browned bits off the bottom. Add lime juice, fish sauce, and rice wine vinegar. Stir.

6. Return short ribs to the Dutch oven, making sure they're fully submerged. Cover and bake for 2 hours, 30 minutes.

7. Uncover and stir in full-fat coconut cream. Add green beans and cauliflower, cover, and bake for an additional 30 to 45 minutes, or until short ribs are tender and falling off the bones.

8. Serve short ribs with vegetables and broth, and top with fresh basil.

Thinly sliced flank steak is piled high with caramelized onions and peppers on these open-faced sandwiches.

Philly Cheesesteak

Prep Time: **10 mins** Cook Time: **30 mins** Yield: **2 cheesesteaks** Serving Size: **1 cheesesteak**

Ingredients

- 3 TB. mayonnaise
- ½ tsp. granulated garlic
- 1 tsp. Worcestershire sauce
- ¼ cup ghee
- 2 large portobello mushroom caps, stems and gills removed
- ½ tsp. sea salt
- 6 oz. (170g) beef flank steak
- ¼ tsp. freshly ground black pepper
- ½ yellow onion, thinly sliced
- ½ medium green bell pepper, sliced into thin strips
- 2 oz. (55g) provolone, sliced

Nutrition per Serving

Fat **79%** Net Carb **4%**
Protein **17%** Ratio **1.7:1**

Calories **662**
Fat **58g**
Protein **28g**
Total Carbohydrate **9g**
Dietary Fiber **2g**
Net Carbohydrate **7g**

1 In a small bowl, combine mayonnaise, granulated garlic, and Worcestershire sauce. Set aside.

2 Heat a large skillet over medium heat. Add 2 tablespoons ghee and wait until melted.

3 Place portobello mushroom caps, smooth side down, in the skillet. Cook for 2 to 3 minutes, or until lightly browned.

4 Turn caps and cook for an additional 2 to 3 minutes, occasionally spooning ghee over top. Remove caps from the skillet and place on a paper towel smooth side down. Sprinkle with ¼ teaspoon sea salt.

5 Reheat the skillet over medium heat. Add 1 tablespoon ghee.

6 Season beef flank steak with remaining ¼ teaspoon sea salt and black pepper.

7 Place steak in the hot skillet. (It should sizzle.) For medium doneness, cook for 3 to 4 minutes, turn over, and cook for an additional 1 to 2 minutes.

8 Remove steak from the skillet and let rest for 5 minutes before thinly slicing.

9 While steak rests, reheat the skillet over medium heat. When the skillet is hot, add remaining 1 tablespoon ghee.

10 Add yellow onion and green bell pepper, and sauté, stirring occasionally, until softened and well browned, about 7 to 10 minutes.

11 To assemble cheesesteaks, spread mayonnaise mixture on inside of mushroom caps. Top with steak slices, onion and bell pepper mixture, and provolone. Broil on high for 2 to 4 minutes or until cheese is golden brown. Serve immediately.

An opulent mushroom and cream sauce with tender beef is served over sweet golden ribbons of spaghetti squash.

Beef Stroganoff

Prep Time: **10 mins** Cook Time: **35 mins** Yield: **9 cups** Serving Size: **1½ cups**

Ingredients

- 1 small spaghetti squash (about 3 lb.; 1.5kg)
- 1¼ lb. (565g) beef sirloin steak, thinly sliced
- 1 tsp. sea salt
- ½ tsp. freshly ground black pepper
- 6 TB. ghee
- ½ cup yellow onion, diced
- 8 medium white button mushrooms, sliced (about 8 oz.; 225g)
- 2 cups beef broth
- 1 cup heavy cream
- 2 cups sour cream

Nutrition per Serving

Fat **70%** Net Carb **10%**
Protein **20%** Ratio **1.0:1**

Calories **645**
Fat **50g**
Protein **33g**
Total Carbohydrate **19g**
Dietary Fiber **3g**
Net Carbohydrate **16g**

1 Preheat the oven to 375°F (190°C).

2 Cut spaghetti squash in half lengthwise. Remove and discard seeds. Place squash, cut side down, in a baking dish with ½ cup water. Bake for 30 to 35 minutes, or until soft to the touch.

3 Meanwhile, season beef sirloin steak with sea salt and black pepper.

4 Heat a heavy-bottomed skillet or Dutch oven over medium-high heat. When the skillet is hot, add 2 tablespoons ghee.

5 When ghee melts, add beef and brown on all sides, about 4 to 6 minutes. Remove beef from the skillet and set aside.

6 Add remaining 4 tablespoons ghee to the hot skillet. Add yellow onion and white button mushrooms and sauté, stirring occasionally, for 4 to 6 minutes, or until browned and fragrant.

7 Reduce heat to medium. Pour beef broth into the hot skillet and stir, scraping up any browned bits from the bottom of the skillet.

8 Add heavy cream and browned beef to the pan. Simmer for 15 minutes, or until beef is tender.

9 Remove the skillet from heat and stir in sour cream.

10 When spaghetti squash is tender, carefully remove halves from the baking dish (hot steam will escape from underneath). Using a metal fork, loosen and scrape squash strands from shell (about 6 cups total).

11 Spoon beef sauce over spaghetti squash strands to serve.

Prep Time: **20 mins** | Cook Time: **1 hr, 30 mins** | Yield: **1 loaf** | Serving Size: **1/10 loaf**

Ingredients

- ¼ cup pure lard
- ¾ cup yellow onion, diced
- ½ cup celery, diced
- 2 garlic cloves, minced
- 1 TB. Worcestershire sauce
- 1 TB. salt-free Cajun spice blend
- 1 TB. sea salt
- ½ cup evaporated milk
- ½ cup sugar-free catsup or tomato sauce
- 1½ lb. (680g) ground beef
- ½ lb. (225g) ground pork
- 2 large eggs, beaten
- ¼ cup coconut flour
- ½ lb. (225g) thin-sliced bacon (about 15 slices)
- 1 to 2 TB. hot pepper sauce
- 1 cup mayonnaise

Nutrition per Serving

Fat **76%** Net Carb **3%**
Protein **21%** Ratio **1.4:1**

Calories **511**
Fat **43g**
Protein **27g**
Total Carbohydrate **6g**
Dietary Fiber **2g**
Net Carbohydrate **4g**

1 Preheat the oven to 375°F (190°C). Heat a medium skillet over medium-high heat. When the skillet is hot, add lard and let melt.

2 Add yellow onion, celery, garlic, Worcestershire sauce, Cajun spice blend, and sea salt. Sauté, stirring occasionally, for 4 to 5 minutes, or until onion softens and begins to brown.

3 Remove the skillet from heat. Add evaporated milk and catsup and stir until well blended. Transfer onion-spice mixture to a smaller container and put in the freezer to cool for 10 minutes.

4 Using freshly washed hands, combine beef, pork, eggs, onion-spice mixture, and coconut flour in a large bowl and mix gently until blended.

5 Line a 4×10-inch (10×25cm) loaf pan with parchment paper. Transfer mixture to the pan and press sides of meatloaf down around the edges of the pan.

6 Place bacon slices over meatloaf, overlapping slightly, and tuck ends down the sides of the pan. Cover the pan with foil.

7 Place the pan into the oven and bake for 35 minutes. Remove the foil and bake an additional 40 minutes, or until a thermometer inserted into middle of loaf reads 350°F (180°C).

8 Meanwhile, whisk hot pepper sauce, to taste, and mayonnaise in a small bowl. Refrigerate.

9 Let loaf cool for 10 minutes before slicing and serving alongside spicy mayonnaise.

If you'd like to make your own Cajun spice blend, you can find a recipe for it in the sidebar for Gumbo.

This hearty meatloaf with fierce Cajun spices is wrapped in bacon and served with a hot pepper mayonnaise.

Cajun Meatloaf

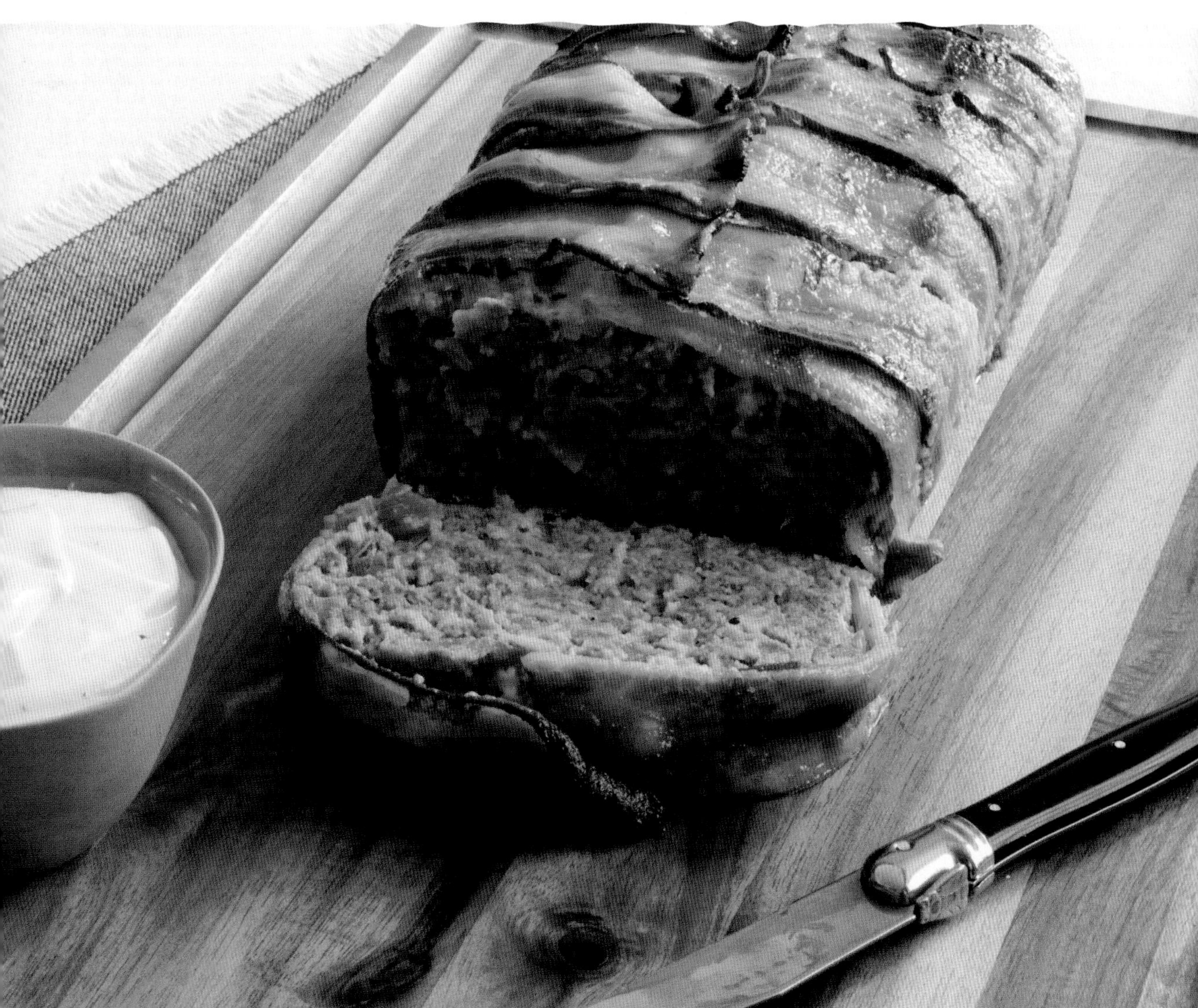

Pork Mains

Bacon, pork chops, and pork belly—they're all delicious and include rich, flavorful fat. This means they're absolutely allowed on a keto diet. From spiced pork belly with ginger and cilantro, to apple and hazelnut-stuffed pork chops, to sausage crust pizza, this chapter offers many fantastically flavorful pork-based recipes that are both incredibly satisfying and 100 percent keto compliant.

Pork belly is slow cooked in fragrant spices until tender and served with a sweet honey pan sauce and crisp slaw.

Spiced Pork Belly with Ginger and Cilantro

Prep Time: **10 mins**
Cook Time: **3 hrs**

Yield: **4 slices**
Serving Size: **1 slice**

Ingredients

- 2 TB. peanut oil
- 1 lb. (450g) boneless pork belly, sliced into 4 equal parts
- ¼ cup yellow onion, diced
- 2 garlic cloves, minced
- 2 tsp. fresh ginger root, grated
- ½ tsp. ground cumin
- 2 TB. raw honey
- 2 TB. tamari
- 1 tsp. fish sauce
- 2 cups chicken broth
- 1 cinnamon stick
- 2 whole star anise
- 2 whole cloves
- 2 Thai chilies, halved
- 2 cups purple cabbage, sliced thin
- 2 medium carrots, grated
- ½ cup fresh cilantro, chopped

Nutrition per Serving

Fat **85%** Protein **7%** Net Carb **8%** Ratio **2.5:1**

Calories **711**
Fat **67g**
Protein **13g**
Total Carbohydrate **16g**
Dietary Fiber **2g**
Net Carbohydrate **14g**

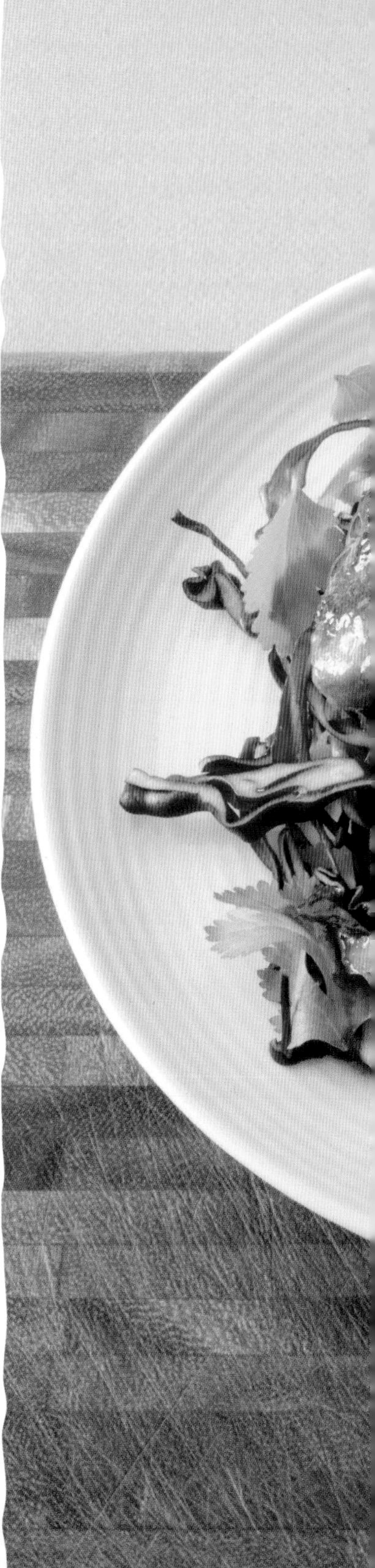

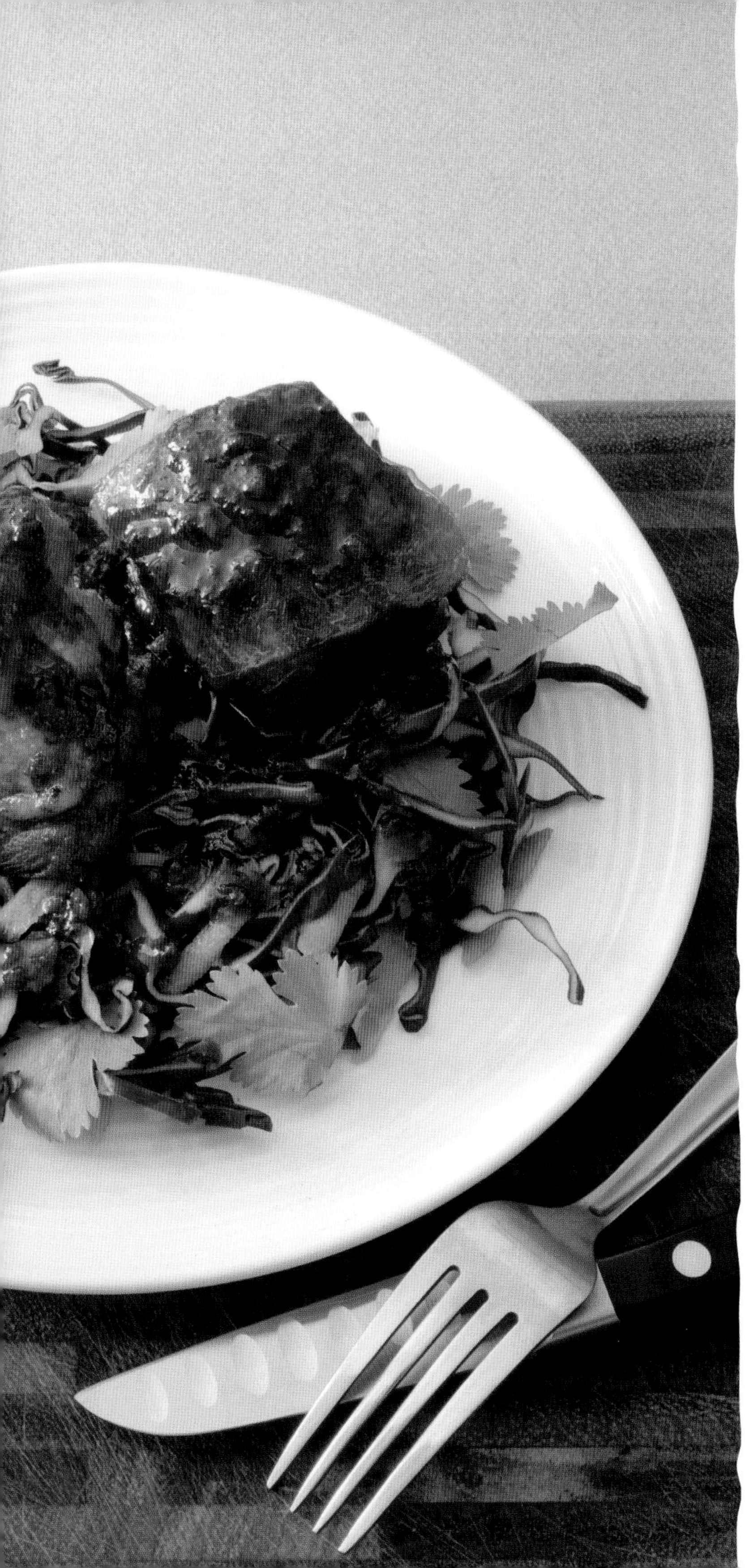

1 Preheat the oven to 250°F (120°C). Heat a Dutch oven or braising pan over medium heat. When hot, add peanut oil and wait for 30 seconds.

2 Place pork belly in hot oil and brown well on all sides, about 2 minutes per side. Remove from the Dutch oven. Add yellow onion, garlic, and ginger root to hot oil and cook, stirring frequently, for 2 to 3 minutes, or until fragrant.

3 Add cumin, raw honey, tamari, and fish sauce and cook for 1 minute, stirring constantly to prevent burning.

4 Pour chicken broth into the Dutch oven and stir, scraping up any browned bits from the bottom of the Dutch oven.

5 Add cinnamon stick, star anise, cloves, Thai chilies, and browned pork belly. Cover and place in the oven for 2 hours to 2 hours, 30 minutes, or until pork is tender. Remove pork from the Dutch oven and set aside.

6 Heat the Dutch oven over high heat on the stovetop to bring remaining juices to a boil. Boil for 15 to 18 minutes, or until reduced by half. Remove and discard star anise, cinnamon stick, and cloves.

7 To serve, toss purple cabbage, carrots, and cilantro together; place pork belly on top; and drizzle with pan sauce.

Slow-cooked pork shoulder is shredded and served in a creamy tomato sauce over thin zucchini ribbons.

Pork Shoulder Ragu

Prep Time: **10 mins** Cook Time: **3 hrs, 15 mins** Yield: **6 cups** Serving Size: **1½ cups**

Ingredients

- 1¼ lb. (565g) pork shoulder or butt roast
- ½ tsp. sea salt
- ½ tsp. freshly ground black pepper
- 4 TB. unsalted butter
- 4 TB. extra-virgin olive oil
- 2 TB. shallots, minced
- 1 garlic clove, minced
- ½ cup dry red wine
- ½ cup diced tomatoes, with juice
- 2 cups beef broth
- ½ tsp. fennel seeds
- ½ tsp. thyme or 5 sprigs fresh thyme
- ¼ tsp. crushed red pepper flakes
- 3 medium zucchini, trimmed
- ¼ cup shaved Parmesan

1 Preheat the oven to 325°F (170°C). Sprinkle pork roast on all sides with sea salt and black pepper.

2 Heat a large Dutch oven over medium-high heat. When hot, add 2 tablespoons unsalted butter and 2 tablespoons extra-virgin olive oil.

3 Place roast in hot oil. Brown on all sides, about 5 to 8 minutes. Remove roast from the Dutch oven and set aside.

4 Reheat the Dutch oven over medium-high heat. Add remaining 2 tablespoons butter and remaining 2 tablespoons olive oil.

5 Add shallots and sauté, stirring occasionally, for 1 to 2 minutes, or until slightly translucent. Add garlic and cook for an additional 1 minute.

6 Add dry red wine, scraping up any browned bits off the bottom of the Dutch oven. Add tomatoes, beef broth, fennel seeds, thyme, and crushed red pepper flakes and stir.

7 Place browned roast back into the Dutch oven. Cover, place in the oven, and braise for 2 to 3 hours, or until roast is tender enough to fall apart.

8 While roast braises, use a vegetable peeler to make long strips or ribbons of zucchini. Refrigerate.

9 Remove roast from the oven. Using 2 forks, shred roast into small pieces. Stir shredded pork back into sauce formed in the Dutch oven.

10 Stir zucchini ribbons into sauce to warm through. Top with Parmesan to serve.

Nutrition per Serving

Fat **72%** Net Carb **5%**
Protein **23%** Ratio **1.2:1**

Calories	Fat	Protein	Total Carbohydrate	Dietary Fiber	Net Carbohydrate
561	45g	32g	9g	2g	7g

Layers of fresh vegetables, seasoned sausage, and a creamy Alfredo sauce make this low-carb lasagna worth the effort.

Spinach Alfredo Lasagna

Prep Time: **25 mins** Cook Time: **1 hr, 15 mins** Yield: **1 lasagna** Serving Size: **1⁄12 lasagna**

Ingredients

- 1¼ lb. (565g) ground mild Italian sausage
- 5 TB. unsalted butter
- 1½ cups heavy cream
- ½ tsp. ground cardamom
- ½ tsp. white pepper
- 1½ cups grated Parmesan
- 2 TB. extra-virgin olive oil
- 10 medium mushrooms, diced
- 3 garlic cloves, minced
- 3 medium zucchini
- 30 oz. (850g) ricotta, divided into 2 equal portions
- 2 medium carrots, grated
- 2½ cups shredded provolone
- 1 (10-oz.; 285g) pkg. frozen spinach, thawed and squeezed to remove liquid
- ½ cup chopped fresh basil

1 Preheat the oven to 350°F (180°C). Heat a large skillet over medium-high heat. When hot, add sausage and cook for 5 to 7 minutes, or until crumbled and cooked through. Remove sausage and set aside.

2 Reheat the skillet over medium heat. Add unsalted butter to the hot skillet. When butter is melted, add heavy cream, cardamom, and white pepper, and bring to a simmer. Simmer for 3 minutes. Whisk in Parmesan and simmer for 2 to 3 minutes, or until thickened.

3 Heat a large saucepan over medium-high heat. When hot, add extra-virgin olive oil and wait for 30 seconds. Add mushrooms and garlic and sauté, stirring occasionally, for 4 to 6 minutes, or until mushrooms soften and garlic is fragrant. Set aside.

4 Trim zucchini. Cut lengthwise into thin slices. (Alternately, use a mandolin for even slices.)

5 Line a 9×13-in. (22×33cm) casserole dish with an even layer of zucchini slices. Top with half of ricotta, half of sausage, carrots, ¾ cup Alfredo sauce, and 1 cup provolone.

6 Add another layer of zucchini slices, remaining ricotta, spinach, remaining sausage, mushrooms, remaining Alfredo sauce, basil, and remaining provolone.

7 Bake, uncovered, for 45 to 50 minutes, or until vegetables are tender and cheese is golden and bubbly. Let cool 15 minutes before slicing and serving.

Nutrition per Serving

Fat **75%** Net Carb **5%**
Protein **20%** Ratio **1.4:1**

Calories	Fat	Protein	Total Carbohydrate	Dietary Fiber	Net Carbohydrate
585	49g	29g	9g	2g	7g

Succulent boneless pork loin is rolled in a crackling crust of golden pork belly, rubbed with garlic, rosemary, and sage.

Porchetta Roast

Prep Time: **30 mins** Cook Time: **3 hrs, 30 mins** Yield: **1 roast** Serving Size: **1⁄16 roast**

Ingredients

- 4 garlic cloves, minced
- 4 TB. fresh rosemary, minced
- 4 TB. fresh sage, minced
- ¼ cup extra-virgin olive oil
- 4 tsp. sea salt
- 2 tsp. freshly ground black pepper
- 4 lb. (2kg) pork belly
- 2 lb. (1kg) boneless pork loin

Nutrition per Serving

Fat **86%** Net Carb **1%**
Protein **13%** Ratio **2.7:1**

Calories **681**
Fat **65g**
Protein **23g**
Total Carbohydrate **1g**
Dietary Fiber **0g**
Net Carbohydrate **1g**

1 Preheat the oven to 500°F (260°C). In a small bowl, combine garlic, rosemary, sage, extra-virgin olive oil, 2 teaspoons sea salt, and 1 teaspoon black pepper. Set aside.

2 Place pork belly fat side up on a sturdy surface. Use a paring knife to score fat in a diamond pattern. Make sure to score about ¼ inch (.5cm) deep.

3 Turn belly over. Spread herb mixture evenly over belly.

4 Place pork loin in the center and roll belly around loin. Tie rolled belly crosswise with undyed kitchen twine every ½ inch (1.25cm), starting in the center of roast and working toward the edges.

5 Place tied roast rack in a roasting pan. Season outside of roast with remaining 2 teaspoons sea salt and remaining 1 teaspoon black pepper. Add 2 cups water, or enough to cover the bottom of the pan.

6 Roast for 20 minutes. Reduce the oven temperature to 300°F (150°C) and continue to roast for 1 hour, 30 minutes, to 2 hours, or until internal temperature reaches 145°F (65°C).

7 Let rest for 20 minutes before thinly slicing to serve.

Pork loin is higher in fat and a much wider cut than tenderloin. Tenderloin is excellent cooked quickly, while loin needs a longer cooking time to tenderize. Therefore, it's a good idea to familiarize yourself with both cuts to avoid confusion.

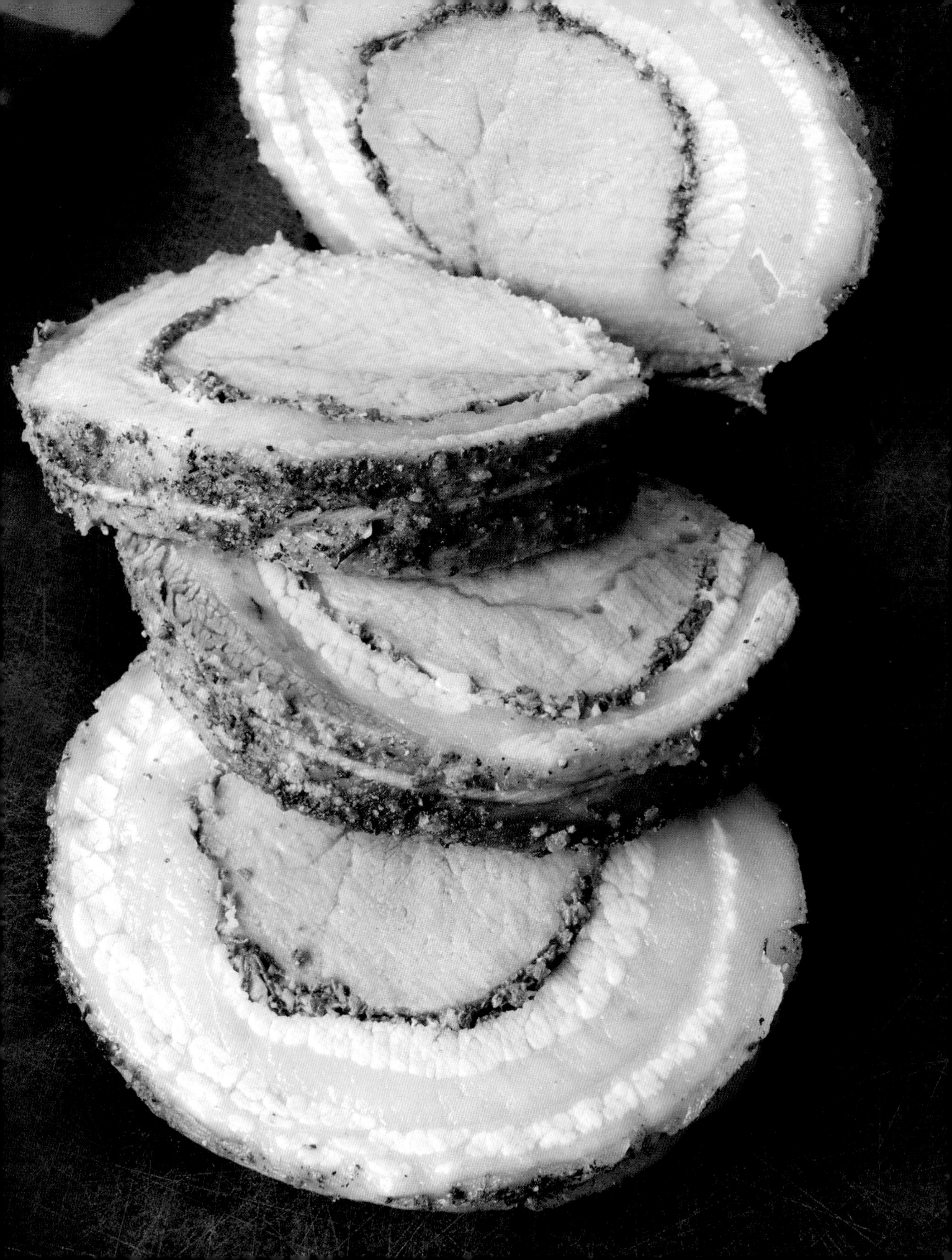

Pork cutlets are breaded and fried and served with a rich mushroom cream sauce, accented with garlic and rosemary.

Fried Pork Cutlets with Mushroom Sauce

Prep Time: **15 mins** | Cook Time: **20 mins** | Yield: **4 cutlets** | Serving Size: **1 cutlet**

Ingredients

- 4 (4 oz.; 110g each) boneless pork loin cutlets or chops
- ½ tsp. sea salt
- ½ cup almond flour
- 2 TB. tapioca flour
- ½ tsp. granulated garlic
- 1 large egg, beaten
- 2 TB. lard
- 2 TB. unsalted butter
- 1 clove garlic, minced
- 1 TB. fresh rosemary, minced
- 6 cremini mushrooms, thinly sliced
- ¾ cup chicken stock
- ¾ cup heavy cream
- ¼ tsp. freshly ground black pepper
- 5 tsp. cornstarch
- 5 tsp. cold water

1. Using a meat tenderizer or mallet, pound pork loin cutlets until ¾ inch (2cm) thick. Season with ¼ teaspoon sea salt and let sit for 5 minutes.

2. In a shallow dish, combine almond flour, tapioca flour, and granulated garlic. Dip each cutlet into egg. Dredge in almond flour mixture to coat.

3. Heat a large skillet over medium-high heat. Add lard. When lard is hot, carefully place cutlets into the skillet (they should sizzle, but not smoke).

4. Fry for 4 to 5 minutes, or until nicely browned. Turn and cook for 4 to 5 minutes, or until cooked through. Remove from the skillet and set on a wire rack.

5. Wipe the skillet clean and reheat over medium-high heat. Add unsalted butter. When melted, add garlic, rosemary, and mushrooms and sauté for 3 to 4 minutes, or until garlic is fragrant and mushrooms soften.

6. Pour chicken stock and heavy cream into the skillet and stir, scraping up any browned bits from the bottom of the skillet. Season with remaining ¼ teaspoon sea salt and black pepper. Bring to a light simmer.

7. Meanwhile, mix cornstarch with cold water. Pour slurry into simmering sauce, whisking until thickened, about 1 to 2 minutes. Remove from heat. Drizzle pork cutlets with mushroom sauce to serve.

Nutrition per Serving

Fat 69% | Net Carb 8% | Protein 23% | Ratio 1.0:1

Calories	Fat	Protein	Total Carbohydrate	Dietary Fiber	Net Carbohydrate
524	40g	30g	13g	2g	11g

Rich and creamy carbonara sauce is tossed with thick, chewy bacon lardons and curly spiralized zucchini noodles.

Zucchini Noodle Carbonara

Prep Time: **10 mins** | Cook Time: **15 mins** | Yield: **8 cups** | Serving Size: **2 cups**

Ingredients

- 3 medium zucchini, trimmed
- ¼ tsp. sea salt
- ½ lb. (225g) bacon lardons or diced thick-sliced bacon
- 2 garlic cloves, minced
- ½ cup yellow onion, diced
- ¾ cup heavy cream
- 2 large eggs, beaten
- ¾ cup grated Parmesan

1. Spiralize zucchini to create noodles. (Alternately, use a vegetable peeler to create long ribbons.)
2. Sprinkle zucchini with sea salt and gently massage to coat. Place in a colander to drain.
3. Heat a large skillet over medium-high heat. Add bacon lardons and cook for 5 to 8 minutes, or until browned and crisp, turning as needed. Remove lardons and place on a paper towel.
4. Reheat the skillet over medium heat and add garlic and yellow onion. Sauté in bacon fat, stirring occasionally, for 4 to 6 minutes, or until browned.
5. Gently squeeze zucchini to release any liquid. Place in the skillet and toss for 30 seconds to heat through. Remove the skillet from heat.
6. Add heavy cream, eggs, and Parmesan and continuously stir for 30 seconds, or until a creamy sauce forms. Top with lardons to serve.

Some people love peas in carbonara. When you're able to add additional carbs, feel free to toss in ⅓ cup shelled peas.

Nutrition per Serving

Fat **73%** Net Carb **4%**
Protein **23%** Ratio **1.2:1**

Calories	Fat	Protein	Total Carbohydrate	Dietary Fiber	Net Carbohydrate
601	49g	34g	8g	2g	6g

Italian sausage makes the perfect keto pizza crust for garlicky mushrooms, plenty of mozzarella, and black olives.

Sausage Crust Pizza

Prep Time: **10 mins**
Cook Time: **30 mins**

Yield: **1 (12-in.; 30.5cm) pizza**
Serving Size: **¼ pizza**

Ingredients

- 4 TB. extra-virgin olive oil
- 1 lb. (450g) mild Italian ground sausage
- 6 white button mushrooms, sliced
- 2 garlic cloves, minced
- 1 tsp. dried oregano
- 2 cups grated mozzarella
- ½ cup black olives, sliced
- 2 cups arugula

Nutrition per Serving

Fat **77%**
Net Carb **5%**
Protein **18%**
Ratio **1.5:1**

Calories **599**
Fat **51g**
Protein **28g**
Total Carbohydrate **9g**
Dietary Fiber **2g**
Net Carbohydrate **7g**

It's important to use a pizza pan with a rimmed edge. The sausage crust releases quite of bit of grease, so you want to be sure it stays in the pan and doesn't drip into the oven.

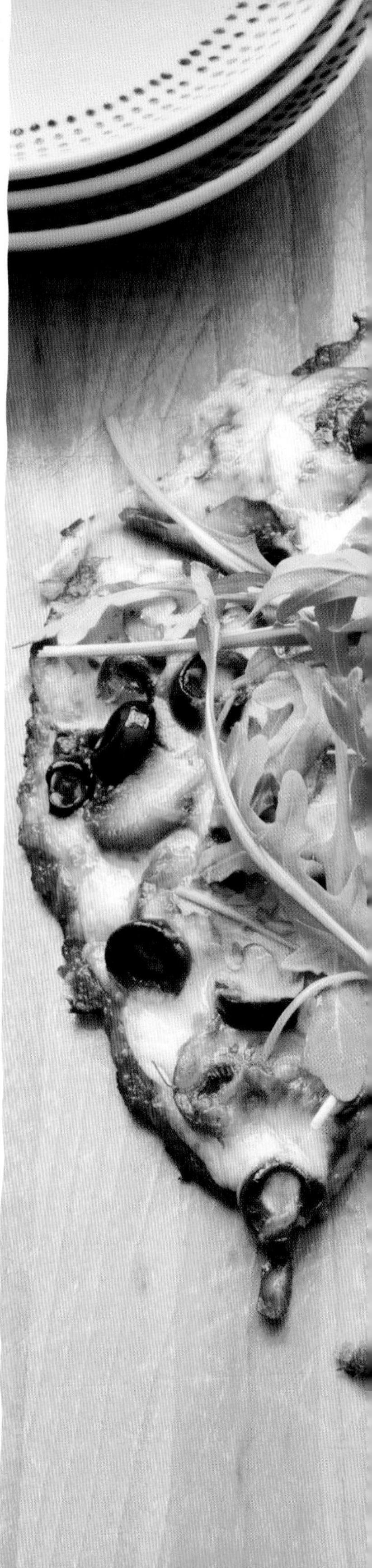

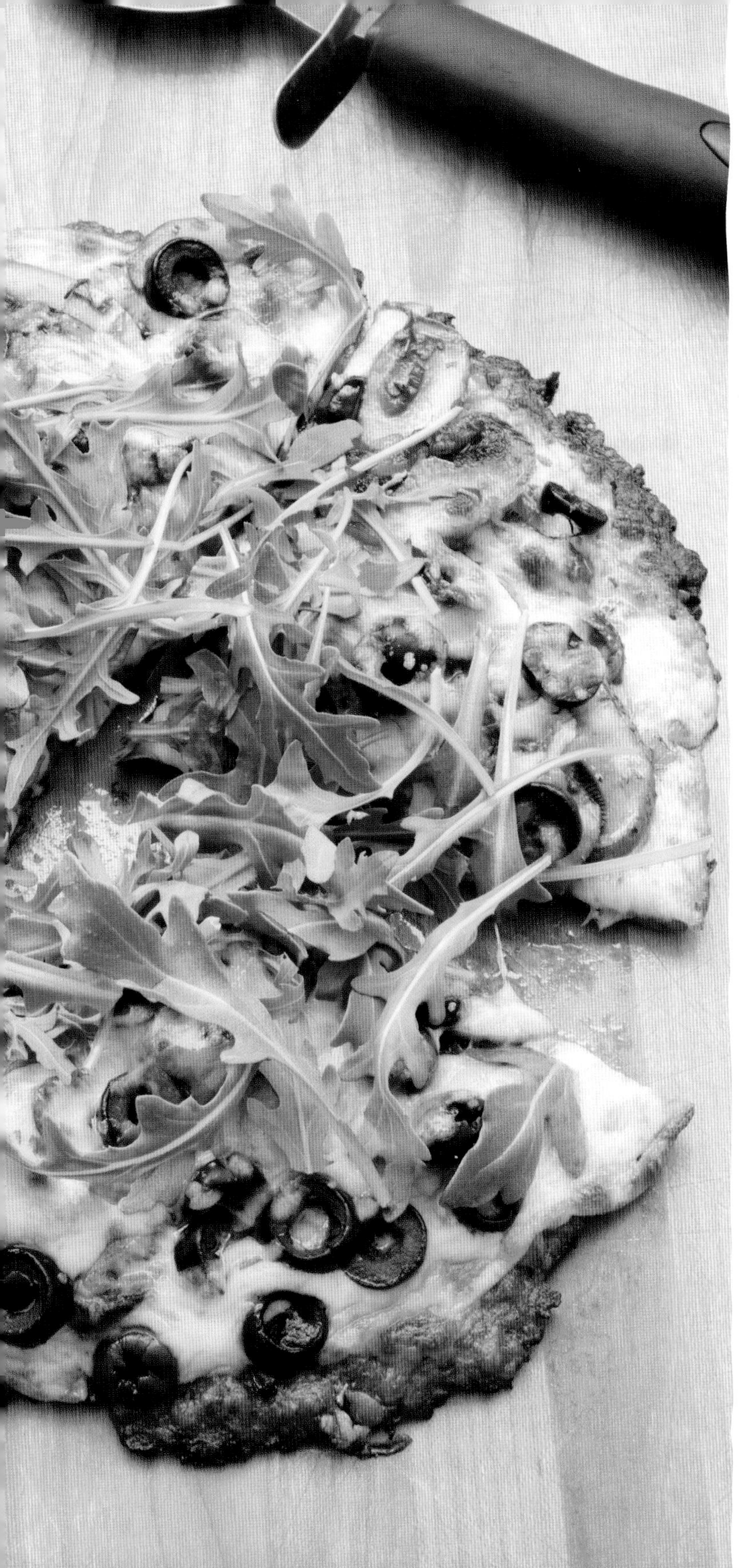

1 Preheat the oven to 400°F (200°C). Lightly grease a round, rimmed pizza pan with 1 tablespoon extra-virgin olive oil.

2 Gently flatten Italian sausage toward the edges of the pan in a thin layer. (It may help to cover sausage with a square of parchment paper and roll toward the edges.) Bake for 12 minutes.

3 While crust bakes, heat a medium skillet over medium-high heat. Add remaining 3 tablespoons olive oil to it.

4 Add button mushrooms and sauté, stirring occasionally, for 4 minutes. Add garlic and oregano and continue to cook for 1 to 2 minutes, or until garlic is fragrant and golden brown.

5 Spread mushroom mixture over sausage crust. Sprinkle with mozzarella and black olives. Return to the oven and bake for 10 to 12 minutes, or until sausage is cooked through and cheese is browned and bubbly.

6 Let pizza rest for 5 minutes. Sprinkle with arugula before slicing into wedges to serve.

Variation: To make a **Pepperoni Crust Pizza,** replace Italian sausage crust with 1 pound (450g) sliced pepperoni. Line the pizza pan with a thin layer of pepperoni, add toppings, and bake as instructed.

Sauerkraut takes on the fragrance of juniper, caraway, and bay as it's cooked with baby back ribs, bacon, and kielbasa.

Choucroute Garnie

Prep Time: **20 mins** Cook Time: **2 hrs** Yield: **9 cups** Serving Size: **1½ cups**

Ingredients

- ½ lb. (225g) thick-sliced uncured bacon, cut into 1-in. (2.5cm) pieces
- ¼ cup duck fat
- ½ cup yellow onion, diced
- 2 garlic cloves, minced
- ½ cup dry white wine
- 1½ lb. (680g) sauerkraut, drained
- 10 whole juniper berries
- 2 bay leaves
- ½ tsp. caraway seed
- ¼ tsp. freshly ground black pepper
- 1½ cups chicken broth
- 1 lb. (450g) baby back pork ribs
- 1 lb. (450g) smoked kielbasa, cut into 1-in. (2.5cm) pieces
- ¼ cup fresh tarragon, chopped (optional)
- 2 TB. Dijon or spicy mustard (optional)

1 Preheat the oven to 300°F (150°C). Heat a large Dutch oven or heavy bottomed braising pan over medium-high heat. Add bacon and cook for 4 to 6 minutes, or until crisp. Remove bacon from the Dutch oven and set aside.

2 Reheat residual bacon fat and add duck fat. When melted, add yellow onion and garlic and sauté for 5 to 7 minutes, or until softened and fragrant.

3 Pour dry white wine into the the Dutch oven and stir, scraping up any browned bits from the bottom of it.

4 Add sauerkraut, juniper berries, bay leaves, caraway seed, black pepper, and chicken broth. Stir to combine.

5 If baby back pork ribs are in still in a whole rack, slice between each bone to separate into individual ribs. Tuck ribs into sauerkraut and bring to a boil.

6 Cover and bake for 1 hour to 1 hour, 30 minutes, or until ribs are tender.

7 Remove bay leaves. Add kielbasa and cooked bacon. Stir, cover, and bake for an additional 10 to 15 minutes, or until meats are warmed through.

8 To serve, divide sauerkraut into bowls. Top with pieces of rib, kielbasa, and bacon. Sprinkle with fresh tarragon (if using) and serve with a side of Dijon mustard (if using) for dipping kielbasa.

Nutrition per Serving

Fat 71% Net Carb 6%
Protein 23% Ratio 1.1:1

Calories	Fat	Protein	Total Carbohydrate	Dietary Fiber	Net Carbohydrate
569	45g	33g	11g	3g	8g

Thick, juicy, bone-in pork chops are stuffed with sweet apple, crunchy hazelnuts, and flavorful bacon.

Apple and Hazelnut–Stuffed Pork Chops

Prep Time: **10 mins** Cook Time: **30 mins** Yield: **4 chops** Serving Size: **1 chop**

Ingredients

- 4 oz. (110g) uncured bacon, diced
- ½ medium sweet apple (such as Fuji or Honey Crisp), cored, peeled, and grated
- ⅓ cup raw hazelnuts, chopped
- 5 oz. (140g) frozen spinach, thawed and squeezed to remove liquid
- ½ tsp. granulated garlic
- 6 TB. unsalted butter, at room temperature
- 4 (5 oz.; 140g each) bone-in pork rib chops
- ½ tsp. sea salt
- ¼ tsp. freshly ground black pepper

1. Preheat the oven to 375°F (190°C).

2. Heat a large cast-iron skillet over medium heat. Add uncured bacon and cook, stirring occasionally, for 4 to 5 minutes, or until browned and crisp.

3. Spread bacon out on a paper towel to cool and reserve bacon fat in the skillet.

4. Place cooled bacon, apple, hazelnuts, spinach, granulated garlic, and unsalted butter in a food processor. Pulse for 30 seconds to 1 minute, or until fully blended.

5. Carefully slice a horizontal slit into meaty side of each pork rib chop to make a deep pocket. Stuff opening full of butter mixture and secure with a toothpick.

6. Reheat remaining bacon fat in the skillet over medium-high heat.

7. Sprinkle stuffed pork chops with sea salt and black pepper. Place pork chops in hot bacon fat and brown for 1 to 2 minutes per side.

8. Cover the skillet with aluminum foil and bake for 20 minutes, or until chops reach an internal temperature of 145°F (65°C). Serve immediately.

Nutrition per Serving

Fat **70%** Net Carb **3%**
Protein **27%** Ratio **1.1:1**

Calories	Fat	Protein	Total Carbohydrate	Dietary Fiber	Net Carbohydrate
512	40g	34g	7g	3g	4g

Rich and hearty, this savory pork sauce has enough fat to balance tomatoes, carrots, onions, and zucchini noodles.

Pork Bolognese

Prep Time: **15 mins**
Cook Time: **1 hr, 30 mins**

Yield: **12 cups**
Serving Size: **2 cups**

Ingredients

2 oz. (55g) uncured bacon, minced
3 TB. extra-virgin olive oil
½ cup yellow onion, finely diced
¼ cup carrot, finely diced
¼ cup celery, finely diced
1 garlic clove, sliced
1 tsp. dried thyme
1½ lb. (680g) ground pork
1½ cups chicken broth or stock
2 TB. tomato paste
½ cup tomato sauce
¼ cup dry white wine
1 bay leaf
½ tsp. sea salt
3 medium zucchini, trimmed
1 cup heavy cream
3 oz. (90g) grated Parmesan

Nutrition per Serving

Fat **78%**
Net Carb **1%**
Protein **21%**
Ratio **1.5:1**

Calories **626**
Fat **54g**
Protein **33g**
Total Carbohydrate **9g**
Dietary Fiber **2g**
Net Carbohydrate **2g**

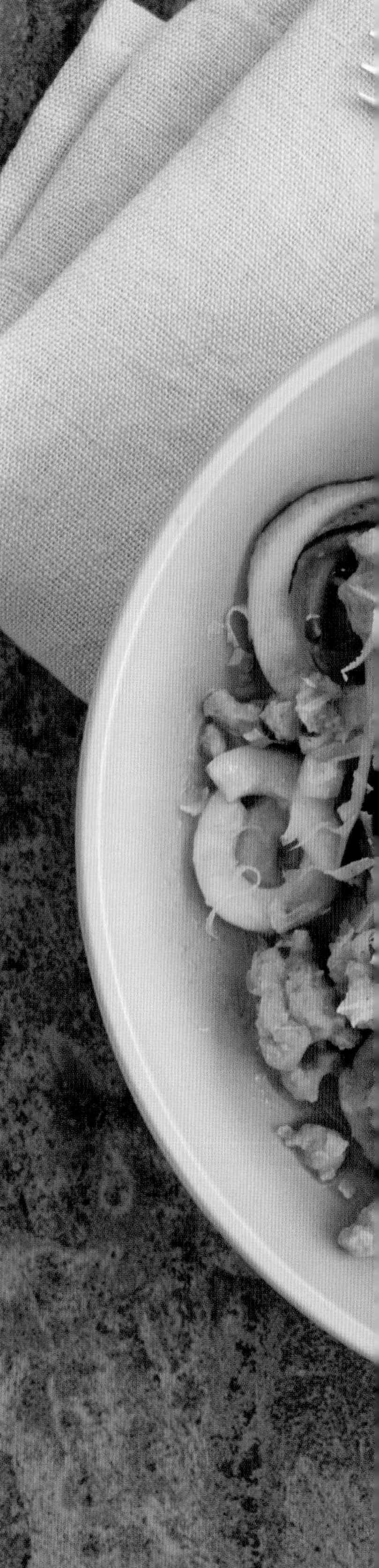

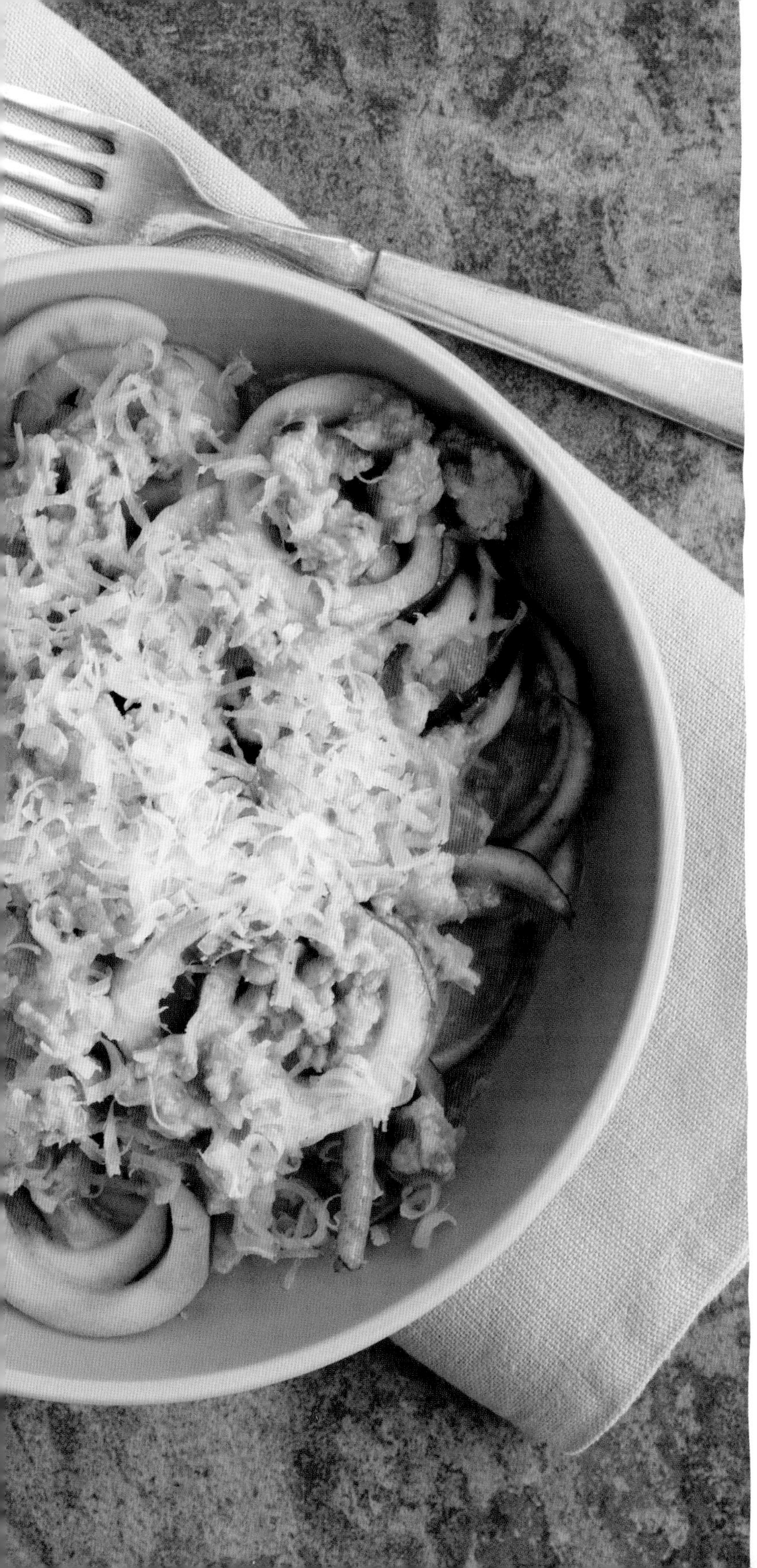

1 Heat a large saucepan or Dutch oven over medium heat. Add uncured bacon and cook for 4 to 6 minutes, or until lightly browned. Add extra-virgin olive oil and wait for 15 seconds.

2 Add yellow onion, carrot, celery, garlic, and thyme and cook, stirring occasionally, for 2 to 3 minutes, or until softened.

3 Add pork and break up into smaller pieces in the pan. Cook for 3 to 5 minutes, or until pork breaks into crumbles and begins to brown.

4 Add chicken broth and stir, scraping up any browned bits from the bottom of the pan.

5 Add tomato paste, tomato sauce, dry white wine, bay leaf, and sea salt. Stir and reduce heat to medium-low. Simmer, uncovered, for 1 hour, or until reduced by half.

6 While sauce cooks, spiralize zucchini to create noodles. (Alternately, use a vegetable peeler to create long ribbons.)

7 Stir heavy cream into sauce and bring back to a simmer. Taste and season with additional sea salt, if desired. Remove and discard bay leaf.

8 Stir zucchini noodles into hot sauce and cook for 30 seconds to warm through. Divide into bowls and top with Parmesan to serve.

Seafood Mains

Seafood provides the heart-protective, brain-boosting health benefits of omega-3 fatty acids. Even if you're not a big seafood lover, it's so versatile and easy to prepare, you're sure to find a few options in this chapter you'll love. From crab legs to salmon, the recipes in this chapter will elevate your keto diet to a whole new level of sophistication and flavor.

Succulent, sweet crab legs are dunked in golden yellow drawn butter for a truly decadent entrée.

Crab with Drawn Butter

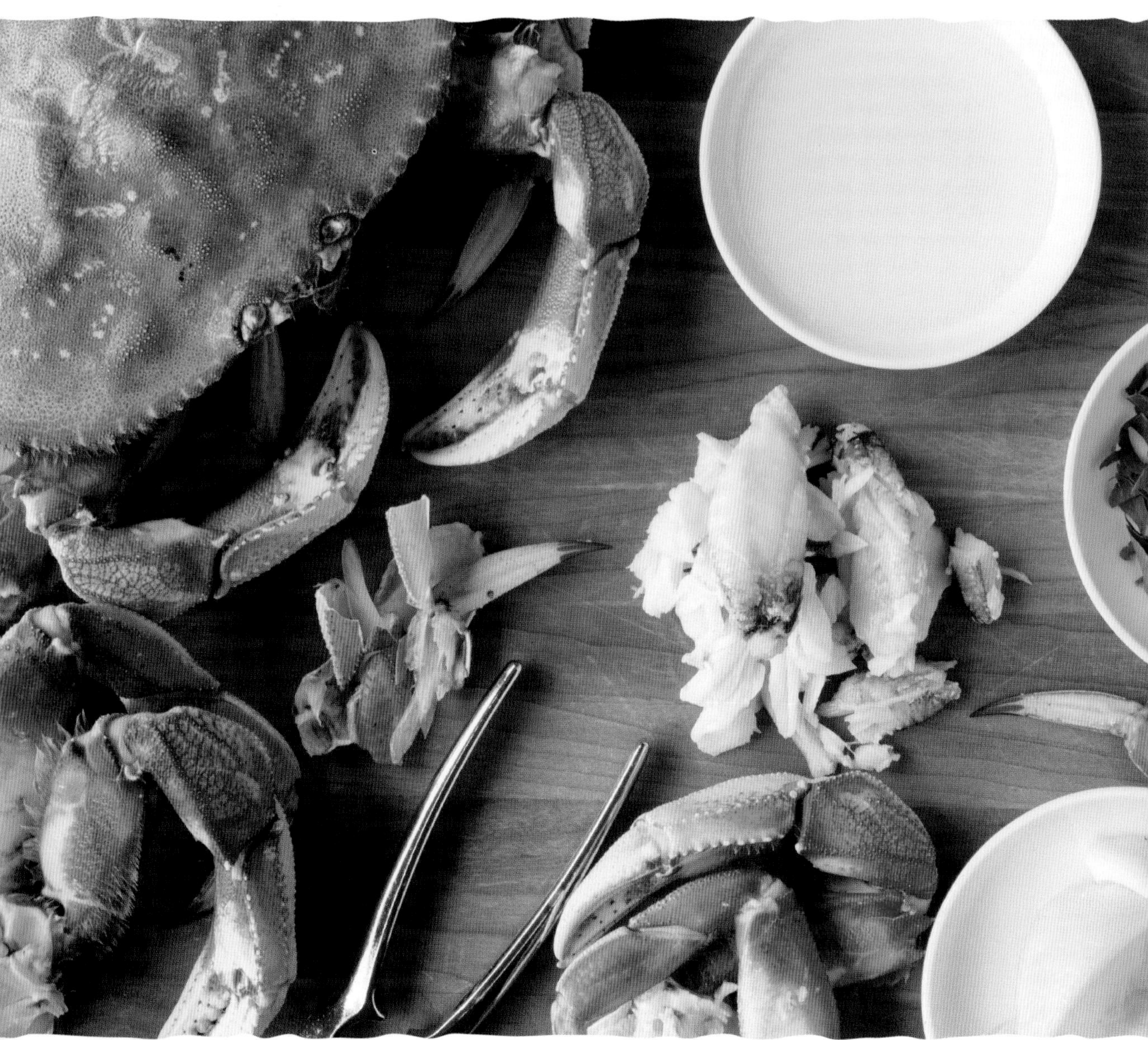

Prep Time: **10 mins** | Cook Time: **10 mins** | Yield: **16 legs** | Serving Size: **4 legs**

Ingredients

¼ cup sea salt

1 cup salted butter, cut into cubes

3 lb. (1.5kg) crab legs

4 lemon wedges

2 TB. fresh parsley, chopped

1 Fill a 2-gallon (2l) pot ½ full of water. Add sea salt. Cover, place over high heat, and bring to a boil.

2 While water comes to a boil, heat a small saucepan over low heat. Add salted butter.

3 Wait for butter to melt and foam, about 2 to 4 mintues. When foaming stops, remove butter from heat.

4 Using a spoon, carefully skim off and discard cloudy white foam from melted butter. Keep warm.

5 When water boils, add crab legs, cover pot, and cook for 2 minutes. Remove crab legs from the pot.

6 Pour drawn butter into 4 ramekins and place on 4 plates. Place lemon wedges and parsley in 2 separate bowls. Serve crab legs whole with an extra bowl for shells.

7 To eat, break legs at each joint. Use seafood crackers and picks to carefully remove crab meat from shells. Squeeze lemon juice over crab meat, dip in drawn butter, and sprinkle with fresh parsley.

If you can find live crab, this recipe can be adapted for two 2-lb. (1kg) crabs. Cook them for 14 minutes.

Nutrition per Serving

Fat **47%** Net Carb **0%**
Protein **53%** Ratio **0.4:1**

Calories **950**
Fat **50g**
Protein **125g**
Total Carbohydrate **0g**
Dietary Fiber **0g**
Net Carbohydrate **0g**

Variation: If you're cooking for a crew, you can make a **Cajun Crab Boil.** Add ¼ cup crushed red pepper flakes; ½ cup Old Bay seasoning blend; 2 large yellow onions, quartered; 1 pound (450g) Andouille sausage links, cut into 2-inch (5cm) sections; and 1 pound (450g) Manila clams into the boiling water along with crab legs. Boil until clams open (discard any that remain closed). Serve with extra drawn butter. Serves 8 to 10.

Prep Time: **15 mins** | Cook Time: **10 mins** | Yield: **4 cups** | Serving Size: **2 cups**

Ingredients

- 3 cups cauliflower florets
- 3 TB. unsalted butter or coconut oil
- ¼ cup yellow onion, diced
- ¼ cup carrot, diced
- 1 oz. (25g) uncured bacon, diced
- 1 tsp. freshly grated ginger root
- 2 TB. toasted sesame oil
- 1 large egg, beaten
- 2 TB. wheat-free tamari
- 4 oz. (110g) cooked shrimp, peeled
- 2 green onions, thinly sliced
- ¼ cup cashews

1 Place cauliflower florets in a food processor. Pulse several times, scraping down the sides of the bowl occasionally, until cauliflower resembles the coarse texture of rice. Set aside.

2 Heat a large skillet over medium-high heat. When the skillet is hot, add unsalted butter and wait for 15 seconds.

3 Add yellow onion, carrot, and uncured bacon, and cook, stirring occasionally, for 3 to 4 minutes, or until onion and carrot have softened. Add cauliflower rice and ginger, and cook for an additional 3 to 4 minutes.

4 Push vegetables to the sides of the skillet to create an opening at the center. Pour toasted sesame oil into opening, and then immediately add egg. Stir egg continuously for about 30 seconds, or until scrambled.

5 Add wheat-free tamari, shrimp, green onions, and cashews and stir to combine. Cook for 30 seconds to 1 minute, or until shrimp are warmed through. Serve immediately.

Variation: You can easily switch out the shrimp for another protein in this recipe. To make **Chicken Fried Cauliflower Rice,** use 4 ounces (110g) skinless, boneless chicken thighs, diced, instead of shrimp. Dice chicken and cook with onion, carrot, and bacon. You may need to extend the cooking time by a few minutes to be sure the chicken is cooked through before adding cauliflower rice and ginger.

You can add ¼ cup peas into this meal in step 3 once you begin to increase your carbs for the maintenance phase.

Nutrition per Serving

Fat **71%** Net Carb **9%**
Protein **20%** Ratio **1.1:1**

Calories	Fat	Protein	Total Carbohydrate	Dietary Fiber	Net Carbohydrate
547	43g	27g	18g	5g	13g

Cauliflower "rice" is fried in butter and packed with plump shrimp, crunchy cashews, and familiar fried rice flavors.

Shrimp Fried Cauliflower Rice

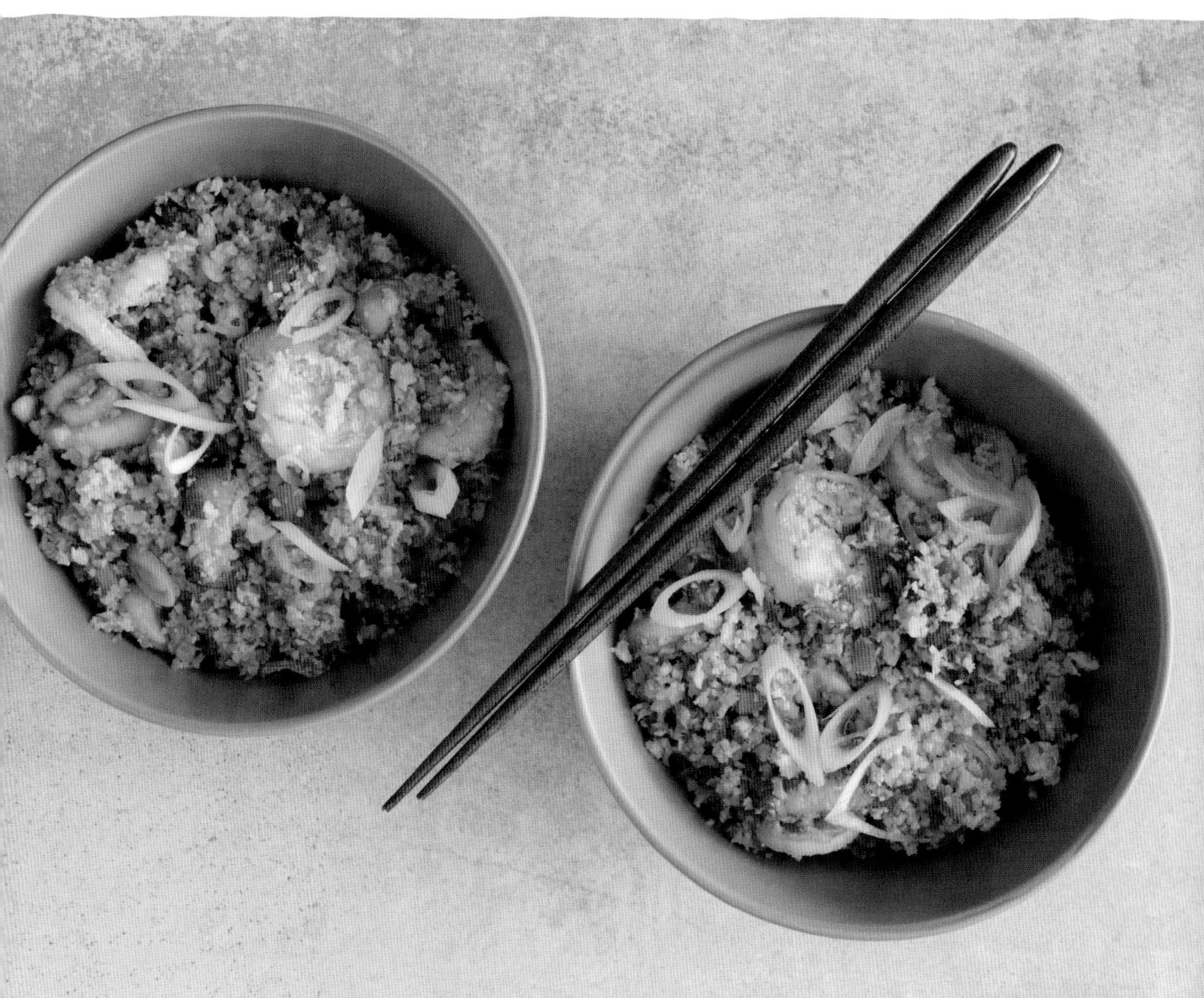

Flaky trout is pan-fried and drenched in a golden brown butter and garlic sauce with nutty almonds.

Trout Almondine

Prep Time: **5 mins** | Cook Time: **15 mins** | Yield: **1 fillet** | Serving Size: **½ fillet**

Ingredients

- ¼ cup blanched almond slices
- 6 TB. salted butter
- 6 oz. (170g) trout fillet
- ⅛ tsp. freshly ground black pepper
- 2 garlic cloves, minced
- 1 tsp. lemon juice
- 2 TB. fresh parsley, chopped

1. Place almond slices in a medium skillet over low heat. Stirring constantly, gently toast almonds for 4 to 5 minutes, or until fragrant. Transfer almonds to a plate.
2. Reheat the skillet over medium-high heat. Add 2 tablespoons salted butter to the skillet.
3. Sprinkle both sides of trout fillet with black pepper.
4. When butter melts, add trout fillet. Cook for 1 to 2 minutes per side, until a golden crust forms and fish flakes easily with a fork. Divide fillet in half and place on 2 plates.
5. Reheat the skillet over medium-high heat. Add remaining 4 tablespoons salted butter and garlic. Cook for 1 to 2 minutes, or until butter is browned and garlic is crisp. Remove from heat.
6. Stir lemon juice into butter-garlic mixture. Drizzle over trout. Top with toasted almonds and parsley to serve.

You could also substitute an oily fish like salmon; however, the delicate flavor of trout works best with this dish.

Nutrition per Serving

Fat **81%** Net Carb **2%**
Protein **17%** Ratio **1.9:1**

Calories	Fat	Protein	Total Carbohydrate	Dietary Fiber	Net Carbohydrate
532	48g	22g	5g	2g	3g

Tender white fish fillets are fried in crunchy almond meal and Parmesan, and served with a dollop of tartar sauce.

Almond-Crusted Fish with Tartar Sauce

Prep Time: **10 mins** Cook Time: **10 mins** Yield: **2 fillets** Serving Size: **½ fillet**

Ingredients

- ¾ cup mayonnaise
- 1 TB. sweet pickle, chopped
- 1 TB. capers, rinsed
- 1 green onion, minced
- 1 tsp. whole-grain mustard
- 2 tsp. lemon juice
- ½ tsp. sea salt
- ½ tsp. freshly ground black pepper
- ½ cup almond meal
- ½ cup finely grated Parmesan
- 1 large egg
- 4 TB. ghee or other high-temperature oil
- 2 (4 oz.; 110g each) whitefish fillets

1 In a small bowl, mix mayonnaise, sweet pickle, capers, green onion, whole-grain mustard, lemon juice, ¼ teaspoon sea salt, and ¼ teaspoon black pepper. Refrigerate tartar sauce.

2 In a shallow dish, combine almond meal and Parmesan.

3 In a separate shallow dish, beat egg, remaining ¼ teaspoon sea salt, and remaining ¼ teaspoon black pepper until well blended.

4 Heat a medium nonstick frying pan over medium heat. When the pan is hot, add ghee.

5 Dip whitefish fillets in egg mixture, and then coat with almond meal mixture. Place coated fillets in hot ghee. Cook for 2 to 4 minutes per side, or until fillets are cooked through.

6 Serve hot fillets with a generous portion of tartar sauce.

In the process of making ghee, the milk solids are removed, making it a fat that won't smoke when used at higher temps.

Nutrition per Serving

Fat **85%** Net Carb **2%**
Protein **13%** Ratio **2.4:1**

Calories	Fat	Protein	Total Carbohydrate	Dietary Fiber	Net Carbohydrate
650	61g	22g	5g	2g	3g

Tender sea scallops make a quick dinner when served with an aromatic sauce of sizzling butter and brined capers.

Scallops with Brown Butter and Capers

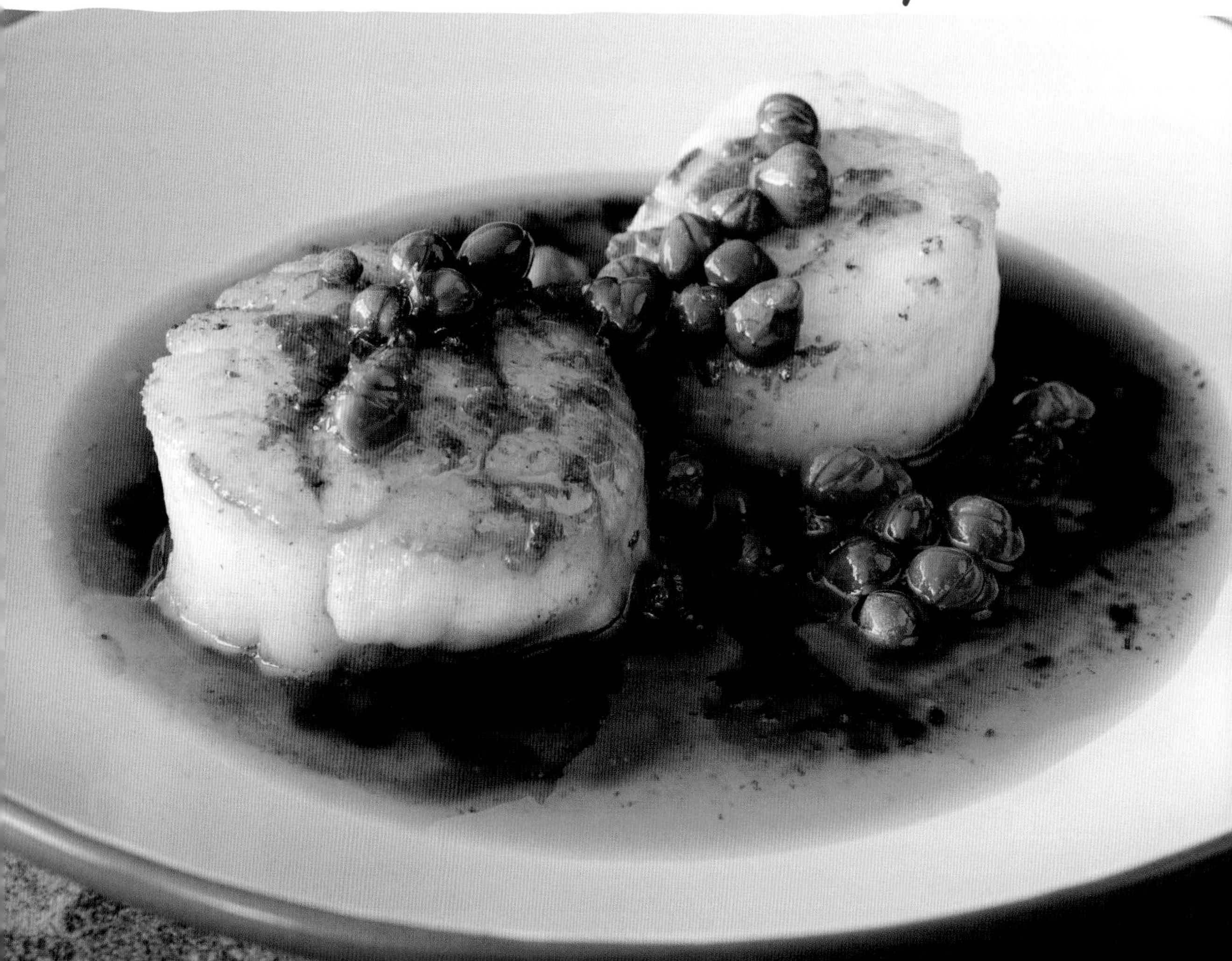

Prep Time: **10 mins** | Cook Time: **15 mins** | Yield: **4 scallops** | Serving Size: **2 scallops**

Ingredients

- 4 jumbo fresh dry pack sea scallops (about 6 oz.; 170g)
- 6 TB. unsalted butter
- 2 TB. grapeseed oil
- ½ cup dry white wine
- 1 tsp. lemon zest
- ¼ tsp. sea salt (optional)
- 1 TB. capers, rinsed

It's important to use an oil with a high smoke point to sear food. For a neutral taste, avocado, sunflower, safflower, or grapeseed oil are all excellent choices.

1. Rinse sea scallops and pat dry with a paper towel. Set aside.

2. Heat unsalted butter in a heavy-bottomed skillet over medium-low heat. Cook for 3 to 4 minutes, watching constantly and stirring frequently, until butter turns a light brown and has a slight nutty aroma. (You'll notice some small particles of milk solids in the bottom of the skillet that will also turn light brown.)

3. Immediately remove butter from the skillet and place in a bowl to cool. (If any milk solids turned dark brown, simply pour off and reserve butter on top and discard solids.)

4. Reheat the skillet over high heat. Add grapeseed oil to the skillet and wait for oil to shimmer (just before smoking), about 15 to 30 seconds.

5. Place scallops into oil. Without moving, cook for 2 to 3 minutes, or until a caramel crust forms. Turn scallops and cook for an additional 3 to 4 minutes, or until browned.

6. Remove scallops from the skillet and set aside.

7. Reheat the skillet over medium-high heat. Add dry white wine and scrape up any browned bits from the bottom of the skillet. Simmer for 1 minute.

8. Whisk in lemon zest, sea salt (if using), and browned butter. Cook, stirring constantly, for 1 minute. Stir in capers.

9. Drizzle scallops with warm sauce and serve immediately.

Variation: This recipe can be made with many types of seafood. To make **Tuna with Brown Butter and Olives,** replace sea scallops with 6 ounces (170g) boneless tuna steak and use ¼ cup pitted, chopped Kalamata olives instead of capers. Cook tuna an additional 1 minute per side.

Nutrition per Serving

Fat **89%** Net Carb **2%**
Protein **9%** Ratio **3.5:1**

Calories	Fat	Protein	Total Carbohydrate	Dietary Fiber	Net Carbohydrate
497	49g	11g	3g	0g	3g

Tuna, peas, sharp cheddar, and creamy mushroom gravy rest atop cauliflower florets in this keto twist on the classic.

Tuna Casserole

Prep Time: **15 mins** | Cook Time: **40 mins** | Yield: **1 casserole** | Serving Size: **1/8 casserole**

Ingredients

- ¼ cup extra-virgin olive oil
- ½ cup yellow onion, diced
- ½ cup celery, diced
- 5 white button mushrooms, diced
- 1½ cups heavy cream
- 1 cup sour cream
- ½ tsp. freshly ground black pepper
- 2 cups grated sharp cheddar cheese
- ½ cup frozen peas
- 6 cups cauliflower florets, cut into small pieces
- 2 (5-oz.; 140g) cans tuna in olive oil, drained
- 2 tsp. Old Bay seasoning

1 Preheat the oven to 375°F (190°C). Heat a large heavy-bottomed skillet over medium heat. Add extra-virgin olive oil and wait for 30 seconds.

2 Add yellow onion, celery, and white button mushrooms and cook, stirring occasionally, for 5 to 6 minutes, or until softened.

3 Add heavy cream, sour cream, and black pepper. Stir to combine and bring to a simmer. Simmer for 2 minutes, stirring frequently.

4 Stir in 1 cup sharp cheddar cheese and peas and stir until thickened. Remove from heat and set aside.

5 Place cauliflower florets in the bottom of a 9-inch (22cm) square covered casserole dish. Spread tuna over cauliflower.

6 Pour cream sauce evenly over top. Sprinkle with remaining 1 cup sharp cheddar cheese and Old Bay seasoning.

7 Cover and bake for 15 minutes. Remove cover and continue to cook for 10 to 15 minutes, or until cheese is golden and cauliflower is tender. Serve immediately.

If you can find fried pork rinds without any added fillers or artificial ingredients, you can crumble 1 cup on top of the dish.

Nutrition per Serving

Fat 77% | Net Carb 6% | Protein 17% | Ratio 1.5:1

Calories	Fat	Protein	Total Carbohydrate	Dietary Fiber	Net Carbohydrate
481	41g	21g	9g	2g	7g

Vegetables abound in this quick curry, loaded with scrumptious shrimp, velvety coconut milk, and fresh basil.

Coconut Shrimp Curry

Prep Time: **20 mins** Cook Time: **15 mins** Yield: **4 cups** Serving Size: **2 cups**

Ingredients

- 3 TB. coconut oil
- ¼ cup yellow onion, chopped
- 1 TB. curry powder
- 1 tsp. ground coriander
- 2 tsp. grated fresh ginger
- 1 (14-fl.-oz.; 400ml) can full-fat coconut milk
- 2 cups cauliflower florets
- 4 oz. (110g) pea pods
- ½ medium red bell pepper, seeded and sliced
- 1 tsp. high-quality fish sauce
- 1 tsp. lime juice
- ¼ tsp. sea salt
- 6 oz. (170g) cooked shrimp, peeled and deveined
- ¼ cup fresh basil, chopped

1. Heat a large skillet over medium-high heat. When the skillet is hot, add coconut oil and wait for 15 seconds.

2. Add yellow onion, curry powder, coriander, and ginger, and sauté, stirring occasionally, for 3 to 4 minutes, or until onion softens and spices are fragrant.

3. Add coconut milk, cauliflower florets, pea pods, red bell pepper, fish sauce, lime juice, and sea salt. Stir to combine.

4. Reduce heat to low, cover, and steam for 8 to 10 minutes, or until vegetables are softened but firm.

5. Add shrimp and stir. Cook for 1 minute, or until shrimp are warmed through. Serve with basil.

Made from salted and fermented anchovy juice, fish sauce is a great way to add a deeper flavor to seafood dishes.

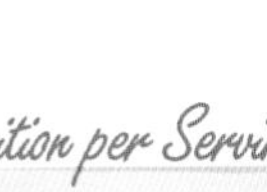

Fat 76% Net Carb 8%
Protein 16% Ratio 1.4:1

Calories	Fat	Protein	Total Carbohydrate	Dietary Fiber	Net Carbohydrate
765	65g	30g	22g	7g	15g

Bright pan-fried salmon fillets are served with a softened spoonful of savory herb-infused butter.

Salmon with Herb Butter

Prep Time: **5 mins** Cook Time: **7 mins** Yield: **2 fillets** Serving Size: **1 fillet**

Ingredients

- 4 TB. salted butter, at room temperature
- 1 TB. fresh chives, chopped
- 1 TB. fresh parsley, chopped
- 1 tsp. fresh rosemary, chopped
- 1 tsp. fresh tarragon, chopped
- ½ tsp. granulated garlic
- ¼ tsp. freshly ground black pepper
- 1 TB. safflower oil
- 2 (4 oz.; 110g each) boneless salmon fillets
- 2 cups steamed greens, to serve (optional)

1 In a small bowl, combine salted butter, chives, parsley, rosemary, tarragon, granulated garlic, and black pepper and mix until well blended. (Alternately, use a small food processor to purée ingredients.) Set aside.

2 Heat a medium frying pan over medium-high heat. When the pan is hot, add safflower oil and wait for 30 seconds.

3 Place salmon fillets, skin side down, in hot oil. Cook for 3 to 4 minutes, or until golden brown and crisp. Carefully turn over fillets and cook for an additional 2 to 3 minutes, or until firm to the touch.

4 Spoon herb butter over hot salmon fillets just before serving to soften. Serve alongside steamed greens (if using) for a complete meal.

Variation: Compound butters are a great way to add extra fat to meals. To make a **Dill and Caper Butter,** blend butter with 1 tablespoon chopped fresh dill, and then add 2 teaspoons rinsed and chopped capers and 1 teaspoon lemon zest.

Nutrition per Serving

Fat **78%** Net Carb **1%**
Protein **21%** Ratio **1.5:1**

Calories **429**
Fat **37g**
Protein **23g**
Total Carbohydrate **1g**
Dietary Fiber **0g**
Net Carbohydrate **1g**

Nutrition per Serving (with Greens)

Fat **73%** Net Carb **3%**
Protein **24%** Ratio **1.2:1**

Calories **466**
Fat **38g**
Protein **28g**
Total Carbohydrate **8g**
Dietary Fiber **5g**
Net Carbohydrate **3g**

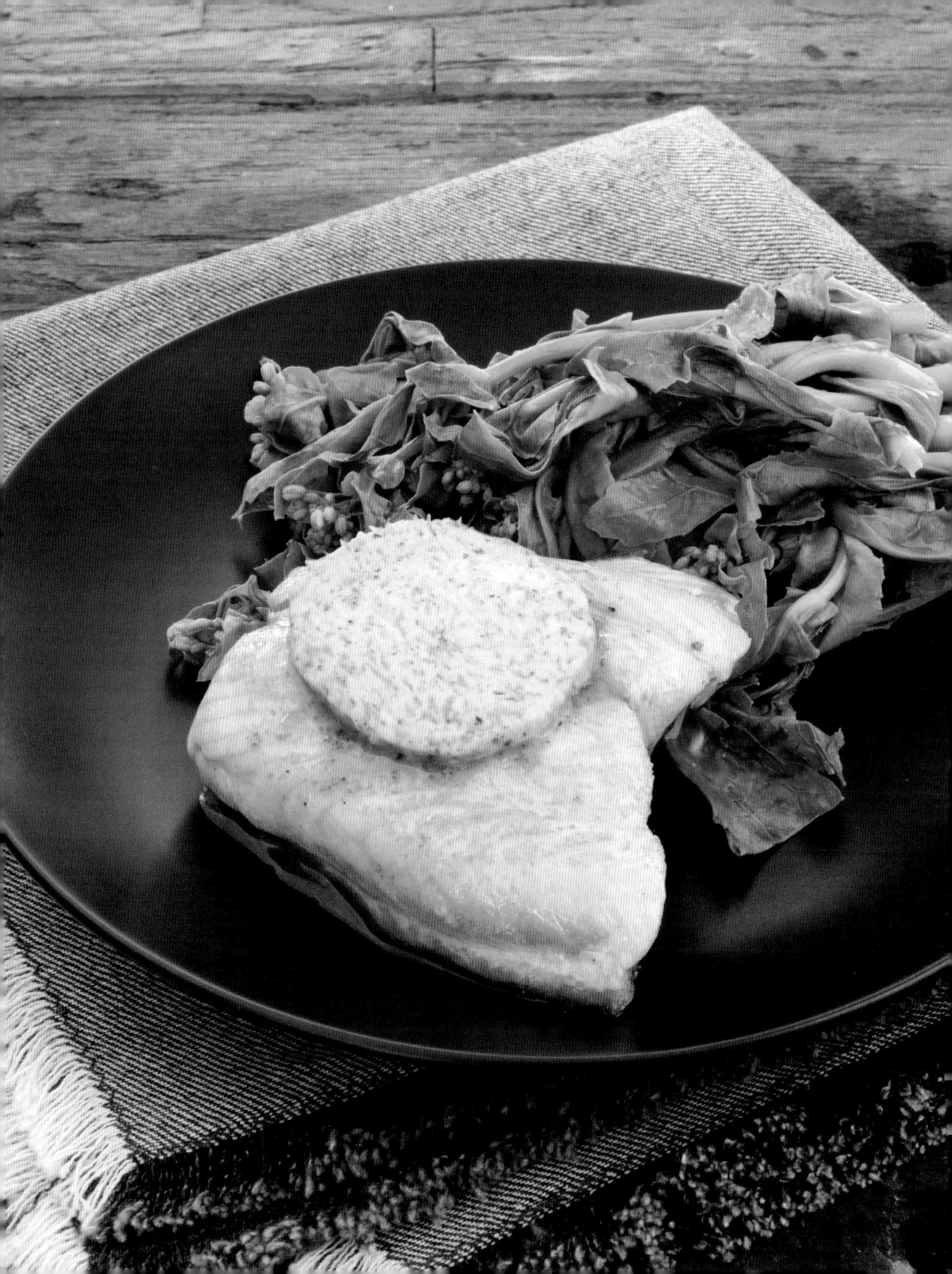

Sides

What's a main dish without a fabulous side? A well-paired side dish can turn your entrée into an interesting, more well-rounded experience. From green bean casserole to a simple side salad, the easy and versatile sides in this chapter provide the perfect keto-friendly accompaniments to the broad range of main dishes in the previous chapters of this book.

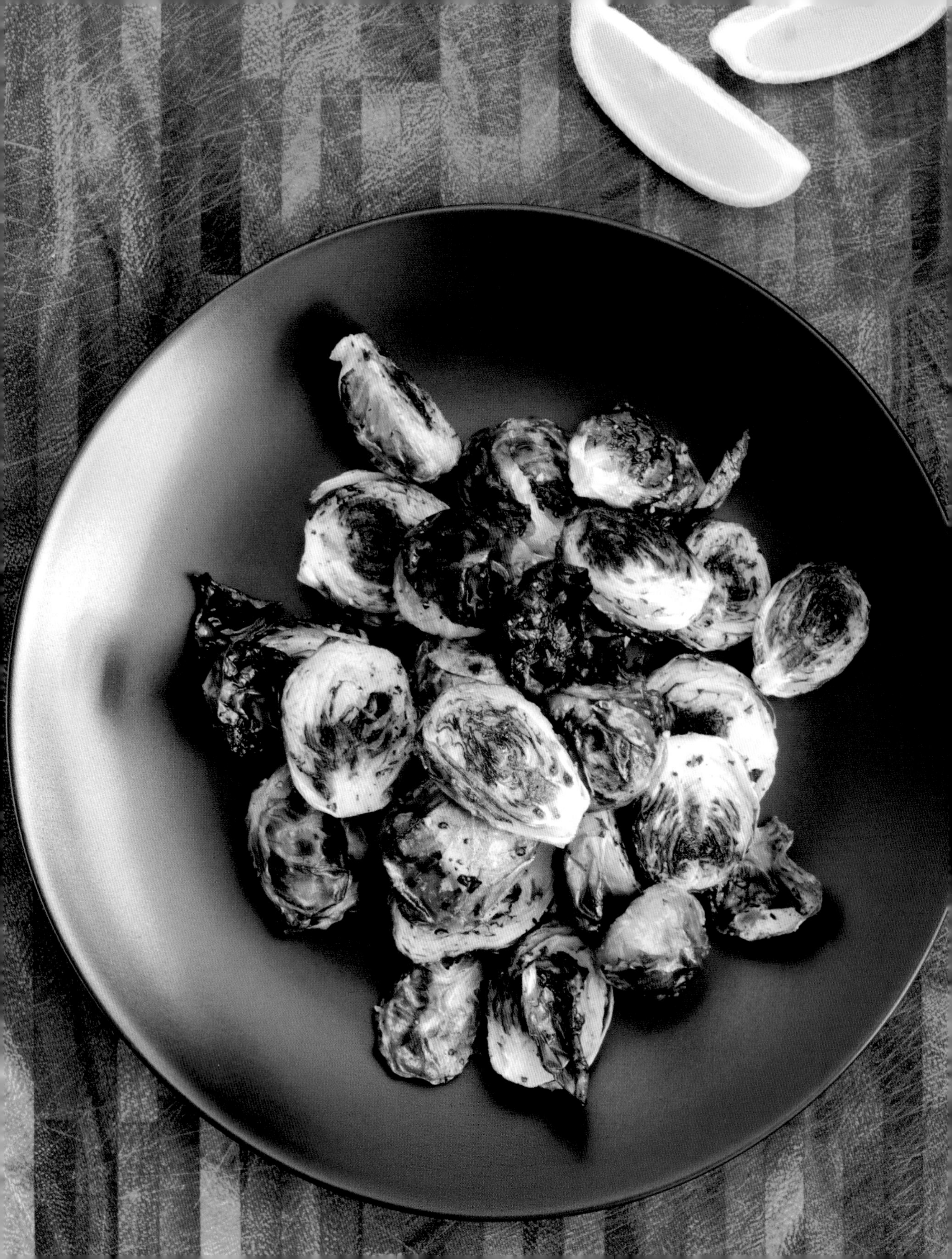

Rich, palate-coating duck fat smothers brussels sprouts that are sweet and caramelized from roasting.

Duck Fat–Roasted Brussels Sprouts

Prep Time: **10 mins** | Cook Time: **25 mins** | Yield: **3 cups** | Serving Size: **½ cup**

Ingredients

- 1 lb. (450g) brussels sprouts
- ½ cup pure duck fat
- ½ tsp. sea salt
- ½ tsp. freshly ground black pepper
- 1 tsp. granulated garlic
- 1 tsp. dried thyme
- 1 TB. fresh-squeezed lemon juice

1 Preheat the oven to 450°F (230°C). Trim stem ends and any loose leaves from brussels sprouts. Cut each in half and place halves in a mixing bowl.

2 Warm duck fat in a small skillet over low heat (or in the microwave for 15 to 30 seconds) until melted. Pour duck fat over brussels sprouts. Add sea salt, black pepper, granulated garlic, and thyme and toss to evenly coat sprouts.

3 Transfer mixture to a rimmed metal baking sheet. Arrange brussels sprouts so each sprout is face down on the baking sheet.

4 Bake for 15 to 20 minutes, or until brussels sprouts are tender but still firm. Sprinkle with lemon juice just before serving.

These brussels are just as tasty with coconut oil. Try to find a virgin or extra-virgin variety for more sweet coconut flavor.

Variation: You can use up extra bacon grease by making **Bacon Fat–Roasted Brussels Sprouts.** Simply replace duck fat with ½ cup warmed bacon fat and replace thyme with ½ teaspoon smoked paprika.

Nutrition per Serving

Fat **83%** Net Carb **11%**
Protein **6%** Ratio **2.1:1**

Calories 185
Fat 17g
Protein 3g
Total Carbohydrate 8g
Dietary Fiber 3g
Net Carbohydrate 5g

Romanesco broccoli is drizzled in garlic and rosemary–infused olive oil and sprinkled with toasty pine nuts.

Romanesco with Rosemary and Garlic

Prep Time: **10 mins**
Cook Time: **25 mins**

Yield: **2 cups**
Serving Size: **½ cup**

Ingredients

- 1 medium head Romanesco, cut into florets (about 2 cups)
- 6 TB. extra-virgin olive oil
- 1 garlic clove, minced
- 1 TB. fresh rosemary, chopped
- ¼ tsp. sea salt
- ¼ tsp. freshly ground black pepper
- 3 TB. pine nuts, lightly toasted

Nutrition per Serving

Fat **95%** Net Carb **2%**
Protein **3%** Ratio **9.7:1**

Calories **246**
Fat **26g**
Protein **2g**
Total Carbohydrate **3g**
Dietary Fiber **2g**
Net Carbohydrate **1g**

To toast pine nuts, heat a small skillet over low heat. Add pine nuts to the skillet. Stirring constantly, toast for 2 to 3 minutes.

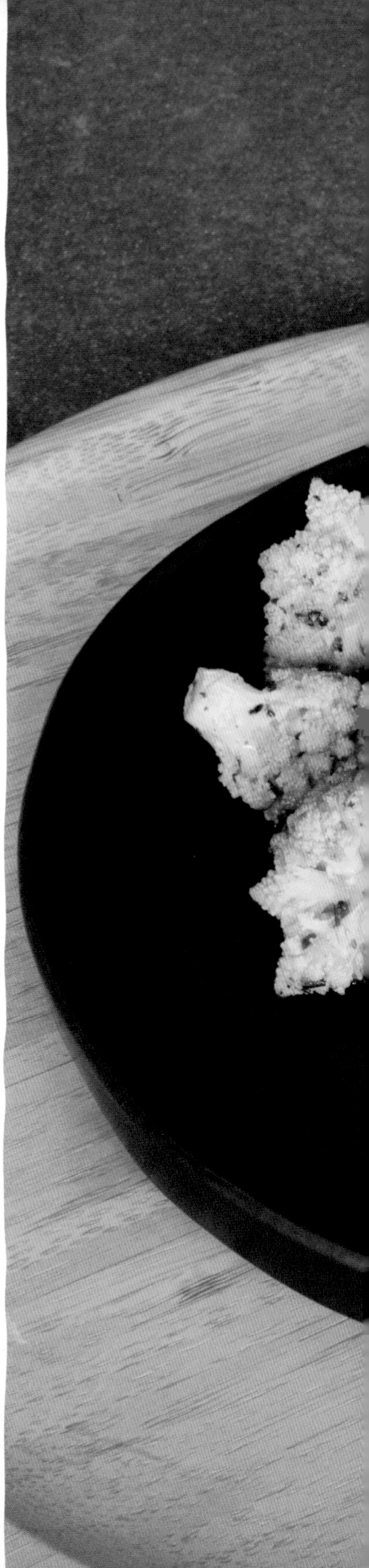

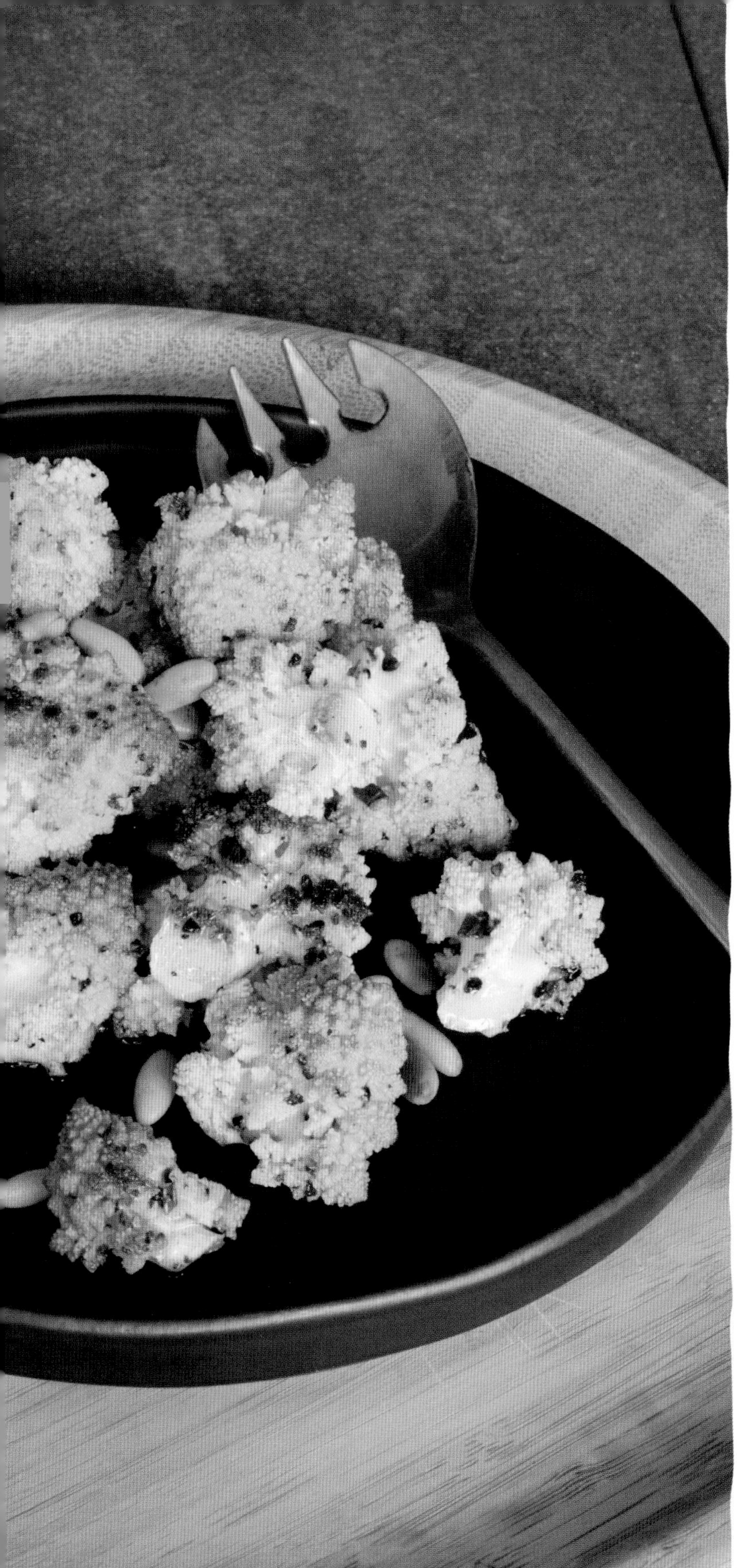

1 Preheat the oven to 400°F (200°C). Spread Romanesco on a rimmed metal baking sheet. Drizzle with 2 tablespoons extra-virgin olive oil.

2 Bake for 20 to 25 minutes, or until golden brown and tender but still firm.

3 Meanwhile, heat a small skillet over medium heat. Add remaining 4 tablespoons extra-virgin olive oil and wait for 30 seconds.

4 Add garlic and rosemary and cook, stirring occasionally, for 1 to 2 minutes, or until fragrant and lightly browned. Remove from heat.

5 When Romanesco is done, remove baking sheet from the oven. Pour oil over top, sprinkle with sea salt and black pepper, and gently stir to coat all sides of florets.

6 Sprinkle toasted pine nuts over Romanesco to serve.

Variation: To make **Cauliflower with Spiced Garlic Butter,** replace Romanesco with 2 cups cauliflower florets and use 1 teaspoon paprika, 1 teaspoon garam masala, and 1 teaspoon ground cumin in place of rosemary.

Tender bok choy and earthy shiitake mushrooms are sautéed in toasted sesame oil with garlic and tamari.

Sesame Bok Choy and Shiitake Mushrooms

Prep Time: **5 mins** | Cook Time: **10 mins** | Yield: **3 cups** | Serving Size: **1½ cups**

Ingredients

- 3 TB. toasted sesame oil
- 4 oz. (110g) fresh shiitake mushrooms, sliced
- 1 garlic clove, minced
- 1 lb. (450g) baby bok choy, trimmed and sliced
- 1 TB. wheat-free tamari or coconut aminos
- ¼ tsp. sea salt
- 1 TB. toasted sesame seeds

1 Heat a large skillet over medium-high heat. When the skillet is hot, add toasted sesame oil and wait for 15 seconds.

2 Add shiitake mushrooms and sauté, stirring occasionally, for 3 to 5 minutes, or until golden. Add garlic and cook for an additional 2 minutes.

3 Add baby bok choy, wheat-free tamari, and sea salt, and cook for 2 to 3 minutes, or until greens are wilted. Sprinkle with toasted sesame seeds to serve.

For an alternate version, sauté vegetables in sweet virgin coconut oil and add a pinch of cayenne.

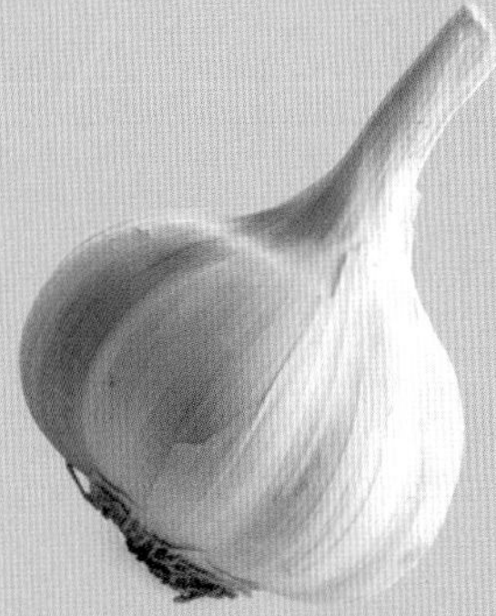

Nutrition per Serving

Fat 81% | Net Carb 9% | Protein 10% | Ratio 1.9:1

Calories	Fat	Protein	Total Carbohydrate	Dietary Fiber	Net Carbohydrate
255	23g	6g	11g	5g	6g

Tender mashed cauliflower is loaded up with sour cream, cream cheese, sharp cheddar, bacon bits, and ranch.

Loaded Cauliflower

Prep Time: **10 mins** Cook Time: **35 mins** Yield: **8 cups** Serving Size: **1 cup**

Ingredients

1 large head cauliflower, cut into florets

1 cup heavy cream

1 cup sour cream

4 oz. (110g) full-fat cream cheese

½ tsp. dried parsley

½ tsp. granulated garlic

½ tsp. onion powder

½ tsp. dried dill

½ tsp. freshly ground black pepper

½ tsp. sea salt

4 oz. (110g) grated sharp cheddar cheese

6 oz. (170g) uncured bacon, diced

¼ cup fresh chives, chopped

1 Preheat the oven to 350°F (180°C).

2 Place cauliflower florets in a large microwave-safe bowl with 1 inch (2.5cm) water at the bottom of the bowl.

3 Cover the bowl and microwave for 3 to 10 minutes, or until cauliflower is very tender. Drain.

4 Transfer cauliflower to a food processor. Add heavy cream, sour cream, cream cheese, dried parsley, granulated garlic, onion powder, dried dill, black pepper, and sea salt, and pulse until puréed.

5 Transfer mixture to a 9×13-inch (23×33cm) ceramic baking dish or Dutch oven and spread evenly in the pan.

6 Cover with sharp cheddar cheese. Bake for 15 to 20 minutes, or until cheese is golden and bubbly.

7 While cauliflower cooks, heat a medium skillet over medium heat. When the skillet is hot, add bacon and cook for 4 to 5 minutes, or until crisp. Place bacon on a paper towel to drain.

8 Remove cauliflower from the oven and let rest for 5 minutes. Sprinkle with bacon and chives to serve.

Nutrition per Serving

Fat **81%** Net Carb **7%**
Protein **12%** Ratio **1.9:1**

Calories	Fat	Protein	Total Carbohydrate	Dietary Fiber	Net Carbohydrate
321	29g	9g	8g	2g	6g

Cremini mushrooms and creamy leeks float in a rich Gruyère cheese sauce, scented with thyme and nutmeg.

Mushrooms Au Gratin

Prep Time: **10 mins**
Cook Time: **55 mins**

Yield: **4 cups**
Serving Size: **½ cup**

Ingredients

8 TB. unsalted butter

2 medium leeks, thinly sliced

2 garlic cloves, minced

1 lb. (450g) cremini mushrooms, trimmed and quartered

1 cup heavy cream

1 tsp. fresh thyme

¼ tsp. freshly grated nutmeg

¼ tsp. freshly ground black pepper

¼ tsp. sea salt

4 oz. (110g) Gruyère, grated

½ cup almond meal

½ cup grated Parmesan

Nutrition per Serving

Fat **81%** Net Carb **8%**
Protein **11%** Ratio **1.9:1**

Calories **356**
Fat **32g**
Protein **10g**
Total Carbohydrate **9g**
Dietary Fiber **2g**
Net Carbohydrate **7g**

While cremini mushrooms add an earthy flavor to this dish, you can also use white button mushrooms. Better yet, use a variety of wild mushrooms from your local farmer's market.

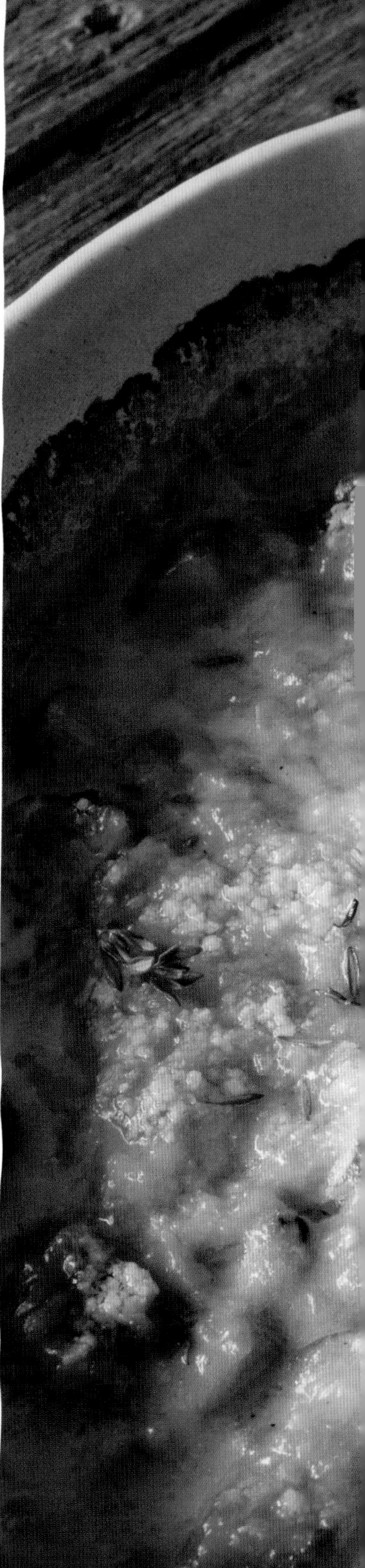

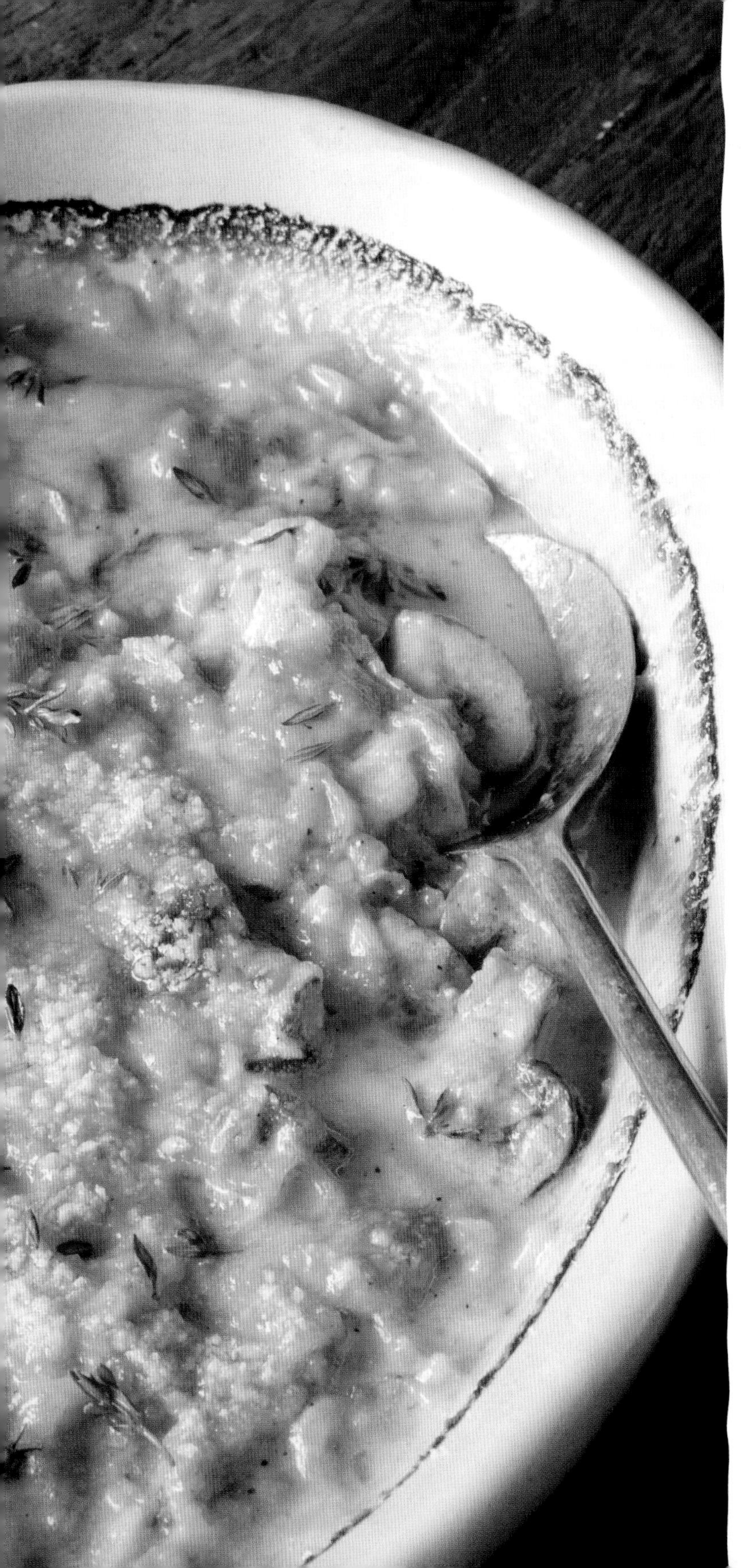

1. Preheat the oven to 400°F (200°C).

2. Heat a medium skillet over medium heat. When the skillet is hot, add 3 tablespoons unsalted butter.

3. Add leeks and cook for 8 to 10 minutes, or until softened.

4. Add garlic and cremini mushrooms and cook for 5 to 7 minutes, or until garlic is fragrant. Remove from heat.

5. Heat a small saucepan over medium heat. When the pan is hot, add remaining 5 tablespoons unsalted butter.

6. Stir in heavy cream, thyme, nutmeg, black pepper, and sea salt and bring to a light simmer. Simmer for 2 minutes, stirring occasionally.

7. Whisk in Gruyère and simmer until thickened, about 1 to 2 minutes.

8. Transfer mushrooms to an oven-proof ceramic or glass baking pan. Pour cheese sauce over mushrooms and top with almond meal and Parmesan.

9. Bake, uncovered, for 20 to 30 minutes, or until cheese is golden and bubbly. Let sit for 5 minutes before serving.

This classic is made with fresh green beans, a mushroom and Parmesan cream sauce, and crispy fried shallots.

Green Bean Casserole

Prep Time: 20 mins | Cook Time: 35 mins | Yield: 1 casserole | Serving Size: ⅙ casserole

Ingredients

- 1 lb. (450g) fresh green beans, trimmed and halved
- ¼ cup almond flour
- 2 TB. tapioca flour
- ½ tsp. sea salt
- 2 medium shallots, thinly sliced into rings
- 1 large egg, beaten
- ¼ cup safflower oil
- 3 TB. unsalted butter
- 8 medium white button mushrooms, sliced (about 8 oz.; 225g)
- 1 garlic clove, minced
- 1 cup heavy cream
- 1 cup grated Parmesan

1. Preheat the oven to 400°F (200°C). Fill a large pot with water and bring to a boil over high heat.
2. Add green beans and boil for 3 to 5 minutes, or until tender but firm. Immediately drain from water and run under cold water. Set aside.
3. In a small bowl, combine almond flour, tapioca flour, and sea salt. Dip shallot rings in egg. Dredge in flour mixture.
4. Heat a 10-inch (25cm) cast-iron skillet over medium-high heat. When the skillet is hot, add safflower oil. Wait for 15 seconds.
5. Add shallots to cover the bottom of the skillet. Fry, turning once, until shallots are deep brown and crispy, about 2 to 4 minutes. Remove and set on a paper towel.
6. Reheat the skillet over medium heat. Add unsalted butter and wait until melted.
7. Add white button mushrooms and garlic and sauté, stirring occasionally, for 4 to 6 minutes, or until softened and fragrant.
8. Pour heavy cream into the skillet, scraping up any browned bits from the bottom of the skillet. Lightly simmer, stirring frequently, for 2 minutes.
9. Stir Parmesan into cream and cook for an additional 1 minute. Remove from heat.
10. Stir green beans into cream sauce. Sprinkle with shallots. Bake for 15 to 20 minutes, or until green beans are tender. Serve immediately.

Nutrition per Serving

Fat 80% Net Carb 12%
Protein 8% Ratio 1.8:1

Calories	Fat	Protein	Total Carbohydrate	Dietary Fiber	Net Carbohydrate
417	37g	9g	15g	3g	12g

With bright broccoli smothered in a thick cheese sauce, this time-honored combination fits the keto profile wholly.

Broccoli with Cheese Sauce

Prep Time: **5 mins** Cook Time: **15 mins** Yield: **6 cups** Serving Size: **1 cup**

Ingredients

- 1 lb. (450g) broccoli florets
- 2 TB. unsalted butter
- 1 cup heavy cream
- 2 cups grated mild cheddar cheese
- ½ tsp. sea salt
- ½ tsp. smoked paprika (optional)

1 Fill a large pot with 1 inch (2.5cm) water. Place a steamer basket in the bottom of the pot. Cover and bring to a boil over high heat.

2 When water boils, remove lid and carefully place broccoli florets in the steamer basket. Replace cover and steam for 4 to 6 minutes, or until florets are bright green and tender.

3 Meanwhile, heat a small saucepan over medium-high heat. Add unsalted butter.

4 When butter melts, add heavy cream and bring to a light simmer. Simmer for 2 minutes.

5 Stir in mild cheddar cheese until thickened. Add sea salt and smoked paprika (if using) and stir. Spoon sauce over broccoli to serve.

This recipe can be modified for fresh cauliflower. Also, if you're pinched for time, you can use frozen florets instead of fresh.

Variation: To make **Broccoli with Yeast Gravy,** cook broccoli as instructed. Instead of using cheese sauce, melt 6 tablespoons salted butter. Stir 2 tablespoons nutritional yeast into butter and then drizzle over broccoli.

Nutrition per Serving

Fat 82% Net Carb 4%
Protein 14% Ratio 2.0:1

Calories	Fat	Protein	Total Carbohydrate	Dietary Fiber	Net Carbohydrate
352	32g	12g	6g	2g	4g

Emerald baby spinach is braised in silky coconut milk with a hint of nutmeg and cayenne and some crunchy cashews.

Coconut Creamed Spinach

Prep Time: **5 mins** | Cook Time: **5 mins** | Yield: **3 cups** | Serving Size: **¾ cup**

Ingredients

- 3 TB. coconut oil
- 1 garlic clove, minced
- 1 lb. (450g) baby spinach, coarsely chopped
- ¾ cup full-fat coconut milk
- ¼ tsp. freshly ground nutmeg
- ⅛ tsp. cayenne pepper (optional)
- ½ tsp. sea salt
- ½ cup cashews

1 Heat a large frying pan or skillet over medium-high heat. Add coconut oil and wait for 15 seconds.

2 Add garlic and cook for 30 seconds, or until fragrant. Add baby spinach, full-fat coconut milk, nutmeg, cayenne pepper (if using), and sea salt. Stir until wilted, or about 2 to 3 minutes.

3 Add cashews and stir to combine. Season with additional sea salt, if desired. Serve hot.

Variation: To make **Coconut Creamed Chard,** replace baby spinach with 1 pound (450g) Swiss chard, leaves chopped and stems finely chopped. Use 1 tablespoon minced shallot instead of garlic, and sauté the stems a few minutes before adding the leaves.

You can vary this recipe by using other spices, such as curry power or cardamom, to season the spinach.

Nutrition per Serving

Fat 82% Net Carb 10%
Protein 8% Ratio 2.0:1

Calories	Fat	Protein	Total Carbohydrate	Dietary Fiber	Net Carbohydrate
286	26g	6g	10g	3g	7g

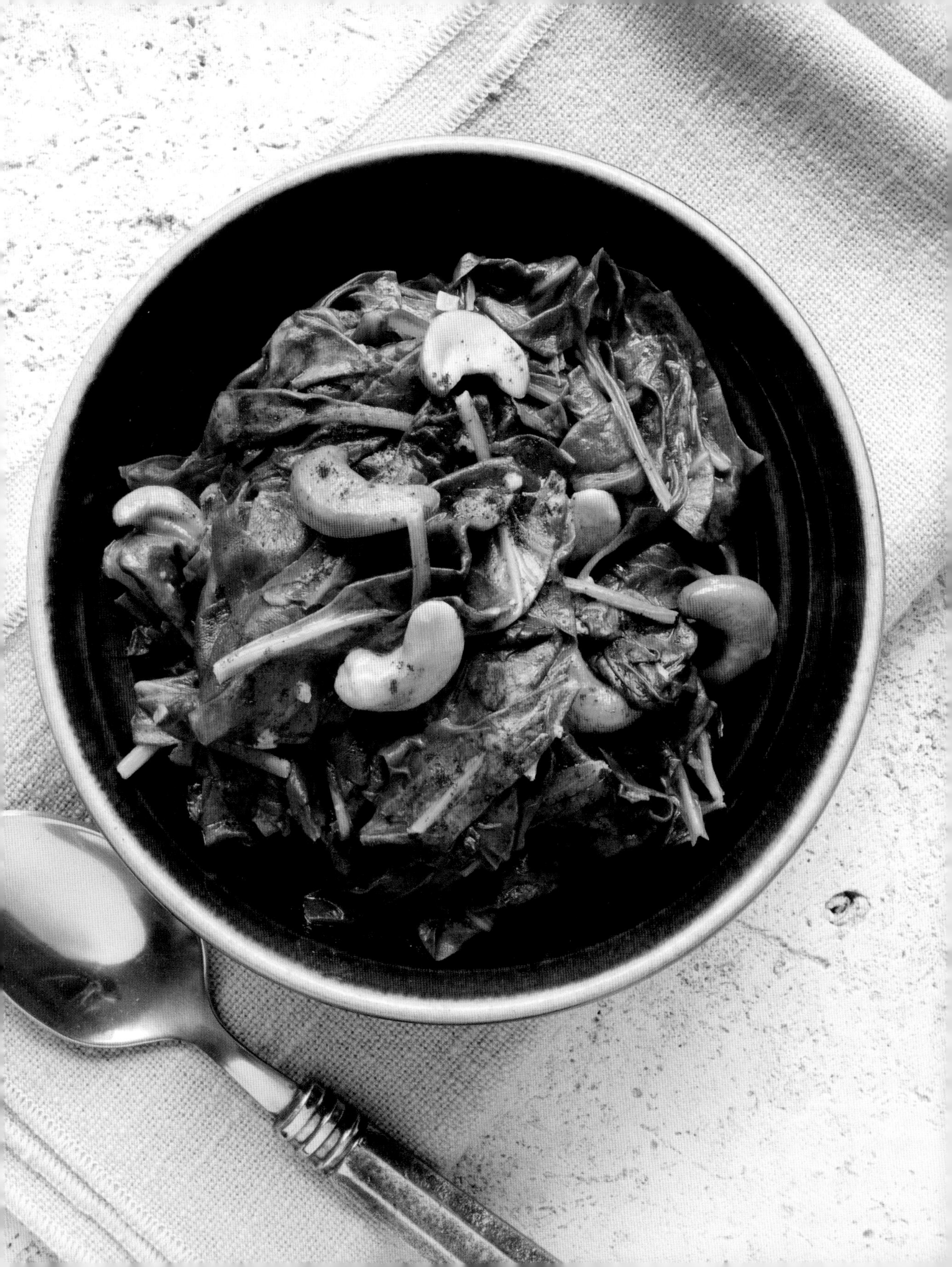

This colorful salad is a blend of crisp cabbage and sweet carrot, covered in a cider vinegar and Dijon dressing.

Creamy Coleslaw

Prep Time: **15 mins** Chill Time: **3 hours** Yield: **6 cups** Serving Size: **1 cup**

Ingredients

- 1 cup mayonnaise
- 1 TB. Dijon mustard
- 2 TB. apple cider vinegar
- 1 tsp. celery salt
- 1 TB. red onion, minced
- 1 large carrot, grated (about ½ cup)
- 5 cups green or purple cabbage, grated

1. In a large bowl, whisk mayonnaise, Dijon mustard, apple cider vinegar, celery salt, and red onion.
2. Add carrot and green cabbage and toss to combine. Refrigerate for 2 to 3 hours before serving.

Variation: Add 2 tablespoons hot pepper sauce instead of Dijon mustard and 1 teaspoon smoked paprika to the dressing mixture to make **Smoky Red Slaw.**

This coleslaw can be made up to 48 hours ahead of time, making it a great choice for holiday gatherings or parties.

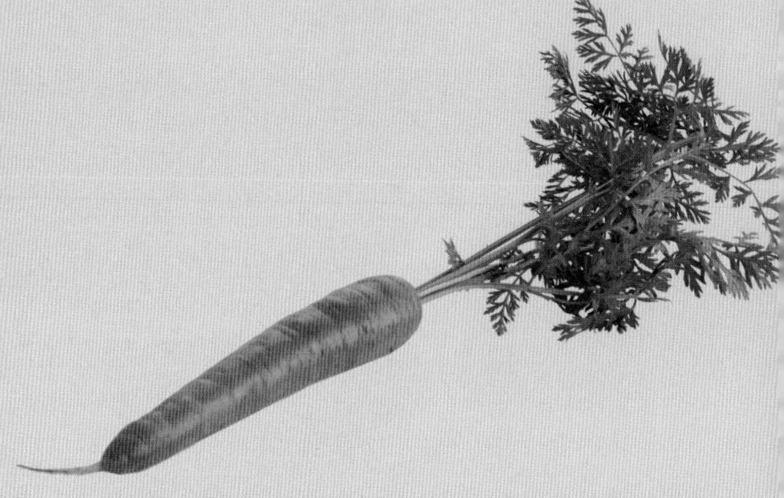

Nutrition per Serving

Fat 95% Net Carb 3%
Protein 2% Ratio 9.3:1

Calories	Fat	Protein	Total Carbohydrate	Dietary Fiber	Net Carbohydrate
264	28g	1g	6g	4g	2g

This simple side salad is quick and easy, with mixed greens, creamy avocado, and a super-fast oil and vinegar dressing.

Keto Side Salad

Prep Time: **10 mins**	Cook Time: **none**	Yield: **2 salads**	Serving Size: **1 salad**

Ingredients

- 3 cups mixed greens
- 2 TB. extra-virgin olive oil
- 1 TB. balsamic vinegar
- ¼ tsp. sea salt
- ½ medium avocado, diced
- 2 green onions, thinly sliced
- 2 TB. raw sunflower seeds
- 2 oz. (55g) chèvre, crumbled

1 In a large bowl, combine mixed greens, extra-virgin olive oil, balsamic vinegar, and sea salt. Toss to coat.

2 Divide greens into 2 bowls. Top with avocado, green onions, raw sunflower seeds, and chèvre and serve.

For a more kid-friendly version, you can use lemon juice instead of balsamic vinegar, replace the chèvre with ½ cup grated mild cheddar cheese, and eliminate the green onions.

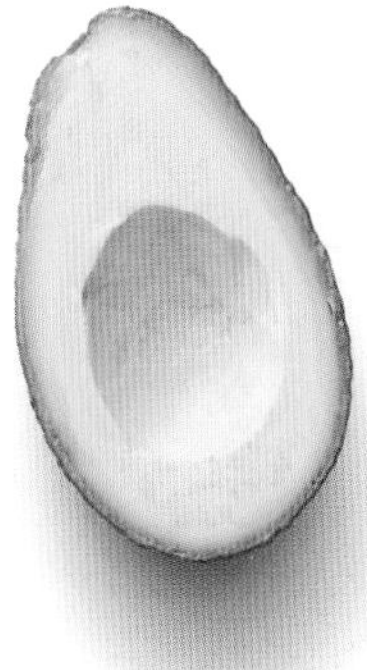

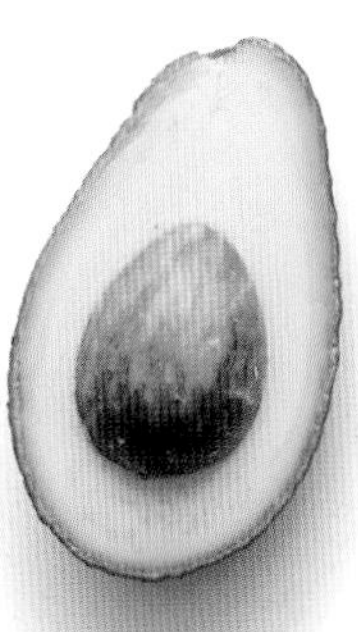

Nutrition per Serving

Fat	82%	Net Carb	6%
Protein	12%	Ratio	2.0:1

Calories	Fat	Protein	Total Carbohydrate	Dietary Fiber	Net Carbohydrate
330	30g	10g	11g	6g	5g

Tender asparagus spears are roasted with salty Serrano ham and drizzled with a rich Mahón cheese sauce.

Serrano-Wrapped Asparagus with Mahón

Prep Time: **10 mins** Cook Time: **20 mins** Yield: **12 spears** Serving Size: **3 spears**

Ingredients

6 thin Serrano ham slices (about 3 oz.; 85g)

12 asparagus spears

1 TB. extra-virgin olive oil

¾ cup heavy cream

4 oz. (110g) Mahón, grated

½ tsp. smoked paprika

¼ tsp. freshly ground black pepper

1 Preheat the oven to 400°F (200°C). Cut Serrano ham slices in half lengthwise to create 2 long strips from each slice.

2 Wrap each asparagus spear with Serrano ham. Place on a baking sheet and drizzle with extra-virgin olive oil.

3 Place the baking sheet in the oven and bake for 10 to 12 minutes, or until asparagus is tender.

4 Meanwhile, heat a small saucepan over medium-high heat. Add heavy cream and bring to a boil. Boil, stirring constantly, for 1 minute.

5 Add Mahón. Cook, stirring constantly, for 3 to 5 minutes, or until a smooth consistency forms. Remove from heat.

6 To serve, drizzle Mahón sauce over baked asparagus spears and then sprinkle with smoked paprika and black pepper.

If you have trouble finding Serrano ham and Mahón, you can substitute prosciutto and Gouda, respectively.

Nutrition per Serving

Fat **82%** Net Carb **3%**
Protein **15%** Ratio **2.1:1**

Calories	Fat	Protein	Total Carbohydrate	Dietary Fiber	Net Carbohydrate
352	32g	13g	4g	1g	3g

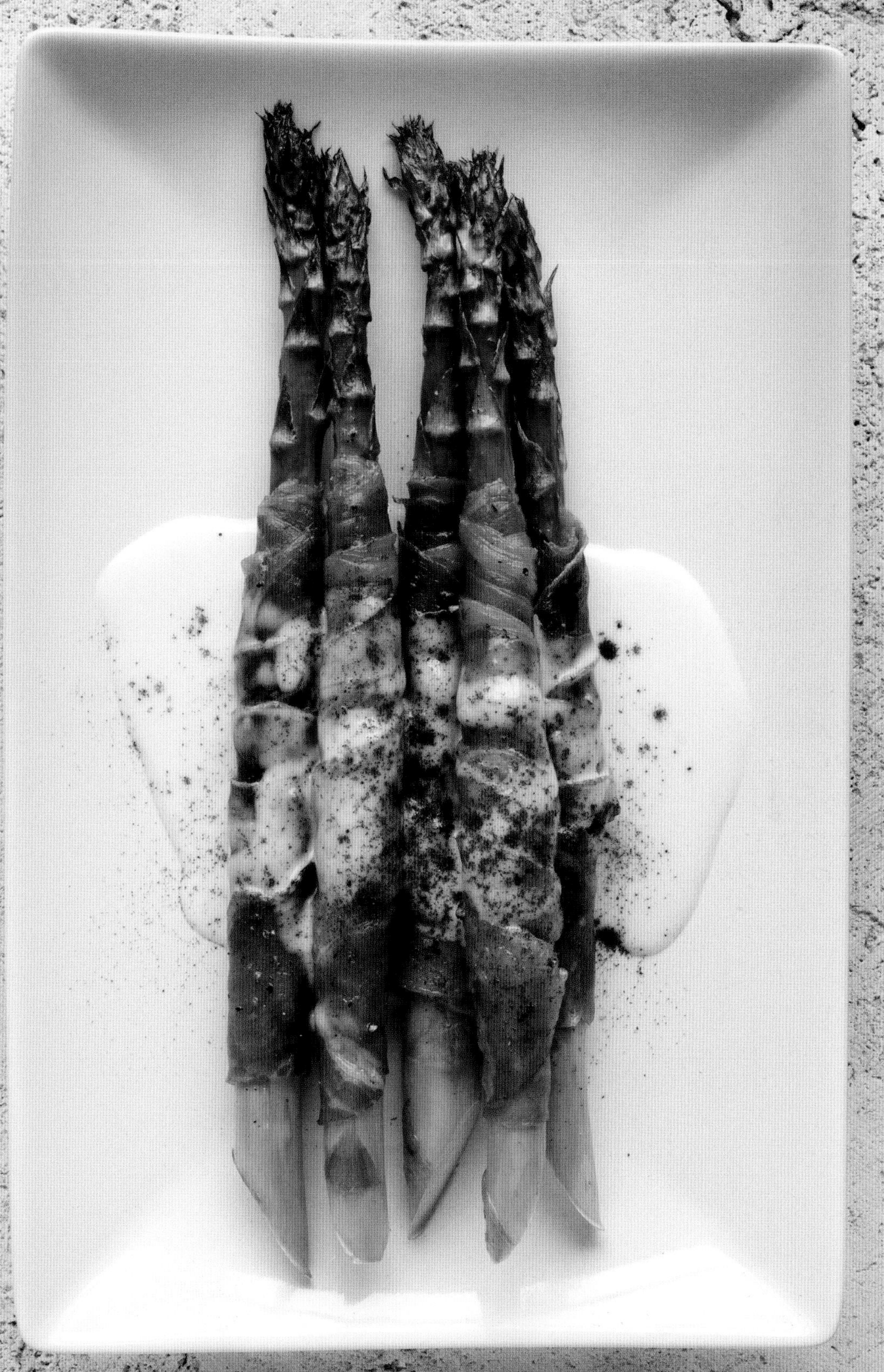

Desserts

If you enjoy dessert, you've probably thought a low-carb diet is not for you. While you'll find your cravings for sweets may change and level off as you adapt to the keto diet, you don't have to deprive yourself of the occasional sweet treat. In fact, you can enjoy some pretty decadent desserts while on this diet. From almond truffles to mini-cheesecakes, the rich recipes in this chapter satisfy even the most powerful sweet tooth.

These enticing toasty coconut bites have a hidden almond center and a lavish dark chocolate coating.

Coconut Almond Bites

Prep Time: **40 minutes** | Cook Time: **12 mins** | Yield: **16 bites** | Serving Size: **2 bites**

Ingredients

- 2 large egg whites
- 2 tsp. raw honey
- 1 tsp. pure almond extract
- 2 cups unsweetened shredded coconut
- 16 whole almonds
- 4 oz. (110g) 85 percent cacao dark chocolate bar
- 1 TB. coconut oil

1 Preheat the oven to 350°F (180°C). Line a rimmed metal baking sheet with a piece of parchment paper. (Alternately, use a silicone baking mat to prevent sticking.)

2 In a medium bowl, whisk egg whites, raw honey, and almond extract. Add unsweetened coconut and mix until combined.

3 Form coconut mixture around 1 whole almond to make a round ball about 1½ inches (3.75cm) in diameter. Place on the parchment paper. Repeat with remaining almonds to make 16 balls.

4 Bake for 10 to 12 minutes, or until coconut is a deep golden brown. Remove from the oven and cool completely.

5 When bites have cooled, chop or break dark chocolate bar into small pieces. Place chocolate and coconut oil in a heavy-bottomed saucepan over low heat.

6 When chocolate begins to melt, stir constantly to prevent scorching until completely melted, about 1 minute. Remove from heat.

7 Drizzle chocolate over coconut bites. Let cool completely before serving or storing in an airtight container.

If you really love chocolate, you can dip the coconut bites into it instead of just drizzling it on top.

Nutrition per Serving

Fat **81%** Net Carb **13%**
Protein **6%** Ratio **1.8:1**

Calories **268**
Fat **24g**
Protein **4g**
Total Carbohydrate **14g**
Dietary Fiber **5g**
Net Carbohydrate **9g**

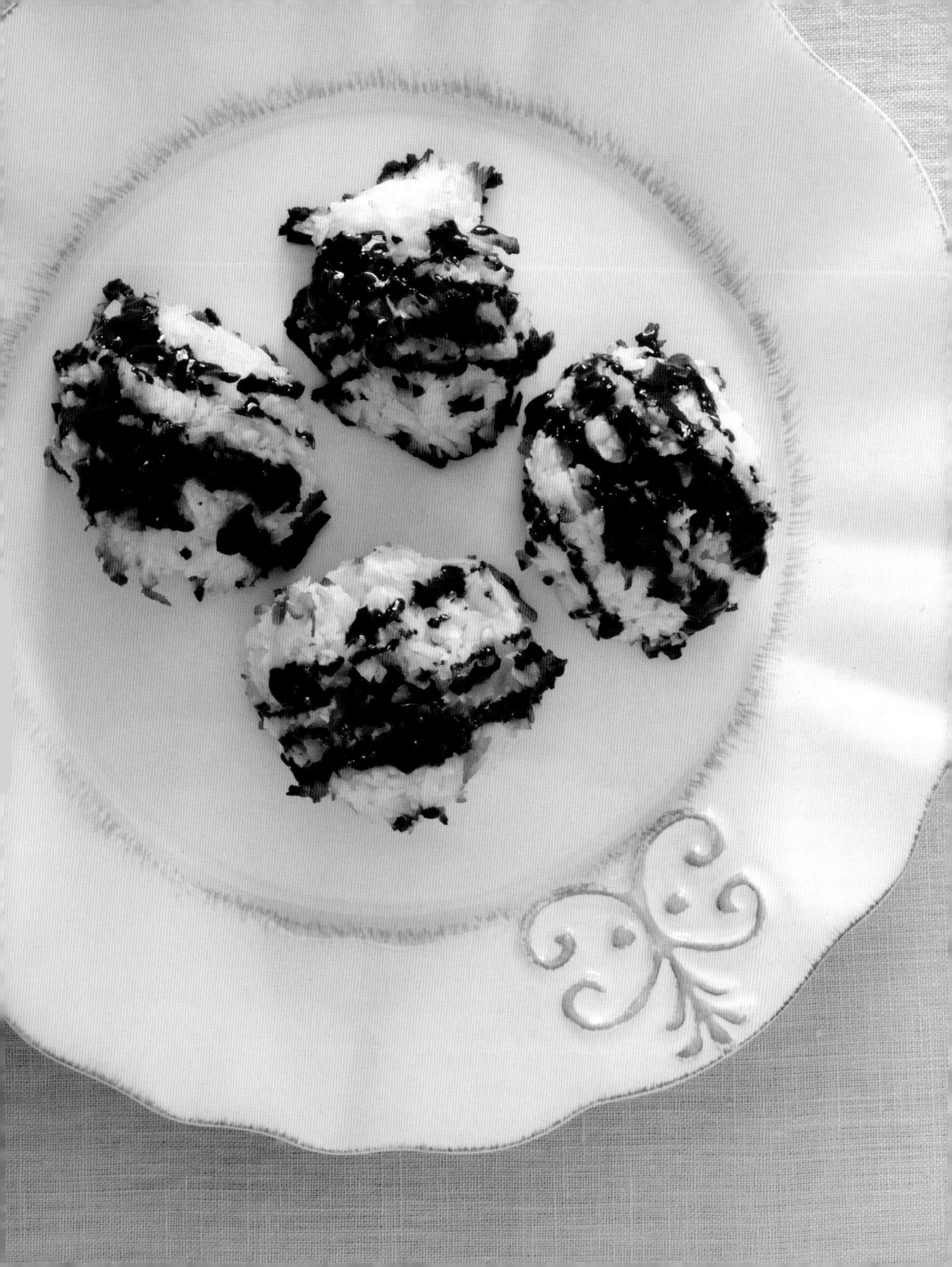

These colorful mini-cheesecakes—topped with fluffy whipped cream and fresh berries—are real crowd-pleasers.

Mini-Cheesecakes with Fresh Berries

Prep Time: 1 hr, 10 mins
Cook Time: 30 mins
Yield: 12 mini-cheesecakes
Serving Size: 1 mini-cheesecake

Ingredients

- 1½ cups pecans
- 4 TB. unsalted butter, melted
- ⅛ tsp. sea salt
- 2½ tsp. powdered stevia
- 3 (8-oz.; 225g) pkg. cream cheese, at room temperature
- 1½ tsp. pure vanilla extract
- 2 large eggs, beaten
- 1 cup heavy whipping cream
- 1 tsp. liquid stevia
- ¾ cup fresh berries of choice

Nutrition per Serving

Fat 90%
Net Carb 4%
Protein 6%
Ratio 3.8:1

Calories 422
Fat 42g
Protein 6g
Total Carbohydrate 6g
Dietary Fiber 1g
Net Carbohydrate 5g

What is stevia? Stevia is a natural sugar substitute from the leaves of the stevia plant. While it's much sweeter than sugar, it doesn't adversely affect your blood glucose level.

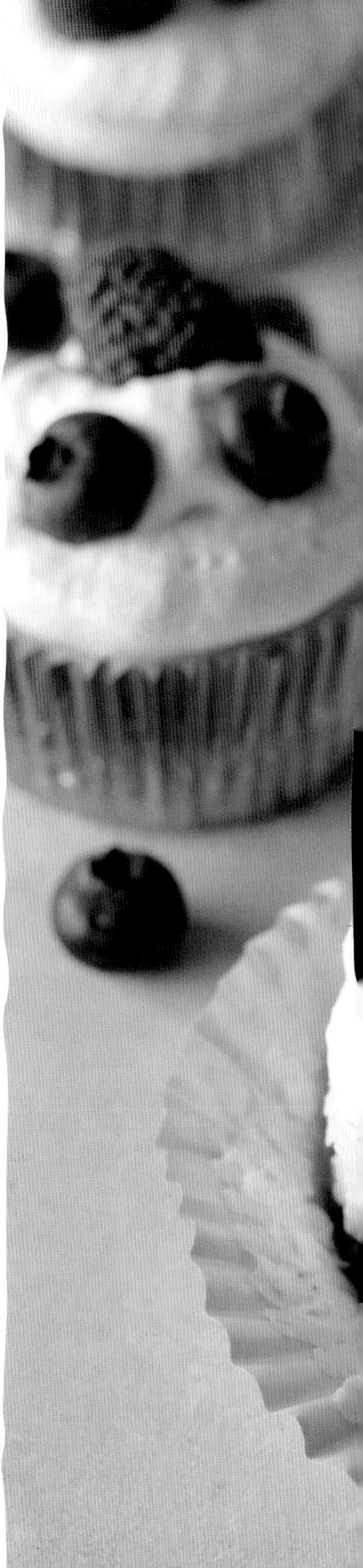

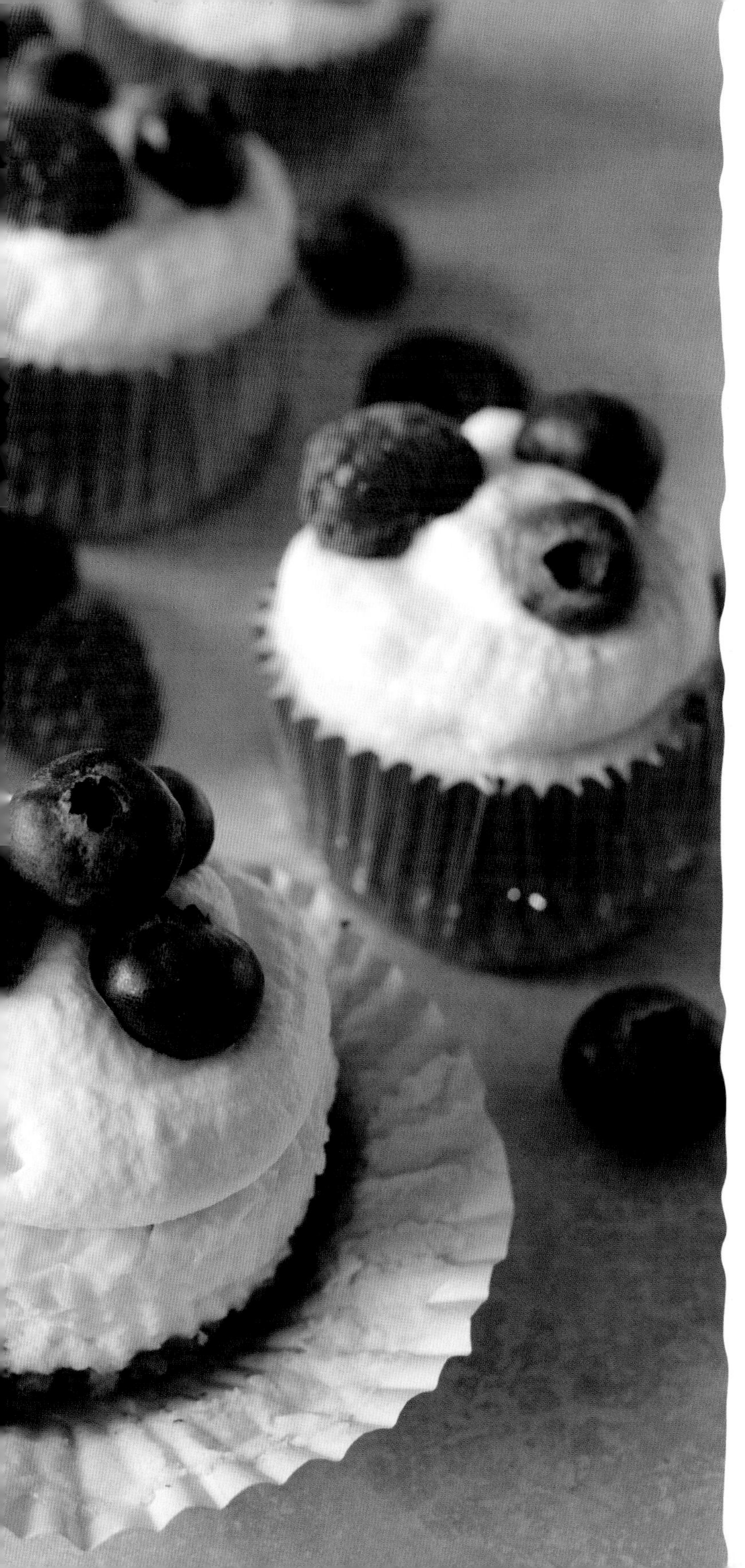

1. Preheat the oven to 350°F (180°C).

2. Place pecans in a food processor and pulse until finely chopped.

3. Combine pecans, unsalted butter, sea salt, and ½ teaspoon powdered stevia and mix until fully blended.

4. Place 12 paper muffin cups in a muffin tin. (Alternately, you can use a silicone muffin pan without the paper liners.)

5. Divide pecan mixture evenly into the muffin cups. Press into the bottom of each cup. Bake for 5 minutes.

6. In a stand mixer, beat cream cheese, 1 teaspoon vanilla extract, and remaining 2 teaspoons powdered stevia until light and creamy. Add eggs and beat just until incorporated.

7. Pour or scoop cream cheese mixture evenly into muffin cups over baked crusts. Bake for 20 to 25 minutes, or until set in the middle. Remove from the oven and chill for at least 1 hour.

8. Shortly before serving, whip heavy whipping cream, liquid stevia, and remaining ½ teaspoon vanilla extract until soft peaks form. Frost chilled cheesecakes with whipped cream and top with fresh berries to serve.

Honey-sweetened peanut butter is surrounded by dark chocolate in this nod to a dessert favorite.

Chocolate Peanut Butter Cups

Prep Time: **20 mins** Chill Time: **2 hrs** Yield: **12 muffin cups** Serving Size: **1 muffin cup**

Ingredients

- 7 oz. (200g) 85 percent cacao chocolate bar
- ¼ cup coconut oil
- ¾ cup unsweetened peanut butter
- 2 TB. raw honey
- ⅛ tsp. sea salt

1. Break chocolate bar into small pieces. Heat a small saucepan or double boiler over low heat. Add chocolate pieces and coconut oil and stir occasionally until melted, about 3 to 5 minutes.

2. Line a 12-cup muffin tin with paper liners. Pour a ⅛-inch (3mm) layer of chocolate in the bottom of each paper liner. Place in the freezer for 10 minutes.

3. Meanwhile, in a medium bowl, combine unsweetened peanut butter, raw honey, and sea salt and mix well.

4. Remove chocolate cups from freezer. Spoon peanut butter mixture into the cups, and then drizzle with remaining chocolate (You may need to reheat chocolate slightly and whisk to remove clumps.)

5. Refrigerate for 2 hours, or until chocolate hardens. Serve cold, and keep refrigerated to store.

If you can't or don't eat peanut butter, you can substitute unsweetened almond or cashew butter instead.

Nutrition per Serving

Fat **75%** Net Carb **17%**
Protein **8%** Ratio **1.3:1**

Calories	Fat	Protein	Total Carbohydrate	Dietary Fiber	Net Carbohydrate
240	20g	5g	13g	3g	10g

Sweet diced mango flavors this creamy coconut and chia pudding, topped with a pop of toasted sesame seeds.

Mango Coconut Pudding

Prep Time: **5 mins** | Chill Time: **8 hrs** | Yield: **2 cups** | Serving Size: **½ cup**

Ingredients

- 1 (14-fl.-oz.; 400ml) can full-fat coconut milk
- ⅓ cup white chia seeds
- 1 cup mango, diced
- 1 TB. toasted sesame seeds (optional)

1. In a medium bowl, combine coconut milk, white chia seeds, and mango and mix well.
2. Cover the bowl and refrigerate for at least 8 hours or until gelled and thickened.
3. Sprinkle with toasted sesame seeds (if using) to serve.

Variation: To make **Chocolate Raspberry Pudding,** replace mango with 1 cup fresh or frozen raspberries, and add ¼ cup unsweetened cocoa powder and ½ teaspoon almond extract. Eliminate toasted sesame seeds.

If mango isn't in season when you're making this recipe, you can replace it with fresh peach or strawberry slices.

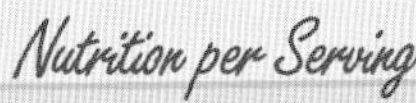

Fat 81% Net Carb 12%
Protein 7% Ratio 1.9:1

Calories	Fat	Protein	Total Carbohydrate	Dietary Fiber	Net Carbohydrate
299	27g	5g	15g	6g	9g

These decadent truffles boast elegant flavors of dark, bittersweet chocolate and pure almond extract.

Almond Truffles

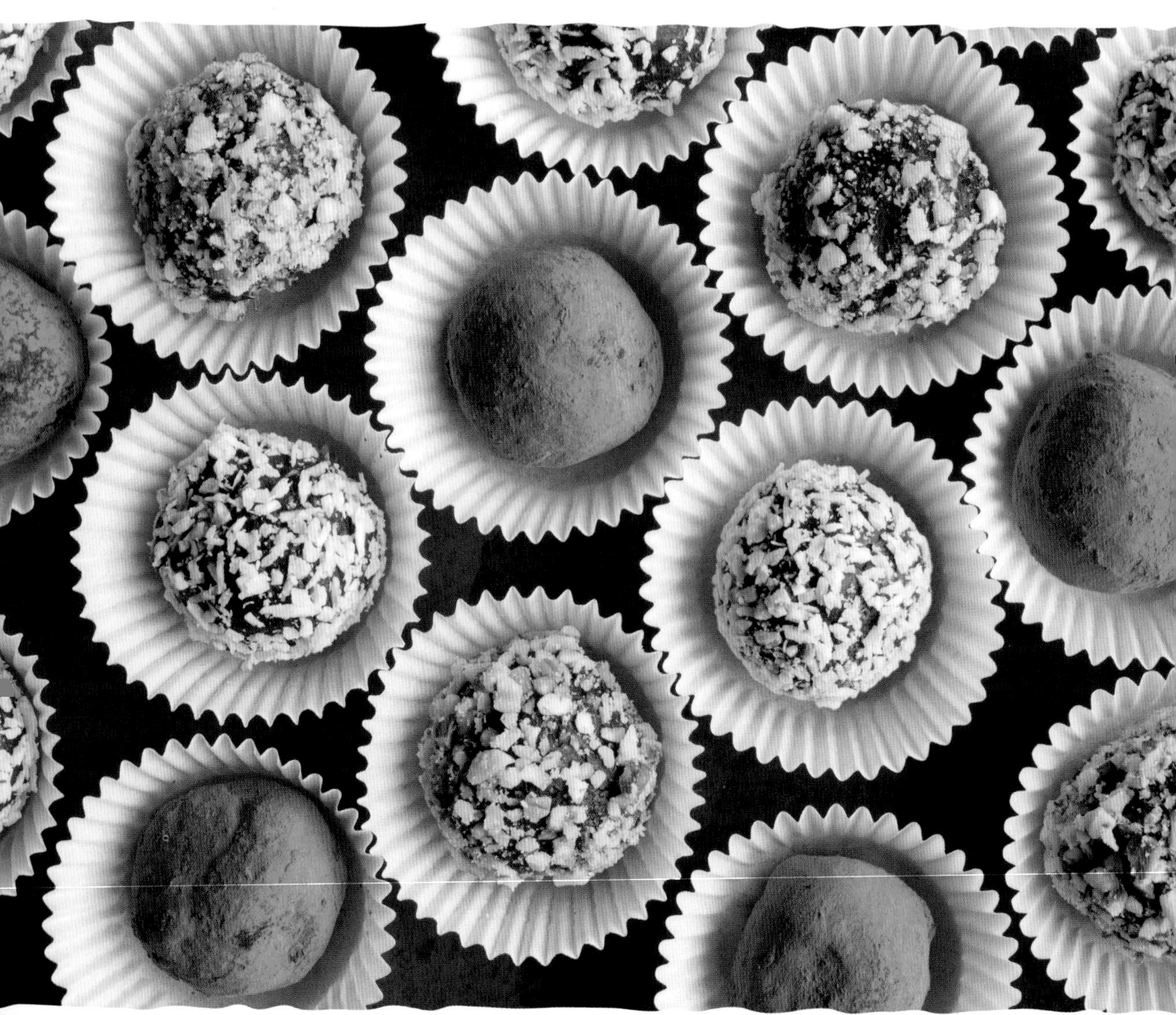

Prep Time: **1 hr, 15 mins** Cook Time: **5 mins** Yield: **24 truffles** Serving Size: **4 truffles**

Ingredients

- 8 oz. (225g) 75 percent or higher chocolate
- 4 fl. oz. (120ml) heavy cream (about ½ cup)
- 1 tsp. almond extract
- ¼ cup unsweetened cocoa powder

1. Chop chocolate into very small pieces. Place in a medium bowl.
2. Heat a small heavy-bottomed saucepan over low heat. Add heavy cream and bring to a simmer, occasionally scraping down the edges of the pan with a rubber scraper. Add almond extract and stir. Remove from heat.
3. Pour hot cream over chocolate pieces. Wait for 1 minute and vigorously whisk until chocolate is fully melted and smooth.
4. Spread chocolate in a thin layer on a parchment-lined baking sheet. Refrigerate for 1 hour.
5. Using a sturdy metal spoon, scoop 1-inch (2.5cm) mounds of chocolate. Use your hands to quickly roll each mound into a smooth ball.
6. Immediately roll each ball in unsweetened cocoa powder. Place each in a small paper or foil wrapper, or store on a clean sheet of parchment.
7. Serve truffles immediately or store in the refrigerator.

The truffles are only as good as the chocolate you use. Look for high-quality bars of at least 75 percent cacao.

Nutrition per Serving

Fat **79%** Net Carb **15%**
Protein **6%** Ratio **1.7:1**

Calories **136**
Fat **12g**
Protein **2g**
Total Carbohydrate **8g**
Dietary Fiber **3g**
Net Carbohydrate **5g**

Variation: To make **Cherry Hazelnut Truffles,** replace almond extract with 1 teaspoon cherry extract and roll truffles in chopped hazelnuts. Or you can make **Vanilla Coconut Truffles** by using 1 teaspoon vanilla extract and coating truffles in shredded unsweetened coconut flakes.

Smooth pumpkin custard is sweetened with maple syrup and topped with vanilla whipped cream.

Pumpkin Custard Cups

Prep Time: **10 mins** Cook Time: **35 mins** Yield: **8 custard cups** Serving Size: **1 custard cup**

Ingredients

- 3 eggs, beaten
- 2 cups heavy cream
- 1 (15-oz.; 420g) can cooked, puréed pumpkin
- ½ tsp. ground cinnamon
- ½ tsp. freshly ground nutmeg
- ¼ tsp. ground cloves
- ⅛ tsp. sea salt
- 3 TB. pure grade B maple syrup
- 1 tsp. pure vanilla extract

1 Preheat the oven to 350°F (180°C). In a large bowl, combine eggs, 1 cup heavy cream, puréed pumpkin, cinnamon, nutmeg, cloves, sea salt, 2 tablespoons grade B maple syrup, and ½ teaspoon vanilla extract. Beat with a stand or hand mixer until smooth.

2 Pour batter evenly into 6 small 1-cup oven-proof baking cups or ceramic crocks.

3 Bake for 25 to 35 minutes, or until a toothpick inserted into the center comes out clean. Remove from the oven and cool completely.

4 Shortly before serving, in a medium bowl, whip remaining 1 cup heavy cream, remaining ½ teaspoon vanilla extract, and remaining 1 tablespoon maple syrup until fluffy.

5 Serve cooled custard in the baking cups, topped with a dollop of whipped cream.

To adapt this recipe for 12 muffin cups, place 12 paper liners in the pan and reduce the time by 5 to 10 minutes.

Nutrition per Serving

Fat 81% Net Carb 13%
Protein 6% Ratio 1.8:1

Calories	Fat	Protein	Total Carbohydrate	Dietary Fiber	Net Carbohydrate
268	24g	4g	11g	2g	9g

Thick slabs of rich coconut and macadamia nut "fudge" are sweetened with maple syrup and loaded with walnuts.

Maple Walnut and Macadamia "Fudge"

Prep Time: **10 mins** Chill Time: **3 hours** Yield: **12 bars** Serving Size: **1 bar**

Ingredients

- 1 cup raw macadamia nuts
- ½ tsp. maple extract
- 2 TB. pure grade B maple syrup
- ¾ cup virgin coconut oil, melted
- ¼ tsp. sea salt
- ½ cup walnuts, chopped

1. In a small food processor, pulse raw macadamia nuts until a dough texture forms.
2. Add maple extract, grade B maple syrup, virgin coconut oil, and sea salt and purée until blended.
3. Line a small 5¾×3¼×2-inch (14.5×8.25×5cm) loaf pan with parchment paper. (Alternately, line a 12-cup muffin tin with paper liners.)
4. Spread walnuts evenly in the bottom of the loaf pan. Pour fudge over top.
5. Refrigerate for 2 to 3 hours, or until firm. Cut into 12 equal slices and serve.

Maple extract gives this fudge a unique flavor, but if you have trouble finding it, you can use ½ tsp. vanilla extract instead.

Nutrition per Serving

Fat 92% Net Carb 5%
Protein 3% Ratio 5.0:1

Calories	Fat	Protein	Total Carbohydrate	Dietary Fiber	Net Carbohydrate
245	25g	2g	4g	1g	3g

Sweet coconut sugar stars in this silky coconut cream pie, served in a crisp almond flour crust.

Coconut Cream Pie

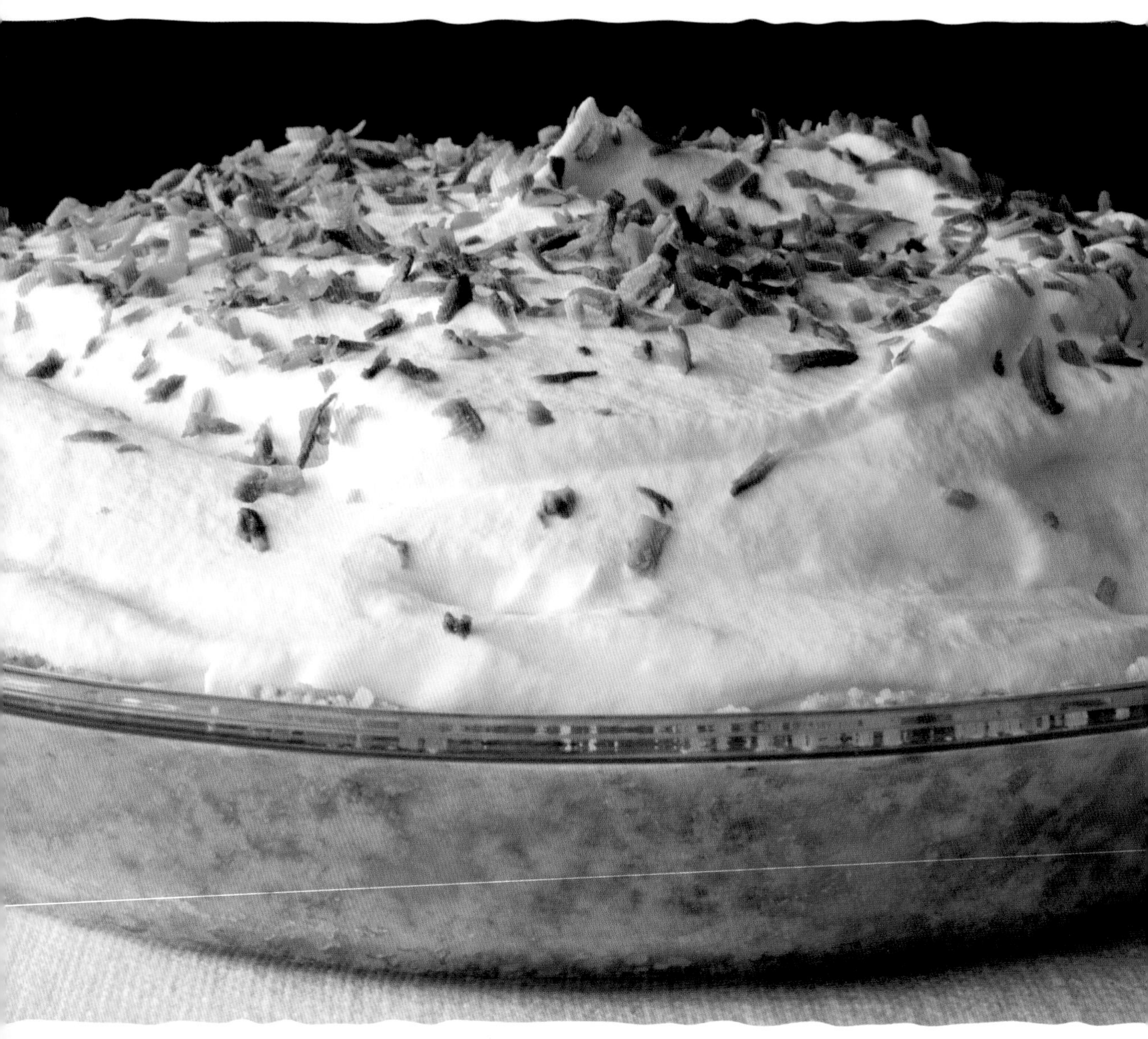

Prep Time: **1 hr, 15 mins** Cook Time: **15 mins** Yield: **1 pie** Serving Size: **1/12 pie**

Ingredients

- 1¼ cups almond flour
- 8 tsp. coconut sugar
- 3 TB. salted butter, melted
- ¾ cup unsweetened shredded coconut
- 1 (14-fl.-oz.; 400ml) can full-fat coconut milk
- 1 tsp. pure vanilla extract
- 1 (1.8g) pkg. powdered gelatin (about 1 scant TB.)
- 2 cups heavy cream
- 1 TB. raw honey

Nutrition per Serving

Fat **84%** Net Carb **10%**
Protein **6%** Ratio **2.4:1**

Calories **362**
Fat **34g**
Protein **5g**
Total Carbohydrate **11g**
Dietary Fiber **2g**
Net Carbohydrate **9g**

1. Preheat the oven to 350°F (180°C). In a medium bowl, mix almond flour, 2 teaspoons coconut sugar, and salted butter until fully combined. Press into the bottom of a 9-inch (23cm) pie pan. Bake for 10 minutes or until golden brown. Remove crust and cool for 10 minutes.

2. While crust bakes, spread ¼ cup unsweetened shredded coconut on a rimmed metal baking sheet. Bake alongside crust for 2 to 4 minutes, or until browned and toasted. (Watch carefully so coconut does not burn!) Remove from the oven and cool for later use.

3. In a medium saucepan, combine full-fat coconut milk, ½ teaspoon vanilla extract, remaining 6 teaspoons coconut sugar, and remaining ½ cup unsweetened shredded coconut over medium heat. Heat until coconut sugar dissolves, stirring occasionally, for about 5 minutes. Do not boil.

4. Mix gelatin with 2 tablespoons cold water. Whisk until gelatin dissolves. Stir mixture into warm coconut milk and whisk until fully dissolved. Pour coconut cream filling into cooled pie crust. Chill for at least 1 hour to set gelatin.

5. Shortly before serving, whip heavy cream, raw honey, and remaining ½ teaspoon vanilla extract for 2 to 4 minutes, or until soft peaks form.

6. Spread whipped cream in an even layer over chilled pie. Sprinkle with coconut to serve.

Variation: To make **Chocolate Coconut Cream Pie,** add ¼ cup unsweetened cocoa powder to the filling mixture in step 3. Sprinkle pie with ¼ cup miniature bittersweet chocolate chips, along with the ¼ cup toasted coconut.

Index

A

B

C

D

M–N–O

P–Q

R

S

T–U–V

W–X–Y–Z

About the Authors

Molly Pearl is a writer, recipe developer, and food photographer living in Portland, Oregon. She is the author of *Idiot's Guides: Mediterranean Paleo Cookbook* and *Idiot's Guides: Paleo Slow Cooking,* and has contributed recipes to *The Complete Idiot's Guide to Eating Paleo*. She was the recipe and meal plan creator for Paleo Plan (paleoplan.com) for 5 years, has written recipes for Jimmy Moore's Livin' Low-Carb Meal Plan, and collaborated with others to develop meal plans and recipes for Mark Sisson's Primal Blueprint website. She and her husband, Jason, currently write for Knives and Pearls: Primal Recipes for the Civilized Cook (knivesandpearls.com).

Kelly Roehl, MS, RD, LDN, CNSC, is a registered dietitian and nutritionist at Rush University Medical Center in Chicago, Illinois. Well-known in the keto community, Kelly specializes in ketogenic diet therapy for both adult and pediatric patients for the treatment of epilepsy and other neurological conditions, as well as weight loss. Kelly has presented her award-winning research on the benefits of the ketogenic diet at multiple international conferences and is an avid keto-dieter herself.

Acknowledgments

Molly Pearl: Thanks to my husband, Jason, for his ceaseless support and encouragement, as well as his creative eye in styling and photographing this book. Jason, you are my co-author. Thanks for walking alongside me on this project.

Thanks to the Owen family in Wisconsin and the Peters family in Nebraska for giving us so many Midwest recipes to draw inspiration from.

Kelly Roehl: Thank you to my family, friends, and colleagues for your unconditional love and support. Thanks as well to my patients, clients, and students, who inspire me every day!

HELEN PLUM MEMORIAL LIBRARY
3 1502 00792 1685

Y
796
.32364
CHICAGO

Please check all items for damages
before leaving the Library.
Thereafter you will be held
responsible for all injuries
to items beyond reasonable wear.

Helen M. Plum Memorial Library

Lombard, Illinois

A daily fine will be charged for
overdue materials.

JAN 2015

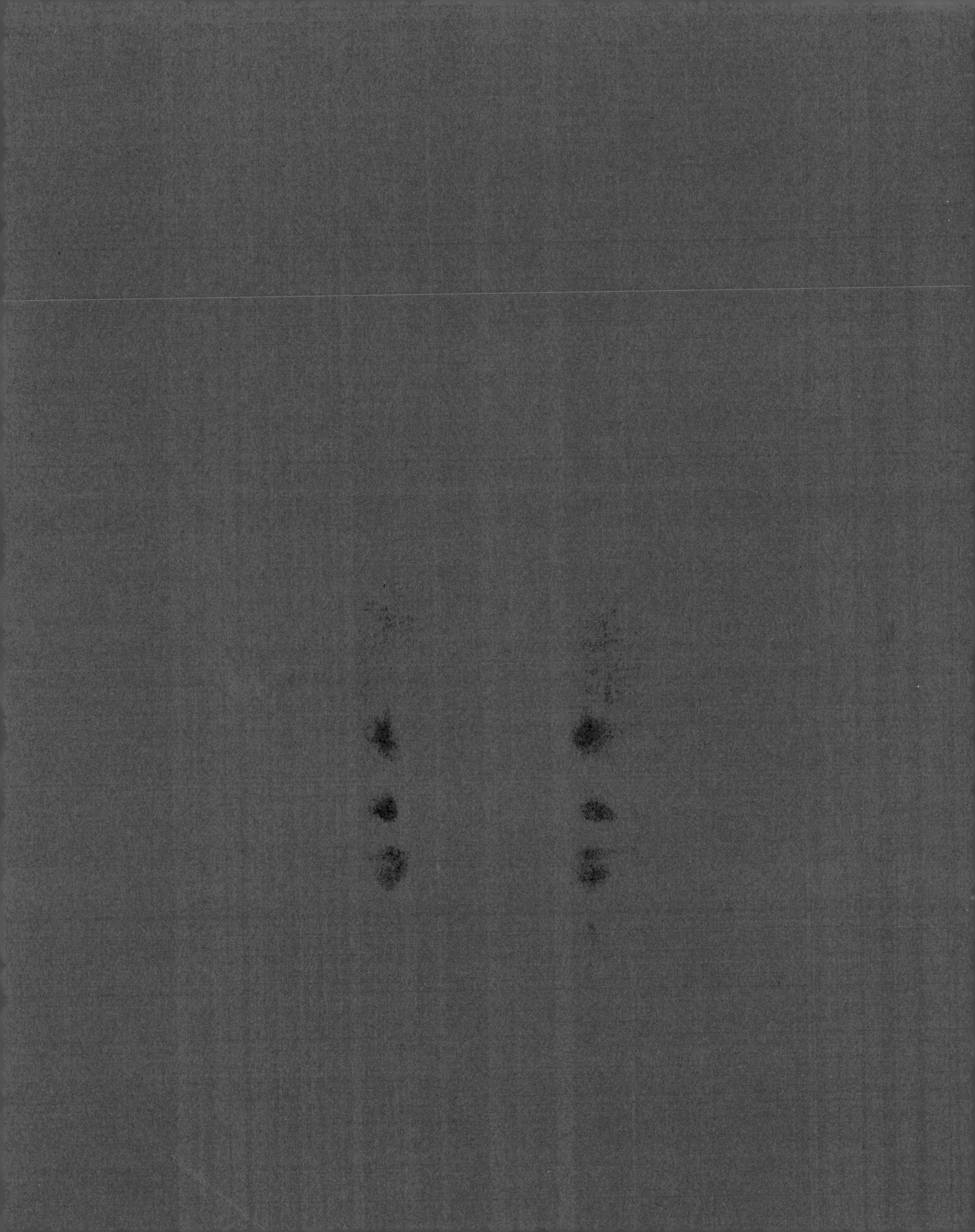

THE STORY OF THE CHICAGO BULLS

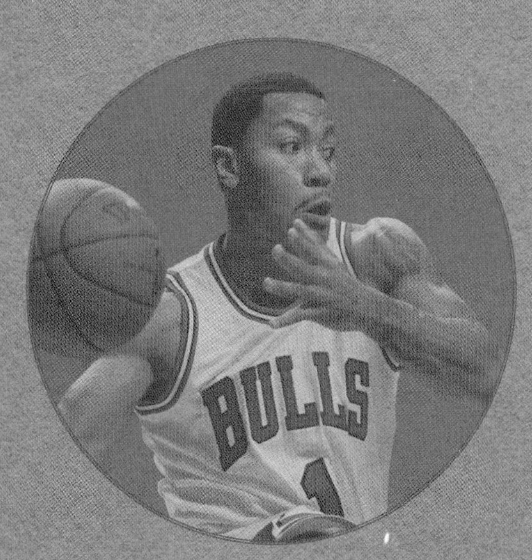

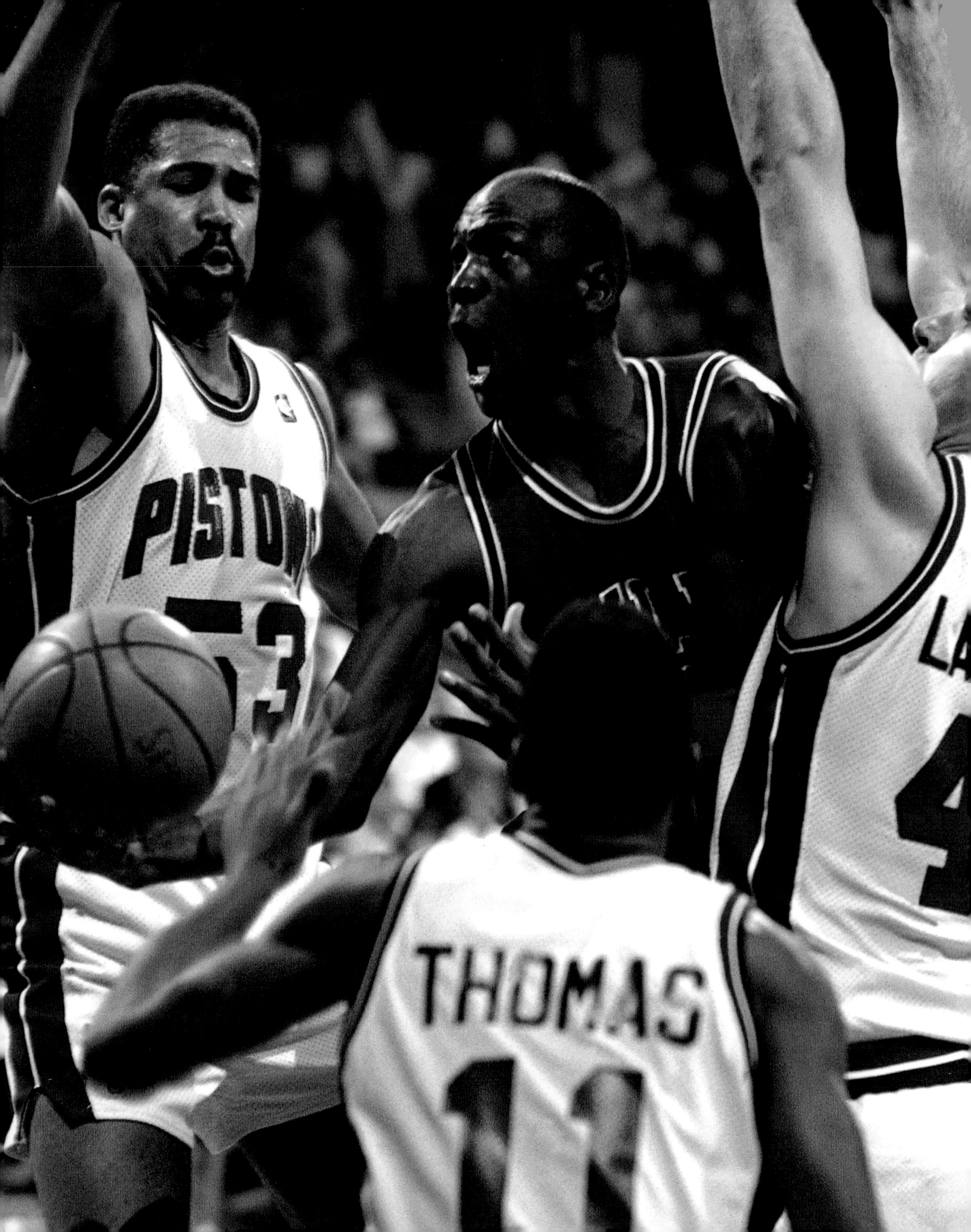
THOMAS

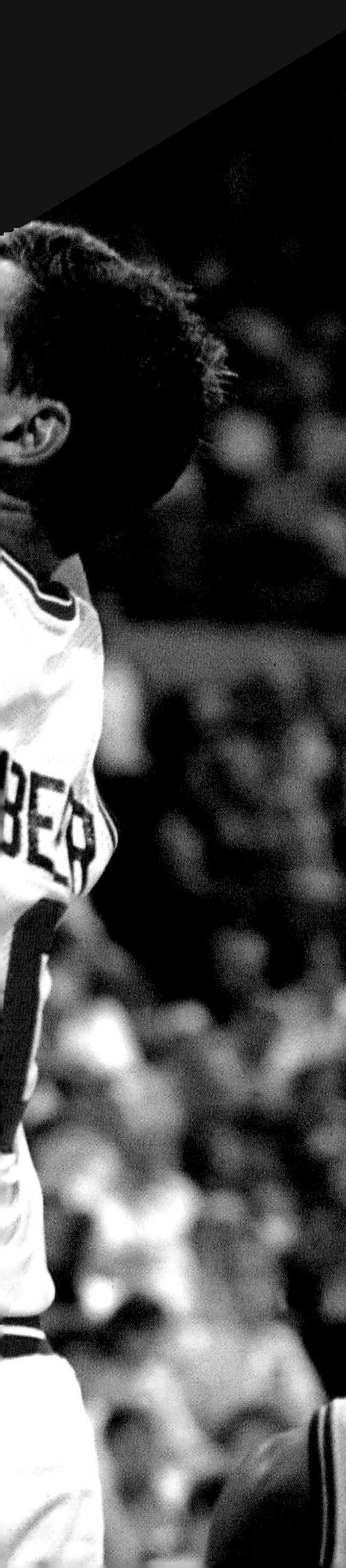

THE NBA:
A HISTORY
OF HOOPS

THE STORY OF THE CHICAGO BULLS

NATE FRISCH

CREATIVE EDUCATION

HELEN PLUM LIBRARY
LOMBARD, IL

Published by Creative Education
P.O. Box 227, Mankato, Minnesota 56002
Creative Education is an imprint of The Creative Company
www.thecreativecompany.us

Design and production by Blue Design
Art direction by Rita Marshall
Printed in the United States of America

Photographs by Corbis (Steve Lipofsky), Getty Images (Randy Belice/NBAE, Andrew D. Bernstein/NBAE, John Biever/Sports Illustrated, Nathaniel S. Butler/NBAE, Jonathan Daniel, Focus on Sport, John Iacono/Sports Illustrated, Adam Jones, Heinz Kluetmeier/Sports Illustrated, David E. Klutho/Sports Illustrated, Fernando Medina/NBAE, Manny Millan/Sports Illustrated, Layne Murdoch/NBAE, Joe Murphy/NBAE, Paul Natkin/WireImage, NBA Photos/NBAE, Robert Abbott Sengstacke, Rick Stewart/Stringer), Newscom (BRIAN KERSEY/UPI, TANNEN MAURY/EPA, Ting Shen/Xinhua/Photoshot)

Copyright © 2015 Creative Education

International copyright reserved in all countries. No part of this book may be reproduced in any form without written permission from the publisher.

Library of Congress Cataloging-in-Publication Data
Frisch, Nate.
The story of the Chicago Bulls / Nate Frisch.
p. cm. — (The NBA: a history of hoops)
Includes index.
Summary: An informative narration of the Chicago Bulls professional basketball team's history from its 1966 founding to today, spotlighting memorable players and reliving dramatic events.
ISBN 978-1-60818-425-5
1. Chicago Bulls (Basketball team)—History—Juvenile literature. I. Title.

GV885.52.C45F76 2014
796.323'640977311—dc23 2013037444

CCSS: RI.5.1, 2, 3, 8; RH.6-8.4, 5, 7

First Edition
9 8 7 6 5 4 3 2 1

Cover: Guard Derrick Rose
Page 2: Guard Michael Jordan
Pages 4–5: Guard Derrick Rose (right), center Joakim Noah (#13)
Page 6: Forward Bob Love

3 1502 00792 1685

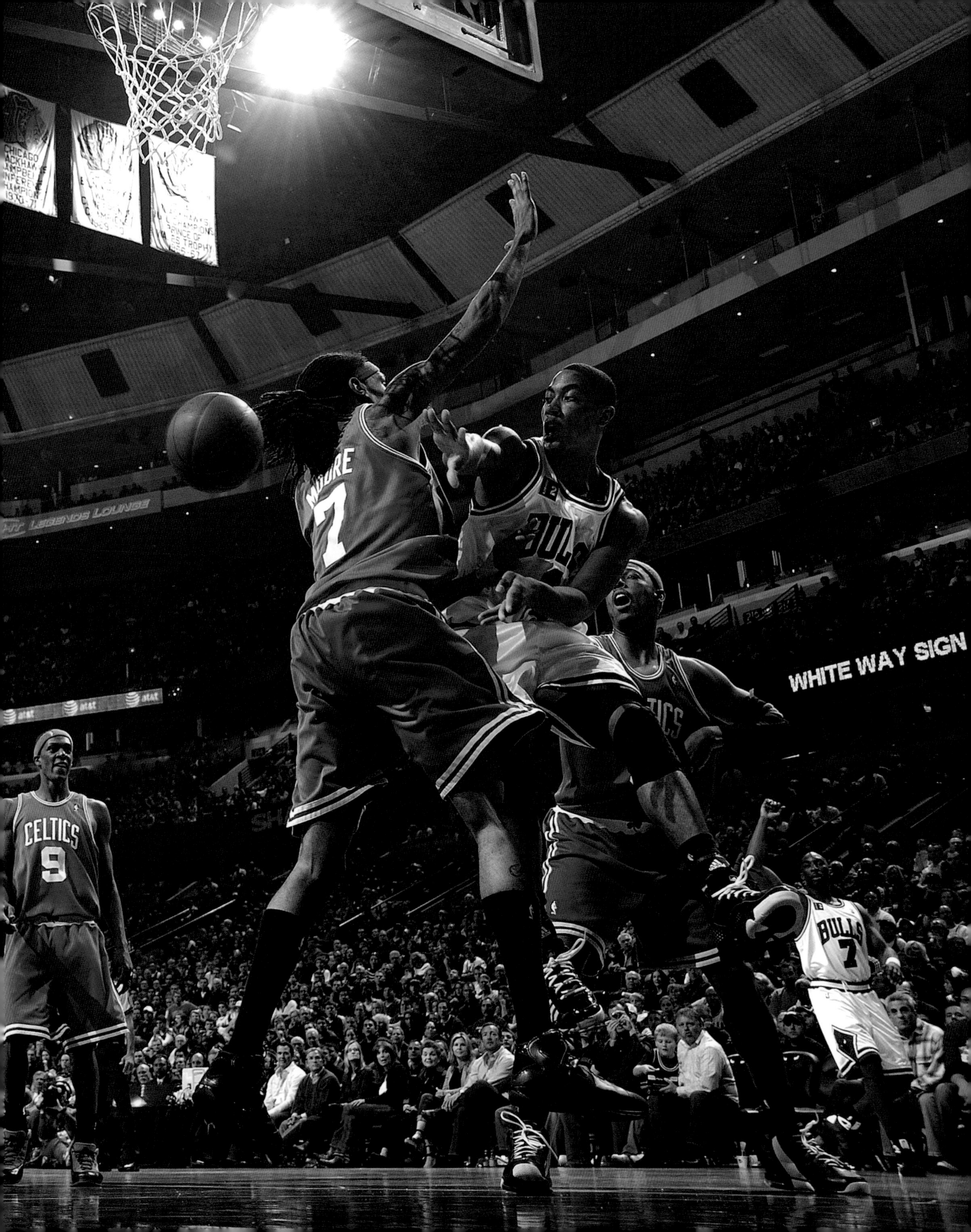

WHITE WAY SIGN
LEGENDS LOUNGE
MOORE
7
BULLS
CELTICS
9
BULLS
7

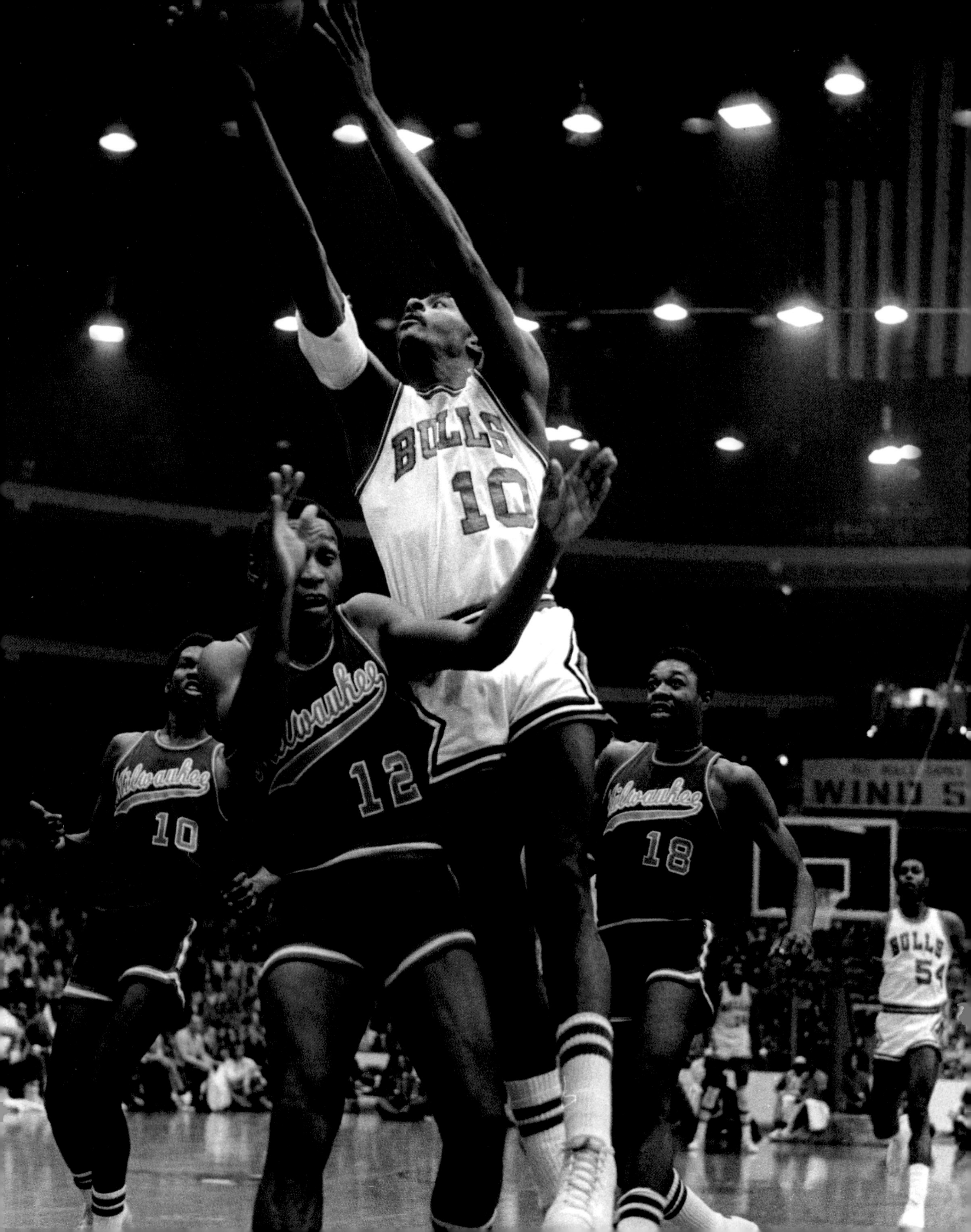
BULLS
10
12
Milwaukee
10
Milwaukee
18
BULLS
54

TABLE OF CONTENTS

COURTSIDE STORIES

INTRODUCING...

BULLISH DETERMINATION

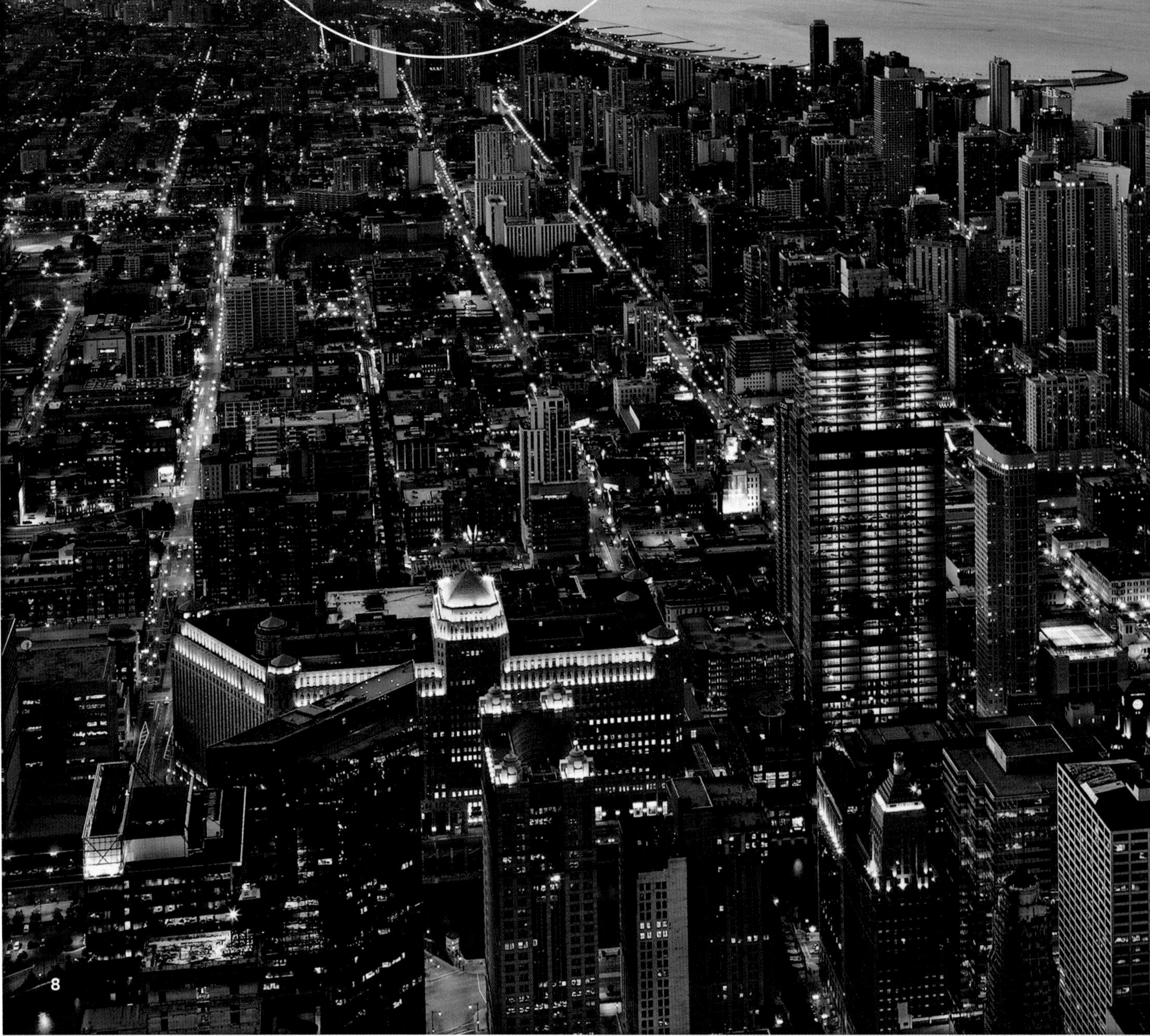

THE CITY OF CHICAGO (NOT INCLUDING THE METRO AREA) IS HOME TO 2.7 MILLION PEOPLE.

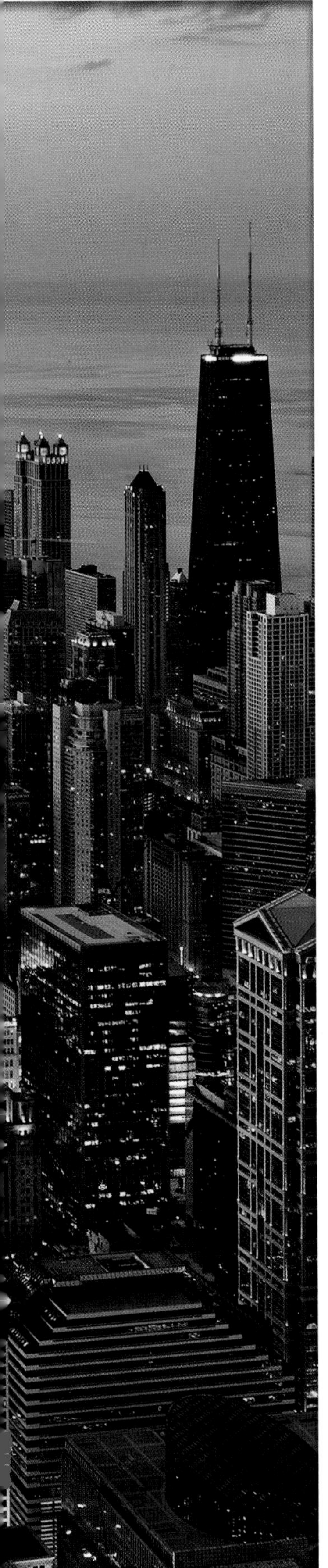

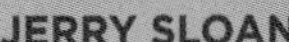

JERRY SLOAN

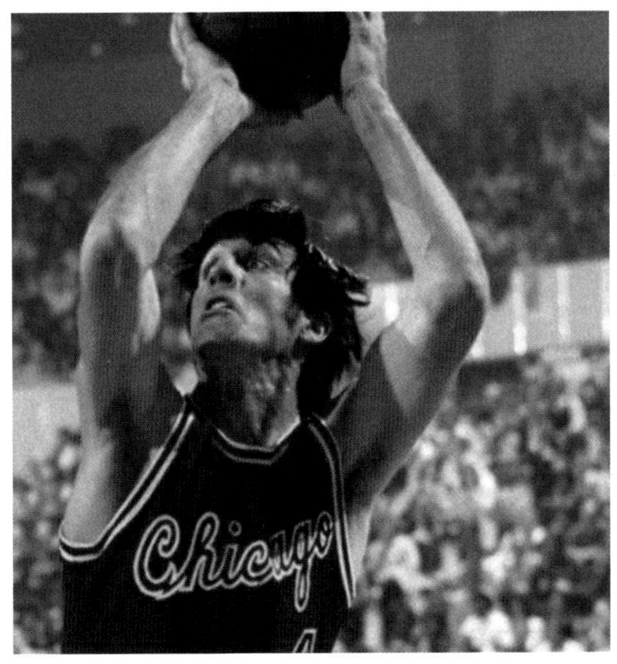

Beginning in the mid-1800s and continuing for more than a century, the bellowing of cattle and squealing of hogs rang out in the city of Chicago, Illinois. Home to the Union Stock Yards, Chicago was a focal point of the United States' meat-packing industry. The city's location along the shore of Lake Michigan made it a logical site for processing livestock of the Midwest and transporting it by boat or railway to the rest of the country. Today, Chicago has evolved into America's third-largest city, and major international companies such as McDonald's call the area home.

"The Windy City"—nicknamed for the gusts that come off Lake Michigan—has a long, proud history of professional sports. Football's Bears, baseball's Cubs, and hockey's Blackhawks are all among the oldest franchises (pre-1930) in their respective leagues. However, the more intricate

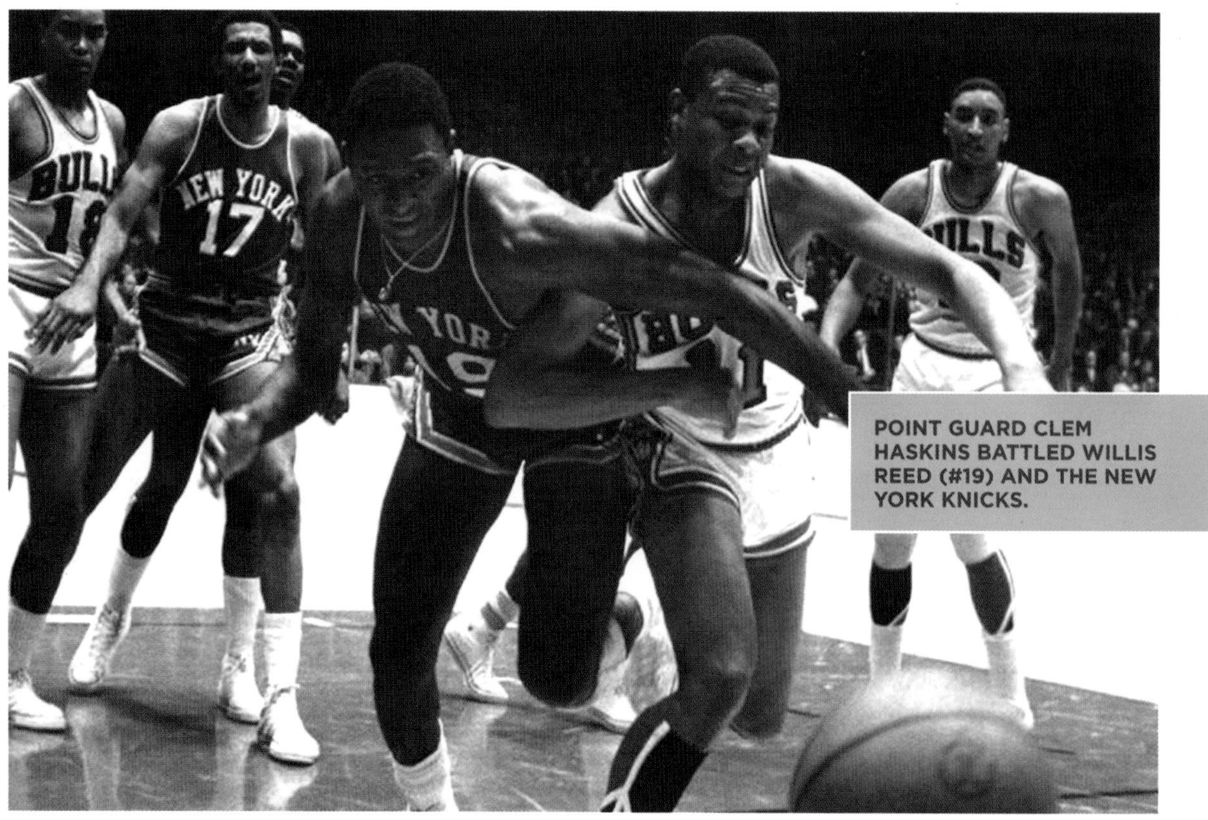

POINT GUARD CLEM HASKINS BATTLED WILLIS REED (#19) AND THE NEW YORK KNICKS.

game of basketball was slower to catch on. A local team called the Stags started playing in 1946, and when the National Basketball League (NBA) began in 1949, the Chicago Stags became one of the league's first teams. Failing to gain a foothold, they folded after only one season. It would be 17 years before another NBA franchise would test its welcome in Chicago. Drawing upon the city's meat-packing history, that new team was named the Bulls. The title also suggested explosive power and aggression—beneficial traits on the hardwood.

Playing in a city that had previously shown little interest in pro hoops, the Bulls were determined to make a strong first impression. So they hired head coach Johnny "Red" Kerr. Kerr had spent his high school playing days in Chicago and competed collegiately at the University of Illinois. They also brought in Illinois native Jerry Sloan, a second-year swingman who epitomized hustle and basketball intelligence. In the Bulls' inaugural 1966–67 campaign, Sloan paired up with efficient scoring forward Bob Boozer and slick-passing guard Guy Rodgers. The trio led Chicago to three straight wins to open the season and eventually, took the team into the NBA playoffs. The Bulls were quickly dispatched in the postseason, but

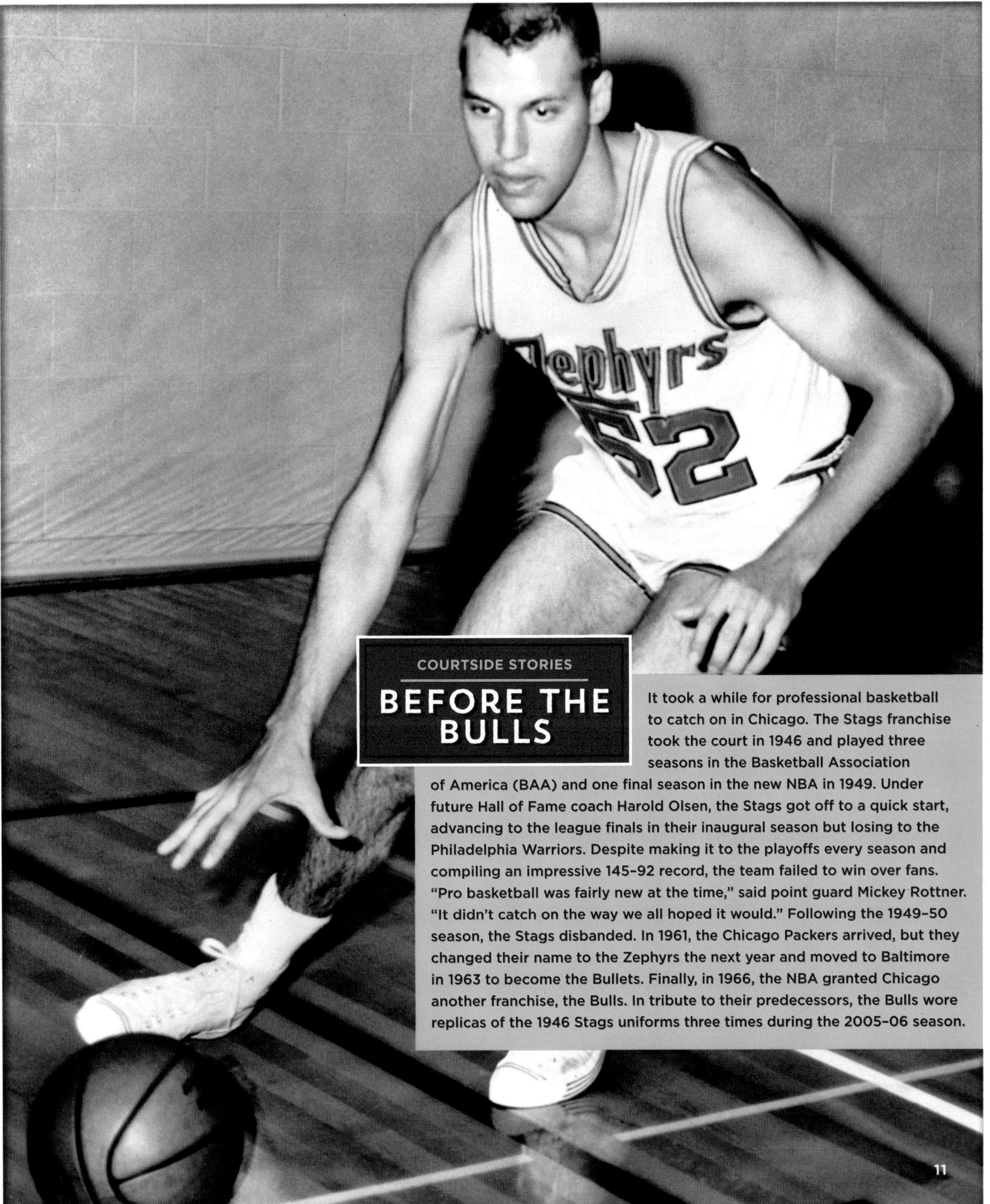

COURTSIDE STORIES

BEFORE THE BULLS

It took a while for professional basketball to catch on in Chicago. The Stags franchise took the court in 1946 and played three seasons in the Basketball Association of America (BAA) and one final season in the new NBA in 1949. Under future Hall of Fame coach Harold Olsen, the Stags got off to a quick start, advancing to the league finals in their inaugural season but losing to the Philadelphia Warriors. Despite making it to the playoffs every season and compiling an impressive 145–92 record, the team failed to win over fans. "Pro basketball was fairly new at the time," said point guard Mickey Rottner. "It didn't catch on the way we all hoped it would." Following the 1949–50 season, the Stags disbanded. In 1961, the Chicago Packers arrived, but they changed their name to the Zephyrs the next year and moved to Baltimore in 1963 to become the Bullets. Finally, in 1966, the NBA granted Chicago another franchise, the Bulls. In tribute to their predecessors, the Bulls wore replicas of the 1946 Stags uniforms three times during the 2005–06 season.

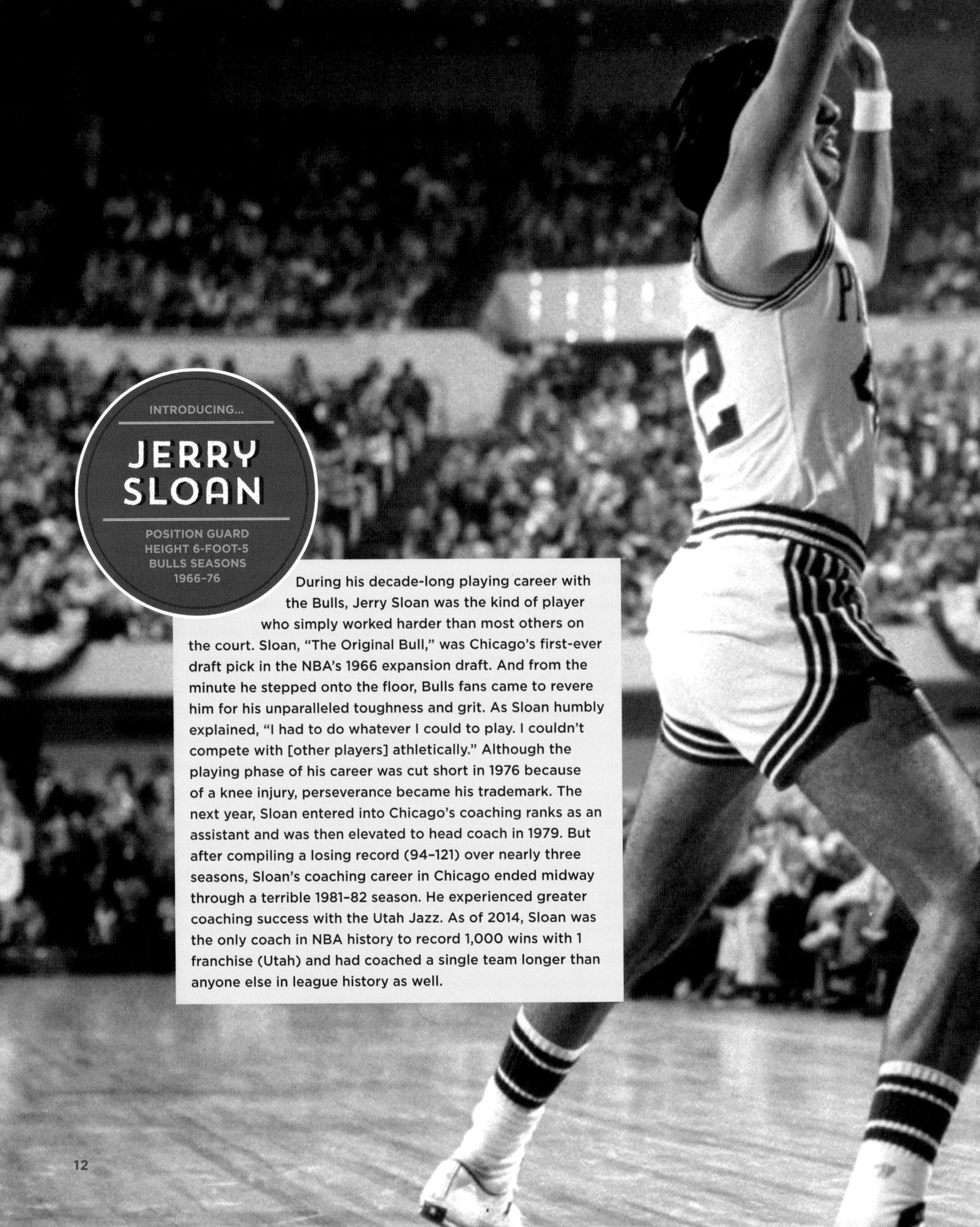

INTRODUCING...

JERRY SLOAN

POSITION GUARD
HEIGHT 6-FOOT-5
BULLS SEASONS
1966–76

During his decade-long playing career with the Bulls, Jerry Sloan was the kind of player who simply worked harder than most others on the court. Sloan, "The Original Bull," was Chicago's first-ever draft pick in the NBA's 1966 expansion draft. And from the minute he stepped onto the floor, Bulls fans came to revere him for his unparalleled toughness and grit. As Sloan humbly explained, "I had to do whatever I could to play. I couldn't compete with [other players] athletically." Although the playing phase of his career was cut short in 1976 because of a knee injury, perseverance became his trademark. The next year, Sloan entered into Chicago's coaching ranks as an assistant and was then elevated to head coach in 1979. But after compiling a losing record (94–121) over nearly three seasons, Sloan's coaching career in Chicago ended midway through a terrible 1981–82 season. He experienced greater coaching success with the Utah Jazz. As of 2014, Sloan was the only coach in NBA history to record 1,000 wins with 1 franchise (Utah) and had coached a single team longer than anyone else in league history as well.

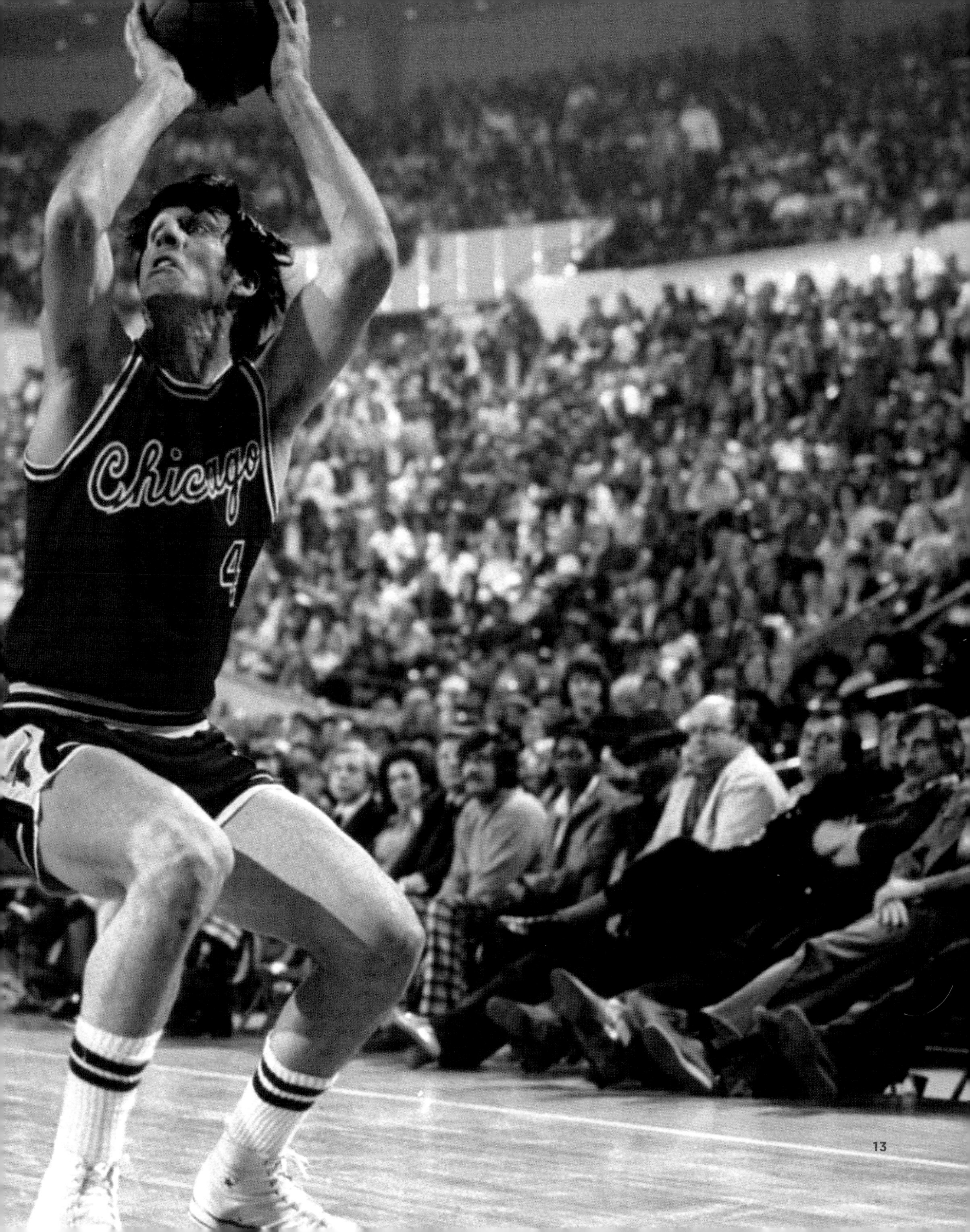
Chicago
4

"PLAYING THE BULLS IS LIKE RUNNING THROUGH A BARBED WIRE FENCE. YOU MAY WIN THE GAME, BUT THEY'RE GONNA PUT LUMPS ON YOU."

— LAKERS GUARD GAIL GOODRICH

they had taken the first steps to becoming a permanent fixture in Chicago.

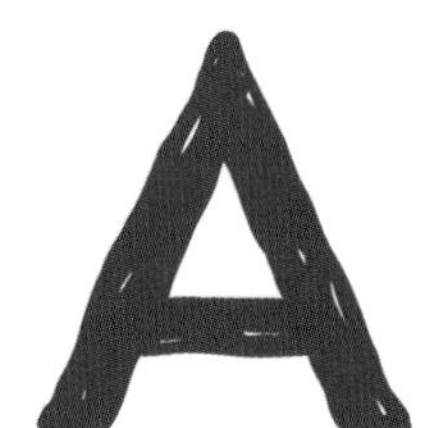

fter another early dismissal from the playoffs the following season, Kerr resigned, and Dick Motta took over coaching duties. Improvement was marginal the first two seasons, but in 1970–71, Motta's Bulls posted an impressive 51–31 record, good enough to rank second in the Western Conference's Midwest Division. However, they could not match the Los Angeles Lakers in the playoffs, who bested them not only in that postseason but in the next two as well.

By 1972–73, the Bulls had built a starting lineup that included scrappy point guard Norm Van Lier and hulking, seven-foot center Tom Boerwinkle. And Sloan had proven to be one of the league's best defenders. The offensive punch in this defensive powerhouse came courtesy of forwards Chet Walker and Bob Love. "Playing the Bulls is like running through a barbed wire fence," said Lakers guard Gail Goodrich. "You may win the game, but they're gonna put lumps on you."

A huge drop in the team's performance in 1975–76 cost Motta his job. New coach Ed Badger took over for the 1976–77 season, the same year the team acquired center Artis Gilmore, a player known as "The A-Train" because of his enormous size and strength. That year, Gilmore led the team in scoring and rebounding and remade the Bulls into a winner. Despite Gilmore's consistently impressive numbers, a championship eluded him during his six seasons with the team. Following the 1981–82 season, the Bulls decided to rebuild with younger players, and Gilmore was traded to the San Antonio Spurs. "It's a shame we couldn't put a better team around Artis," noted Van Lier. "He did everything he could, but when we lost, he always got the blame."

Despite the rebuilding efforts, Chicago was in disarray. Between 1976 and 1982, the team hired and fired six coaches, including former fan favorite Sloan. The club was reassigned to the Eastern Conference's Central Division in 1980–81, and standouts such as guard Reggie Theus and forward Orlando Woolridge provided steady play in the early 1980s, but the Bulls lacked competitiveness. Fortunately, a huge gust of Air was on the way to help turn the team's fortunes around.

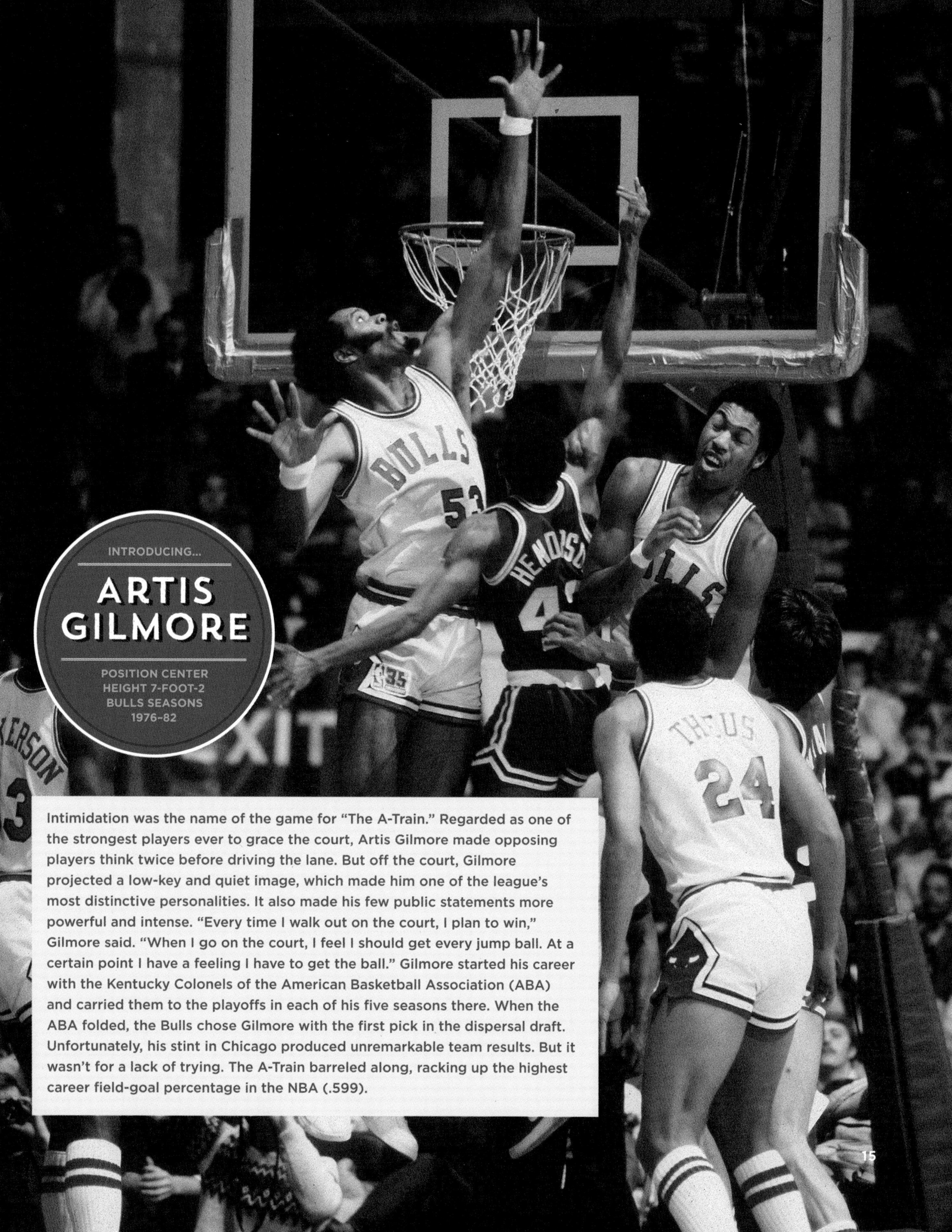

INTRODUCING...

ARTIS GILMORE

POSITION CENTER
HEIGHT 7-FOOT-2
BULLS SEASONS
1976–82

Intimidation was the name of the game for "The A-Train." Regarded as one of the strongest players ever to grace the court, Artis Gilmore made opposing players think twice before driving the lane. But off the court, Gilmore projected a low-key and quiet image, which made him one of the league's most distinctive personalities. It also made his few public statements more powerful and intense. "Every time I walk out on the court, I plan to win," Gilmore said. "When I go on the court, I feel I should get every jump ball. At a certain point I have a feeling I have to get the ball." Gilmore started his career with the Kentucky Colonels of the American Basketball Association (ABA) and carried them to the playoffs in each of his five seasons there. When the ABA folded, the Bulls chose Gilmore with the first pick in the dispersal draft. Unfortunately, his stint in Chicago produced unremarkable team results. But it wasn't for a lack of trying. The A-Train barreled along, racking up the highest career field-goal percentage in the NBA (.599).

CHANGING WINDS

NORM VAN LIER EARNED THE NICKNAME "STORMIN' NORMAN" FOR HIS FIERCENESS.

ED NEALY

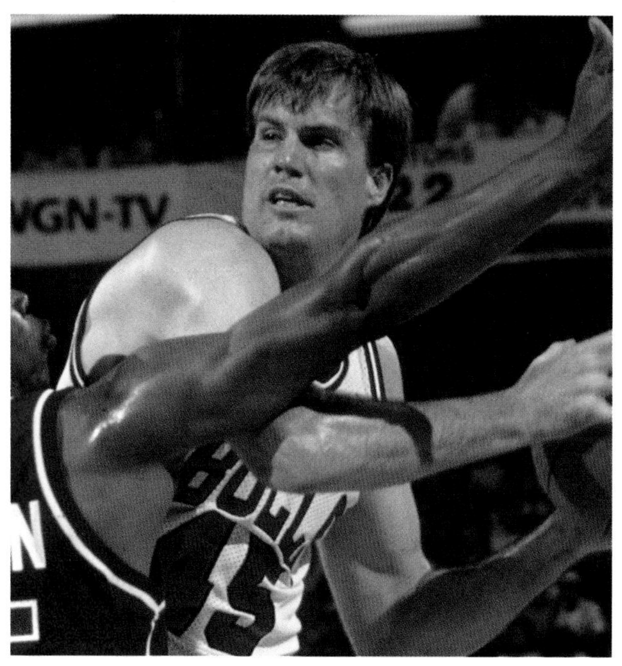

A new era began in 1984 when Chicago White Sox owner Jerry Reinsdorf began negotiations to purchase the Bulls. George Steinbrenner, principal owner of the New York Yankees, was also a part owner of the Bulls at the time. By chance, Steinbrenner mentioned to Reinsdorf that he was embarrassed by the Bulls and wanted to sell his stake. So a deal was quickly put together that allowed Reinsdorf to acquire more than half the team's stock, and he became the team's chairman in March 1985. The Bulls were coming off 4 consecutive losing seasons and averaging little more than 6,300 fans per game at Chicago Stadium. But Reinsdorf was determined to put a winner on the floor, and the team had a great player around whom it could rebuild—a dynamic rookie shooting guard named Michael Jordan.

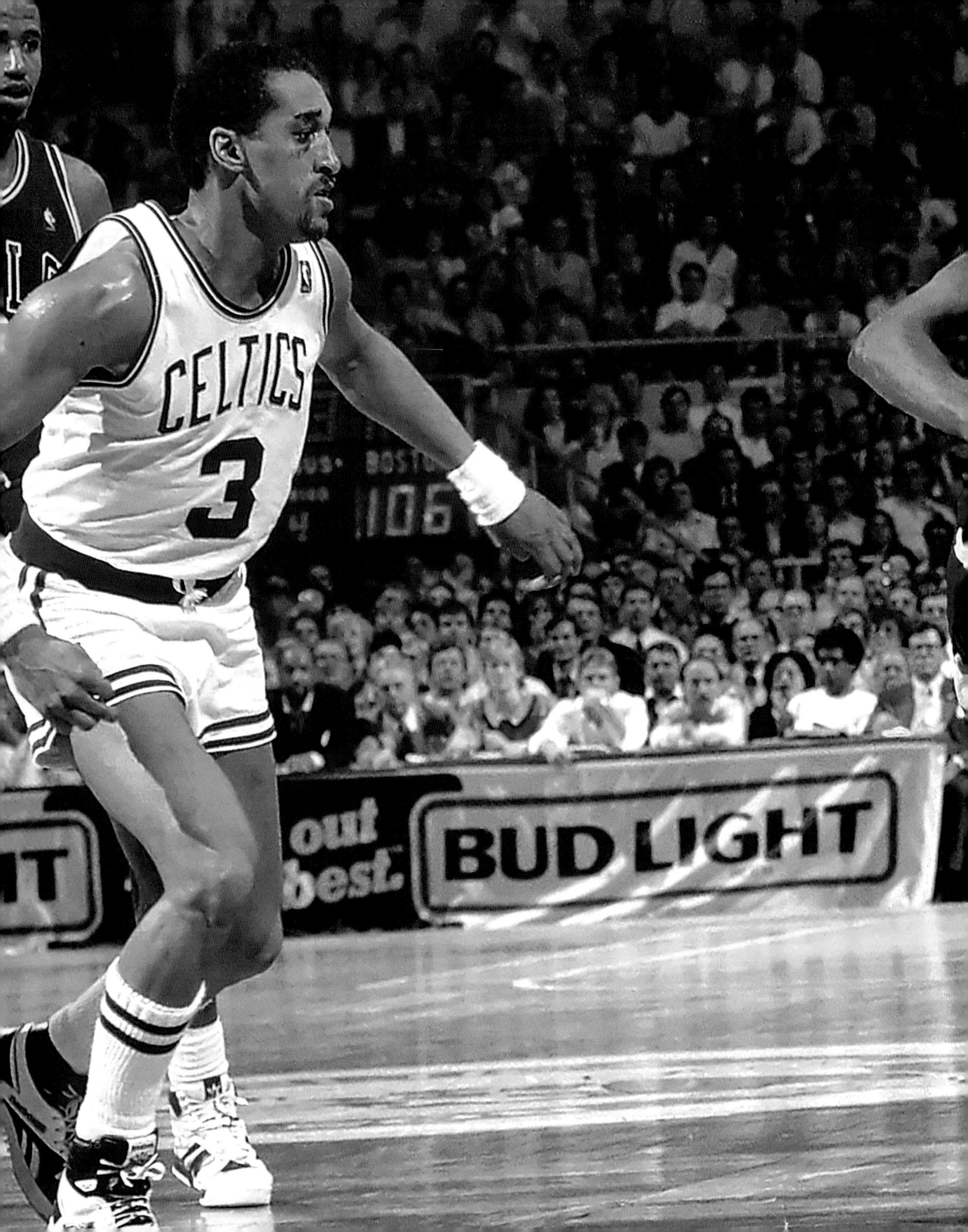
CELTICS
3
106
BUD LIGHT

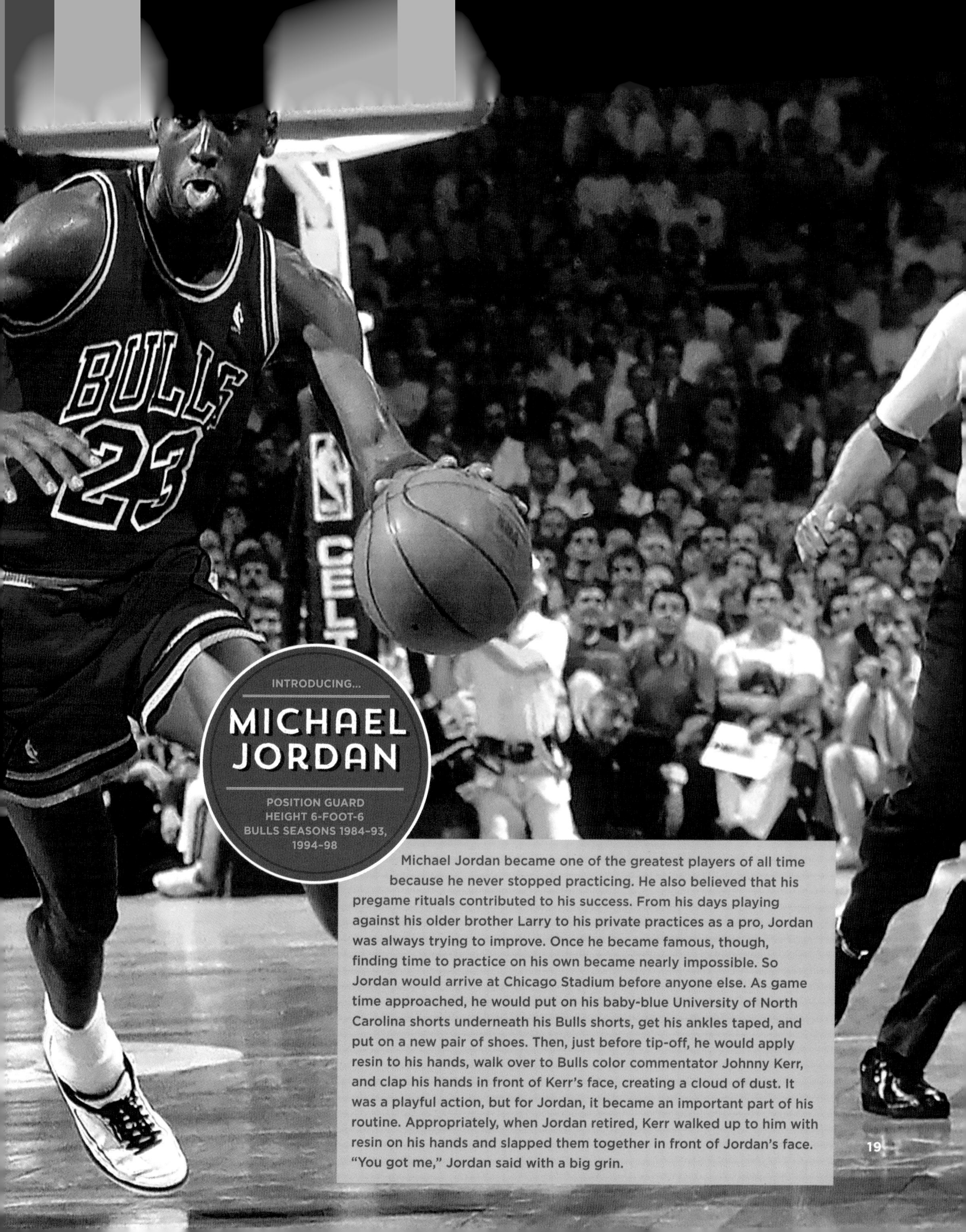

INTRODUCING...

MICHAEL JORDAN

POSITION GUARD
HEIGHT 6-FOOT-6
BULLS SEASONS 1984–93, 1994–98

Michael Jordan became one of the greatest players of all time because he never stopped practicing. He also believed that his pregame rituals contributed to his success. From his days playing against his older brother Larry to his private practices as a pro, Jordan was always trying to improve. Once he became famous, though, finding time to practice on his own became nearly impossible. So Jordan would arrive at Chicago Stadium before anyone else. As game time approached, he would put on his baby-blue University of North Carolina shorts underneath his Bulls shorts, get his ankles taped, and put on a new pair of shoes. Then, just before tip-off, he would apply resin to his hands, walk over to Bulls color commentator Johnny Kerr, and clap his hands in front of Kerr's face, creating a cloud of dust. It was a playful action, but for Jordan, it became an important part of his routine. Appropriately, when Jordan retired, Kerr walked up to him with resin on his hands and slapped them together in front of Jordan's face. "You got me," Jordan said with a big grin.

"IT MUST BE GOD DISGUISED AS MICHAEL JORDAN."

– LARRY BIRD ON JORDAN'S NBA PLAYOFF-RECORD 63 POINTS

Jordan sent shockwaves throughout the league as soon as he joined Chicago as the third overall pick in the 1984 NBA Draft. With unstoppable moves, explosive quickness, and unrivaled leaping ability, "Air" Jordan soared to dizzying heights, leading the Bulls in every major statistical category. He was the runaway choice as 1985 NBA Rookie of the Year and became an instant All-Star. But still, Chicago remained a losing team.

In Jordan's second season, he missed 64 games with a broken foot. The team urged him to sit out the remaining games, but after Jordan accused management of not wanting to make the playoffs so that the Bulls could obtain a better draft pick, he was reluctantly allowed to return. With just 15 games to go in the regular season, he worked alongside rugged forward Charles Oakley to carry the Bulls into the playoffs. Although they were swept by the Boston Celtics in 3 games, Jordan established himself as a major force in Game 2 by scoring an NBA playoff-record 63 points. His performance was so miraculous that Celtics forward Larry Bird commented, "It must be God disguised as Michael Jordan."

The 1986–87 season signaled a major turning point for the Bulls' fortunes. The team solidified its coaching regime with the talented but untested Doug Collins, and general manager Jerry Krause was determined to get Jordan some help. So in the 1987 NBA Draft, Chicago selected forward Horace Grant and traded for little-known forward Scottie Pippen from the University of Central Arkansas. "I never heard of him or his school," Jordan at first said of Pippen. But the rookie's skills quickly opened Jordan's eyes. Behind the unstoppable duo of Jordan and Pippen, Chicago became a powerhouse in the Eastern Conference and won 50 games during the regular season.

However, Chicago's quest for a championship was thwarted by the rough-and-tumble Detroit Pistons in the second round of the 1988 playoffs. Detroit coach Chuck Daly and his All-Star cast of "Bad Boys," such as center Bill Laimbeer and forward Dennis Rodman, developed "The Jordan Rules," a strategy for containing Jordan. They felt that Jordan's superstar status led referees to give him preferential treatment over opposing guards, so the Pistons got physical with Jordan and tried to throw him off balance with different

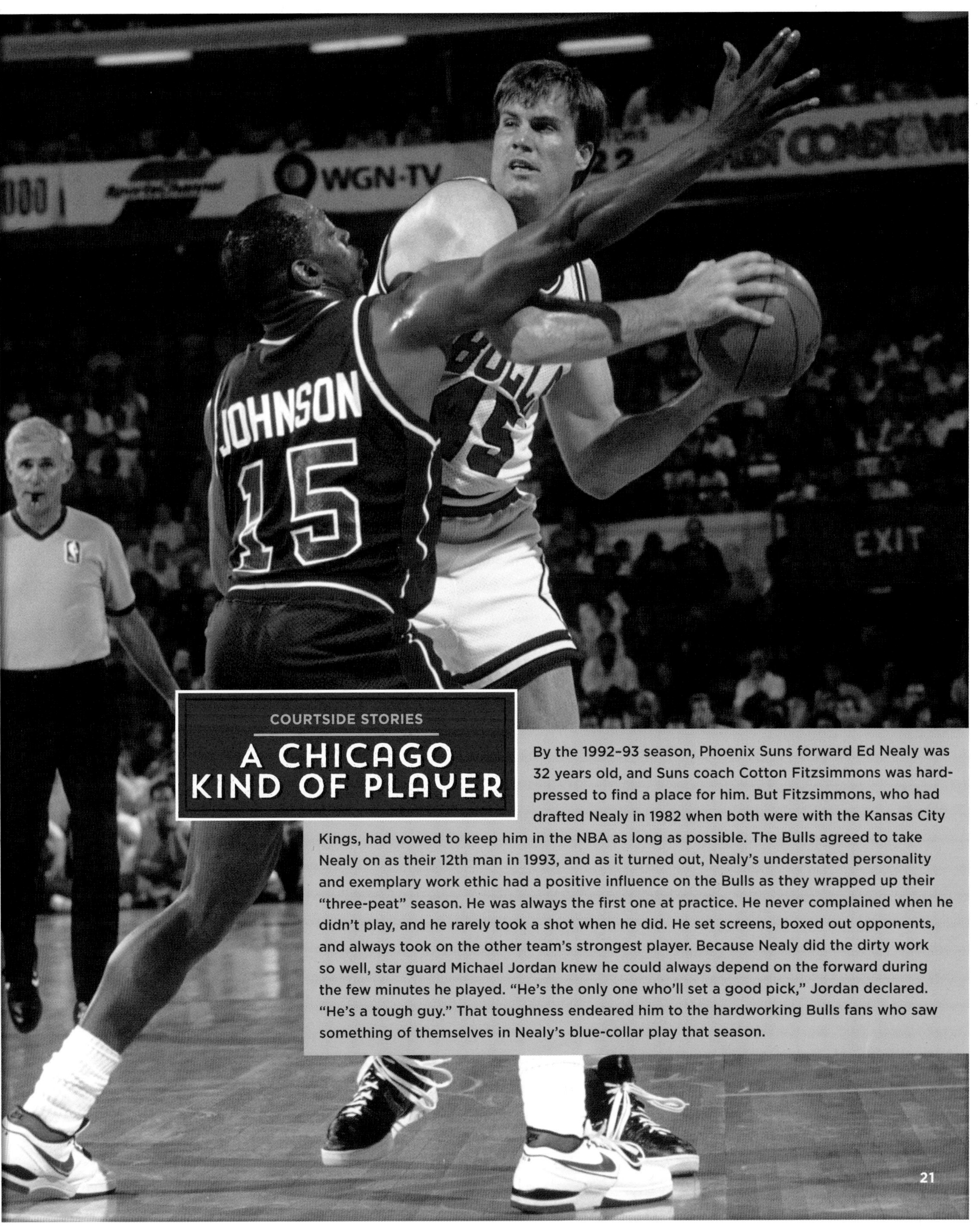

COURTSIDE STORIES

A CHICAGO KIND OF PLAYER

By the 1992–93 season, Phoenix Suns forward Ed Nealy was 32 years old, and Suns coach Cotton Fitzsimmons was hard-pressed to find a place for him. But Fitzsimmons, who had drafted Nealy in 1982 when both were with the Kansas City Kings, had vowed to keep him in the NBA as long as possible. The Bulls agreed to take Nealy on as their 12th man in 1993, and as it turned out, Nealy's understated personality and exemplary work ethic had a positive influence on the Bulls as they wrapped up their "three-peat" season. He was always the first one at practice. He never complained when he didn't play, and he rarely took a shot when he did. He set screens, boxed out opponents, and always took on the other team's strongest player. Because Nealy did the dirty work so well, star guard Michael Jordan knew he could always depend on the forward during the few minutes he played. "He's the only one who'll set a good pick," Jordan declared. "He's a tough guy." That toughness endeared him to the hardworking Bulls fans who saw something of themselves in Nealy's blue-collar play that season.

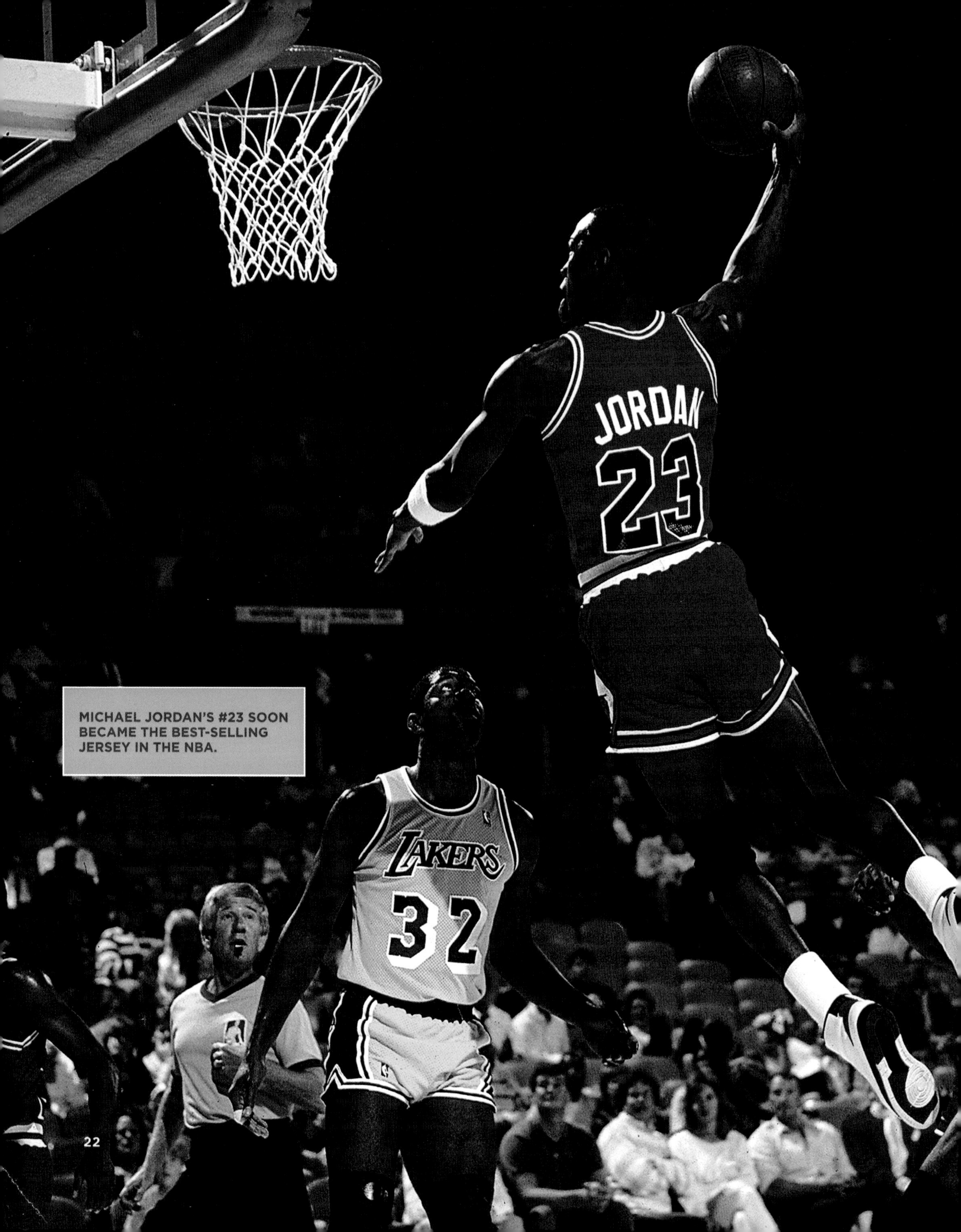

MICHAEL JORDAN'S #23 SOON BECAME THE BEST-SELLING JERSEY IN THE NBA.

"[JORDAN] IS THE GREATEST COMPETITOR I'VE EVER SEEN, AND THEN HE GOES TO STILL ANOTHER LEVEL IN THE BIG GAMES."

– ASSISTANT COACH JOHN BACH ON MICHAEL JORDAN

defensive formations and hard fouls. "You hear about [The Jordan Rules] often enough—and the referees hear it, too—and you start to think they have something different," said Chicago assistant coach John Bach. "It has an effect, and suddenly people think they aren't fouling Michael, even when they are."

After adding veteran center Bill Cartwright before and shooting guard Craig Hodges during the 1988–89 season, the Bulls finished near the bottom of the Central Division but defeated the Cleveland Cavaliers in the first round of the playoffs. Jordan, now playing point guard, had promised that the Bulls would win the Cleveland series, and he contributed to the effort with averages of 39.8 points, 8.2 assists, and 5.8 rebounds in 5 games. With time about to expire in Game 5, he drove to his left at the top of the key and hit a hanging jumper to give the Bulls a one-point victory. "[Jordan] is the greatest competitor I've ever seen," Bach said afterwards, "and then he goes to still another level in the big games." But once again, it was all for naught. Although Chicago went on to beat the New York Knicks in the second round, the Pistons eliminated the Bulls in six games in the Eastern Conference finals.

The 1989–90 season was a momentous one. Collins was let go, and one of his assistants, Phil Jackson, was named head coach. The move proved to be an excellent one as the Bulls rolled up a regular-season record of 55–27, and then charged back for a conference finals rematch with Detroit. It took seven games, but Detroit dispatched Chicago again en route to its second straight NBA championship.

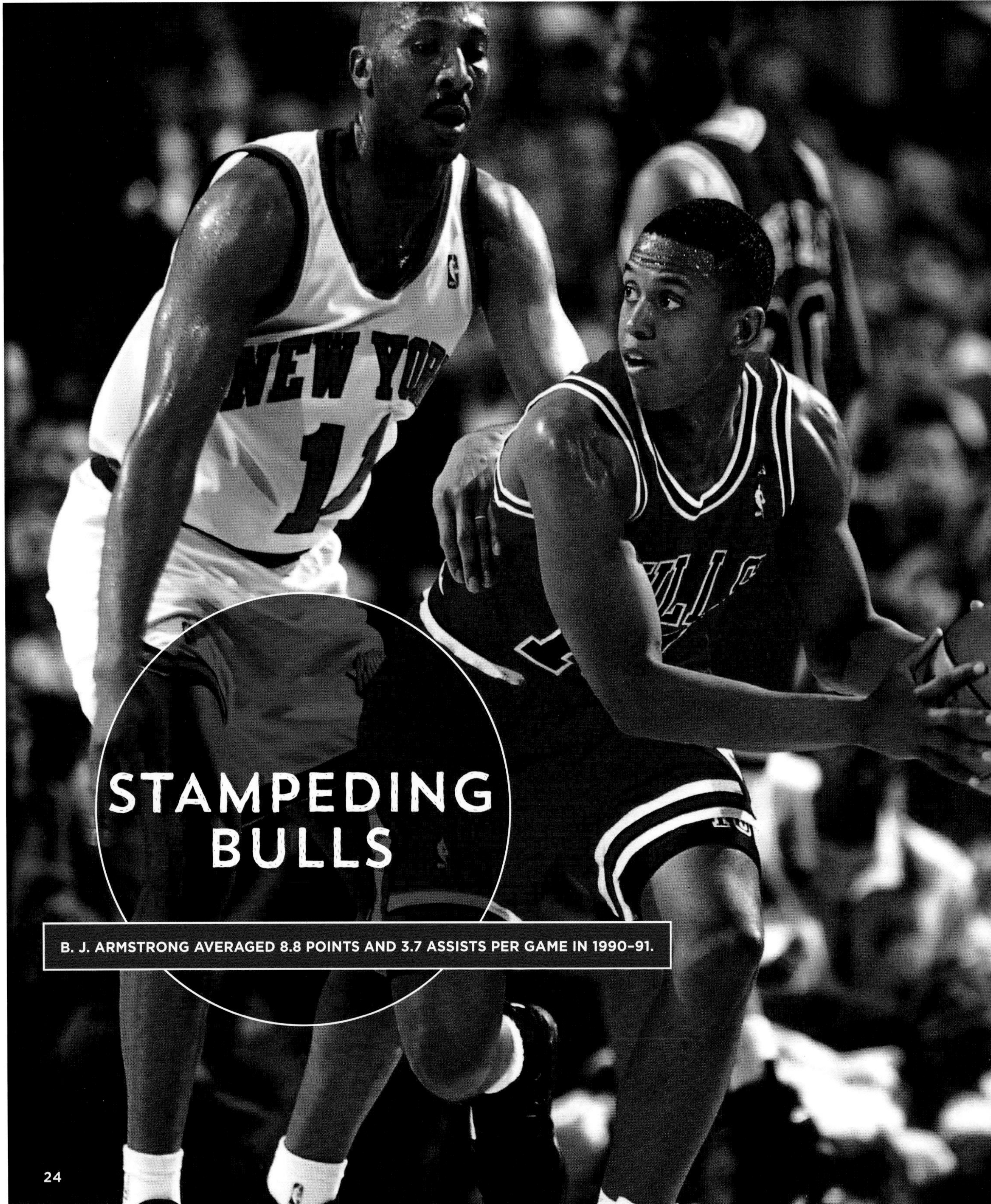

STAMPEDING BULLS

B. J. ARMSTRONG AVERAGED 8.8 POINTS AND 3.7 ASSISTS PER GAME IN 1990–91.

TONI KUKOC

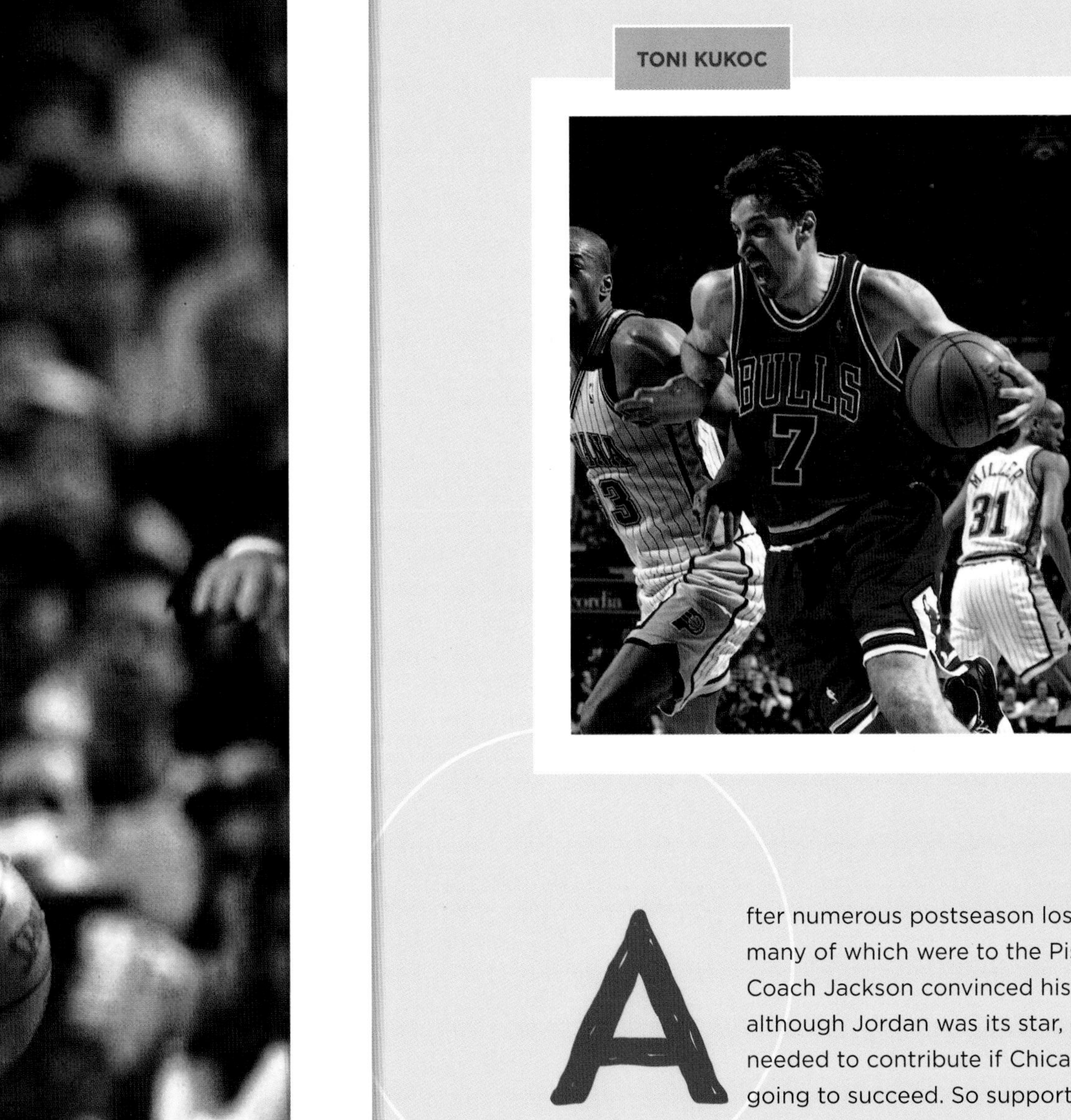

After numerous postseason losses—so many of which were to the Pistons—Coach Jackson convinced his team that, although Jordan was its star, everyone needed to contribute if Chicago was going to succeed. So supporting players such as sharpshooter John Paxson and baby-faced guard B. J. Armstrong stepped up their efforts. And when the 1990–91 season opened, the Bulls were confident that their time had come.

Chicago reached the end of the regular season with a 61–21 record. In the second round of the playoffs against the Philadelphia 76ers, Jordan's performance was simply unbelievable: he propelled Chicago to victory by averaging 33.4 points, 7.8 assists, and 8 rebounds per game. Lying in wait was Detroit, Chicago's old nemesis, but this time, the Bulls were not intimidated and proved it by sweeping the

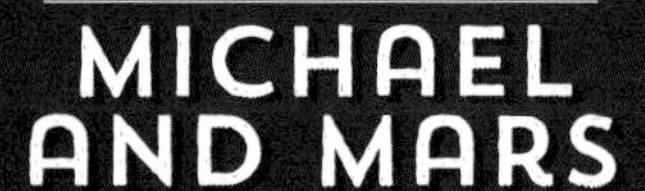

MICHAEL AND MARS

In the early 1990s, Michael Jordan's sensational style of play made him one of the most famous people in the world. Another element of Jordan's fame was his participation in advertisements for Nike's "Air Jordan" basketball shoes. As Nike chairman Phil Knight explained in 1992, Jordan's image made the shoes into a status symbol. "Not every player has the style of Michael Jordan, and if we tried to make 'Air Jordan' appeal to everyone, it would lose its meaning," Knight said. "We had to slice up basketball itself." The black-and-white "Air Jordan" commercials featured Jordan with Mars Blackmon, an alter ego for filmmaker Spike Lee, who got his point across by using repetition to explain how great a player Jordan was. In one commercial, Blackmon said: "Nobody in the world can cover my main man, Michael Jordan. Nobody, nobody, nobody." Jordan, who had been dunking baskets in the background, then came over to cover Blackmon's mouth. These brief and humorous commercials, seen by a wide television audience, further increased Jordan's celebrity status outside of basketball.

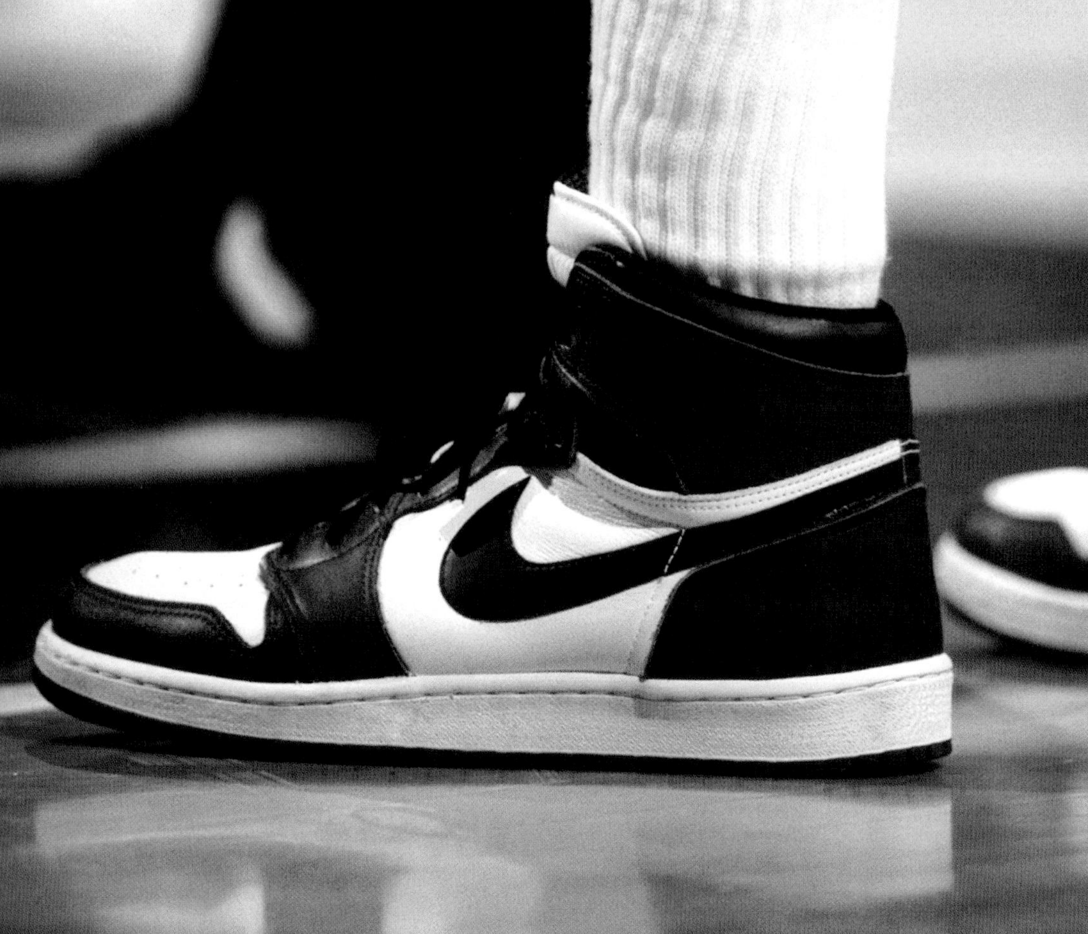

Pistons in four games. "They got in our head with the physical stuff," admitted Pippen. "But in doing it, the Pistons taught us the toughness we needed." Chicago so frustrated the Pistons that many of Detroit's stars walked off the court in the final game before the last seconds had even ticked off the clock. The Bulls then advanced to the long-elusive NBA Finals, where they faced the Lakers.

The Lakers and star guard Magic Johnson surprised the Bulls by winning the first game, but Chicago took the next four straight. In doing so, the team proved Jackson's theory correct—although Jordan confirmed his superstar status, it was his strong supporting cast that helped Chicago win its first-ever NBA championship.

The critics had said Jordan was the phenom who couldn't win a title. Now, not only had he and his team won, but he had done it in the way he had always dreamed—as the Finals' Most Valuable Player (MVP). Jordan was chosen unanimously, and 1 of the 11 electors even tried to refuse the ballot, saying, "Who else could it be?" The morning after that final victory, Jordan couldn't put the championship trophy down, and he slept with it all the way from Los

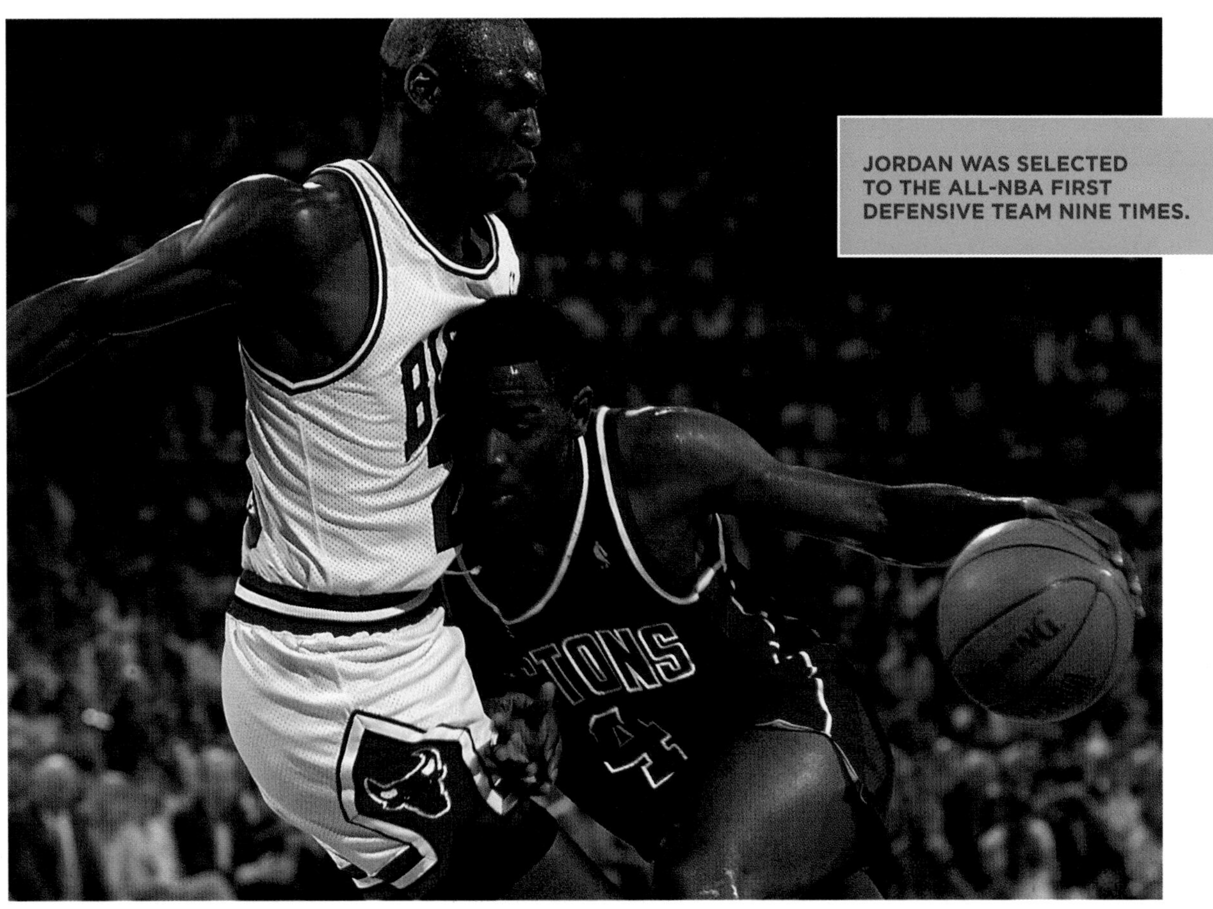

JORDAN WAS SELECTED TO THE ALL-NBA FIRST DEFENSIVE TEAM NINE TIMES.

Angeles back to Chicago.

Chicago would not have to wait so long for the second title. The next season, the Bulls rumbled to a team-record 67–15 mark, breezed through the playoffs, and throttled the Portland Trail Blazers in six games in the NBA Finals. The Bulls then "three-peated" in 1993 by beating star forward Charles Barkley and the Phoenix Suns in six games, thanks in part to some sharp three-point shooting by veteran guard Trent Tucker. Then Jordan, who was at the top of his game with nothing more to prove, suddenly decided to retire—a decision prompted in part by the murder of his father, James, in a 1993 robbery. At age 30, the NBA's best player walked away to pursue a career in professional baseball.

With Pippen now leading the way, the Bulls won more games than they lost in the next two seasons, but their horns were dulled without the presence of their star. Jordan, too, was feeling low. Although he was improving as a baseball player for the minor league Birmingham (Alabama) Barons, his dream of making the major leagues looked dim.

In August 1994, Chicago opened the United Center, a new arena that would house both the Bulls and the National Hockey League's Blackhawks. With its exterior designed to look like old Chicago Stadium, it became known as "The House that Jordan Built" and featured a statue of the Hall-of-Famer out front. Several months after its opening, Jordan returned

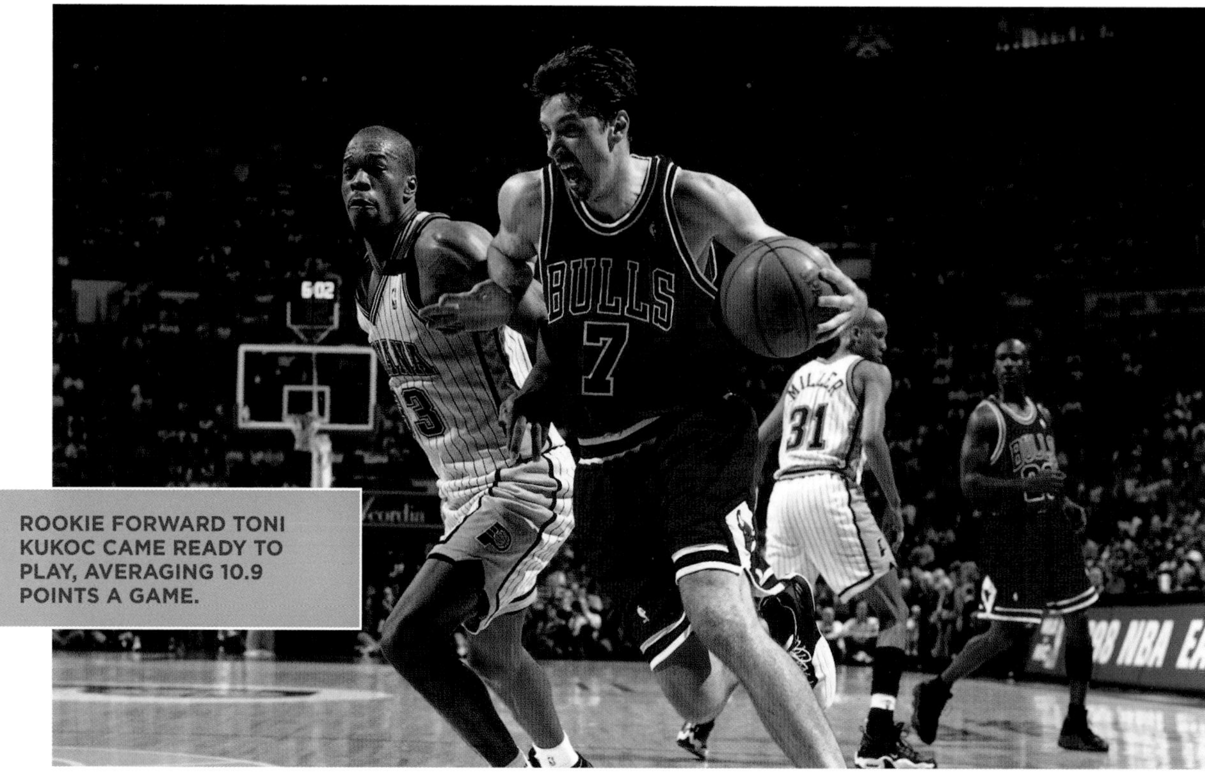

ROOKIE FORWARD TONI KUKOC CAME READY TO PLAY, AVERAGING 10.9 POINTS A GAME.

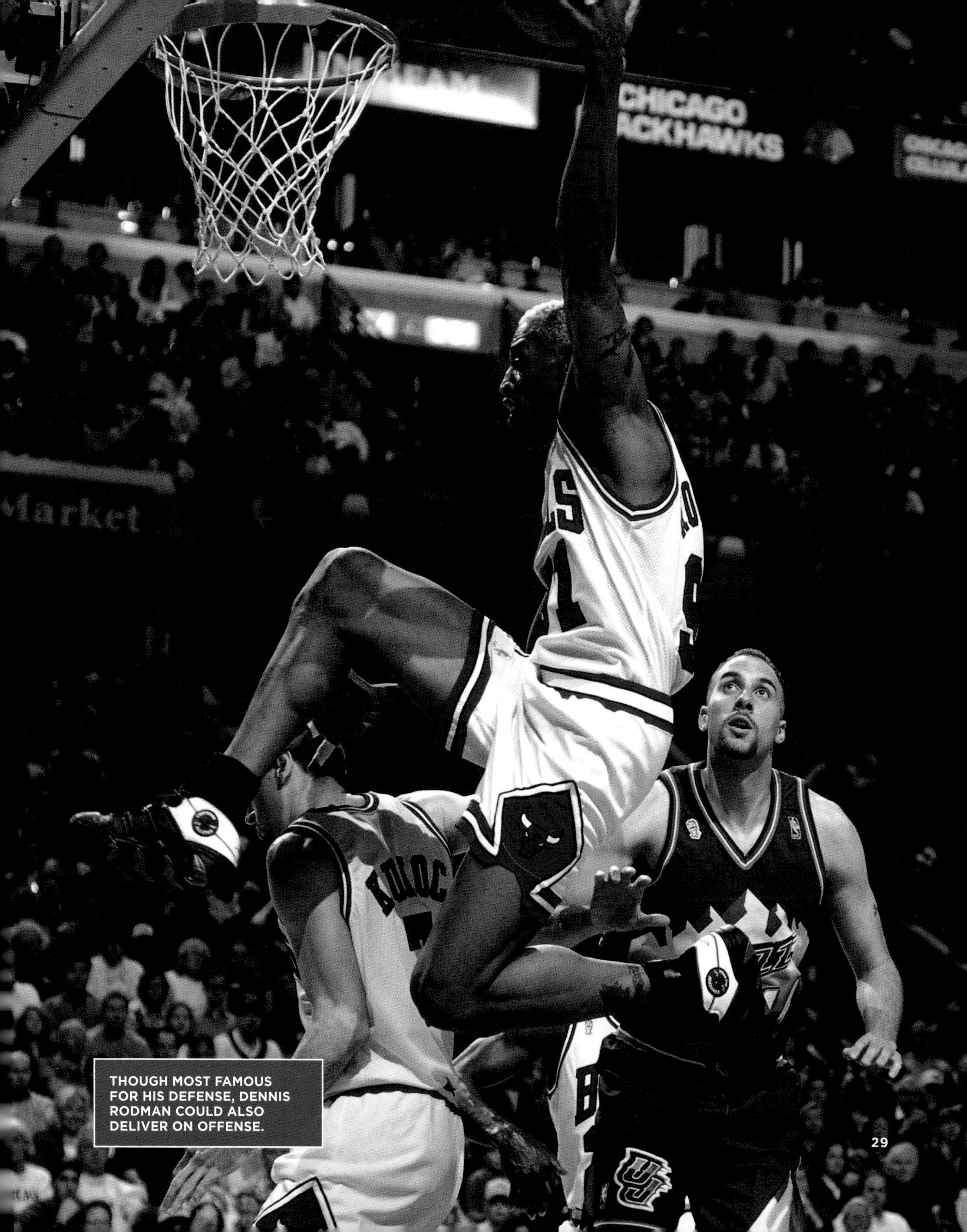

THOUGH MOST FAMOUS FOR HIS DEFENSE, DENNIS RODMAN COULD ALSO DELIVER ON OFFENSE.

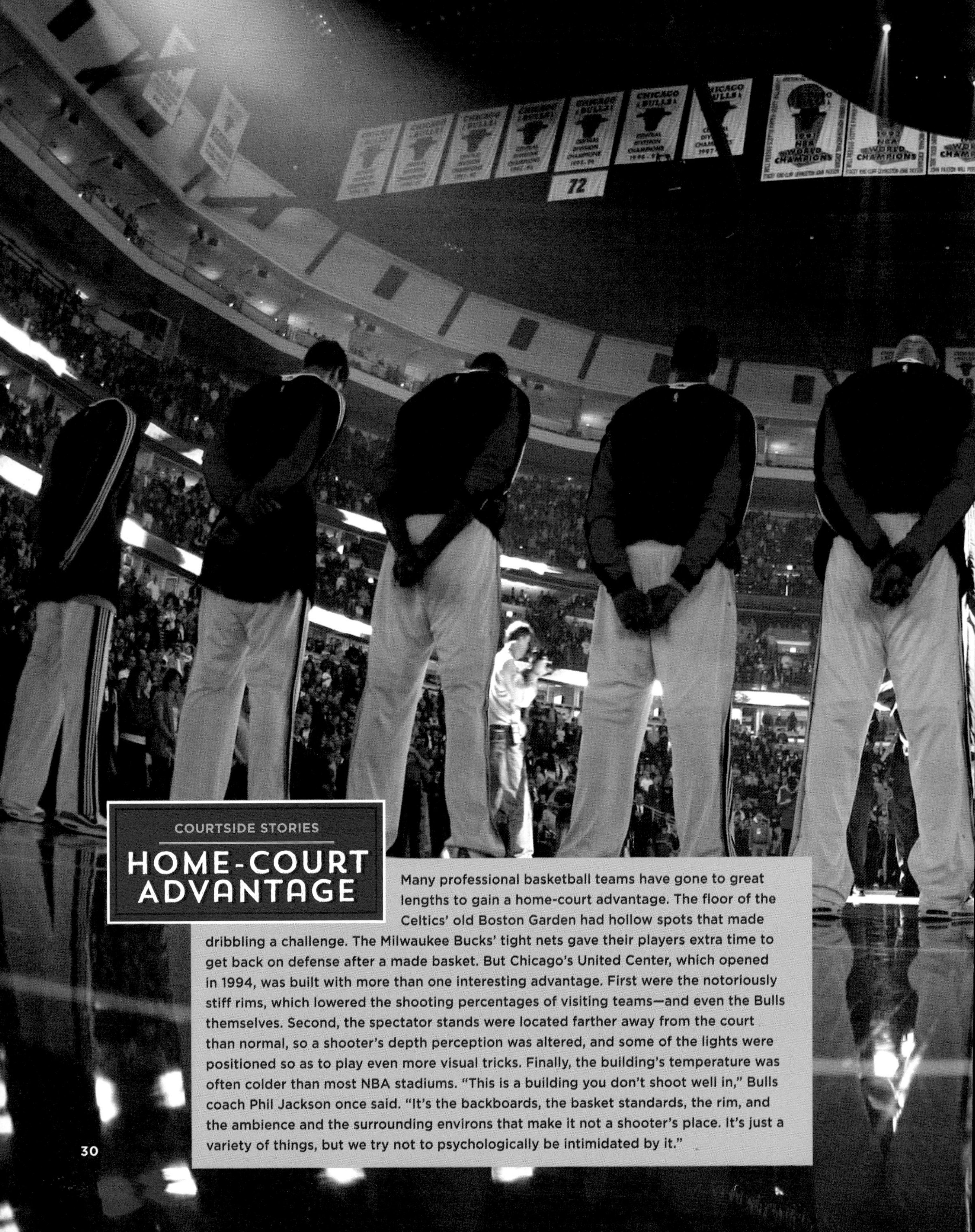

COURTSIDE STORIES

HOME-COURT ADVANTAGE

Many professional basketball teams have gone to great lengths to gain a home-court advantage. The floor of the Celtics' old Boston Garden had hollow spots that made dribbling a challenge. The Milwaukee Bucks' tight nets gave their players extra time to get back on defense after a made basket. But Chicago's United Center, which opened in 1994, was built with more than one interesting advantage. First were the notoriously stiff rims, which lowered the shooting percentages of visiting teams—and even the Bulls themselves. Second, the spectator stands were located farther away from the court than normal, so a shooter's depth perception was altered, and some of the lights were positioned so as to play even more visual tricks. Finally, the building's temperature was often colder than most NBA stadiums. "This is a building you don't shoot well in," Bulls coach Phil Jackson once said. "It's the backboards, the basket standards, the rim, and the ambience and the surrounding environs that make it not a shooter's place. It's just a variety of things, but we try not to psychologically be intimidated by it."

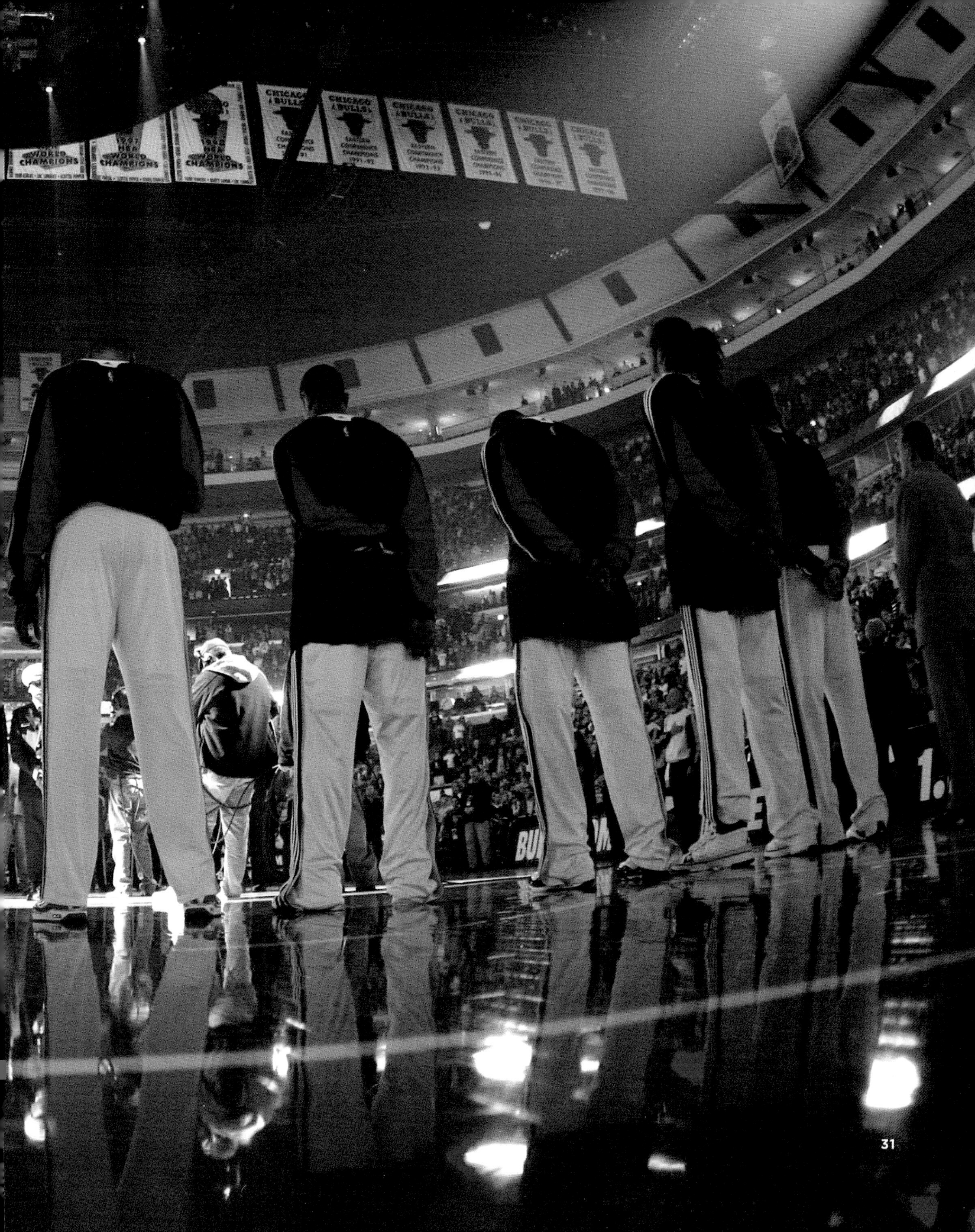
WORLD CHAMPIONS
1997 NBA WORLD CHAMPIONS
NBA WORLD CHAMPIONS
CHICAGO BULLS
CHICAGO BULLS EASTERN CONFERENCE CHAMPIONS 1991-92
CHICAGO BULLS EASTERN CONFERENCE CHAMPIONS 1992-93
CHICAGO BULLS
CHICAGO BULLS
CHICAGO BULLS

"THIS MEANS A LOT TO ME. PEOPLE DOUBTED US. WE PROVED THEM WRONG."

– MICHAEL JORDAN ON THE 1996 NBA CHAMPIONSHIP

home to suit up once more. He elected to wear jersey number 45, since his former number, 23, had already been retired by the team. In the 1995 playoffs, Jordan and the Bulls fell to the Orlando Magic. Afterwards, Orlando guard Nick Anderson told reporters that the new Jordan wasn't equal to the old. "That number 45, he isn't Superman," Anderson said. "Number 23 was, but this guy isn't."

Stung by that loss, Jordan took his old jersey number out of retirement. The Bulls then added Dennis Rodman, a heavily tattooed forward known for his energetic rebounding skills, to the lineup. In 1995–96, Chicago's 72–10 regular-season mark set an NBA record for most wins in a season. The Bulls then proved unstoppable in the playoffs, charging to their fourth NBA championship in six years by defeating the Seattle SuperSonics in the Finals. "This means a lot to me," said an emotional Jordan. "People doubted us. We proved them wrong."

Over the next two seasons, no one doubted the Bulls as they stampeded to two more NBA championships. Jackson's thoughtful coaching and a scrappy supporting cast that included center Luc Longley, guard Steve Kerr, and Croatian forward Toni Kukoc kept the Bulls rolling. In Game 6 of the 1998 NBA Finals—his last game in a Bulls uniform—Jordan poured in 45 points, including the game-winning basket, to top the Utah Jazz for the Bulls' sixth championship in eight years.

After a 13-season career in which he won 5 NBA MVP awards and 6 NBA Finals MVP awards and completely rewrote Chicago's record books, Jordan again retired from the Bulls. Shortly after that, Pippen was traded away, Rodman was released, and Coach Jackson left the team to join the Lakers. One of the greatest dynasties in NBA history had ended.

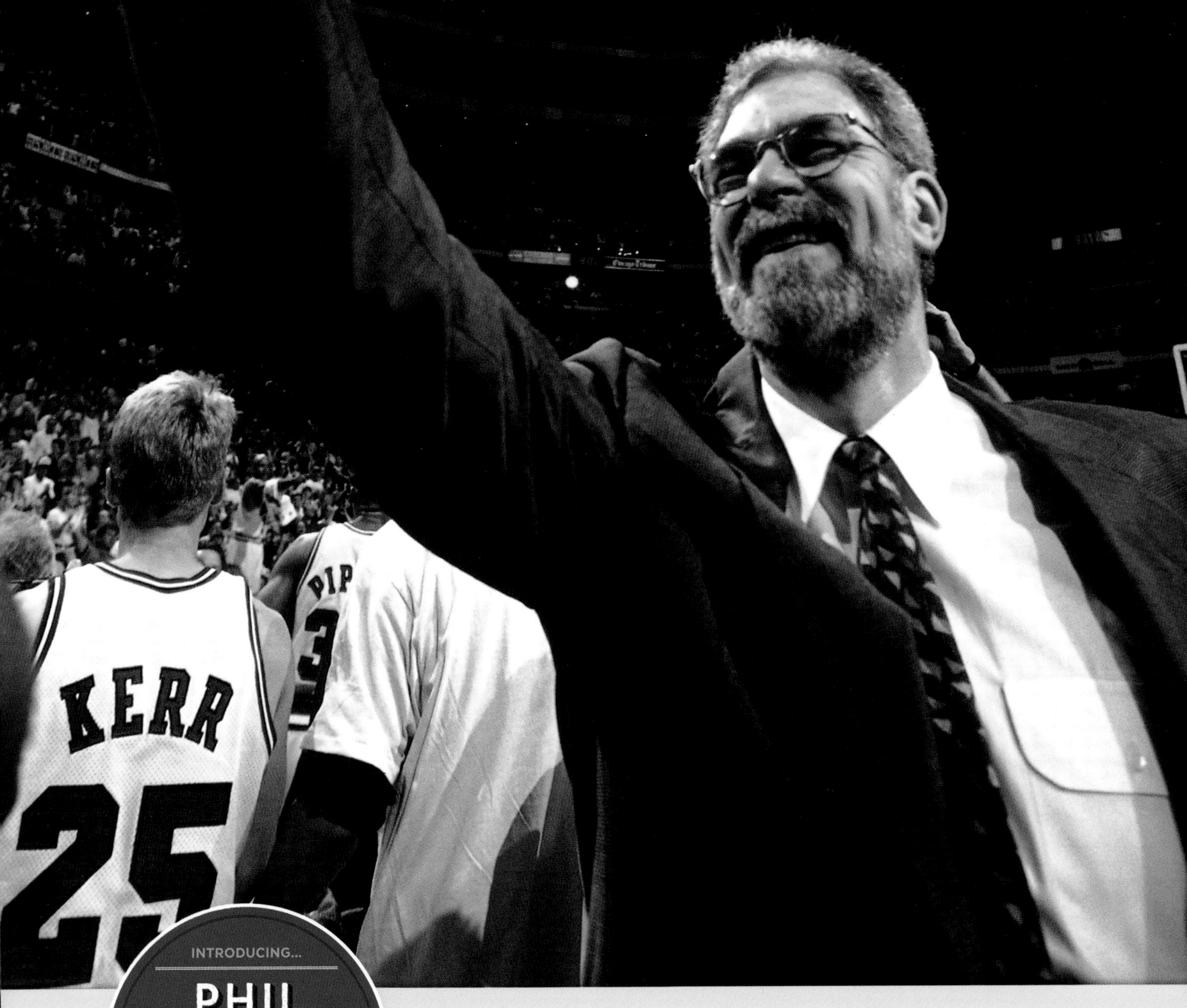

INTRODUCING...

PHIL JACKSON

COACH
BULLS SEASONS
1989–98

Following trusted mentors was a recurring theme in Phil Jackson's basketball career. It began in the fifth grade in Great Falls, Montana, with "Babe," a coach who spent extra practice time teaching Jackson how to shoot a step hook. In the seventh grade, Jackson started to learn every position on the basketball court. That's when 4-H agent Don Hotchkiss, who started a six-county basketball league in Montana and North Dakota, discovered Jackson's skills. The 4-H slogan, "Learn by doing," would later help form Jackson's unique, Zen style of coaching. He kept things simple, from pregame pep talks such as "Do what you were prepared to do," to his adoption of NBA coach Red Holzman's game philosophy: hit the open man and quickly get back on defense. Eventually, one of his most effective methods of getting his message across became silence. Once, when the Bulls were lagging behind in points and not heeding his directions, Jackson called a timeout and stood silently staring at his players. "The message was pretty clear," assistant coach John Bach said. "You're not listening, so solve it yourself." By the time he retired in 2011, Jackson had won 11 NBA championships as coach: 6 with the Bulls and 5 with the Los Angeles Lakers.

THE NEW HERD

SWINGMAN RON HARPER EFFECTIVELY SHUT DOWN OPPONENTS FROM THE PERIMETER.

LUOL DENG

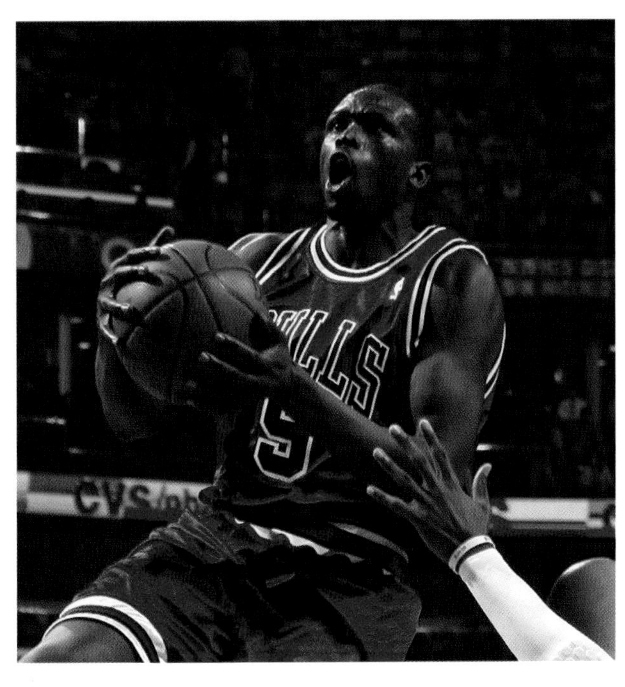

The Bulls plummeted from 62–20 in 1997–98 to 13–37 in a lockout-shortened 1998–99 season. Aside from the big-name players, Longley and Kerr were gone. Former college coach Tim Floyd took Jackson's seat on the bench. Among the few recognizable returnees were Kukoc and guard Ron Harper, but they too would soon be gone, and the club got even worse each of the next two seasons, bottoming out at 15–67, the worst record in franchise history. Floyd resigned after a 4–21 start to the 2001–02 campaign, and former Bulls center Bill Cartwright took over as coach for the remainder of that season and 2002–03. There was little Cartwright could do, though. The team simply lacked continuity and talent. Players came and went in one- and two-year stints. Draft selections either flopped or were traded away before their potential was realized.

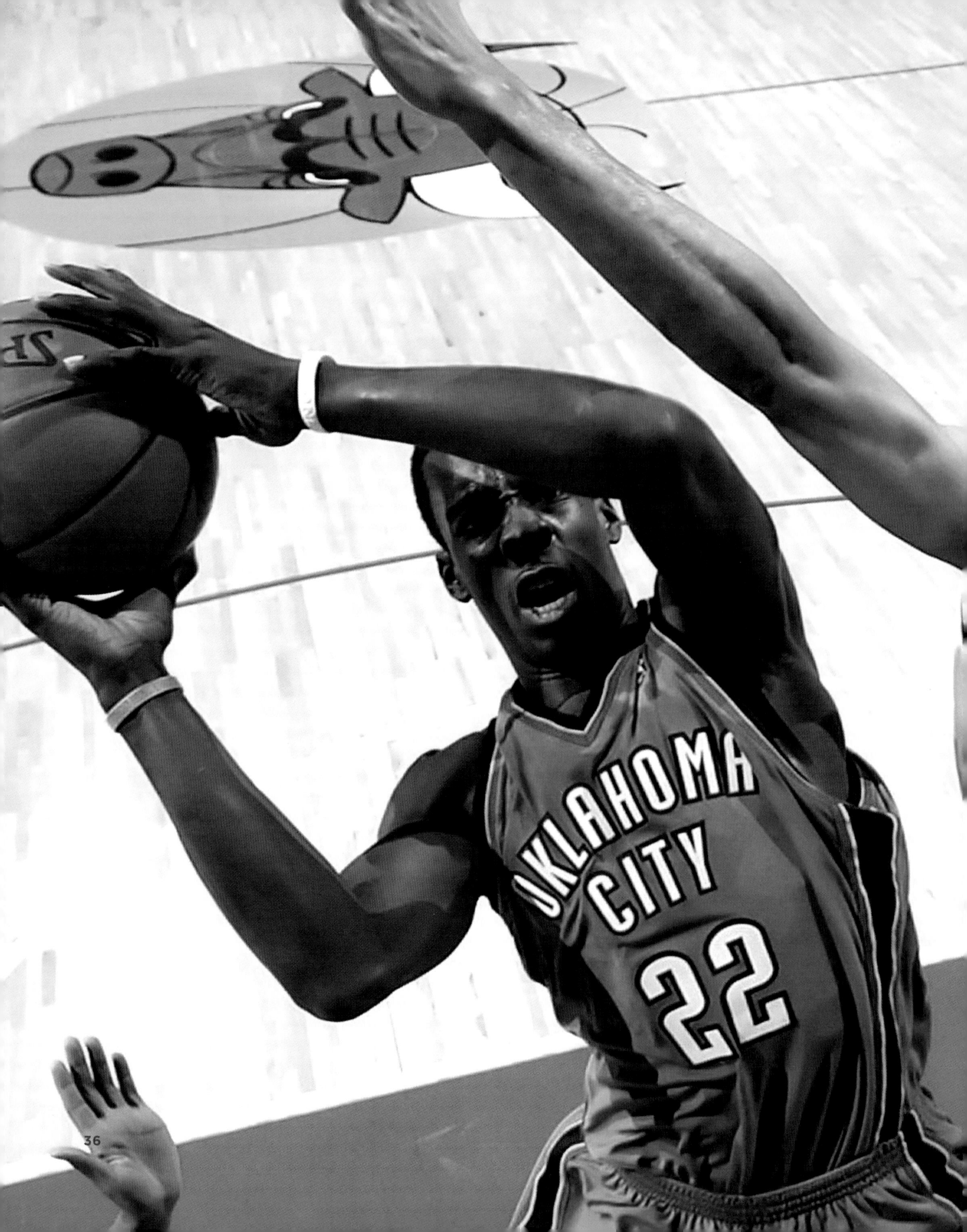
OKLAHOMA
CITY
22

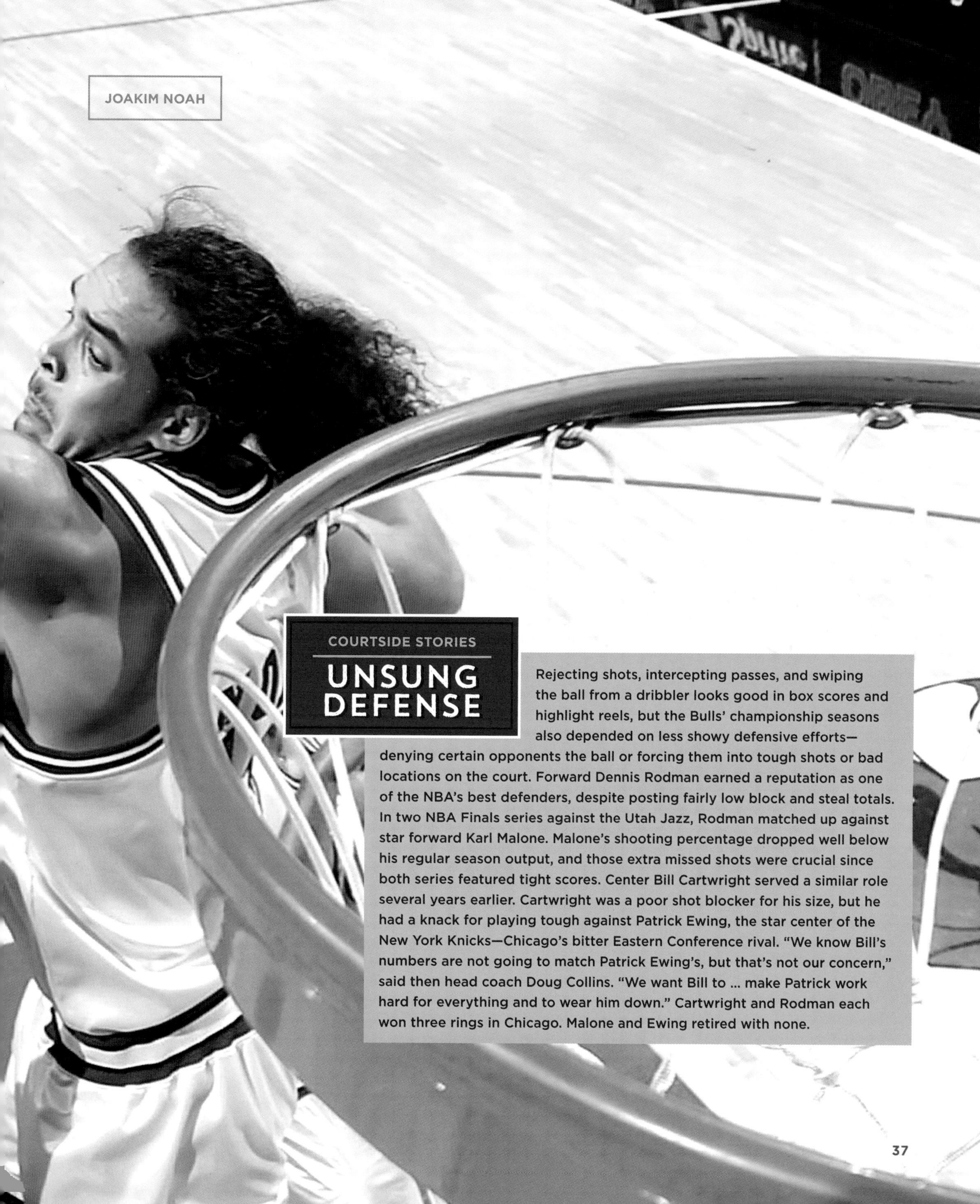

JOAKIM NOAH

COURTSIDE STORIES

UNSUNG DEFENSE

Rejecting shots, intercepting passes, and swiping the ball from a dribbler looks good in box scores and highlight reels, but the Bulls' championship seasons also depended on less showy defensive efforts—denying certain opponents the ball or forcing them into tough shots or bad locations on the court. Forward Dennis Rodman earned a reputation as one of the NBA's best defenders, despite posting fairly low block and steal totals. In two NBA Finals series against the Utah Jazz, Rodman matched up against star forward Karl Malone. Malone's shooting percentage dropped well below his regular season output, and those extra missed shots were crucial since both series featured tight scores. Center Bill Cartwright served a similar role several years earlier. Cartwright was a poor shot blocker for his size, but he had a knack for playing tough against Patrick Ewing, the star center of the New York Knicks—Chicago's bitter Eastern Conference rival. "We know Bill's numbers are not going to match Patrick Ewing's, but that's not our concern," said then head coach Doug Collins. "We want Bill to ... make Patrick work hard for everything and to wear him down." Cartwright and Rodman each won three rings in Chicago. Malone and Ewing retired with none.

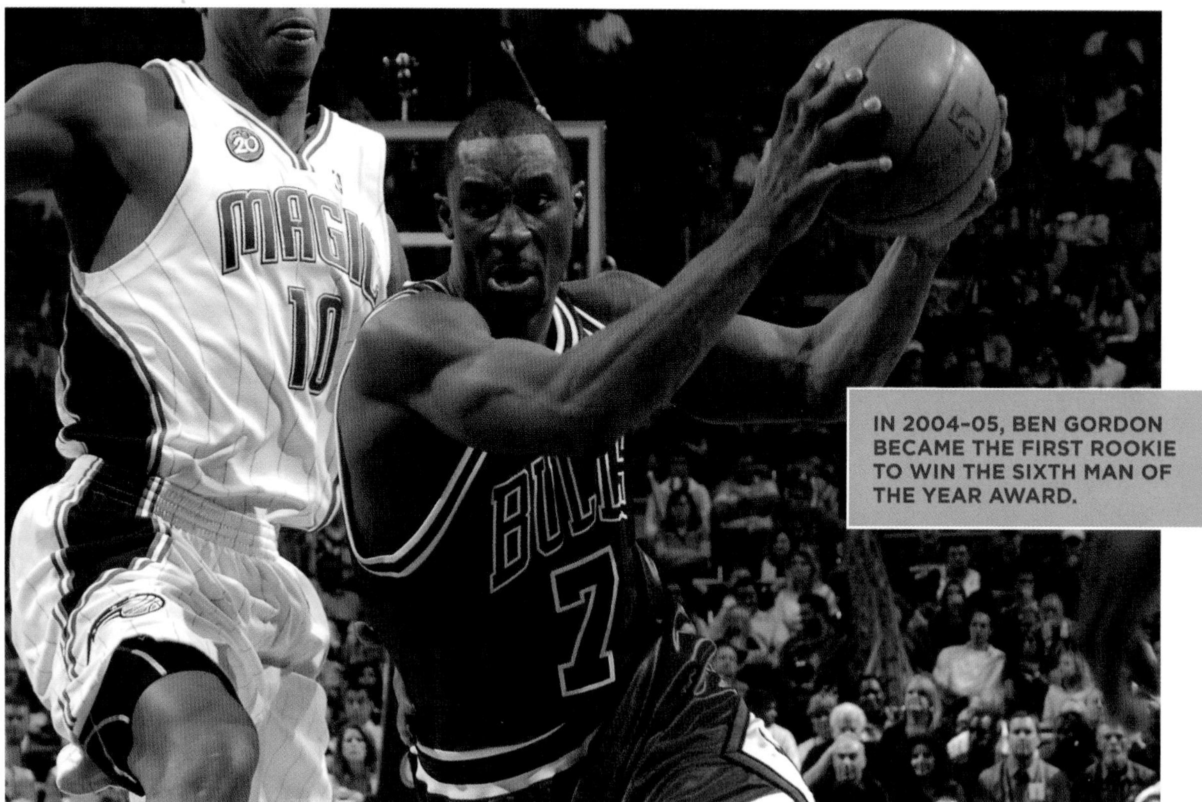

IN 2004-05, BEN GORDON BECAME THE FIRST ROOKIE TO WIN THE SIXTH MAN OF THE YEAR AWARD.

Personnel decisions seemed to start improving in the 2003 off-season with the drafting of steady guard Kirk Hinrich. The following season, Scott Skiles, a former NBA point guard known for his heart and hustle, took over coaching duties. The Bulls' record still stunk, but winds were changing in Chicago. Before the 2004–05 season, the Bulls drafted shifty guard Ben Gordon to pair up with Hinrich in the backcourt and added long, multipurpose forward Luol Deng. "They are good," Skiles said of his rookies. "You are never really sure what you are going to get, even though they played big games in college."

What the Bulls got initially was nine straight losses to start the season, but then things started to click. Seven-footers Eddy Curry and Tyson Chandler, both of whom had joined the club in 2001 straight out of high school, were starting to bloom three years later. Suddenly, the Bulls had a young, talented, well-balanced team that became known as "The Baby Bulls." The youngsters proved tough the duration of the season, finishing with a 47–35 record and reaching the playoffs for the first time since Jordan had left town. Despite losing four games out of the six-game series, Chicago's future looked bright.

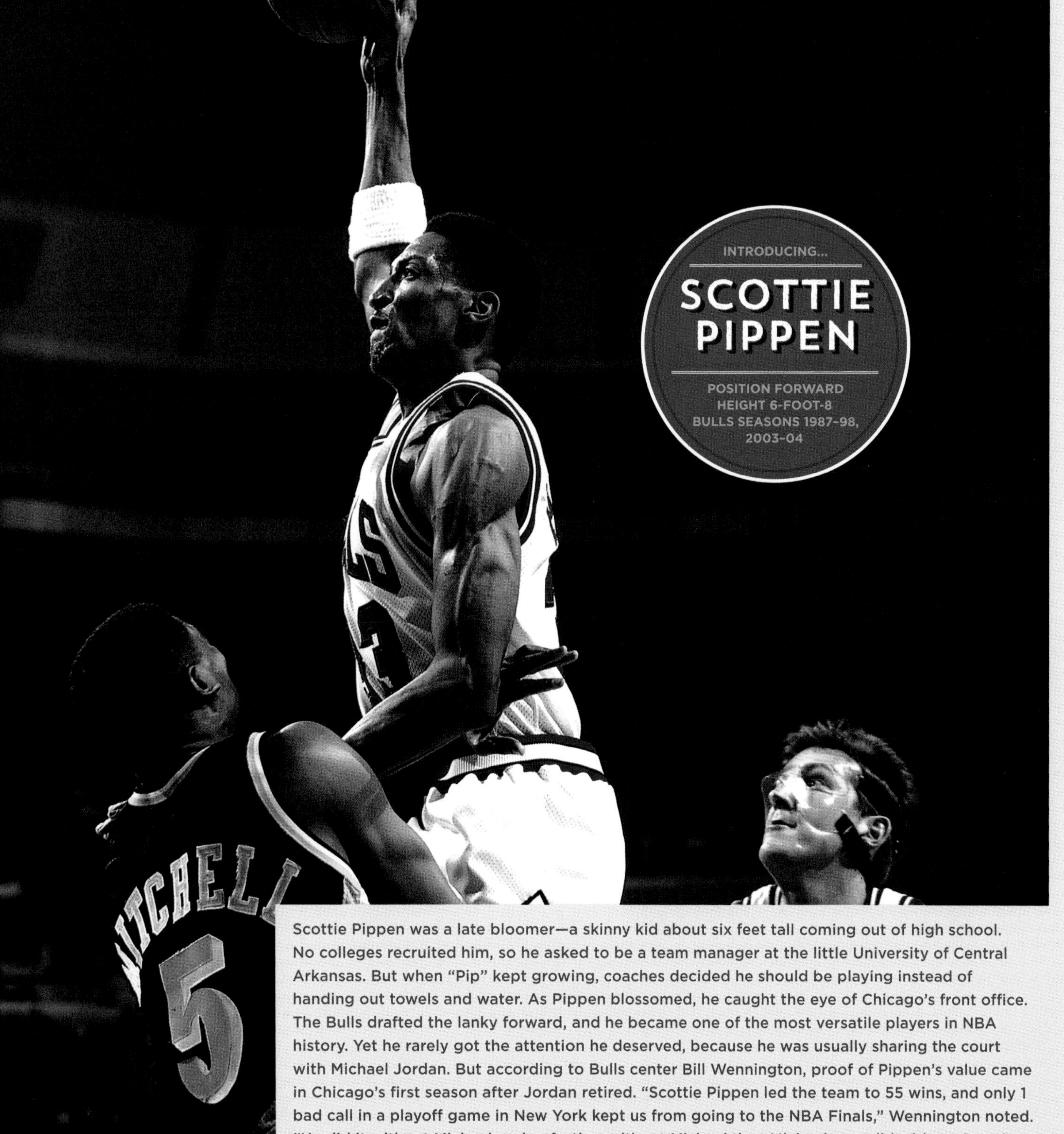

INTRODUCING...

SCOTTIE PIPPEN

POSITION FORWARD
HEIGHT 6-FOOT-8
BULLS SEASONS 1987–98, 2003–04

Scottie Pippen was a late bloomer—a skinny kid about six feet tall coming out of high school. No colleges recruited him, so he asked to be a team manager at the little University of Central Arkansas. But when "Pip" kept growing, coaches decided he should be playing instead of handing out towels and water. As Pippen blossomed, he caught the eye of Chicago's front office. The Bulls drafted the lanky forward, and he became one of the most versatile players in NBA history. Yet he rarely got the attention he deserved, because he was usually sharing the court with Michael Jordan. But according to Bulls center Bill Wennington, proof of Pippen's value came in Chicago's first season after Jordan retired. "Scottie Pippen led the team to 55 wins, and only 1 bad call in a playoff game in New York kept us from going to the NBA Finals," Wennington noted. "He did it without Michael, going further without Michael than Michael ever did without Scottie. ... That season was an indication of what Scottie was capable of doing as a team leader." Pippen played a vital role in six NBA titles and, in 2010, was inducted into the Basketball Hall of Fame.

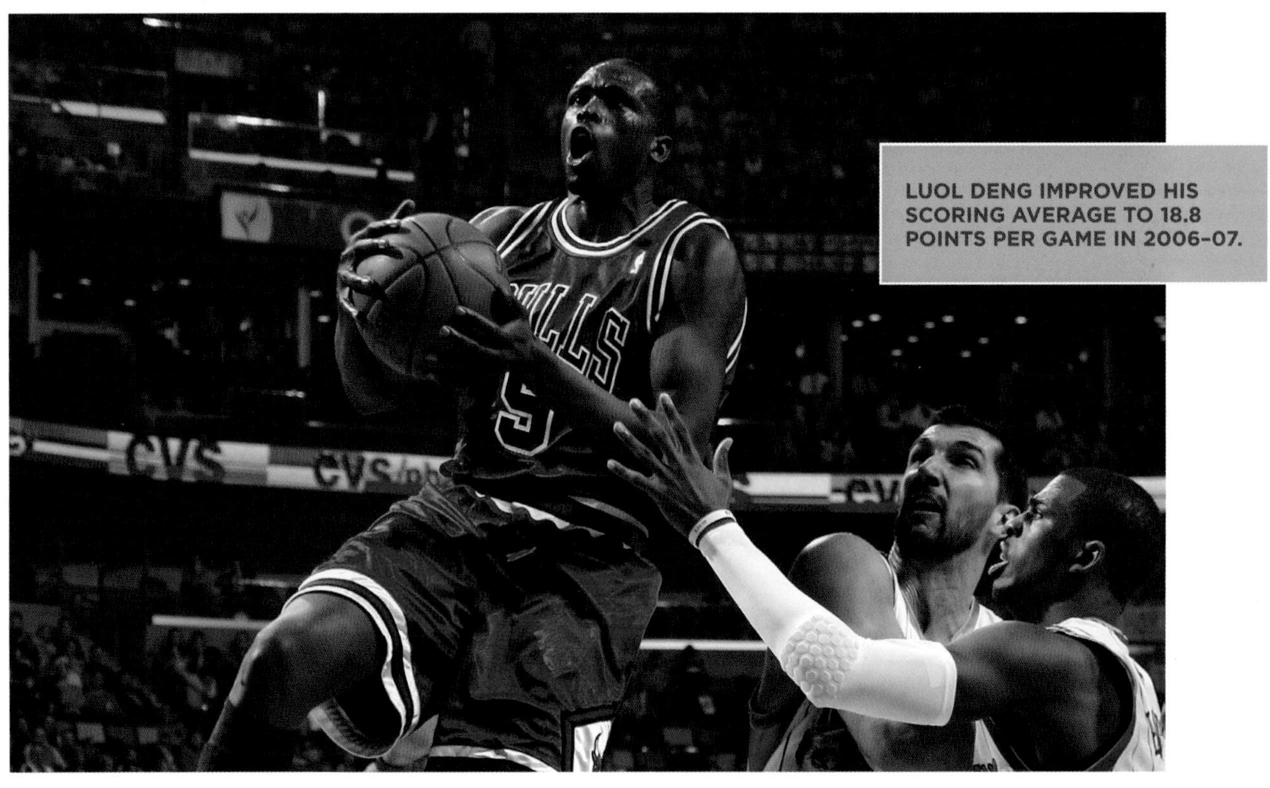

LUOL DENG IMPROVED HIS SCORING AVERAGE TO 18.8 POINTS PER GAME IN 2006-07.

Fans were disappointed when the club dropped to 41–41 in 2005–06 and were again bounced from the opening round of the playoffs. Prior to the 2006–07 season, Chandler was traded, and Chicago signed veteran forward/center Ben Wallace from the rival Pistons. Wallace wasn't especially tall or much of an offensive threat, but he had been named NBA Defensive Player of the Year four times and twice had led the league in rebounds. He added grit to a team that was becoming increasingly polished offensively, and the Bulls stormed into the 2006–07 playoffs, sweeping the defending NBA champion Miami Heat in the first round. The Pistons got the best of them in round two, however.

Even after they added high-energy rookie center Joakim Noah to the roster, the 2007–08 Bulls slipped to 33–49. New head coach Vinny Del Negro took over in 2008–09, and Chicago added another calf to the corral—explosive rookie point guard Derrick Rose. The backcourt-oriented Bulls made the most of their seven nail-biting postseason games, forcing the defending NBA champion Celtics into overtime in four of the contests—a first for an NBA playoff series—before ultimately losing the thrilling series. The

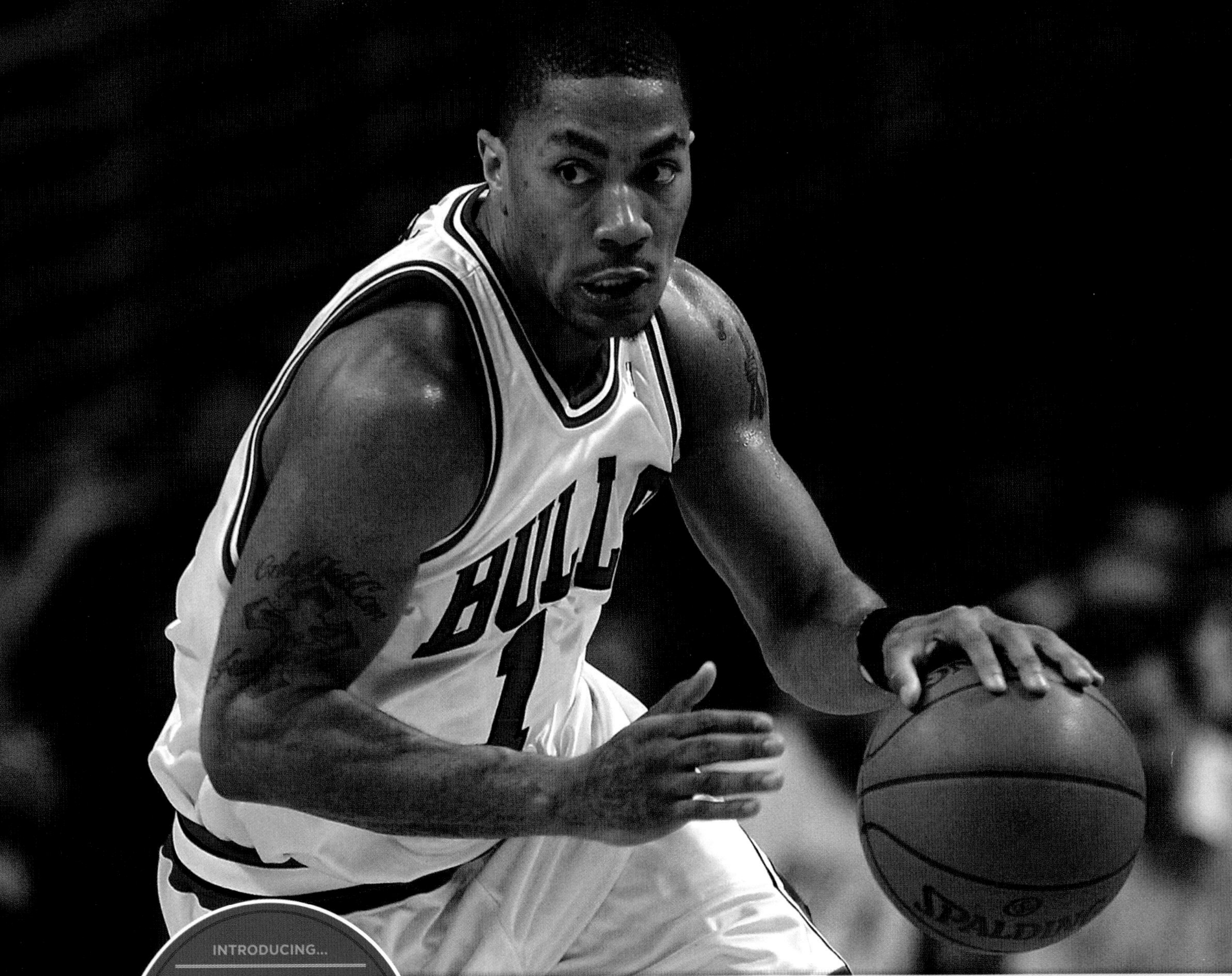

INTRODUCING...

DERRICK ROSE

POSITION GUARD
HEIGHT 6-FOOT-3
BULLS SEASONS
2008–PRESENT

Conventional wisdom says that the paint is the domain of towering centers and burly forwards. Derrick Rose didn't accept conventional wisdom, and the 6-foot-3 point guard made a habit of attacking rim. Ankle-breaking quickness and dribbling skills allowed Rose to blow past nearly any perimeter defender, and, once he was in the lane amongst the trees, he'd leap and hang in the air for an impossibly long time, double clutching and windmilling the ball around defenders on his way to spectacular assists, layups, scoop shots, and floaters. Other times, he'd forego the evasive maneuvers and just dunk the ball in the face of the opposition. Rose was not only lightning-quick, but he hardly ever took a seat on the bench, meaning he'd often torment the competition for the entirety of the game. That sort of tenacity made Rose the NBA's 2011 MVP and drove opponents nuts. Indiana Pacers forward Danny Granger compared Rose's doggedness to a "crazy stalker ex-girlfriend. Every time you tell her you don't want to talk to her, she'll show up at your door again."

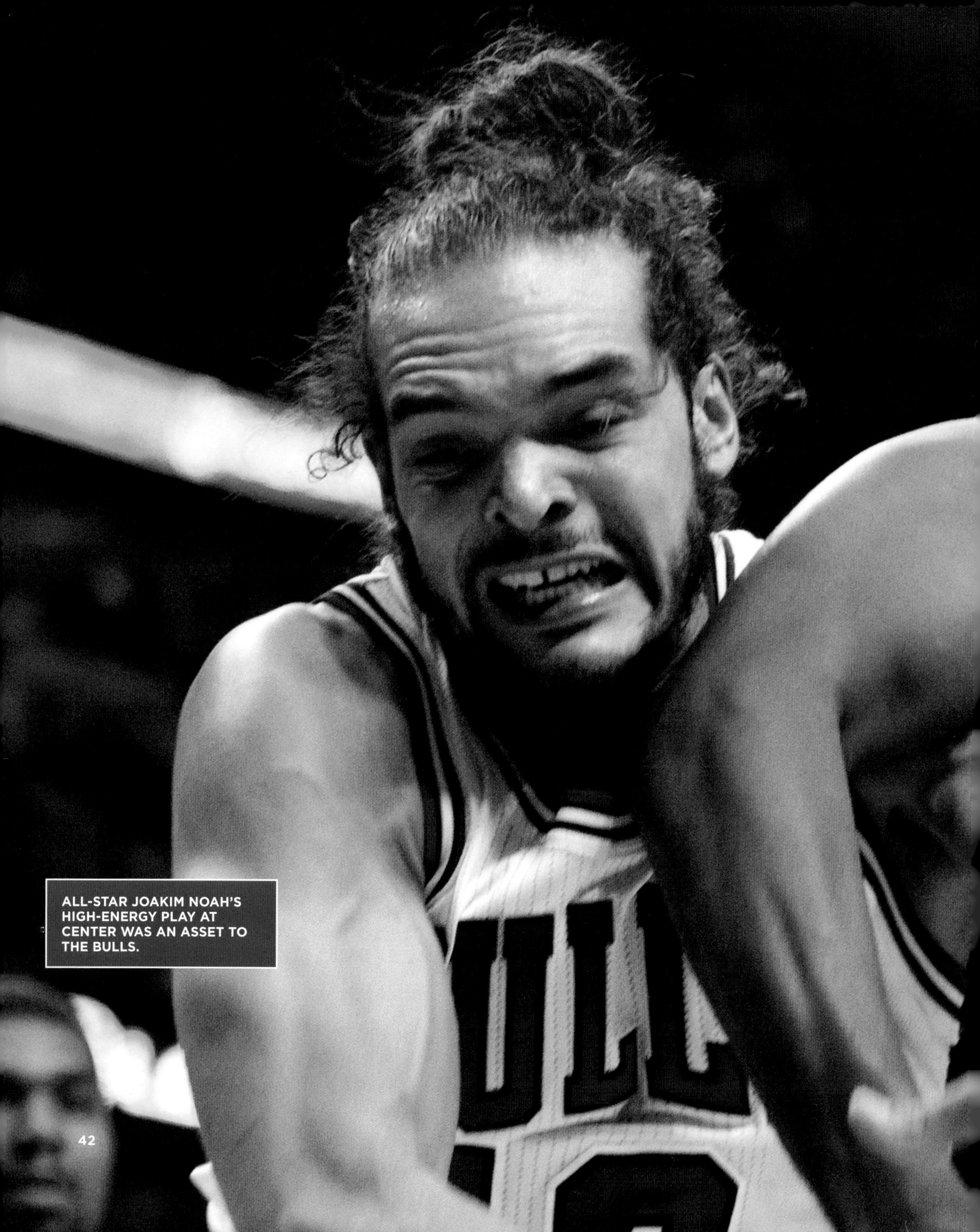

ALL-STAR JOAKIM NOAH'S HIGH-ENERGY PLAY AT CENTER WAS AN ASSET TO THE BULLS.

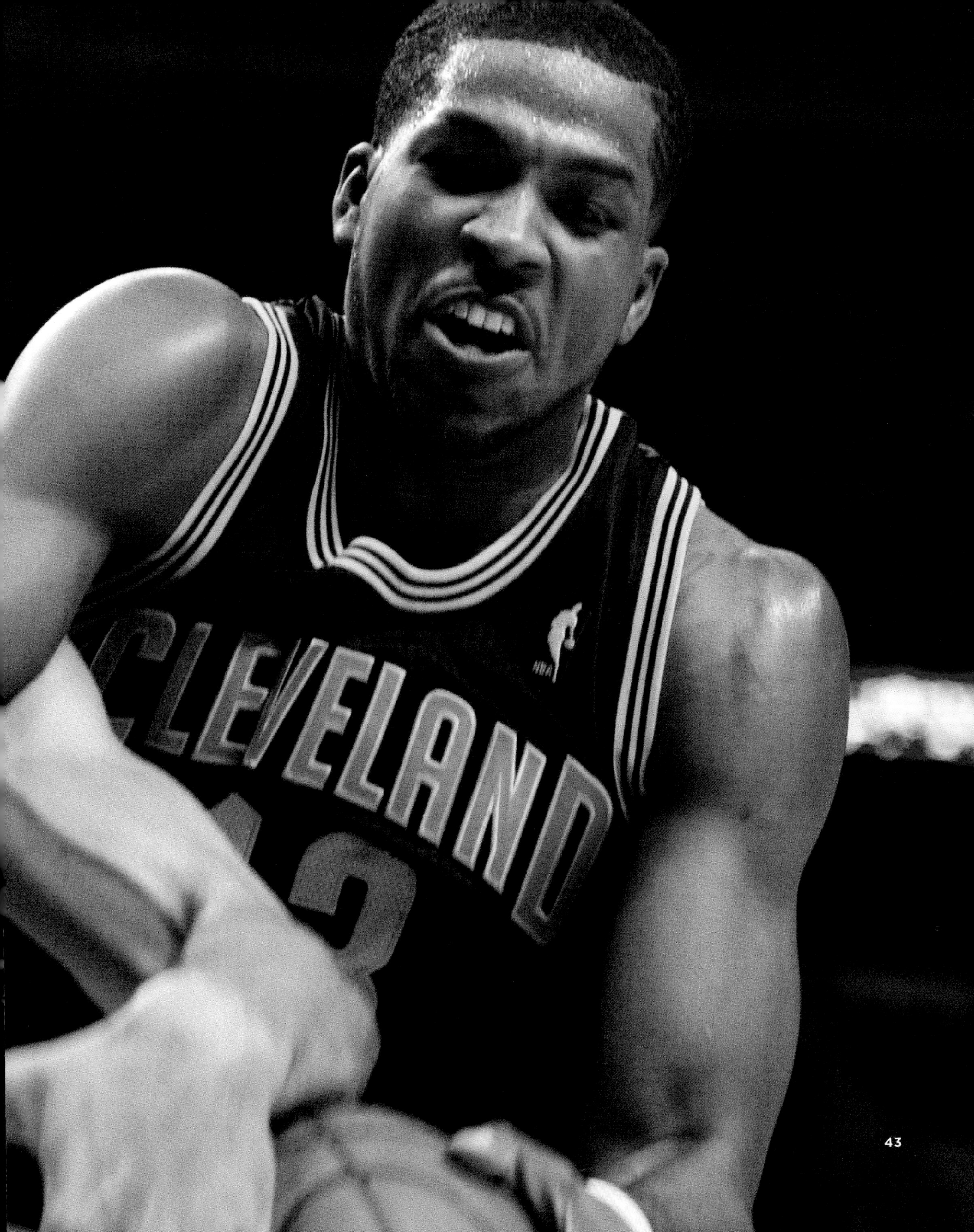
CLEVELAND

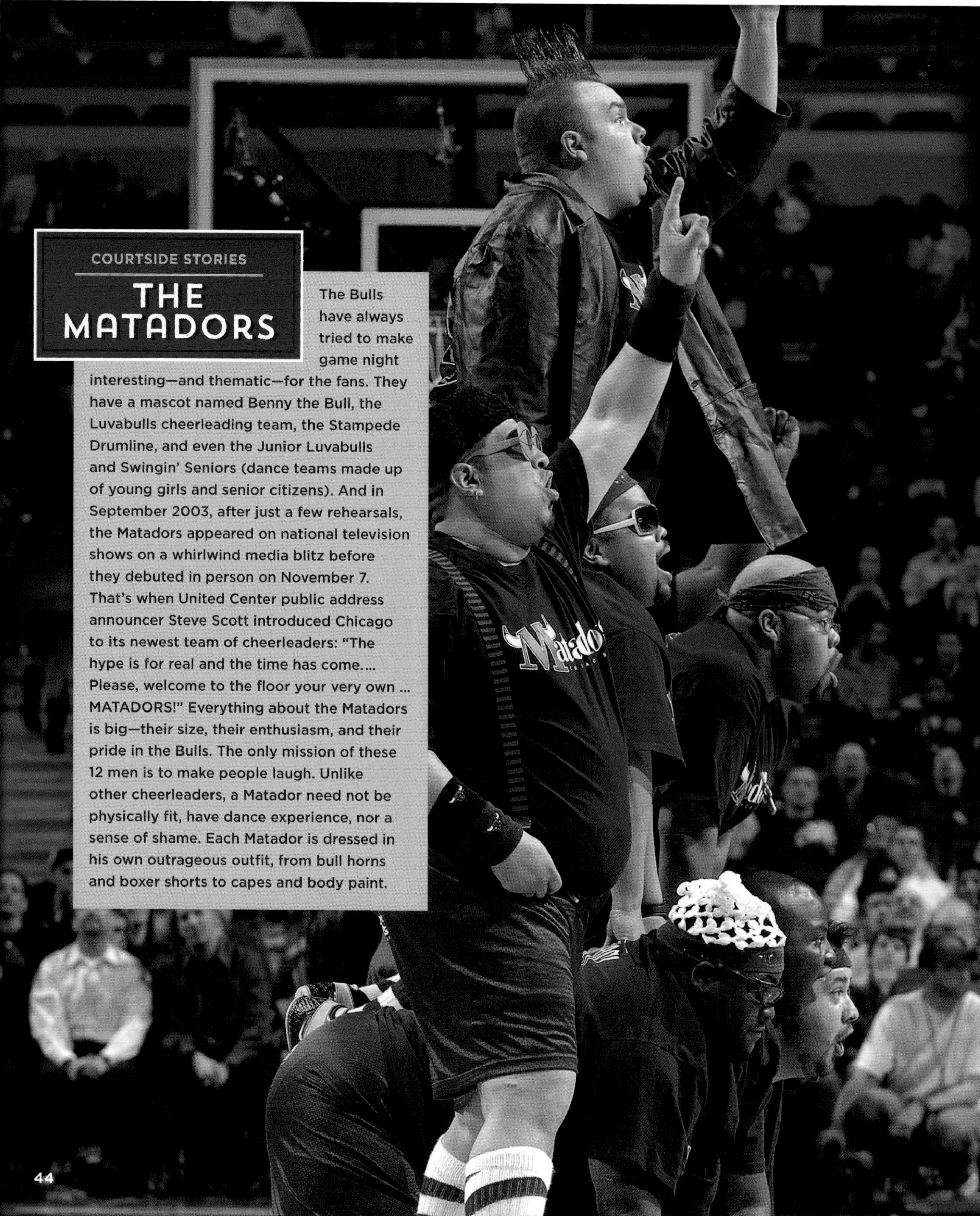

COURTSIDE STORIES

THE MATADORS

The Bulls have always tried to make game night interesting—and thematic—for the fans. They have a mascot named Benny the Bull, the Luvabulls cheerleading team, the Stampede Drumline, and even the Junior Luvabulls and Swingin' Seniors (dance teams made up of young girls and senior citizens). And in September 2003, after just a few rehearsals, the Matadors appeared on national television shows on a whirlwind media blitz before they debuted in person on November 7. That's when United Center public address announcer Steve Scott introduced Chicago to its newest team of cheerleaders: "The hype is for real and the time has come.... Please, welcome to the floor your very own ... MATADORS!" Everything about the Matadors is big—their size, their enthusiasm, and their pride in the Bulls. The only mission of these 12 men is to make people laugh. Unlike other cheerleaders, a Matador need not be physically fit, have dance experience, nor a sense of shame. Each Matador is dressed in his own outrageous outfit, from bull horns and boxer shorts to capes and body paint.

Bulls duplicated their season record of 41–41 in 2009–10 and suffered another first-round postseason knockout, this time at the hands of superstar forward LeBron James and his squad of Cavaliers.

Determined to make more noise the following season, Chicago appointed Tom Thibodeau as coach, and he shifted the team back toward a balanced offense. Beefy forward/center Carlos Boozer, a scoring threat and a tough rebounder, was brought in to help Chicago catch fire. Rose emerged as an all-around threat, tallying 25.0 points and 7.7 assists per game. Boozer, Noah, and Deng also proved versatile, and each made solid contributions to scoring, rebounding, and defense, as the Bulls won their first division title since 1998.

In the postseason, the Bulls kept the wins coming, dispatching first the Indiana Pacers and then the Atlanta Hawks. In Game 1 of the Eastern Conference finals, Chicago thumped Miami, but it seemed to lack balance in the following games, losing all four. The final game was particularly heartbreaking, as the Bulls blew a 12-point lead in the last few minutes. "I do think experience helps," Thibodeau said of his young team later. "Tonight, we had the lead, and we couldn't hold on to it. Hopefully, we learn from that, move on. I think you use this experience to drive you so you can improve for next year."

Chicago looked intent on improving the next season and once again finished first in its division. The Bulls were the overwhelming favorites in their first-round playoff matchup against the 76ers, but near the end of a Game 1 victory, Rose collapsed in agony after driving toward the basket. Fans held their collective breath while he clutched his knee. The injury would sideline Rose for more than a year. Without their dynamic floor leader, the deflated Bulls went on to lose the series.

In the 2012–13 campaign, Deng, Noah, and Boozer battled to hold down the fort in Rose's absence. Chicago's offense slowed down, but stingy defense earned the 45–37 Bulls their fifth playoff berth in a row. The Bulls went the full seven games to defeat the Brooklyn Nets in the first round before losing to the eventual champion Miami Heat, four games to one.

Chicago received bad news just 10 days into the 2013–14 campaign when Rose sustained another season-ending injury. By then, the team was used to playing without the star and seemed more focused than ever. Veteran guard D. J. Augustin, swingman Jimmy Butler, and sixth-man forward Taj Gibson stepped up to fill the scoring gap left by Deng, who was traded midseason, as the Bulls finished with a winning record. Noah was happy with how his teammates played, saying, "To be known as the team that goes out there and gives it everything they got every night, that's a good feeling."

Several decades now separate Chicago from its days as a livestock town. The cattle of the old stockyards have faded into memory as generations of Chicago Bulls, led by the likes of Sloan, Gilmore, Jordan, and Rose, have helped create a new identity for the city. Today's Bulls aim to display the power and aggressive spirit that will earn them their next NBA title and leave their fans bellowing for more.

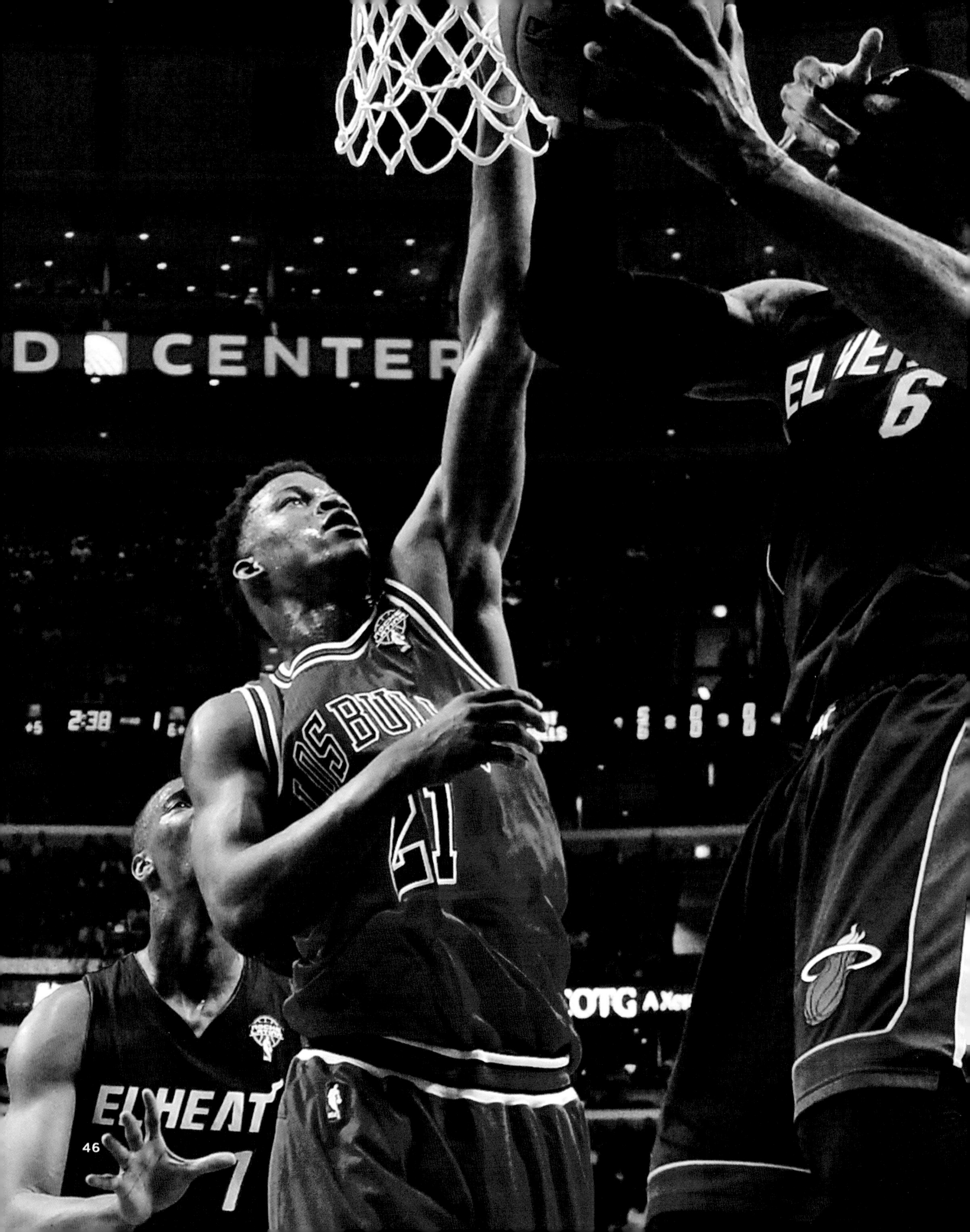

JIMMY BUTLER (#21) AND TAJ GIBSON (#22) FEARLESSLY SHIELDED THE BASKET AGAINST LEBRON JAMES.

INDEX

2053 49
W9-BZY-206

BEAVERTON CITY LIBRARY
Beaverton, OR 97005
Member of Washington County
COOPERATIVE LIBRARY SERVICES

DRAMA *for Students*

DRAMA *for Students*

Presenting Analysis, Context and Criticism on Commonly Studied Dramas

Volume 4

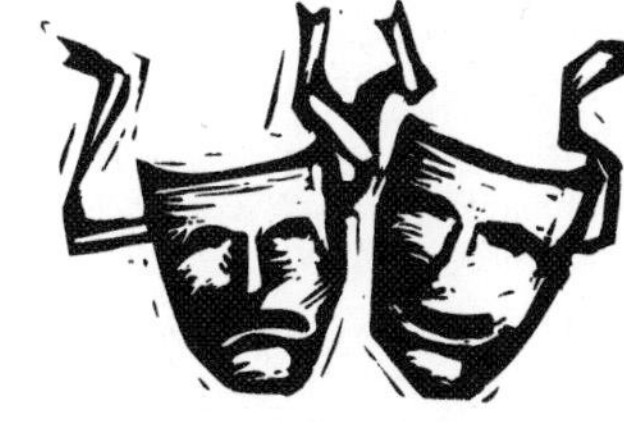

David Galens, Editor

Dale Allender, English Instructor at West High School, Iowa City, Iowa, and liaison officer for Iowa Council of Teachers of English Language Arts, Advisor

Carolyn Tragesser, English Instructor, Moscow Junior High School, Moscow, Idaho, liason for National Council of English Teachers, Advisor

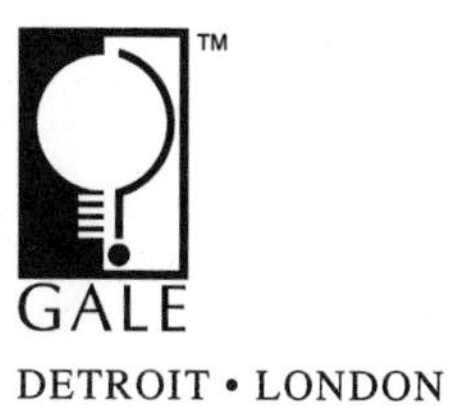

GALE

DETROIT • LONDON

Drama for Students

Staff

Editorial: David M. Galens, *Editor.* Terry Browne, Christopher Busiel, Clare Cross, John Fiero, David M. Galens, Carole Hamilton, D. L. Kellett, Erika Kreger, Sheri Metzger, Daniel Moran, Terry Nienhuis, Arnold Schmidt, William P. Wiles, Etta Worthington, *Entry Writers.* Elizabeth Cranston, Catherine V. Donaldson, Kathleen J. Edgar, Jennifer Gariepy, Dwayne D. Hayes, Joshua Kondek, Tom Ligotti, Scot Peacock, Patti Tippett, Pam Zuber, *Contributing Editors.* James Draper, *Managing Editor.* Diane Telgen, *"For Students" Line Coordinator.* Jeffery Chapman, *Programmer/Analyst.*

Research: Victoria B. Cariappa, *Research Team Manager.* Andy Malonis, Barb McNeil, *Research Specialists.* Julia C. Daniel, Tamara C. Nott, Tracie A. Richardson, Cheryl L. Warnock, *Research Associates.* Phyllis P. Blackman, Jeffrey D. Daniels, Corrine A. Stocker, *Research Assistants.*

Permissions: Susan M. Trosky, *Permissions Manager.* Kimberly F. Smilay*Permissions Specialist.* Steve Cusack and Kelly A. Quin, *Permissions Associates.*

Production: Mary Beth Trimper, *Production Director.* Evi Seoud, *Assistant Production Manager.* Shanna Heilveil, *Production Assistant.*

Graphic Services: Randy Bassett, *Image Database Supervisor.* Robert Duncan and Michael Logusz, *Imaging Specialists.* Pamela A. Reed, *Photography Coordinator.* Gary Leach, *Macintosh Artist.*

Product Design: Cynthia Baldwin, *Product Design Manager.* Cover Design: Michelle DiMercurio, *Art Director.* Page Design: Pamela A. E. Galbreath, *Senior Art Director.*

Copyright Notice

Since this page cannot legibly accommodate all copyright notices, the acknowledgments constitute an extension of the copyright notice.

While every effort has been made to secure permission to reprint material and to ensure the reliability of the information presented in this publication, Gale Research neither guarantees the accuracy of the data contained herein nor assumes any responsibility for errors, omissions, or discrepancies. Gale accepts no payment for listing; and inclusion in the publication of any organization, agency, institution, publication, service, or individual does not imply endorsement of the editors or publisher. Errors brought to the attention of the publisher and verified to the satisfaction of the publisher will be corrected in future editions.

This publication is a creative work fully protected by all applicable copyright laws, as well as by misappropriation, trade secret, unfair competition, and other applicable laws. The authors and editors of this work have added value to the underlying factual material herein through one or more of the following: unique and original selection, coordination, expression, arrangement, and classification of information. All rights to this publication will be vigorously defended.

Copyright © 1998
Gale Research
835 Penobscot Building
645 Griswold
Detroit, MI 48226-4094

All right reserved including the right of reproduction in whole or in part in any form.

∞™ This book is printed on acid-free paper that meets the minimum requirements of American National Standard for Information Sciences—Permanence Paper for Printed Library Materials, ANSI Z39.48-1984.

ISBN 0-7876-2753-4
ISSN 1094-9232
Printed in the United States of America

10 9 8 7 6 5 4 3 2 1

Table of Contents

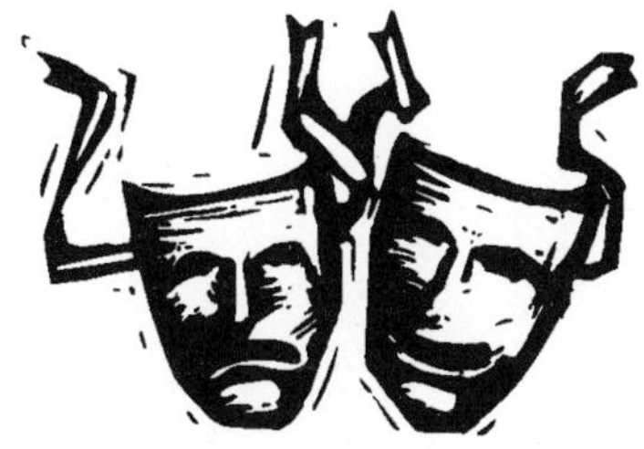

The Study of Drama

We study drama in order to learn what meaning others have made of life, to comprehend what it takes to produce a work of art, and to glean some understanding of ourselves. Drama produces in a separate, aesthetic world, a moment of being for the audience to experience, while maintaining the detachment of a reflective observer.

Drama is a representational art, a visible and audible narrative presenting virtual, fictional characters within a virtual, fictional universe. Dramatic realizations may pretend to approximate reality or else stubbornly defy, distort, and deform reality into an artistic statement. From this separate universe that is obviously not "real life" we expect a valid reflection upon reality, yet drama never is mistaken for reality—the methods of theater are integral to its form and meaning. Theater is art, and art's appeal lies in its ability both to approximate life and to depart from it. By presenting its distorted version of life to our consciousness, art gives us a new perspective and appreciation of reality. Although, to some extent, all aesthetic experiences perform this service, theater does it most effectively by creating a separate, cohesive universe that freely acknowledges its status as an art form.

And what is the purpose of the aesthetic universe of drama? The potential answers to such a question are nearly as many and varied as there are plays written, performed, and enjoyed. Dramatic texts can be problems posed, answers asserted, or moments portrayed. Dramas (tragedies as well as comedies) may serve strictly "to ease the anguish of a torturing hour" (as stated in William Shakespeare's *A Midsummer Night's Dream*)—to divert and entertain—or aspire to move the viewer to action with social issues. Whether to entertain or to instruct, affirm or influence, pacify or shock, dramatic art wraps us in the spell of its imaginary world for the length of the work and then dispenses us back to the real world, entertained, purged, as Aristotle said, of pity and fear, and edified—or at least weary enough to sleep peacefully.

It is commonly thought that theater, being an art of performance, must be experienced—that is, seen—in order to be appreciated fully. However, to view a production of a dramatic text is to be limited to a single interpretation of that text—all other interpretations are for the moment closed off, inaccessible. In the process of producing a play, the director, stage designer, and performers interpret and transform the script into a work of art that always departs in some measure from the author's original conception. Novelist and critic Umberto Eco, in his *The Role of the Reader: Explorations in the Semiotics of Texts,* explained, "In short, we can say that every performance offers us a complete and satisfying version of the work, but at the same time makes it incomplete for us, because it cannot simultaneously give all the other artistic solutions which the work may admit."

Thus Laurence Olivier's coldly formal and neurotic film presentation of Shakespeare's *Hamlet* (in which he played the title character as well as directed) shows marked differences from subsequent adaptations. While Olivier's Hamlet is clearly entangled in a Freudian relationship with his mother, Gertrude, he would be incapable of shushing her with the impassioned kiss that Mel Gibson's mercurial Hamlet (in director Franco Zeffirelli's 1990 film) does. Although each of the performances rings true to Shakespeare's text, each is also a mutually exclusive work of art. Also important to consider are the time periods in which each of these films were produced: Olivier made his film in 1948, a time in which overt references to sexuality (especially incest) were frowned upon. Gibson and Zeffirelli made their film in a culture more relaxed and comfortable with these issues. Just as actors and directors can influence the presentation of drama, so too can the time period of the production affect what the audience will see.

A play script is an open text from which an infinity of specific realizations may be derived. Dramatic scripts that are more open to interpretive creativity (such as those of Ntozake Shange and Tomson Highway) actually require the creative improvisation of the production troupe in order to complete the text. Even the most prescriptive scripts (those of Neil Simon, Lillian Hellman, and Robert Bolt, for example), can never fully control the actualization of live performance, and circumstantial events, including the attitude and receptivity of the audience, make every performance a unique event. Thus, while it is important to view a production of a dramatic piece, if one wants to understand a drama fully it is equally important to read the original dramatic text.

The reader of a dramatic text or script is not limited by either the specific interpretation of a given production or by the unstoppable action of a moving spectacle. The reader of a dramatic text may discover the nuances of the play's language, structure, and events at their own pace. Yet studied alone, the author's blueprint for artistic production does not tell the whole story of a play's life and significance. One also needs to assess the play's critical reviews to discover how it resonated to cultural themes at the time of its debut and how the shifting tides of cultural interest have revised its interpretation and impact on audiences. And to do this, one needs to know a little about the culture of the times which produced the play as well as the author who penned it.

Drama for Students supplies this material in a useful compendium for the student of dramatic theater. Covering a range of dramatic works that span from the fifth century B.C. to the 1990s, this book focuses on significant theatrical works whose themes and form transcend the uncertainty of dramatic fads. These are plays that have proven to be both memorable and teachable. *Drama for Students* seeks to enhance appreciation of these dramatic texts by providing scholarly materials written with the secondary and college/university student in mind. It provides for each play a concise summary of the plot and characters as well as a detailed explanation of its themes and techniques. In addition, background material on the historical context of the play, its critical reception, and the author's life help the student to understand the work's position in the chronicle of dramatic history. For each play entry a new work of scholarly criticism is also included, as well as segments of other significant critical works for handy reference. A thorough bibliography provides a starting point for further research.

These inaugural two volumes offer comprehensive educational resources for students of drama. *Drama for Students* is a vital book for dramatic interpretation and a valuable addition to any reference library.

Source: Eco, Umberto, *The Role of the Reader: Explorations in the Semiotics of Texts,* Indiana University Press, 1979.

Carole L. Hamilton
Author and Instructor of English
Cary Academy
Cary, North Carolina

Introduction

Purpose of Drama for Students

The purpose of *Drama for Students* (*DfS*) is to provide readers with a guide to understanding, enjoying, and studying dramas by giving them easy access to information about the work. Part of Gale's ''For Students'' literature line, *DfS* is specifically designed to meet the curricular needs of high school and undergraduate college students and their teachers, as well as the interests of general readers and researchers considering specific plays. While each volume contains entries on ''classic'' dramas frequently studied in classrooms, there are also entries containing hard-to-find information on contemporary plays, including works by multicultural, international, and women playwrights.

The information covered in each entry includes an introduction to the play and the work's author; a plot summary, to help readers unravel and understand the events in a drama; descriptions of important characters, including explanation of a given character's role in the drama as well as discussion about that character's relationship to other characters in the play; analysis of important themes in the drama; and an explanation of important literary techniques and movements as they are demonstrated in the play.

In addition to this material, which helps the readers analyze the play itself, students are also provided with important information on the literary and historical background informing each work. This includes a historical context essay, a box comparing the time or place the drama was written to modern Western culture, a critical overview essay, and excerpts from critical essays on the play. A unique feature of *DfS* is a specially commissioned overview essay on each drama by an academic expert, targeted toward the student reader.

To further aid the student in studying and enjoying each play, information on media adaptations is provided, as well as reading suggestions for works of fiction and nonfiction on similar themes and topics. Classroom aids include ideas for research papers and lists of critical sources that provide additional material on each drama.

Selection Criteria

The titles for each volume of *DfS* were selected by surveying numerous sources on teaching literature and analyzing course curricula for various school districts. Some of the sources surveyed included: literature anthologies; *Reading Lists for College-Bound Students: The Books Most Recommended by America's Top Colleges;* textbooks on teaching dramas; a College Board survey of plays commonly studied in high schools; a National Council of Teachers of English (NCTE) survey of plays commonly studied in high schools; St. James Press's *International Dictionary of Theatre;* and Arthur Applebee's 1993 study *Literature in the Secondary School: Studies of Curriculum and Instruction in the United States.*

Input was also solicited from our expert advisory board (both experienced educators specializing in English), as well as educators from various areas. From these discussions, it was determined that each volume should have a mix of ''classic'' dramas (those works commonly taught in literature classes) and contemporary dramas for which information is often hard to find. Because of the interest in expanding the canon of literature, an emphasis was also placed on including works by international, multicultural, and women playwrights. Our advisory board members—current high school teachers—helped pare down the list for each volume. If a work was not selected for the present volume, it was often noted as a possibility for a future volume. As always, the editor welcomes suggestions for titles to be included in future volumes.

How Each Entry Is Organized

Each entry, or chapter, in *DfS* focuses on one play. Each entry heading lists the full name of the play, the author's name, and the date of the play's first production or publication. The following elements are contained in each entry:

- **Introduction:** a brief overview of the drama which provides information about its first appearance, its literary standing, any controversies surrounding the work, and major conflicts or themes within the work.
- **Author Biography:** this section includes basic facts about the author's life, and focuses on events and times in the author's life that inspired the drama in question.
- **Plot Summary:** a description of the major events in the play, with interpretation of how these events help articulate the play's themes. Subheads demarcate the plays' various acts or scenes.
- **Characters:** an alphabetical listing of major characters in the play. Each character name is followed by a brief to an extensive description of the character's role in the plays, as well as discussion of the character's actions, relationships, and possible motivation.

  Characters are listed alphabetically by last name. If a character is unnamed—for instance, the Stage Manager in *Our Town*—the character is listed as ''The Stage Manager'' and alphabetized as ''Stage Manager.'' If a character's first name is the only one given, the name will appear alphabetically by the name.

  Variant names are also included for each character. Thus, the nickname ''Babe'' would head the listing for a character in *Crimes of the Heart,* but below that listing would be her less-mentioned married name ''Rebecca Botrelle.''

- **Themes:** a thorough overview of how the major topics, themes, and issues are addressed within the play. Each theme discussed appears in a separate subhead, and is easily accessed through the boldface entries in the Subject/Theme Index.
- **Style:** this section addresses important style elements of the drama, such as setting, point of view, and narration; important literary devices used, such as imagery, foreshadowing, symbolism; and, if applicable, genres to which the work might have belonged, such as Gothicism or Romanticism. Literary terms are explained within the entry, but can also be found in the Glossary.
- **Historical and Cultural Context:** This section outlines the social, political, and cultural climate *in which the author lived and the play was created.* This section may include descriptions of related historical events, pertinent aspects of daily life in the culture, and the artistic and literary sensibilities of the time in which the work was written. If the play is a historical work, information regarding the time in which the play is set is also included. Each section is broken down with helpful subheads.
- **Critical Overview:** this section provides background on the critical reputation of the play, including bannings or any other public controversies surrounding the work. For older plays, this section includes a history of how the drama was first received and how perceptions of it may have changed over the years; for more recent plays, direct quotes from early reviews may also be included.
- **For Further Study:** an alphabetical list of other critical sources which may prove useful for the student. Includes full bibliographical information and a brief annotation.
- **Sources:** an alphabetical list of critical material quoted in the entry, with full bibliographical information.
- **Criticism:** an essay commissioned by *DfS* which specifically deals with the play and is written specifically for the student audience, as well as excerpts from previously published criticism on the work.

In addition, each entry contains the following highlighted sections, set separate from the main text:

- **Media Adaptations:** a list of important film and television adaptations of the play, including source information. The list may also include such variations on the work as audio recordings, musical adaptations, and other stage interpretations.
- **Compare and Contrast Box:** an "at-a-glance" comparison of the cultural and historical differences between the author's time and culture and late twentieth-century Western culture. This box includes pertinent parallels between the major scientific, political, and cultural movements of the time or place the drama was written, the time or place the play was set (if a historical work), and modern Western culture. Works written after the mid-1970s may not have this box.
- **What Do I Read Next?:** a list of works that might complement the featured play or serve as a contrast to it. This includes works by the same author and others, works of fiction and nonfiction, and works from various genres, cultures, and eras.
- **Study Questions:** a list of potential study questions or research topics dealing with the play. This section includes questions related to other disciplines the student may be studying, such as American history, world history, science, math, government, business, geography, economics, psychology, etc.

Other Features

DfS includes "The Study of Drama," a foreword by Carole Hamilton, an educator and author who specializes in dramatic works. This essay examines the basis for drama in societies and what drives people to study such work. Hamilton also discusses how *Drama for Students* can help teachers show students how to enrich their own reading/viewing experiences.

A Cumulative Author/Title Index lists the authors and titles covered in each volume of the *DfS* series.

A Cumulative Nationality/Ethnicity Index breaks down the authors and titles covered in each volume of the *DfS* series by nationality and ethnicity.

A Subject/Theme Index, specific to each volume, provides easy reference for users who may be studying a particular subject or theme rather than a single work. Significant subjects from events to broad themes are included, and the entries pointing to the specific theme discussions in each entry are indicated in **boldface.**

Each entry has several illustrations, including photos of the author, stills from stage productions, and stills from film adaptations.

Citing Drama for Students

When writing papers, students who quote directly from any volume of *Drama for Students* may use the following general forms. These examples are based on MLA style; teachers may request that students adhere to a different style, so the following examples may be adapted as needed.

When citing text from *DfS* that is not attributed to a particular author (i.e., the Themes, Style, Historical Context sections, etc.), the following format should be used in the bibliography section:

"Our Town," *Drama for Students.* Ed. David Galens and Lynn Spampinato. Vol. 1. Detroit: Gale, 1997. 8–9.

When quoting the specially commissioned essay from *DfS* (usually the first piece under the "Criticism" subhead), the following format should be used:

Fiero, John. Essay on "Twilight: Los Angeles, 1992." *Drama for Students.* Ed. David Galens and Lynn Spampinato. Vol. 1. Detroit: Gale, 1997. 8–9.

When quoting a journal or newspaper essay that is reprinted in a volume of *DfS,* the following form may be used:

Rich, Frank. "Theatre: A Mamet Play, 'Glengarry Glen Ross'." *New York Theatre Critics' Review* Vol. 45, No. 4 (March 5, 1984), 5–7; excerpted and reprinted in *Drama for Students,* Vol. 1, ed. David Galens and Lynn Spampinato (Detroit: Gale, 1997), pp. 61–64.

When quoting material reprinted from a book that appears in a volume of *DfS,* the following form may be used:

Kerr, Walter. "The Miracle Worker," in *The Theatre in Spite of Itself* (Simon & Schuster, 1963, 255–57; excerpted and reprinted in *Drama for Students,* Vol. 1, ed. Dave Galens and Lynn Spampinato (Detroit: Gale, 1997), pp. 59–61.

We Welcome Your Suggestions

The editor of *Drama for Students* welcomes your comments and ideas. Readers who wish to suggest dramas to appear in future volumes, or who have other suggestions, are cordially invited to contact the editor. You may contact the editor via E-mail at: **david.galens@gale.com.** Or write to the editor at:

David Galens, *Drama for Students*
Gale Research
835 Penobscot Bldg.
645 Griswold St.
Detroit, MI 48226-4094

Literary Chronology

c. 496 B.C.: Sophocles is born in Colonus, near Athens, Greece.

c. 484 B.C.: Euripides is born in Athens, Greece.

c. 414 B.C.: *Iphigenia in Taurus* is presented at the Athenian Dionysia.

c. 409 B.C.: *Electra* debuts at the annual Dionysia festival in Athens, Greece.

c. 406 B.C.: Sophocles dies in Athens.

406 B.C.: Euripides dies in Macedonia.

c. 1572: Ben Jonson is born near London, England.

1610: *The Alchemist* has its debut performance.

1637: Ben Jonson dies in London. He is buried in Westminster Abbey.

1751: Richard Brinsley Sheridan is born in Dublin, Ireland, in September (though some sources cite October). He is christened on November 4.

1777: London's Drury Lane Theatre (of which playwright Sheridan is a co-owner) presents the debut of *School for Scandal* in May. The play is an immediate success.

1816: Richard Brinsley Sheridan dies on July 7 in London, England. He is buried in the Poet's Corner of Westminster Abbey.

1854: August Strindberg is born Johan August Strindberg on January 22, in Riddarholm, Stockholm, Sweden.

1854: Oscar Wilde is born on October 15 (though some sources cite October 16), 1854 (some sources cite 1856) in Dublin, Ireland.

1867: Luigi Pirandello is born on June 28 in Girgenti, Sicily, Italy.

1888: Eugene O'Neill is born on October 16, in New York City.

1888: Strindberg's *Miss Julie* is first published. The frank sexual content shocks readers across Europe. While the play is privately produced in the following years, it is not until 1906 that it receives a public production in the author's native country of Denmark.

1888: T. S. Eliot is born September 26, in St. Louis, Missouri.

1895: *The Importance of Being Earnest* is a success upon its London debut in February, running for eighty-six performances.

1897: Thornton Wilder is born in Madison, Wisconsin, on April 17.

1898: Bertolt Brecht is born Eugen Bertolt Friedrich Brecht on February 10 in Augsburg, Germany.

1898: Federico Garcia Lorca is born on June 5 near Granada, Spain.

1900: Wilde dies in Paris, France.

1909: Eugene Ionesco is born in Slatina, Romania, on November 26.

1912: August Strindberg dies from stomach cancer on May 14. He is buried in New Church Cemetery, Solna, Sweden.

1921: The original production of *Six Characters in Search of an Author* is staged in Rome, Italy, on May 10. Subsequent productions are mounted in Milan, London, and New York. The popularity of the play continues into the middle of the decade as Pirandello's own production company stages a worldwide tour in 1925.

1922: The Provincetown Players stage the debut performance of *The Hairy Ape* on March 9.

1925: Emilio Carballido is born in Cordoba, Veracruz, Mexico, on May 22.

1928: *The Threepenny Opera* stages its debut performance.

1929: John Osborne is born on December 12, in Fulham, South West London, England.

1935: *Murder in the Cathedral* debuts at the Canterbury Festival.

1936: *The House of Bernarda Alba* is completed. Garcia Lorca's last play is not produced until March 8, 1945, at the Teatro Avendia in Buenos Aires, Argentina.

1936: Federico Garcia Lorca is executed on August 19 by fascist rebels. An early casualty of the Spanish Civil War, he is buried in an unmarked grave.

1936: Luigi Pirandello dies in Rome, Italy, on December 10.

1937: Lanford Wilson is born in Lebanon, Missouri, on April 13.

1940: Mark Medoff is born in Mount Carmel, Illinois, on March 18.

1942: Ariel Dorfman is born in Buenos Aires, Argentina, on May 6.

1942: Following warm-up performances in New Haven and Baltimore, the Broadway debut of *The Skin of Our Teeth* is staged at the Plymouth Theatre on November 18. The play is an enormous success, running for 355 performances and eventually winning the Pulitzer Prize.

1945: David Hare is born in St. Leonard's, Sussex, England, on June 5.

1950: First production of *The Bald Soprano.*

1953: O'Neill dies from complications of pneumonia on November 27, 1953, in Boston, Massachusetts.

1956: The fledgling English Stage Company debuts its third production, *Look Back in Anger,* on May 8 at the Royal Court Theatre.

1956: Bertolt Brecht dies from coronary thrombosis on August 14 in East Berlin (now Berlin), East Germany (now Germany).

1965: T. S. Eliot dies January 4 in London, England. He is buried in Westminster Abbey.

1965: *I, Too, Speak of the Rose* is published. The play makes its staged debut the following year at Mexico City's Teatro Jimenez Rueda.

1975: Thornton Wilder dies of a heart attack on December 7 in Hamden, Connecticut.

1978: The debut performance of *Plenty* is staged on April 7 at London's Lyttelton Theatre.

1979: *Children of a Lesser God* debuts. The play wins the Tony Award the following year.

1987: *Burn This* debuts in Los Angeles, California, on January 22.

1991: *Death and the Maiden* debuts as a workshop production in Santiago, Chile. The play has its world premiere in July at London's Royal Court Upstairs Theatre.

1994: Eugene Ionesco dies on March 28.

1994: John Osborne dies of heart failure on December 24, in Shropshire, England.

Acknowledgments

The editors wish to thank the copyright holders of the excerpted criticism included in this volume and the permissions managers of many book and magazine publishing companies for assisting us in securing reproduction rights. We are also grateful to the staffs of the Detroit Public Library, the Library of Congress, the University of Detroit Mercy Library, Wayne State University Purdy/Kresge Library Complex, and the University of Michigan Libraries for making their resources available to us. Following is a list of the copyright holders who have granted us permission to reproduce material in this volume of ***Drama for Students.*** Every effort has been made to trace copyright, but if omissions have been made, please let us know.

COPYRIGHTED EXCERPTS IN *DFS,* VOLUME 4, WERE REPRODUCED FROM THE FOLLOWING PERIODICALS:

Classical Quarterly, v. 38, 1988 for "Pelopid History and the Plot of Iphigenia in Taurus" by Michael J. O'Brien. Reproduced by permission of Oxford University Press and the author. —***Commonweal,*** v. XXXVII, December 4, 1942; v. CXIII, September 26, 1986; v. CXIV, December 18, 1987; v. CXIX, May 8, 1992. Copyright 1942, © 1986, 1987, 1992 Commonweal Publishing Co., Inc. All reproduced by permission of Commonweal Foundation. —***Drama Survey,*** v. 4, Spring, 1965 for "The Averted Crucifixion of Macheath," by Bernard F. Dukore. Copyright 1965 by The Bolingbroke Society, Inc. Reproduced by permission of the author. —***The Explicator,*** v. 43, Winter, 1985; v. 55, Fall, 1996; v. 55, Spring, 1997. Copyright © 1985, 1996, 1997 Helen Dwight Reid Educational Foundation. All reproduced with permission of the Helen Dwight Reid Educational Foundation, published by Heldref Publications, 1319 18th Street, NW, Washington, DC 20036-1802. —***The Hudson Review,*** v. XLI, Spring, 1988. Copyright © 1988 by The Hudson Review, Inc. Reproduced by permission.—***Modern Drama,*** v. 10, February, 1968; v. XXXIII, September, 1980. © 1968, 1980 University of Toronto, Graduate Centre for Study of Drama. Both reproduced by permission. —***Ms.,*** v. XIV, October, 1985 for "A One-Man Revival of Great Women's Roles: David Hare's 'Wetherby' and 'Plenty'," by Molly Haskell. Copyright © 1985 by Molly Haskell. Reproduced by permission of Georges Borchardt, Inc. for the author. —***The Nation,*** v. 185, October 19, 1957. © 1957 The Nation magazine/ The Nation Company, Inc. © renewed 1985. Reproduced by permission. —***The New Republic,*** v. 182, June 7, 1980. © 1980 The New Republic, Inc. Reproduced by permission of *The New Republic.* —***New York,*** Magazine, v. 25, March 30, 1992. Reproduced by permission. —***The New York Times,*** November 19, 1942; March 4, 1947; March 3, 1956; October 2, 1957. Copyright 1942, 1947, © 1956, 1957 by The New Yorker Magazine, Inc. All reproduced by permission. —***Theatre Journal,*** v. 39, October, 1987; v. 40,

October, 1988. © 1987, 1988 University College Theatre Association of the American Theatre Association. Both reproduced by permission of The Johns Hopkins University Press. —*Time,* v. LXXXI, February 1, 1963. Copyright 1963. Time Warner Inc. Renewed November 1991 by Time, Inc. All rights reserved. Reproduced by permission from *Time.*

COPYRIGHTED EXCERPTS IN *DFS,* VOLUME 4, WERE REPRODUCED FROM THE FOLLOWING BOOKS:

Brustein, Robert. From ***The Third Theatre.*** Alfred A. Knopf, 1969. Copyright © 1969 by Robert Brustein. All rights reserved. Reproduced by permission of Random House, Inc.—Clurman, Harold. From ***Lies like Truth: Theatre Reviews and Essays.*** Macmillan, 1958. © Harold Clurman 1958. © renewed in 1986 by Juleen Compton. All rights reserved. Reproduced by permission of Macmillan, a division of Simon & Schuster, Inc.—Freedman, Morris. From ***The Moral Impulse: Modern Drama from Ibsen to the Present.*** Southern Illinois University Press, 1967. Copyright © 1967 by Morris Freedman. All rights reserved. Reproduced by permission of Southern Illinois University Press.—Rokem, Freddy. From ***Strindberg's Dramaturgy.*** Edited by Goran Stockenstrom. University of Minnesota Press, 1988. Reproduced by permission.—Skinner, Eugene R. From "The Theater of Emilio Carballido" in ***Dramatists in Revolt: The New Latin American Theater.*** Edited by Leon F. Lyday and George W. Woodyard. University of Texas Press, 1976. Reproduced by permission of the publisher and the author.

PHOTOGRAPHS AND ILLUSTRATIONS APPEARING IN *DFS,* VOLUME 4, WERE RECEIVED FROM THE FOLLOWING SOURCES:

A view of the Greek Theatre at Bradfield College in Berkshire with the audience watching a performance of Goethe's play ***Iphigenia in Taurus,*** by Euripides, photograph. Hulton-Deutsch Collection/Corbis. Reproduced by permission.—Actor John Gielgud as Joseph Surface in ***School for Scandal,*** by Richard Brinsley Sheridan at the Queen Theatre, 1937, photograph by Gordon Anthony. Hulton-Deutsch Collection/Corbis. Reproduced by permission.—Actress Constance Collier in Sheridan's ***The School for Scandal,*** by Richard Brinsley Sheridan, photograph. Hulton-Deutsch Collection/Corbis. Reproduced by permission.—Alec Guinness as Abel Drugger in Ben Jonson's play ***The Alchemist,*** May 10, 1957, photograph. Hulton-Deutsch Collection/Corbis. Reproduced by permission.—Brecht, Bertolt, photograph. Bettmann/UPI Bettmann. Reproduced by permission.— ***Death and the Maiden,*** by Areil Dorfman, from a movie still with Ben Kingsley and Sigourney Weaver, 1994, photograph by Francois Duhamel. Fine Line. Courtesy of The Kobal Collection. Reproduced by permission.— ***Death and the Maiden,*** by Ariel Dorfman, from a movie still with Ben Kingsley, and Stuart Wilson, 1994, photograph by Francois Duhamel. Fine Line. Courtesy of The Kobal Collection. Reproduced by permission.—From a theater production of Oscar Wilde's ***The Importance of Being Earnest.*** Mander & Joe Mitchenson Theatre Collection. Reproduced by permission.—From a theater production of Thornton Wilder's ***The Skin Of Our Teeth,*** presented by the Department of Theater Arts, directed by Richard Corley at the Beigel Theater, Spingold Theater Center at Brandeis University in Waltham, MA, April, 1996, photograph by Eric Levenson. Brandeis University. Reproduced by permission.—From a theatre production of Bertolt Brecht and Kurt Weill's, ***The Threepenny Opera,*** directed by Ron Daniels at the Loeb Drama Center, May 1995, photograph by T. Charles Erickson. AMERICAN REPERTORY THEATRE. Reproduced by permission of the photographer.—From a theatre production of Eugene Ionesco's, ***The Bald Soprano,*** directed by Andrei Belgrader at the American Repertory Theatre and Institute for Advanced Theatre Training, November, 1989, photograph by Richard Feldman. AMERICAN REPERTORY THEATRE. Reproduced by permission of the photographer.—From a theatre production of Federico Garcia Lorca's ***The House of Bernarda Alba,*** with Amanda Root as Adela, Joan Plowright as La Poncia, Christine Edmonds as Magdalena, and Deborah Findlay as Martinio at The Lyric Theatre, London, September, 1986, photograph. Donald Cooper, London. Reproduced by permission.—From a theatre production of Federico Garcia Lorca's ***The House of Bernarda Alba,*** directed by Beth McGee and Francine Hart at Case Western Reserve University, Design by Russ Borski, 1994/1995 season, with Saritha Bhat, Ivettza Sanchez, Emily Smauda, Sarah Morrison, and Rachel Fink, photograph by Mike Sands. Case Western University. Reproduced by permission.—From a theatre production of Lanford Wilson's, ***Burn This,*** directed by Trish Hawkins, Iowa Summer Rep, 1991, The University of Iowa, photograph by Tom Jorgensen. University of Iowa. Reproduced by permission.—From a theatre production of Luigi Pirandello's, ***Six Characters in Search of a Author,*** directed by Robert Brustein at the American Repertory Theatre and Institute for Advanced Theatre Training, December 3-January 14, 1996-97 revival, photograph by Richard Feldman. AMERICAN REPERTORY THEATRE. Reproduced by permission of the photographer.—From a theatrical production with Veronica Linford and James Daly of ***Miss Julie,*** by August Strindberg, photograph. Springer/Corbis-Bettmann. Reproduced by permission.—Garcia Lorca, Federico, photograph. Archive Photos/Popperfoto. Reproduced by permission.—Hare, David, photograph by Daniel Locus. © Daniel Locus. Reproduced by permission of the photographer.— ***Look Back in Anger,*** by John Osborne, Jimmy Porter played by Kenneth Haigh (l) dances with his friend Cliff (Alan Bates) whilst his wife Alison does the ironing, 1956, photograph by Slim Hewitt. Hulton-Deutsch Collection/Corbis. Reproduced by permission.—Matlin, Marlee, photograph. UPI/Corbis-Bettmann. Reproduced by permission.—Medoff, Mark, photograph. AP/Wide World Photos. Reproduced by permission.— ***Murder in the Cathedral,*** by T. S. Eliot with John Westbrook as Thomas Becket being murdered at Canterbury Cathedra, September 23, 1970, photograph. Hulton-Deutsch Collection/Corbis. Reproduced by permission.—O'Neill, Eugene, photograph. AP/Wide World Photos. Reproduced by permission.—Osborne, John, photograph. AP/Wide World Photos. Reproduced by permission.—Pirandello, Luigi, photograph. AP/Wide World Photos. Reproduced by permission.— ***Plenty,*** by David Hare, from a movie still with Meryl Streep and Charles Dance, 1985, photograph. 20th Century Fox. Courtesy of The Kobal Collection. Reproduced by permission.— ***Plenty,*** by David Hare, from a movie still with Meryl Streep and Sting, 1985, photograph. 20th Century Fox. Courtesy of The Kobal Collection. Reproduced by permission.—Sophocles, photograph of a illustration. Archive Photos, Inc. Reproduced by permission.—The actress Mrs. Patrick Campbell in a production of Sophocles's tragedy ***Electra,*** 1908, photograph. Hulton-Deutsch Collection/Corbis. Reproduced by permission.— ***The Hairy Ape,*** by Eugene O'Neill, from a movie still with William Bendix, Susan Hayward, John Loder, and Dorothy Comingore, directed by Alfred Santell, 1944, photograph. United Artists. Courtesy of The Kobal Collection. Reproduced by permission.—Wilde, Oscar, photograph. AP/Wide World Photos. Reproduced by permission.—Wilder, Thornton, photograph. AP/Wide World Photos. Reproduced by permission.—Wilson, Lanford, photograph. AP/Wide World Photos. Reproduced by permission.—Dorfman, Ariel, photograph by Jerry Bauer. © Jerry Bauer. Reproduced by permission.

Contributors

Terry Browne: Professor in the School of Performing Arts, State University of New York, Geneseo. Entry on *Look Back in Anger.*

Christopher Busiel: Doctoral candidate, University of Texas, Austin. Entries on *Death and the Maiden* and *The House of Bernarda Alba.*

Clare Cross: Doctoral candidate, University of Michigan, Ann Arbor. Entry on *Miss Julie.*

John Fiero: Professor of Drama and Playwriting, University of Southwestern Louisiana. Entry on *The Bald Soprano.*

Carole Hamilton: Freelance writer and instructor at Cary Academy, Cary, North Carolina. Entries on *Iphigenia in Taurus* and *The Threepenny Opera.*

D. L. Kellett: Freelance writer. Entry on *Plenty.*

Erika Kreger: Doctoral Candidate, University of California at Davis. Entry on *Skin of Our Teeth.*

Sheri Metzger: Freelance writer, Albuquerque, NM. Entries on *The Alchemist, Burn This,* and *School for Scandal.*

Daniel Moran: Educator and author, Monmouth Junction, NJ. Entry on *Murder in the Cathedral.*

Terry Nienhuis: Associate Professor of English, Western Carolina University. Entry on *Six Characters in Search of an Author.*

Arnold Schmidt: Ph.D. affiliated with the English department at California State University, Stanislau. Entries on *Electra* and *The Importance of Being Earnest.*

William P. Wiles: Freelance writer, Rutland, VT. Entry on *Children of a Lesser God.*

Etta Worthington: Freelance writer, Oak Park, IL. Entries on *The Hairy Ape* and *I, Too, Speak of the Rose.*

The Alchemist

BEN(JAMIN) JONSON

1610

The Alchemist is one of Ben Jonson's more popular comedies. Cony-catching or swindling (a cony was another word for dupe, gull, or victim) was as popular in the seventeenth century as it is in the twentieth. The con or swindle was a familiar theme and one which Jonson found to be a natural topic for comedy. There is little known about audience reaction to any of Jonson's plays. There were no theatre reviews and no newspapers or magazines to report on the opening of a play. The little that is known is drawn from surviving letters and diaries. But Jonson was not as popular with theatre-goers as William Shakespeare. In general, Jonson's plays were not well received by audiences, but *The Alchemist* appears to have been more popular than most, probably because of its topic.

Jonson differed from other playwrights of his period in that he did not use old stories, fables, or histories as the sources for his plays. Instead, Jonson used a plot "type" as the basis for most of his drama. In *The Alchemist* the plot is the familiar one of a farce. The characters are common, a man or men and a woman who set up the swindle. The victims offer a selection of London society. Like the characters from Geoffrey Chaucer's *Canterbury Tales,* there are religious men, a clerk and a shopkeeper, a widow, a knight, and a foolish young man. Jonson's characters are not well-defined, nor do they have any depth. Instead, they are "types" familiar to the audience. The initial popularity of *The Alchemist* diminished in subsequent years; by

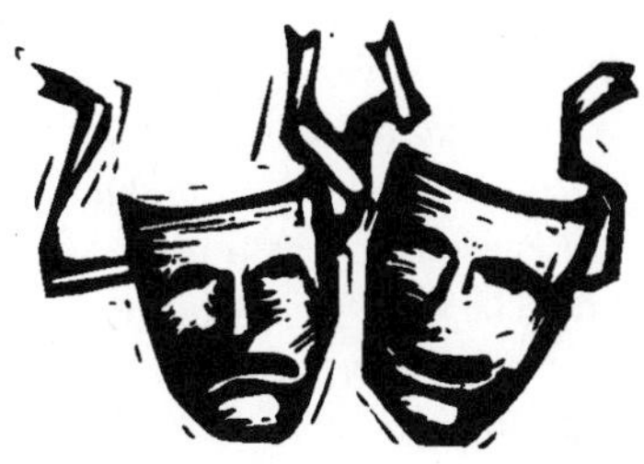

the eighteenth century the play was rarely being produced. As is the case with most of Jonson's plays, *The Alchemist* has been rarely produced outside of England during the twentieth century.

AUTHOR BIOGRAPHY

Jonson was born in about 1572. The date is uncertain, since Elizabethans were very casual about the recording of exact dates. He was a scholar, a poet, and a dramatist. Jonson was born near London shortly after the death of his father. He was educated at Westminster School and for a brief period worked as a bricklayer for his stepfather. Jonson was briefly in the military where he killed an enemy in combat.

In his next career as an actor, Jonson also wrote additional dialogue for some of the works in which he performed. After killing another actor in a duel, Jonson was arrested but released after claiming benefit of clergy, which meant that he was an educated man. Jonson converted to Roman Catholicism during this period, and although he escaped hanging, he was still labeled a felon after his release.

Jonson's first play, *Every Man in His Humour,* was written in 1598, with William Shakespeare playing one of the roles on stage. Jonson continued with a new play every year for the next few years: *Every Man out of His Humour* (1599), *Cynthia's Revels* (1600), and *Poetaster* in 1601. Perhaps best known for his court masques, Jonson wrote the first of many, *The Masque of Blackness,* in 1605.

Although Jonson became well established as a playwright with works such as *Volpone* (1606), *Epicene, or the Silent Woman* (1610), *The Alchemist* (1610), *Bartholomew Fair* (1614) and *The Devil was an Ass* (1616), he is also well known as a poet. Jonson was not formally appointed England's poet laureate, but he was awarded a pension in 1616 by King James I, thus acknowledging that the author was essentially performing that function.

Also in 1616, Jonson became the first poet or dramatist to publish a folio edition of his *Works.* Since not even Shakespeare had published a compilation of his work, Jonson received some criticism for this action. He was also awarded with an honorary degree from Cambridge University in 1616. Among Jonson's patrons was the Sidney family for whom he wrote one of his most famous poems, *''To Penshurst,''* one of the best known poems to celebrate an estate and family. The beauty of this poem and the skill with which Jonson composed it is evident to visitors who abandon the road to approach Penshurst from the back of the estate.

Jonson was not always popular with audiences, who while attending his plays, were often verbally critical of the writer. During the height of his creativity, Jonson was as popular a writer as Shakespeare, who was also Jonson's friend. But he saw much of his popularity diminish later in his life while Shakespeare's continued to grow. Although Jonson was largely responsible for the publication of the first folio of Shakespeare's work in 1623, for which he wrote a poem, Jonson was less generous with his praise in private. Still, there is no doubt that Jonson both liked and admired Shakespeare. While Jonson was a talented writer, his misfortune was to be writing plays during the same period as a talent as enormous as Shakespeare. Jonson spent the last nine years of his life bedridden after suffering a stroke. He died in 1637 and was buried in Westminster Abbey

PLOT SUMMARY

Act I

The scene is London in 1610. This is a plague year and wealthy people have fled London for the safer countryside. Lovewit has departed until the plague is over and has left his butler, Jeremy, to care for the house. As the play begins, Jeremy and Subtle are arguing over their relative importance to the swindle they are organizing, and each is claiming a larger share of the profit. Dol, who realizes that the two could ruin everything with their loud quarreling, tries to quiet the two men.

At that moment, the first victim, Dapper, arrives at the house. Dapper has come to the astrologer, Subtle, to find a way to win at gambling. After paying the two men all his money, Dapper is assured that he was born under a lucky star and that he will win. He is also told that the Queen of Fairy will help him win. The next victim, Drugger, arrives and is told that he, too, will be very wealthy and a great success.

Act II

Sir Epicure Mammon, accompanied by Pertinax Surly arrive at the house. Mammon is promised the philosopher's stone which will turn all base metals into gold. His companion, Surly is not as innocent and suspects Subtle of being a thief. Mammon has great plans for the stone that include having great wealth and power. Surly is not convinced and sneers as Mammon tries to convince him of the power of the stone. Mammon accidentally sees Dol and is told that she is a Lord's sister who is suffering from madness. Subtle and Jeremy get rid of Surly by sending him on an errand. Mammon leaves with the promise that he will send many of his household goods to Subtle to be turned into gold.

The next visitor is Ananias, who, when he reports that he cannot get more money to invest, is turned away by Subtle. Drugger calls again to bring tobacco and to tell Subtle that the Widow Pliant wishes to have her fortune told. He also agrees to bring Pliant's brother to the house so that his wishes can also be fulfilled.

Act III

Ananias returns with Wholesome, who when told of a way to turn pewter into coins, is concerned with the morality of counterfeiting, even to benefit the church. They both agree to purchase Mammon's household goods, and both leave to consider the legality of the counterfeiting problem. Surly returns to the house disguised as a Spaniard, Kastril arrives with Drugger and is so impressed with Subtle that the two young men leave to bring Dame Pliant back.

Dapper returns to meet the Queen of Fairy. Dapper is undressed and his money taken in an elaborate ritual during which he meets Dol disguised as the Queen of Fairy. When Mammon knocks on the door, Dapper, who is tied up and blindfolded, has a piece of gingerbread stuffed in his mouth. He is locked in the privy.

Act IV

Mammon is ushered in to meet Dol, who is disguised as an aristocratic lady suffering from madness. Mammon is warned that he should not speak of religion, as it will bring on the woman's madness. As others arrive, Dol and Mammon are moved into another room of the house. Dame Pliant arrives and is placed in the garden to walk with the Spaniard. Soon, Dol assumes a guise of madness, and Mammon is told that he has caused this because of his moral laxity, and thus, the completion of the stone is certainly delayed.

While this is occurring, Surly, disguised as the Spaniard, has revealed to the widow that Subtle and Face/Lungs/Jeremy are swindlers. Surly also proposes marriage to the widow. Her brother, who has been learning the art of quarreling in another part of the house, is told that since the Spaniard is an impostor, Kastril should challenge Surly to a duel. The two Puritans reappear and announce that they have decided that the church's need for money meant that counterfeiting, although against the king's law, was certainly not against God's law. Surly is so disgusted that he leaves the house. The scene ends with Lovewit's reappearance.

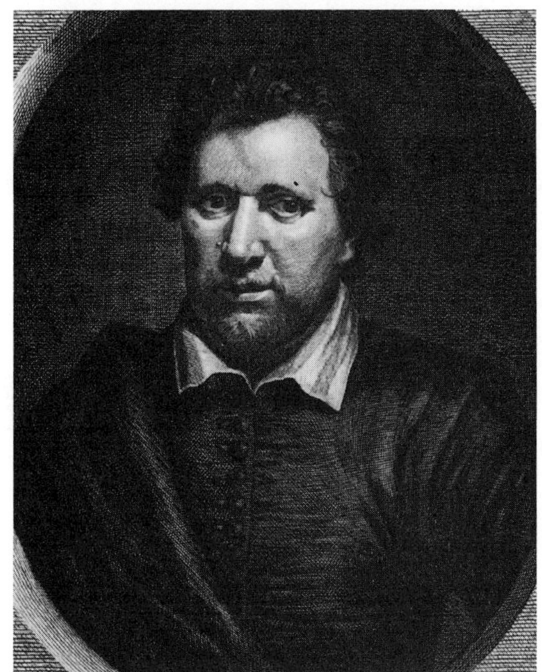

A portrait of Ben Jonson

Act V

Jeremy goes to the door and tries to detain Lovewit long enough for Subtle and Dol to escape. Jeremy's attempts to convince his master that the neighbors are wrong about the activities that have occurred in the house fails when Mammon and Surly return to expose Subtle and Dol. Jeremy decides to confess his role in the game to his master, who decides to forgive the butler when he promises to deliver Dame Pliant to Lovewit as wife.

In the back of the house Dapper has been freed and has received what he thinks is a guarantee that he will be a winner at gambling. Subtle and Dol are forced to flee without their reward and Drugger is tricked out of his fiance. After Lovewit weds Dame Pliant, he convinces the remaining characters that they have been victims of their own greed. Kastril is pleased that his sister has made a good match and is no longer interested in a duel. The plays ends with Jeremy in control and safe from retribution.

CHARACTERS

The Alchemist

See Subtle

Ananias

Ananias is one of the holy Brethren of Amsterdam. He is a Puritan who seeks out the swindlers so that he might secure possession of the philosopher's stone. He hopes to increase his influence through possessing the stone. But when Ananias tells the alchemist that the Brethren will not invest any more money in the stone, Subtle drives the Puritan from the house. Later he returns with another elder, Tribulation Wholesome, and the promise to pay more money. He is zealous and quarrelsome, an idealist who rejects Christmas as too Catholic but who decides that counterfeiting is not really a crime if it benefits his congregation. In the Bible, Ananias is a man who was struck dead for lying.

Jeremy Butler

Jeremy is Master Lovewit's butler. He is known to his friends as Face, while Lungs is the persona Jeremy assumes as the alchemist's assistant. Knowing that while the plague continues to claim victims Lovewit will remain absent, Jeremy decides to offer the home and his services to an acquaintance, Subtle and his partner Dol, so that they can prepare an elaborate swindle. He is smart and inventive. In his disguise as Face, he is able to recruit new victims to the house and the swindle.

When Lovewit returns unexpectedly, Jeremy offers marriage to the rich Widow Pliant as a means of escaping punishment. Lungs is an appropriate name for one who assists an alchemist with the dark and shadowy process of turning base metals into gold. His name conjures up the smoky furnace of the alchemist's laboratory. Since alchemy is also associated with Satan, Lungs also suggest the fires and smoke of hell. Face is symbolic of the many faces, names, and characters that Jeremy can assume depending on his need and audience.

Dol Common

Dol Common is a prostitute, a friend of Jeremy and Subtle, and a partner in their con game. She disguises herself as the Queen of Fairy as part of the swindle of Dapper. She also assumes the persona of a great scholar who is seeking a rest cure as part of the swindle of Mammon.

Dol is the cool, level-headed partner, the one who keeps the other two under control when their arguing gets too loud. Her name offers two clues to her identity. Dol suggests doll, an artificial plaything that can become whatever its owner or holder wishes. Common represents the nature of the prostitute, lower class and too readily or easily available.

Dapper

Dapper is a law clerk who gambles and who hopes to learn how to win at games of chance. Jeremy met Dapper at the Dagger and the young law clerk comes to the house seeking assistance and a means to win at racing and gambling. Dapper pays Subtle and is told that a rare star was aligned at his birth, a good fairy, who will help him win. When Dapper returns prepared to meet his fairy, he is stripped, his mouth is stuffed with gingerbread, and he is locked in an outhouse as a more important customer arrives at the house.

The word dapper was identified with young men who present themselves as neat, trim, and smart in appearance, but was also often associated with littleness or pettiness.

Deacon

See Ananias

Abel Drugger

Drugger is a tobacconist who is also a victim of the swindlers. Drugger is seeking a magic that will tell him where to place the doors of his new shop and where to store certain goods so that he can make more money and be successful in his enterprise. The swindlers tell Drugger that it will be his fortune to enjoy great success and that he will achieve a position beyond his youthful years. Drugger returns to the swindlers a second time with a story about a rich young widow who would like her fortune told. He hopes that Subtle will assist with a match between the tobacconist and the widow.

The smoking of tobacco in London began with the importation of the product from the New World. Since Drugger was used to refer to someone who dealt in drugs or who functioned as a druggist, Jonson's use of the name may suggest that he viewed tobacco as a drug.

Elder

See Ananias

Face

See Jeremy Butler

Kastril

Kastril, brother to Dame Pliant, has recently inherited money, and he wants to learn to be quarrelsome so that he might be a gentleman and a gallant. He is referred to as the angry boy. He is given a lesson in quarreling by Subtle. At the play's conclusion, Kastril is very impressed with Lovewit's ability to quarrel and so consents to his sister's marriage to Lovewit. According to *The Oxford English Dictionary,* the word, Kastril, is thought to be an derivative of Kestrel, a type of small hawk that is most noted for its ability to hold itself in the same place in the air with its head turned into the wind.

Lovewit

Lovewit is master of the house. Because of the plague that has hit London in 1610, he has left town and taken refuge in the country. He returns home earlier than expected and interrupts the swindle that his butler, Jeremy, has undertaken. He decides to forgive his butler in exchange for his assistance in marrying a rich widow who will make him feel seven years younger. Lovewit's departure from London permits the knavery to begin; his return brings the trickery to a close. He forgives his butler for allowing his master's house to be used in the deceptions, hence the love origin of Lovewit's name.

Lungs

See Jeremy Butler

Epicure Mammon

Mammon is a disreputable knight who is guilty of avarice and lechery. He is a great believer in alchemy. He anticipates being able to transform all the base metals in his house into gold and precious metals. He has grandiose plans to be wealthy and to acquire all the lead, tin, and copper available, which he will then turn into gold. He also thinks he can turn old men young, cure all disease, and eliminate the plague. Mammon even pays more money for the extra promises the stone offers. He expects to have many wives and mistresses, silk clothing, and wonderful perfumes.

After Mammon catches a glimpse of Dol, he is enamored and wants to marry her. As is true for so many of the swindler's victims, Mammon is foolish and greedy and an unsympathetic victim of his own avarice. The explosion of the alchemist's furnace wipes out Mammon's investment in the scheme. Mammon's origination is as a Greek word for riches. In Medieval English, Mammon is thought to be the name of the devil who covets riches. Its use in Jonson's play describes the nature of the character.

Widow Pliant

See Dame Pliant

Dame Pliant

Dame Pliant is a soft and buxom widow, who just happens to be rich and whom Drugger seeks to marry. Surly also wishes to marry her, but in the end, Dame Pliant weds Lovewit. Although she is engaged to Drugger she is willing to marry another man, hence the meaning of her name (''pliant'' meaning flexible).

The Spaniard

See Pertinax Surly

Subtle

Subtle is a swindler who poses as an alchemist. He is disreputable and uses his persuasive abilities to cheat his gullible victims. Subtle has a talent for language and so presents a sort of pseudo-science that convinces his willing victims to part with their money. When Lovewit returns, Subtle is forced to flee without his gains. Subtle fits the definition of his name: he is cunning and crafty, difficult to discern or perceive, and a skillful, clever liar.

Pertinax Surly

Surly is experienced with swindlers and he immediately suspects that Face, Dol, and Subtle are conducting a swindle. He is unconvinced at the evidence, and so Sir Mammon attempts to persuade Surly with documents. Surly, however, is unconvinced. He is finally sent off on an errand. When Surly returns in Act IV, he is dressed as a Spaniard who cannot speak English. The swindlers heap insults upon Surly when they think he cannot understand English. When left alone in the garden with Dame Plaint, Surly reveals the swindlers' purpose and purposes marriage to the widow.

As his name suggests, Surly is a menacing threat to Subtle and his partners. He is unfriendly and rude, and as his first name (probably derived from pertinacious) alludes, he is tenacious in his quest to expose the swindlers.

Tribulation Wholesome

Wholesome is a church elder who accompanies Ananias on his second trip to the see the swindlers. He promises more money and when he is told that he and Ananias might transform pewter into money, he finds he must debate the ethics of coining foreign money. Like Ananias, Wholesome represents Jonson's use of satire to poke fun at Puritanism. Wholesome is the opposite of his name. He is much more willing that Ananias to forget ethical concerns when the question becomes one of compromise and profit or conscience.

THEMES

Appearances and Reality

What the victims of the three swindlers perceive as reality is not the truth of the play. Each one thinks that he will receive wealth or power as a reward gained through little effort. The reality is that each will be left with less wealth and no more power than they had initially.

Change and Transformation

The theme of transformation is crucial to this play. The plot revolves around the chance and expectation that Subtle can change base metals into gold. A belief in alchemy was still firmly held at the beginning of the seventeenth century. Queen Elizabeth investigated the possibility of using alchemy to increase her worth and even Sir Isaac Newton believed in the principle. In *The Alchemist,* alchemy is the basis for a con game, a means to swindle unsuspecting victims. The only transformation that occurs is a lightening of their purses.

Deception

The plot of Jonson's play is based on deception. Each of the three swindlers uses deception for financial gain. But the victims are also self-deceiving. Their willingness to believe allows the game to succeed. Surly assumes a disguise to reveal the deception, but his disguise is in itself a deception. Jeremy disguises himself as Face to lure victims to the house and later he becomes Lungs, the alchemist's assistant. Dol pretends to be the Queen of Fairy and a mad aristocrat as part of the game, and Subtle is an astrologer and an alchemist. Each deception is dependent on none of the victims meeting one another. Thus, beginning with the middle of Act IV when the victims comings and goings reach a level of unanticipated activity, the deception becomes more difficult to control.

Greed

It is the victim's greed that allows the swindles to occur. Each man seeks more power or wealth than he has earned or deserves. And each returns to be further swindled as their greed escalates. The loss of goods and money increases as each victim fails to be satisfied with his lot and each desires even more wealth.

Morality

The play's resolution creates some questions about morality. The sting of loss is eased in the victims as they learn their lessons; their lives are better knowing the ill-effects caused by excessive greed. When Subtle and Dol are forced to flee the house without the money and goods gained from their efforts, it is also clear that there is no reward for dishonesty. But Jeremy escapes any punishment for his role in the swindles, and so, the concept of justice is questioned. Traditionally, the audience wants to see the bad guys punished and the good characters rewarded. That resolution is denied when Jeremy is forgiven by his master, and the end of the play leaves Jeremy victorious.

Order and Disorder

These two ideas are tied to the exit and entrance of Lovewit. When Lovewit leaves London and his house in Jeremy's care, disorder is the result. This is especially evident in Act IV when the victims begin amassing at the house, each seeking more help and more wealth. Order is finally restored when Lovewit returns to the house. The swindlers flee the house and the victims are forced to restore order to their lives when they accept their losses.

Religion

The two Puritans are important symbols of Jonson's intent to satirize extreme religious practice. When Subtle tells the two that they need more money, he also suggests that they can ''make'' more money by transforming pewter to coin. The initial concern is the legality of transforming foreign coin. But this is all a deceptive debate about counterfeiting. The two Deacons decide that their need for money is necessary to fulfill God's work.

TOPICS FOR FURTHER STUDY

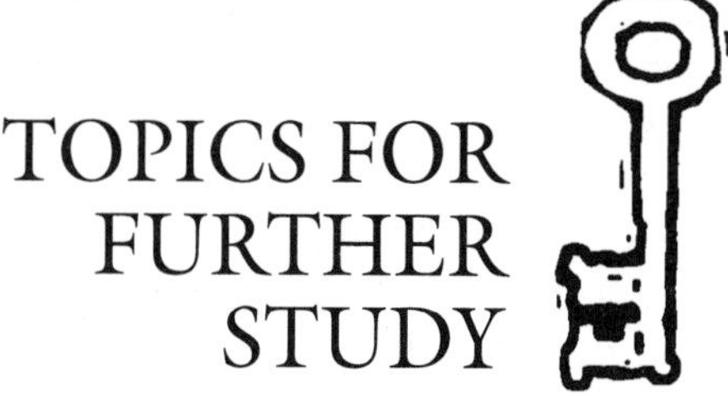

- Research the use of character names to represent traits or ideology. When did playwrights first begin this practice? Research contemporary characters in theater, film, and literature. How do their names reflect their character?
- Religion was very important to English social structure during the seventeenth century. Roman Catholics were forbidden from receiving degrees from the universities and also banned from holding many political offices. Puritans were often the object of derision and many fled to the New World seeking religious freedom. Examine the role of religion during this period and try to resolve some of the references to religion that you find in Jonson's play.
- At the end of the play, Subtle and Dol have fled without any reward for their knavery and only Jeremy seems to have profited from the three weeks his master has been gone. Jeremy is forgiven when he offers the widow in marriage. Nearly four hundred years after the play was written, changing social values would condemn such an arrangement and insist that Jeremy be punished rather than having the widow ''sold'' in exchange for his master's forgiveness. Considering those issues, do you think the play is still effective? Do you find that it condemns ''get rich quick schemes'' or that it offers an effective satire of the artificial nature of men's morals. Consider who you think really benefits from the play's resolution.
- Critics sometimes argue that Jonson's play lacks a comedic plot and that it is really just a series of short episodes strung together, thus it is not really a comedy. Traditionally, comedies of this period were defined as such if they ended with a happy marriage. If you compare *The Alchemist* to other comedies of the period, what is it lacking? Because of the public's exposure to television sitcoms, do you think a modern audience might be more receptive to the structure of this play?

Accordingly, the needs to God outweigh the laws of man or, in this case, the laws of the king.

In effect, the Puritans compromise their religion and their ethics in the name of God's work. Jonson uses the two Puritans to illustrate what he sees as one of the problems of organized religion, the inability of some zealots to recognize that civil laws are important in the function of a society and cannot be discarded to satisfy religious need.

Victim and Victimization

The Alchemist put the definition of victim and victimization to the test. The victims of the swindlers are victims because they have been willing to cheat, to gain from magic or dishonesty what they have not earned. The issue, then, becomes whether they are victimized by Subtle, Jeremy, and Dol or if they are victims of their own greed. Since in the end, all, except Jeremy, become victims, the audience concludes that each character has arrived at their destination due to their own actions; they have only victimized themselves and have reaped what they deserve.

STYLE

Act

A major division in a drama. In Greek plays the sections of the drama signified by the appearance of the chorus were usually divided into five acts. This is the formula for most serious drama from the Greeks to the Romans and to Elizabethan playwrights like William Shakespeare. The five acts denote the structure of dramatic action. They are exposition, complication, climax, falling action, and catastrophe. The five act structure was followed until the nineteenth century when Henrik Ibsen combined some of the acts.

The Alchemist is a five act play. The exposition occurs in the first act when the audience learns of Subtle and Face's plan and meets the first of the victims. By the end of Act II, the complication, the audience has met the rest of the victims. The climax occurs in the third act when the victims all begin to arrive and Dapper must be gagged and locked in the privy. The near misses as each of the victims is targeted by the swindlers in a separate part of the house provides the falling action, and the catastrophe occurs in the last act when Lovewit arrives to restore order and each victim discovers the extent of the trickery.

Character

A person in a dramatic work. The actions of each character are what constitute the story. Character can also include the idea of a particular individual's morality. Characters can range from simple stereotypical figures to more complex multi-faceted ones. Characters may also be defined by personality traits, such as the rogue or the damsel in distress. ''Characterization'' is the process of creating a life-like person from an author's imagination. To accomplish this the author provides the character with personality traits that help define who he will be and how he will behave in a given situation.

The Alchemist differs slightly from this definition, since each character is little more than a ''type.'' The audience does not really know or understand the character as an individual. For instance, Drugger is recognizable as a representative the new merchant class. He is a shopkeeper who hopes to use magic to be more successful than other shopkeepers.

Genre

Genres are a way of categorizing literature. Genre is a French term that means ''kind'' or ''type.'' Genre can refer to both the category of literature such as tragedy, comedy, epic, poetry, or pastoral. It can also include modern forms of literature such as drama novels, or short stories. This term can also refer to types of literature such as mystery, science fiction, comedy, or romance. *The Alchemist* is a comedy.

Plot

This term refers to the pattern of events. Generally plots should have a beginning, a middle, and a conclusion, but they may also sometimes be a series of episodes connected together. Basically, the plot provides the author with the means to explore primary themes. Students are often confused between the two terms; but themes explore ideas, and plots simply relate what happens in a very obvious manner. Thus the plot of *The Alchemist*is the story of three swindlers to try to cheat some gullible victims of their money. But the theme is that of greed.

Setting

The time, place, and culture in which the action of the play takes place is called the setting. The elements of setting may include geographic location, physical or mental environments, prevailing cultural attitudes, or the historical time in which the action takes place. The location for Jonson's play is London and the house of Master Lovewit. The action is further reduced to three weeks during 1610.

Satire

Satire attempts to blend social commentary with comedy and humor. Satire does not usually attack any individual but rather the institution he or she represents. The intent is to expose problems and create debate that will lead to a correction of the problem. In *The Alchemist,* the two Puritan Deacons are the object of satire because they represent an over-zealous approach to religion.

HISTORICAL CONTEXT

Religion and Society

In 1610, James I had been king for seven years. And the Anglican church, firmly re-established with the reign of Elizabeth I, was only one of several religious influences at work in Renaissance England. Among these different religions, the Puritans were of major importance to theatre-goers. Puritans opposed the theatre, since they viewed it as deceitful. Actors were, after all, assuming a role other than their own. For Puritans, acting was analogous to lying.

Accordingly, it is easy to understand why Jonson might target Puritans for satire in *The Alchemist.* It is also important to understand that plays were subject to censure and were reviewed by the Master of Revels, who could force revisions and censure content. Unlike twentieth-century works, seventeenth-century plays were not reviewed for sexual content or obscene language. Instead, the issue of review was religion and politics, theology governed

COMPARE & CONTRAST

- **1610:** The plague, which is a reoccurring problem for congested London, hits especially hard.

  Today: The plague, while not completely eradicated, is no longer a major threat to London or other major cities of the world. Today's modern plague continues to be HIV and AIDS.

- **1610:** The New World is being settled with Jamestown colonists preparing to abandon their colony after a particularly difficult period. They are convinced to stay and try again when more colonists arrive.

  Today: Those British colonies, whose tenuous survival were once in doubt, have become a major military and economic force, the United States.

- **1610:** Henry Hudson makes another attempt to find a Northwest Passage. Backed by English investors, Hudson succeeds only in entering the strait that will bear his name.

  Today: The twentieth-fifth anniversary of the last manned lunar landing is celebrated, and NASA announces that another exploration of the moon is planned.

- **1610:** Shakespeare has enjoyed nearly twenty-five years of success as a playwright. After 1610, he will write *The Tempest* and collaborate on two more plays, *All Is True (Henry VIII)* and *The Two Noble Kinsmen.*

  Today: Shakespeare is enjoying a Renaissance in film and theatre. Nearly a dozen of his plays have been filmed in the last ten years or are in the planning stages. In addition, scenes or plots have been adapted to other popular film use.

politics in many cases. In addition, the depiction of the king, who was a representative of God, and as such, was head of the Anglican Church, was especially important.

The hierarchy that began with God and moved to the King, was also analogous to the structure of the family, with the order descending from man to woman to child. England was still a largely agrarian society at the beginning of the seventeenth century. Most men labored outside the house and most women functioned primarily as wife, mother, cook, housekeeper, and sometimes nurse. Few men and even fewer women could read. Society was very class-defined.

For most purposes, there were two classes: the aristocratic land-owners and those who worked for them. In a society where few people could read, men and women were largely dependent on the church for their information. The clergy used church services as an opportunity to teach lessons and morals, and so the English had a knowledge of the Bible that few twentieth-century church-goers can appreciate.

The Theatre

The first permanent theatre was built c. 1576 and this led to a greater social status for theatre people. By 1600, some actors and playwrights like William Shakespeare also owned an interest in a theatre and earned a comfortable income. Most theatres were located just outside town due to religious problems, especially with Puritans. Plays were performed outside, during the day, and many patrons stood during the entire performance.

The theatres were open at the top, shaped in a circle or octagon, with rows of seating along the perimeter. The seats were protected by a covered gallery, but there was a large area in front of the stage where spectators stood that was open to the elements. If the weather was cooperative and a play was to be performed, a flag was displayed to notify the audiences of a performance. Since working people were not usually free to attend plays during the day, the audience consisted largely of gentlemen who paid about 1 pence for the more expensive seats, while those who could afford the less costly center area crowded before the stage. Respectable women could attend if accompanied by a male escort. Prostitutes also attended to increase trade. All roles were played by male actors, with younger boys assuming the roles of female characters.

Although many in the audience were uneducated, stage presentation and performance usually overcame those shortcomings, and the ideas of the plays were often familiar enough to be easily grasped by the audience. There were no curtains or dimming of lights to signal the end of an act; the act was finished when all actors in the scene had left the stage. There was no intermission and no scenery and none of the time or location indicators that are so familiar to today's audiences. There was only the text, which was often in verse.

Jonson's plays were frequently performed in the Globe, the theatre in which Shakespeare was part owner. Plays were very popular, but thirty years after Jonson's play, Puritans finally succeeded in closing down the theatres. They would remain closed until the Restoration in 1660.

CRITICAL OVERVIEW

There is little information about how Ben Jonson's *The Alchemist* was received by critics and the public. Most scholars acknowledge that Jonson's plays were not generally well received. The audience was often loudly critical, and Jonas Barish noted that several of Jonson's plays were hissed from the stage. This is not necessarily because the plays were not entertaining or topical, but rather, the play's reception reflected the audience's acceptance of the author. Jonson is usually described as arrogant and difficult; that may be a generous report. Jonson inspired little neutral comment. Critics and contemporaries either loved and worshipped Jonson or they hated and scorned him.

Since plays were not reviewed during the period in which this play was composed, response to a play may be determined by examining how often it has been produced in the years since its creation. Another way to gauge a play's popularity is through anecdotal evidence, letters, diary, and journal entries from the period. Unfortunately, in the case of *The Alchemist,* there is little evidence of this kind available. There is also little information about how long any play remained in production and on the stage during the early part of the seventeenth century. Although all plays were licensed by a government official, the Master of Revels, these records have not survived. The details of performance that are so readily available in the twentieth century, length and dates of performance and the theatre in which a production played, are not available for the period during which Ben Jonson wrote.

The topic of *The Alchemist* was a familiar one to Elizabethan audiences. The idea of a con man or swindler who, with or without a partner, seeks to part a gullible fool from his or her property derives from an old tradition in literature. It is a well-known story in Geoffrey Chaucer's *Canterbury Tales.* The most familiar of Chaucer's stories of a fool conned by a woman and man is ''The Miller's Tale,'' the narrative of a young wife and her lover who swindle a greedy older husband of his wife's fidelity. Thus, the plot of *The Alchemist* would have been anticipated and enjoyed by Jonson's audience. Indeed *The Alchemist* proved to be popular during the seventeenth century.

Alvin Kernan observed in *Jonson & Shakespeare,* that this Jonson play reappeared on stage throughout the seventeenth century and into the eighteenth. But by the middle of the eighteenth century, the play's language and its allusions had become too alien for audiences. During the nineteenth century the play was rarely performed, but many of Jonson's plays have been reappearing on stage during the twentieth century.

Most often, the reasons cited for not performing Jonson's work center on the difficulty of the language and the obscure nature of the references. It is interesting to note that while William Shakespeare's plays are enjoying a resurgence of interest on film (they have never been gone long from the stage), none of Jonson's plays has ever been filmed and few are produced on stage outside England. Shakespeare was Jonson's friend, but he was also his greatest rival. That appears to be just as true four hundred years later.

The Alchemist was not Jonson's only use of the con game as a play's primary topic. In *Volpone* (written five years before *The Alchemist*), Jonson creates an elaborate swindle devised by a man and his servant. The premise is the duping of several individuals who, thinking they will be left a substantial estate, shower the charlatan with expensive gifts. Of course the protagonist is not dying, the victims will not inherit anything, and the entire plot is revealed and order is restored in the conclusion.

The central idea, the farce, needs only a full compliment of cheaters and victims to be successful.

Like *The Alchemist, Volpone* is set in contemporary London. This is one way in which Jonson differed from his contemporaries, especially Shakespeare. Shakespeare's plots were drawn from stories and from history. They were set in another time or in another land, but they did not relate the events of the London outside the theatre's walls. It is difficult to assert exactly why Jonson's popularity with theatre audiences lagged so far behind Shakespeare's. But Jonson was enormously popular with James I and Charles I. Jonson's masques (masques differed from plays because they were characterized by elaborate costumes, scenery, and stage machinery; they were very expensive to produce) were very successful, and Jonson is best known for revitalizing a genre that dated from the Medieval period and reintroducing it in the seventeenth century. It is ironic that the excessive and progressively expensive cost of the masques were one element of what ultimately led to the closing of the theatres (in 1642) and the deposition of Charles I during the English Revolution.

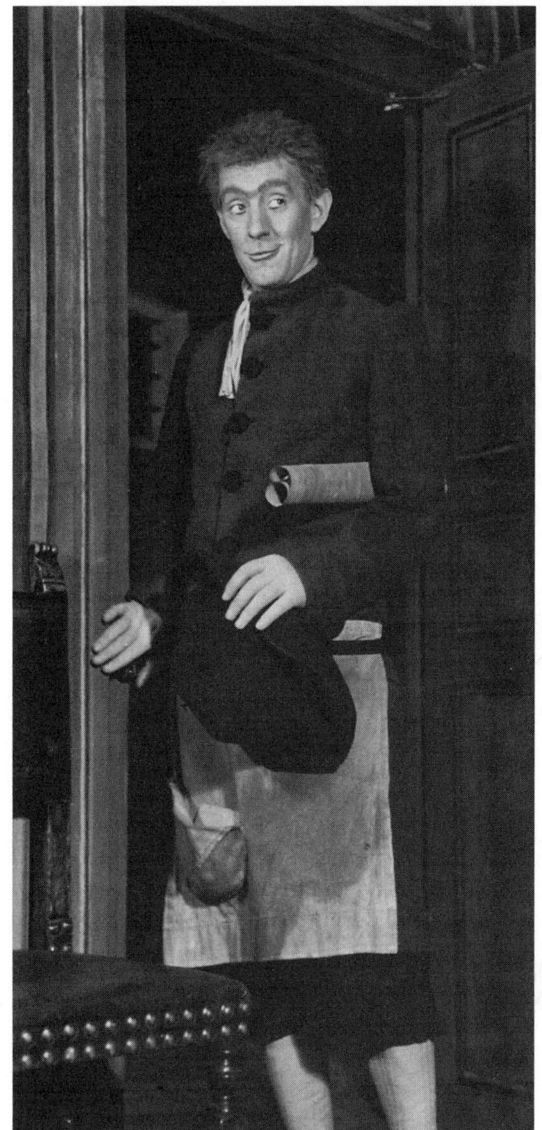

Alec Guiness as Abel Drugger in a 1957 production of The Alchemist

CRITICISM

Sheri Metzger

In this essay, Metzger discusses Jonson's symbolic use of the plague to satirize social dysfunction.

In 1610, London suffered another bad plague year. Those who could, left their city homes and fled to the clean air and relative safety of country life. It is this partial desertion of London that provides the time and setting for *The Alchemist.* Unlike his friend and contemporary, William Shakespeare, Ben Jonson incorporated topical locations and issues into his plays. When Lovewit leaves his home in the care of his butler, Jeremy, and flees to the country, thus setting up the action of the play, the master's actions are similar to those that were occurring in London at the time.

The importance of setting is the focus of Cheryl Lynn Ross's examination of *The Alchemist* in *Renaissance Quarterly.* Ross explained that "the world of Ben Jonson's *Alchemist*—its setting, its rogues and their victims, the structure of the play, and the moral judgments both inherent in the text and on its margins—is the world of London during a plague." The plague grants Jeremy a freedom he would not otherwise enjoy. Ross argued that it is this freedom, common enough during a plague year, that provides Jeremy with the unstructured time to assume other identities. He is free to roam the city as Face, to go into taverns and seek out victims, and to transform himself into Lungs, the alchemist's assistant.

The plague also provides an empty house in which the three knaves can centralize their plot and the action. Victims can be invited back to the house to be conned at the thieves' leisure. This is another

- Ben Jonson's *Volpone,* written in 1605, is another play that uses the farce or the con game as a plot device. In this case a wealthy man pretends to be dying so that he can con expensive gifts from everyone who thinks he or she might benefit from his will.
- Geoffrey Chaucer's "The Miller's Tale" is another parable about greed. As he did elsewhere in his *Canterbury Tales,* written c. 1387, Chaucer uses an old man's greed and lust to reveal the vulnerability of men.
- *Twelfth Night,* by William Shakespeare, was first presented in 1600. Although the plot is not about a swindle, it does involve the use of disguise and trickery to bring about order and resolution. Since Shakespeare was a contemporary of Jonson's, his comedies provide a useful contrast to Jonson's.
- *The Merchant of Venice,* also by Shakespeare, was first presented in 1596. This play also involves disguise and deceit, but it is interesting because the ending creates many questions about the definition of comedy. Like *The Alchemist,* a complete moral resolution is missing, but in the case of this Shakespearean play, the plot raises more complicated questions about racism and honesty. The character of Portia also provides a contrast to Dol and Dame Pliant for those who are interested in the depiction of female characters in comedies of this era.
- Volume 11 of *Ben Jonson,* written by C. H. Herford and Percy and Evelyn Simpson (published 1925-52), provides the most complete information about Jonson and his plays. Vol. 10 also provides some of the history of *The Alchemist*'s production.

glimpse of the plague than that traditionally offered in historical accounts. The increase in crime due to increased opportunity is clearly established in Jonson's comedy and is just one element of the connection between Jonson's location and his theme. The observation that crime in *The Alchemist* is an opportunistic disease is only one small part of the satire that Jonson employs to provide laughs at the expense of his victims: the clergy, scientists, philosophers, and merchants of London.

One important element of satire is its ability to poke fun at institutions and ideas rather than individuals. This occurs in *The Alchemist* when the plague that visits the city becomes a part of Lovewit's house. As sickness envelops the real London, Jonson uses the symbols of sickness to illustrate the infection (in the form of con games and dishonesty) that threatens London. During the height of the plague, men abandoned their wives, mothers, and children, and neighbors became enemies. Fear became a motivating force in the destruction of social relationships.

Ross concluded that this betrayal of humanity is another part of the sickness that accompanies the plague. Jonson illuminates the problem by transforming it into a plot about three scheming knaves who try to bilk other Londoners out of their money. Of these characters, Ross stated that "from Drugger to Mammon, the characters represent a society suffering a thoroughgoing contagion of immorality." It is not the plague that makes them sick; it is their lack of morality. Ross continued with "[these characters] absolute selfishness is a symptom of moral sickness that the plague characteristically and unerringly uncovered, tearing away at relationships of love and trust, pitting neighbor against neighbor, parent against child, subject against ruler."

Indeed, *The Alchemist* exemplifies the moral rottenness of London. It is little wonder that Jonson was unpopular with his audience. His picture of London society was not a flattering one. Ross insisted that to cure the city of its moral plague, Jonson subverts the usual ending of the plague—the return to the city of those who had fled to the safety of the country. Rather than have Lovewit return to the house and restore order to the play, and by representation, to London, Jonson uses Lovewit to illustrate a different ending. Ross noted that "with Lovewit's entrance, the play changes its appearance. . . . For Lovewit does not return London to its original, pre-plague state; he does not restore Subtle's booty to its rightful owners. Instead, he appropriates it himself, turning Subtle's productive efforts to his own advantage."

Jonson's ending denies his audience the tidy resolution they expect. The moral ambiguity of a master who seizes the victims' property and who forgives his butler for such acts of deception raises some questions. Ross would argue that Jonson is only illuminating the moral decay of London society. But that interpretation is dependent on a close reading of the final act.

It is this interpretation of the final act that interested G. D. Monsarrat, who argued in *Cahiers Elisabethans* that an understanding of Lovewit is completely dependent on how the last three scenes are read. Monsarrat provided a close reading of the final scenes and concluded that Lovewit is not a dishonest rogue as is his butler; instead, Lovewit is provided only the briefest information that Jeremy has confessed to his master. Traditional readings of the last act assume that Jeremy confesses everything to Lovewit offstage. On-stage, the audience learns only that Jeremy asks that Lovewit "pardon me th' abuse of your house."

To help make this forgiveness easier, Jeremy offers his master the Widow Pliant as an incentive. When Jeremy tells Dol and Subtle that Lovewit knows all, the audience assumes that the butler has confessed everything offstage. But it is also possible that Jeremy offers Lovewit's knowledge and forgiveness as a means of convincing Subtle and Dol that the master of the house is in control, and with him lies the authority of the law. Monsarrat pointed out that "even if Lovewit does not know everything Jeremy must make them believe that he does, otherwise they themselves might reveal *all* to Lovewit. Thus, Jeremy has a lot at stake if he cannot convince Dol and Subtle to leave quickly and quietly.

Although the audience knows that Jeremy is a liar, Monsarrat noted that Jeremy does not have an opportunity to meet Lovewit offstage, and accordingly, the audience should not believe Jeremy's warning to Subtle and Dol.

"THE OBSERVATION THAT CRIME IN *THE ALCHEMIST* IS AN OPPORTUNISTIC DISEASE IS ONLY ONE SMALL PART OF THE SATIRE THAT JONSON EMPLOYS TO PROVIDE LAUGHS AT THE EXPENSE OF HIS VICTIMS: THE CLERGY, SCIENTISTS, PHILOSOPHERS, AND MERCHANTS OF LONDON."

Lovewit is further absolved of complicity, according to Monsarrat, when he fails to ask Jeremy whether he has gotten rid of Subtle and Dol. The critic argued that "if Jeremy and Lovewit were partners the natural thing for Lovewit to do would be to inquire whether Jeremy has got rid of Subtle and Doll. But Lovewit does not ask any questions, and Jeremy volunteers no information, precisely because they are not partners." Lovewit's failure to question Jeremy about his partners indicates that the master has no knowledge of them. When Lovewit invites the officers to search the house, it is because he has no reason not to.

As Monsarrat pointed out, Lovewit says that butler has "let out my house / . . . To a Doctor and a Captain: who, what they are, / Or where they be, he knows not." On stage, Jeremy has only confessed to the abuse of the house, and yet Lovewit states that the house was let to a doctor and captain. This information is not provided on stage and appears to contradict Monsarrat's argument, since Lovewit is either embellishing Jeremy's story to protect his butler or Jeremy has talked to Lovewit offstage. Monsarrat assumed that Jeremy has told his master this information, but it creates a loose end that weakens the argument.

In his discussion of the disposition of the goods, though, Monsarrat does offer some interesting observations that help diminish Lovewit's appearance of guilt. Mammon claims the goods as his. But Subtle has sold them to Ananias and Tribulation, who also claim the goods as theirs. Lovewit does what any good magistrate might: he asks Mammon to prove his ownership. Monsarrat argued that "whatever Lovewit's personal motives, it seems evident that he also fulfills a judicial function . . . the officers never intervene, and therefore do not object to Lovewit's behaviour.''

Mammon appears to accept Lovewit's judgment, since he acknowledges that the loss of his dreams is a greater disaster than the loss of his household goods. The goods do not represent great wealth. They are the pewter and tin that Mammon has sent to be changed into gold. The wealth lies with the widow. In marrying her, Lovewit acquires more wealth, but he also acquires a younger wife who will help keep him young. She is the real prize. Monsarrat made one last point that is an important observation about Jonson's use of language in naming his characters. Lovewit's name does not suggest deception, as does Subtle or Face. In a play, such as *The Alchemist,* where the character's name reveals his or her personality and temperament, Lovewit's name reveals only innocent traits, not deceptive ones.

Monsarrat's argument provided a very different glimpse of Lovewit than the one offered by Ross. Ultimately, only the reader's close examination of the text will reveal the Lovewit each reader believes Jonson intended.

Source: Sheri Metzger, for *Drama for Students,* Gale, 1998.

Nathan Cervo

In this essay, Cervo discusses the allusions to odors—particularly offensive ones—that characterize the emotional content of a scene in The Alchemist.

In the spat between Face and Subtle, the alchemist, that opens Jonson's play, Subtle is described as having been very much down on his luck before Face met him:

> Piteously costive, with your pinch'd-horn-nose, And your complexion of the Roman wash, Stuck full of black and melancholic worms, Like powder-corns shot at th' artillery-yard. (1.1.28–31)

Glossing ''Roman wash,'' Brooke and Paradise suggest ''a wash of alum water,'' that is, an emetic. Face apparently returns to this odious metaphor when he calls Subtle ''The vomit of all prisons—.'' However, the phrase ''Piteously costive'' introduces the motif of constipation to the passage that seems to point to a conflation of sewer and stomach contents, such as occurs in the *Curculio* of Jonson's chief comedic model, Plautus.

In *Curculio* (corn-worm, weevil), Platus uses the word *cloaca* (a sewer, drain) to describe the stomach of a drunken woman.

Vomit and excrement may be equally offensive to one's ''nose,'' and Face knows, in retrospect, that Subtle was a charlatan waiting to explode. In the spat, Subtle resorts to a kind of halo-effect defense/attack, berating Face as a ''scarab,'' that is, a dung beetle, and ''[t]he heat of horse's dung.'' Jonson's irony here centers on the fact that the scarab held a privileged place in esoteric alchemy, signifying the survival of the stag (Christ) in a world the morality and thought processes of which amounted to little more than vomit and excrement.

In addition to being known as the dung beetle, the scarab is also known as the stag beetle because of the peculiarity of the structure of its antennae. *Cervo volante,* ''the flying stag,'' is Italian for scarab. Whereas Christ's flying may be linked to resurrection and ascension, comparable to the ascension of the illuminated man in esoteric alchemy, Subtle's ''flying'' is a swindle, consisting in the ''Selling of flies,'' that is, familiar spirits, to gullible clients. Consequently, Jonson's parodic irony is positively vitriolic when he has Face exclaim to Dapper, a mark, in reference to Subtle, ''Hang him, proud stag, with his broad velvet head''—velvety like the dung beetle's antennae and broad with relatively enormous pincers.

The element of the cloaca is essential to Jonson's larger satirical meaning. In the passage cited above, it seems clear that Jonson is punningly acknowledging the *Curculio* (the corn-worm) as his contextual source: ''worms'' and ''corns'' point to Plautus. Clyster and emetic combine to produce Subtle's moral character.

Source: Nathan Cervo, ''Jonson's *The Alchemist*'' in the *Explicator,* Volume 55, no. 3, Spring, 1997, pp. 128–29.

Robert Brustein

In this excerpt from his book The Third Theatre, *Brustein reviews a performance of* The Alchemist. *While he complains of the lackluster production, Brustein does note that Jonson's play is ''one of the three most perfect plays in literature''—a fact that is not diminished by mundane performances and staging.*

Jules Irving had two possible alternatives when he decided to stage Ben Jonson's *The Alchemist*—either to find some modern equivalent for the action which might point its relevance to contemporary

America or to choose a more traditional mode of presentation and offer the work frankly as a revival. Irving made the latter option, setting the play near its own time (the seventeenth century) and adopting a style common on the English stage about fifteen years ago: measured pace, lots of props, elocutionary delivery. The initial decision was honorable enough—it is a pleasure to see a work as brilliantly conceived as *The Alchemist* either in a new framework or an old—but within that option, the production is not successful. For all the farcical frenzy and frenetic activity on the stage of the Vivian Beaumont, there is no real speed in the performance, with the result that some inner vitality has been lost and one of the fastest works in the English language now seems like one of the slowest.

It is difficult to account for the longueurs of the evening: certainly the playwright is not at fault. The con games Jonson provided for his three central characters are still as fresh and inventive as the day they were conceived, and if alchemy is no longer exactly a popular hipster racket, why then politics and advertising can easily be substituted. Tribulation Wholesome and Ananias, those fanatical Puritan elders, have been replaced by more glib but no less dubious personalities like Oral Roberts and Billy Graham; the gigantic hedonism of Sir Epicure Mammon is now being realized by the kick-seeking Hollywood and Bohemian aristocracy; and open-mouthed suckers—like Jonson's gullible Dapper—are still looking for shortcuts to fortune with the horses or the numbers. Kastril, the angry boy who lives to quarrel, is personified today by those who try to prove their manhood through persistent violent encounters, and Abel Drugger, who wants his tobacco shop blessed with magical charms, is no more absurd than those who put religious icons in their automobiles. As for Jonson's amiable con artists, Subtle and Face, they have become as indigenous to American life as Mom and apple pie—indeed, Melville took the confidence man to be an archetypal national figure. Perhaps the ideal actors in these roles would have been W. C. Fields and Groucho Marx, perhaps the ideal epigraph of the play a common Americanism: never give a sucker an even break.

Then, Jonson's manipulation of his complex action is absolutely masterly: Coleridge was correct to call this one of the three most perfect plays in literature. The author keeps at least six distinct plots bustling simultaneously, not to mention countless secondary plots, and enormous energy is unleashed through this method—none of the strands allowed

"THE CON GAMES JONSON PROVIDED FOR HIS THREE CENTRAL CHARACTERS ARE STILL AS FRESH AND INVENTIVE AS THE DAY THEY WERE CONCEIVED, AND IF ALCHEMY IS NO LONGER EXACTLY A POPULAR HIPSTER RACKET, WHY THEN POLITICS AND ADVERTISING CAN EASILY BE SUBSTITUTED."

to touch until the conclusion, when they are rolled into a tight ball with the appearance of Face's master, Lovewit, returning to London.

Why then does the Repertory Theatre production seem so dull? The company is considerably more accomplished than previous casts at Lincoln Center, James Hart Stearn's setting captures the atmosphere of the Jacobean theatre without sacrificing the spaciousness or ingenuity of the modern one, and George Rochberg's brassy score has a fine dissonant, and occasionally electronic, raucousness. But the evening suffers from much too much production, as if the budget for the show were a large one and every penny had to be spent. Points which should be made through character are made through the use of expensive props; a huge steam-producing machine, with a female figurehead, is pumped for laughs whenever the action flags; the costumes, though handsome, do not look as if they had ever been worn by human beings; and none of the actors manages to make a vivid imprint on his part.

The failure of the actors to rise above the production is the most disappointing aspect of the evening, for most of these performers have been extremely impressive in previous roles. Perhaps they are hamstrung by the casting—I certainly found it strange. Epicure Mammon, for example, possibly the most extravagant and voluptuous figure in dramatic literature, is reduced, by George Voskovec, to a mincing courtier with nervous mannerisms and minor appetites. Mammon's desires are so immense that even his speech is a form of gorging: note how, in his description of the banquets and orgies he intends to give after achieving the philosopher's stone, the sibilant consonants make him sound as if he were slobbering over his words:

> I myself will have The beards of barbels served, instead of sallads: Oil'd mushrooms; and the swelling unctuous paps Of a fat pregnant sow, newly cut off, Drest with an exquisite, and poignant sauce . . .

Mammon is a Marlovian figure who wishes not to conquer the world but to swallow it; Voskovec turns him into a hungry Middle European who would be perfectly satisfied with a few scraps in a restaurant not even endorsed by Michelin.

The actors playing Subtle and Face also seem to be miscast, since each would have been more effective in the other's role. Michael O'Sullivan—a galvanic actor with Beatle bangs and a marvelous dental smirk—is too light for the weighty Subtle, while Robert Symonds—a heavy presence with the sonorous chuckle of Frank Morgan—is too earthbound for the quicksilver Captain Face. Both Symonds and O'Sullivan are extremely inventive performers who are perfectly capable of managing the numerous impersonations called for by the text (*The Alchemist* is based on the varying of shapes), but since it is makeup and costume that is forced to do the job, one goes away remembering not so much alterations in character as changes in wigs, cloaks, and beards. Philip Bosco, an actor who looks like Redgrave and sounds like Gielgud, is solid and authoritative as Lovewit, and Nancy Marchand, as Dol Common, maintains a solid, vulgar, brawling quality which suggests more than anything the low-life character of the play. But the actors as a whole simply cannot hold one's attention for more than moments at a time, or wake one from a state of semi-somnambulism.

The production, finally, is without risk, and without the fine ensemble work that might divert attention from the lack of risk. Oh, there is one playful textual innovation—Tribulation Wholesome is played by a woman. Aline MacMahon, who plays the part, is a charming, warmhearted actress, but charm and warmth are hardly appropriate qualities for this smooth, unctuous hypocrite, and considering what the Puritans thought about the ''monstruous regement of woman,'' it is not very likely that a female preacher would have been accepted into the ranks of the Anabaptists. Ultimately, then, the production is the result neither of good antiquarian research nor of a new vision, and that may be why, for all its intermittent moments of vitality, it gives the impression of having entombed the play.

Source: Robert Brustein, ''Sepulchral Odors at Lincoln Center'' in his *The Third Theatre,* Knopf, 1969, pp. 173–77.

SOURCES

Ferreira-Ross, Jeanette D. ''Jonson's Satire of Puritanism in *The Alchemist''* in *Sydney Studies in English,* Vol. 17, 1991-92, pp. 22-42.

Fotheringham, Richard. ''The Doubling of Roles on the Jacobean Stage'' in *Theatre Research International,* Vol. 10, no. 1, September, 1985, pp. 18-32.

Harp, Richard. ''Ben Jonson's Comic Apocalypse'' in *Cithara: Essays in the Judaeo Christian Tradition,* Vol. 34, no. 1, November, 1994, pp. 34-43.

Kernan, Alvin B. ''Shakespeare's and Jonson's View of Public Theatre Audiences'' in *Jonson & Shakespeare,* edited by Ian Donaldson, Humanities, 1983, pp. 74-78.

Kernan, Alvin B., Editor. *The Alchemist,* Yale, 1974.

Mares, F. H. ''Comic Procedures in Shakespeare and Jonson: *Much Ado about Nothing* and *The Alchemist*'' in *Jonson & Shakespeare,* edited by Ian Donaldson, Humanities, 1983, pp. 101-18.

Monsarrat, G. D. ''Editing the Actor: Truth and Deception in *The Alchemist,* V.3-5'' in *Cahiers Elisabethans: Late Medieval and Renaissance Studies,* Vol. 23, April, 1983, pp. 61-71.

Raw, Laurence J. A. ''William Pole's Staging of *The Alchemist''* in *Theatre Notebook,* Vol. 44, no. 2, 1990, pp. 74-80.

Ross, Cheryl Lynn. ''The Plague of *The Alchemist''* in *Renaissance Quarterly,* Vol. 41, no. 3, Autumn, 1988, pp. 439-58.

FURTHER READING

Ford, Boris, Editor. *The Cambridge Cultural History of Britain* Vol. 4: *Seventeenth-Century Britain,* Cambridge, 1989.

This book provides an easy to understand history of England in the seventeenth century. The book is divided into separate sections on literature, art, and music. An introductory section provides a historical context.

Fotheringham, Richard. ''The Doubling of Roles on the Jacobean Stage'' in *Theatre Research International,* Vol. 10, no. 1, September, 1985, pp. 18-32.

This short essay provides an interesting examination of the doubling of roles on stage. Most playwrights wrote with an eye to how few actors would have to be paid to play the roles. Thus scenes and lines were constructed with the anticipation that one actor might be playing several roles, thus entrances and exits were planned accordingly.

Herford, C. H., Percy and Evelyn Simpson, Editors. *Ben Jonson,* Vols. I-XI, Oxford, 1925-52.

This eleven volume work includes a biography of Jonson and introductions to each of the plays. This text of the plays is a reprint of the 1616 folio that Jonson printed. There is also some information about the public's reception of the plays and a great deal of information dealing with almost every aspect of Jonson's life and work.

Hill, Christopher. *The Century of Revolution 1603-1714,* Norton, 1961.

Hill is a well-known author of Renaissance books that examine the cultural and historical background of English literature. Hill has provided an well-organized examination of the economic, religious, and political issues of the seventeenth century. The events that led up to the English Revolution, the Revolution, and the Restoration that followed were crucial incidents that shaped the literature of this period and that which followed.

Maclean, Hugh, Editor. *Ben Jonson and the Cavalier Poets,* Norton, 1974.

This text provides a good selection of Jonson's poetry. Because a selection of his contemporary's poetry is also included, Maclean offers readers and students an easy way to study and compare the poetry of the period.

The Bald Soprano

EUGENE IONESCO

1950

In 1948, Eugene Ionesco began writing *The Bald Soprano,* as he later confessed, almost in spite of himself, for by that time he had come to despise the theater that he had much loved in his youth. What did intrigue him was the banality of the expressions used in an English-language phrase book. These phrases were the inspiration for this anti-play or parody, ''a comedy of comedies.'' Although he set out to show how human discourse had devolved into a collection of empty platitudes and self-evident truisms, something that he believed was very distressing, his friends found his play very amusing, and they encouraged him to find a theater that would stage it. One of these friends, Monique Saint-Come, showed the work to Nicolas Bataille, the director of a group of avant-garde actors working in Paris.

It was under Bataille's direction that *La Cantatrice chauve* was first produced in French at the Theatre des Noctambules in Paris on May 11, 1950. In rehearsal, the company had first tried staging the play as parody but had soon discovered that it worked best if presented as wholly serious drama, in the realistic mode of Ibsen. They had also experimented, trying several different endings, for example. Essentially, even after it opened, *La Cantatrice chauve* remained a work in progress.

The first staging was poorly received. Only the dramatist Armand Salacrou and the critic Jacques Lemarchand praised it. However, the negative re-

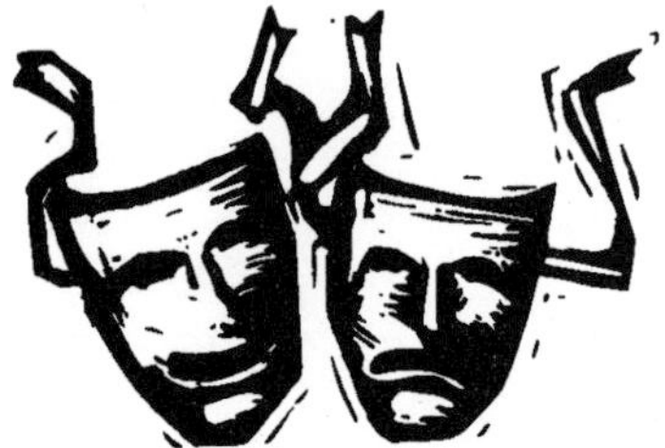

sponses mattered little to Ionesco, who "suddenly . . . realized that it was his destiny to write for the theatre." He began a series of "anti-plays" that within a decade established his place in the new French theater, the group of avant-garde playwrights that included Samuel Beckett, Arthur Adamov, and Jean Genet. In the 1950s, *La Cantatrice chauve* was translated into various languages and widely staged; by 1960, in the United States, where it had been translated and produced as *The Bald Soprano,* it was already being recognized as a modern classic, an important seminal work in the theater of the absurd, which by then was first coming into vogue in America.

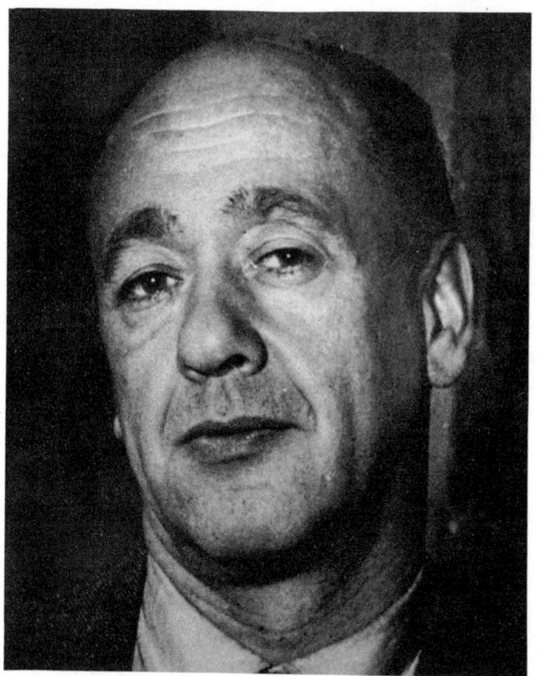

Eugene Ionesco

AUTHOR BIOGRAPHY

Eugene Ionesco (Ionescu) was born in Slatina, Romania, on November 26, 1909, the son of a municipal official and a French mother working as a civil engineer for a Romanian railway company. Ionesco's early childhood was spent in Paris, where in 1912 his father took the family when he began studying law. A quarrelsome, choleric man, Ionesco's father treated his wife badly, leading to her attempted suicide and to Ionesco's life-long distaste for brutal authority figures.

In 1916, when Germany declared war on Romania, Ionesco's father left to return to Bucharest. He lost contact with the family. Without support, Ionesco's mother had to take a factory job, leaving her son to spend lonely months in a cheerless children's home near Paris. However, in 1922, at age thirteen, Ionesco had to return to Romania. His father had secretly divorced his mother, remarried, and gained legal custody of Eugene and Marilina, Ionesco's younger sister. The uprooting was traumatic, for it required that Ionesco learn a new language and once more live with his tyrannical father, whom he despised, both for his familial violence and his devious political fence straddling.

At the age of seventeen, Ionesco fled his father's house, finding work as a French tutor; in 1928 he entered the University of Bucharest to study French literature. During his studies, Ionesco made connections in Romanian literary circles and established a reputation as a poet and a critic. His work focused on novelists, poets, and philosophers rather than playwrights. He claimed, in fact, that the great French classical dramatists held little interest for him, though Shakespeare did. He would later come to writing plays almost by accident.

In 1938, Ionesco and his wife went to France so that he could complete a doctoral thesis on French poetry, and though World War II forced him to return to Romania, in 1942, having obtained an exit visa, he returned to France, living near poverty in Marseilles. At the war's end, he moved back to Paris, where he found work as a proofreader. Three years later, in 1948, the year his father died, Ionesco wrote *The Bald Soprano,* the first of his "anti-plays." The work was inspired by a language primer that Ionesco had used to learn English. At first writing in Romanian, Ionesco set out to parody the inane phrasing of the book's dialogue, but he recast it in French, giving it the title *La Cantatrice chauve.* In 1950, the year he acquired French citizenship, Ionesco was able to have the play produced at the Theatre des Noctambules in Paris before a small, largely unenthusiastic audience.

The work marked the debut of Ionesco as one of the new playwrights of the avant-garde theater centered in Paris and quietly launched a dramatic career that by the 1960s, his most prolific period, brought him world-wide acclaim. In 1970, he was elected to the Academie Francaise. Along with Samuel Beckett, Jean Genet, and Arthur Adamov, Ionesco is now honored as a major seminal figure in the absurdist movement in France. He died on March 28, 1994.

PLOT SUMMARY

The Bald Soprano, a one-act ''anti-play,'' opens in a ''middle-class English'' interior, furnished with typically English furniture and a typically English couple, Mr. and Mrs. Smith, whose first names remain unknown. It is an English evening, and the pair is engaged in English activities. He reads a newspaper while she darns socks. The silence is broken by an English clock that strikes seventeen times, prompting Mrs. Smith to remark that ''it's nine o'clock.''

Mrs. Smith recounts what the pair had for dinner, mentally wandering from the menu to the pair's children while Mr. Smith continues to read and click his tongue. He finally responds when she concludes that one Dr. MacKenzie-King was to be trusted because he underwent a liver operation before performing the same operation on a patient. They start a mild quarrel over the issue because the doctor's patient died, prompting Mr. Smith to conclude that the doctor was not conscientious.

After the clock strikes seven times, then three more times, Mr. Smith announces that Bobby Watson has died, something, presumably, that he has learned from the newspaper's obituaries. In the ensuing dialogue, the couple disclose that Bobby Watson was married to Bobby Watson, and, further, that there is whole clan of Bobby Watsons. Threaded through the Watson discussion are several inconsistencies and contradictions, so it is never clear, for example, whether the first named Bobby Watson had died recently, or one, or two, or three, or even four years before.

The discussion leads into a brief altercation. Mr. Smith accuses his wife of asking ''idiotic questions,'' while she complains that men do nothing but sit around smoking and either powdering their noses and putting rouge on their lips or drinking heavily. Mr. Smith, apparently deaf to what Mrs. Smith has just said, asks her what she would say if she saw men behaving like women, powdering their noses, using rouge on their lips, and consuming whiskey. When Mrs. Smith complains about his kind of joking, and in a snit throws socks across the room, Mr. Smith tries to placate his ''little ducky daddles'' with a suggestion that they turn off the lights and ''go bye-byes.''

Mary enters to explain that she is the maid and has just spent the afternoon with a male companion, and, further, that the guests, the Martins, have arrived. After complaining that Mary should not have gone out, the Smiths leave to dress while Mary greets the Martins. After complaining about the Martins' lack of punctuality, Mary also exits, leaving the guests alone.

The Martins sit facing each other and, after an uncomfortable silence, begin a polite exchange in which, through elaborate, lengthy deduction, they come to the belief that they are, in fact, husband and wife, though neither can actually recall knowing the other. Among other ''curious'' coincidences are the revelations that they both originally came from the city of Manchester and that they had left just five weeks previously, had ridden the same train, and had even shared the same compartment. Since then they have lived in the same London apartment and have even slept in the same bed. Further, they are named Donald and Elizabeth, the names of their respective husband and wife, and have a child named Alice who has one red and one white eye. As the clock strikes one, they embrace, sit in the same armchair and promptly fall asleep.

Mary re-enters to confide a secret to the audience—that the Martins are not really Donald and Elizabeth. She claims that their whole deduction collapses because of a single contradictory detail, that, based on the discrepancies in the color of Alice's right and left eyes, they are not the girl's parents. She suggests, however, that this fact remain a secret, then leaves, confiding that her ''real name is Sherlock Holmes.''

After the Martins awake, the Smiths enter to welcome them. Mrs. Smith is effusive in her greetings, but her husband ungraciously complains about their tardiness. The Smiths then sit facing the Martins, who have returned to their original seats. They attempt to engage in conversation, but their efforts are punctuated with silences that precede each rather pointless remark. Mrs. Smith is finally able to break the ice by encouraging the Martins to relate what ''interesting things'' they have seen during their travels. Mrs. Martin then tells of seeing a man bend over to tie his shoe lace, an event that the rest consider rather extraordinary.

The ringing doorbell then interrupts the conversation, but when Mrs. Smith goes to the door to see who has arrived, nobody is there. That fact leads to an argument between Mr. and Mrs. Smith. After a second ring with a similar outcome, Mrs. Smith takes the position that a ringing doorbell indicates that there is no one there, and when it rings a third time, she refuses to go to the door. The argument, becoming slightly heated, is interrupted with the arrival of the Fire Chief, who appears when Mr. Smith opens the door after the fourth ring.

The Fire Chief, in uniform and wearing a huge shining helmet, greets everyone and is quickly drawn into the controversy over the significance of the ringing doorbell. After conceding that both Smiths are partly right, he sits down, announcing that he has no time to stay. He is under orders to put out all fires in the city. The Smiths deny that there is a fire in their house, prompting the Chief to announce that things are not going well, that fires have been few and minor, limiting profits. After remarking that he has no right to extinguish the fires of clergymen and that naturalized citizens are not entitled to fire protection, he offers to tell the others some stories.

There follows a series of incongruous tales, told in turn by the Chief, Mr. Smith, Mrs. Smith, and the Chief again. The stories provoke both irrelevant and irreverent remarks from the listeners, though none of the stories makes any sense. Because Mrs. Martin loses the thread of the Chief's last story, she requests that he retell it, but before he can begin, the maid interrupts, asking that she also be allowed to tell a story. The Smiths and Martins are annoyed by her temerity, but the Fire Chief recognizes her, and he and Mary have a joyous but brief reunion. The Chief defends Mary's behavior against the others' disapproval. Mary, over Mrs. Smith's objections, recites her poem in honor of the Fire Chief, even as the Smiths push her offstage. The Chief remarks that the poem was "marvelous," then prepares to leave the party, first asking after the bald soprano. The question occasions a brief embarrassment before Mrs. Smith confirms that the soprano "always wears her hair in the same style."

After the Chief departs, the Smiths and Martins begin an exchange of increasingly nonsensical and discontinuous statements, full of phrases characteristic of language phrase books. Some of the statements are platitudes, like "charity begins at home," but others, like "I'd rather kill a rabbit than sing in the garden," are pure nonsense. As sense breaks down into repeated word fragments—mere syllables—the four characters grow increasing hostile and aggressive, until they are all angrily screaming. Then, after the lights go out and come back on, the play begins again, with the Martins taking the place of the Smiths in the opening moment, speaking the very same lines.

CHARACTERS

The Fire Chief

The Fire Chief appears midway through *The Bald Soprano,* ostensibly on official business. He is looking for fires, under orders to put out any that he finds. He observes that the fire-extinguishing business is not good, that profits are down. Although a little more brusque than the others, like the Martins and Smiths he is superficially polite. He takes the role of an adjudicator and confessor, trying to restore peace between Mr. and Mrs. Smith, who have engaged in a nonsensical argument over whether or not a ringing doorbell indicates that there is actually someone at the door.

He is also a raconteur, though his stories are wholly nonsensical, without logical continuity, unity, or intelligible point. One of them is a shaggy-dog saga that meanders aimlessly along, confusing everybody. When Mary enters, she and the Fire Chief embrace, revealing that they were engaged in a former relationship. That disturbs the Martins and Smiths who are class conscious and find the affair inappropriate. After Mary recites her cataclysmic fire verse, the Fire Chief, having provided "a truly Cartesian quarter of an hour," departs with his oddly incongruous remarks about a bald soprano.

Donald Martin

Like his host, Mr. Smith, and the two wives, Donald Martin is distinguished only by having no distinguishing qualities at all. When he and Mrs. Martin first enter, they begin their inane exchange of information from which they deduce that they are husband and wife. The two mirror each other in their banal, excessively polite language and their ridiculous inability to make a logical leap to the conclusion that their tediously repetitive banter finally draws them. These are mechanical puppets or interchangeable parts, not pliable humans.

MEDIA ADAPTATIONS

- The only feature film in English adapted from an Ionesco play is *Rhinoceros,* which was released in 1974. An American Film Theatre production, it was directed by Tom O'Horgan and starred Karen Black, Zero Mostel, and Gene Wilder. Ionesco was one of the screenwriters. The stage play did not translate well into film, and most critics consider it a failure. It not currently available on video.
- An audio tape of *Rhinoceros,* featuring the same leading actors as the film version, was released by Harper Audio on cassette in 1973. It is out of print, but used copies are sometimes available from such services as Amazon.com.
- *La Vase* (*The Slough*), a film made at La Chapelle-Anthenaise in 1970, was written by Ionesco and features him in its single role. In 1971, the film played briefly at a Latin Quarter cinema in Paris, but it was poorly received. It is not currently available in the United States.
- A reading of *The Chairs* was recorded and released by Caedmon Records in 1963, featuring Siobhan McKenna and Cyril Cussack. It was re-released on audio cassette by Harper Audio but is not generally available.

The Martins are so shallow as to be unable to recognize each other when they enter the Smiths' home, even though they have come in together. When the Smiths re-enter, the two couples engage in further pleasantries, a pastiche of non sequiturs consisting of vapid observations and tidbits of very conventional wisdom. All seem to grow excited over the most mundane behavior, such as a man bending over to tie his shoe or reading a newspaper. Their responses seem artificial, their words ludicrously inappropriate to the situation.

Like the others, Mr. Martin also seems utterly without any important convictions. He is timorous and excessively apologetic. He can not even take a side in the silly doorbell argument between Mr. and Mrs. Smith. The only times that he seems in the least genuine in the expression of his feelings are when he airs his class-conscious biases against Mary, some sexist remarks about women, and in the cacophonous exchange of verbal nonsense in which the characters heatedly engage just before the end of the play.

Elizabeth Martin

Like her husband, Elizabeth Martin is a human cipher. In their initial exchanges, her speech, except in the nouns of address, is virtually indistinguishable from that of Mr. Martin. They simply echo each other, using the same phrases and words repeatedly, especially variations on the exclamation "how curious it is." Like him, she also seems at times to have no grasp of the most obvious things, though at other times she finds the most mundane and obvious behavior extraordinary.

For example, she is apprehensive about disclosing that she saw the man who bent over to tie his shoe for fear that she will not be believed. Mrs. Martin cautiously sides with Mrs. Smith in her doorbell argument with Mr. Smith, even though Mrs. Smith concludes that when the doorbell rings it means that there is nobody at the door. Mrs. Martin claims that her husband is also "obstinate," yet when the Fire Chief actually appears the fourth time the bell is rung, she stubbornly maintains that the fourth time does not count because she will not allow experience to invalidate Mrs. Smith's claim that a ringing doorbell means that there is nobody at the door.

Like the other characters, at odd moments Mrs. Martin offers bizarre observations that seem out of character because they glimpse beyond the inane dialogue that generally suggests no intelligence at all. For example, it is she who thanks the Fire Chief for the ''truly Cartesian quarter of an hour'' that he has spent at the Smiths'. Otherwise, she mirrors the character of her husband and the Smiths, revealing the same social prejudices and rigid ineptitude. That she is almost identical to Mrs. Smith is made apparent when at the end of the play she replaces Mrs. Smith in the repeated opening of the play, using the same dialogue but with the Martins as the prospective host and hostess.

Mary

Mary is the Smiths' maid, which she announces when she first enters, presumably to inform the audience of her role. She has just returned from spending the afternoon at the cinema and having milk and brandy with a male friend. At first she is very matter-of-fact in her manner, but suddenly breaks into laughter, then tears, announcing ''I bought me a chamber pot,'' as if that fact explained her emotional instability. When the Smiths go off to dress for their guests, Mary lets the Martins in, upbraiding them for being late. She then exits, but returns on tiptoe after the Martins fall asleep, exhausted from their protracted verbal voyage on which they have discovered that they are man and wife. Mary then lets the audience in on the secret that despite the extensive logical deduction of Donald Martin, the Martins are not really the parents of their alleged common child and are, therefore, not really who they claim to be. She exits after confiding that she, in reality, is Sherlock Holmes. Mary reappears during the visit of the Fire Chief, requesting, to the chagrin of Martins and Smiths, that she also be allowed to tell a story. She and the Chief recognize each other, overcome with wonder that they should be reunited in the Smiths' home. When he explains that Mary had helped him put out his earliest fires, she tells him, ''I am your little firehose.'' The Martins and Smiths become irritated by Mary's familiarity, but can not prevent her from reading her poem honoring the Fire Chief as the Smiths push her offstage.

Mr. Smith

Mr. Smith, the host, is a *reductio ad absurdum* parody of a complacent, middle-class British suburbanite and husband, one confident in his ignorance and stupefyingly dull in his observations. In the first part of the play, he merely reads and clicks his tongue while his wife gives her account of who they are and what they consumed at dinner. When he finally talks, he does so to take issue with his wife, whom he mildly bullies with a ridiculously smug sense of having superior reasoning powers, when in fact neither is capable of logical discourse or even meaningful communication.

Smith and his wife may talk, but neither seems to really listen to the other or even to their own previous observations. In their mostly-quiet, polite game of one-upmanship, they often contradict themselves, oblivious to their illogicality. They share no love or genuine concern for each other, only a mutual shallowness covered with a thin veneer of verbal civility that sometimes breaks down, as, for example, when Mr. Smith angrily upbraids the Martins for having arrived so late, and when he calls Mrs. Smith ''disgusting'' for having interrupted his interruption of Mrs. Martin's aborted account of a man she saw outside a cafe.

Most of the time, however, Mr. Smith is simply boring, incapable of sustaining any original thought or meaningful discussion on any topic broached. Only in his trivial argument with Mrs. Smith over the import of the doorbell does he come close to maintaining a consistent stance. Like his wife and the Martins, he generally makes incongruous, irrelevant, or contradictory pronouncements that frustrate all attempts at rational discourse.

Mrs. Smith

Mrs. Smith, a parody of a stuffy, middle-class British housewife, is the appropriate counterpart to Mr. Smith. Like his, her speech is basically a litany of incoherent trivia often couched in pat phrases and class-reflective cliches. At the beginning of the play, she presents a virtual monologue in which she gives a tedious, detailed account of what she and Mr. Smith consumed for dinner. She also reveals that the couple have children and hints that Mr. Smith lacks sufficient sexual vigor, which she obliquely continues to target in the pair's put-down game.

That she and her husband are otherwise virtually indistinguishable in outlook and temperament is borne home by their discussion of the Watsons, a husband and wife, both named Bobby, who were so much like each other as to confuse acquaintances. Although they take opposite tacks, as in their silly doorbell argument and the manner in which they first greet the Martins, they sound so like each other as to suggest that they take their stances not from conviction but from spite for each other. The spite sometimes erupts, as when Mrs. Smith bares her teeth and hurls some socks across the stage, or when she attacks her husband as a boor. It also takes other forms, flirtation with Mr. Martin and the Fire Chief, for example.

Like her husband and the Martins, Mrs. Smith seems driven by underlying but non-specific anxieties that partly account for the bizarre observations that each of them makes. Her insecurities seem to be centered on sex, health, and mortality; normal concerns, certainly, but ones which remain mostly subliminal in the superficially polite conversation that blocks all attempts at honest communication.

THEMES

Absurdity

Absurdist themes are pervasive in *The Bald Soprano.* In fact, the work is often critically mined to illustrate absurdist ideas and motifs. Chief among them in Ionesco's play is the concept of entropy, or the tendency of order to decay into chaos. This collapse is reflected in the speech of the characters, which, in the course of the play, becomes increasingly dysfunctional, resulting in the total breakdown of language as a viable tool of human communication.

Entropy is also conveyed by the characterizations, or, more accurately, the lack of them. Humankind is reduced to the Smiths and Martins, who, at times, behave very much like some of those contemporary dolls that issue pat, random expressions when their recordings are activated by pulling a string or pressing some part of their plastic anatomy. Like the dolls, the Smiths and Martins are soulless and hollow remnants of character reduced to exhibiting only a sort of vestigial anxiety about their missing or confused identities.

The general breakdown of language-borne sense and logic gives *The Bald Soprano* a facade of nonsense, sometimes even an infantile silliness. The remarks of the characters are often inappropriate, contradictory, or completely devoid of meaning, especially towards the end, when, as language decays into word fragments, the Martins and Smiths become almost manic in their anger. What they reveal is one of the most important absurdist themes: the modern inability of humans to relate to each other in either an authentic or honest fashion.

Language and Meaning

The Bald Soprano is a "tragedy of language" dealing with the gradual loss of its communicative function and its final fossilization into inane phrases and meaningless cliches. At first there is at least a thread of logic in the characters' conversation, but it is often interspersed with contradictory and inconsistent statements, as when, for example, Mr. Smith first says he learned of Bobby Watson's death in the newspaper, then claims that it had happened three years earlier, and that he "remembered it through an association of ideas."

It is, in fact, a sort of free association that takes the characters off on ever-widening tangents, their statements jumping completely off contiguous mental tracks onto barely relevant sidings. For example, in her opening monologue, Mrs. Smith meanders through a series of simple sentences that have no cohesive point at all. She moves cursorily from a description of what the Smiths consumed for dinner towards her pronouncements about Dr. Mackenzie-King's virtues as a physician.

Towards the end of the play, the mental track-shifting accelerates. The dialogue breaks into a series of non sequiturs, suggesting that rational discourse has become impossible, that relevant thought can not even be sustained past a single sentence or two. The Martins and Smiths simply cascade through unrelated and inane phrase-book cliches before breaking into a sort of syllabic babble. Words degenerate into mere objects, thrown about like pies in a comic free-for-all.

Alienation and Loneliness

In his parodist's treatment of his bourgeois non-characters, the Smiths and Martins, Ionesco stresses both the loss of a personal identity and social and familial estrangement. His characters are alienated, not because they are sensitive beings in a hostile or impersonal world, but because they have no individuality at all. They are no longer merely threatened by machines; they have become like them, manufactured on a sort of class assembly line and engineered to conform to middle-class values as codified in hackneyed expressions and rigid patterns of behavior. They are too similar to have personal identities, thus it hardly matters whether, like the Smiths, they have no first names, or, like the various Watsons, they all have the same one. Their alienation has everything to do with a total lack of a personal identity, which even their language inhibits them from establishing. They have simply been rendered incapable of incisive, individual thought.

Identity

At the opening of *The Bald Soprano,* Ionesco stresses the typicality of his characters in his repeated insistence that they and their surroundings are "English." The first characters encountered are named "Smith," a very common English patronymic also suggesting the couple's conventional nature. These are figures who have no discrete sense of self.

Moreover, Ionesco continually drives his characters' lack of self-awareness beyond even a simple stereotype. The Martins, for example, cannot even recognize each other as husband and wife, and have to go through their distended and repetitive deductive process to establish their relationship. Even then their identities are called into question by what Mary discloses, leaving the audience somewhat mystified. However, the playwright's point is that the truth, if there is any, does not matter, for the Martins can serve as wholly suitable surrogates for the "real" Donald and Elizabeth Martin because they are almost their perfect clones.

The only hints of a different identity are drawn along sexual and class lines, and even these are deliberately blurred. While Mrs. Smith is responsible for homemaking duties, she hints about Mr. Smith's inadequacies as a male, while, he, in his turn, complains about women behaving like men. Throughout the play, the characters' anxieties seem to center on threats, not to their individuality, but only to their roles as determined by gender and class.

Time

If language gradually loses all significance in *The Bald Soprano,* time, as measured by the Smiths' English clock, immediately becomes so erratic as to mean nothing at all. Before Mrs. Smith first speaks, the clock strikes seventeen times, prompting her to announce that it is nine o'clock. Thereafter, it strikes as few as one and as many as twenty-nine times, in a random, jumbled order. Finally, according to the stage directions, it "strikes as much as it likes," as if it were an animate or sentient object, entirely out of human control.

Time in the play has lost its purpose—it no longer represents a logical sequence in a spatial dimension. The strokes, rather than conveying a sense of progression, act like a neurotic chorus reinforcing the absurdity of the dialogue. Like the words, the strokes participate in the centripetal decay or entropy that describes both the play's basic movement and its central theme.

Gender Roles

Even a reliable identity based on gender is undermined in *The Bald Soprano.* The Smiths and Martins may voice or evidence some commonplace gender-based biases, but role distinctions erode in the course of the play. Early on, Mr. Smith accuses his wife of asking stupid questions, indicating his belief that his mind is superior to hers and that her powers of reasoning are severely limited because she is a woman, an irrational "romantic." However, during the Fire Chief's visit Mr. Smith concedes that his wife is more intelligent than he is, and even "much more feminine," suggesting that there is a feminine side to his character and behavior. Mrs. Smith says as much when she complains about men who use rouge on their lips and sit around all day

TOPICS FOR FURTHER STUDY

- Investigate the basic existential tenets of the French philosophers and writers Jean Paul Sartre and Albert Camus and their impact on Ionesco's absurdist drama.
- Compare the dramatic techniques of an existential drama such as Sartre's *No Exit* or Camus's *The Misunderstanding* with those of *The Bald Soprano.*
- Investigate the work of Alfred Jarry and the science of pataphysics, relating your discoveries to Ionesco's anti-plays.
- Research the impact of Charlie Chaplin and other film comedians on the absurdists, including Ionesco.
- Research surrealism as a movement in art and drama, noting its influence on Ionesco's *The Bald Soprano.*

and drink. She also suggests that Mr. Smith lacks the ''salt'' of the evening's soup, an oblique slur on her husband's deficient masculinity. Further, she is the more sexually aggressive of the two. She flirts with both the Fire Chief and Mr. Martin, suggesting her need to establish a sexual identity denied her by her emasculated husband.

Class Conflict

The Smiths and Martins have a class-consciousness challenged by Mary, the Smiths' maid. Mary presents a threat to them because she is willful and disrespectful, and does not seem to know her place. The couples grow testy and self-righteous when, during the Fire Chief's visit, Mary requests that she be allowed to tell a story. They find her request presumptuous and inappropriate, and though Mary manages to recite her poem in honor of the Chief, she is forced off stage in the process.

STYLE

Setting

The setting of *The Bald Soprano* is so typically ''English'' as to be a reductio ad absurdum. The interior, the furnishings, the characters' dress and manners are all ''English,'' at least in the sense of epitomizing a national stereotype. The setting is the modern interior of a middle-class London couple's home, while the characters are a husband and wife who evidence those qualities attributed to the type, a sort of stoic stiffness and reserve and superficial cheeriness and civility.

The actual furnishings may be realistic enough, but the behavior of the Smiths and their visitors most certainly is not. Nor is the English clock, which, from the outset, indicates that the action within the seemingly real surroundings is to be distorted through the lens of a parodist.

Structure

Billed as an ''anti-play,'' *The Bald Soprano* parodies the well-made problem play of the realistic tradition. Rather than develop on a linear, causal path towards a climax and denouement, Ionesco's work progresses haphazardly, and though it becomes increasingly frenetic near the end, as if approaching an emotional climax, it finally folds back on itself and starts all over again. Its cyclical structure suggests that an infinite and tedious replay is possible but is aborted, not because there is an Aristotelian end, but simply from practical necessity. Even an anti-play has to finish.

Although it may be described as a fairly long one-act play, there is no formal division of *The Bald Soprano* into either acts or scenes. The entrances and exits of characters mark episodic changes that do not carry forward any causal or thematic links. Basically, there are five major episodes or ''French scenes'': first the Smiths are alone, arguing over trivial matters and discussing the Bobby Watsons; next the Martins are alone, tediously discovering that they are husband and wife; then the Martins and Smiths are together, exchanging empty observations and arguing over the significance of the ringing doorbell; next the Fire Chief arrives, visiting with the two couples, telling stories; and finally, after the maid's interruption and the Chief's exit, the Smiths and Martins are alone again, engaging in a nonsensical verbal ruckus. Thereafter the anti-play shifts into a combination epilogue and prologue, starting all over again.

Anti-Characters

The Bald Soprano is also an ''anti-play'' because its characters are anti-characters. The Smiths and Martins are entirely lacking distinct or consistent personalities; they are indistinguishable, virtually interchangeable, and essentially characterless. They speak alike, often echoing each other's phrases, as evidenced in the dialogue between the Martins. They are unable to begin and sustain meaningful discourse, for they are defined by the cliches of their class, from which they can not depart and which they never transcend. They are anti-heroes not because they are physically disabled or have weak minds or experience extraordinary bad luck but because they have no minds at all. None of them serves as a protagonist or main character in any traditional sense.

There are hints of potential character, conveyed in the vague anxiety that afflicts these figures, something lying outside the ability of their language to express it, except perhaps in isolated moments of oblique word play. Characters seem compelled to say things, to cover a silence that would expose their vulnerability. When the Martins and Smiths first sit down to talk, they must overcome an embarrassing silence, an uncomfortable moment in which the realization that they have nothing to say threatens to expose their hollowness. The silence is broken, first with hemming and hawing, then with pointless pleasantries, but the silence keeps returning with its disturbing presence. The silence seems to be a more authentic act of communication than the silly and self-evident comments the Smiths and Martins make.

Nonsense

The Bald Soprano may have a serious theme, but it uses nonsense and buffoonery to advance its idea that language has become denuded of its majesty and affective power. The physical slapstick of classic farce, used to beat the comic stooge, has been transformed into a verbal counterpart, noisy but ineffective.

Words are depleted of force in various comic ways. One way is through tedious repetition. For example, the words "bizarre," "coincidence," and "curious," used in the first exchange between the Martins, are worn down to pointlessness through repetition. Words are also misapplied, such as when the Martins and Smith find the most mundane or trivial act to be "something extraordinary" or "incredible." Words also go limp when they appear in doughy lumps or hackneyed expressions, randomly inserted in dialogue that goes nowhere because it is simply a meandering stream of non sequiturs. Words deprived of meaning become mere objects, to be thrown about like brickbats in a comic but nonsensical free-for-all.

There are also some nonverbal farcical elements in *The Bald Soprano,* although they seem of less importance. Characters sometimes act in ways diametrically opposed to what they say they will or will not do, as, for example, when the Fire Chief announces that he has no time to sit down and then proceeds to do so, or when the Smiths retire to change their clothes but return to greet the Martins without having done so. Buffoonery is also evident in their dress itself, notably in the large, shiny helmet the Chief wears, and in such classic clowning routines as shoving an intruder offstage, as the Smiths do to Mary while she recites her poem, and in Mrs. Smith's repeated trips to the door to find that no one has rung the doorbell. This silliness has a purpose, serving as a visual concomitant to the basic breakdown of sense in language that is the play's central concern.

HISTORICAL CONTEXT

In the period between 1948, when Ionesco began writing *The Bald Soprano,* and 1956, when Peter Wood directed the play's first production in English at the Arts Theatre in London, the split that divided the world into two hostile super powers deepened and widened. Ionesco, who obtained French citizenship in 1950, the year the work was first performed, was cut off from his homeland, Romania, which by then was firmly within the Soviet bloc of communist satellite states.

The Cold War arms race began in earnest in that same period. The "police action" in Korea, starting in 1950, heated up the war, pitting North Korea and its Communist Chinese allies against South Korea and United States and other United Nations forces. The prospects of spreading hostilities loomed large, prompting fears at home and abroad of a new world war that would employ weapons of vast destruction, like the thermonuclear device that was detonated at the Bikini Atoll in the Pacific Ocean in 1954. America's first hydrogen bomb, the device was hundreds of times more powerful than the more primitive atomic bombs dropped on Japan in 1945.

In the United States, congressional investigations of suspected communists continued, although the excesses of Senator Joseph McCarthy, censured for misconduct in 1954, were slowly turning the tide of public opinion against the investigations. Many felt the inquiries had turned into a hysterical witch hunt, as Arthur Miller had suggested in *The Crucible,* his 1952 drama based on the Salem witchcraft trials of the seventeenth century. It was also in 1954 that, at a conference of world powers meeting in Geneva, Vietnam was divided into two separate states, setting the stage for the Vietnam War.

In France, Ionesco's adopted country, the conservative government fell in June, 1954, bringing to the premiership Pierre Mendes-France, leader of the Radical-Socialist party. Among other leftist policy changes, Mendes-France favored an end to French colonialism in North Africa and Indochina. Algerian nationalists, hoping to hasten their independence, revolted against France the following October, creating a national crisis.

Winds of political and social change were also shifting in the United States. In the momentous 1954 *Brown v. Board of Education* decision, the Supreme Court ruled that racial segregation in public schools was unconstitutional, effectively overturning laws based on the "separate but equal" ruling of a much earlier Court. The landmark decision was the legal basis for the civil rights movement of the next two decades.

By the early 1950s, television had become the principal medium of popular culture in the United

COMPARE & CONTRAST

- **1950s:** There is a growing concern about the misuse and abuse of language, particularly as an instrument of propaganda. Words are used to sway public and political opinion, particularly by the powers waging the Cold War. As communication technology advances, concerns arise over the negative effects on the human mind. Some believe that media advances make a sort of massive brain washing possible, a danger reflected in both nonfiction and fictional works, including George Orwell's *1984* (1949) and Vance Packard's *The Hidden Persuaders* (1957).

  Today: Many critics argue that in stressing the need for "political correctness" the media and various public agencies are currently engaged in social engineering through the manipulation of language, even if the aim, multi-cultural understanding and tolerance, is praiseworthy.

- **1950s:** In the traditional stereotype of the middle-class family, the roles of husband and wife are primarily limited to the husband as "bread winner" and the wife as "nurturer." World War II temporarily altered this pattern as women replaced military-bound men in factory jobs. After the war, the pattern resumed, but many women discovered they were dissatisfied with a life confined to the domestic sphere.

  Today: Women are much more active in the work force. They have also made significant inroads in the military, with many serving in combat roles.

- **1950s:** The Cold War is a global pressure cooker threatening an uneasy peace with heated words and threats. Although *The Bald Soprano* remains free of any reference to the ideological struggle, Ionesco's "anti-play" is the first of several in which he deliberately neglects current affairs for his more abstract ends, leaving the international crisis conspicuous only by its total absence.

  Today: With the Cold War over, Ionesco's unwillingness to use drama to promote partisan views seems intellectually justified, as does his concern with the debasement of language.

States, supplanting the radio and offering a major challenge to the motion picture industry. Prices for black and white television sets with nineteen-inch screens had dropped to an average of $187 by 1954, bringing them within the affordable means of the average family. In that same year, RCA introduced the first color television set, and though the quality was poor and unreliable, within six years, with improved technology, color television began replacing black and white television as the household standard. A "hot" medium, television would soon begin purveying popular artistry, such as the new and revolutionary style of music known as rock and roll, including the work of Elvis Presley, who cut his first commercial recording in 1954.

In the American theater, the principal playwrights were Arthur Miller, Tennessee Williams, and a rediscovered Eugene O'Neill. Although all three used non-realistic elements in their drama, they largely worked within the tradition of the well-made play and shared a similar focus on social and psychological problems affecting realistic characters. Compared to the Broadway and West End fare of 1954—plays like Herman Wouk's *The Caine Mutiny Court-Martial* and Terrence Rattigan's *Separate Tables*—Ionesco's *The Bald Soprano* and Samuel Beckett's *Waiting for Godot* represented a new, bold, and highly controversial use of theater. Their influence in the American theater would first be felt in the United States in the off-off Broadway movement of the late 1950s.

Like much of absurdist drama, *The Bald Soprano* seems detached from the real world. It is virtually free of any topical allusions to current affairs. It goes down its own sort of metaphysical rabbit hole, creating a world in which there is no verisimilitude, no link to actuality. It does make reference to several real persons, to Benjamin Franklin, Robert Browning, and Rudyard Kipling, for example, but these are anachronistic names invoked in the muddle of verbal nonsense that dominates the last part of the play. Except in the most abstract sense, Ionesco's purpose is not political. He is not dealing with a social or even an ethical wrong. He is lamenting the death of language, a tragedy of such magnitude that it renders the current state of world affairs trivial and irrelevant.

CRITICAL OVERVIEW

At the time Ionesco wrote *The Bald Soprano,* serious French theater was under the domination of writers who wrote very literate plays with serious, intellectual themes. Among them were Jean-Paul Sartre and Albert Camus, who, although they shared a philosophical kinship with Ionesco, chose to write in a traditional mode. There were a few dissenters, particularly Antonin Artaud. In *The Theatre and Its Double* (1938), he had clamored for something new, an overpowering drama that would have an impact analogous to that of the Black Death on medieval Europe. Few outside small avant-garde circles listened, however, and the new theatrical revolution preached by Artaud, which Ionesco's anti-play helped promote, began far less dramatically than Artaud had hoped. On May 11, 1950, *The Bald Soprano* opened before an audience of three people who sat under a leaky roof at the dilapidated Theatre des Noctambules on Paris's Left Bank.

The audience never grew very large during the play's brief run. The work was simply too different for the established tastes of most patrons, some of whom hooted indignantly, outraged by the audacity of the piece. To them and most reviewers, *The Bald Soprano* was contrary to the very idea of theater. Few saw any merit in the play, and despite the cast and playwright's energetic efforts to drum up new audiences, the house soon went dark from lack of interest.

The chilling reception of *The Bald Soprano* did not discourage Ionesco, however. His fascination with theater rekindled, he continued writing his series of anti-plays, undeterred by the hostile or indifferent welcome of his early French audiences. The reactions even seemed to support the implications of his play, that the bourgeoisie was incapable of fresh judgments. It was the very discomfort of Ionesco's audiences that amused an early supporter, the French critic Jacques Lemarchand, who, in his "Preface to Eugene Ionesco," confessed that he found great pleasure in the "insults" and "grunts and ironic laughter of the notables in the audience."

Because he shared their distrust of rationalism, Ionesco won immediate approval by some surrealists, including the playwright Armand Salacrou, one of the three members of the play's first audience. However, it took the support of establishment critics and writers to break through the barrier of public aversion. The tide of public opinion really began to turn in 1954 with the revival of Ionesco's third produced play, *The Chairs.* It had played to sparse audiences in 1952, when it was first produced, and though it prompted a serious defense in the magazine *Arts,* it fared little better than *The Bald Soprano* had two years earlier. However, the revival became a significant success when France's premier dramatist, Jean Anouilh, openly deemed it a masterpiece, a classic in the avant-garde theater. Ionesco soon found a niche in the front rank of the new French playwrights, some of whom, like him, were expatriates living in Paris, notably Samuel Beckett and Arthur Adamov.

There were those who complained that Ionesco's anti-plays advanced no causes, that the playwright lacked the kind of political commitment of dramatists like Bertolt Brecht. A major controversy arose after, in translation, Ionesco's plays made their way onto the British stage, starting with *The Bald Soprano* in November, 1956. Within two years, the so-called "London Controversy" started when an extremely influential leftist critic and early defender of Ionesco, Kenneth Tynan, began a celebrated debate with the playwright over what Tynan believed was Ionesco's linguistic nihilism, his distrust of language as a viable tool for human advancement. Several important persons were eventually drawn into the controversy, including Philip Toynbee and Orson Welles. In the intellectual fur flying, Ionesco made it clear that he saw little difference between the totalitarian regimes on the left and the fascist regimes on the right, and he openly attacked leftist apologists, among whom he numbered Jean-Paul Sartre, Bertolt Brecht, John Osborne, and Arthur Miller. To Ionesco, drama had little to do with doctrines, as he had endeavored to show in his early diary entries explaining his purpose in *The Bald Soprano* and *The Lesson.* His aim was to create "pure drama" that was "anti-thematic, anti-ideological, anti-social-realist, anti-philosophical, anti-boulevard-psychology" and "anti-bourgeois."

His was to be a new, "abstract" theater, liberated from any sort of doctrinal adhesion.

Throughout the 1960s, with a growing worldwide reputation, Ionesco remained a prolific dramatist. His achievement, recognized by his election to the conservative Academe Francaise in 1970, was exceptional, but his influence on avant-garde theater was gradually waning. Some of his most ardent earlier admirers were frustrated by his inflexible opposition to didactic drama. Ironically, he had become increasingly partisan in his adherence to non-partisanship, a paradox that he himself pointed out. According to Deborah Gaensbauer in *Eugene Ionesco Revisted,* during the Cold War, many "French intellectuals and critics . . . became devotees of Brecht," who had been one of Ionesco's major targets in his debate with Tynan. As a result, he alienated some of his original followers, becoming "cast once more as a pariah in an all-too-familiar irrational discourse."

By the 1970s, Ionesco had simply become too familiar, like an old hat worn too often. Though still honored for his first contributions to the new French theater, he was criticized for lacking the profundity of Beckett, the rebellious zeal of Genet, and the courage needed to take new artistic risks. Ionesco, stung by the rebukes, turned increasingly away from theater to fiction, criticism, and painting.

Ironically, the end of the Cold War helped restore some of Ionesco's diminished reputation as a playwright and thinker, for as Gaensbauer noted, in the 1980s "many of Ionesco's political claims were vindicated," making him a kind of prophet, a "modern Tiresias, shunted aside for seeing uncomfortable truths." Still, as Martin Esslin suggested in *The Theatre of the Absurd,* Ionesco's ultimate place in "the mainstream of the great tradition" remains uncertain, although his plays, including *The Bald Soprano,* have made "a truly heroic attempt to break through the barriers of human communication."

CRITICISM

John W. Fiero

Fiero is a professor of English at the University of Southwestern Louisiana, where he teaches drama and play writing. In this essay he discusses the interrelationship of Ionesco's anti-play elements in The Bald Soprano, *including character, language, and structure.*

The Bald Soprano (1950) is Eugene Ionesco's first "anti-play," conceived and created as a deliberate spoof or parody of the plays then in vogue in Paris. Ionesco was attempting to create "a new free theatre," one devoid of theme, ideology, social realism, philosophy, and the thin "boulevard" psychology then pervading French drama. His targets were the complacent bourgeoisie and intellectual drones who went to see plays that fed them nothing to challenge their smug certainty that such matters as social injustice could be ameliorated through political convictions and rational discourse. For Ionesco, the very efficacy of language was in question, something far more fundamental and troubling than the passing concerns of political ideologies, no matter what their flavor.

Ionesco's method was to weave together trite expressions pilfered from an English-language primer that he had used while learning English. He translated these for his trenchant caricature of the bourgeoisie, whom he saw as prattlers of an endless stream of mindless expressions and hackneyed slogans. As he confides in *Notes and Counter Notes,* the process proved unsettling. While writing the work, he "felt genuinely uneasy, sick and dizzy," because, perhaps, he glimpsed from the outset that what he was writing "was something like the *tragedy of language!*"

The Bald Soprano may have tragic implications, but on the surface it is pure comedy, almost farce. In fact, Ionesco was aware of the seeming contradiction, for he also dubbed his anti-play a "comedy of comedies." He set out in artistic defiance of the Aristotelian notions of plot, character, diction, and thought—the elements of the "well-made" play—designing a new drama as free of such conventional elements as he could make it. His main characters, the Martins and Smiths, are robotic ninnies, so much alike as to be indistinguishable, either in language or function. Their diction is largely pre-masticated cant, made up of self-evident observations and the various insincere pleasantries that polite but empty civility requires. The Martins and Smiths are middle-class English couples, though they could just as well be of any nationality in Europe or North America.

Hemmed in by their hollow platitudes, these anti-characters never seem to progress much beyond a pre-cognitive ritual of acknowledging the

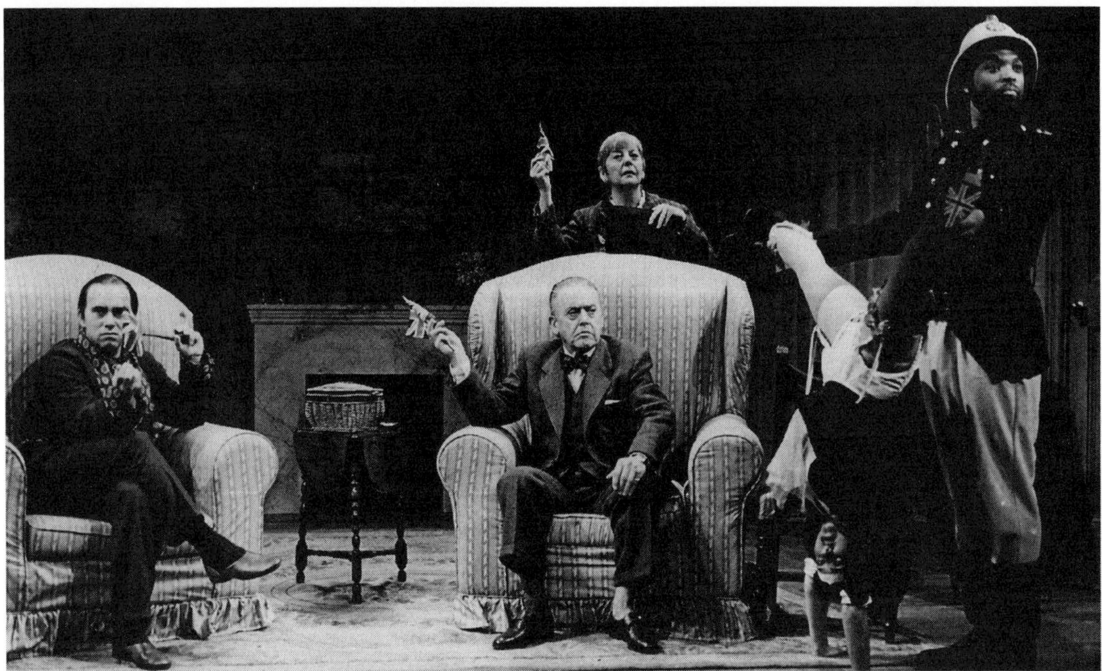

A production of The Bald Soprano *with Thomas Derrah, Jeremy Geidt, Tresa Hughes, Deborah Lewin, and Rodney Scott Hudson.*

existence of each other. Even that much is resisted by Mr. Smith when, at the play's opening, he reads and clicks his tongue while Mrs. Smith jabbers incoherently. Empty niceties and insincere expressions of awe lock out any understanding or insight, resulting, for example, in the ludicrous discovery by the Martins that they are actually husband and wife. Or so they agree to believe.

These are characters who either cannot think for themselves because they have no selves or have no selves because they cannot think. That is the ironic implication of Mrs. Martin's farewell thanks to the Fire Chief, with whom she says she has "passed a truly Cartesian quarter of an hour." In essence, the Smiths and Martins have provided the negative corollary to Descartes' famous principle, *cogito ergo sum* ("I think therefore I am"). They do not think; therefore they are not. They have no discreet identities, thus it is no wonder that Mr. and Mrs. Martin cannot recognize each other when they first enter the Smiths' home. The amnesia they suffer is a condition of non-being.

When a real thought threatens to invade the consciousness of these anti-characters, it is usually too evanescent to have any sticking power. It comes and is immediately lost, forcing discourse into a crazy-quilt pattern of incongruous observations, many of which are self-evident or indisputable truisms, like the fact that a week consists of seven days or that the ceiling lies above and the floor below, snippets of inane conversation that Ionesco took from his English phrase book. Still, throughout the first half of *The Bald Soprano,* there are a few occasions in which a sense of anxiety breaks through the barriers erected by the polite platitudes. Angst is revealed in the characters' inability to endure silence and in a few hostile remarks that disclose, at least in the Smiths, fears of sexual inadequacy and the resulting threat to any last remnants of a meaningful identity. It is only at such points that characters, however crudely, use language creatively rather than merely mechanically. There is, for example, Mrs. Smith's early quip that although the soup of the evening meal "was perhaps a little too salty," it was "saltier" than Mr. Smith.

For the most part, as George Wellwarth remarks in "Beyond Realism: Ionesco's Theory of the Drama," the Smiths and Martins use language "as decorative verbiage to cover over the subconsciously felt fear of being in a reasonless void, of being an effect without a cause." Such isolated wordplay as Mrs. Smith's, indicative of an echo of

WHAT DO I READ NEXT?

- *Waiting for Godot* (1952) is Samuel Beckett's best known play and shares top billing with Ionesco's *The Bald Soprano* as the most important works in the theater of the absurd. It was written at about the same time but not produced until 1953.
- *The Chairs* (1952), Ionesco's third staged anti-play, which many consider his best, also depicts a collapse into nothingness, partly through words but also through the crowding of the stage with empty chairs and invisible characters.
- *1984* (1949), George Orwell's dystopian study of Oceana, depicts a futuristic society gone amok. Mind control is partly achieved through Newspeak, a diminished version of English which attempts to limit proletariat thinking to government-sanctioned ideas.
- *Fahrenheit 541* (1953) is Ray Bradbury's science fiction novel of future society in which books, including the great classics of literature, are banned and people are spoon fed verbal and visual images by the government.
- *The American Dream* (1960), by Edward Albee, is the first real foray into the absurdist technique by a major American playwright. It shares Ionesco's concern with the debasement of language.
- *The Myth of Sisyphus* (1942) is Albert Camus's inquiry into the value of life in an absurd world—one devoid of purpose or meaning. A major proponent of existentialism, Camus provides insight into the philosophical basis of absurdist drama.

---

an intuitive ability, is both faint and rare. In fact, in the final moments, just before the play starts over again, the hostile anger that emerges as the play's strongest emotion grows in potency as any semblance of meaning expressed in language breaks down. Discourse simply implodes into babble, word fragments strung together by sounds, not by the association of ideas. Words lose their symbolic value altogether, thus language utterly fails, leaving the Smiths and Martins in frustrated rage. The basis of that rage is completely lost in a torrent of nonsense. At that point, as Richard Coe says in *Ionesco: A Study of His Plays,* ''language is used almost physically, as a kind of bludgeon or blunt instrument'' and the audience is ''physically assaulted by the barrage of quasi-meaningless sounds emitted by the characters on stage.''

Formal logic and inductive reasoning, tools of rational discourse, are also assaulted in the playwright's scathing parody. Like the surrealists, Ionesco had a distrust of rational thought, widely regarded by Western thinkers from Aristotle forward as the principal means to human understanding. Ionesco mimics the rational process even as he mocks it, clearly defying it with highly improbable or random occurrences and contradictions. For example, the Smiths, masking sexual fears, engage in futile arguments built on ever-shifting premises. Like the clock, which finally strikes whatever it wants, the characters say whatever does or does not move them.

As in dreams, in Ionesco's world a ringing doorbell might announce the presence of someone at the door; then again, it might not. It is a random and arbitrary world, in which causal reasoning is at best unreliable. There can be no certainty. The Martins, having determined through their lengthy and comically tedious deductive process that they are married to each other, are actually deceived, if Mary can be trusted as accurate. Moreover, it makes no difference, for like the proliferated Bobby Watsons, one Mr. Martin or Mrs. Martin is basically the same as the next.

For Ionesco, causal argument badly misrepresents reality by putting too much faith in artificially ordered and focused conscious thought. He targeted the plays of the social realists because they told stories with events chained together in a logical, interlocking pattern that falsified true experience through drastic oversimplification and distortion. To reveal the deficiencies of such a causal pattern, he has the Smiths and Martins attempt to apply its principles to the more chaotic and less predictable world of the inner being. He does it, as Richard Schechner says in "*The Bald Soprano* and *The Lesson:* An Inquiry into Play Structure," by "stripping away" the usual order, "the causative world," and thereby revealing the true "rhythms" of the theater. These more faithfully reflect that same inner being.

The basic structural paradigm for the linear, causally-developed, well-made play is an isosceles triangle, sometimes referred to as "Freytag's pyramid," after the nineteenth-century German writer who devised its schema. It reflects a unified structural pattern in which action rises from a stasis or equilibrium to a climax, then falls in denouement to an end. Theoretically, that sequence describes not only the entire structure but each dramatic "moment" or "beat."

Scrapping this artificial structure, Ionesco had to find a way to bring *The Bald Soprano* to closure. His first working solution, arrived at in rehearsal, was to end the action abruptly, using a sort of *deus ex machina* device in which the performance was closed down by "the Superintendent of Police and his men, who open fire at the rebellious audience" and simply order the theater vacated. The actors and playwright considered other possibilities but rejected them as too problematic. Then they came up with the clever idea of simply letting the play begin again, giving the work its cyclical structure. The play was already up and running when, as a final structural refinement, Ionesco substituted the Martins for the Smiths in the repeated opening.

Perhaps the Ouroboros, a snake devouring its own tail, can serve as the new structural paradigm. It suggests an endless, tedious, and futile cycle. It is, therefore, an appropriate structural symbol for much of the avant-garde drama influenced by Existentialism, representing the absurd condition of man explored by Albert Camus in *The Myth of Sisyphus.* With variations, it would be used again by Ionesco, in, for example, his very next play, *The Lesson* (1951). Sensing that tedious and pointless labor was appropriate to the absurd condition, Samuel Beckett used a parallel structure in the two acts of *Waiting for Godot* (1952).

"FOR IONESCO, THE VERY EFFICACY OF LANGUAGE WAS IN QUESTION, SOMETHING FAR MORE FUNDAMENTAL AND TROUBLING THAN THE PASSING CONCERNS OF POLITICAL IDEOLOGIES, NO MATTER WHAT THEIR FLAVOR."

As a complement to the infolding or collapsing structure, Ionesco employs a centripetal design in which language seems to go berserk. Everything speeds up. Words proliferate, then break into mere cacophonous fragments just prior to the blackout that divides round one from round two in the interminable main event. That pattern of acceleration and proliferation, whether of words or objects, characterizes most of Ionesco's anti-plays. It remains his indelible artistic signature and a hallmark by which his plays are easily recognized.

Source: John W. Fiero, for *Drama for Students,* Gale, 1998.

John V. McDermott

McDermott examines Ionesco's use of inane, meaningless dialogue as a means of criticizing small talk or conversation with very little content. Ionesco felt that such discourse prevented people from thinking and talking about subjects that were truly important.

In his play *The Bald Soprano,* Eugene Ionesco objected to mundane, peripheral talk "to diversions that tempt us to avoid thinking about or talking about the only things that really matter—the meaning of existence and the inevitability of death." Ionesco was agitated because he felt that "words no longer demonstrate: they chatter. . . . They are an escape. They stop silence from speaking. . . . They wear out thought, they impair it."

In relation to the idea that words no long "mean," Mrs. Martin remarks near the end of the play "We have passed a truly Cartesian quarter of an hour," which implies that those with her all knew that they existed because they were thinking. But since Ionesco parodies to the extreme their so-

> "IONESCO WAS AGITATED BECAUSE HE FELT THAT 'WORDS NO LONGER DEMONSTRATE: THEY CHATTER. . . . THEY ARE AN ESCAPE. THEY STOP SILENCE FROM SPEAKING. . . . THEY WEAR OUT THOUGHT, THEY IMPAIR IT."

called thinking, they are not truly considering who they are or the reason for their existence; they are not truly living. All they wish to consider is how to pass the time as comfortably as possible.

Picking up on Mrs. Martin's inane remark, the Fire Chief incongruously blurts out the most enigmatic phrase of the play: "Speaking of that—the bald soprano?" The phrase is met with "embarrassment" and dumb "silence" by the Smiths and the Martins. The silence is termed "general," for it is all-pervasive; it is not the silence that speaks. This phrase is Ionesco's happy solution to the problem cited by Coe: It is "the phrase whose very essence is meaningless insignificance but which must become significant without thereby becoming meaningful. . . . It must reveal its own absurdity" [Coe, Richard, *Eugene Ionesco,* Grove, 1961]. And so it does; it is the epiphanic phrase by which Ionesco chose to reveal the complete *de*signification of the *word.* In its having no connection to anything spoken heretofore, in its isolation from predication, this phrase is worse than any of the banal platitudes that have preceded it. It is the nonexistent "prima donna" that does not appear in the play, for as Ionesco said when asked why he had given the play this title, "One of the reasons . . . is that no prima donna appears in the play. This detail should suffice." And so it does, for the phrase which the playwright liked because of its sound signified his belief that words had become nothing but meaningless sounds.

Following the "general" silence that follows the Fire Chief's meaningless phrase, Mrs. Smith remarks, "She always wears her hair in the same style." This vapid attempt at humor is not used to cover any embarrassment she may feel over her ignorance of what possible meaning the phrase may have; rather it points up her indifferent attitude toward the idea of *thought,* for in her world words no longer signify anything.

That "the bald soprano" was an inadvertent remark or "slip of the tongue" by the actor who played the part of the fire chief, is an appropriate seed that must have struck Ionesco in its inappropriate relation to anything else in the play. The phrase served Ionesco's purpose well in signaling the final collapse of the *word*—sound without meaning, without significance—the way of the world.

Source: John V. McDermott, "Ionesco's *The Bald Prima Donna*" in the *Explicator,* Volume 55, no. 1, Fall, 1996,p. 40.

Rosette C. Lamont

In this essay Lamont provides an overview of Ionesco's play, chronicling reaction to its premiere as well as the playwright's motivations and inspirations for writing this masterpiece of farce.

The curtain rises on a middle-class English couple, Mr. and Mrs. Smith: the wife is a non-stop chatterbox who has nothing to say beyond praising the cooking of their maid, Mary, while Mr. Smith is content with clicking his tongue from behind his opened newspaper. He is busy scanning the obituary page where a notice appears about the death of one Bobby Watson. Confusion pervades the exchange between husband and wife as to the gender of the dead person since both husband and wife were called Bobby. The clock strikes seven, three, then five, as Mrs. Smith wonders when the two Bobby Watsons plan to get married. The time is definitely "out of joint." These speculations, which also include the little Bobby Watsons, are interrupted by Mary who comes in to announce the arrival of Mr. and Mrs. Martin. As the Smiths rush out to change, their guests settle in the vacant armchairs. Although Mr. and Mrs. Martin have come down on the same train from Manchester, they do not seem at first to know one another. Step by step they reconstruct their lives, becoming convinced that they are man and wife. Mary, the self-proclaimed "Sherlock Holmes" of the play, blows up their pyramid of evidence by stating that the little girl they assume to be their child cannot be their offspring: ". . .whereas it's the right eye of Donald's child that's red and the left eye that's white, it's the left eye of Elizabeth's child that's red and the right eye that's white." There are no certainties in Ionesco's world. With the unexpected arrival of the Captain of the Fire Brigade, the maid's erstwhile lover, matters disintegrate further. The Fireman's absurdist tales unleash a kind of madness. The play ends with the Smiths and Martins dancing round and round like cannibals, hurling invectives or hissing syllables at one another. At the end, the Martins and Smiths trade roles and places. Everything starts all over again.

When *The Bald Prima Donna* was presented by Nicolas Bataille in 1950 on the tiny stage of the now defunct Theatre des Noctambules, the one-act sketch was received as a witty prank, the kind of show one might expect to see in a cabaret. The title appeared to be a joke since no bald diva was seen on the stage. The audience was unaware that the Fire Chief had slipped up in rehearsal, substituting the words "bald prima donna" for another group of nonsense terms, and as a result Ionesco decided that this chance twist of the tongue would determine the play's title. Such a solution was in keeping with the tradition of Dadaism, a school whose own title came from flipping open a dictionary and choosing a word at random. Ionesco, the admitted heir of Tristan Tzara, welcomed the intrusion of chance as an element of his aesthetic.

Ionesco likes to say that in composing *The Bald Prima Donna* he was not quite certain of what he had produced. He assumed that it was "something like the tragedy of language," and was therefore amazed to hear the audience laughing. Later, when he had had time to reflect upon this non-psychological, apolitical work, he came to see it as pure structure, like a musical composition or an architectural construction. Although Ionesco claimed the text of the play was "dictated" to him by the characters from a conversation book, *English Made Easy,* a careful analysis reveals that it is crafted with minute precision, that the rhythm of the play gathers momentum and reaches a crescendo. Although Ionesco sub-titles this sketch an "anti-play," pointing out its parodic intent, it must be seen as a lampoon that pays homage to the genre it mocks.

Most French critics made the mistake of considering this comedy to be social satire, a way of poking fun at bourgeois French society by means of a cartoon version of the British middle class. However, Ionesco is quick to declare: "I'm a good bourgeois myself!" If any joke was intended, it was at the expense of boulevard melodrama in the style of Henri Bernstein. Nicolas Bataille claims to have imitated this style in directing his actors, just as he ordered his set designer to recreate the decor of *Hedda Gabler.* Ionesco suggests that his play must be understood to be the satire of bourgeois mentality, not bourgeois customs. He says that he makes fun of a universal petite-bourgeoisie, of men of fixed ideals, who live by slogans, using mechanical language without ever questioning it.

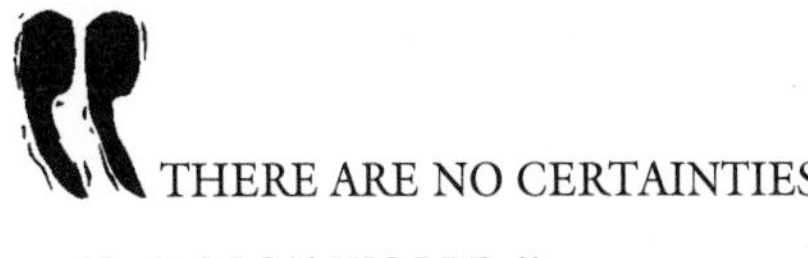

THERE ARE NO CERTAINTIES IN IONESCO'S WORLD."

There are six characters in the *Bald Prima Donna.* The Smiths and the Martins are interchangeable, and in the end they do change places. The Maid and the Fire Chief, her erstwhile lover, are no less indistinct, but they are colorful rather than gray. Ionesco's Mary is the Bacchante of Dionysus/The Fire Chief whom she celebrates by reciting a paean to fire. Of course the Fire Chief is enchanted with this celebration of his "conception of the world." It seems that being worshipped in this manner frees his own creative impulses; he manifests a gift for story telling. Both Mary's paean and her lover's surrealist fables constitute the dynamite charge that brings down the walls of convention. The play's rhythm intensifies, grows delirious. What becomes obvious is that the flat, cartoon-like characters are made of words, not of flesh and blood.

Ionesco's first play is still his favorite because of its simple abstract quality. It has been running at the Theatre de La Huchette in the Latin Quarter for over 35 years. It is also widely performed in university campuses in the United States. The *Bald Prima Donna* has ushered in the leading dramatic form of the second half of the 20th century, the metaphysical farce.

Source: Rosette C. Lamont, "*The Bald Prima Donna*" in *The International Dictionary of Theatre I: Plays,* edited by Mark Hawkins-Dady, St. James Press, 1992, p. 47.

SOURCES

Coe, Richard N. *Ionesco: A Study of His Plays,* Methuen & Co., 1971, p. 60.

Esslin, Martin. *The Theatre of the Absurd,* 2nd edition, Penguin, 1968, pp. 135, 138, 351.

Gaensbauer, Deborah B. *Eugene Ionesco Revisited,* Twayne, 1996, pp. 13-14, 17.

Ionesco, Eugene. *Notes and Counter Notes,* translated by Donald Watson, Grove, 1964, pp. 179-81, 184-85.

Lemarchand, Jacques, "Preface to Eugene Ionesco," *Theatre I,* Gallimard, 1954, p. 9.

Schechner, Richard. "*The Bald Soprano* and *The Lesson:* An Inquiry into Play Structure," in *Ionesco: A Collection of Critical Essays,* edited by Rosette C. Lamont, Prentice Hall, 1973, p. 22.

Wellwarth, George E. "Beyond Realism: Ionesco's Theory of the Drama," in *The Dream and the Play: Ionesco's Theatrical Quest,* edited by Moshe Lazar, Undena Publications, 1982, p. 34.

FURTHER READING

Hayman, Ronald. *Eugene Ionesco,* World Dramatists Series, Frederick Ungar, 1976.

Written in 1973, after Ionesco virtually turned away from theater, Hayman's study concludes that the playwright's best work was written in the 1950s, which he deems superior to that of the 1960s. The work provides a chronology of stage and broadcast pieces through 1973 and a play-by-play analysis of dramas up through *Macbett.* Hayman claims that Ionesco's greatest weakness is structural. Includes an interview with Ionesco.

Killinger, John. *World in Collapse: The Vision of Absurd Drama,* Dell, 1971.

Aids in the interpretation of absurdist drama, explaining the philosophical base for the structural designs and thematic motifs in the plays of Ionesco and other absurdists.

Lamont, Rosette C. *Inonesco's Imperatives,* University of Michigan, 1993.

A major resource text for further study, this work reflects thorough research into Ionesco's historical and political milieu. It features valuable aids, including a rich chronology and notes on productions.

Pronko, Leonard C. *Eugene Ionesco,* Columbia Essays on Modern Writers, Columbia University Press, 1965.

A brief pamphlet, this work provides a quick overview of Ionesco's plays of the 1950s and early 1960s. It provides information about the playwright's techniques and artistic aims in his earliest works.

Burn This

LANFORD WILSON

1987

Burn This opened in Los Angeles, California, on January 22, 1987. Wilson's play is a contemporary romantic drama, but it is not a happy romance, and even the resolution cannot be described as entirely happy. The two romantic leads, Anna and Pale, do not find love easy, and it is not easy for the audience to witness. Early reviews of the play were mixed. Although reviewers commended Joan Allen and John Malkovich's performances, some critics questioned the credibility of an attraction between Anna and Pale. Nevertheless, the play has been generally well-received because the characters are interesting, particularly Larry, Anna's homosexual roommate, who is funny and endearing. In a 1986 interview with David Savron, Wilson explained that *Burn This* is a love story different from any other love story because the characters do not say, "I love you"; they say, "I don't want this." This conflict, argued Wilson, makes the love story contemporary. Wilson spent time studying modern dance so that he could incorporate the atmosphere and style into his character of Anna. *Burn This* is Wilson's thirty-eighth play, and he was willing to wait for nearly a year to put it on stage because he wanted John Malkovich to play Pale. He has stated that with this play he wanted to recapture the convoluted plotting of his earliest plays. Wilson relies upon dialogue to reveal the plot, and thus, the audience must pay close attention in order to follow the action. *Burn This* was not as commercially or critically successful as were Wilson's *Talley's Folly* or *Hot l Balti-*

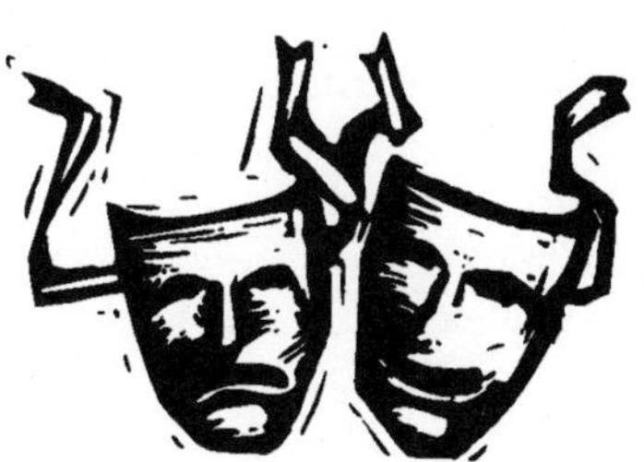

more, but it has been widely discussed as a depiction of a contemporary love story.

AUTHOR BIOGRAPHY

Lanford Wilson was born in Lebanon, Missouri, on April 13, 1937. He was five when his parents divorced. His father moved to California, and Wilson lived with his mother until 1956. Wilson attended Southwest Missouri State College from 1955 to 1956 and San Diego State College from 1956 to 1957; he planned on being an artist, although he had done some acting in high school. When he was nineteen, Wilson moved to Chicago, where he was employed as an illustrator at an advertising agency. He had been writing stories on his lunch hours and gathering rejection slips, when he suddenly realized that the story he was writing was not a story but a play. He has considered himself a playwright ever since.

Since he had no real knowledge about the writing of plays, Wilson enrolled at the University of Chicago to learn about plays and playwriting. After he moved to New York in 1962, Wilson became an active participant in the Off-Off Broadway theatre community. Several of his early plays were produced at the Caffe Cino or at La Mama Experimental Theatre, including *The Madness of Lady Bright* (1964) and *Home Free* (1964). These early one-act plays were followed by a succession of full-length works, beginning with *Balm in Gilead* (1965). In 1968, Wilson was a cofounder of the Circle Repertory Company, where most of his works have since premiered. Strong character development has become a hallmark of Wilson's work. His characters often exist on the fringes of society, but as the play progresses, they demonstrate that they are capable of growth and change.

Burn This (1987) is Wilson's thirty-eighth play. In a December, 1986, interview, Wilson stated that he considers *Burn This* to be the best work he has ever done. But he also explained that it is difficult to decide on a favorite, as his opinion sometimes changes when new productions of his works are staged. Wilson has been the recipient of several awards, including the New York Drama Critics' Circle award in 1973 for *Hot l Baltimore* and in 1980 for *The Migrants.* Wilson also received the American institute of Arts and Letters Award in 1974, and in 1980, he received the Pulitzer Prize for Drama, the Theatre Club, Inc. Medal, and the Brandeis University Creative Arts Award for *Talley's Folly.* Wilson has received Tony Award nominations for *Fifth of July* (1979), *Talley's Folly* (1980), and *Angels Fall* (1983). *The Migrants* (a collaboration with Tennessee Williams), *Fifth of July, Lemon Sky, The Rimers of Eldritch, The Sand Castle, Wandering,* and *The Mound Builders* have all been produced on television. Wilson has also written two original television plays, *Stoop: A Turn* and *Taxi. Hot l Baltimore* was adapted as a television series in 1975. Wilson received a Ph.D. in 1985 from University of Missouri.

PLOT SUMMARY

Act I, scene 1

Burn This opens just after the death and funeral of Robbie, Anna and Larry's roommate. The action takes place in the roommates' loft, and as the play begins Anna is huddled on the sofa smoking, a drink in her hand. Burton arrives at the loft and is admitted. In the conversation that follows, the audience learns that Robbie and his partner, both of whom were gay, were killed recently in a boating accident. Anna was unable to reach Burton, who was out of town, and he has come to the apartment upon returning to New York and hearing the news. When Larry enters with groceries, the audience learns even more about the events of the past few days. The audience also learns about the nature of Anna and Burton's relationship. Although he is supposed to be her boyfriend, he could not be reached by phone when she needed him, and his initial interaction with Anna seems distant. Both Larry and Anna take turns describing Robbie's funeral and his family's reaction to his death. The audience learns that Robbie and Anna worked closely together and that she had recently changed careers from dancer to choreographer. Robbie was an integral part of Anna's new career, and his dancing was also a part of her choreography work. Thus, she has not only lost a friend and roommate, she has lost an artistic partner. Anna tells Burton that Robbie's family, none of whom had never seen him dance, did not acknowledge that he was gay. Instead, they assigned Anna the role of Robbie's girlfriend and treated her as his grieving widow. Both Larry and Anna are upset at this treatment by Robbie's family, and the dialogue serves an important purpose of establishing this family's background before the arrival of Pale, Robbie's older brother, who appears at the loft later in Act I. Anna, Larry, and Burton also talk about Burton's recent trip, the purpose of which was to help him find sources and inspiration for his next screenplay. Burton makes a great deal of money for the sale of his scripts, but apparently feels no great loss at their sale and would just as soon not know how Hollywood uses his material.

Act I, scene 1

The scene opens with a pounding on the door; it is the middle of the night. Pale, enters the loft; he is loud and obnoxious. His speech makes little sense to Anna and is filled with obscenities. It is revealed that Pale is twelve years older than Robbie and that it has been a month since the funeral. Pale creates so much noise that Larry is awakened but returns to bed. The conversation between Pale and Anna is confrontational and unpleasant. At times neither seems to be listening to the other person and the speech becomes almost a monologue. As he has been speaking, Pale has also been undressing. When he breaks down, Anna tries to comfort him. Pale lies down on the sofa; his conversation is peppered with sexual innuendo, and the lights fade. When the stage lights come back up in a few moments, it is morning. The conversation between Anna and Larry reveals that Pale slept in Anna's bed. Anna states that Pale was like a bird with a broken wing that needed healing. Pale is anxious to leave and almost bolts from the loft, but first he tells Anna that he has a wife and children.

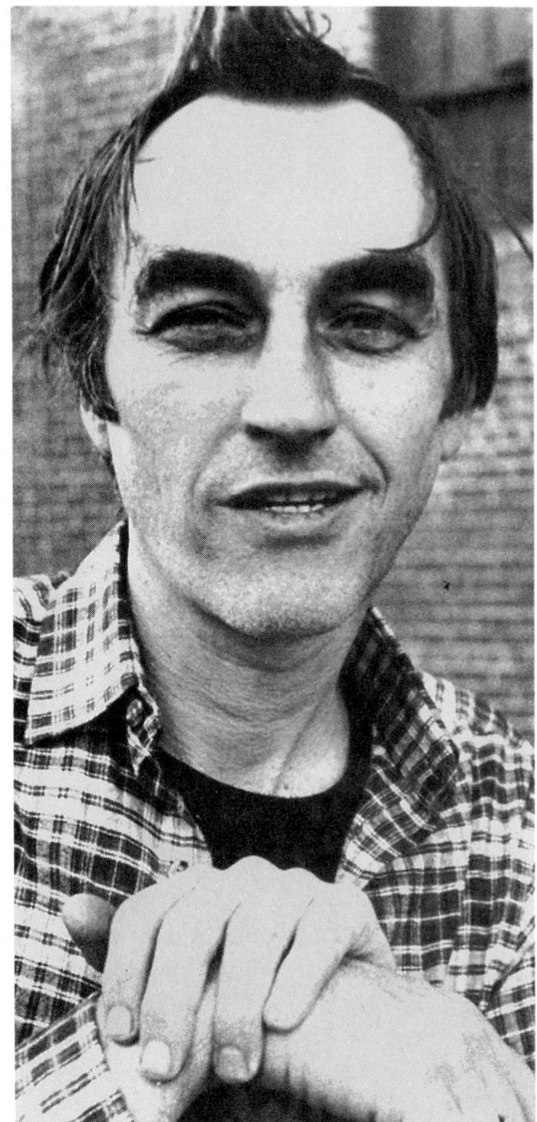

Lanford Wilson

Act II, scene 1

It is almost two months later, New Year's Eve. Anna and Burton are together. They are discussing their recent work when Larry returns early from a trip, interrupting what was obviously planned intimacy between Anna and Burton. The three begin talking and Burton tells a story about an anonymous quasi-homosexual experience he once had during a snow storm. The conversation ends when Larry opens the door and a very drunk Pale falls into the room. Pale is as rude as he was during his first visit to the loft, and a confrontation erupts between Pale and Burton, which escalates into a fight. Anna throws Burton out; she would like to throw Pale out, but he is too drunk. Anna and Larry leave the stage as each goes to bed; a sleeping Pale is left lying to the side of the stage. But before the lights fade, the audience sees Pale walking toward Anna's bedroom. When the lights come back up, Larry is preparing coffee. Pale emerges and begins making tea, and finally Anna comes out of her bedroom. Anna states that she and Pale are like apples and oranges that do not belong together. Pale makes an effort to convince her that they do belong together, but she is determined to have him leave. Anna reveals that she is frightened of a serious emotional commitment. The scene ends with Pale leaving the loft and Anna leaving to be alone.

Act II, scene 2

Burton and Larry are alone on stage. Burton appears dejected and is holding his new script. It has been a month since the confrontation on New Year's Eve. Larry reveals that Anna has been working on a new dance, but that she has not seen Pale. Burton

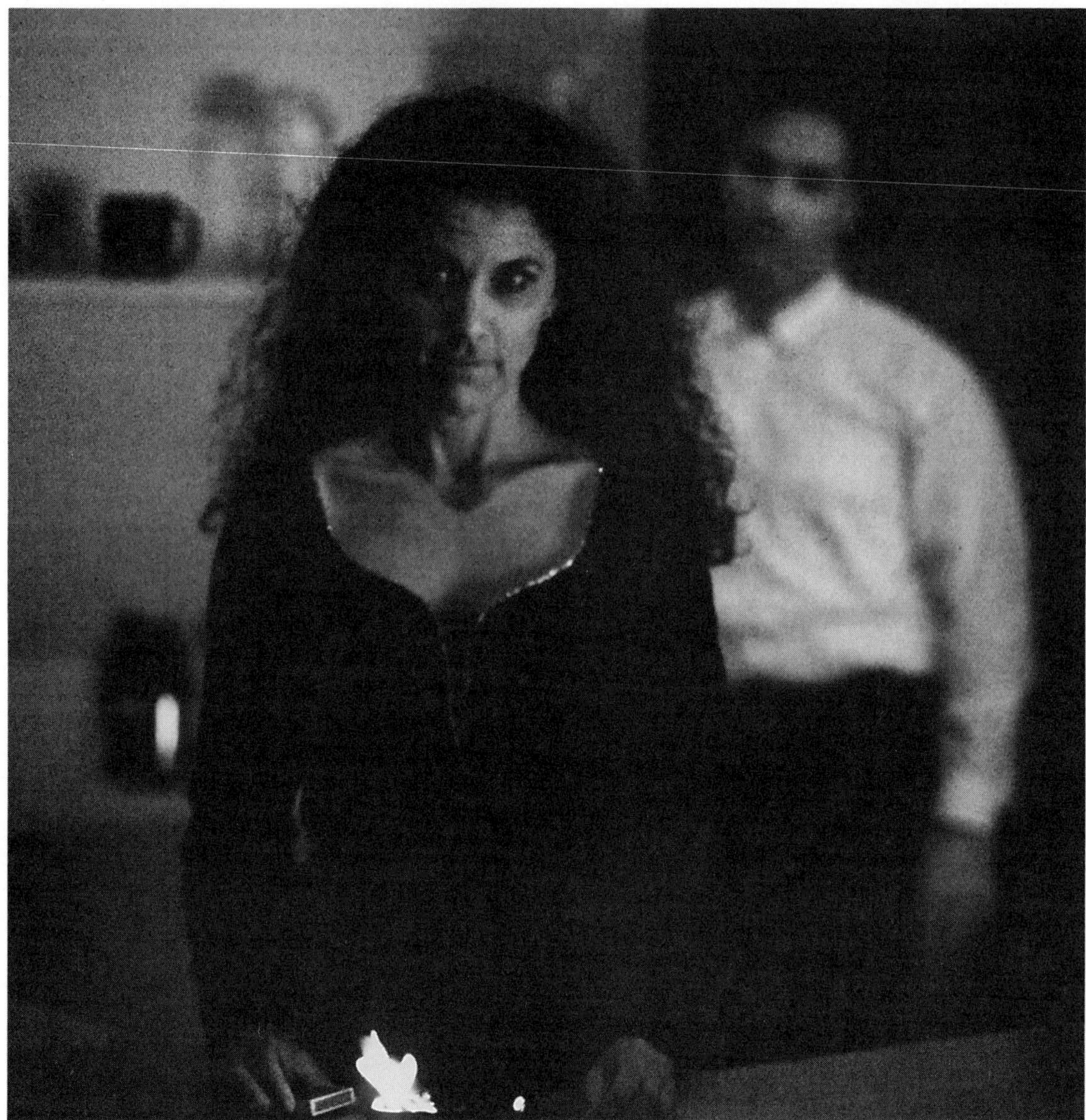

Anna in a scene from a 1991 production at the University of Iowa

says that he has never had to deal with loss before; he had a privileged childhood and has always had what he wants. Burton cannot understand why Anna has thrown Pale out and then created a dance about him. Burton leaves his new screenplay with Larry to read and then leaves. The stage fades to black and when the lights come up in a few moments it is night and Pale is waiting as Anna enters and turns on the lights. Pale reveals that Larry invited him to see Anna's new dance and that Larry gave Pale a key and a note asking him to come to the loft. Larry also gave Anna a note asking her to meet Larry there. Both Anna and Pale understand that Larry has set them up, and although Anna says that she does not want this, the play ends with the burning of Larry's notes and Anna and Pale's embrace.

CHARACTERS

Anna

Anna is a thirty-two-year-old dancer and aspiring choreographer. She is beautiful, tall, and strong. When the play begins she is grief-stricken at the recent death of her gay roommate, Robbie, who has just died in a boating accident. At the funeral, Anna is mistaken for Robbie's girlfriend, since his family either did not know or refused to acknowledge that he was gay. In the opening scene, she is exhausted from the experience, is drinking, and has resumed smoking. When Pale appears in the middle of the night a month later, Anna comforts him, and after an initially rocky start the two share her bed. After Pale leaves, it is clear that Anna has not been left unaffected by his visit. The next act takes place two months later, with Anna, who has been thinking about marriage and motherhood, celebrating New Year's Eve with Burton. After Pale once again spends the night, Anna asks him to leave and admits that she is frightened. For the next weeks she escapes into work, but what she creates is a dance about Pale. In the last scene of the play, Anna and Pale are reunited and both admit their feelings.

Burton

Burton is tall, athletic, and good-looking. He is a successful screenwriter and Anna's boyfriend. In the opening scene, Burton is consoling Anna, but since she could not reached him earlier (he was in Canada), Anna attended the funeral without him. He is very focused on his work and appears to view screenwriting as a way of making a great deal of money rather than as an artistic pursuit. When a screenplay is sold, Burton never concerns himself with how it is produced. In the second act, when Pale's sudden arrival interrupts Anna and Burton's celebration of New Year's Eve, he and Pale fight, and Burton learns that Pale and Anna were intimate. During the confrontation that follows, Burton is rejected by Anna and asked to leave the apartment. The next morning, Burton calls Anna, but when Pale interrupts the conversation, Burton hangs up. He reappears at the beginning of the next scene, and tells Larry that Anna has not returned any of his calls or responded to his messages. Burton admits he was a privileged child and that he has never lost anything important before. His loss of Anna is difficult for him to accept or to understand.

Jimmy

See Pale

Larry

Larry is another of Anna's roommates. He is twenty-seven, very intelligent, and gay. Larry works in advertising. He is Anna's good friend and confidant, and is aware of Anna's love for Pale long before she is ready to admit it. Larry provides some light comedy that helps dispel the tension of the play. He also recognizes that Anna loves Pale, and so Larry arranges for Pale to see the premier of a dance she has choreographed. Larry finally uses a note as a means of bringing the two lovers together.

Pale

Pale is Robbie's older brother who appears in the second scene to collect Robbie's belongings. He manages a restaurant, but is vague and misleading about his life. He is separated from his wife and children, but does not admit it until later in the play. Pale is thirty-six and is described as very sexy in a blue-collar working-class kind of way; his language is filled with obscenities. He admits that he knew that Robbie was gay but is initially contemptuous and sarcastic about his brother's lifestyle. Pale initially appears loud, rude, and obnoxious, but Anna thinks he is trying to disguise his pain at his brother's loss. When he breaks down finally, Anna invites him into her bed. After spending the night with Anna, Pale rushes out the next morning. He returns two months later to interrupt Anna's date with Burton. After the two men fight, Burton is forced to leave, and Pale spends the night. The next morning, Anna asks Pale to leave, and he does so reluctantly. Following his attendance of Anna's dance premier, during which he realizes that the dance is about himself and Anna, Pale returns to Anna's apartment after Larry provides him with the keys. In the final scene he admits to Anna his feelings for her.

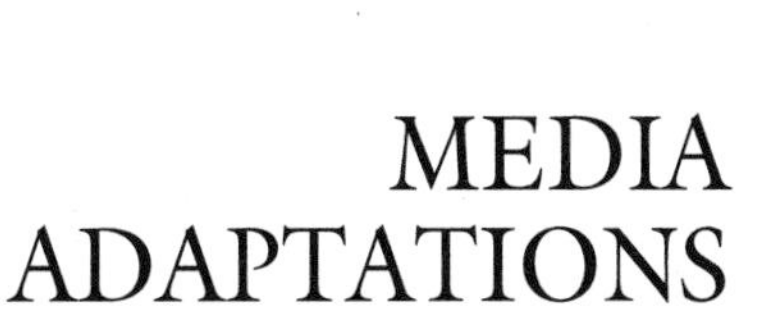
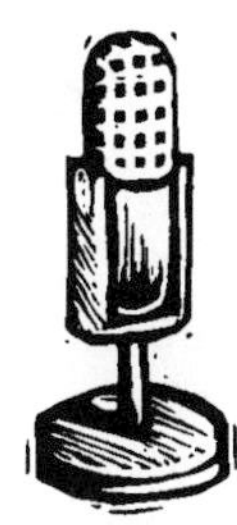

MEDIA ADAPTATIONS

- There are no media adaptations of *Burn This.* A few of Lanford Wilson's plays have been produced for television. These include: *Stoop: A Turn* (New York Television Theatre, 1969), *Fifth of July* (Showtime, 1982), and *The Migrants* (with Tennessee Williams; CBS, 1973).

THEMES

Art

Three of the characters in *Burn This* have artistic careers. Anna has been a dancer, and as the play begins, she is trying to draw upon her experience as a dancer in a new career as a choreographer. Anna uses art as the creative outlet of her emotions and experiences. The new dance she creates in the last act is based on her relationship with Pale. For Burton, art leads to financial reward; he is not willing to take risks for art. He uses his experiences and the environment around him to create screenplays, but Burton's attachment to his art is less personal than Anna's. He easily sells his work and dismisses his creative attachment to it once the sale is completed. Larry is a graphic artist for an advertising firm. He acknowledges that he sells his creative talents and that the intended purpose of his art is to make money and sell products. All of these characters in *Burn This* find a use for art, but art means something different to each one.

Death

It is Robbie's death that leads Pale to Anna. Wilson asks the audience to believe that Pale's rude and socially inept behavior is camouflage for his grief at his brother's death. In a very real sense, it is death that leads these two characters to re-evaluate their respective lives. Without Robbie's death, the audience is led to believe that Anna, who is feeling the desire to marry and have children, would have chosen Burton. Pale's emergence in her life forces her to confront her fear of emotional intimacy.

Friendship

The friendship between Anna and Larry is the anchor in her life. It is Larry's line, "Now you show up," that reveals to the audience that Burton was not available to comfort Anna when she needed him, and so Larry creates the first questions about the nature of Anna and Burton's relationship. It is Larry who helps Anna deal with Robbie's death, and it is Larry who appears when he thinks that Anna needs rescuing from Pale. Most importantly, Larry seems to recognize, even before Anna, the growing importance of Pale in her life. And it is Larry who finally resolves the impasse, by using notes to bring Pale and Anna together.

Human Condition

Larry represents humanity's attempt to confront modern life. One of the first examples of this is revealed in the story he tells about designing a Christmas card for Chrysler that must be so politically correct that the only thing that everyone can believe in is a car. Larry is cynical about his nieces and nephews, and he sees all these children as a result of a woman's need to become a "baby machine." Larry notes that all the wrong people reproduce, as has been the case throughout history. Anna represents humanity's effort to confront prejudice. Her outrage at how Robbie's family had removed themselves from his life establishes Anna's sensitivity to her friend's pain. But she is also trying to prevent more pain by distancing herself from any serious emotional involvement. Anna says she is sick of the age she is living in, that she is feeling ripped off and scared. While Pale can only curse at the indignities of urban life, both Anna and Larry are trying to find a deeper understanding of life and love and the demands of modern existence, which make uninvolvement more desirable.

Prejudice and Tolerance

An important theme is that of prejudice. Robbie's family cannot acknowledge his homosexuality and so they negate his existence. They must create a fantasy life for him that is different from the one he actually led. Robbie is assigned Anna as a girlfriend and his career as a dancer is ignored. No member of Robbie's family had ever seen him dance. Pale is concerned that Robbie's death might be a criminal mob punishment for Robbie's sexuality. Later in the play, Larry relates an experience from his recent plane trip in which a seat-mate lectured him on the sanctity of the American home and family. Burton, who is heterosexual, relates an experience he had with another man while crouched in the a doorway. Burton's story is meant to establish that he is open-minded and tolerant. That he must attach a disclaimer to the story to assert that the experience did not mean anything also establishes the influence of social prejudice.

STYLE

Act

In Greek plays the sections of the drama were signified by the appearance of the chorus and were usually divided into five acts. This is the formula for most serious drama from the Greeks to the Romans,

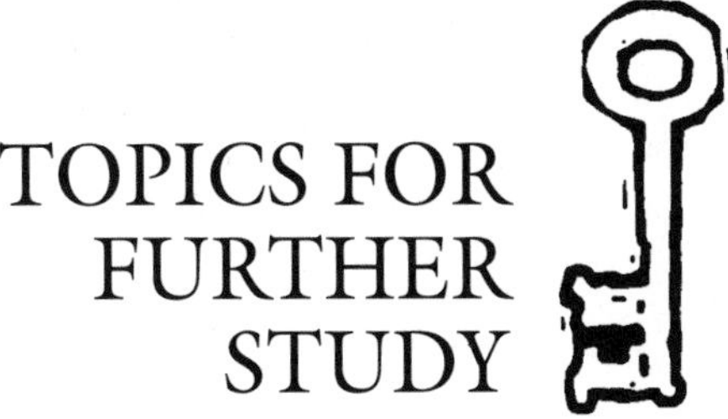

TOPICS FOR FURTHER STUDY

- Wilson's play relies upon his carefully crafted dialogue to carry the performance. Since there is little action on stage to define the characters, the audience is forced to listen to the words very closely. What does the dialogue in *Burn This* reveal about each character's life, dreams, and fears?
- Anna, Pale, and Burton each change and grow during the three months during which the play is set. Their relationships evolve and alter in several ways. What do you think these characters learn about themselves? About each other?
- Research what it means to be a choreographer. What is required? Is schooling enough, or is experience as a dancer more important? Is this a difficult career choice requiring much sacrifice? What are the rewards?
- It used to be argued that small towns were disappearing from the map because people were moving to the big cities. In recent years this trend is being reversed. How does living in the city differ from living in the country? Note the references to the small town in which Robbie grew up. What are those references meant to signify if Wilson is also lamenting the lack of humanity in a modern world?
- Explore Wilson's references to an alienating modern civilization. Are people required to fight progress so that they can preserve their humanity? Exactly what does technology mean to humanity?

and for Elizabethan playwrights like William Shakespeare. The five acts denote the structure of dramatic action. They are exposition, complication, climax, falling action, and catastrophe. The five act structure was followed until the nineteenth century when Henrik Ibsen combined some of the acts. *Burn This* is a two-act play. The exposition occurs in the first act when the audience learns of Robbie's death and the family history. The complication also occurs in this act when it becomes clear that Anna cares about Pale. The climax occurs at the beginning of the second act when Burton and Pale fight, and Anna throws Burton out and chooses Pale. The falling action, which is the result of the climax, occurs later in act two when Anna admits that she is frightened of emotional involvement. In the catastrophe, an old word for conclusion, Larry unites the two lovers.

Characters

The actions of each character are what constitute the story. Character can also include the idea of a particular individual's morality. Characters can range from simple stereotypical figures to more complex multi-faceted ones. Characters may also be defined by personality traits, such as the rogue or the damsel in distress. "Characterization" is the process of creating a life-like person from an author's imagination. To accomplish this the author provides the character with personality traits that help define who he will be and how he will behave in a given situation. *Burn This* provides characters whose dialogue reveals their temperament and identity. For example, Larry uses comedy to confront life. It is a means of easing life's pain.

Plot

Generally plots should have a beginning, a middle, and a conclusion, but they may also sometimes be a series of episodes connected together. Basically, the plot provides the author with the means to explore primary themes. Students are often confused between the two terms; but themes explore ideas, and plots simply relate what happens in a very obvious manner. Thus the plot of *Burn This* is the story of Anna and Pale's romance.

Setting

The time, place, and culture in which the action of the play takes place is called the setting. The elements of setting may include geographic location, physical or mental environments, prevailing cultural attitudes, or the historical time in which the action takes place. The location for Wilson's play is a loft in New York City.

HISTORICAL CONTEXT

Sexuality and Disease

When Lanford Wilson was writing *Burn This,* the Acquired Immune Deficiency Syndrome (AIDS) epidemic was a major issue for homosexuals. But Wilson never refers to AIDS; instead the play is a heterosexual love story. But AIDS was not far from the news in 1987; AZT, a drug to treat AIDS, was approved by the FDA. Although AZT was expensive, predicted to cost at least $10,000 per year per patient, it was the first treatment that offered hope for AIDS victims. Another effort to halt the AIDS epidemic was suggested by the United States Surgeon General C. Everett Koop, who argued that condom commercials should be permitted to air on television. Koop's suggestion was greeted with shock by those groups who argued that condom advertisements would encourage more illicit sexual activity. Some religious groups, who interpreted AIDS as God's punishment of homosexuals, wanted total abstinence to be the official government position in terms of public service campaigns about the disease. Attempts to raise government spending on AIDS research created controversy, although homosexuals did demonstrate in Washington to demand that the federal government increase funding for AIDS. But President Ronald Reagan failed to act until he was forced to recognize that AIDS presented a risk to the heterosexual population as well as to gays. The sexual revolution that had begun in the mid– to late–1960s, and which had continued through the 1970s and into the early 1980s, finally peaked when it became clear that AIDS was more than a rare, ''gay man's disease.'' By the end of the 1980s, fear of AIDS was making more people cautious about sexual relationships. Consequently, when Anna and Pale, who barely know one another, engage in a sexual relationship, the play's 1987 audience was likely considering the risk involved in their behavior.

Art

In many cases art was imitating life in 1987. Theatre and film releases echoed newspaper headlines. Racial and sexual intolerance and the growing perception that big business was uncaring and dishonest provided ample subject matter for entertainment. Although *Burn This* does not deal overtly with prejudice, one of its primary themes is intolerance. Wilson devotes a significant part of the text to establishing the intolerance of Robbie's family. Later, Larry relates the story of his plane trip and the intolerant attitude of a seat-mate who expounds upon the importance of the American family. In the years just before 1987, prejudice against homosexuality had become more visual, fed in part because of the increase in the number of people afflicted with Human Immunodeficiency Virus (HIV) and AIDS. Fear motivated much of this intolerance, but the effect was an increase in hate crimes against homosexuals. When *Burn This* debuted, two other plays that dealt with discrimination were also first presented. August Wilson's drama *Fences* looked at how discrimination could destroy a man's hopes and dreams, and Alfred Uhry's *Driving Miss Daisy* demonstrated that people could rise above the social constraints placed upon them based on their class, race, and religion. On Wall Street, a rash of insider trading scandals provided material for both the front pages of newspapers and the entertainment page as *Wallstreet* became a hit Hollywood film. The film's star, Michael Douglas, won an academy award for his portrayal of a cold-hearted businessman who is willing to sacrifice the American worker to increase personal wealth. 1987 brought inflation and depression as American farmers lost their livelihood. With the perception that life was out of control, that inflation, depression, business, and disease were eroding the American dream, all of these plays and this film end with the promise of justice and the hope of a better life. This was a period in which entertainment provided escape with films such as *Moonstruck, Babette's Feast,* and *The Untouchables.* In 1987, American audiences were in desperate need of hope, either real or perceived.

CRITICAL OVERVIEW

Reviews for *Burn This* have been mixed: most have noted strong performances by actors appearing in the productions, but they have also faulted the play as weak in elements of plot and character development. Wilson has stated in interviews that he waited

COMPARE & CONTRAST

- **1987:** Homosexuals protest in Washington, D.C., to demand an end to discrimination and to demand more federal funding for research of AIDS.

  Today: Homosexuality remains a basis for discrimination in many areas of life. In the military, homosexuality is a leading reason for general discharges, in spite of President Clinton's "don't ask, don't tell" policy.

- **1987:** AZT wins FDA approval for the treatment of AIDS. The treatment will cost $10,000 a year, but it is not a cure and its side effects mean that many AIDS victims will not be able to take the drug.

  Today: The most recent AIDS treatment, a protease inhibitor, though initially promising, still fails to provide a cure. And, as has been the case with so many other treatments, newer drug combinations fail to help some patients while proving to be prohibitively expensive for many.

- **1987:** U.S. Surgeon General C. Everett Koop asks that commercials for condoms be shown on television.

  Today: Although they are boycotted in some areas, a few condom commercials have aired on national television. However, there still remains a great deal of public resistance to the commercials.

- **1987:** India and Sri Lanka sign a treaty designed to end the ethnic violence that has persisted for four years. But the violence continues even with the treaty.

  Today: Ethnic violence in Bosnia continues to draw American troops to the area. Atrocities, especially against women, have been an central part of the Croatian-Serb War.

- **1987:** *Beloved,* a novel by Toni Morrison which details the story of a slave girl, is published.

  Today: Television host and actress Oprah Winfrey is scheduled to release the film adaptation of *Beloved.*

to premier *Burn This* until John Malkovich was available to play the role of Pale, and in reviews of the play it was Malkovich's performance that was cited as one of the play's strengths. Frank Rich, writing for *The New York Times,* assessed Malkovich as a "combustive figure on stage, threatening to incinerate everyone and everything around him with his throbbing vocal riffs, bruising posture and savage, unfocused eyes." Rich continued to describe Malkovich, whom he declared, "delivers the firepower ... while he is equally busy tossing a mane of long dark hair, hoping to arouse the carnal interest of the very pretty young woman." But Rich was not complimenting Wilson's character development; he was complimenting Malkovich's performance. And after he devoted an entire column to celebrating the actor, Rich admitted that Malkovich's performance "yanks us through this always intriguing, finally undernourishing three-hour play ... more muddled than pointed." One of the problems with the play, according to Rich, is that there is no real reason for Anna to choose Pale over Burton. The script offers little reason for her shift in interest from Burton to Pale, and since any sexual charge between Joan Allen and John Malkovich was missing, the audience remained unconvinced. Instead, Rich suggested that the almost happy ending was more a result of Anna's biological clock forcing her to choose Pale. Rich did note that Larry gets to speak Wilson's funniest lines and that the character is played with "warmth and wry intelligence." Larry's job is to comment upon the actions and lives of the other three characters. This character's voyeurism and disconnectedness, asserted Rich, "seem to say more about the playwright's feelings of loss and longing than the showier romance at center stage.'' Finally, Rich pronounced Wilson's play as self-indulgent with excisable blind alleys and containing small details that substitute for plot contrivances.

Edwin Wilson, who reviewed *Burn This* for *The Wall Street Journal,* focused less on Malkovich's performance and more on the plot; he also found fault with the playwright Wilson's plotting of the romance. One of the major difficulties, explained critic Wilson, ''is the shaky premise that Pale, underneath his rough exterior, is really a tender, caring man who has a healthy effect on others.'' Anna is able to create her first successful dance after she spends two nights with Pale. Yet, ''Pale's behavior is so brutish that Anna discredits herself by taking to him.'' Wilson noted in his review that Pale's purpose may be to shake up people, especially Anna and Larry, who have a ''basic grudge against the philistine, insensitive, materialistic straight world that rejects artists and homosexuals.'' By having Anna choose Pale, Wilson suggested, the playwright may be suggesting that ''art is not enough, that homosexuality is incomplete, that a woman like Anna is really hiding from her true nature with homosexual roommates, that a macho creature like Pale is, underneath it all, a real man and just what Anna needs.'' Wilson concluded his review by citing the play's direction, the witty dialogue, and Malkovich's performance as the play's strong points.

Newsweek reviewer Jack Kroll commended the play's ''voracious vitality and an almost manic determination to drive right into the highest voltage that life can register,'' but also pointed to errors in logic and false leads as a problematic. In a mostly favorable evaluation of *Burn This,* Daniel Watermeier focused on the characters, whom he stated, are grounded against particular archetypes. Although he acknowledged that the ending is only ''tentatively happy,'' Watermeier characterized the romance as more satisfying than had Rich or Wilson, declaring: ''*Burn This* explores the nature of *eros* in contemporary American culture, its relationship to death and to renewal and creativity in both life and art.'' Watermeier considered *Burn This* to be Wilson's ''most complex, sophisticated, and daring play.'' Finally, Martin Jacobi declared that Wilson is really only pointing out that sometimes men and women can only achieve limited happiness. Jacobi's interpretation of the play allows for a more generous evaluation of the romance between Anna and Pale, and it makes the perceived inconsistencies of plot less important.

CRITICISM

Sheri Metzger,

Metzger is an adjunct professor at Embry-Riddle University. In this essay she examines the question of whether it is believable that Anna would choose to be with Pale rather than Burton.

In Lanford Wilson's *Burn This,* the feminine hero, Anna, chooses Pale as her lover/partner rather than Burton. Setting aside the argument that love can sometimes make little sense of emotion, audiences, and especially women, are left wondering why she would make such a choice. Indeed, some of the play's male reviewers noted the unlikeliness of this choice as well. In his review of *Burn This,* Frank Rich noted that Anna and Pale lack the depth of passion of other great romantic theatrical pairings. Wilson's lovers ''don't fight to the death,'' instead they ''slowly settle down to make the choices facing those New York couples who inhabit the slick magazines,'' Rich remarked. ''What begins as a go-for-broke sexual struggle trails off into sentimental conflicts between love and career, unbridled passion and intellectual detachment, a loft life style and the biological clock.''

The question implied by Rich's comments is why Anna would choose Pale. In their first meetings, he is rude, obnoxious, confrontational, emotionally unstable, and drunk. If her desire to have children is a factor, as Rich asserted, would not Burton make the better choice? He is wealthy, steadily employed in an artistic profession that compliments Anna's own, emotionally stable, and in love with her. In recent years, biological anthropologists have insisted that women's reproductive choices focus on a male's ability to support a family, as well as physical attractiveness. If Anna's concern is her biological clock, and the text bears this out, then Burton appears the more likely choice.

Pale is unemployed by the play's end and his emotional instability should make him a less attractive choice. So why does Anna make this unlikely selection? In the stage directions for *Burn This,* Burton is described as tall, athletic, and good-looking. Pale is described as well-built and sexy. Clearly, Wilson intended that Anna's choice should reflect a grand passion, a sexual intensity that she cannot resist; but, the dialogue of the play fails to supply the necessary ingredients. Rich described Anna and Pale's relationship as ''mechanical'' and defined by ''predictable conventions of breezy ro-

WHAT DO I READ NEXT?

- *Talley's Folly,* one of Wilson's most successful plays, was first performed in 1979. Set in 1944, this play is about the romance between a thirty-one-year-old Midwestern spinster and a forty-two-year-old Jewish tax accountant.
- Wilson's *Gingham Dog,* written in 1969, is the story about the end of a marriage. Vincent and Gloria are an interracial couple and the end of their marriage focuses on issues of social change.
- *Serenading Louie,* Wilson's 1976 play, is about alienation, estrangement, and death. The focus is on two couples, neighbors who are enduring a crisis in each couple's lives.
- August Wilson's *Fences,* written in 1987 but set in 1957, examines the effects of discrimination on a family. Although the discrimination that takes place in *Fences* is based on race, the idea of how love can survive in a world filled with pain and death is similar to the subject of *Burn This.*
- Mordaunt Shairp's *The Green Bay Tree,* written in 1933, was one of the first plays to deal with homosexuality. The play focuses on the relationship between a wealthy older man who adopts an attractive, working-class youth and seduces him with a life of luxury.
- Harvey Fierstein's 1978 play *Torch Song Trilogy,* is about a gay man who wants to be loved. The play, which won several awards, was later made into a successful film.
- Fierstein's *On Tidy Endings* (1987) is a short play about relationships. The play is not about AIDS, but it does focus on the loss that results from AIDS.

mantic comedies.'' However, the problem is that *Burn This* is not a breezy romantic comedy. It is a drama that Wilson intends be taken seriously, but its center is a romance that simply is not believable.

Rich is not the only reviewer to question the believability of Anna and Pale's romance. In a review written for *The Wall Street Journal,* Edwin Wilson also pointed out the inconsistency of the romantic plot. E. Wilson declared that ''[o]ne problem with *Burn This* is the shaky premise that Pale, underneath his rough exterior, is really a tender, caring man.'' It is a significant problem, since there is absolutely no reason for Anna to think that Pale is anything other than what he initially seems to be.

The few moments in Act I in which Pale seems to break down are inconsistent with the rest of his dialogue. Rather than mourning Robbie, Pale's tears appear to be more an act of feeling sorry for himself. Most of his comments about his brother are unfeeling and derisive. There is nothing to indicate that Pale is anything more than a drunk engaged in a crying jag. After she sleeps with him, Anna admits her attraction to Pale is a symptom of the ''bird-with-the-broken-wing-syndrome.''

When Pale appears a second time, he is just as rude, just as drunk, and just as confrontational. And yet Anna throws Burton out and chooses Pale. Wilson noted that ''Anna discredits herself in taking to him [Pale].'' That assessment appears accurate, especially in the absence of any dialogue that would support Anna's decision. Why Anna should love Pale remains one of the biggest problems in Lanford Wilson's play.

In a critical essay on *Burn This,* Daniel J. Watermeier maintained that Wilson's play is ''concerned with how and why an unlikely pair 'fall in love'; an ironic, sometimes uncomfortable, love story with a resolution that is only tentatively happy.'' It is clear from his essay that Watermeier is an enthusiastic supporter who finds it difficult to offer negative criticism of Wilson, and yet he cannot ignore the difficult romantic story that lies at the heart of the play. This love story is not only uncomfortable for Anna and Pale, it is uncomfortable for

> "*BURN THIS* IS NOT A BREEZY ROMANTIC COMEDY. IT IS A DRAMA THAT WILSON INTENDS BE TAKEN SERIOUSLY, BUT ITS CENTER IS A ROMANCE THAT SIMPLY IS NOT BELIEVABLE."

the audience as well. And since, as Watermeier acknowledges, the play is about how and why these two fall in love, problems with that "how and why" cannot be ignored.

If the unlikeliness of Anna and Pale's romance is a problem for the audience, Anna's depiction of a modern woman trying to confront issues and make choices that plague her contemporaries presents special issues for women theatre-goers. In writing about the problems of gender in telling a woman's story, Carolyn G. Heilbrun argued that women live the stories they read, that women use literature as a model for behavior. Thus, if as Heilbrun asserted, "What matters is that lives do not serve as models; only stories do that," then women who view *Burn This* take something away that is cause for concern.

When Lanford Wilson has Anna choose Pale, he appears to be embracing the fiction that women don't want nice or good men, that they are looking for "bad" boys to save. Heilbrun contended that "[i]t is a hard thing to make up stories to live by. We can only retell and live by the stories we have read or heard. We live our lives through texts." But if women live by the stories they hear or read, is the image of Anna the story that women want as a model for their own lives? Anna is a woman who functions by emotion. Perhaps Wilson is making a statement about the artistic temperament, but he may also be embracing a dogma as old as man, which is essentially that women are emotionally-based creatures who do not make decisions based upon reason.

Mary Anne Ferguson echoed Heilbrun's argument. Ferguson contended that "[l]iterature both reflects and helps to create reality. It is through their preservation in works of art that we know what the stereotypes and archetypes have been and are; in turn, knowing the images influences our view of reality and even our behavior." Is Wilson reflecting real women in Anna? Male reviewers admit that there is no logic to explain her behavior and this, again, reinforces old debates (going back nearly two thousand years to early theology), that seek to restrict women's choices by arguing that women are without logic.

The problem with depictions of feminine heroes such as Anna is, as Ferguson interpreted it, that "the popularization of literary images has increased their influence so that the distinction between imaginary characters and real people has become blurred in the minds of many readers." This is, of course, a common phenomenon for movie and television stars, who find their audience unable to separate the real from the imaginary. But it can also be applied to literature and theatre. If educators are concerned with the development of self-image in young girls, and they claim to be, then *Burn This* might be accompanied by a disclaimer that young women should in no way find Anna's choice to be a reflection of reality or appropriateness.

Women readers and audience members who question the romance between Anna and Pale should ask themselves, "Is this how a woman would speak? Is this what she would say and do? Does Wilson write a credible woman?" The answer would seem to be no. Julie Brown asserted that in reading the texts of women creative writing students, she has observed that readers too rarely question the authenticity of voice. Does a character's voice reflect reality? Once again, the answer with Anna is no. Instead, Anna may reflect how Wilson thinks women behave, how he thinks they react. Anna may reflect what Wilson thinks women want from life.

My intent is not to question Wilson's right to claim that he can create romantic fiction. Instead the question is whether he can create a real, credible woman, a woman other women would acknowledge as a model. He has failed to do this with Anna. As Brown noted, feminism is not concerned with challenging an author's right to create a story, only with his or her ability to tell the story correctly. Brown's concern is with her female writing students: the problem with male-generated texts is in their influence on the next generation of women writers, who have only the male text as models. Brown echoes the observations of Heilbrun and Ferguson that women use literary texts as models of behavior, and Lanford Wilson's Anna fails as a realistic model for women.

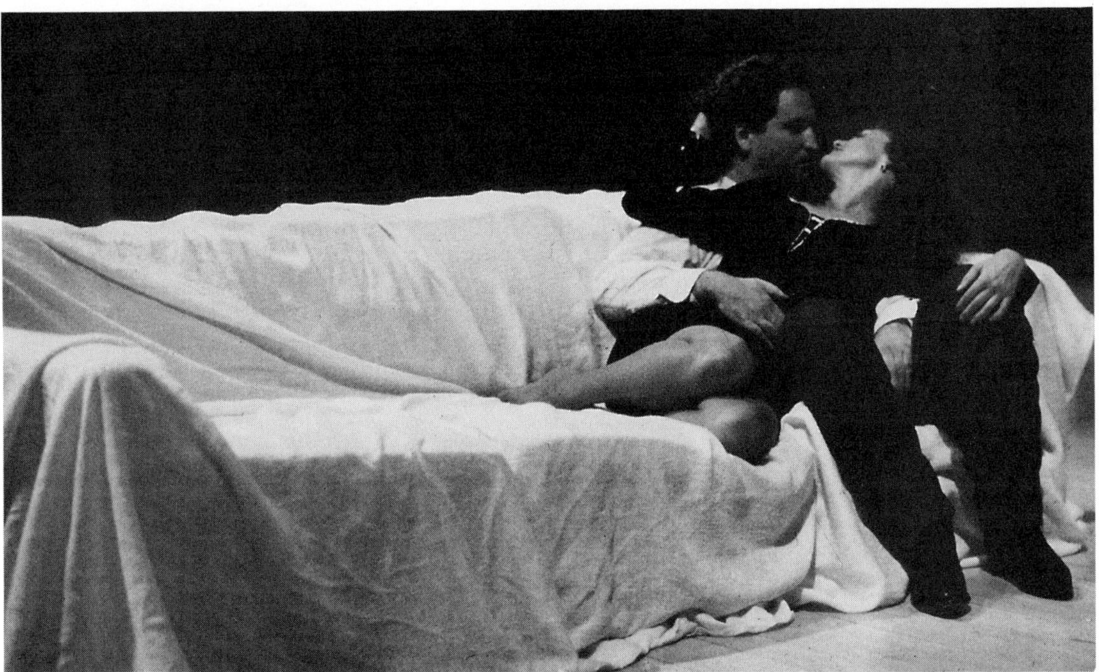

A scene from a 1991 Iowa Summer Repertory production

Source: Sheri Metzger, for *Drama for Students,* Gale, 1998.

Richard Hornby

Hornby offers a mixed review of Wilson's play, finding much to like about the cast and production and less to favor in the playwright's actual words.

Lanford Wilson's *Burn This* concerns three young people—two dancers and a copywriter—who share a Soho loft. The male dancer, a homosexual, has just died in a boating accident, and it becomes clear, in their grief, that the two remaining roommates were in love with him. The female dancer has a boyfriend, a successful screenwriter, whom she likes but does not really love; when the dead roommate's brother arrives, a bizarre, drunk, long-haired, foul-mouthed individual, she falls into a passionate affair with him, despite their obvious differences in temperament and basic dislike for each other. In the end, the woman's remaining roommate (the advertising writer) has moved out, leaving a scornful note ending with the words, "Burn this"; her ex-boyfriend has gone to Hollywood; her new lover has lost his job as maitre d'hotel in a New Jersey restaurant and separated from his wife and family; and the two mismatched sweethearts are left alone with each other in dismay and despair.

Burn This displays the narrowness of scope and looseness of structure so typical of realistic American playwriting today. What elevates Wilson above similar writers like David Mamet, Marsha Norman, Michael Weller, or Tina Howe is his surer literary sense; behind the apparently shapeless slices of life in his plays are traditional literary devices that invigorate what would otherwise be tame pieces of reportage. The brother in *Burn This* is a traditional intruder figure going back to Aristophanic comedy, an *alazon,* or boaster and spoilsport, who tries to gain access to the feast; in *Burn This* he even interrupts a champagne supper between the young woman and the screenwriter. The love triangle, and the general movement from death and separation to a new union, are typical of Western comedy over the past two millennia.

Furthermore, Wilson gives all the traditional archetypes a sardonic twist. The intruder, who seems so bohemian, actually has a very middle-class job plus a wife and family, just as the dancers and writers, whom we would expect to have an unconventional lifestyle, seem very staid and bourgeois. The "happy" ending, with the couple united, is so bitter that it does not seem comic at all except in the ironic sense. Other white American playwrights today—whether commercial, serious, or avant-

"WHAT ELEVATES WILSON ABOVE SIMILAR WRITERS LIKE DAVID MAMET, MARSHA NORMAN, MICHAEL WELLER, OR TINA HOWE IS HIS SURER LITERARY SENSE; BEHIND THE APPARENTLY SHAPELESS SLICES OF LIFE IN HIS PLAYS ARE TRADITIONAL LITERARY DEVICES THAT INVIGORATE WHAT WOULD OTHERWISE BE TAME PIECES OF REPORTAGE."

garde—are either all surface or all depth; Wilson's plays have both an engaging surface and intriguing depths. He is not a great writer; he usually shrinks from even indirect treatment of major existential or social themes, and his dialogue lacks the distinction found, for example, in our black playwrights like August Wilson, whose *Fences* I reviewed here last fall. But he is a good minor playwright, which is about all he seems to want to be.

John Malkovich is so explosive as the brother that he has been compared to the young Marlon Brando in *A Streetcar Named Desire.* Like Brando, he comes on so strong that he threatens to overwhelm the play. In this case, however, the rest of the cast balances him beautifully. Joan Allen is sensitive, intelligent, and emotionally powerful; she also has the bodily control to convince you that she is a professional dancer. Jonathan Hogan gives a superbly detailed yet spontaneous performance as the screenwriter, and Lou Liberatore, as the third roommate, knows how to play a background role with skill and insight without ever calling undue attention to himself. Marshall W. Mason, one of our best directors of original plays, directed with his usual skill and care; John Lee Beatty's magnificent setting of the loft with its cast-iron columns, set against a backdrop of windows showing a huge trompe l'oeil of a hazy skyline, deserves all the awards it will probably win.

Source: Richard Hornby, review of *Burn This* in the *Hudson Review,* Volume XLI, no. 1, Spring, 1988, pp. 187–88.

Gerald Weales

Weales reviews Wilson's play, praising it for its off-kilter performances and dark humor. While he appreciated the play text, Weales's greatest plaudits went to the cast, particularly Joan Allen as Anna.

There is another darkly happy ending in Lanford Wilson's *Burn This,* and another closed, self-protective heroine who must be pried open by a relentless and relentlessly vocal male. Anna is a modern dancer, who was taking her first steps toward becoming a choreographer when the death of her friend, her mentor, her roommate brought her to a mourning standstill. Her grief and her apartment are invaded by Pale, the dead man's brother, eloquently foul-mouthed in his denunciation of New York City and the world at large, as outraged—on the surface, at least—by the absence of parking space as by the death of his brother. Pale, who is about as artificial as grand grotesques tend to be, is some kind of natural force, simply riding over the other characters in the play—Anna's more conventional boyfriend, her other homosexual roommate—and carrying the protesting Anna off to bed every time he (or the drink) bring him to her door. At the end, having agreed to separate, they are brought back together through the good offices of the roommate, a gay Mary Worth, and they accept what both suspect will be a union as disastrous and painful as it is necessary. Beneath this meeting of contraries, there is a subtheme about love, loss, and art. The dance that Anna creates out of the loss of her partner and the sexual energy of her nights with Pale is said to be forceful, commanding, a work of genius alongside the tepid exercises of the other choreographers on the same program, poor would-be professionals who presumably are unlost and underlaid. At the same time, Anna's less vital boyfriend, a screenwriter who thinks that all movies are bad, writes the serious script he has always wanted to do, a contemporary love story (presumably *Burn This*) which the pain of his loss of Anna makes possible.

This recycled romantic myth of creativity need not be taken too seriously, for the heart of the play beats in Pale and Anna, less as characters than as roles for John Malkovich and Joan Allen. Malkovich is outrageous and totally fascinating. He roars, rages, and flutes his way through his part, modulating only to demonstrate how to make a proper pot of tea or to suggest that his hurricane temperament can calm into tenderness. Walter Kerr in a recent column (*New York Times,* November 15) suggested that Malkovich is wrecking Wilson's play, and a playwright who shall remain nameless asked me the other day if I thought Malkovich would ever make his performance mesh with the rest of the cast. I think that Malkovich is the Pale that Wilson wanted, that his unmeshed excess is realizing not trashing the playwright's intention. I miss only the note of vulnerability in the character, for the chinks in Pale's armor, as Malkovich shows them, seem as calculated as most of the rest of the performance. That calculation, however, belongs as much to the character as the actor, for Pale is a self-created figure, always conscious of his costume, his gestures, his rhetoric. For me, the odd thing about Malkovich's performance, which has received so much praise and blame, is that my attention regularly moved from him to Joan Allen. Not all that odd perhaps, because I watched her instead of Kathleen Turner whenever they were on screen together in *Peggy Sue Got Married* and I was startled at what a substantial character she made of Ann in the recent television production of *All My Sons.* Her Anna in *Burn This* often sits silently, her sentences broken off by Pale's verbal avalanche. The play of reactions across her face is a joy to behold. It is her amusement, her impatience, her disbelief that gives force to Pale's fury of words. Less is more in *Burn This,* as it is in *Frankie and Johnny,* and Joan Allen, like Kathy Bates, makes her play particularly worth seeing.

Source: Gerald Weales, ''Send in the Clowns'' in the *Commonweal,* Volume CXIV, no. 22, December 18, 1987, pp. 749–50.

"THERE IS ANOTHER DARKLY HAPPY ENDING IN LANFORD WILSON'S *BURN THIS,* AND ANOTHER CLOSED, SELF-PROTECTIVE HEROINE WHO MUST BE PRIED OPEN BY A RELENTLESS AND RELENTLESSLY VOCAL MALE."

SOURCES

Brown, Julie. ''The Great Ventriloquist Act: Gender and Voice in the Fiction Workshop,'' in *Associated Writing Programs Chronicle,* September, 1993, pp. 7-9.

Bryer, Jackson R. ''Lanford Wilson,'' in *The Playwright's Art: Conversations with Contemporary American Dramatists,* Rutgers University Press, 1995, pp.277-96.

DiGaetani, John L. ''Lanford Wilson,'' in *A Search for a Postmodern Theatre: Interviews with Contemporary Playwrights,* Greenwood Press, 1991, pp. 285-93.

Ferguson, Mary Anne. *Images of Women in Literature,* Houghton Mifflin, 1977.

Heilbrun, Carolyn G. *Writing A Woman's Life,* Ballantine, 1988, pp. 33-47.

Jacobi, Martin J. ''The Comic Vision of Lanford Wilson,'' in *Studies in the Literary Imagination,* Vol. 21, No. 2, 1988, pp. 119-134.

Rich, Frank. Review of *Burn This,* in *The New York Times,* October 15, 1987.

Savran, David. ''Lanford Wilson,'' in *In Their Own Words: Contemporary American Playwrights,* Theatre Communications Group, 1988, pp. 306-20.

Watermeier, Daniel J. ''Lanford Wilson's *Liebestod:* Character, Archetype, and Myth in *Burn This,*'' in *A Lanford Wilson Casebook,* edited by Jackson Bryer, New York, 1990.

Wilson, Edwin. ''Hot and Bothered: Malkovich on Fire,'' in *The Wall Street Journal,* October 21, 1987.

FURTHER READING

Busby, Mark. *Lanford Wilson,* Boise State University, 1987.
This short book—52 pages—is a biography of Wilson.

Byer, Jackson. *A Lanford Wilson Casebook,* Garland, 1990.
This collection of critical essays examine several of Lanford's plays.

Gonzales, Doreen. *AIDS: Ten Stories of Courage,* Enslow, 1996.This book contains brief biographies of some of the more famous victims of AIDS.

Shilts, Randy. *And The Band Played On,* St. Martin's Press, 1987.
This book traces events related to the AIDS epidemic. It was made into a cable television movie in 1993.

Children of a Lesser God

MARK MEDOFF

1979

Mark Medoff wrote *Children of a Lesser God* specifically for the actress Phyllis Frelich. The play is important historically because it includes a lead role for a deaf performer in a drama designed for the hearing theater audience. Unlike some of Medoff's earlier plays, such as *The Wager* and *When You Comin Back, Red Ryder?, Children of a Lesser God* examines communication problems, psychological stress, and emotional abuse, but does so without the threat of physical violence or guns. The play earned Medoff a Tony award in 1980. In 1986, a film version of the play, written by Medoff, was released; the film starred William Hurt as James and Marlee Matlin, who earned an Academy Award for her performance as Sarah.

Sign language is integral to the play. Sarah signs but does not speak aloud until the climactic scene toward the end of the play. When conversing with Sarah, James will often echo her part of the conversation and sign and speak his own responses.

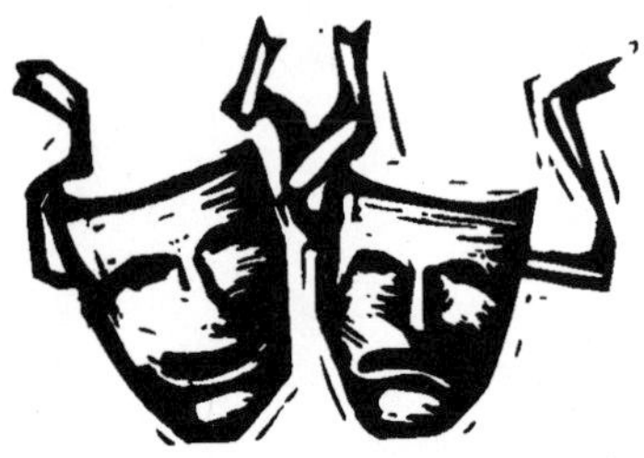

AUTHOR BIOGRAPHY

Mark Howard Medoff was born in Mount Carmel, Illinois, on March 18, 1940. His father, Lawrence, was a physician, and his mother, Thelma, a psychologist. He earned a B.A. in 1962 from the University of Miami, and an M.A. in English from

Stanford in 1966. Medoff has held a number of academic appointments at New Mexico State University, Las Cruces, including the position of dramatist-in-residence and chair of the theater arts department. He and his wife, Stephanie, have three daughters.

Medoff has received several awards and honors for his work. In 1974, he won a Guggenheim fellowship in playwriting. He received the Outer Critics Circle Award in 1974 for *When You Comin' Back, Red Ryder?* and again in 1980 for *Children of a Lesser God.* Also in 1980 Medoff won the Tony Award for *Children of a Lesser God;* in 1987 he earned an Academy Award nomination for his screenplay based on the stage play. Gallaudet College, the only liberal arts college for the deaf in the world, recognized Medoff's achievement for *Children of a Lesser God* with an honorary Doctor of Humane Letters degree in 1981.

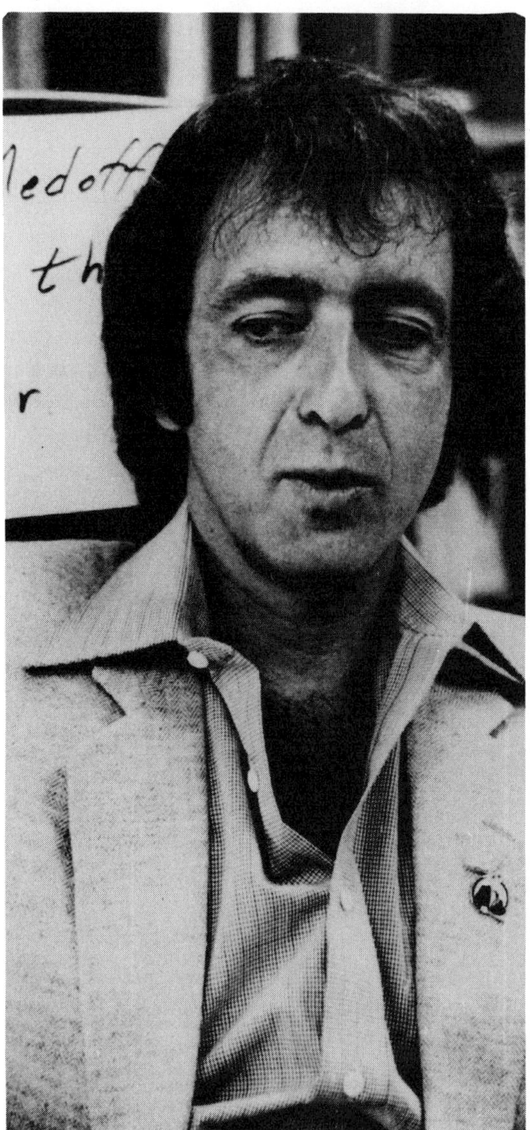

Mark Medoff in his office at New Mexico State University in 1980, just after Children of a Lesser God *won the Tony Award for best play*

PLOT SUMMARY

Act I

The primary action of *Children of a Lesser God* takes place inside the mind of James Leeds. Time is not linear during the play, and characters "step from his memory for anything from a full scene to several lines," and place changes rapidly on a bare stage that holds "only a few benches and a blackboard." James is a speech teacher at a State School for the Deaf. He meets Sarah Norman, a cleaning woman who has been deaf from birth and has resided at the school since the age of five.

Two other students meet with James for speech therapy on a regular basis: Orin, a contemporary of Sarah who has become an apprentice teacher at the school, and Lydia, a girl in her late teens who develops a crush on James. As the relationship between Sarah and James grows, Orin distances himself from James, while Lydia becomes more infatuated with her teacher.

Sarah's mother, known only as Mrs. Norman in the play, appears at first to be a bitter woman, one whose husband left at the same time her daughter was sent away to the State School for the Deaf. Later, James brings Sarah to her mother's house and forces a reunion. The two women reconcile and Mrs. Norman attends James and Sarah's wedding.

Act II

The second act begins with a bridge party at the newlyweds' home attended by Franklin, James's supervising teacher, and Mrs. Norman. Sarah delivers a splendid performance, suggesting that she has become integrated into the middle-class hearing world, but later tells James "I feel split down the middle, caught between two worlds." James also experiences this struggle to feel comfortable in both worlds because he becomes exhausted serving as

Sarah's translator and finds it impossible to enjoy music because Sarah cannot share it with him.

When Orin enlists Sarah's help in a campaign to charge the State School for the Deaf with discrimination for not hiring enough deaf teachers, the personal differences between James and Sarah become part of a larger political issue. Edna Klein, a lawyer brought in by Orin to help with the case against the school, illustrates the misconceptions and mistakes made by well-meaning people from the hearing community. Sarah begins to realize that Edna wants to speak before the commission "for all deaf people," and that James wants to speak for her. Sarah explains that everyone has always assumed that because she cannot hear, she is unable to understand and is incapable of speaking for herself. Her own identity as a separate individual has been ignored by the hearing world in general, by Edna, and by her husband. Sarah declares: "Unless you let me be an individual, an *I,* just as you are, you will never truly be able to come inside my silence and know me. And until you do that, I will never let myself know you. Until that time, we cannot be joined. We cannot share a relationship."

After a climactic argument in which James holds her arms at her side and forces her to speak, Sarah leaves James. James experiences remorse and begins to realize more clearly her position, but Sarah refuses to return. In order for them to be able to reconcile their differences, Sarah maintains that she and James "would have to meet in another place; not in silence or in sound but somewhere else. I don't know where that is now." The play ends with the hope that James and Sarah will be joined once again.

CHARACTERS

Orin Dennis

Orin is two years younger than Sarah and has been a student with her at the State School for the Deaf since he was a young child. Orin, however, has some residual hearing and practices both his lip-reading and his speech. He is described as "the guardian of all . . . deaf children because he [is] an apprentice teacher and speaks." He is also described as someone who "wants to lead a revolution against the hearing world and thinks [the deaf] can hardly wait to follow him."

Orin is angry that Sarah appears to have abandoned him and the deaf world in favor of James and the hearing world. But he enlists both of them to join him in a complaint against the Equal Employment Opportunity Commission that alleges discriminatory hiring practices against teachers who are deaf. He is single-minded in pursuit of his goal, convincing a lawyer, Ms. Klein, to advise them about the case. He wants Sarah to leave her "little romance" and fight with him for deaf rights. Because of his lip-reading and speaking skills, Orin acts as a bridge between the two worlds, although it is apparent from his thoughts and actions that he feels more comfortable in the deaf community.

Mr. Franklin

Mr. Franklin is the Supervising Teacher at the State School for the Deaf. He is one of the "Great White Fathers" of deaf education. He takes a condescending attitude toward everyone. He views all the deaf, even the adults like Orin and Sarah, as needy children who need his protection and guidance. However, his compassionate, benevolent pretense is weakened when he says to James: "Mr. Leeds . . . we don't fornicate with the students. We just screw them over. If you ever get the two confused . . . you're gone." Later, when James goes to him to attempt to broker a settlement in the discrimination case, Mr. Franklin refers to the deaf as his "subjects," and promises that no matter what the commission might decide, he will make Orin and Sarah take him to court, and if they are successful there, he will appeal the ruling, tying them up in litigation for years.

Edna Klein

Ms. Klein is a lawyer who helps Orin with his claim of discrimination against the State School for the Deaf. She does not know how to sign or how to communicate with Orin or Sarah. She plans to read a speech that she has written before the commission but is accused by Sarah of writing "the same old shit"—that deaf people are helpless and need hearing people to get along in the world. Ms. Klein is well-intentioned, but recognizes neither Sarah or Orin as human beings who can speak for themselves.

James Leeds

The play takes place in the mind of James Leeds. As happens to Willy Loman in *Death of a Salesman,* characters step from James's memory "for anything from a full scene to several lines." James Leeds is a speech teacher at a State School for the Deaf. He is bright and articulate, but struggles throughout the play to understand the ''other language'' of Sarah and her deaf counterparts. A former Peace Corps volunteer, James is attracted to support occupations ''because it feels good to help people.'' For the whole length of the play, James tries to ''help'' Sarah, to make her value speech. James wrestles with his motives, struggling to determine whether they stem from a desire to help or a desire to control.

Lydia

Lydia is a State School for the Deaf student in her late teens. She, like Orin, has some residual hearing, and she faithfully practices her speech and lip-reading skills. However, she is not as mature as Orin and throws herself at James throughout the play. As one of James's students, Lydia has frequent contact with him, but that contact turns into a schoolgirl crush. After James and Sarah marry, Lydia is given Sarah's former job as ''maid.'' Lydia often appears at the Leeds's residence to ''watch TV'' and be closer to James. She wants to appear ''hearing,'' and even chides James after Sarah has left: ''You need a girl that doesn't go away. You need a girl that talks.''

Mrs. Norman

Mrs. Norman is Sarah's mother, a hearing woman whose husband left her not long after Sarah was sent to the State School for the Deaf. Mrs. Norman appears to be a bitter woman at the beginning of the play. She has been frustrated and challenged in trying to parent a deaf child, and seems disinterested in what James has to say to her about Sarah and her intellectual capabilities. She complains of ''feeling like another mandatory stop in some training program for new teachers at the school.'' Mrs. Norman does reconcile with Sarah after James forces a visit between the two women. She attends their wedding and joins James and Sarah as Mr. Franklin's partner for the bridge game at the beginning of Act II. She welcomes Sarah with open arms after she leaves James.

Sarah Norman

Sarah is a woman in her mid-twenties who has been deaf from birth; she works as a cleaning woman at the State School for the Deaf. She refuses to speak and rejects James's attempts at therapy because ''I don't do things I don't do well.'' Sarah signs throughout the play, speaking only in the final climactic scene. She uses American Sign Language (ASL; a conceptual, pictorial expression) rather than the Signed English (a word-by-word, grammatical rendition) technique favored by James.

The physicality of the language itself provides a certain eloquence to the dialogue that speech alone cannot deliver. Even though Sarah turns in a splendid performance at the card party at the beginning of Act II that tests her integration into the hearing world, she confesses to James: ''I feel split down the middle, caught between two worlds.'' This is the central problem for Sarah. Like Nora in Henrik Ibsen's *A Doll's House,* she declares her own identity as a separate person, telling James: ''Until you let me be an individual, an *I,* just as you are, you will never be able to come inside my silence and know me. And until you do that, I will never let myself know you. Until that time, we cannot be joined. We cannot share a relationship.''

MEDIA ADAPTATIONS

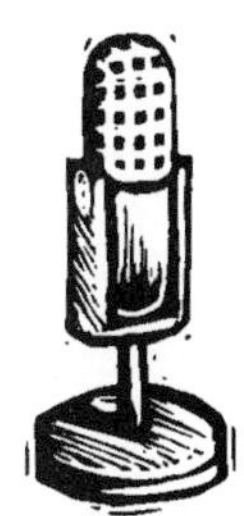

- *Children of a Lesser God* was adapted as a film in 1986. The screenplay was written by Medoff and Hesper Anderson. Randa Haines directed, and the film starred William Hurt as James Leeds, Marlee Matlin in an Oscar-winning performance as Sarah Norman, and Piper Laurie as Mrs. Norman. It is available through Facets Home Video in both VHS and Laser-Disc formats.

THEMES

Language and Meaning

Children of a Lesser God forces its audience to struggle with the problem of language, specifically resulting from the differences between spoken English and American Sign Language (ASL) and those who employ these languages. James becomes ex-

TOPICS FOR FURTHER STUDY

- Research the following and discuss the contribution of each to the world of theater: The National Theater of the Deaf, Louie Fant, Bernard Bragg, and Phyllis Frelich.
- Alexander Graham Bell was a teacher of the deaf long before he invented the telephone. He is well known for devising ''Bell's Visible Speech.'' Find out more information on this topic and pay particular attention to the chart, if available.
- Through the years there has been an ongoing argument between the oralists (those who favor speech and lip-reading only) and the manualists (those who support the learning of sign language). The Clarke School for the Deaf in Massachusetts and the John Tracy Clinic in California are good sources of information for the oral point of view. Gallaudet University in Washington, DC, is an excellent resource for the sign language camp. Consult these resources and use the information you obtain to show how Sarah's character has been influenced by the two opposing factions.
- Just as there are dialects in spoken language (the southern drawl, the New England twang), there are dialects and differing ways to say the same thing in sign language. Research American Sign Language (ASL) and the varying forms of signed English. Show how these signing dialects play an important role in the play.
- Compare the characters of James and Anne Sullivan (from William Gibson's *The Miracle Worker*). How does each approach the role of teacher? How do their teaching strategies compare?

hausted trying to act as bridge between the two. Mrs. Norman lost her daughter for eight years because of the misunderstandings and lack of communication between herself as a hearing person and her deaf daughter. Mr. Franklin is skilled at ASL but refuses to use it, especially in social situations. Orin and Lydia seem to abandon ASL for speech. Sarah refuses to speak and converses only in ASL. And Ms. Klein is confused when people seem less than enthusiastic about her having learned three signs.

English has its own grammatical structure, its own rules, its own way of putting thoughts into communication. ASL has a different grammatical structure, one that linguists say is more like Chinese than English. ASL follows a different set of rules, rules more often made by the speakers themselves than by teachers and writers. ASL uses the entire body to bring the thoughts of its user to the world at large.

Much of the conflict in this play comes from an unwillingness to accept the language system of ''the other.'' James signs, but he is always trying to get Sarah to speak, to use *his* language. At the end of the play, he forces Sarah not to use her hands. Sarah then realizes that even though she loves James and he loves her, James at some level refuses to accept her as she is. ''Am I what you want me to be?'' Sarah speaks in her own barely intelligible voice. There is a hope for reconciliation at the conclusion of the play, but for the moment the chasm separating the spoken and the signed word is too wide to be bridged.

Search for Self

Sarah's mother demanded that her other daughter's boyfriends' friends act as companions to Sarah when the girls were younger. She enthusiastically recalls: ''These boys really liked Sarah, treated her the same way they treated Ruth, with respect, and . . . and if you didn't know there was a problem, you'd have thought she was perfectly normal.'' Mrs. Norman did not realize that none of these boys were interested in Sarah herself, but only in how she could meet their needs; their sole reason for going out with her was to engage in sexual intercourse, which she was willing to provide.

Sarah says that she has always been seen as less than valuable, that, because she cannot hear, she is somehow defective, ''and that's bad.'' When everyone tries to speak for her at the hearing before the commission, Sarah realizes that the integrity of her own identity as a distinct, separate individual human being has been ignored. She expresses this when she says: ''Unless you let me be an individual, an *I,* just as you are, you will never truly be able to come inside my silence and know me. And until you do that, I will never let myself know you. Until that time, we cannot be joined. We cannot share a relationship.'' When Sarah leaves James, she does so with the knowledge that she can say that she hurts and ''won't shrivel up and blow away.'' She will have to ''go it alone.''

Manipulation and Control

James is a speech therapist. He works with Orin and Lydia to improve their speaking skills. (He even corrects Orin's pronunciation of ''sushi'' when Orin expresses his anger that he too has eaten ''hearing food.'') James's job becomes convincing Sarah to speak. But Sarah has an agenda of her own, and does not place any value on learning to speak in order to appear ''normal.''

Mrs. Norman would go to great lengths for Sarah to appear normal: demanding her other daughter's male friends become companions to Sarah, forcing Sarah to attend lip-reading and speech classes, even signing Ricky Nelson's name to a pin-up photo she put in Sarah's room. James's mother used a religion ''heretofore unknown to mankind'' to control her son.

Ms. Klein, the lawyer, assumes that she will speak for the deaf at the commission hearing and has already drafted her remarks. Orin attempts to learn the tools of the hearing world so that he can ''change this system that sticks us with teachers who pretend to help but really want to glorify themselves.''

James pins Sarah's arms to her sides and demands that she speak. In the same manner that others might have used violence or sex to control a partner in a relationship, James makes language a weapon of control. Sarah rebels against this blatant attempt at control and leaves to ''go it alone.''

STYLE

Setting

Children of a Lesser God is a drama set ''in the mind of James Leeds.'' Characters in the play step from his memory for a few lines or an entire scene. There are two ''places'' where the action occurs: the State School for the Deaf and James Leeds's house across the road. In Act I, time is ''fluid.'' Scenes from past and present blend together often without the audience realizing what has happened. In Act II, the sense of time is more linear, although not completely so; there is more of a sense that one scene comes to a conclusion before another scene begins. The audience is better able to follow plot movement as the action progresses from the card party to James's frustration of serving as Sarah's constant interpreter to the complaint before the Commission to the climactic scene in which James forces Sarah to speak. The lack of a set and the use of few props beyond a chalkboard and some benches allow characters to come and go easily.

Flashback

Because the action of the play takes place ''in the mind of James Leeds,'' time does not always move forward. Scenes from the past, like the visit to Mrs. Norman's house in Act I, weave themselves into the fabric of the action. The entire play can be seen as a flashback: the actions and words of the beginning of the play come back again near the end.

Imagery

''Deafness isn't the opposite of hearing. . . . It is a silence full of sounds.'' This is the central image of the play. Sarah tries to show James that the relationship between the deaf and hearing worlds is not an ''either-or'' situation, but rather one with its own distinct and unique possibilities and components.

Much of the imagery of this play is not contained in the words of the characters but rather in the sign language they employ. Sign language in this play provides both visual and verbal imagery for the same idea. ''Join, unjoined'' is the principal sign image, used at both the beginning and end of the action (and also graphically represented on the cover of some print editions of the text of the play).

Language

The story that takes place in *Children of a Lesser God* is told primarily using two languages,

COMPARE & CONTRAST

- **Early 1980s:** Deaf schools are run by hearing administrators, many of whom know no sign language.

  Today: Many schools for the deaf, including Gallaudet University, now have deaf leaders.

- **Early 1980s:** People with hearing handicaps are routinely discriminated against for jobs, in housing, and in access to services.

  Today: With the passage of the Americans with Disabilities Act, hearing impaired individuals have the necessary leverage to find success in the job market, obtain decent housing, and utilize a wide range of services to assist them in pursuit of their goals.

spoken English and American Sign Language (ASL), although a third variety, Signed English, is present as well. ASL is a conceptual and pictorial language, and Signed English is more grammatical and dependent on word order—one sign equals one word—for meaning.

When Sarah ''speaks'' her lines in this play during conversations with James, James provides a simultaneous translation from ASL to spoken English. However, when James speaks to Sarah, he signs what he says (unless he is purposely excluding her from the conversation) using Signed English. When James speaks to Orin and Lydia who can both lip-read, James does not sign; he enunciates carefully. Mr. Franklin, who as the supervising teacher at the State School for the Deaf is a competent signer, refuses to sign for Sarah's benefit, forcing James into the role of continual interpreter. Mrs. Norman has struggled to learn sign language but has not been successful.

Edna Klein knows no sign language and is quite proud that she has learned to sign ''How. Are. You?'' and ''I. Am. Fine''; Sarah, Orin, and James are unimpressed by her efforts. James points out that Edna must be precise in her hand placement or she will say the opposite of what she intended. This illustrates that hearing people often view ASL as ''cute,'' a diversion along the lines of a party game. Sarah's reaction to this particular scene (''More cuteness?'') underscores the feeling deaf people have that their language is not taken seriously.

HISTORICAL CONTEXT

Deafness is a unique condition; its effects are not immediately visible. Individuals whose bodies bear an outward sign of impairment or disability are recognizable in the world at large. And the community recognizes, more or less, what should be done to assist these people to fuller participation in the larger society. How does society as a whole include the deaf in its activities and discussions? That question has had a variety of answers since the 19th century.

In the mid-1800s, two camps argued over how to include the deaf in the wider community: the oralists, who opposed sign language and forbade children in their schools and programs from using it, advocated teaching deaf individuals the skills needed for success in the hearing and speaking world; conversely, manualists held that communication was paramount, and fostered the use of sign language in both instructional and social settings. ''Culture wars'' erupted between the two factions, the remnants of which exist to the present day.

In all of the battles concerning the deaf, one constant remained—hearing people were the ones who made the decisions. Deaf people were viewed as incapable of speaking their own minds or making their own decisions. Most states established residential schools for deaf children, most of whom attended from the age of five to the age of 18, leaving only for Christmas breaks and summer vacations. These schools were run by hearing men (like Mr. Franklin), many of whom had attended teacher-training programs together. These autocratic educators, referred to in some circles as the ''Great White Fathers,'' ruled every aspect of the lives of the students in their charge. Most teachers were hearing and had little knowledge or expertise in sign language. Deaf people were not considered capable of teaching children because they would not be able to teach speech. Occasionally those deaf people who were able to speak well—like Orin—were allowed to become teachers, but those—like Sarah—who did not speak or lip-read were relegated to jobs as kitchen helpers, laundry workers, and maids at these schools. A series of scandals in the 1970s rocked several of these residential schools; as a result, new people from outside the closed circle of selected hearing people who worked with the deaf were brought in to manage these schools. More deaf students were encouraged to pursue post-secondary educational courses of study, including teacher preparation programs.

CRITICAL OVERVIEW

Robert Brustein, writing in *The New Republic,* called *Children of a Lesser God* a "supreme example of a new Broadway genre—the Disability Play," in which, regardless of our defects, the audience learns that we all share a common humanity. He further noted that speech in this drama "operates not to inform and reveal but rather to manipulate emotions and reinforce conventional wisdom." Paul Sagona declared in *Dictionary of Literary Biography* that Medoff "exploits a stark, absolute communication problem," but does so "without the threat of physical violence" or guns. Sagona identified Medoff's plays, especially *Children of a Lesser God,* as addressing the problem of "self-isolated personalities making themselves felt without disintegrating."

Other critical commentary centers on how the characters' inability to communicate with one another works as an effective means of illustrating the both the problems caused by prejudice and those caused by language. Some critics have expressed reservations about Medoff's dramatic work, citing his tendency toward gratuitous use of violence or overly sentimental plot devices and dialogue. *Children of a Lesser God* has been singled out as an example of Medoff's best work, in large part because of Medoff's ability to present the demoralization of the deaf population by a generally ignorant society that assumes that those who cannot hear are somehow mentally or otherwise inferior. The stark reality and emotional intensity of the play have been praised by critics who affirm that *Children of a Lesser God* is evidence of Medoff's exceptional talent as a playwright.

CRITICISM

William P. Wiles,

Wiles is a teacher with over twenty years of experience in secondary education. In the following essay, he explores the characters' individual attitudes toward hearing, speech, and deafness in Children of a Lesser God.

"In the beginning, there was only silence," James Leeds says at the very beginning of *Children of a Lesser God,* "and out of that silence there could come only one thing: Speech. That's right. Human speech. So, *speak!*" he could not have been more wrong.

In this opening speech, James appears to establish silence, and by extension deafness, as "bad," and speech and sound (and hearing) as "good." This is the distinction which most deaf people learn at a young age. Sarah learned this distinction from her mother and her teachers, but chose as an adult to reject this explanation and establish a definition of her own: "Deafness [is] a silence full of sounds . . . the sound of spring breaking up through the death of winter." The words that make this phrase are beautiful; the signs that give this phrase life are deeply moving.

The struggle, then, throughout the play becomes one of making those who have ears, however residual their hearing might be, able to hear. Orin and Lydia have some hearing—not enough to allow them to function in the hearing world without assistance but some hearing nonetheless. Lydia has a crush on James and refuses to listen to anything but her own heart strings. She is oblivious to how her behavior affects Sarah and she will not listen to James's voice or Sarah's signs when they not so indirectly talk to her about watching television.

Orin is deaf to anything that does not fit his vision of protecting the deaf. As a deaf man who speaks relatively clearly and reads lips, Orin is a good candidate for one to bridge the deaf and hearing worlds. But, he is entirely wrapped up in his "cause": deaf teachers for deaf children. When James takes Sarah out to dinner for the first time, Orin becomes jealous and begins to refuse to listen to James. What had once been a vibrant student-teacher relationship disintegrates into posturing and jockeying for position. Orin is so consumed with his "cause" that he turns a deaf ear (pun intended) to Sarah as she tries to explain what it is that she wants to say.

WHAT DO I READ NEXT?

- *The Miracle Worker,* a play by William Gibson, explores the early education of Helen Keller and her teacher, Anne Sullivan. The play confronts the issues of the link between language and communication, and the struggles of both student and teacher to make that link.
- Brian Clark's play *Whose Life Is It Anyway?* examines the idea of allowing individuals who are impaired to make decisions for themselves through the story of Ken Harrison, a sculptor. After he is involved in a car accident and is paralyzed from his neck down, all Harrison can do is talk. He says he wants to die; in the hospital, he makes friends with some of the staff, and they support him when he goes to trial to be allowed to make his own decisions, even if those decisions include ending his life.
- *In This Sign,* a novel by Joanne Greenberg, is the story of a deaf couple and their hearing daughter and their struggle through life. The characters are neither heroic or extraordinary, but they are very real and very human.
- Based on the true story of John Merrick, a 19th-century Englishman afflicted with a disfiguring congenital disease, Bernard Pommerance's *The Elephant Man* explores the issue of the integrity of one's identity. With the help of kindly Dr. Frederick Treves, Merrick attempts to regain the dignity he lost after years spent as a side-show freak.
- In the play *A Doll's House* by Henrik Ibsen, Nora Helmer committed a forgery in order to save the life of her authoritarian husband Torvald. She is blackmailed, and lives in fear of her husband discovering her crime and of the shame such a revelation would bring to his career. But when the truth comes out, Nora is shocked to learn where she really stands in her husband's esteem. Nora's confrontational scene with her husband is echoed in *Children of a Lesser God.*

Mr. Franklin, the supervising teacher, is one of the hearing people whose job it should be to hear what his charges have to say about issues that affect them, but none of the deaf people in this play have any respect for the man. Franklin does nothing to earn that respect, either. He is a skilled signer; he reads Sarah's signing at the bridge party. But throughout the play he refuses to sign in the presence of any of the deaf people, particularly Sarah, always forcing someone else to sign for him. His patronizing attitude will not allow him to hear what Sarah or anyone else (including the Commission) has to say.

Poor Ms. Klein walks into what she thinks is a routine appearance before the Equal Opportunity Commission and finds herself in the middle of a four-way argument about who doesn't listen to whom and who will do the talking for whom. She means well and has none of the mean-spiritedness that seems to come from Franklin, but for all practical purposes in this situation, she is utterly clueless. She fails to hear Orin and Sarah as they try to assert their position. Granted, Klein has limited experience with the deaf population compared to the rest of the characters, but it takes Sarah calling her speech the "same old shit" and threatening to walk away from the Commission hearing to get Klein to hear what she and Orin have to say.

Mrs. Norman has struggled for 26 years with Sarah and her deafness. Her early attempts at "normalcy" for Sarah were pathetic. She wrote on a pin-up photo of singer Ricky Nelson in her own handwriting: "To Sarah. Good Luck. From Ricky." She demanded that Sarah's sister, Ruth, ask her boyfriends to find companions for Sarah. To Mrs. Norman, the steady stream of male companions meant that Sarah appeared "normal." In reality, the boys came for sex, which Sarah was willing to provide. When Sarah and James decide to marry, Mrs. Norman and Sarah attempt a reconciliation. Each appears to accept the other at face value, and, at the end of the play when Sarah leaves James, she goes to her mother's house. Mrs. Norman has stopped trying to make Sarah into something she is not and relates to her on a more human level.

James is the most complex character of the drama. He is the detached intellectual who falls in love. He cannot shape this woman into an image that suits him. He cannot make her accept speech and sound. As a speech teacher, James's professional responsibility is to work diligently with the population of the State School for the Deaf. He has achieved outstanding success with both Orin and Lydia; even Mr. Franklin recognizes that Orin never worked that hard for him. But with Sarah, James faces a challenge that he cannot overcome. That is because Sarah is a human being with dignity and integrity and individuality who refuses to play the "deafie" game.

James falls in love with Sarah, in some part because of her feisty nature. In a kind of role reversal, it is the man who thinks he can change the woman into the prize, the perfect middle-class housewife. Sarah's success at the bridge party appears to prove James right. It is when Sarah decides that she will "speak" for herself at the Commission hearing that James's vision of the perfect housewife begins to crumble. In frustration, he clamps her arms to her side and demands that she speak: "Shut up! You want to talk to me, then you learn *my* language! . . . Now come on! I want you to speak to me. Let me hear it. Speak! Speak! Speak!"

James's call for speech from Sarah's silence destroys the relationship he had built with Sarah. The insistence that she speak creates a rift so deep that not even love can mend it. Sarah realizes that even though she loves him, she cannot stay with him. Maybe, she muses, they will be able to meet somewhere "not in silence or in sound but somewhere else. I don't know where that is now."

Out of that silence came speech but it was forced and pained. Out of that silence also came love, strength, self-knowledge, and beauty. James's demand that Sarah be "normal" refuses to acknowledge the idea that normalcy is in the mind and eye of the beholder.

Source: William P. Wiles, for *Drama for Students,* Gale, 1998.

Tom O'Brien

O'Brien reviews the film adaptation of Children of a Lesser God, *which Medoff cowrote. While he praises the performances, the critic was less pleased with the translation from stage to screen, feeling that certain elements of Medoff's original text were misused for the screenplay.*

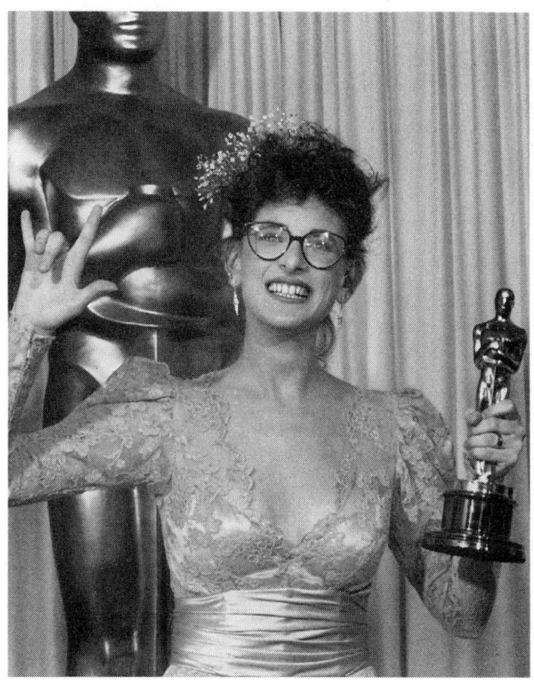

Actress Marlee Matlin after receiving the Academy Award for her portrayal of Sarah Norman in the film adaptation of Medoff's play

Children of a Lesser God both moves and disappoints. Directed by Randa Haines, whose television experience includes *Hill Street Blues* and the film about incest, *Something about Amelia, Children* provides a bare-bones story about an angry young deaf woman (Marlee Martin) and a teacher (William Hurt) determined to get her to speak. Their romance is compelling, especially because of the verve and pain of their "dialogue" through sign language. But Haines makes their love stand too much alone, leaving a thin feel. The movie never delivers what it promises.

Partly this results from changes made in Mark Medoff's play—changes which he presumably approved as co-screenwriter. Of course, what works as a play doesn't always work as film. A play has to be opened up, dialogue simplified, scenes added, etc. Nevertheless, both stage play and screenplay require a strong, rich story, and it is unfortunate that Medoff succumbed to pressures to simplify his,

"JAMES'S DEMAND THAT SARAH BE 'NORMAL' REFUSES TO ACKNOWLEDGE THE IDEA THAT NORMALCY IS IN THE MIND AND EYE OF THE BEHOLDER."

which has been adapted, not into a film, but into *television* film, with a lowest-common-denominator plot, reduced list of characters, and pro forma happy end. As a result, it lacks the ambition, rawness, and hard-earned optimism not just of its source, but its prototype, *The Miracle Worker.*

Hurt and Martin make the film worth seeing. As with his Oscar-winning role in *Kiss of the Spider Woman,* Hurt took a pay cut to make this film. He is at his best in classroom scenes with deaf students, when he tries to coax them from negativism via an idealism that Hurt, both by age and look, seems to have memorized from the 1960s. He also has a hard task to master: since Marlee Martin won't speak, he has to interpret her rapid (often tempestuous) sign language in a deadpan fashion to avoid stealing any of her thunder. Martin has remarkably severe black and white coloring, and taut, expressive cheekbones. She also uses her thick black boots for punctuation and to embody frustration. Between her and Hurt some real heat gets generated, especially in one scene of angry lovemaking where she vehemently overwhelms him.

But they are limited by the thinness of the plot. Hurt's egoism is introduced, but never explored, so that he comes across as too pure a hero. Martin can rely on no more than petulant perfectionism (or as she explains in sign language, ''I won't do anything I don't do well'') to explain her refusal to vocalize. Some strong minor characters, like the school principal (Phillip Bosco) and Martin's mother (Piper Laurie), are also left undeveloped, as though Haines had to hold the story to a strict diet of characterization.

Moreover, Haines uses landscape symbolism unevenly. At first her touch is light, with mood scenes showing Hurt's trip by ferry to the peninsula where the school is located. The water imagery is deepened, poetically, with some beautiful scenes of Martin's nude swimming; the suggestion is even made that she has developed other, extraordinarily sensuous capacities as compensation for deafness. But the water imagery is overdone, especially in a stupid scene where Hurt ''descends'' into her pool. Save us.

Also uneven is Haines's use of music. Hurt's love of Bach and his attempt to teach some of his students rock music through rhythmic vibrations are deftly exploited. But the script is over-heavy with rock songs and teenage behavior. There is a line between appealing to adolescents and pandering to them. There is also a line between adaptation and dilution. Unfortunately, *Children of a Lesser God* often crosses both lines.

Source: Tom O'Brien, ''Adaptation Loss: Minor Miracle Worker'' in *Commonweal,* Volume CXIII, no. 16, September 26, 1986, pp. 500–01.

Robert Brustein

In the following review of Children of a Lesser God*'s original Broadway run, Brustein offers a positive review of Medoff's play. The critic categorizes the work as part of a dramatic subgenre that he terms the ''disability play''—a drama whose intentions are so well-placed and politically correct that a viewer feels morally compelled to speak positively of it.*

Mark Medoff's *Children of a Lesser God* (Longacre) is a supreme example of a new Broadway genre—the Disability Play. The origin of the species, I suppose, was William Gibson's *The Miracle Worker,* written 20 years ago—but only following the success of such recent extensions of the formula as *The Elephant Man* and *Whose Life Is It Anyway?,* has the Disability Play taken Broadway by storm as its dominant ''serious'' drama. It's not hard to understand the success of the genre, since it has everything going for it: 1) Unforgettable Characters, including spastics, paraplegics, the deaf, and the blind; 2) Intriguing Conflict, between the handicapped protagonist and the ''normal'' person who invites contempt by trying to help; 3) Love Reversal, the moment the conflict between these two characters ends in an embrace; 4) Terrific Breakthrough, when the protagonist reveals that he/she can speak/feel/read lips/walk; and 5) Inspirational Theme, after we learn we all share a common humanity, regardless of our defects. The impact of this on the tear ducts is dynamite. I haven't seen audiences leaving a theater with such glistening faces since the last revival of Bette Davis in *Dark Victory,* or perhaps since Peter Sellers rose from his wheelchair in *Doctor Strangelove* (after a ferocious struggle with his mechanical hand) to announce to the American president, "Mein Führer, I can walk."

The other built-in success factor is that the species is really a subgenre of a time-tested Broadway artifact—The Play You Are Not Allowed to Dislike. In the past, this used to be a political drama—people resisting a corrupt political system, or fighting for the loyalist cause during the Spanish Civil War. More recently, it has featured almost exclusively ethnic and sexual minorities, thus increasing the quota of moral extortion. To fail to respond to plays about blacks or women or homosexuals, for example, is to be vulnerable to charges of racism, sexism, homophobia, or getting up on the wrong side of the bed. Now that the handicapped have organized themselves into another minority pressure group, they have access to the same kind of blackmail. Meanwhile, the theater becomes another agency for consciousness raising, with audiences being alternately tutored and entertained for considerably less than a healthy contribution to an effective rehabilitation program.

Medoff's version of this formula is partly successful because it combines the features of two current offerings you are forbidden to dislike: the disability play and the feminist play. Its male hero is James Leeds, a speech therapist who works in a clinic for the "non-hearing" (the word *deaf* having been consigned to the same dusty lexicon of archaic English as *Negro* and *Mrs.*). One of his charges is a feisty woman named Sarah Norman, deaf and dumb since birth, who absolutely refuses to learn to speak or read lips (they communicate entirely through signing). Not only this, she dislikes everybody who does, including the baffled Leeds, who can't understand why the recalcitrant Sarah continues to refuse his help. Nevertheless, he continues to offer it, and, endlessly, to discuss it (*help* is the most frequently uttered word of the play). A former Peace Corps officer, he is attracted to support occupations "because it feels good to help people." When he goes to bed with Sarah, it feels even better, and his efforts at helping enter a new phase.

Eventually, they get married. Leeds, who leans toward pop psychoanalysis, concludes that Sarah's hatred of "hearing" people is related to her hatred of herself, while she confesses that she has refused his therapy because "I don't do things I don't do well." Although sex is not among these (she has had an active history before she married him), the two soon fall to quarreling. He hasn't turned on his

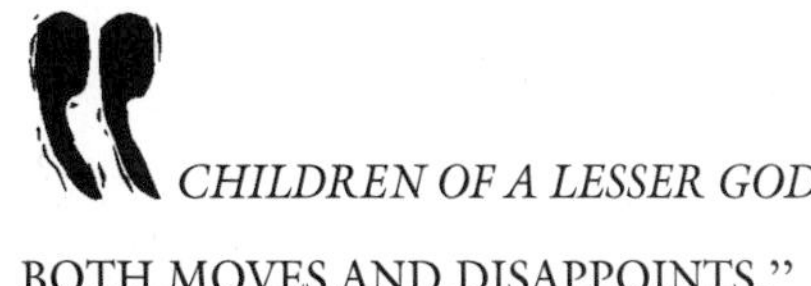

CHILDREN OF A LESSER GOD BOTH MOVES AND DISAPPOINTS."

stereo in months, and she seems more interested in fighting for the rights of "non-hearing" people than in the marriage. These personal battles lead to two dramatic revelations. His is an admission that he feels guilty over the suicide of his mother, not surprisingly since it occurred right after he announced to the unfortunate woman that if he lived with her for one more day, he would put a gun to one of their heads. Hers arrives when he forces her to utter sounds, and she confesses that she has been reading lips for years. In a scene you may recognize from about 50 other plays (beginning with *A Doll's House*), she then tells her husband that until she becomes an "individual," "we cannot be joined, we cannot share a relationship." The payoff comes when Leeds, after trying to help Sarah for the whole length of the play, is forced to admit his own dependency ("Help me—teach me . . . be brave, but not so brave that you don't need me anymore"). She leaves anyway. Will she return? Tune in tomorrow. In the ambiguous conclusion, Sarah reaches out to James in a half-light, signing, "I'll help you if you help me," following which the spectators helped themselves to their handkerchiefs and I helped myself to my coat.

Obviously, only a stony heart could remain cold to such a story, especially when it is delivered with such conviction by the two principal actors, John Rubenstein and Phyllis Frelich. Rubenstein, who has the sharp angular features of a young Fred Astaire, carries the burden of virtually the entire play on his talented shoulders, since he not only speaks his own lines but translates Miss Frelich's signs as well. This double task he discharges with such wit and passion that he almost succeeds in forcing some suppleness into the cardboard goody two shoes he is forced to impersonate. As for Miss Frelich, she is an accomplished mime, with a mischievous smile and an instinct for deviltry that remind one of Harpo Marx, and she demonstrates how well spiritual beauty and intelligence can be manifested without the aid of speech. Indeed, the whole play is a good argument for the return of the silent film. Expertly crafted, and directed with considerable skill (by Gordon Davidson), it successful-

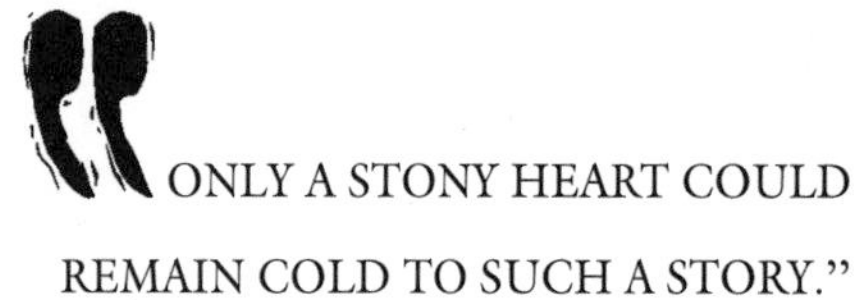

ONLY A STONY HEART COULD REMAIN COLD TO SUCH A STORY."

ly disguises its soap-opera origins by being a chic compendium of every extant cliché about women and minority groups, where speech operates not to inform and reveal but rather to manipulate emotions and reinforce conventional wisdom. . . .

Source: Robert Brustein, ''The Play You Are Not Allowed to Dislike'' in the *New Republic,* Volume 182, no. 23, June 7, 1980, pp. 23–24.

SOURCES

Adams, Elizabeth. ''Mark Medoff'' in *Contemporary American Dramatists,* edited by Jim Kamp, St. James Press, 1994, pp. 443-45.

Brustein, Robert. Review of *Children of a Lesser God* in the *New Republic,* Vol. 187, no. 23, June 7, 1980, pp. 23-24.

Sagona, Paul. ''Mark Medoff'' in *Dictionary of Literary Biography,* Volume 7: *Twentieth Century American Dramatists,* edited by John MacNicholas, Gale, 1981, pp. 82-86.

FURTHER READING

Gallaudet University Home Page, http://www.gallaudet.edu.
This home page to the largest and best-known school of higher learning for the deaf provides information on deafness and links to a variety of sites associated with deaf culture.

DeafNation Links Page, http://www.deafnation.com/Deaflinks.html.
An extensive compilation of links related to deafness and deaf culture.

Deaf World Web & ASL Dictionary Online, http://dww.deafworldweb.org/asl/.
Among other things, contains a dictionary of signs grouped alphabetically and categorically.

Death and the Maiden

ARIEL DORFMAN

1991

Ariel Dorfman's *Death and the Maiden* is a moral thriller about a woman, Paulina, who believes that a stranger who comes to her home is the doctor who, under a military dictatorship, tortured and raped her many years before. (The play's title is taken from a piece of music by Franz Schubert; Paulina loved the piece but grew to revile it when it was played repeatedly during her torture sessions.) Dorfman began writing the play in the mid-1980s, when he was in exile from Chile, a country under the rule of the military dictator General Augusto Pinochet. It was not until Chile's return to democracy in 1990 that Dorfman returned to the play and "understood ... how the story had to be told." A workshop production of *Death and the Maiden* was staged in Santiago, Chile, opening in March, 1991, and in July of that year the play had its world premiere at London's Royal Court Upstairs. In November the production, which received the London *Time Out* Award for best play of 1991, moved to the Royal Court Mainstage. Reception of the play was positive, critics finding it both dramatically engaging as well as historically timely (given the number of societies around the world facing painful legacies of repressive regimes).

The play had its Broadway premiere on March 17, 1992, directed by Mike Nichols and starring Glenn Close as Paulina (a performance for which she received an Antionette "Tony" Perry Award), Richard Dreyfuss as Gerardo, and Gene Hackman as Miranda. The casting of three Anglo actors in

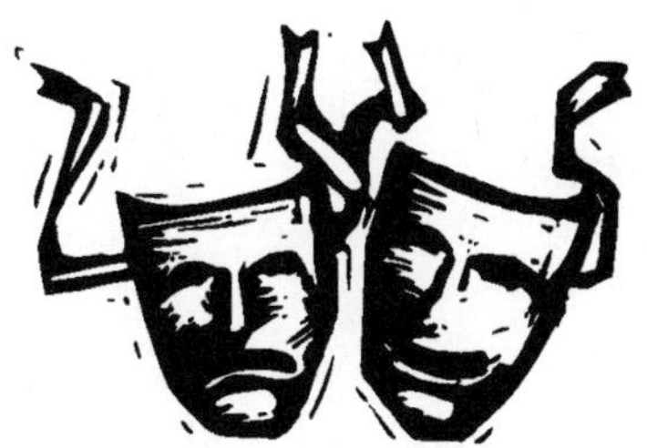

a play with a Latin American context was protested by Latino organizations and the Actors' Equity Association (the union for American actors). Dorfman's play, ultimately, did not receive as high praise in the United States as it had in England but did create enough interest to inspire a film adaptation in 1994. *Death and the Maiden* is valued as a dramatic work that examines the psychological repercussions of human rights abuses.

AUTHOR BIOGRAPHY

Playwright, essayist, novelist, poet, and short story writer Ariel Dorfman was born in Buenos Aires, Argentina, on May 6, 1942, the son of an economist and a literature teacher. His life illustrates the fragmented experience of the modern Latin American exile. At the age of two, his family was forced to flee to the United States because of his father's opposition to the Argentine government of Juan Peron. Dorfman's father was one of the architects of the United Nations, and the family lived in New York for ten years before leaving in 1954, during the McCarthy era, to settle in Chile. Completing a University education, Dorfman became a naturalized Chilean citizen in 1967. Working for the next several years as a journalist and activist, he published several works, including a study of the plays of Harold Pinter (*The Homecoming*).

A supporter of Chilean President Salvador Allende, Dorfman was forced into exile after a military coup led by General Augusto Pinochet seized control of the country in 1973. He intermittently lived in Argentina, France, the Netherlands, and eventually settled in the United States (in 1980), holding a variety of academic posts in each of the countries. In 1984 he became a professor at Duke University in Durham, North Carolina, where he maintains a part-time residence. Remaining active in Chile's political and social affairs while in exile, Dorfman first tried to return home to Chile in 1983 yet felt uncomfortable in the environment there. He tried a part-time return in 1986, but the following year, he was stopped at Santiago airport, detained, and then deported. Dorfman returned to Chile again in 1989. Following Pinochet's abdication to a popularly-elected president in 1990, the playwright attempted to re-establish a semi-permanent residence in his adopted homeland.

Dorfman's writings have been translated into over twenty languages. Like many other Latin American authors, he is also a social critic who investigates the relationship between politics and culture. He is the author of important essays and works of cultural criticism—*How to Read Donald Duck: Imperialist Ideology in the Disney Comic* (1975), *Culture and Resistance in Chile* (1978) and *The Empire's Old Clothes* (1980)—which argue that popular literatures promote capitalist and neo-imperial ideology and encourage passivity. Dorfman has additionally written literary works in a variety of forms. His collections of short stories include *The Medicine Goes Down* (1985) and *My House Is on Fire* (1979) which examines how people retain a sense of hope living under an oppressive military regime. Dorfman's novels have been praised for their highly original narrative techniques. *The Last Song of Manuel Sendero* (1987) combines several different perspectives, including those of cartoon characters and the unborn. *Mascara* (1988) explores human identity and the paranoia created by authoritarian regimes. Dorfman's many collections of poetry include *Missing* (1982) and *Last Waltz in Santiago and Other Poems of Exile and Disappearance* (1986). In the theater—besides his success with *Death and the Maiden* (1991)—Dorfman has created stage adaptations of his novel *Widows* (1981) and his short story "Reader" (1979).

PLOT SUMMARY

Act I

When the play opens, "The time is the present and the place, a country that is probably Chile but could be any country that has given itself a democratic government just after a long period of dictatorship." At the Escobar's secluded beach house it is late at night and an uneaten dinner is laid out on the table. Paulina sits on the terrace, startled by the sound of an unfamiliar car motor. She takes a gun from the sideboard, and stands listening as her husband, Gerardo, speaks to the driver of the car and then enters the house. Paulina is disturbed by the unusual occurrence, and Gerardo explains that he had a flat tire on the way home and accepted a ride from a passing motorist. He blames Paulina for the spare tire being flat and for the jack being gone (Paulina lent it to her mother). The couple argue about these details and then discuss Gerardo's meeting with the country's president, from which he has just returned.

Gerardo has been named to a commission examining human rights abuses under the country's previous government, a military dictatorship. (It is revealed through dialogue that Paulina was arrested and tortured while attending medical school during this dictatorship.) Paulina has mixed feelings; she is suspicious of the commission, which is only to investigate cases of abuse that ended in death. A case like Paulina's own abduction, therefore, would not fall within the commission's jurisdiction. Paulina is still traumatized by the memory of being raped and tortured, but she has never discussed details of her experience with her mother or other people close to her.

Gerardo agrees with Paulina that the power of the commission is limited, but he believes nevertheless that "there is so much we can do. . . ." Gerardo makes a point of appearing to ask for Paulina's permission to sit on the commission, but the first scene ends with his admission that he has already accepted the president's appointment. An hour later, a knock at the door rouses the Escobars. Gerardo is ill at ease until he opens the door to admit Doctor Roberto Miranda, the man who earlier drove him home. Miranda apologizes for the intrusion, and as the two men speak, Paulina edges closer, listening in on their conversation. As she listens, the sound of Miranda's voice appears to greatly upset her. Miranda explains that he heard a news story about the commission on the radio, only then realizing who Gerardo was, and felt he had to return to congratulate him on the appointment. Miranda appears very enthusiastic about the commission, although he also realizes that the investigations are unlikely to conclude with punishment. Miranda prepares to leave, promising to pick Gerardo up the next morning and help him retrieve his car, but Gerardo insists that Miranda stay the night.

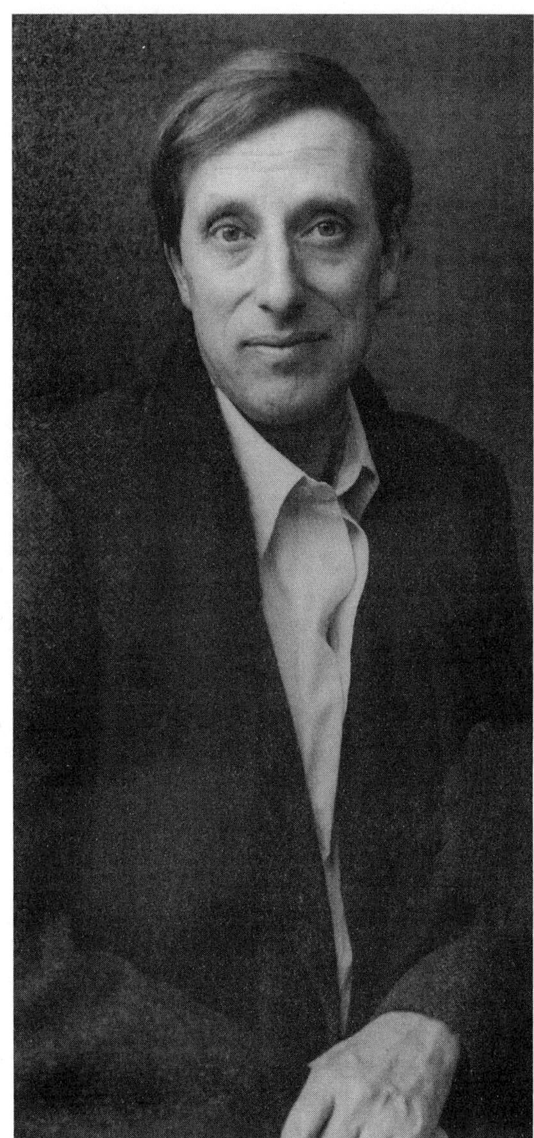

Ariel Dorfman

The third scene is a brief interlude a short time later, in which Paulina is seen dragging Miranda's unconscious body into the room and tying him to a chair. She gags him with her own underwear, then takes his car keys and leaves. When dawn rises on the fourth scene, Paulina has returned and sits with her gun, watching Miranda. When he awakens, she speaks to him for a long while, playing a cassette of Schubert's quartet *Death and the Maiden* which she found in Miranda's car. This music has painful associations for Paulina; it was played while she was in captivity, and Paulina takes Miranda's cassette—along with the familiarity of his voice—as proof that he is the doctor who tortured her. Gerardo enters, aghast at the scene he finds. Paulina explains her discovery, and Gerardo's first conclusion is: "You're sick." Gerardo makes a move to untie Miranda, and Paulina fires the gun wildly. She explains that she has already called a mechanic, and when the latter arrives, she ushers Gerardo out of the house to retrieve their car. The act ends with Paulina's cool statement, "We're going to put him on trial, Gerardo, this doctor. Right here, today."

Act II

The time is midday; Miranda is still tied and Paulina speaks to him intimately about her captivity and the night of her release. Gerardo enters after

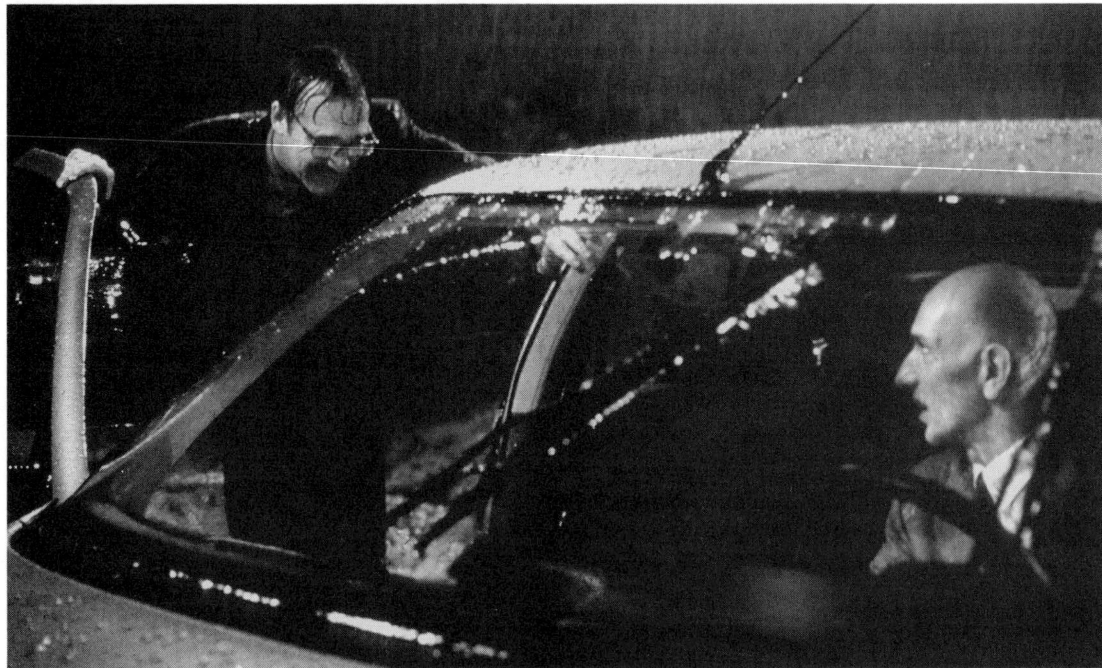

Gerardo (Stuart Wilson) is offered a ride by Roberto Miranda (Ben Kingsley) in director Roman Polanski's film adaptation of Dorfman's play. Miranda's kind gesture will set the play's conflict in motion

retrieving the car, with a new resolve to talk his wife into releasing Miranda. Gerardo appeals to an ideal of law, implying Paulina is no better than the military regime if she will not allow Miranda to defend himself. Paulina says she has every intention of allowing the doctor to argue his case. She was only waiting for Gerardo's return, having decided that her husband will act as a lawyer for the accused. When Paulina removes his gag, Miranda claims never to have seen Paulina before, calling her ''extremely ill, almost prototypically schizoid.''

Gerardo continues to plead with his wife, and as they argue it becomes evident that Gerardo has difficulty speaking about Paulina's experience. If she can prove beyond a shadow of a doubt that Miranda is the same doctor, Paulina asks, would Gerardo still want her to set him free. Gerardo replies, ''If he's guilty, more reason to set him free.... Imagine what would happen if everyone acted like you did.'' Gerardo argues that if Miranda is guilty of the crimes, they should turn him over to the proper authorities. His wife, however, believes that while the new government calls itself a democracy, many of the same men who were part of the dictatorship are still active in the government. Not only does she contend that the authorities would immediately release Miranda, she states her belief that the doctor is part of the current government and that his encounter with Gerardo was no coincidence.

Paulina explains that at one point she wanted retribution from Miranda but says that now she merely wants him to confess and she will let him go. ''What can he confess if he's innocent?'' wonders Gerardo. The scene ends on Paulina's reply, ''If he's innocent? Then he's really screwed.''

The second scene is at lunch. Paulina watches from the terrace as Gerardo feeds Miranda and the two men talk. Gerardo stresses that a confession, even a false one, is Miranda's only hope of escaping unharmed, while Miranda emphasizes that he is only in his current situation because he stopped to pick up Gerardo and now depends on the lawyer to get him out of this mess. After another threatening appearance by Paulina, Miranda accuses Gerardo of not being as impartial as he has claimed to be: ''She plays the bad guy and you play the good guy . . . to see if you can get me to confess that way.'' The two men argue but eventually admit they are both scared, and the act ends with Miranda asking

Gerardo's help in fabricating a convincing confession for Paulina.

Act III

The final act opens just before evening. Miranda is still bound, and Gerardo, with a tape recorder on his lap, pleads with Paulina to tell him the details of her abduction before he has to hear them from Miranda. Paulina reminds him that she had attempted to tell him these details before, just after she was released, when they were interrupted by the woman with whom Gerardo was involved during Paulina's absence. This memory is a severe blow to Gerardo, and he eventually persuades Paulina to speak instead of her abduction. When she gets to the point in her story of first meeting the doctor and hearing Schubert in the darkness, the lights fade and her voice overlaps with that of Miranda. The lights come up to reveal Miranda making his confession into the tape recorder. He claims that the music was an attempt to alleviate the suffering of the prisoners. He describes how a ''brutalization took over my life,'' and he began to enjoy the torture with a detached curiosity ''partly morbid, partly scientific.''

The confession over, Paulina sends Gerardo to retrieve Miranda's car. After his departure, however, she changes her tone, saying she was entirely convinced by the doctor's confession and now ''could not live in peace with myself and let you live.'' She informs him that she inserted small errors in her own taped account, which Miranda apparently corrected of his own accord; now Paulina says she will kill him ''because you haven't repented at all.'' On Paulina's unanswered question, ''What do we lose by killing one of them?'' the action freezes and the lights go down on the scene.

A giant mirror descends in front of the characters, ''forcing,'' as the stage directions state, ''the members of the audience to look at themselves.'' The lights come up on the final scene of the play, in a concert hall several months later. Gerardo and Paulina enter, elegantly dressed, and sit down facing the mirror. When the music ends they rise as if at intermission, and Gerardo speaks to a number of well-wishers who have gathered around him. Paulina observes Miranda entering (''or he could be an illusion,'' the directions read.) The three characters are seated as the performance recommences, and Schubert's ''Death and the Maiden'' is heard. Paulina and Miranda lock eyes for a moment, then she looks ahead into the mirror as the music plays.

MEDIA ADAPTATIONS

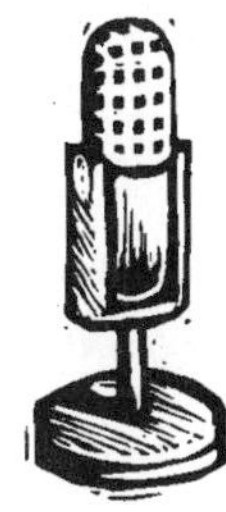

- *Death and the Maiden* was adapted as a film in 1994, directed by Roman Polanski, and starring Sigourney Weaver as Paulina, Ben Kingsley as Miranda, and Stuart Wilson as Gerardo. Novelist Rafael Yglesias (*Fearless*) and Dorfman wrote the screenplay based on the original play.

CHARACTERS

Gerardo Escobar

Paulina's husband, he is a lawyer about forty-five years of age. Gerardo has recently been appointed by the president to a commission that will examine human rights abuses during the military dictatorship. Gerardo has a high ideal of justice which he invokes in an attempt to persuade his wife to release Miranda. Paulina is ethically motivated, too, but she stresses repeatedly that corruption in the country's legal system leaves considerable doubt that the military's abuses will be properly rectified. Gerardo maintains his faith in the government's ability to do the best it can do under the circumstances, while Paulina feels pushed to take matters into her own hands. Undoubtedly, her more personal resolve is the product of her abduction and torment, which Gerardo seems to find almost unfathomable on a personal level, despite the nature of his work.

Gerardo has always had great difficulty discussing Paulina's experience, a guilt that is compounded by the fact that when Paulina went to him following her release, she discovered that he had been having an affair in her absence. Gerardo's suggestion that Paulina make a tape recording may be a way of addressing his problem, putting words to something he has not wanted to face.

Doctor Roberto Miranda

A doctor, around fifty years old. Roberto—Doctor Miranda—remains indignant at Paulina's accusations. He repeatedly reminds Gerardo of his place on the human rights commission and that it is his duty in that capacity to command his wife to release Miranda. The doctor denies having had any role in torturing military abductees and offers a confession that he claims to have fabricated in the hopes that Paulina will release him unharmed. Miranda, however, corrects details in the narrative of Paulina's experience which she recorded for Gerardo; this is enough proof for Paulina that her prisoner is the doctor who raped and tortured her. Miranda does not succeed in convincing her to the contrary but without having to make a direct and true confession he does somehow convince Paulina to spare his life with his plea, ''Oh Paulina—isn't it time we stopped?''

Miranda is a mysterious character who Dorfman never fully reveals to the audience. While there is considerable evidence presented that seems to incriminate the doctor, the possibility remains that it is merely coincidence that he fits the profile of Paulina's tormentor. His guilt appears to be further cemented by his decision not to report his kidnapping to the authorities, yet his silence may be attributed to a fear that Gerardo may use his position on the commission to discredit Miranda. Dorfman does not offer explanations for any of these situations. Miranda's fate at the play's conclusion is ambiguous: he may be a guilty man tormented by the atrocities he committed during wartime, or he may be an innocent man terrified by the threat of an unbalanced woman.

Paulina Salas

As a young student in the early days of the military dictatorship that ruled her country (the specific location is never given), Paulina worked with Gerardo helping people seek asylum in embassies and smuggling them out of the country. Paulina's activism, and her medical studies, were cut short, however, when she was arrested by the government. She was tortured and raped repeatedly before finally being released. This devastating experience which so altered her life continues to affect her seventeen years later, when the action of the play occurs.

Paulina has suppressed the worst details of her incarceration. Her paranoia has prevented her from sharing this information with Gerardo or her mother—for fear that the knowledge might place them in danger. While her country has replaced the dictatorship with a free, elected government, she suspects that many in power are from the military and only pretending to be democratic and fair-minded. She lives with acute fear, as can be seen from her defensive actions when Roberto Miranda's unfamiliar car first pulls up to the house. Since her ordeal, Paulina has also stifled a great deal of anger, which surfaces with the opportunity to exact revenge on the man she believes was her primary tormentor. Sure of herself after ''trying'' Miranda, Paulina appears set to kill the doctor but ultimately chooses to be merciful. This action seems to suggest that she ultimately rejects the idea of an eye for an eye. Yet her humane gesture comes at a price to her piece of mind. The tense final image of the play suggests that Paulina may never be able to achieve a satisfying resolution to her lingering pain.

THEMES

Atonement and Forgiveness

While there exists no acceptable rationale for the violence of the military regime, Paulina implies that she can forgive the individual for being fallible: she promises to release Miranda if he will confess to torturing and raping her. Miranda does not genuinely appear to ask for forgiveness; he does so only in the context of a confession which may be falsified. Paulina, although she ultimately chooses not to kill Miranda, does not forgive him, either. The play suggests that despite the lingering pain of political oppression, there is no concrete act that can atone for past wrongs.

Death and the Maiden

The title of Dorfman's play comes from the quartet by Schubert which Paulina associates with her abduction and torture. She finds a cassette of this music in Miranda's car. The piece, String Quartet No. 14 in D minor (D. 810), takes the name ''Death and the Maiden'' from a Schubert song that is quoted in it. The theme is common in folk music such as the English song ''Death and the Lady,'' in which a rich lady who has failed to bribe Death into granting her a few more years of life sings of having been betrayed by him. The theme of the song (hence the dramatic context for Schubert's quartet) is reflected in the characters themselves, with the shadowy doctor who raped and tortured Paulina existing as a kind of Death figure in her memory. However, Dorfman's play presents a reversal on the theme—if the audience agrees that Paulina has found the right doctor, that is—for in the present circumstance it is the Maiden (Paulina) who holds the power of life over Death (Miranda).

Doubt and Ambiguity

Paulina does not doubt that Roberto Miranda is the doctor who tortured and raped her years before or that he deserves to be tried and punished for these crimes. She is also convinced that she is the only person who can administer a punishment to fit the crime. One of the related themes of *Death and the Maiden,* however, is the lingering ambiguity which troubles a society attempting to rectify wrongs from a turbulent era in its past. Nagging questions remain: who can be sure the correct people are being tried, and what constitutes just punishment? The play examines the consequences of such justice, provoking questions as to the effects such a process will have not only on the accused but on the accuser.

Freedom

The play contrasts the present era to the repressive military regime which has recently ended. At the same time, it makes the complex point that in this fragile period of political transition, the legacy of the past still haunts people, preventing them from being truly free. Paulina mockingly questions the value of freedom in a society which has only provisionally returned to democracy: "Isn't that what this transition is all about? The Commission can investigate crimes but nobody is punished for them? . . . There's freedom to say anything you want as long as you don't say everything you want?" While political freedom is one major issue in the play, there is also the theme of emotional freedom. "You're still a prisoner," Gerardo tells Paulina, "you stayed behind with them, locked in that basement." Gerardo encourages her to "free yourself from them" in order to put her mind at rest. Paulina, however, is insulted by the implication that her only option is to forget her pain. Yet her solution is no less absolute: she feels she can only put her mind at rest by seeking punishment for her tormentors. In the end, however, she stops short of administering the ultimate punishment of death. It has been speculated that while this action does not liberate her from the pain of her torture and rape, it does grant her freedom from the savagery that afflicted her tormentors.

Justice and Injustice

Death and the Maiden contrasts ideal and practical concepts of justice. Both Paulina and Gerardo perceive the considerable injustices exerted by the former military regime, but they differ in their ideas of how justice can best be served under present circumstances. Gerardo believes in the efficacy of the commission to which he has been appointed, feeling that justice will be served by faithfully investigating human rights abuses and then turning the findings over to the country's courts. Paulina, however, is suspicious of the loyalties of those "same judges who never intervened to save one life in seventeen years of dictatorship." To her mind, justice cannot possibly be served through the channels which presently exist, so she resolutely takes the law into her own hands. The brutality of her past experience is undoubtedly at the root of her position; when Gerardo pleads with her at one point to be "reasonable," she bitterly responds: "You be reasonable. They never did anything to you."

TOPICS FOR FURTHER STUDY

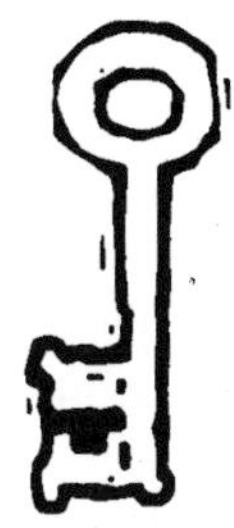

- Summarize the evidence presented that Roberto Miranda is the doctor who raped and tortured Paulina. Does the play offer convincing evidence for his guilt or innocence?
- Compare director Roman Polanski's film adaptation to Dorfman's original text. Screenwriters Dorfman and Rafael Yglesias altered the play's ending, providing further evidence that Miranda is guilty. Do you think this detracts from the play's original vision?
- How do the life roles or careers of each of the characters seem to be reflected in their actions and beliefs?
- Analyze the different ways the characters view the idea of revenge in the play. In what ways is it presented as satisfying or dissatisfying?
- Research the recent work of human rights tribunals in countries like Chile or Argentina. How do accounts of this process suggest that the individuals involved balance the ethical issues presented in this play?
- Analyze the theatrical device of the mirror which is lowered near the conclusion of the play. What effect(s) does this image achieve?

Memory and Reminiscence

Dorfman commented in an interview with Carlos Reyes on the Amnesty International homepage: ''Memory is a constant obsession for me,'' observing that a memory of the past is a counter against those, like the military rulers, ''who would obliterate others, who would forget them, ignore them, neglect them, erase them from the earth.'' Dorfman's ''obsession'' shows in his characterization of Paulina, whose strong memories of being raped and tortured still haunt her and provide a challenge to the historical revisionists who would claim that such events did not take place. Establishing a history of the victims will be an important step towards national reconciliation, but the question of just how satisfying such a process can be to Paulina and others like her is one of the more difficult issues presented in the play.

Morality and Ethics

The immorality of the past military regime is not debated in *Death and the Maiden;* the discussion of Paulina's torment and the mention of other cases of extra-judicial abduction, torture, and murder are enough to establish the context. The central ethical issue of the play is whether Paulina, by choosing to try—and punish—Miranda herself, is merely replicating the same injustices of the military regime. ''We can't use their methods,'' Gerardo comments. Paulina agrees in concept but feels that the circumstances are different. She also argues that she is giving Miranda the opportunity to defend himself, a privilege she was not granted.

STYLE

Death and the Maiden is highly realistic in form and structure, with a plot that rapidly unfolds in linear progression, characters that are fully-realized individuals, and a fixed, recognizable setting. Dorfman breaks with this basic structure only at the end of the play, when the setting jumps to a concert hall several months later. At this point, the playwright introduces an expressionistic device, a mirror aimed at the audience, to bring thematic unity to the piece. A fully realistic play would present some kind of resolution to the dramatic conflict but this is hardly possible in *Death and the Maiden.* Indeed, the play suggests precisely the difficulty of resolving the social issue which is at its heart: how can a society reconcile itself with its violent past and, somehow, move forward?

While it is the tendency of most theater critics to compare the work of different playwrights in order to give their readers a point of reference for a particular work, this has rarely been the case in the published criticism of *Death and the Maiden.* Critics have not been so focused on applying labels to Dorfman's theatrical technique, perhaps because they do not consider Dorfman—an intellectual and academic internationally known for his essays, novels, and poetry—to be primarily a playwright. Additionally, the content and political context of *Death and the Maiden* being so novel to English and American audiences, critics have focused more on these elements than on categorizing Dorfman's dramatic style.

As an exception to this tendency, one playwright with whom Dorfman is often related is Harold Pinter. The British playwright has remained an important touchstone for Dorfman; his first book was an academic study of the politics of oppression in Pinter's early play *The Room,* and he dedicates *Death and the Maiden* to Pinter. The connections between the two writers, however, are related more to their political investments than their dramatic techniques. An article by Stephen Gregory in *Comparative Drama,* for example, suggested how a retrospective reading of Dorfman's study of Pinter illustrates ''how it anticipates both the concerns of his later work on Latin America and the issues that will unite the two writers some twenty years after its publication.'' Dorfman hardly works in the style of Pinter, a playwright associated with the Theatre of the Absurd.

Literally meaning ''out of harmony,'' the term absurd was the existentialist Albert Camus's designation for the situation of modern men and women whose lives lack meaning as they drift in an inhuman universe. *Death and the Maiden* explores a political context which could properly be described as absurd, as a military regime prevents individuals from exerting any control over their own destiny. In terms of theatrical technique, however, Dorfman's play remains realistic in form without the stylistic exaggeration of Pinter's work, or that of other playwrights, such as Samuel Beckett (*Waiting for Godot*) and Eugene Ionesco (*The Bald Soprano*), who are usually labeled as absurdists.

While *Death and the Maiden* resists comparison with the work of contemporary playwrights, many have observed that it functions something like Greek tragedy. ''More than one critic,'' wrote John Butt in the *Times Literary Supplement,* ''has commented on this production's formal perfection, the way it unwinds with a remorseless inevitability that recalls the finest classical tragedy.'' In form, of course, the play differs from tragedy on many levels: it lacks, for example, the downfall and death of a hero or heroine and the ''anagnorisis'' or self-recognition on the part of that character about the mistake that led to his or her demise. Still, the parallels exist; Mimi Kramer noted in the *New Yorker* that ''the play observes classical rules about unity of time and place, and about offstage violence.''

Dorfman himself has used the term tragedy to refer to the work, responding to the suggestion that the play functions as political propaganda by saying in *Index on Censorship* that ''tragedies are never propaganda, ever.'' This comment is merely a suggestion of the thematic and dramatic complexity of the work, but Dorfman has explored the idea of tragedy further by examining the concept of catharsis, the social function of classical tragedy by which audiences would purge themselves of certain emotions. ''The play,'' Dorfman stated in the same article, ''is not just a denunciation of how bad torture is. It aims to help purge ourselves of pity and terror.'' In Greek society, the catharsis of tragedy helped to unify people, and Dorfman implies a hope that his play might serve the same role in Chilean society, further enabling the process of reconciliation with that country's past atrocities.

The device of the mirror at the conclusion of the play contributes most strongly to the process of catharsis. In an interview in the London *Times,* Dorfman said, in reference to the audience, that *Death and the Maiden* ''is not a play about somebody else, it's a play about them.'' The mirror coming down is a device which implicates them in the moral dilemma. ''People are going to watch themselves and ask: 'what would I do, who am I in the midst of all this?''' The mirror is also the element which separates the play from its realistic form and structure; it leaves the audience with a powerful image at the conclusion of a play whose central conflict remains otherwise unresolved.

HISTORICAL CONTEXT

Ariel Dorfman carefully specifies in his stage directions that *Death and the Maiden* is set in ''a country that is probably Chile but could be any country that has given itself a democratic government just after a long period of dictatorship.'' There is both a specificity and a universality to the play, as many critics have noted, making it extremely topical in the late-twentieth century era of tentative political transformation. Frank Rich of the *New York Times,* for example, called the play a ''mousetrap designed to catch the conscience of an international audience at a historic moment when many more nations than Chile are moving from totalitarian terror to fragile freedom.'' John Butt similarly found the play ''timely,'' saying that it catches the audience ''in a neat moral trap'' by making them ''confront choices that most would presumably leave to the inhabitants of remote and less favoured countries.''

Among the many Latin American countries which in recent decades have similarly experienced periods of military rule (Guatemala, Brazil, Bolivia), Argentina and Chile are often compared to one another because of their shared history and close geographical proximity in the ''Southern Cone'' of South America. Both Chile, following Augusto Pinochet's military coup, and Argentina, in the years of the military's ''Dirty War,'' were characterized by civil repression, extra-judicial abductions and ''disappearances,'' torture, and murder. Familiarity with the modern history of these two countries provides a good basis of understanding for the context of *Death and the Maiden.*

Throughout the first half of the twentieth century in Chile, the political climate swung often between right and left with no government strong enough to effect large scale change. Infrastructure developed slowly and rural poverty became an increasing problem, along with rapid urbanization as desperate populations flooded the city. Some social reforms were achieved in the 1960s, but Chile's politics became increasingly polarized and militant. Salvador Allende crept to presidential victory in 1970 with a leftist coalition of socialists, communists, and extremists. Allende's sweeping economic reforms included the state takeover of many private enterprises; the United States was angered by the confiscation of U.S.-controlled copper mines and Chile's openly friendly relationship with Cuba, a country with whom America had ceased diplomatic and economic ties.

The Chilean military, in a coup orchestrated by General Augusto Pinochet, seized power on September 11, 1973, using air force jets to bomb the presidential palace. (U.S. support of the coup through the Central Intelligence Agency [CIA] has been documented.) Allende died, apparently a suicide, and thousands of his supporters were killed. Pinochet,

COMPARE & CONTRAST

- **1992:** Augusto Pinochet, who handed over the Chilean presidency in 1990 to democratically-elected Patricio Aylwin Azocar, remains commander in chief of the army.

  Today: Pinochet has stepped down as army commander but in March, 1998, was bestowed the title of senator for life, despite widespread protest.

- **1992:** With Pinochet still their commander in chief, the Chilean armed forces continue to wield a good deal of autonomous power in Chilean society.

  Today: There is still considerable tension between the government and the military concerning the human rights violations of the Pinochet era. Although current president Eduardo Frei has accelerated human rights tribunals and inquiries into Chile's "disappeared," punishment of the perpetrators remains extremely difficult.

- **1992:** The era of Apartheid is gradually drawing to a close in South Africa, with whites voting two to one in a referendum to give President F. W. de Klerk a mandate to end white-minority rule. A June massacre in a black township, however, and charges of police involvement in the case, suggest the pressing need for more rapid transformation.

  Today: While many political, social, and economic difficulties remain for South Africa, the peaceful transfer of power to President Nelson Mandela makes the country an excellent example of how a society can make the difficult transition to democracy.

- **1992:** Peru's President Alberto Fujimori suspends the Constitution April 5, and assumes dictatorial powers in the fight against corruption and Maoist guerrilla group Sendera Luminosa ("Shining Path"). The United States suspends aid to Peru.

  Today: On April 22, 1997, President Fujimori orders a military attack against a group of leftist guerrillas who have held hostages for several months in the Japanese embassy in the capitol of Lima. All fourteen of the guerrillas are killed, along with two soldiers, and one of the hostages; many others are wounded. Fujimori's actions are celebrated internationally, but nagging issues remain, including damaged relations with Japan (who had pushed for a peaceful negotiation to end the standoff), and accusations that Fujimori has used government intelligence forces to investigate political opponents. Throughout Latin America, the continued existence of guerrilla activity combined with hard-line government policies suggest the continued fragility of many of the region's democracies.

at the head of a four-man ruling junta (a group or council that controls a government), dissolved Chile's congress and repressed—often violently—political opposition. His government maintained power for the next decade and a half, frequently resorting to terror (including the abduction/tortures to which Paulina was subjected) in order to suppress dissent.

A peaceful transfer of presidential power was achieved in 1990 but considerable tension continued between the military and the government concerning the human rights violations of the Pinochet era. Under a constitution written during his regime, Pinochet himself remained army commander until stepping down in March, 1998. Yet after that time he still retained congressional influence with the title of senator for life. Chilean society continues to struggle with the violent legacy of its past, although current president Eduardo Frei has sped the process of reconciliation by accelerating human rights tribunals and inquiries into Chile's "disappeared" (through commissions like the one to which Gerardo has been appointed in *Death and the Maiden*).

Chile's neighbor, Argentina, has likewise seen frequent suppression of democratic processes. The country experienced its first coup in 1930, the government falling to a coalition of military officers and civilian aristocrats who established a semi-fascist state following the growing trend of fascism in Europe. The military undertook a more forceful coup in 1943, one which set out to restructure Argentine culture totally. The goal this time was not the mere suppression of political radicals but the complete eradication of civilian politics. There were to be five more coups between 1943 and 1976, the year in which the military initiated the brutality known as the Dirty War. During this period, Argentina's most influential ruler was Colonel Juan Peron, first elected to the presidency in 1946.

Peron was different from his military predecessors in that he sought to integrate the urban working class into his party, although his government retained a strong hand on more hard-line radicalism. Peron's partner in everything during the early years of his presidency was his mistress, later his wife, Eva Duarte—known popularly as Evita (composer Andrew Lloyd Weber and lyricist Tim Rice would immortalize her in their 1978 musical *Evita*). She had cunning political instinct, upon which Peron grew to rely. When the military threw Peron over in 1955, many of the social changes he and Evita had initiated remained in place. The legacy of Evita (she died of cancer in 1952), combined with the knowledge that Peron was alive in exile, empowered many to adhere to Peronist ideals, despite the military's attempts to suppress them. Peron was resurrected in 1973 as the economic situation in Argentina continued to worsen, and the public, looking for some positive way out of the military regimes, enthusiastically welcomed his return; he died a mere eight months into his new term as president.

A coup on March 24, 1976, overthrew Peron's widow Isabel, president since his death, and a military junta composed of the three commanders in chief of the armed forces installed itself as the government. In the years between the coup and the resumption of democratic elections in 1983, the military fought a vicious and covert war against the people of Argentina, totally restructuring society to eradicate any political consciousness. A system of clandestine concentration camps, numbering over three hundred at their peak, provided the center of an all-out policy of abduction, torture, murder, and disposal. Estimates of the dead run as high as thirty thousand, and the lives of the survivors were left destroyed in other ways. As in Chile, following a tenuous return to democracy Argentine society at large continues to struggle with the issue of how to rectify the violence of the past. Activists such as Las Madres de Plaza de Mayo (who daringly initiated protests against the military government while it was still in power) maintain pressure on the current government to investigate human rights abuses, although punishment for many of the perpetrators remains unlikely.

CRITICAL OVERVIEW

From the time of its debut, the international reception of *Death and the Maiden* was largely positive, extending Dorfman's reputation as an important writer and intellectual. Reviews of the Broadway production were less enthusiastic, but critics differ on whether the weaknesses were the result of failings in the play, the performances (Glenn Close, Richard Dreyfuss, and Gene Hackman), or the direction of Mike Nichols. English and American audiences lacked the political experience of a recent return to democracy, shared by so many emerging nations in this era, yet the play is easily accessible to them. Matt Wolf wrote in the *Times* of London that the play was an unlikely success given its topic, but "Dorfman argues that its time is now. 'It clearly has touched some sort of nerve, some sort of centre.'" As "a play about the empowerment of women," *Death and the Maiden* grounds the anger of Paulina in concrete historical circumstances, yet universalizes it. "Her rage," Dorfman stated to Wolfe, "comes out of something . . . that can be understood as the product of a system. At the same time, she is clearly speaking for more than torture victims."

Also inspired by the excellence of the London production, Andrew Graham-Yooll commented in *Index on Censorship,* "The conflict between the three characters, the suspect's denial, the woman's search for revenge, and the husband's need for justice, create gripping, thrilling and intense theatre." The *Times Literary Supplement*'s Butt, meanwhile, called the play "harrowing." He observed that *Death and the Maiden* might draw some criticism for failing to provide any solutions to the moral dilemma it presents, any "easy answers to the question of how the new democracies should deal with the criminals in their midst." The critic, however, found this dramatic choice to be more true to experience and a real strength of the play: "In fact, the play's depressing message is that none of the three characters can offer a solution because all are still re-living the past.''

In citing negative aspects of the Broadway production, Frank Rich of the *New York Times* nevertheless praised the strength of Dorfman's play. What makes it ''ingenious,'' he wrote, is the playwright's ''ability to raise such complex issues within a thriller that is full of action and nearly devoid of preaching.'' Rich found that despite the heavy star power of the Broadway production, its light tone diminished the inherent strengths of Dorfman's complex play. Rich wrote that ''it is no small feat that the director Mike Nichols has managed to transform 'Death and the Maiden' into a fey domestic comedy. But what kind of feat, exactly?'' Rich found the direction and characterizations flat and one-dimensional, producing an ironic and ''tedious trivialization of Ariel Dorfman's work.'' Nichols took a similar approach in his film version of Edward Albee's *Who's Afraid of Virginia Woolf?* noted Rich but there produced a ''funnier though still valid alternative'' to the play. ''But what exactly,'' wondered Rich about the current production, ''is the point of his jokey take on a play whose use of the word death in the title is anything but ironic?''

Mimi Kramer in the *New Yorker* similarly criticized the Broadway production in comparison to the London one but found the inadequacies to be a product of Dorfman's ''obvious'' and ''flaccid'' play. ''The questions raised by 'Death and the Maiden' have been oft before but ne'er so ploddingly explored,'' she wrote. The play takes too long to set up its central conflict, Kramer felt, dwells too long on the irony of Paulina contemplating doing just what her tormentors did to her, and ''never gets much beyond that idea.'' Thomas M. Disch of the *Nation* also found that the weaknesses of the play and of the production reflected one another. ''The plot is all too simple,'' he wrote, the characters ''generic and hollow,'' and Dorfman ''neither engages one's emotions nor thinks through the situation with any rigor.'' The director cannot be blamed for the result, Disch concluded, ''nor yet can the cast, who do no more and no less than Hollywood stars usually do—play themselves, for lack of any better-defined roles.''

In concert with Kramer, John Simon identified weaknesses in Dorfman's play. He wrote in *New York* magazine of the ''unconvincing'' devices which establish the dramatic situation in the play, and other flaws of technique. ''Yet these are small matters,'' he continues, ''compared to the basic insufficiency of reducing a national and individual tragedy to a mere whodunit.'' For Simon, the play fails because of this trivialization. And whereas Butt found the lack of resolution in the play to be a strength, Simon argued that because the play ''avoids coming satisfactorily to grips with the one question it raises,'' it cannot succeed as a whodunit, either.

Jack Kroll of *Newsweek* also argued that Dorfman lessened the impact of his play by turning it into a ''whodunnit.'' One effect of his choice was that it allowed the director, quoted as saying ''God preserve us all from a true political play,'' to turn the production into a ''domestic imbroglio.'' Kroll's assessment falls somewhere in between Simon, who found the play a failure, and Rich, who argued its strength despite the nature of the Broadway production. *Death and the Maiden* remains ''a fiercely political play,'' Kroll commented, and if Dorfman had only forced his character Miranda to face his own guilt, this one change could have produced the ''masterwork'' that many critics have called the play, and enabled the star actors ''to reach an emotional focus that they only glancingly hit in this production.''

Apart from reviews of the premiere productions and interviews with Dorfman, there exists yet little criticism of *Death and the Maiden.* Most articles and other extended works on Dorfman focus on his novels, poetry, or his experience as a critic and artist in exile. One exception is Stephen Gregory's lengthy article for *Comparative Drama,* which explores parallels between Dorfman and British playwright Harold Pinter.

CRITICISM

Christopher G. Busiel

Death and the Maiden *is a play fundamentally concerned with memory, exploring the relationship (and occasional conflict) between personal and institutional memories. In this essay, Busiel examines these and other issues.*

Ariel Dorfman observed in an interview with Carlos Reyes on the Amnesty International website, ''Memory is a constant obsession for me. I deal often with people who are fighting against those who would obliterate others, who would forget them, ignore them, neglect them, erase them from the earth.'' Memory becomes an obsession in the context of a society confronting the legacy of a

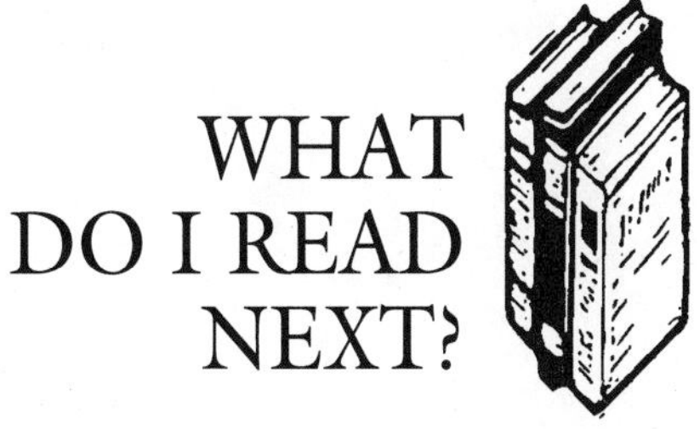

WHAT DO I READ NEXT?

- *Widows,* a 1981 novel by Dorfman, later adapted into a play of the same name. *Widows* focuses on a group of thirty-seven women who suspect that their missing husbands have been abducted and killed by authorities of their government. Dorfman set the novel in occupied Greece in the 1940s to avoid censorship but changed the setting to Chile when he created the stage adaptation. Depicting the experience of people seeking justice under a repressive regime, *Widows* provides an interesting counterpoint to *Death and the Maiden.*
- *How to Read Donald Duck: Imperialist Ideology in the Disney Comic,* an early work of criticism by Dorfman, which illustrates his argument that forms of popular literature such as comic books have historically been used to promote capitalist ideology and encourage passivity, specifically for the benefit of American business interests in Latin America.
- *La casa de los espiritus* (1982), the first novel by Isabel Allende, now one of the world's most widely read Hispanic writers, whose father was first cousin to Chilean President Salvador Allende (the novel was translated by Magda Bogin as *The House of the Spirits* and published by Knopf, 1985). Allende, like Paulina in *Death and the Maiden* helped transport people to avoid military repression after Pinochet's coup. The events she witnessed, ''the dead, the tortured, the widows and orphans, left an unforgettable impression on my memory,'' and were incorporated into this work.
- *Allende: A Novel,* by Fernando Alegria, is a biography of Salvador Allende cast in a novel form, illustrating ''how fiction and history occasionally ''collide, then merge, enriching and refining each other.''
- *Chilean Writers in Exile: Eight Short Novels,* edited by Fernando Alegria (Crossing Press, 1981) presents ''an expression of a group of writers who, in spite of all the hardships of life in exile, are producing vigorous statements on behalf of the Chilean people.'' The collection, which contains Dorfman's *Putamadre,* offers the opportunity to compare different perspectives on Chilean politics and life in exile, as expressed in fiction.
- *Extremities,* by William Mastrosimone, a contemporary American play about a woman victimized by a rapist in her own home, who manages to turn the tables and trap her attacker. The play (which was made into a film in 1986 starring Farah Fawcett) makes an interesting contrast to *Death and the Maiden* because of the revenge theme and the different ways in which it is played out.

---

repressive regime, where painful individual memories of past injustices are often eradicated by a government which wants to forget the past or even deny that such violence ever occurred.

In Dorfman's *Death and the Maiden,* it is years after Paulina's abduction and torment, yet her memory of the experience remains crystal clear. She concludes without a doubt in her own mind that Roberto Miranda is the doctor who tortured and raped her, drawing on particular details such as the Schubert quartet, Miranda's quoting of Nietzsche, his smell, his voice, and the feel of his skin. Gerardo questions the value of Paulina's evidence and Miranda calls her memories ''fantasies of a diseased mind,'' but Paulina remains resolute. While a few details of her experience had initially appeared fuzzy, Paulina reveals in the course of the play that she obscured information in order to protect her loved ones from pain or possible danger. Gerardo, for example, has always believed that Paulina does not remember how many times she was raped in captivity: ''I didn't count, you said.'' But Paulina

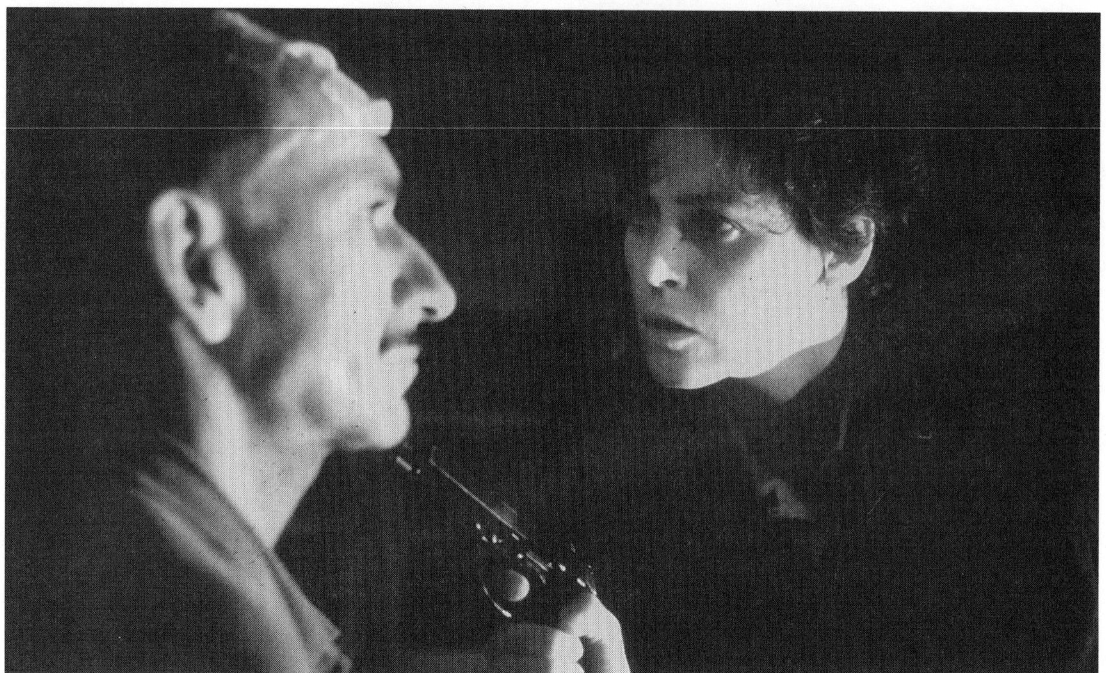

Miranda and Paulina (Sigourney Weaver) in a tense moment

confronts him with the fact that she always knew exactly—she merely hid the fact from Gerardo because he was so obviously uncomfortable with the details of her experience.

Death and the Maiden unfolds simultaneously forward and in reverse; in fact there is very little forward movement of plot in comparison to the unfolding of the past which occurs in the course of the play. Dorfman's primary theme of the past affecting the present is also a central stylistic device built into his play's technique. The two threads are intricately bound: just as a country cannot move forward by forgetting its history, the play's present tense narrative depends utterly on the events of the past. There is the painful legacy of Paulina's abduction and the question regarding Miranda's role in her rape and torture; Gerardo's affair with another woman while Paulina was in captivity is another painful memory that is revealed as the play's narrative progresses. Paulina's perception of the past is clear, but she struggles with the issue of just how she should remedy these injustices. Indeed, John Butt observed in the *Times Literary Supplement* that "the play's depressing message is that none of the three characters can offer a solution because all are still re-living the past." Like the society of which they are a part (probably, but not exclusively, Chilean), all three must find a productive way to move forward.

In a play contrasting the ideal and the practical, Paulina and Gerardo differ in their respective concepts of justice under the present circumstances. Consequently, they also differ in their notions of how both individuals and society at large can address their painful memories of the past and what, exactly, can be done with this knowledge. Gerardo believes in the efficacy of the commission (and the country's new "democratic" government) to which he has been appointed, feeling that justice will be served by faithfully investigating human rights abuses and then turning the findings over to the country's courts. He sees Paulina as emotionally trapped by memories that she must somehow put behind her. "You're still a prisoner," Gerardo tells Paulina, "you stayed behind with them, locked in that basement." Gerardo encourages her to "free yourself from them" in order to put her mind at rest.

While the play is not largely sympathetic to Gerardo or his point of view, Dorfman explained in the Amnesty International interview that he can understand the political value of Gerardo's perspective: "In a transition to a democracy as in Chile, Bolivia, South Africa, there are different reasons why people do not want to remember. They say,

'Look, if we keep on stirring up the past it's going to destroy us.' This includes many who were themselves repressed, hurt or part of the resistance.'' Seeking to turn the page and move into a productive future, individuals like Gerardo hope that their society can reach a consensus and doing so often requires ''excluding those who continue to remember.''

Paulina is insulted by Gerardo's implication that her only option is to forget her pain; in her mind, justice cannot possibly be served through the channels which presently exist, so she takes the law into her own hands. To Gerardo, Paulina's actions ''open all the wounds,'' but Paulina's wounds have been festering for years, and her action is the beginning of a process of healing. She mocks Gerardo's suggestion that she merely let Miranda go, so that years from now ''we see him at the Tavelli and we smile at him, he introduces his lovely wife to us and we smile and we all shake hands and we comment on how warm it is this time of the year.'' Gerardo, meanwhile, perceives himself as realistic and does not mean to trivialize Paulina's pain and anger when he states: ''basically, yes, that is what we have to do'' in order for *society* to begin its process of healing.

The question of whether Miranda is the doctor who tortured and raped Paulina is the central dramatic conflict in *Death and the Maiden,* but the play contains the larger thematic issue of how a society should confront a violent and repressive past, specifically reconciling conflicting memories of what occurred in this era. Establishing a history of the victims will be a valuable step towards national reconciliation, and the tape recording Paulina makes for Gerardo is an important trial run for his work on the commission. It is an interview much like the ones he will conduct in a professional capacity, but the process also has strong implications for the couple putting their own personal demons to rest. ''That's the way,'' Gerardo states, ''that's how we'll get out of this mess—without hiding a thing from each other, together.'' Dorfman himself believes in the importance of truth commissions such as the one to which Gerardo has been appointed, for even if they have little or no power to punish the guilty, they do establish a social or institutional memory. ''The previous regime,'' Dorfman told Reyes, ''lived by telling this falsity: This never happened to you.'' The commissions can be crucial, therefore, because they ''are able to establish certain truths in a public way, to become part of official history.'' Just how satisfying such a process can be

"JUST AS A COUNTRY CANNOT MOVE FORWARD BY FORGETTING ITS HISTORY, *DEATH AND THE MAIDEN*'S PRESENT TENSE NARRATIVE DEPENDS UTTERLY ON THE EVENTS OF THE PAST."

to Paulina and others like her, however, lingers as one of the more difficult issues presented in the play.

When the mirror is lowered near the conclusion of *Death and the Maiden,* a powerful image is introduced which implicates the audience in the play's central social conflict. ''The point about the play is that it works in the grey zone of ambiguity,'' Dorfman related to Andrew Graham-Yooll in *Index on Censorship.* ''It allows each person in the audience, or each reader, to ask themselves who they are in relation to each character.'' To assess one's own investment is part of the process of rectifying different memories, conflicting narratives of what occurred in the past. ''In Chile, everybody has lived that situation. How do you make the truth, how do you pervert one truth to bring out another?'' Certainly, the image of the mirror functions somewhat ambiguously, as indeed does the conclusion of the play itself. Dorfman's characters are forced to move forward, putting the past at rest without necessarily resolving it. What is a personal issue for them is reflected in the social quandary faced by countries like Chile or Argentina, in which the process of investigation goes on despite the promise of a clear resolution any time in the near future.

Dorfman commented to Matt Wolf in the London *Times* that the impact of *Death and the Maiden* stems largely from the fact that ''there are few plays about the real difficulties of the transition to democracy and few plays about violence and memory that work in this way.'' Indeed, it is a tribute to the strength of the play, and to Dorfman's experience as a novelist as well, that the playwright was able to explore the implications of the past so fully while still meeting the theatre's requirements for an exciting and dramatically viable plot. The play's intriguing treatment of memory is thus at the center of

> "AS A WHODUNIT, *DEATH AND THE MAIDEN* FAILS BECAUSE IT AVOIDS COMING SATISFACTORILY TO GRIPS WITH THE ONE QUESTION IT RAISES."

both its current political topicality and its lingering literary value.

Source: Christopher G. Busiel, for *Drama for Students,* Gale, 1998.

John Simon

In this unfavorable review, Simon feels that Dorfman fumbles an opportunity to expound upon the subjects of dictatorships and human rights violations. Death and the Maiden, *he feels, is nothing more than a contrived mystery.*

Ariel Dorfman, the Chilean writer, brings us his *Death and the Maiden,* a drama set in a country that, the program coyly tells us, "is probably Chile." A long era of dictatorship has yielded to a new democracy, and Gerardo Escobar, a lawyer, has been appointed to the presidential commission investigating political crimes. Driving back to his beach house, he blows a tire and, having neither a spare nor a jack (much is made of these two unconvincing circumstances), gets a stranger, Dr. Miranda, to give him a lift home. By an even less persuasive device, Miranda drops in after midnight, and Gerardo's wife, Paulina, recognizes him (or so she thinks) as the man who, fifteen years ago, participated in torturing her and repeatedly raped her. But she keeps mum.

Miranda accepts Gerardo's invitation to spend the night (more stretching of credibility), and while he sleeps, Paulina knocks him out, drags him into the living room, ties him to a chair, and gags him. In the morning, she is seated beside him with a gun. She tells her flabbergasted husband that they will hold a trial; Gerardo is to be the defense, Paulina the witness, prosecutor, and judge. Miranda, when he does get a chance to speak, flatly denies being *that* doctor. Paulina, we gather, has been mentally unbalanced since those terrible events: Is she capable of determining what's what? And how will she deal with Miranda if he is found guilty?

But we do not get enough of the Escobars' home life to infer just how crazy Paulina is. Or enough about this society to deduce whether Miranda's loving Schubert's famous quartet and quoting (or misquoting) Nietzsche constitute enough grounds for identifying a person. We don't even know what to make of the fact that former evildoers are to be ferreted out but granted amnesty. Yet these are small matters compared to the basic insufficiency of reducing a national and individual tragedy to a mere whodunit. For despite the little grace (or disgrace) notes of humorous squabbles and troubled personal relationships, the play is really all is-he-or-isn't-he, did-he-or-didn't-he: too trivial for the amount of suffering on which it is predicated. Can you imagine *Hamlet* if its only real concern were whether Claudius did or did not poison his brother?

Yet even as a whodunit, *Death and the Maiden* fails because it avoids coming satisfactorily to grips with the one question it raises. Would Agatha Christie leave a murder unresolved and then pride herself on her ambiguity? And it isn't as if the wit, pathos, or language here were good enough to carry the play or even a half-pound paperweight. Mike Nichols's direction does not seem to achieve more than anyone else's would, and the acting does rather less. Gene Hackman is a believable Miranda, perhaps because he is spared the excesses of Dorfman's fancy writing. But Richard Dreyfuss's lawyer is only Richard Dreyfuss, take it or leave it. As for Glenn Close, she is not exactly bad but seems, as usual, miscast. For Miss Close is almost always a bit too much this or not enough that; with rare exceptions, her performances leave you undernourished or overstuffed. Personally, I would have loved to see Mary Beth Hurt or Laila Robins in the part, or indeed Lizbeth Mackay, Miss Close's talented standby.

Curiously, Tony Walton, perhaps having shot his wad on *Baboons,* has under—or misdesigned—the scenery, which is sparse and a bit bewildering. And Jules Fisher's lighting (no doubt at Nichols's behest) turns illicitly stylized for a naturalistic play. But Ann Roth's costumes are suitably understated. Last time, I reviewed a terrible play by Richard Caliban. Here, despite an Ariel and a Miranda, things are not appreciably better.

Source: John Simon, "The Guary Apes," in *New York,* March 30, 1992, pp. 87–88.

Gerald Weales

Weales offers a mixed appraisal of the 1992 New York production of Dorfman's play, finding the play's ambiguous ending frustrating. The critic did note, however, that the work deals with important issues and makes for adequate entertainment.

Somewhere beneath the slick and enervating surface of Ariel Dorfman's *Death and the Maiden,* there are serious themes struggling to get out. The play is set in ''a country that is probably Chile,'' one that has recently emerged from a dictatorship and has become, tentatively, a democracy. The question—one that is asked every day in Eastern Europe, in South and Central America, in Africa—is whether the new nearly democratic health of a country depends on the recognition and punishment of the oppressors from the past or whether the present is better served—as Mussolini's sexpot granddaughter was saying on television recently—by dismissing all that ugliness as history. In Dorfman's play there are advocates of recognition and of punishment, although not necessarily of both. Gerardo Escobar (Richard Dreyfuss) is a lawyer who has been named to a commission, with minimal power, that will investigate charges of wrongdoing—very wrongdoing—in the past. His wife, Paulina Salas (Glenn Close), who was raped and tortured in an attempt to extract information from her, is understandably obsessed by what happened to her and aches to punish the villains. Circumstances provide an occasion. Roberto Miranda (Gene Hackman), who has earlier rescued Escobar, stranded on the road by a plot device, drops by in the middle of the night to congratulate Escobar or perhaps to soften him up in case his name should come up in the hearings. Paulina recognizes (or thinks she does) Miranda as the Schubert-loving doctor who led her torturers; she ties him up, demands a mock trial, threatens to be judge and executioner.

Escobar is potentially the most interesting character. Miranda either is or is not the torture doctor; Paulina either will or will not kill him. Escobar finally sides with Miranda and feeds him information, which he may not need, for the confession Paulina demands. Escobar's motivation is nicely unclear. His distress at Paulina's homemade vengeance may result from his belief in proper legal proceedings, even though he knows that the judiciary is still shot through with appointees of the old regime; after all, *we* do not want to be like *them.* He may be afraid that Paulina's irrational behavior will

"IN DORFMAN'S PLAY THERE ARE ADVOCATES OF RECOGNITION AND OF PUNISHMENT, ALTHOUGH NOT NECESSARILY OF BOTH."

wreck his career, stain his growing importance within the new government. It may be a bit of male bonding; we learn that while Paulina was under arrest, risking her life to protect Escobar's name, he was having an affair.

In the next to last scene, Escobar having been sent offstage, Paulina listens to Miranda's confession and decides to kill him anyway. After an impassioned speech about the way victims are expected to act in a civilized way (''And why does it always have to be people like me who have to sacrifice''), she holds a gun to his head and. . .blackout. In the published play, Dorfman asks for a mirror to descend so that the audience can see itself while a spotlight picks out one playgoer after another. This effect would presumably generalize the theme, take the play away from Paulina, who may or may not be mad, and prepare for the final scene. There, the three principals, formally dressed, arrive at a concert to hear a little Schubert. Dorfman may intend a final ambiguity to an ambiguous play—a testimony to Paulina's unwillingness to act as her torturers did, an indication that the past is to be smoothed over by social ritual, or, given the look exchanged between Paulina and Miranda, a confession that the questions the play presumably faces are questions still.

If this sounds like an interesting—even an important—play, it certainly did not seem so in the theater. Part of the problem lies with Dorfman. Although moral problems can certainly be carried by a thriller or a mystery, here the emphasis is on the is-he-or-isn't-he of Miranda and the possibility that Paulina may have been driven mad by her experience. More of the blame lies with director Mike Nichols. That blackout on the gun-wielding Paulina is a case in point. It comes across not as her hesitation, but as a directorial tease, an attempt to pump suspense into a flaccid melodrama. The three stars, all of whom have done admirable work elsewhere, seem simply to be going through the motions of performance. Everything is as elegant and sterile as Tony Walton's set. I found I did not believe in any of the characters nor care about their dilemmas which meant that it was also difficult to dig for the half-buried serious themes.

Source: Gerald Weales, ''Go Ahead, Shoot,'' in *Commonweal,* Volume CXIX, no. 9, May 8, 1992 , p. 21.

SOURCES

Butt, John. ''Guilty Conscience?'' in the *Times Literary Supplement,* February 28, 1992, p. 22.

Disch, Thomas M. Review of *Death and the Maiden* in the *Nation,* May 11, 1992, pp. 640-43.

Dorfman, Ariel. Afterword to *Death and the Maiden,* Penguin (New York), 1992, pp. 71-75.

Kramer, Mimi. ''Magical Opportunism'' in the *New Yorker,* March 30, 1992, p. 69.

Kroll, Jack. ''Broadway Mind-Stretchers'' in *Newsweek,* March 30, 1992, p. 65.

Reyes, Carlos, and Maggie Patterson. ''Ariel Dorfman on Memory and Truth'' on the Amnesty International Home Page, http://www.oneworld.org/textver/amnesty/journal_july97/carlos.html.

Rich, Frank. ''Close, Hackman and Dreyfuss in 'Death and the Maiden''' in the *New York Times,* March 18, 1992, p. C15.

Simon, John. ''The Guary Apes'' in *New York,* March 30, 1992, pp. 87-88.

Wolf, Matt. ''Power Games at Home'' in the *Times* (London), November 4, 1991, p. 14.

FURTHER READING

Contemporary Literary Criticism, Gale: Vol. 48, 1988, Vol. 77, 1993.

This resource compiles selections of criticism; it is an excellent starting point for a research paper on Dorfman. The selections in these two volumes span Dorfman's career up to 1993 (criticism of *Death and the Maiden* is found in Volume 77). Dorfman is also covered in *Hispanic Writers, Hispanic Literary Criticism,* and Volume 130 of *Contemporary Authors.*

Graham-Yooll, Andrew. ''Dorfman: A Case of Conscience'' in *Index on Censorship,* Vol. 20, no. 6, 1991, pp. 3-4.

An interview with Dorfman in which the playwright discusses Chile's transition to democracy and his own plays *Reader* and *Death and Maiden.*

Gregory, Stephen. ''Ariel Dorfman and Harold Pinter: Politics of the Periphery and Theater of the Metropolis'' in *Comparative Drama,* Vol. 30, no. 3, 1996, pp. 325-45.

An article that fleshes out the ''string of contingencies'' between these two writers. Gregory's article presents ''a summary of the writers' respective political involvements and commitments,'' continues with an analysis of several plays (including *Death and the Maiden*), and concludes ''with a retrospective political reading of Dorfman's study of Pinter to show how it anticipates both the concerns of his later work on Latin America and the issues that will unite the two writers some twenty years after its publication.''

Guzman, Patricio. *The Battle of Chile* (re-release), First Run/Icarus Films, 1998.

A documentary, produced in the years 1973-1976, which is still banned in Chile to this day. The film presents a leftist perspective on Salvador Allende's presidency, the coup of Pinochet, and the first ''years of terror'' following the installation of the dictatorship. Guzman's more recent work also includes the film *Chile: The Persistent Memory.*

Skidmore, Thomas E. and Peter H. Smith. *Modern Latin America,* fourth edition, Oxford University Press (New York), 1997.

A comprehensive, general resource on the interrelated political histories of this vast region. It is particularly useful in understanding the context of Dorfman's play, applicable to Chile as well as to a number of other Latin American countries who have experienced periods of military repression. Students interested specifically in the history of modern Chile may investigate some of the many books on the topic, such as Mark Falcoff's *Modern Chile, 1970-1989: A Critical History* (published by Transaction, 1989).

Electra

SOPHOCLES

c. 409 B.C.

Sophocles's *Electra,* written around 409 B.C., is based on the legend of the House of Atreus, a story which contemporary Greek audiences would have known from childhood. The major themes of this story concern retribution for crimes committed within the family of Atreus, who was Electra's grandfather. Electra's duty in the play is to avenge her father's murder, but this involves killing her own mother, another crime which will have consequences down the line.

Sophocles's tragedy deals with the fate of mortals such as Electra and her brother Orestes, who act out lives which seem on the one hand to be determined by the gods, yet on the other hand are shaped by decisions made by seemingly autonomous individuals. One reason why Sophocles's plays were so successful was that he was able to articulate this complex and problematic relationship between humans and gods in a probing yet eloquent manner. His audiences responded to Electra's filial duty to avenge her father's death, for this was an honorable deed, and they were affected by the tragic consequences which it involved.

The powerful characters in *Electra* express many emotions with which Athenian audiences identified. Many of these themes still prove captivating centuries later, for they are universal human feelings of love and hate, suffering and triumph. Critics have noted that in other versions of the same story, such as Aeschylus's *Oresteia* trilogy, events

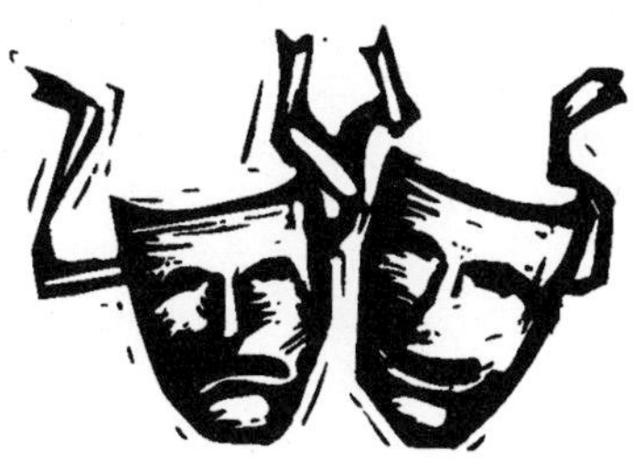

are presented as the result of destiny, whereas Sophocles brings the action down to the human sphere and causes his audience to wonder at the level of responsibility which man has for his own actions.

AUTHOR BIOGRAPHY

Sophocles was born in Colonus, near Athens, Greece, circa 496 B.C. The son of a prosperous family, he was well-respected in his day for his dramatic writings as well as for his civic and religious service. When Athens defeated the Persians in the naval victory at Salamis in 480 B.C., the sixteen-year-old Sophocles led an important choral performance in a ceremony celebrating the Athenian victory. A friend of Athenian leader Pericles, he served as a general in the Samian War (440-439 B.C.). He was also a priest of the minor deity Amynos and demonstrated religious devotion by taking the sacred snake of Asclepius (the god of healing and medicine) into his house while a shrine was being prepared for it.

Sophocles studied tragedy under Aeschylus, defeating his mentor in the Great Dionysia of 468 B.C. The Dionysia were yearly festivals held in Athens in honor of the god Dionysus and featured drama competitions between rival playwrights. Sophocles won first prize in 468 B.C. with his *Triptolemos,* one of his many lost plays, and is said to have won first prize more than twenty times at the festival. He never placed below second in these competitions, an unequaled record. Of his work which survives, there are seven complete tragedies and fragments of ninety other plays or poems; he was believed to have written one hundred and twenty-three plays in total. The best-known of his works are the plays *Antigone* (c. 442 B.C.), *Oedipus the King* (c. 430 B.C.), and *Electra* (c. 409 B.C.).

Much of Sophocles's success can be attributed to his innovations in the theater. Perhaps the most important of these modifications was the introduction of a third actor in his tragedies, which allowed for more complex dialogue and interactions between the characters. Traditionally, there had been only two actors in each episode of a play, along with the chorus. Sophocles also altered the composition of the chorus, reducing its size to fifteen members (compared to the fifty members that Aeschylus used). Additionally, he brought an element of realism to the stage itself by introducing painted scenery, addtional props, and more expressive masks (the masks were worn by actors to differentiate characters).

Sophocles died c. 406 B.C. in Athens. His death nearly coincided with the end of Athens's dominance of Greek culture, when the powerful city-state was defeated in the Peloponnesian War (431-404 B.C.). Indeed, his life spanned Athens's Golden Age, and his plays contributed significantly to the rich cultural life of his time. After his death, a cult was founded to honor him as a hero.

PLOT SUMMARY

The play opens at dawn in Mycenae, where Paidagogos and Orestes stand before the palace of the slain Agamemnon, discussing how best to revenge the murdered king. The god Apollo instructed Orestes to seek revenge, not by ''shield nor army'' but ''secretly'' and with his own hand. Orestes plans to have Paidagogos enter the palace carrying an funeral urn full of ashes and announce that Orestes has been killed in a chariot race.

Electra enters alone, mourning the fate of her murdered father, Agamemnon, and hoping for the arrival of her brother, Orestes, so together they can seek revenge. A Chorus of Myceneaen women enters, singing a ''kommos,'' or song of lament. The Chorus suggests that Electra accept her fate, reminding her that the weak cannot destroy the strong and offering stoic advice to accept life's troubles—after all, everyone dies. Above all, they urge her to be reasonable, advising her: ''Do not feed your frenzy.''

Electra's sister Chrysothemis enters, and Electra urges her to help revenge their father's murder. Chrysothemis refuses, seeming at times both reasonable and cowardly. Chrysothemis leaves, and Electra continues her lamentation, as the Chorus continues urging her to be reasonable—though they concede the justice of her vengeful intentions.

Chrysothemis re-enters, telling Electra that when their mother's new husband, Aegisthos, returns, he plans to hide Electra away to punish her for her public mourning. Chrysothemis tells Electra about their mother's dream. Upset by the dream, Clytemnestra ordered Chrysothemis to put offerings on the grave of Agamemnon.

Clytemnestra appears and argues with Electra, attempting to justify Agamemnon's murder, done in part to avenge the death of their daughter Iphigeneia, whom Agamemnon sacrificed to the gods. Like her father, however, Electra saw the sacrifice as necessary to appease the will of the gods, who would have prevented the Athenic fleet from sailing to Troy unless Iphigeneia was offered. Also, Electra asks why, if revenge for Iphigeneia was her sole motivation, Clytemnestra has married her husband's killer?

Paidagogos enters, disguised as a traveler who offers the false news of Orestes's death. Clytemnestra's feelings are mixed: she is sad that her child has been killed but relieved that her husband's avenger is no longer pursuing her. Electra is distraught over the news of her brother's death and again the Chorus urges acceptance. Clytemnestra is relieved she has no revenge to fear from Electra.

Chrysothemis enters, telling Electra the good news that their brother Orestes has arrived. Chrysothemis has found offerings to Agamemnon at the grave, which she assumes were left by Orestes. Electra tells her Orestes has been killed, and now they both mourn. This is tragic irony, as both mourn for Orestes who is alive and nearby.

Orestes enters, disguised as a traveler who tells Electra about Orestes's death. Overcome by his sister's outpouring of grief, however, Orestes reveals his true identity and his plan for revenge. Orestes and Paidagogos perform a ritual purification, then enter the palace, followed by Electra. The Chorus narrates the action as Clytemnestra is killed.

Aegisthos returns, happy to hear the news of Orestes's death. He enters the palace to see Orestes's body but uncovers instead the body of Clytemnestra. The play ends as Orestes leads him offstage to be killed.

CHARACTERS

Aegisthos

Son of Thyestes, Aegisthos is Clytemnestra's former lover (and now husband) who conspired with her to murder Agamemnon.

Chorus of Mycenaean Women

The Chorus provide background information and narrates the off-stage violence. While they recognize the justice of Electra's cause, they urge her to take a stoic position. They deplore Clytemnestra's crime but advise Electra, rather than

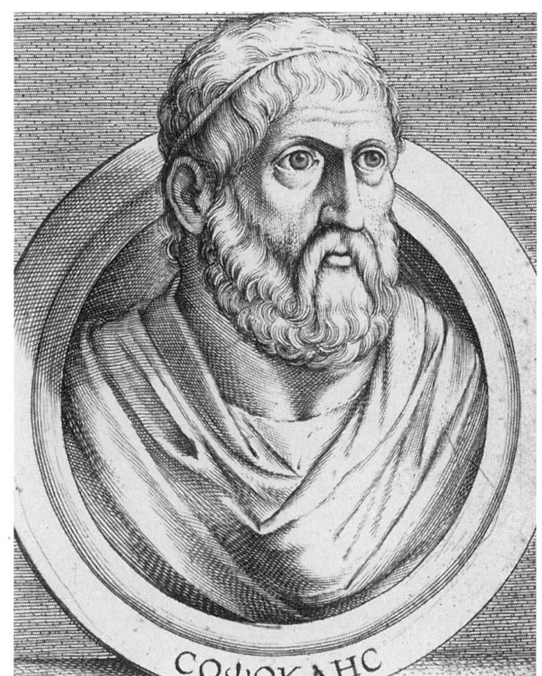

Sophocles

seek revenge, to leave revenge to the gods and to accept the fact that all people, being mortal, die.

Chrysothemis

Daughter of Agamemnon and Clytemnestra, Chrysothemis is the sister of Electra and Orestes. She refuses to help Electra with her planned revenge against their mother, Clytemnestra, for murdering their father. Chrysothemis urges Electra to be reasonable, though Electra accuses her sister of cowardice.

Clytemnestra

Agamemnon's wife, who, along with her lover Aegisthos, killed her husband, because of the role Agamemnon played in sacrificing their daughter, Iphigeneia.

Electra

The daughter of Agamemnon and Clytemnestra, Electra's sister is Chrysothemis and her brother is Orestes. Iphigeneia, whom her father sacrificed to the gods, was also her sister. Electra is a strong character, determined and directed, though she is incapable of heeding the moderating voice of the Chorus or the explanations of her mother. She publicly mourns her father's death and her mother's marriage to his murderer. When she believes that Orestes is dead, she mourns for him but is overjoyed to learn he is alive and participates in his revenge against Clytemnestra and Aegisthos.

Orestes

Son of Agamemnon and Clytemnestra, Orestes is brother to Electra and Chrysothemis. After her father's murder, Electra protected Orestes by sending him off to Phocis, where he was raised by Paidagogos. Orestes fakes his own death to gain access to the palace, then kills his mother Clytemnestra and her husband Aegisthos. The play ends here, but according to myth, Orestes was pursued and punished by the Furies for his act of matricide.

Paidagogos Prism

A loyal friend of Agamemnon, Paidagogos hid, protected, and raised Orestes when, after his father's murder, Electra entrusted her brother into his care. Paidagogos returns to help Orestes and Electra avenge Agamemnon's murder, first pretending to be a traveler with news of Orestes's death and later helping Orestes storm the palace.

THEMES

Revenge

Revenge drives all of the action in *Electra.* The family history involves a horrific crime and most of the tragedies which follow are crimes committed to compensate for an earlier crime. Agamemnon sacrifices Iphigeneia, for which Clytemnestra kills him. For her crime, Orestes kills his mother, for which he is pursued by the Furies (although this aspect of the legend is not addressed in Sophocles's drama).

Public vs. Private Life

Since tragedy, according to Aristotle's definition in his *Poetics,* involves a central figure of more than common stature, key figures are often kings or other prominent political or national figures. Consequently, this makes it possible to interpret tragedies as both explorations of private psychology and public politics. For example, William Shakespeare's *Hamlet* is about murder, revenge, and madness, but it is also about the failure of proper political succession and ill-gotten power (Hamlet's uncle murders his brother the king, marries his widow, and assumes the throne, bypassing Hamlet's birthright of ascendancy). The same is true of *Electra,* where, after Agamemnon's death, his son, Orestes should have assumed the throne. The play then becomes one about the usurpation of power, and in that sense, merges public and private action.

Guilt and Innocence

The issue of guilt in *Electra* depends on the perspective from which one evaluates the actions. Is Clytemnestra guilty of murdering Agamemnon for political/romantic reasons (so she may marry Aegisthos who will assume her dead husband's monarchy) or is she simply avenging her daughter's sacrifice? Is Orestes guilty of Clytemnestra's murder for similar political reasons or is he merely executing her for murdering his father, Agamemnon? Ultimately, guilt or innocence is central to the world of Greek tragedy, where characters are destined by the gods but also act freely.

Duty and Responsibility

This theme becomes particularly complex in *Electra,* where various characters often have contradictory, even mutually exclusive responsibilities. For example, as a father, Agamemnon must protect his daughter, Iphigeneia, but as a king, his duty is to sacrifice her for the good of his kingdom. As a son, Orestes must love his mother, but also as a son, he must avenge his father's murder.

STYLE

Stichomythia

A series of short—usually one line—dialogue exchanges between or among characters. The words are often confrontational and language seems to act as a substitutes for physical violence. Originating in Greek tragedy, stichomythia occurs in Roman (i.e. Senacan) tragedies and also in the Elizabethan plays influenced by classical predecessors such as in Shakespeare's *Hamlet* and *Richard III.* In *Electra,* stichomythic dialogue takes place between Electra and Chrysothemis early in the play and between Electra and Orestes during the revelation scene.

Tragic Irony

Irony is a sophisticated rhetorical strategy whereby a character is led to believe one thing, when in fact, the opposite is true. While it serves a dramatic function, it also serves a thematic one, reminding the characters and audience of the limitations of

TOPICS FOR FURTHER STUDY

- The question of how much of human action is directed by free will and how much is determined by fate has fascinated people from the Greeks to the present. Think about this issue in historical terms, considering the impact of the natural sciences on this debate or in philosophical terms, researching the ideas of Existentialist writers like Jean Paul Sartre and Albert Camus.
- In many ways, Electra is a powerful woman and can be seen as someone driven toward a higher purpose by her profound inner strength. How do her actions fit into the Greek definition of hero? Is that definition different for a woman that it would be for a man? You might research classical mythology generally (reading Ovid's *Metamorphosis,* for example) or Homer's *Odyssey.* Or you could compare Electra with another of Sophocles's titular heroines, Antigone.
- The cycle of plays of which *Electra* can be seen as a part raise important issues about the relationship between divine law to human law. Try to develop an independent standard of criteria by which people might act ethically. You might look at classical writers like Aristotle (the *Ethics* or *Politics*) or you might research into the relationship between law and literature.
- Critics have argued that while Sophocles's play is entitled *Electra,* Electra herself is not really central to the play's action. They contend that she stands around speaking while those around her act. Do you agree?

---

human knowledge: what we know to be certain may not be; and the uncertainty of human circumstances—what we know to be good may turn out badly, while assumed evils may result in good.

In *Electra,* there are several examples of tragic irony. One occurs when Electra thinks that Orestes is dead (while Chrysothemis thinks him alive) when he is alive all along. It recurs later, when Orestes, in disguise, tells Electra of his own death, until her grieving makes him confess the truth.

Tragedy

In his *Poetics,* Aristotle defines a tragedy as a play which recounts the fall or destruction of a person of elevated position. In Classical and Renaissance tragedy, the person is usually a king, though tragedy can befall anyone elevated in politic, ethical, or spiritual terms. For example, Christopher Marlowe's *Dr. Faustus* is tragic, for, though Faustus is not a noble, he is socially elevated as a great scholar and falls by his own hand in the service of his intellectual pride.

Tragic heroes fall in part because of fate, but their fall is usually not due to destiny alone but rather is complicated by some character flaw; ''hubris'' or pride usually precipitates such a fall. In the case of King Oedipus in Sophocles's *Oedipus Rex,* it is his desire to know the cause of the plague that afflicts his kingdom; the plague was brought on when he killed his father and married his mother. In the case of Hamlet, it is his inaction and hesitation. Because of the offenses of her ancestors, Electra's family is cursed to suffer. This fate or destiny generally dictates her tragedy, but the specific cause is her failure to balance passion (grief at her father's murder) with reason (her mother's guilt is partially mitigated by the role Agamemnon played in their daughter Iphigeneia's death).

HISTORICAL CONTEXT

Athens and the City-states

Although the exact date of Sophocles's *Electra* is not known, it was probably written and first performed around 409 B.C. (at that year's Dionysia), when the playwright was in his eighties. At this

COMPARE & CONTRAST

- **The Athenian Age:** Greece has a legal system based largely on revenge. Later, during the high point of Athenic culture in the fifth century B.C., a more complicated system of law develops, one on which many modern legal concepts are based.

  Today: Legal systems prevent people from seeking revenge individually (acting as vigilantes). Rather, injuries are remedied by way of the courts.

- **The Athenian Age:** It is a sign of respect to cremate the dead and keep their ashes in urns. These are large vessels decorated with graphics that identify the deceased, relating key events from their lives. For warriors, the urns might recount their most celebrated battles.

  Today: While some people are cremated, many are buried in caskets below the ground.

- **The Athenian Age:** Greeks' lives are largely dictated by what they believe the gods intend. Worship of multiple gods, who represent such aspects of life as war, music, love, and agriculture, is commonplace.

  Today: Monotheistic religion (the worship of one god) dominates world religion. While some still believe their destinies are controlled by a higher power, many more believe that humankind shapes and directs its own fate.

time, the Greek states were battling one another in the Peloponnesian War. The city-state of Athens had established itself as the dominant region in Greece, following its decisive role in the defeat of the Persians in the battle of Salamis in 480 B.C.

After the Persians were expelled from Greece, the city-states banded together to form the Delian League. This alliance ensured the mutual protection of each state and was ostensibly a confederacy of equals. Each city paid an annual tribute to maintain the strength of the alliance. However, Athens gradually became the leader of the Delian League, and Pericles, head of the Athenians, used the surplus tribute to rebuild the Athenian Acropolis rather than for the common good of all the states.

Under Pericles, the Parthenon and other architectural masterpieces were constructed on the Acropolis at this time (approximately 450 to 405 B.C.). Predictably, members of the other Greek states were angered at Pericles for using their tribute money to beautify his own city. Because of this and other affronts, they waged war against Athens in the Peloponnesian War of 431-404 B.C. Athens ultimately fell to the military strength of Sparta.

Greek Drama

Tragedies such as *Electra* were presented in the annual Dionysia festivals in Athens, where playwrights competed with each other for a prize. At the Dionysia, each writer presented a group of four plays: three tragedies, which often formed a trilogy on a given subject—such as Sophocles's Oedipal trilogy (*Antigone, Oedipus at Colonus,* and *Oedipus Rex*)—and a satyr-play, which was a form of comic relief. The tragedies concerned mortals who were at the mercy of their fate and who evoked pity from the audience. Greek audiences expected to be moved by the drama unfolding before them, experiencing a catharsis, or a purging (purification) of the emotions of pity and fear. These emotions were associated with the fall of a great person, the tragic hero.

In contrast to the cathartic effect of the tragedies, the satyr-plays provided a lighthearted antidote. In these plays, the chorus dressed as satyrs, figures who were half-man and half-beast, and performed rough but witty routines which can be likened to later forms of light entertainment such as slapstick or vaudevillian comedy. The third genre of Greek drama, comedy, was not performed at the Dionysia. However, there are many surviving comedies from the fifth century B.C., and these seem to have served the function of providing an emotional release also. In addition, comedies were directly political and provided a vehicle for authors to offer thinly-veiled commentary on the happenings of the day.

The Legend of the House of Atreus

Electra concerns one part of the story of the House of Atreus, a doomed family which was cursed from its inception. According to legend, the patriarch Atreus was the grandson of Tantalus, who killed his own son and served the pieces of his body to the gods at a feast. Because this was an atrocious crime, the gods sentenced Tantalus to eternal punishment in the underworld. They also restored his son, Pelops, to life. Pelops, a favorite of the god Poseidon, won a chariot race which enabled him to claim the beautiful Hippodamia as his wife. However, he was only able to win the race because Hippodamia bribed the other charioteer to lose on purpose. When the charioteer came to claim his bribe, Pelops killed him and the charioteer uttered a curse on Pelops and his descendants as he died.

Atreus, who became the king of Mycenae, was one of the sons of Pelops and Hippodamia. He was cuckolded by his brother, Thyestes, and, in a fit of anger, killed Thyestes's sons and served them to his brother at a banquet, in a crime similar to that of his forbearer, Tantalus. Thyestes, upon finding out what Atreus had done, cursed him and his house as well. In order to avenge his sons' deaths, Thyestes learned from the Delphic Oracle that he had to father a child by his own daughter Pelopia; the product of this union was Aegisthus.

Atreus, however, believed the boy to be his own son, and raised him as such, since he had in the meantime married Pelopia. But when Aegisthus learned that Thyestes was his true father, he killed Atreus. Thus, Atreus's real sons Agamemnon and Menelaus were forced into exile as Thyestes took over the throne of Mycenae. The rivalry between Agamemnon and Aegisthus, central to the story of *Electra,* had begun.

Agamemnon married Clytemnestra, producing their daughters Iphigeneia and Electra and their son Orestes. When Agamemnon departed for the Trojan War, Clytemnestra took his rival Aegisthus as her lover and plotted to kill her husband when he returned. Clytemnestra and Aegisthus succeeded in murdering Agamemnon, and the plot of *Electra* centers around Electra and Orestes's plans to avenge their father's death by killing their mother and Aegisthus.

Sophocles's audience would have been familiar with the legend of the House of Atreus and would have recognized the disparities between his version of the legend and other plays which dealt with the same cursed family. It was not necessary for the classical audience to be presented with the entire legend in any given play; rather, each play concentrated on one major aspect of the larger story, assuming the audience was already familiar with the general legend.

CRITICAL OVERVIEW

Since the time of their first production in the fifth century B.C., scholars and critics have contended that the tragedies of Sophocles represent Greek drama in its purest and most highly-attained form. Aristotle used elements of Sophoclean tragedy as the main concepts of his general theory of drama in the *Poetics.* According to Aristotle, a tragedy is most successful when the moments of recognition (what he termed anagnorisis) and reversal (peripeteia) occur at the same time. Aristotle claims that a tragedy is not merely the imitation of an individual but of a life. By this he means that an individual's actions are more important to the development of the play than the particulars of his or her character.

Aristotle criticizes plays which include lengthy speeches solely for the purpose of expressing character and praises those works which sacrifice such elements in favor of a meaningful and well-structured plot. Sophocles is considered a master at characterization, particularly in *Electra,* providing just enough necessary information about each character through succinct and direct lines.

The twentieth century writer Edith Hamilton praised Sophocles's characterization, particularly in comparison to his contemporary (and teacher) Aeschylus. In her widely-read book *The Greek Way,* Hamilton claimed that Sophocles surpasses Aeschylus in technical ability, though he falls short in sheer dramatic power. According to Hamilton, when Sophocles wrote a play, it would be done as well as it possibly could be in terms of craftsmanship. In *Electra,* there are no words wasted, no time spent on details which detract from the main thrust of the plot.

Hamilton noted that in this play, Electra's character is conveyed in the terse, compact dialogue exchanged between she and Chrysothemis. The depth of Electra's suffering, expressed in the lament sung between Electra and the chorus, is brought into relief when contrasted with Chrysothemis's compliance and acceptance of her miserable situation. Electra is clearly the stronger and more noble character, striving to avenge their father's murder and not accepting the tyranny of their mother silently. As Hamilton claimed, Sophocles is able to convey the essential elements of his characters and draw the audience into their stories through intense, compressed dialogue which is charged with meaning.

In terms of dramatic power, Hamilton believed that Sophocles does not achieve the emotional heights of which Aeschylus was capable. For example, she wrote that Sophocles passed over the murder of Clytemnestra by her son Orestes, in order to get to the real climax of the play, the killing of Aegisthos. In her opinion, Sophocles missed a moment of great dramatic opportunity. After Orestes kills Clytemnestra, Electra and her brother discuss the deed only briefly before Aegisthos enters and they prepare to kill him as well.

Hamilton concluded that Sophocles made the matricide into punishment for Clytemnestra's own crime, which would have been accepted by the audience and would not have moved them into the higher feelings of pity and awe. She argued that the high passion which could have been invoked by the matricide was beyond the reach of Sophocles's talents and that he knew he could not adequately convey such passion. Therefore, she concluded, he did not attempt to write what he could not do perfectly.

Virginia Woolf wrote a brief essay entitled "On Sophocles' Electra" in 1925 (published in *Sophocles: A Collection of Critical Essays*), in which she commented on the way Electra is presented as a tightly bound character, unable to move or act on her own. Woolf claimed that Electra's cries, even in moments of crisis, are bare and consist of mere expressions of emotion. However, these cries are crucial and shape the movement of the play. Woolf even compared Sophocles's use of dialogue to that of the British novelist Jane Austen (*Pride and Prejudice*), claiming that Austen's female characters, like Electra, are bound and constrained by their social roles yet are able to express much through simple phrases. Though their words may be direct and simple, these women are able to shape the outcome of the drama at hand, even when they themselves are not the most active characters in the story.

Another twentieth century critic writing in the same critical collection on Sophocles (*Sophocles: A Collection of Critical Essays*), Thomas Woodward, also discussed how Sophocles's *Electra* progresses while seemingly bypassing the heroine altogether. Like Woolf, Woodward noted that Electra stands in the midst of a drama which involves the men in the story; she lives in a world of suffering while the men are able to act in a more noble realm. Yet, Electra finds her place in the larger sphere outside of her own feelings, and, according to Woodward, her strength and passion overpower the men's plot; she fully deserves to have the play centered around her.

Though she does not perform the climactic murders herself, Electra is a truly heroic character by virtue of her depths of emotion and her righteous motivation for revenge. Indeed, Sophocles emphasizes her importance by giving her one of the longest speaking parts in Greek tragedy and by having her remain on the stage for nine-tenths of the play. Through all of this, however, the audience is made aware of Electra's isolation as a woman confined to a life inside the palace walls. While Orestes and the other men are able to act on their plans, Electra can only lament. Yet it is perhaps her lamentations which cause the gods to send Orestes back—and so she is able to provoke action, even if she is restricted from acting herself.

Woodward and other modern critics have also asserted the importance of props as dramatic devices in Sophocles's work. In Electra, the urn which Orestes carries when he enters the "recognition" scene dominates the stage. It is the focus of the scene: Electra addresses it in a lament while holding it in her arms, almost as if it were a living actor. It is, in fact, a surrogate for Orestes, until he reveals himself to her. Because of how Electra acts towards the urn, Orestes ceases to conceal his true identity from her. The urn therefore is critical to the tragedy—once Orestes reveals himself to Electra, she is

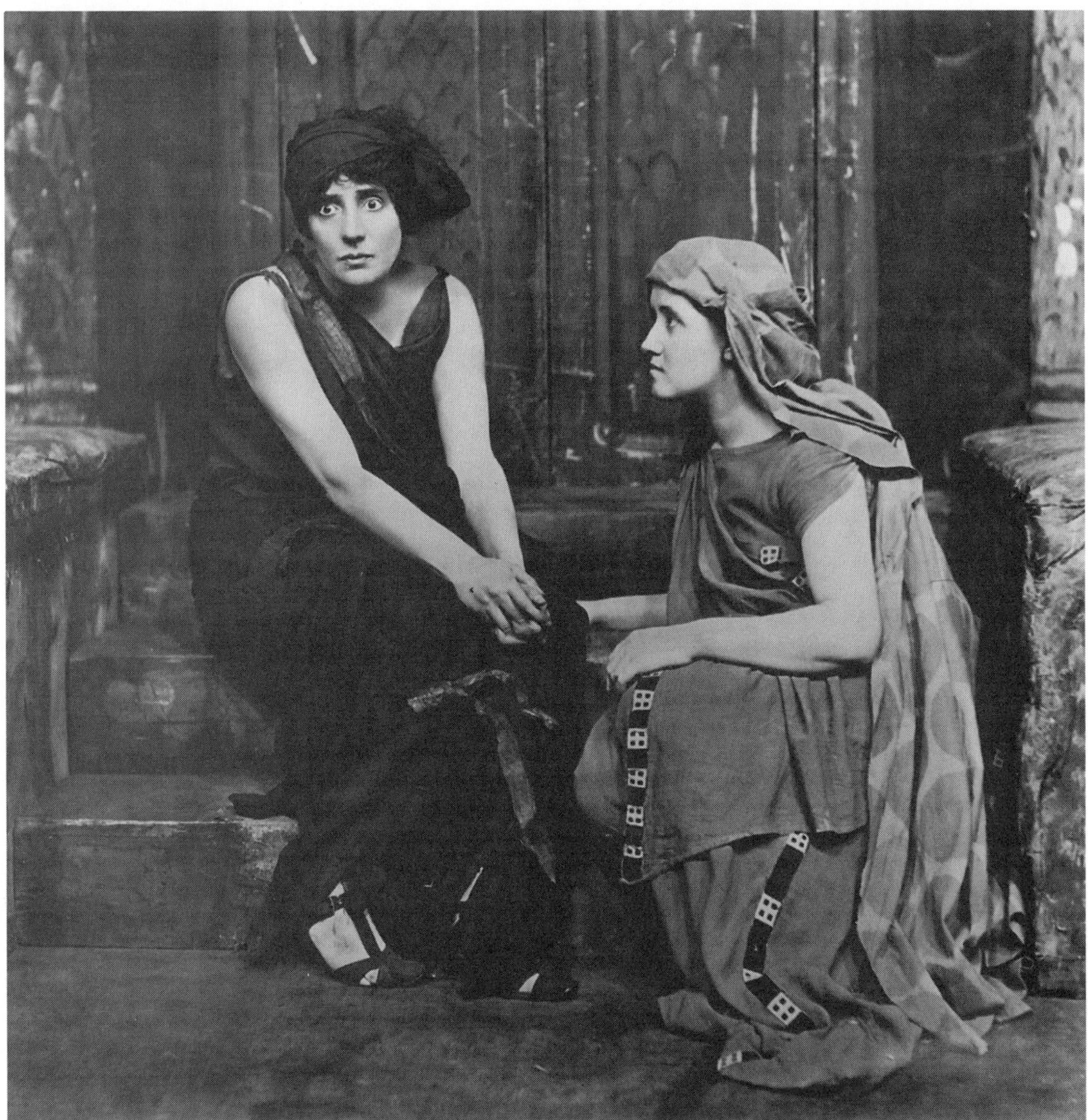

A 1908 production of Electra *shows the title character in black*

released from her sorrows and the play quickly draws to its bloody conclusion.

CRITICISM

Arnold Schmidt

Schmidt received his Ph.D. from Vanderbilt University, where he specialized in literature and drama. Exploring the cycles of violence in Electra *leads him to consider the play as an allegory of the law.*

Ordinarily, a hero is a righteous person who stands on the side of justice, fighting oppression. In many ways, Electra's personality, strong and determined, is admirable and heroic. Her desire to avenge the murder of Agamemnon, her father, regardless of the consequences, is commendable, but her situation is more complicated that of an ordinary hero. In the world of *Electra,* heroism depends on one's point of view. From Agamemnon's perspective, Electra would be heroic, but from Clytemnestra's

WHAT DO I READ NEXT?

- Another of Sophocles's tragedies, *Antigone* tells of a woman's struggle to bury her brother's body against the orders of the king. Like *Electra,* it features a strong female character and involves the conflict between family and politics. *Antigone* is the last play in the Oedipal trilogy.
- In three plays, *Mourning Becomes Electra, Ah! Wilderness,* and *Days without End,*, the Nobel Prize-winning American playwright Eugene O'Neill retells the story of Electra and her family's tragedy.
- William Shakespeare's *Hamlet* bears many similarities with *Electra,* including the murdered father, the widow's marriage to the murderer, and ineffective efforts at revenge.
- For a very different kind of tragedy, consider Arthur Miller's *Death of a Salesman,* which relates the tribulations of an average man whose flaw is a naive obsession with the American Dream.

point of view, her daughter may seem admirable but misguided. The fact that right and wrong change places depending on how the circumstances are considered is significant. It raises the possibility that an absolute standard of justice may elude us. Further, since this is a blood feud with a long history, the rights and wrongs almost fade into the fog of time.

The play's moral high-ground shifts back and forth, as victims of crimes become criminals themselves—and visa versa. The play attempts to distinguish between what was done—the crime—and who was to blame—the criminal—and why they acted as they did. It explores differences between the fact of the crime and the personal guilt or innocence based on premeditation, intention, and free will, for which an individual can be liable. It raises questions not of Justice (is this a crime against the law?), but of Equity (yes, it's against the law but are there extenuating circumstances).

For example, two people steal money. One is a poor man who has never stolen anything before in his life; out of work, he needs money to buy medicine to save his dying daughter's life. The other man is a multi-millionaire who has been convicted of stealing half a dozen times now, who wanted the money because he wanted the money. Yes, they both stole. They're both guilty of breaking the law, but are their crimes the same—in other words, should they be punished identically? They are identical in regard to the letter of the law but in terms of equity—fairness, they differ. The poor man's crime seems understandable and justified—to some extent, at least—while the rich man's criminal act appears motivated solely by greed.

Part of the problem—in the previous example as in *Electra*—stems from a conflict between and among different types of law: divine law or the will of the gods; natural law, based on blood relationships; and human law, ordained by the state. In the world of the play, human law is the weakest of the three. Solutions to grievances depend more on an ethic of revenge rather than on justice. How else can a victim seek remedy for injustice? The answer lies in a society's stages of development.

In primitive society, loyalty to the family surpasses loyalty to the state and without a powerful state government to make and enforce law, vengeance remains necessary. Crime demands retribution and since the intermediary third party, the state, is weak and unable to impose a just settlement, the family seeks revenge. One of the things embedded in Electra's story, though, is an end to this cycle of revenge and the initiation of a modern, rational system of justice.

From Agamemnon's perspective, killing Iphigeneia was just. After all, the king of all gods, Zeus, ordered him to undertake the Trojan War and Agamemnon sacrifices his daughter in the service of that cause, obeying what he believes to be the will of the gods. Agamemnon's actions may violate natural law, a father killing his child, and human law but they seem in accordance with divine law as the Greeks understood it; this is the highest law and Agamemnon obeys.

Clytemnestra privileges natural law, the love of a mother for her child, over divine law, the need to sacrifice Iphigeneia to prosecute the war. Clytemnestra admits to violating human law in killing Agamemnon, but is pleased that Iphigeneia's sacrifice (what she sees as Agamemnon's greater crime) mitigates her guilt. As she tells Electra: "I killed him. . . . Because that man who you still cry for / Was the one Greek who could bear to sacrifice / Your sister," Iphigeneia.

Electra strikes an uneasy balance between natural and divine law. She appeals to natural law in condemning her mother, saying, "You issue yourself remorse and punishment. / For if a killer merits death / You must die next, to satisfy that justice." Electra's position is not pure, however, for she ignores the claims of natural law that called for Iphigeneia's revenge, which Clytemnestra has satisfied in killing her husband. On this point, Electra appeals to divine law, asking what else Agamemnon could do, under orders from the gods to fight the war and believing his daughter's sacrifice was the only way to free his fleet.

Complicating the debate between them is Clytemnestra's marriage with Agamemnon's murderer, Aegisthos. Electra calls her mother's appeal to natural law an "ugly pretext. . . . To join with a mortal enemy in marriage."

Orestes's position is unique, as he finds himself punished by one divine entity, the Furies, for obeying another divine entity, Apollo. By revenging his father and killing his mother at the insistence of the gods, he obeys divine law and violates natural law. After all, Orestes should by nature have been the avenger of his mother's death, except for the fact that he is her murderer. Finding himself persecuted by the Furies, Orestes too feels it is wrong for him to be punished for doing what the gods ordered.

Chrysothemis is a militant centrist, trying to hold a middle ground. She recognizes that Clytemnestra's actions are evil and that Agamemnon should be revenged. She also realizes that she has no real power and is ready to accept necessity. She

"ELECTRA STRIKES AN UNEASY BALANCE BETWEEN NATURAL AND DIVINE LAW."

echoes the position recommended by the Chorus, who see and proclaim against evil but advocate stoic acceptance of life's tribulations. As Chrysothemis says, "be reasonable. . . . Helpless as you are, yield to the strong."

In *Electra,* there are a series of wrongs present: Agamemnon sacrifices his daughter Iphigeneia; Clytemnestra kills Agamemnon; Orestes (aided/supported by Electra) kills Clytemnestra. All are wrong yet all have reasons which justify their actions—and in that sense, all are justly motivated. We might ask: is Orestes his mother's murderer or executioner? Is he murdering her or serving justice to her for killing Agamemnon. She might reply that she did not kill Agamemnon but "executed" him for his role in the sacrifice of their daughter, Iphigeneia. To which Agamemnon might reply, it was the gods who prevented the fleet from moving unless Iphigeneia was sacrificed—is not her death the fault of the gods?

Remaining within the narrative history of a single play in this family drama, it is impossible to escape this cycle of accusation and recrimination. The myth—and the drama—continues in Aeschylus's *Eumenides,* where it can be seen to tell the origin of Attic democracy. After killing Clytemnestra, Orestes flees, pursued by the avenging Furies. He finds solace only in the temple of Athena, who appreciates his predicament. She decides his case cannot be adjudicated by the gods alone and so sets it before a human jury in the Court of Areopagus.

Critics see this symbolizing the birth of the Greek rule of law, a movement from an ethic of revenge to a system of justice and equity (a system that supports and informs modern justice). Based on reason, the decision of human jurors ends this cycle of blood feuding. The story of Electra's family concludes with the classical endorsement of reason's role in moderating passion.

Source: Arnold Schmidt, for *Drama for Students,* Gale, 1998.

J. Michael Walton

Walton provides an overview of Sophocles's Electra *in this essay. He differentiates Sophocles's version of the story from similar works by his Greek contemporaries Euripides (a play also titled* Electra*) and Aeschylus (who chronicles the legend in his trilogy the* Oresteia*).*

Orestes, son of Agamemnon and Clytemnestra, arrives back in Argos from exile to avenge the murder of his father by his mother. A plot is hatched which leads to the death of Clytemnestra and her lover Aegisthus, but the play centres on the character of Electra, Orestes's sister, and her sufferings at the hands of Clytemnestra.

The Electra plays of Sophocles and Euripides share plot and main characters, if not title, with *Libation-Bearers,* the middle play of Aeschylus's *Oresteia.* The relationship between the two *Electra* plays is a subject of constant debate, as no firm date can be assigned to either. The approach is so different that a case can be made for either *Electra* having been written as a riposte to the other. What is not in doubt is that at the time of writing his *Electra* Sophocles and Euripides each knew Aeschylus's *Libation-Bearers* and could be confident that their audience did too.

Sophocles declares his independence from any previous version in the opening scene with the arrival back in Argos of Orestes and Pylades with Orestes's Servant or Tutor, a new character in the story, who is to play a major role in carrying out Orestes's revenge on Clytemnestra and Aegisthus. When Orestes has announced his intentions, the Tutor persuades him to leave before the entrance of Electra. The rest of the play is effectively Electra's; she remains on stage, a picture of mounting desperation, as she continues to mourn her father despite her mother's plans to have her put away. She loses her last hope with the news that Orestes has been killed in a chariot-race. She resolves to take action herself, with or without the help of her sister Chrysothemis. With no more than a quarter of the play to run, she finds herself confronting the urn containing her brother's ashes.

But his death is, in fact, only supposition. The audience know that her brother is alive and holding the urn himself. It was the Tutor who told the story of the fatal race. It is all part of the plot, and only Electra's passionate grief weakens Orestes's resolve to keep her in the dark until he has succeeded in his revenge. Electra's plight runs parallel to Orestes's return, but until late in the play has no effect upon it. Indeed, when brother and sister are reunited their extravagant behaviour almost sabotages the plot.

The recognition scene, which Aeschylus placed early in his *Libation-Bearers,* is delayed by Sophocles so as to provide an emotional climax that the violent end of Clytemnestra and Aegisthus barely matches. The use of a stage-property, in this case the urn, is a device used elsewhere by Sophocles to concentrate and externalise an issue; Ajax's sword in *Ajax,* and the bow of Heracles in *Philoctetes* offer similar examples of the stage power residing in an object. The urn has the extra dimension of being both a mechanism in the plot and a trigger to the release of Electra from her captivity.

The powerful emphasis on Electra's character is at the expense of the moral dilemma of Orestes. Aeschylus based the *Oresteia* on the paradox inherent in the demand of a God that a son avenge his father, when to do so involves the killing of his mother. Euripides in his *Electra* stresses the horror of the act of matricide with an Orestes driven reluctantly to commit an unnatural act. For both of these playwrights the climax was the murder of Clytemnestra—with Aegisthus killed first in order not to distract from the mother and son confrontation.

Sophocles reverses the order of the murders. Aegisthus is away from the palace when the Tutor tells of the chariot-race and when Orestes introduces the urn to confirm the story. Clytemnestra's death is simply an appropriate act accompanied by neither the threat of the Furies which hounded Aeschylus's Orestes, nor the conscience and revulsion which torment him in Euripides's version. For Sophocles, Apollo has authorised Clytemnestra's death and that is enough. When Aegisthus does appear, Clytemnestra is already dead, a sheeted figure he takes for the body of Orestes. The revelation that it is Clytemnestra offers as macabre a moment as any in Sophocles and leads rapidly to the conclusion of the play. Though Orestes and Electra are now united, her oppressors dead, her story continues to run parallel to that of her brother without the two truly overlapping.

By consciously bypassing the issue of matricide Sophocles returns to a Homeric notion of justice. In the *Odyssey* Orestes had been held up as a model of filial behaviour with no questions raised about the rightness of his actions. But in Homer Aegisthus was the principal villain and there was no Electra. Aeschylus had added the moral dimension with the clash between Apollo, demanding that Orestes avenge his father, and the Furies demanding their due for the murder of a mother. Sophocles does not dodge this issue. He deflects it, by introducing new characters and a novel dramatic structure, in order to point to Electra herself. Few Greek plays are as single-minded in their presentation of the individual.

Source: J. Michael Walton, "*Electra*" in *The International Dictionary of Theatre 1: Plays,* edited by Mark Hawkins-Dady, St. James Press, 1992, p. 218.

John A. Hawkins

In this review, Hawkins encapsulates the plot of Electra *and appraises a 1987 production of the play.*

High on the wall of the *scenae frons* for this production of Sophocles' *Electra* is hung a gigantic reproduction of Schliemann's so-called "mask of Agamemnon." This giant face, its mouth rendered much more severe than in the original—so severe that under many of the lighting conditions of the performance, it seems to harden into a scowl—stands as mute witness to this play, with its bizarre remnants of his great Mycenean kingdom. Hanging profusely, even haphazardly, below the face are black curtains which catch the light at certain times in the play, looking at these moments like a blood-streaked shroud, littered with slashes. More significant use might have been made of the face: although it possesses an attitude, we do not sense that the characters do what they do because the face impels them.

At the start of the performance, the center door opens slowly, lit from behind like a great red furnace. It comes up like an automatic garage door, and the slowness and ominousness with which it rises sets the rhythm for the first section of the performance. Then the actors file in through the door in a dumb-show that at first seems too long, too tedious: they seem to be entering merely in order to introduce the characters. They walk in a kind of death march, and their gradual massing on the stage, in the half-light, gives a mounting sense of both grief and fore-boding. The dumb-show ends with a re-enactment, in silence and slow-motion, of the murder of Agamemnon—but done in such a spare manner that we are sure only of the death blow, and the plucking of the crown from the head of the falling figure by the female murderer, as all actors exit. Then the center door slowly closes, and Sophocles' play begins.

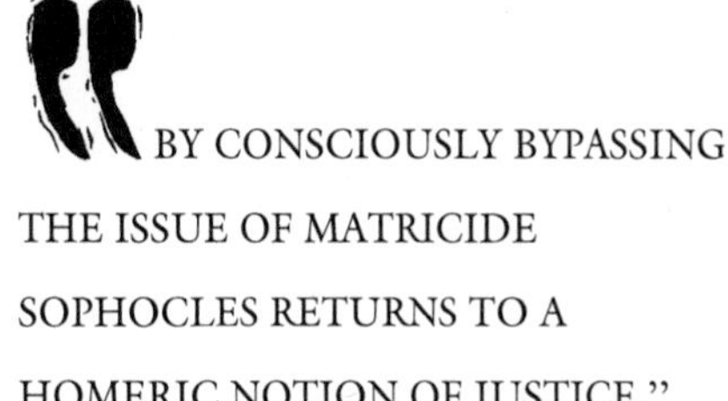

After the brief *prologos,* in which Orestes seems almost bewildered, as if he had wandered in from another play (*Rosencrantz and Guildenstern Are Dead,* perhaps), we have the most striking clue that we are about to witness a remarkable performance: the entrance of Electra. This production, from first to last, is rooted firmly in Marietta Rialdi's startling portrayal of Electra. To begin with, at her entrance, she really does not enter at all. The center door opens, and we see (or think we see, with the light in our eyes) an ambulatory bed, a kind of hospital gurney, at the head of which is a ghostly figure in dark glasses—the attendant, apparently. On the bed is a strange, stunted figure, whose voice we can locate only because of the fluttering of its arms. The figure on the bed is Electra, crying in a kind of hysterical lost-child's voice—exhausted, it seems, from having done this for days, months, years. Has she been confined to this bed because of mental illness, strapped in out of fear that the madwoman will harm herself? She has the shrill demented sound of the profoundly insane.

The remarkable achievement of Rialdi is that she portrays a constant emotional state of being *in extremis*—on one shrill note that seems never to waver, conveying Electra's total commitment to the cause of keeping alive the memory of her slain father—yet *never* tires us. Her cries become a kind of accompaniment that has a stylistic rightness to the events which have given it impulse. She *cannot* relent, and we begin to enter *her* vortex of grief and despair. She moves us easily from vicarious experience—the second-hand experience of the audience—toward an experience that seems direct, that feels like our own. Rialdi keeps us engaged by modulating, phrasing, slightly varying her pace and her pitches, a striking vocal achievement. She seems to draw no breath, and we discover ourselves gasping, taking them for her. She goes from grief to grief without flagging: her speech of despair later on in the play, to the urn supposedly containing the ashes of the dead Orestes, which she embraces fiercely,

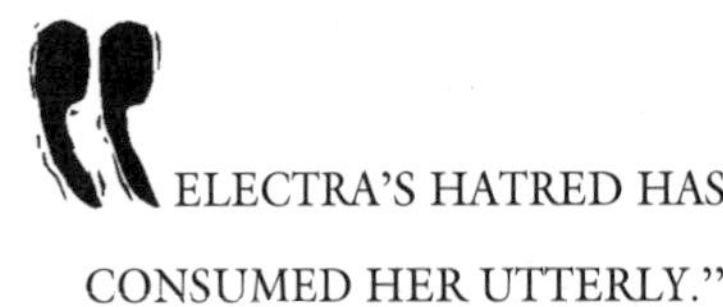

ELECTRA'S HATRED HAS CONSUMED HER UTTERLY."

like a lover, is the most spectacular reminder to us that any true grief is bottomless, wretched, unremitting.

Her entrance sets the tone for all of this. Lying on the gurney, she is only partially visible to us—she remains inside the inner below for a long portion of her speech. We see her forearms flapping, as if to punctuate her speech, but they seem ineffectual, like vestigial wings. Then the gurney is wheeled in to Left Center, and parked there, abandoned. Electra's vocalizations and her emotional extension do not waver through any of this. Continuing her strange aria, she gradually struggles to a sitting position, then throws her legs over the edge of the gurney, then stands on the floor, then waddles away on her own. Rialdi, who is tiny in physical stature, is brilliant throughout this section. Her struggle to walk is inept, uncoordinated. Her body seems to have atrophied from her time in bed, and her limbs seem incapable of response. Her physical appearance is dwarfish, warped.

One is grateful to Rialdi for daring to exhibit herself so unattractively in order to convey with such realism and poignancy the *dementia* of Electra. She gives us much of Hugo von Hofmannstahl's insight into this character, and serves Sophocles with it brilliantly. Her dementia has a further extension: at the moment of Orestes' revelation of his identity to Electra, the audience responds with greater relief and enthusiasm than she does. We are momentarily baffled by Electra's seeming not to notice. She takes in this information only insofar as it means that the revenge can now be resumed. She is so steeped in her own habits of grief and self-pity that she cannot alter her pattern of behavior, even as she is delivered from them. Rialdi's is a thoroughly original performance.

In the important scene between Electra and Clytemnestra, much is revealed to the audience of the similarities between the two women. Electra has waited years for her revenge, as did Clytemnestra, but the latter's hatred has since metamorphosed into fear. As with Electra, the central emotion goes deep, to the core of her self. Rialdi's Electra—the demented soprano—and Thalia Calliga's aging Clytemnestra—all *contralto profundissimo*—argue in a duet skillfully handled in its sustained, slow movements, and deliberate, forceful vocalization. Their passages of stichomythia make sharp contact between the adversaries, as Clytemnestra, edgy and defensive, refuses to face Electra, and stands looking at us—the ambiguity in her face impossible to decipher.

Minor objections aside, the production stands on the achievements of Marietta Rialdi, who has given a startling and bold interpretation of Sophocles' play and of his central character. Her success is in no small measure due to her acting, based as it is upon her willingness to expose the last indignity of Electra. But Rialdi refuses to allow us the comfort of sympathy for her; instead, she makes us face the ugly reality. Electra's hatred has consumed her utterly.

Source: John A. Hawkins, review of *Electra* in *Theatre Journal,* Volume 39, no. 3, October, 1987, pp. 387–89.

SOURCES

Hamilton, Edith. *The Greek Way,* W. W. Norton (New York), 1930, pp. 258-70.

Woodward, Thomas. "The *Electra* of Sophocles" in *Sophocles: A Collection of Critical Essays,* edited by Woodward, Prentice-Hall, 1966, pp. 125-45.

Woolf, Virginia. "On Sophocles's *Electra*" in *Sophocles: A Collection of Critical Essays,* edited by Thomas Woodward, Prentice-Hall, 1966, pp. 122-24.

FURTHER READING

Blundell, Sue. *Women in Ancient Greece,* Harvard University Press, 1995.

This book illuminates the world of women in Sophocles's time, revealing that although their roles were limited, they contributed to the cultural and artistic life of Ancient Greece.

Nardo, Don, Editor. *Readings on Sophocles,* Greenhaven Press, 1997.

This is a collection of critical essays on Sophocles, which also includes a useful appendix on Greek theatrical production and a biography of the playwright.

Woodward, Thomas, Editor. *Sophocles: A Collection of Critical Essays,* Prentice-Hall, 1966.

Woodward's collection of essays includes his own article, "The *Electra* of Sophocles," and Virginia Woolf's essay, "On Sophocles's *Electra.*" The collection also offers an excellent critical overview of many of Sophocles's dramatic works.

The Hairy Ape

EUGENE O'NEILL

1922

Eugene O'Neill's *The Hairy Ape* was first produced on March 9, 1922, by the Provincetown Players, a theatrical group that he co-founded. The work was staged in New York City at the company's own Provincetown Theatre. Publication of the play occurred that same year. By this time O'Neill was already an established playwright, having won two Pulitzer Prizes. *The Hairy Ape* represented something of a departure for him, being an exploration into a more expressionistic style than his previous plays.

The Hairy Ape had been written rather quickly in 1921, and the first production left little time between the final draft and the start of rehearsals. There is some dispute as to who actually directed the first production, with evidence that a triumvirate of Anthony Hopkins, James Light, and O'Neill contributed to the stage direction.

Alexander Woollcot reported in the *New York Times* that this Provincetown production was "a bitter, brutal, wildly fantastic play of nightmare hue and nightmare distortion." Other critics agreed, finding the play to be a powerful commentary on the human toll exacted from America's bumpy transition from an agrarian to industrial nation. Audiences also identified with O'Neill's characters, who represented, in some form, people from their everyday life.

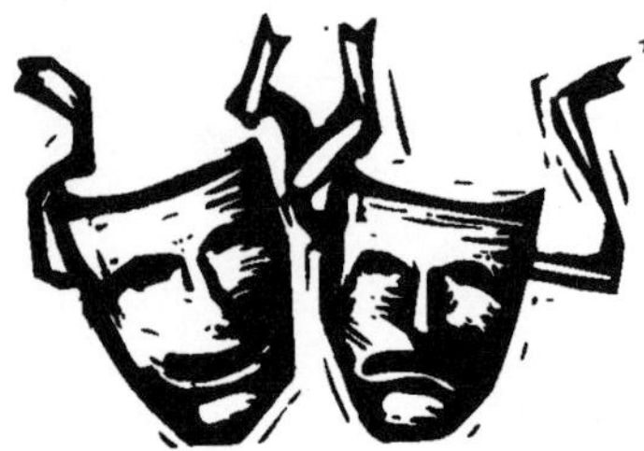

The Hairy Ape's strong condemnation of the dehumanizing effects of industrialization made it appealing to many labor groups and unions, who seized upon its concepts to further their cause for better working conditions. The play also attracted the attention of the Federal Bureau of Investigation (FBI), which had kept a file on O'Neill. The organization's report on the playwright stated that "*The Hairy Ape* could easily lend itself to radical propaganda, and it is somewhat surprising that it has not already been used for this purpose."

The Hairy Ape's New York production faced more concrete bureaucratic interference: an attempt was made by the mayor to close the play down for fear that it would provoke labor disputes or riots. Despite the fears of local and federal governments, the play never became a threat in that sense. Rather audiences and critics embraced it as thought-provoking entertainment. Although Woolcott found fault with the play's initial production, he also concluded his review by stating that he found *The Hairy Ape* to be "a turbulent and tremendous play, so full of blemishes that the merest fledgling among the critics could point out a dozen, yet so vital and interesting and teeming with life that those playgoers who let it escape them will be missing one of the real events of the year." In the years since its debut the play has become one of O'Neill's better-known works and a distinctive exploration of a pivotal period in American society.

AUTHOR BIOGRAPHY

O'Neill was born on October 16, 1888, in New York City, the son of a successful touring actor. His early life was spent on the road, a difficult life for a child. He later criticized the family's constant travelling, suggesting that the stress led to his mother's addiction to drugs as well as heavy drinking by the other family members. O'Neill started his college education at Princeton University, but that came to an abrupt end when he was dismissed for a prank. He married Kathleen Jenkins in 1909, producing a son, but divorced her only three years later. He then spent two years working as a sailor and manual laborer in South American ports.

In 1912 O'Neill was diagnosed with tuberculosis and sent to a sanitarium. Forbidden any strenuous physical activity, he resolved to get serious about his writing. During his recuperation, he became interested in playwrights, in particular the works of August Strindberg (*Miss Julie*). His contact with such literary works convinced him that he wanted to be an artist; he moved to Cambridge, Massachusetts, and began studying at Harvard. He stayed there for a year and then moved on to Greenwich Village in New York. From there, he went to Provincetown, Massachussetts, and met a group of artists and writers that included playwright Susan Glaspell (*Trifles*) and radical journalist John Reed. With these writers, O'Neill started the Provincetown Players, an amateur theater company dedicated to producing independent works. O'Neill's first play, the one-act *Thirst,* was produced in 1916.

O'Neill wrote and was produced regularly throughout his life, earning a worldwide reputation as a premier playwright. He is noted not only for the quality of his work but for the considerable volume of his creations; during his nearly forty years as a professional playwright he produced over fifty works for the stage. Many of his plays are today considered hallmarks of American drama, including *The Hairy Ape* (1922), *Desire under the Elms* (1924), *Mourning Becomes Electra* (1931), *The Iceman Cometh* (1946), and *A Moon for the Misbegotten* (1957). Of the many accolades bestowed upon him, he received four Pulitzer Prizes—for *Beyond the Horizon* (1920), *Anna Christie* (1922), *Strange Interlude* (1928), and *Long Day's Journey into Night* (1957)—and, in 1936, a Nobel Prize for literature.

O'Neill's stature is such that he is regarded as one of America's greatest dramatists, although there were periods during which his work was not held in such high regard. Critical and popular opinion turned firmly to the positive with the 1956 debut of *Long Day's Journey into Night,* an autobiographical work that frankly examines the dysfunction of the O'Neill family. Due to the sensitive nature of the material, the playwright stipulated in his will that the play not be produced until after his death. The emotional power of *Long Day's Journey* prompted a re-examination of O'Neill's earlier work, earning him newfound appreciation among theatergoers and critics.

Despite the great number of works he saw produced during his life, O'Neill died with a number of unfinished or unproduced plays, including a cycle he was completing at the time of his death. A great number of his latter writings—like *Long Day's Journey*—were of a personal nature, and O'Neill ordered them destroyed before his death. A handful of these plays were spared, however, and the collections *The Unknown O'Neill* (1988) and *Ten "Lost" Plays* (1995) resurrected the play-

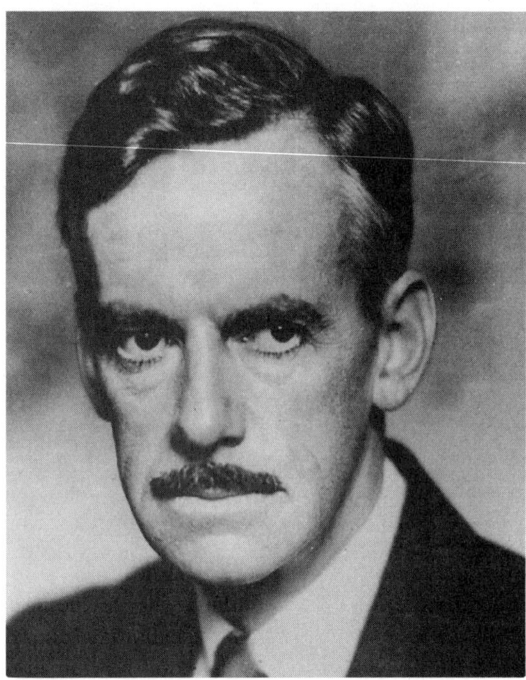

Eugene O'Neill in the 1920s

wright's unpublished work for future reading and production.

O'Neill remarried twice in his life, in 1918 to writer Agnes Boulton (a union that produced two children) and in 1929 to the actress Carlotta Monterey. He died from complications of pneumonia on November 27, 1953, in Boston, Massachusetts.

PLOT SUMMARY

Scene 1

The play opens in a ship's forecastle, the quarters for the crew located in the forward part of the boat. The firemen of the large ocean-going ship are all happily drinking, although there is discernible tension, indicating that the men are capable of violence at a moment's notice. One of the firemen, Yank, declares that beer is sissy and that he only drinks the "hard stuff." Paddy sings a song about whiskey. Yank yells at them, insisting that they are "dead." He says he wants quiet because he's trying to think. Someone sings a sentimental song about home and Yank launches into a verbal attack of home, of emotional connections, and of women.

Long claims they are all really living in hell and blames their miserable conditions on the people in first-class, "the damned Capitalist class." Yank doesn't have the time or attention span for Long's talk of politics. He calls Long yellow and declares that all of the workers are better men than the people in first-class. "Dem boids don't amount to nothing." He gets the group riled up, drowning out Long's speech. Paddy reminisces about the old days, before boats had engines, when man and the sea and the ship became one. Yank says he's crazy, dead even. It takes a real man to work in hell he claims. Yank sees his energy as what drives the ship. "I'm steel," he says, ridiculing the idea that they are slaves. He dismisses Paddy as an outcast, a leftover from a previous age.

Scene 2

On the promenade deck, young Mildred Douglas reclines in a deck chair with her aunt. They engage in small talk and little arguments. Her aunt chides Mildred about her forays into social service and attempts to help the poor. Mildred says she wants "to touch life somewhere," although she has enjoyed the benefits of the wealth produced by her family's steel business.

The aunt points out that Mildred is really quite artificial and that her efforts in helping the poor are actually thinly veiled attempts at some kind of social credibility. Mildred, however, is intent on visiting the stokehole of the ship, to mingle with the common workers and experience their lifestyle. She has received permission from the ship's captain by claiming she had a letter from her father, the chairman of the ship line, who requested that she inspect the vessel. The second engineer escorting her to the stokehole questions her white dress, since she might rub up against dirt or oil; Mildred replies she will throw it out when she comes back up because she has plenty of dresses.

Scene 3

In the stokehole, the men are bare-chested, sweaty, and dirty as they shovel coal into the massive furnace that propels the ship's engines. The heat appears to be oppressive, close to unbearable. Paddy is exhausted. Yank ridicules him and brags about his own ability to face the furnace without tiring. He rallies the men as they put their energy into stoking the furnace.

"He ain't got no noive (nerve)" Yank says of Paddy, and the men respond to his encouragement as he calls on them to feed the baby (the furnace). At the height of their brute physical activity, Mildred enters in her lily-white dress. The whistle sounds, signaling the end of the work shift. The men notice Mildred and are shocked by her incongruous presence. Yank is oblivious to her and continues to work, shaking his shovel at the whistle.

Mildred observes Yank's animal-like force and is appalled by it. Suddenly Yank sees her, sending a venomous, hateful glare at her. She swoons with fear, nearly fainting into her escort's arms. She asks to be taken away, labeling Yank a filthy beast. He is enraged at the insult and throws his shovel at the door through which she has exited.

Scene 4

Yank, unlike the other fireman, has not washed himself after their shift. The men are off-duty and entertaining themselves, while Yank sits, his face covered in coal soot, trying to figure out the previous events in the furnace room. The other men tease him, suggesting he's fallen in love with the stokehole's strange visitor. No, he counters, the feeling he has for Mildred is hate.

Long complains that the engineers put them on exhibition, like they were monkeys. He mentions that Mildred is the daughter of a steel magnate. Paddy suggests her visit was like a visit to the zoo, where they were pointed out as baboons. Paddy says it was love at first sight when she saw Yank, like she had seen a great hairy ape escaped from the zoo. He makes fun of how Yank threw the shovel at her exit.

Yank seems to like the label "Hairy Ape" and imagines that his encounter with Mildred resulted in violence to her. Long says he would have been punished for such an act, but Yank continues this fantasy, feeding his anger over the disparity in his and Mildred's social standing. As Yank shows signs of losing his temper and control, the others pile on him and hold him down. Paddy advises them to give Yank time to cool down before letting him up.

Scene 5

It is some time after the ship's return to port, and Yank and Long walk down Fifth Avenue in New York, talking. Long is once again offering his political rhetoric about the working class while Yank, oblivious to his companion's words, speaks of his growing obsession with teaching the upper class—specifically Mildred—a lesson about human worth. At the same time Yank complains that he doesn't fit in or belong anywhere. They see the jewelry and the furs in the windows of the store and are infuriated at the prices, which are far beyond the means of common men such as themselves. Yank sees a group of wealthy people coming out of a church where they have been making relatively insignificant contributions to the needy. Yank verbally attacks this group saying they don't belong and bragging about his physical prowess, how people like him are the ones who make things work. He challenges them to a fight. Before he can commit any physical violence, however, Yank is restrained by police, who arrest him.

Scene 6

Yank is in jail, angry at being caged like an animal in the zoo. The other prisoners mock him. They ask him what crime he committed, suggesting a domestic argument. Yank explains the root of his anger—Mildred's visit to the stokehole—and his subsequent attack on the rich people. During his rant, he mentions Mildred's last name. The prisoners inform him that her father is president of the Steel Trust. One inmate suggests that Yank join a group of labor activists, the Wobblies, whose efforts are aimed at exacting revenge upon upper class denizens such as Mildred and her father. The inmate gives Yank information about the union. Yank gets very excited that a tangible solution to his problems has presented itself. He talks about the steel bars that are restraining him, imagining himself as a fire that will burn through them. His fervor becomes so intense that he bends the bars and has to be subdued by the guards.

Scene 7

Yank shows up at the Wobblies (the nickname for the International Workers of the World) local union office. He asks to join but has to stop and think when they ask him his real name. The union members are happy to find a fireman from the shipping line who is willing to join their cause. They express an interest in organizing the line's other workers. They want to know why Yank is joining. They ask whether he wants to change the inequality of the world with "legitimate direct action—or with dynamite." He responds that dynamite is the answer and indicates his desire to blow up the Douglas Steel Trust and its president. Quickly sensing that Yank is mentally unstable and dangerous, the union rejects his application. Out on the street, Yank becomes agitated, repeating his belief that there is no place where he truly belongs. A pair of policemen chastise him, believing him to be a drunk.

Scene 8

Yank visits the monkey house at the zoo. He talks to the animals about his experiences in the city. One gorilla responds by pounding on his chest, and Yank decides that they are members of the same club, the Hairy Apes. He wonders how the animals feel, having people look at them in a cage and make fun of them. Pondering the similarities in his and the animals' situations, Yank is so moved that he pries the cage door open. As the gorilla exits, Yank tries to exchange a secret handshake with his newfound friend. The gorilla grabs him in a crushing hug. Yank drops to the ground and, as he dies, realizes that he doesn't even belong with the hairy apes. The monkeys jump and chatter about the stage.

CHARACTERS

Mildred Douglas

Mildred is a vision in white, appropriate for the upper class promenade deck which she inhabits. She is young and idealistic and at the same time oddly aware that her idealism is without real impact or significance. She has a history of social activism and empathy for the lower class in spite of the wealth accumulated by her steel tycoon grandfather and father, whose millions were made by the sweat of workers such as Yank. There is a hint of guilt in her inquiry into the state of the workers, but her interest lacks, as her aunt has criticized, vitality. She shrinks back from the brutal sight of the stokehole and Yank, the quintessential fireman.

Guard

His role is to keep the prisoners in line. He is faced with Yank, a very strong and surprisingly out of control prisoner.

Long

Criticized by Yank for his Socialist leanings, Long still has much in common with Yank. He also sees the dehumanization that is occurring and ties it to the importance of the machine. He agrees with Yank when he sees the people in first class, who represent the ruling class, as being the people who have enslaved the workers by putting them in front of the brutal furnace. While Yank goes off to glory in his position with the furnace, Long proposes socialist solutions to the problem of dehumanization and enslavement. His propositions are rejected by Yank.

Mildred's Aunt

The aunt is accompanying Mildred on the ship and obviously has little sympathy with her niece's charitable tendencies. This lack of sympathy exhibits itself in banter between the two women when the aunt criticizes her niece for being insincere, suggesting that artificiality is a much more natural pose for Mildred.

Paddy

Paddy is a worker on the ship and the voice of the past. He spends his time in reverie, remembering the pleasure he derived from sailing in the old days, when he could feel the wind and the waves; he longs for the simplicity of a time gone by. He has only reluctantly gone on to the new mechanized form of water travel. He is old and tired and wants time to reflect, to sit with his pipe. Paddy acts as a counterpoint to Yank's brute strength and calls to mind an earlier day before industrialized society wrought dehumanized creatures such as Yank and inhuman working conditions such as those found on the ship.

Second Engineer

The Second Engineer takes Mildred to the stokehole, while cautioning her about the dirt she may encounter. He suggests that she change her outfit.

Robert Smith

See Yank

Union Secretary

The Secretary greets Yank with open arms but then is suspicious about his reasons for joining the union. He baits him with questions that Yank is too stupid to circumvent and then throws the brute out, suspecting that he is a plant from the police or the secret service.

Yank

Yank is a foot soldier in the industrial revolution, a fireman (one who tends the massive furnaces that power the ship) who boasts that he loves the hellish heat of the stokehole in which he works. He is a caricature of masculinity, the ultimate macho man—he disdains anything soft or "sissy" and makes fun of anyone he sees as being less than his ideal of a strong man. It is his physical strength that sustains him, the only thing on which he can depend, his only source of pride.

Yank starts the play feeling superior to others because of his physical prowess though he slowly comes to realize that this strength makes him seem like an animal. When he is first introduced to the idea of being a hairy ape he likes it, but he soon finds that the label causes him trouble. He eventually strives to rise above that role, struggling to understand the world and his place in it. For all his efforts at higher thinking, however, he's not successful at figuring it out; his resulting confusion often sends him into uncontrollable rages. Unable to clearly see himself, Yank projects his own doubts and faults on others. When he says others don't belong in society, he is really announcing his own alienation. He only begins to realize his true state as he dies.

MEDIA ADAPTATIONS

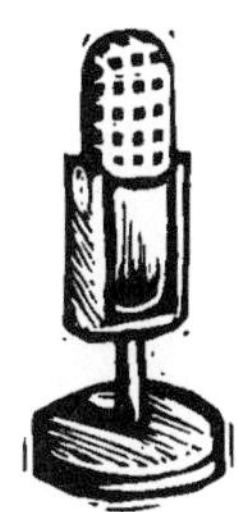

- *The Hairy Ape* was adapted as a film in 1944 with Alfred Santell directing. It stars Susan Hayward as Mildred and William Bendix as Yank. The black and white film was produced by United Artists and is available on videocassette from United American Video Corporation.

THEMES

Class Conflict

Yank is the epitome of the lower class, the working poor. He has the brawn but not the brain. He and his peers put their shoulders to the wheel and make the great capitalist machine run; they provide the sweat and muscle that will push America to the forefront of the industrial age. The system exploits these efforts, reaping great profits for those who own the machines but offering little reward for those who operate them.

Although Yank initially envisions himself above the first-class passengers on the ship—reassuring himself with the knowledge that without people like him the ship would not run—he comes to realize that the rich are getting richer from his efforts while his own rewards remain paltry. It is Mildred's father who owns the steel works and the ship line. And it is people like Mildred who can afford the furs and diamonds on Fifth Avenue. They are living the good life by exploiting the workers.

It is this realization that he is only a cog in the machine and not the center of the industrial universe that plants the first seeds of Yank's disillusion. Before Mildred's appearance in the stokehole, Yank had not been directly exposed to the upper class. While his perception of himself was one of elevated status, he is confronted with the fact that the true mark of high status—money—is in the hands of others. His illusions of importance in question, Yank begins to ponder his exact place in society.

Meaning in Life

Although it is a pose at direct odds with his mental capacities, Yank is seen several times throughout the play in the pose of the "Thinker" (a famous sculpture by Auguste Rodin depicting a man in deep, contemplative thought). What provokes these ponderous episodes is his struggle to understand his role in life. It is a role that he thought he understood. He worked hard, providing the human energy that enabled the massive ship to run its engines. For these efforts he felt he should be viewed as a kind of superhuman, a creature upon whom the rest of society depended. Yet when Mildred nearly faints at his brutish appearance, he is confronted with the possibility that others do not see him in this light.

While his initial reaction to being called an animal—a hairy ape—is one of pleasure, he comes to realize that the distinction is not a positive one. Far from being considered a superman, he is an outcast and an oddity. He is not like his fellow workers and he is certainly not like the first-class passengers.

His first realization that he does not have the social standing he believed provokes growing self-reflection in Yank. Prior to Mildred's visit, he had a firm ideal of his place in society, the meaning of his life. Learning that others do not see him as he sees himself poses the question: where does he fit in? Lacking even the most basic social tools, Yank is an outcast even among the other firemen. Where he

TOPICS FOR FURTHER STUDY

- Think about the character of Yank as a representative for the common laborers who worked in the stokehole. How do these workers compare to laborers in contemporary society? What might you expect to be their (the laborers) take on society and the economic conditions? How is this similar to or different from Yank's attitude?
- How does Yank compare with the character of Willy Loman in Arthur Miller's *Death of a Salesman?* How is he different? How are their fates similar or different?
- Investigate the era of the 1920s. If you were Eugene O'Neill today and wanted to write about the same topic, where would you set this play, what would you title it, and who would you have as main characters?
- Imagine you were a politician in the 1920s. What would you have proposed as political platforms to try and gain the support of laborers such as the firemen on the ship.
- Investigate composers who were producing work in the 1920s. Listen to their music. How does this art form compare with *The Hairy Ape* in style and content? How is it different?

had previously seen this alienation as proof of his superiority, he now begins to question his place among humanity. At the start of the play, Yank is happy—or at least content—with his station in life. The knowledge that reality is far from his perception marks the start of his downfall, his search for a place to belong, and eventually his death.

Socialism and Society in the Industrial Age

While the FBI feared that *The Hairy Ape* would be used as a propaganda tool for those with socialist/communist agendas, the play came to be known more for its study of human nature than for its politics. Socialism, as voiced by the character of Long, argues that the only fair economic system is one that allows ownership by the workers and a more even distribution of wealth among all citizens. While *The Hairy Ape* makes some arguments in favor of better working conditions and an equitable share of profits (it is clear from the play that the firemen are not well compensated for toiling under extreme conditions), it does not aspire, like Clifford Odets's *Waiting for Lefty,* to present an overview of the injustices wrought on the working class.

What O'Neill sought to illustrate was how America's rapid evolution into an industrial nation created personality types that were suited for the necessary tasks. In a form of Darwinian adaptation, those with physical prowess became the workers while those with a sense for money and planning became the upper class. This evolution also created rigid ideals for each social class. O'Neill's interest lay in the development of an extreme social persona such as Yank. Yank's strength and skill as a menial worker allowed him to develop and excel at one thing—stoking an engine furnace. Yet his advancement as a firemen came at a cost to his humanity. He has evolved to an ultra-refined state in which he is as much a machine as human. He can no longer interact with his peers. Beyond criticizing or embracing one system, the play condemns a society—socialist, capitalist, or other—that would allow such an extreme disassociation to take place in the name of progress.

STYLE

Scene vs. Act

Unlike many traditional plays that utilize the act format, O'Neill designed *The Hairy Ape* to be broken up as eight scenes. An act is a demarcation of action in a play that is often comprised of several scenes. Scenes are typically shorter than acts and limited to one or two locations. By structuring his play's action around short episodic scenes, O'Neill is able to encompass a variety of settings that depict Yank's disassociation with both his peers and members of the upper class. The scene format also allows the action of the play to flow quicker, creating a tension that builds to Yank's death in scene 8.

Expressionism and Realism

The Hairy Ape is often categorized as expressionist theater. O'Neill's writing did not exclusively center on this style—in fact, only a handful of the playwright's work fits the definition of expressionistic theater. Dramatic expressionism is a theatrical movement that is largely credited to August Strindberg (author of *Miss Julie* and a significant influence on O'Neill). Within this genre, a playwright can show a very subjective viewpoint on life, one that can be interpreted on a number of levels (which explains why *The Hairy Ape* has variously been viewed as both pro-socialist propaganda and anti-socialist criticism).

With expressionism, the playwright depicts life not as it really is but as he (or his characters) perceives it to be. Often expressionism has found itself connected with social concerns. It also frequently addresses itself to a future, which may or may not ever be experienced in the work (such as Long's utopia of a worker-owned state). The approach is often seen as pessimistic in that it commonly finds society to have serious flaws, yet most expressionistic theater offers some hope for improvement—although a character such as Yank does not reap the benefits of such improvement.

Within the theater, the expressionistic approach opened up the space well beyond the stage and offered the possibility of involving the audience in a much more intimate way. The structure of the play does not have to concern itself as much with a strict chronology of time and sequence, so the playwright has more opportunity to make use of imagination; O'Neill's intent is less concerned with establishing a clear narrative path than painting an impression of Yank's character and dislocation. The playwright can express his views, make use of theatrical devices such as lighting and sound effects, and can distort or exaggerate characters (while realistic in some sense, the hyperbolic Yank is a good example of an extreme expressionist character).

While *The Hairy Ape* has distinct expressionist tendencies, O'Neill infused realistic elements to set off the more extreme action and define his message. The structure of the play is somewhat disjointed and has its surreal moments (particularly the scenes set in the hellish stokehole), yet O'Neill has populated his play with a variety of recognizable character types and settings. Part of the play's success in reaching its audience lies in the familiarity of the people and situations it portrays. By allowing his viewers to identify with facets of his play, O'Neill is able to drive home the more subjective, expressionist aspects of the play. Set against relatively normal characters such as Long and Mildred, Yank appears even more grotesque and out of step with society. Likewise, the relative normalcy of the first-class deck contrasts with the fiery, otherworldly stokehole, emphasizing the vast differences between the classes.

Symbolism

There are some significant and important symbols throughout *The Hairy Ape.* The symbols are employed to reinforce the playwright's ideas and intentions behind the play. Mildred, with her pure white dress, is a symbol of naivete, an unspotted, pure life. This innocence sinks into the depths of the ship, disrupting the equilibrium that had existed among the firemen.

The fire of the furnace is tied into the animal energy of the fireman, who are harnessed to a fever pitch when they feed the ship's engines. The stokehole also symbolizes the hellish nature of the men's lives. It is an underworld that is uncomfortable to all except Yank, who has, symbolically, sold his soul to the ideal of work.

Steel comes up often in the play. Yank claims he is steel. Mildred is the daughter of a man who makes steel. The bars of the prison are steel as are the bars of the gorilla's cage in the zoo. Within the play steel represents that hard and irresistible fact of separation and enslavement. Yank mistakenly sees himself as made of steel but it is the steel of society that holds him apart from the rest of humanity.

The ape is a symbol of the animal and basic nature of man, the evolutionary beginnings of the human race. Yank is a kind of missing link between socialized humans and the wilder animals. His persona is one that is to be harnessed or put behind bars; as evidenced by his attack on the high society group in scene 5, it is something that is not safe out on the streets. Yank's primal state is far from the world of Mildred, who nearly faints when she sees his raw, brutish strength and frightening, ape-like appearance.

HISTORICAL CONTEXT

The 1920s, the decade in which *The Hairy Ape* first appeared, represented an exciting and tumultuous period in American history. It was the age of the flappers (young female socialites intent on dancing and partying), Prohibition, and a massive influx of wealth, often due to stock market speculation. Although the working class saw little change in

COMPARE & CONTRAST

- **1922:** An important textile mill in Manchester, NH, announces that is cutting wages twenty percent and increasing weekly hours from forty-eight to fifty-two. The Railroad Labor Board announces a thirteen percent wage cut.

  Today: While working conditions in many areas have vastly improved, mergers and downsizing have significantly increased the pool of temporary workers. Many corporations rely on the expertise of former employees who are now employed as independent contractors, working long hours with no benefits and with no assurances as to permanency. This situation reduces the overhead of the corporation, which no longer has to pay benefits for these workers.

- **1922:** Henry Ford makes more than $264,000 per day. The Associated Press estimates his wealth to be in the billions.

  Today: Bill Gates, the founder and chair of Microsoft, a dominant computer software company, is reportedly worth billions. His company controls vast portions of the computer market. The Justice Department investigates what many claim are unfair monopolistic practices in Microsoft's day-to-day business.

- **1922:** An enzyme is discovered by Scottish bacteriologist Alexander Fleming. Able to break down the cellular walls of bacteria, the enzyme is named penicillin, a breakthrough drug that will change the way disease is battled and overcome.

  Today: Researchers have devised a protocol of drugs, which when taken regularly in combination can halt or delay the progress of AIDS. Many HIV positive people depend on this cocktail of drugs to preserve their life, waiting for a more definitive cure for the disease.

- **1922:** Prohibition makes illegal the manufacture, sale, and transportation of alcoholic beverages. Despite the law, a lively trade for alcohol exists, resulting in the rise of the organized crime.

  Today: The use of marijuana is illegal, resulting in a major trade in illegal drugs, involving more than marijuana. Some states have legalized the use of marijuana for medicinal purposes, but the drug must be prescribed by a doctor.

their quality of life during this period, there was a growing affluent class who could afford to indulge themselves in such leisure activities as a sea cruise to Europe, as Mildred and her aunt do in O'Neill's play.

For many decades up to and beyond the 1920s, as the upper classes were amassing considerable wealth from its advances, the Industrial Revolution was creating a more demanding and intense work environment for both skilled and unskilled laborers. As scientific technology created more powerful means of industry, such as the steam engine used to power ocean liners and railroads, more workers were needed to maintain the machines, often with little regard for their safety or mental well-being. As the pitch of the revolution became more intense and the need for faster and faster means of production arose, workers were pushed to often unbearable extremes to foster industrial growth.

As working conditions worsened, unions arose. These organizations sought to ensure that laborers were fairly paid for their work—and that work conditions met with safety requirements. The union movement was viewed by business owners with suspicion. The International Workers of the World (the Wobblies represented in the play) represented a growing movement of workers dissatisfied with the status quo who demanded equity. Often this movement was connected with socialism or the communist party, which attained power in Russia with the revolution of 1917. Socialism argues for community ownership of the means of production, with all classes sharing equally in the profits.

While unions enjoyed significant growth in the 1920s, it was also a difficult period in which union organizers were opposed, often violently, by business owners. A basic tactic of the unions was the strike, in which workers would uniformly walk off the job, stalling production, and, hopefully, forcing the owners to meet their demands. Management retaliated by sending in strikebreakers (often these were thugs hired to intimidate union leaders and brutalize workers) and replacement workers (often called "scabs"). Clashes between striking workers and the management's replacements often turned violent.

The 1920s was the lull between the storms. The world had survived World War I. But it had not yet dealt with the side effects of a burgeoning economy. The 1930s would see an economic depression that impacted the world and the lives of both rich and poor.

By 1922, however, World War I had ended, nations were stabilizing, and the industrial machine built to support the war effort was now put into the service of consumerism. Times were very good for the nations on the winning side of the war. Yet in the nations defeated in WWI, this period marked the rise of fascism, particularly the regimes of Benito Mussolini in Italy and Adolf Hitler in Germany. The impact of these dictatorships would come to the fore in the next two decades as the world headed toward a second global battle.

In addition to lubricating the machines of the industrial age, modern science was making significant inroads in human health care. Discoveries in the treatment of diabetes with animal insulin and microorganisms connected to the advent of the antibiotic penicillin gave humankind greater stability and control of its environment. Crippling diseases that once represented a serious impediment to advancement now seemed surmountable; man was learning to control his world.

As the 1920s brought newfound affluence to many parts of society, people had more time and money to spend on arts and leisure. As a result the decade saw the motion picture industry reach its first zenith of commerce and creativity, and there was a surge in significant new music, art, and literature. Novelist James Joyce published the completed version of his landmark work *Ulysses* in 1922. Although the book would never make any bestseller list, Joyce's account of one day in the life of Molly and Leopold Bloom in Dublin, Ireland, was destined to have a significant impact on how fiction (and other literature forms) was written. Joyce's unique stream of consciousness approach eventually influenced the Beats of the 1950s, which included poet Allen Ginsberg and novelists Jack Kerouac and William S. Burroughs.

In music, Jazz came into its own in the 1920s. A distinctly American musical form with roots in numerous styles, Jazz originated in New Orleans and eventually found mass popularity in New York nightclubs such as the Cotton Club. Although embraced to some extent stateside, Jazz music became wildly popular in Europe, where race proved less of an obstacle for the predominantly black musicians.

This expatriatism came to affect a variety of artists in the 1920s, as a significant number of important Americans left the U.S. to live and work in Europe. This group included writers such Gertrude Stein, Ernest Hemingway, and F. Scott Fitzgerald. While these white writers and artists were sitting in sidewalk cafes in Paris, France, African American writers who had migrated to America's northern cities began to express their anger at racism (notably the recent history of slavery and civil rights abuses that followed Abraham Lincoln's Emancipation Proclamation) and to forge an identity for themselves. This movement was called the Harlem Renaissance and includes writers such as Langston Hughes, Claude McKay, and Zora Neale Hurston.

CRITICAL OVERVIEW

O'Neill himself acknowledged that *The Hairy Ape* straddles a number of styles. "It seems to run the gamut from extreme naturalism to extreme expressionism—with more of the latter than the former," he wrote in 1921. The initial response to productions of *The Hairy Ape* focused on the skill of the play's staging and its forceful impact on a viewer. Describing O'Neill's skill with the voice of the working men, Alexander Woollcoot of the *New York Times* said, "Squirm as you may, he holds you while you listen to the rumble of their discontent, and while you listen . . . it is true talk, all of it, and only those who have been so softly bred that they have never really heard the vulgate spoken in all its richness would venture to suggest that he has exaggerated it."

The playwright's intentions in depicting the world of the ship laborers was graphic: O'Neill intended the stokehole as a depiction of Hell. For Yank this isn't a problem. According to Richard Skinner in *Eugene O'Neill: A Poet's Quest,* "There is both splendor and terror at Yank's pride at being at the bottom." This pride, however, takes him through a number of episodes, culminating in the face to face meeting with a real hairy ape. In Yank's monologue directed to the gorilla, Skinner found "the most profound problem of the disjointed and divided soul." The critic continued, "Man is searching for peace in mere animal instinct and finding that then he can not throw off his manhood. The answer? Escape even from thought."

Although many dubbed it a challenging piece of theater, the majority of critics termed *The Hairy Ape* as a success. What the play is about, however, has been a topic of discussion. Some have claimed it is about the capitalist oppression of the masses (the workers) while others have termed it an examination of alienation in human society.

Alienation is a topic on which many critics have focused, the sense of dislocation that affects the firemen. Yank and his peers may believe themselves to be in touch with the world, better than the rich folks on the upper decks. The workers may echo Yank's sentiment that it is they who drive the world. But as Edwin Engel wrote in *The Haunted Heroes of Eugene O'Neill,* Yank enjoys "a false sense of belonging to something, of being part of steel and of machinery, whereas he is actually their slave." This enslavement is one that dawns on Yank slowly as he realizes he doesn't really belong anywhere.

The realization dawns with Mildred's visit to the stokehole. "Mildred has laid him bare," stated Thierry Dubost in *Struggle, Defeat or Rebirth: Eugene O'Neill's Vision of Humanity,* "He does not know where he fits into a world that has become incomprehensible to him, which is the reason for his wandering, his pathetic quest for community where he could be accepted and could at last be himself."

Although Yank was content in the secluded underworld of the stokehole, Mildred's visit shattered that insularity. After her appearance he starts referring to himself as the hairy ape. Despite Yank's tragic end, many critics have not viewed O'Neill's final message as one of permanent despair. "'The Hairy Ape' was to be only a symbol of the dark despair that sometimes sweeps over the soul to disappear later in a triumph of sheer will," stated Skinner.

Where does *The Hairy Ape* fit into the body of works that have prompted many to proclaim O'Neill as the most important American dramatist? O'Neill thought this play was very important, and it may be his most obvious exploration into how human beings are lost from their past and present. How they cope when any semblance of importance is removed from their lives. While *The Hairy Ape* is not considered in the same league as O'Neill's widely regarded masterpiece, *Long Day's Journey into Night,* it is noted as one of the playwright's more significant dramatic works and a highly effective example of expressionist theater.

CRITICISM

Etta Worthington

Worthington is a playwright and educator. In this essay she examines O'Neill's sense of alienation and despair as seen through the experience of Yank.

On the surface *The Hairy Ape* might seem to be a fairly political play. There is the marked contrast of the sweaty fireman whose brute strength propels the ship that provides diversion and pleasure to those privileged class denizens who inhabit the upper decks. There is obvious reference to exploitation of the workers. But *The Hairy Ape,* although laced with references to capitalism, socialism, and other concepts, is really about the existential condition of man, namely that humans rarely feel like they fit in, that they are essentially always alone and separate.

This play, which was a foray into expressionism for the playwright, presents a number of characters who are in essence only stick figures. There is Mildred, the precious princess who cannot face reality, although she flirts with the idea of social activism and charity. Despite her social posturing, her true self is readily apparent: "Be as artificial as you are," her aunt advises. Ultimately, artificial is all Mildred is—although she is well-intentioned and appears to have a good heart. Then there is Long who mouths socialist gospel but has no personality or soul to speak of. And Paddy, a relic from the past, is painted without dimension. It is only Yank, the

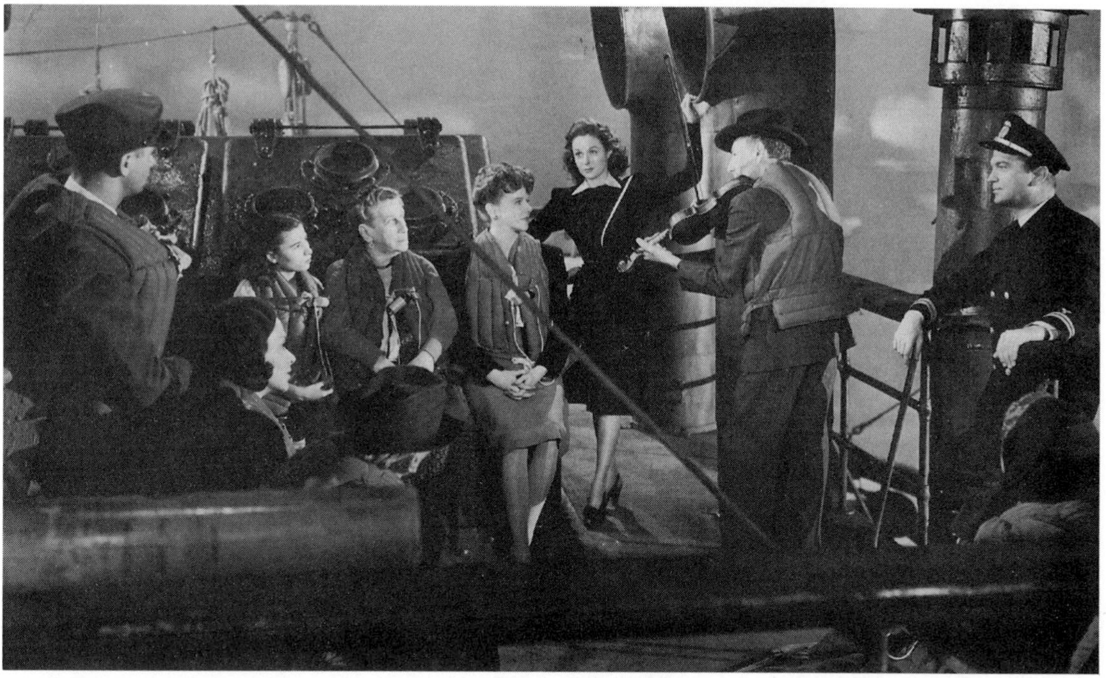

A scene from the 1944 film adaptation of The Hairy Ape. *Mildred (Susan Hayward) is seated to the right of her aunt (Dorothy Comingore)*

swarthy, beastly king of the stokehole, who is a multidimensional character. And it is Yank who personifies O'Neill's examination of the human condition.

"Yank . . . is the only character who really lives, all the others merely serve as background against which he stands out," claimed Andrew Malone in *Contour in Time: The Plays of Eugene O'Neill.*

In the course of the play Yank goes from the cocky leader of the mighty firemen to a heap of a human being, crushed physically and morally. In the sweaty stokehole, Yank possesses a comfortable worldview. He shows disdain for the upper classes that Long criticizes. Yet these supposed oppressors are inconsequential in Yank's view. "They don't belong," he rants again and again. He roars out his defiance toward them, believing his mastery of the furnace defines and raises him above all others.

"In the stokehole, Yank belongs. His credo—that he is the force at the bottom that makes the entire mechanized society move—is right. He is such a force until the meeting with Mildred causes him to doubt himself and sends him out in a frenzied effort to destroy the God of power he has served in his furnace altar." wrote Travis Bogard in *Contour in Time.*

Yank's sense of place is tenuous at best. In what others label as hell, he feels a connection. But this feeling of connection does not extend beyond the stokehole, which for him is the center of the universe, even the pinnacle.

The fateful encounter with Mildred puts his world on edge. He is a man beside himself when her look of horror and revulsion emblazons itself on his psyche. His worldview is shattered as he realizes he is not the king of anything. And he sets out roaring like a wounded beast. Now his only connections are with steel—he has in fact called himself steel: "I'm steel—steel—steel! I'm de muscles in steel, de punch behind it!"—with the fire of the furnace, and with the animals in the zoo (the other hairy apes). He is forced to admit his lack of connection with other humans; he is alienated from society.

This alienation is one that O'Neill underscores throughout the play by employing a number of symbols. The steel, whether it's the clanging door of the furnace, the shovel that is an extension of Yank's arm, or the bars of the prison and the gorilla cage at the zoo, is hard and ultimately isolating. It

WHAT DO I READ NEXT?

- *Emperor Jones* (1920) is another of O'Neill's forays into expressionist theater. It tells the story of a black man who worked as a railroad porter and eventually ends up in the West Indies where, by a bit of fate, raises himself to the role of emperor.
- Arthur Miller's *Death of a Salesman* (1949) chronicles the life of a salesman who, while harboring delusions of grandeur, is ultimately only a cog in the machine of business. The play examines how his failure to grasp reality impacts both his life and the lives of his family.
- John Steinbeck's novel *The Grapes of Wrath* (1939) chronicles the despair of the disenfranchised American worker. The novel deals with the economic period—the Great Depression—that followed the boom era of O'Neill's play.
- *The Great Gatsby,* written by F. Scott Fitzgerald and published in 1925, is a look into the privileged class that before the Great Depression had little care and spent much of its time partying.

reinforces the idea of separation. Even Mildred the unwitting muse (or tormentor) of Yank, represents the metal: she is the daughter of a steel magnate, the offspring of the cold, isolating substance.

Mildred wears white. It is a cold color, one without warmth or hue. Her white dress does not connote pureness or welcome but coolness and distance. The color underscores the gulf between her world and that of the soot-black firemen—and it is Yank who revels in the soot, refusing to wash it off his skin after his work is done. Heightening the contrast, Mildred's complexion, when confronted with the filthy beast-like Yank, turns pale and white.

The sea, which is one of the backdrops for this drama, again reinforces the idea of dislocation. Long a fascination for O'Neill (he worked for a time as a merchant seaman), the sea is always creating distance. The sailors on the ship are disconnected from family and home. Yank himself, drinking with the other firemen, pronounces the lack of importance of home. It was just someplace to get away from for him. "On'y too glad to beat it, dat was me. Home was lickings for me, dat's all." This statement explains his outburst "t'hell wit home."

"No one has understood better than Eugene O'Neill that the soul at war with itself belongs nowhere in this world of realities. The soul that denies or seeks to escape from its own creative powers sinks in misery below the beast," stated Richard Skinner in *Eugene O'Neill: A Poet's Quest.*

Yank first starts to sense this point when he sees Mildred faint at the sight of him. The disturbance that starts to brew in him leaves him confused, trying to think while his drinking companions grow far away from him. The dawning awareness of his disassociation from society comes to a head when Yank is on shore, wandering down Fifth Avenue, gaping at the unattainable luxuries in the glass windows. "De don't belong no more'n she does," he announces. He heckles a group of wealthy church goers exiting a service. He approaches the group, proclaiming that they don't belong. Emphasizing his own place in society (as much for his own benefit as theirs), he shouts: "Look at me, why don't youse dare? I belong, dat's me!" Yank's behavior becomes more erratic as the wealthy people ignore his remarks. Eventually he becomes so violent that the police arrive and arrest him.

Incarcerated, Yank laments his state and obsesses about the woman he believes is responsible for his present condition. "I'll show her who belongs," he vows. But then he explodes with the knowledge that her father has made the steel in the cell that holds him. The guards must come and hose him down, like a wild animal.

Once released from prison, Yank searches out the Wobblies, hoping to find a place in the labor movement, one that will calm his anger and exact the revenge he desires. He's a natural, it seems. A worker with leadership among other workers. But his alienation extends even to this arena as he is ousted by the union. His ideas about blowing up the steel mills are correctly interpreted by the union as a sign of his instability.

Finally, it dawns on Yank that despite his claims of belonging, just the opposite is true. ''Now I ain't steel, and de woild owns me. Aw hell! I can't see—it's all dark, get me? It's all wrong.''

The only place Yank can think to go is the zoo, where he feels an affinity for the gorillas. After all, he is the hairy ape isn't he. Yank struggles to understand what he's been through. He resigns himself to the animal kingdom, believing this is the one place where he will belong. Yet once again, and with tragic finality, he discovers that he doesn't fit in anywhere—even with the animals.

The longing that Yank carries in his breast, this quest for connection and belonging, is, according to some critics, a mystical yearning. Even though it is played out in the arena of social politics, Yank's dilemma, the focus of the play, is ultimately a quest for spiritual fulfillment. While it is ambiguous (in the case of Yank) as to whether the search involves a concrete religion and God, the spiritual theme is one that O'Neill pondered throughout his work.

Explaining the importance O'Neill placed on the spiritual, he once said, ''I suppose that is one reason why I have come to feel so indifferent toward political and social movements of all kinds. Time was when I was an active socialist, and, after that, a philosophical anarchist. But today I can't feel that anything like that really matters.'' While this statement does not explicitly name God, other critics have interpreted the playwright's words to mean that religion in life has far greater weight and import than such trivial and transitory things as social politics. In *Eugene O'Neill: A World View,* Virginia Floyd wrote, ''For O'Neill the quest for the meaning of life, of existence, proves to be religious in nature. His concern is not the relation between man and man but the relation between God and man and between man and his divided soul, seeking, as the playwright himself, for a faith to make it whole.''

Throughout *The Hairy Ape,* we see that Yank's animal nature, which is one of the few things that offers him connection to his world (the stokehole), is grotesque and, ultimately, the cause of his death. He proudly adopts the title of hairy ape and glories in the raw strength of it. But it is Mildred who recognizes the true nature of Yank's brute animal center, and, as a representative of civilized society, the one who rejects and recoils from such traits.

> "YANK'S SENSE OF PLACE IS TENUOUS AT BEST. IN WHAT OTHERS LABEL AS HELL, HE FEELS A CONNECTION. BUT THIS FEELING OF CONNECTION DOES NOT EXTEND BEYOND THE STOKEHOLE, WHICH FOR HIM IS THE CENTER OF THE UNIVERSE."

''I have tried to dig deep in it, to probe in the shadows of the soul of man bewildered by the disharmony of his primitive side,'' O'Neill wrote. That animal or primitive side, which is so near the surface in Yank, is the source of his alienation. Yet, in the final scene, when he makes actual contact with an animal that he believes to be like himself, he is crushed to death, dying with the realization that even among the apes he does not belong. Floyd stated that the final words of the play, which come in the stage directions, are some of the most bitter O'Neill ever wrote. As Yank's lifeless body slumps to the bottom of the gorilla cage, O'Neill writes ''And, perhaps, the Hairy Ape at last belongs.'' Only in complete surrender to alienation and isolation from humanity—which is ultimately death—does Yank find what he wants: to belong to something.

With these enigmatic words concluding his play, O'Neill leads us to assume that the problem of the human condition, the problem of alienation, is one that is never truly solved in life. While some cope with it better than others, no one is exempt. By stating that, in his death, Yank ''at last belongs,'' many have read O'Neill's meaning to be a religious one. While humankind must endure alienation in corporeal life, all will be a part of the heavenly kingdom in their eternal life. Those reading the playwright's intent from a pessimistic point of view, however, have adopted a more organic interpretation of O'Neill's final words regarding Yank. His lifeless form slumped to the ground, it is the earth to which the hairy ape now truly belongs, his decomposing body becoming one with the soil.

Source: Etta Worthington, for *Drama for Students,* Gale, 1998.

Alexander Woolcott

In this review, which was originally published on March 10, 1922, Woolcott states that despite the usual flaws that one comes to expect in the work of O'Neill, The Hairy Ape *is a stunning piece of theatre with at least ''a little greatness'' to it.*

The little theatre of the Provincetownsmen in Macdougal Street was packed to the doors with astonishment last evening as scene after scene unfolded in the new play by Eugene O'Neill. This was *The Hairy Ape,* a bitter, brutal, wildly fantastic play of nightmare hue and nightmare distortion. It is a monstrously uneven piece, now flamingly eloquent, now choked and thwarted and inarticulate. Like most of his writing for the theatre, it is the worse here and there for the lack of a fierce, unintimidated blue pencil. But it has a little greatness in it, and it seems rather absurd to fret overmuch about the undisciplined imagination of a young playwright towering so conspicuously above the milling, mumbling crowd of playwrights who have no imagination at all.

The Hairy Ape has been superbly produced. There is a rumor abroad that Arthur Hopkins, with a proprietary interest in the piece, has been lurking around its rehearsals and the program confesses that Robert Edmond Jones went down to Macdougal Street and took hand with Cleon Throckmorton in designing the eight pictures which the play calls for. That preposterous little theatre has one of the most cramped stages New York has ever known, and yet on it the artists have created the illusion of vast spaces and endless perspectives. They drive one to the conclusion that when a stage seems pinched and little, it is the mind of the producer that is pinched and little. This time O'Neill, unbridled, set them a merry pace in the eccentric gait his imaginings. They kept up with him.

O'Neill begins his fable by posing before you the greatest visible contrast in social and physical circumstance. He leads you up the gangplank of a luxurious liner bound for Europe. He plunges you first into the stokers' pit, thrusting you down among the men as they stumble in from the furnaces, hot, sweaty, choked with coal dust, brutish. Squirm as you may, he holds you while you listen to the rumble of their discontent, and while you listen, also, to speech more squalid than even an American audience heard before in an American theatre. It is true talk, all of it, and only those who have been so softly bred that they have never really heard the vulgate spoken in all its richness would venture to suggest that he has exaggerated it by so much as a syllable in order to agitate the refined. On the contrary.

Then, in a twinkling, he drags you (as the ghosts dragged Scrooge) up out of all this murk and thudding of engines and brawling of speech, to a cool, sweet, sunlit stretch of the hurricane deck, where, at lazy ease, lies the daughter of the President of the line's board of directors, a nonchalant dilletant who has found settlement work frightfully interesting and is simply crazy to go down among the stokers and see how the other half lives aboard ship.

Then follows the confrontation—the fool fop of a girl and the huge animal of a stoker who had taken a sort of dizzy romantic pride in himself and his work as something that was real in an unreal world, as something that actually counted, as something that was and had force. Her horrified recoil from him as from some loathsome, hairy ape is the first notice served on him by the world that he doesn't belong. The remaining five scenes are the successive blows by which this is driven in on him, each scene, as written, as acted and as intensified by the artists, taking on more and more of the nightmare quality with which O'Neill seemed possessed to endow his fable.

The scene on Fifth Avenue when the hairy ape comes face to face with a little parade of wooden-faced church-goers who walk like automata and prattle of giving a ''Hundred Per Cent. American Bazaar'' as a contribution to the solution of discontent among the lower classes; the scene on Blackwell's Island with the endless rows of cells and the argot of the prisoners floating out of darkness; the care with which each scene ends in a retributive and terrifying closing in upon the bewildered fellow—all these preparations induce you at last to accept as natural and inevitable and right that the hairy ape should, by the final curtain, be found dead inside the cage of the gorilla in the Bronx Zoo.

Except for the role of the girl, which is pretty badly played by Mary Blair, the cast captured for *The Hairy Ape* is an exceptionally good one. Louis Wolheim, though now and then rather painfully off the beat in his co-operation with the others, gives a capital impersonation of the stoker, and lesser parts are well managed by Harry O'Neill as an Irish fireman dreaming of the old days of sailing vessels, and Harold West as a cockney agitator who is fearfully annoyed because of the hairy ape's concentrating his anger against this one little plutocrat instead of maintaining an abstract animosity against plutocrats in general.

In Macdougal Street now and doubtless headed for Broadway, we have a turbulent and tremendous play, so full of blemishes that the merest fledgling among the critics could point out a dozen, yet so vital and interesting and teeming with life that those playgoers who let it escape them will be missing one of the real events of the year.

"IN *THE HAIRY APE* WE HAVE A TURBULENT AND TREMENDOUS PLAY, SO FULL OF BLEMISHES THAT THE MEREST FLEDGLING AMONG THE CRITICS COULD POINT OUT A DOZEN, YET SO VITAL AND INTERESTING AND TEEMING WITH LIFE THAT THOSE PLAYGOERS WHO LET IT ESCAPE THEM WILL BE MISSING ONE OF THE REAL EVENTS OF THE YEAR."

Source: Alexander Woolcott, "Eugene O'Neill at Full Tilt" (1922) in *On Stage: Selected Reviews from the New York Times, 1920–1970,* edited by Bernard Beckerman and Howard Siegman, Arno Press, 1973, p. 27.

Marden J. Clark

Clark delineates the dramatic elements of O'Neill's play that qualify the work as a tragedy. Central to the discussion is the main character Yank's transition from an uncomprehending brute to an aware thinker.

The Hairy Ape has been widely praised and widely reprinted. Most reviewers and critics have agreed that it has unusual power and unusual ability to project its sense of tragedy. But critics have disagreed on where that sense of tragedy comes from and, in consequence, on basic matters of interpretation. Early critics saw its power in its brutal naturalism, for a long time hardly noticing the expressionistic techniques—and disregarding O'Neill's explicit instructions that the treatment of the scenes "should by no means be naturalistic." More recently commentators have recognized some of the complex ways in which this comparatively direct and simple play works. I like much of Doris V. Falk's analysis in psychoanalytic and existential terms. She seems especially germane when she suggests that Yank in his "belonging" "has abdicated his manhood, has ceased to be an 'existent' and becomes a passive, vegetative being at the mercy of forces outside himself and beyond his control." [*Eugene O'Neill and the Tragiz Tension,* New Jersey.] However we interpret "belonging," we miss O'Neill's play if we interpret it as good. Yet as late as 1947 Joseph Wood Krutch, perhaps the most sensitive and appreciative of O'Neill's critics, was able to describe Yank as "a man who, however brutalized, remains a man until he loses his sense of 'belonging,' and thereby inevitably becomes an animal." [*American Scholar,* Summer, 1947] The truth, I am convinced, is almost diametrically opposite this. I would describe Yank as a man who, by glorying in his merely belonging, contributes to his own brutalization, who remains a brute until he gets jarred out of that sense of belonging and then inevitably moves toward becoming a man, in the process inevitably destroying himself.

To see this as the direction of the action, we need merely ask at what stage we admire Yank more: when he is the brutal mechanistic ape shoveling coal into the hell-fires to drive faster the mechanism he is part of and exploited by, or when he is talking to himself and to the real ape outside the cage. Yank's movement from the cage and hell of the stokehole to the actual cage involves several different complementary and overlapping threads of action, all but one of them leading downward.

All these threads begin from the dramatic and jarring confrontation of Yank and Mildred in Scene III. Yank has already shown himself not only belonging, but belonging so completely that he neither knows nor needs to know what he rejects in so belonging. He comments "with a cynical grin" on the activity that is to become so important to him: "Can't youse see I'm tryin' to t'ink?" His mates echo the cynicism when they echo the word "Think" and then work it up into almost a chant, "Drink, don't think. Drink, don't think." He has neither a past (like the lost romance and beauty of Paddy's clipper ships) nor a future (not even like the one implied in Long's cheap attacks that look forward to the overthrow of the "damned Capitalist Class"). Yank is all present: "Sure, I'm part of de engines! Why de hell not! Dey move, don't dey? Deyre speed, ain't dey! . . . Steel, dat stands for de whole ting! And I'm steel—steel—steel! I'm de muscles in steel, de punch behind it!" Yank's rhetoric defines a frighteningly blind hubris. He not only belongs to all this; he *is* all of it—crew, ship, motion, steam, money, steel. . . .

Yank not only belongs completely at the beginning of the play, he dominates both his society and the setting. In a way, we admire his sometimes goodnatured, sometimes brutal domination of his mates in the stokehole. But O'Neill carefully controls our response. Though Yank shows a kind of intellect in arriving at the fancy that he is steel, his hubris is hardly an intellectual one: witness the ridicule of his own "trying to t'ink." The first three scenes dramatize the contrast between Yank's pretensions and the reality behind them. That reality is the meaningless stokehole life of the present contrasted with Paddy's clippership life of the past. That reality is the engineer's whistle, a mere sound, which runs Yank. That reality is the money represented by Mildred and her aunt—crass materialism. That reality is Mildred herself, fainting at the sight of "the filthy beast" and being carried up on a stretcher, ironically just as Yank had predicted if one of "dem slobs" came down into the hole. Like that of most tragic heroes, Yank's hubris, especially in the third scene, carries a fine dramatic irony, not too subtle here but powerful. To the first whistle he responds with his "exultant tone of command." To the second he responds "contemptuously": "Take it easy dere, you! Who d'yuh tinks runnin' dis game, me or you? When I git ready, we move. Not before! When I git ready, git me!" To the third he responds with the fierce gestures and curses that Mildred sees and hears. In this scene O'Neill carefully emphasizes Yank's ape-like qualities. All the men shovel "in the crouching, inhuman attitudes of chained gorillas." As Yank curses the engineer, "he brandishes his shovel murderously over his head in one hand, pounding on his chest with the other, gorilla-like." As he becomes conscious of the men watching something behind him, he "whirls defensively with a snarling, murderous growl, crouching to spring, his lips drawn back over his teeth, his small eyes gleaming ferociously." The height of his hubris exactly coincides with the depths of his animality.

Confronted thus with Mildred, from the unknown world behind his own and so diametrically different from him, Yank "feels himself insulted in some unknown fashion in the very heart of his pride." He of course can only feel the insult, not rationalize it, but he feels rightly: it has hit the very heart of his pride. That pride, so intimately associated with his bruteness, is at once the least human and the most human think about Yank, at once the least and the most promising, at once the least and the most admirable. It carries many of the ambiguities and ambivalences of classical hubris. We admire the energy, the confidence, the positiveness. We shudder for the blindness, the swagger, the presumption. Even in associating Yank's pride with his bruteness, O'Neill manages to suggest something of the classical potential for positive development and terrible destruction that can come from hubris, from the all-too human presumption of the godhood that will destroy.

From this confrontation, the movement downward from hubris begins. Also from here, and most important to the tragic effect, the complementary movement upward begins, upward from the depths of Yank's animality. We see the beginnings of his change immediately in the next scene. Still reeling under the impact of Mildred's revulsion, Yank is now "The Thinker"; he shows no self-ridicule, only resentment at interruption when he's "tryin' to tink." O'Neill emphasizes the ironic contrast by having the men echo the work "Think" again, as they did in Scene One. Thinking is nearly always painful; it is especially difficult for this man-brute who has just been shocked out of what was most brute in him. But thinking is a human function: the brute has started to think, and in so doing has started moving toward manhood. A quest also, even for vengeance or for something to belong to, is a human journey. Yank takes that journey, blindly as all men must. Blindly, gropingly, hopelessly (though only at the end can he know that). But his quest aims at the wrong things, is still dictated by the shattered remains of hubris: revenge, he feels, can restore his pride.

Yank may have "fallen in hate," as he insists to Paddy, but his own self, not merely Mildred, is the object of his hate: he cannot stand the self Mildred has revealed to him. But he can sense this only dimly. His "thinking" still remains on the most elementary level. His contemptuous dismissal of "Law," "Government," "God," comes simply from the pragmatic awareness that none of these can solve his problem. And what thinking he has done dissolves into rage as he recognizes Paddy's truth that Mildred had looked "hairy ape" at him even if she had not said the words. The rage subsides momentarily into bewilderment that brings on questions: "Say, who is dat skoit, huh? What is she? What's she come from? Who made her? Who give her de noive to look at me like that? Dis ting's got my goat right. I don't get her. She's new to me. What does a skoit like her mean, huh?" Elementary questions, to be sure, but questions that Yank could not have asked before confronting Mildred. And perhaps not even so elementary. For Yank is really groping toward one of the most fundamental of religious-philosophical questions: the source and meaning of opposites, of Yank and Mildred, of extreme wealth and extreme poverty, of the black animal human and the white effete human, even (though this may seem a big jump) of good and evil. But at this stage Yank can respond only emotionally. His new image of their relationship—"She grinds de organ and I'm on de string, huh"—adds a fine touch to O'Neill's pattern of ironic contrasts between man and ape. With the loss of his hubris, Yank's image of himself shrivels. No longer even the "filthy beast" Mildred had seen, the hairy ape she had "looked" though not said, but just a weak, jabbering monkey on a string. No wonder the image sets off his new "frenzy of rage" and sends him rushing for immediate revenge.

But of course he cannot—and should not—live with the new image of himself. The Fifth Avenue scene shows Yank desperately trying to regain the old image by revenge if not on Mildred herself then on the society she represents. He shows little of his new-found thinking here. But the scene effectively demonstrates the hopelessness of physical revenge and, by implication, of any revenge as a means of restoring the old Yank. The old Yank cannot be restored. But Yank does not know that.

In jail, Yank is "The Thinker" again. He has been given "Toity days to tink it over." But as he says, "Tink it over! Christ, dat's all I been doin' for weeks!" Yank ends this scene with his "appalling" new awareness that Mildred's "old man—president of de Steel Trust—makes half de steel in de world—steel—where I tought I belonged—drivin' trou—movin'—in dat—to make *her*—and cage me in for her to spit on!" We, of course, have seen all this long before, but it is painful new knowledge for Yank. It leads him first to the new image of himself as fire melting steel, "breakin' out in de night—" then to the resultant trouble as he bends the bars and gets the appropriate punishment for fire that has broken out: the fire hose "full pressure."

His encounter with the actual I.W.W., not the demagogue's version, closes the door on the final possibility for revenge. His mad idea to "blow up de steel, knock all de steel in de woild up to the moon" can "belong" no place except in his own wild mind, certainly not in so banal an organization as Yank finds. But being thrown out sets off the thinking again. He sees that the I.W.W. are "in the wrong pew." They want to solve all problems by giving men a dollar more a day and an hour less: "Tree square a day, and cauliflowers in de front yard—ekal rights—a woman and kids—a lousy vote—and I'm all fixed for Jesus, huh?" Bitter irony, this. But Yank has already been forced into a far deeper awarenes of the complexity of human problems, especially his own, than these men will ever reach:

> Dis ting's in your inside, but it ain't your belly. Feedin' your face—sinkers and coffee—dat don't touch it. It's way down—at de bottom. Yuh can't grab it, and yuh can't stop it. It moves, and everything moves. It stops and de whole world stops. Dat's me now—I don't tick, see?—I'm a busted Ingersoll, dat's what. Steel was me, and I owned de woild. Now I ain't steel, and de woild owns me. Aw, hell! I can't see—it's all dark, get me. It's all wrong! (*He turns a bitter mocking face up like an ape gibbering at the moon.*) Say, youse up dere, Man in de Moon, yuh look so wise, gimme de answer, huh? Slip me de inside dope, de information right from de stable—where do I get off at, huh?

I'm not sure that O'Neill plays quite fair with his character here—at the moment of his simple, eloquent rhetoric and his most intense questioning, to describe him as like an ape gibbering at the moon. But the description reinforces the fundamental ironies in the contrasting lines of symbol and action: When most an ape Yank feels himself most a man; now having moved a long way toward manhood he looks most the ape. O'Neill pushes the irony in the brief encounter with the policeman. Yank has two responses, both telling: ''Sure! Lock me up! Put me in a cage! Dat's de ony answer yuh know.'' Underline ''yuh'' and we get the force of this. Yank shows a new kind of unconscious superiority here: he at least knows that the policeman's answer, society's answer, is not enough. And when the policeman asks what Yank's been doing, Yank answers, with a new kind of ironical awareness: ''Enuff to gimme life for! I was born, see? Sure dat's de charge.'' Born, to life in the cage. When Yank asks, ''Say where do I go from here?'' the policeman, *giving him a push—with a grin, indifferently,* answers ''Go to hell.'' The policeman is the last human we see other than Yank. The contrast is telling: the man who has his one answer giving the ape with all his questions a push on the way to hell.

The hell of Yank's finish contrasts tellingly also with the original hell of the stokehole. The zoo is the home of the real ape. As we might expect here, where Yank has come home to belong, he begins by admiring the gorilla's chest and shoulders, the ''punch in eider fist dat'd knock 'em all silly,'' his ability to ''challenge de whole woild.'' But almost immediately he recognizes that he is seeing in the ape what Mildred saw there in the stokehole: ''On'y outa de cage—broke out—free to moider her, see? . . . She wasn't wise dat I was in a cage, too—worser'n yours—sure—a damn sight—'cause you got some chanct to to bust loose—but me—(*He grows confused*) Aw, hell! It's all wrong, ain't it?'' Yes, it is all wrong, on a social and philosophical level. Yank should not have been given the ability to think, without the ability to find some way out for himself. Yank is right on the psychological level, too: he can never find a way out of the cage of himself. At least never so long as he tries merely to belong. But he is wrong about himself on the human, the tragic level. For he *has* busted out of the cage. He *has* begun to think, the distinctively human function. He has even begun to sense beauty, the beauty Paddy had told him of: ''Sure, I seen de sun come up. Dat was pretty, too—all red and pink and green. I was lookin' at de skyscrapers—steel—and all de ships comin' in, sailin' out, all over de oith—and dey was steel, too. De sun was warm, dey wasn't no clouds, and dere was breeze blowin'.'' Here steel no longer cages him in. And he has come to a fine awareness of his own dilemma. All of that is pretty, but he couldn't belong in that: ''It was over my head.'' And so he has hurried over to see the gorilla.

The gorilla (at least Yank has moved back from the monkey-on-a-string image) Yank senses as the only image of himself left after the shock waves set up by the encounter with Mildred have worked themselves this far. Both are, as he puts it, ''members of de same club—de Hairy Apes.'' But especially here with the unthinking gorilla Yank moves gropingly higher in his questioning, toward an increasingly intelligent understanding of himself, though ''tinkin' is hard.'' The gorilla is better off than Yank because he can't think; he can ''sit and dope dream in de past, green woods, de jungle and de rest of it.'' Then he can belong, even though he's in a cage. But Yank ''ain't got no past to tink in, nor nothin' dat's comin', on'y what's now—and dat don't belong.'' Here Yank reaches the high point of his ''tinkin'':

> But I kin make a bluff at talkin' and tinkin;—a'most git away with it—a'most!—and dat's where de joker comes in. (*He laughs.*) I ain't on oith and I ain't in heaven, get me? I'm in de middle tryin' to separate 'em, taken' all de worst punches from bot' of 'em. Maybe that's what dey call hell, huh?

Maybe it is. But it's a new kind of hell, in sharp contrast to the hell of the stokehole. And the policeman who gave him a push toward hell was only repeating in miniature the mighty push given him by Mildred and the lesser shoves by the Fifth Avenue crowd, the guards in prison, and the I.W.W.

And so here is Yank in his hell, without a past to think in or a future to move toward, caught between heaven and earth and trying with his unprepared intellect and emotions to separate them but taking the worst punches from both. And aware of it, able to define it: this is the point. For Yank has moved so far from his original hubris as the figurative steel but the actual human brute that now he is asking, in his own simple language and simple way, the profoundest of questions and defining the profoundest of human dilemmas. For Yank's questions about why he is, what he is, and where he is, are the same questions man has always raised when faced with suffering and injustice and unfulfilled aspirations. His final definition of his situation rings with echoes from the psalmist, from Job, from the Preacher, from Euripides, from Shakespeare. And the Yank that speaks here is a brute-become-man, speaking now with a knowledge earned and tempered in his own demonstrated suffering—a brute reborn a man through the suffering that he has partially brought on himself by denying at first his own humanity.

Such a picture of the new Yank leaves a final question: Why does Yank destroy himself? O'Neill handles this carefully. The new Yank destroys himself, as Sophocles would have him do, by the very fact of his new-found humanity. For the human traits that lead him to the questions also make him despair of answers, and his past has given him no equipment to cope with a universe for which he can find no answers. He releases the gorilla so that together they can "knock 'em often de oith and croak wit de band playin'." Thus release of the ape is a kind of suicide for Yank, an embracing of the animal "brother" or self, which as brute destroys him: the literal hairy ape literally crushing the man, as the symbolic ape had earlier crushed the man in Yank. A kind of suicide, but arrived at not from mere despair, but surely more from his thinking, from having defined his situation and, though finding no other way out, from seeking this as the positive end.

Tragedy is where we find it—even when its author calls it a comedy. I would hardly argue that Yank is noble or tragic in the classical sense. He is no Oedipus caught in a trap the gods have apparently set, no Job craving ultimate understanding, no Lear raving his defiance at the universe and coming to know his own humanity as a result. But I would argue that he is a little bit of all these, reduced at first to the lowest level that still can be called human and forced suddenly to confront on his level the breakup of his universe as all of these had had to confront the breakup of theirs. That the experience should call forth from the brute his humanness, that that humanness should call forth from us our understanding and sympathy and respect, that we should re-experience in Yank's new-found dignity our own sense of human dignity in the face of the inexplicable—these are the sources of the tragic effect in *The Hairy Ape.* And they are sources that reaffirm the power and pertinence and meaning and dignity of tragedy in our age. Even without the mighty heroes of the past, even with heroes reduced to the lowest levels of humanity, man is still man and tragedy still tragedy. And tragedy still speaks to us from the deepest levels of our troubled universe and our troubled spirits. O'Neill and Yank have helped us know all this.

Source: Marden J. Clark, "Tragic Effect in *The Hairy Ape*" in *Modern Drama,* Volume 10, no. 4, February, 1968, pp. 372–82.

SOURCES

Bogard, Travis. *Contour in Time: The Plays of Eugene O'Neill,* Oxford University Press, 1988.

Cargil, Oscar, Editor. *O'Neill and His Plays: Four Decades of Criticism,* New York University Press, 1961.

Dubost, Thierry. *Struggle, Defeat, or Rebirth: Eugene O'Neill's Vision of Humanity,* McFarland, 1997.

Engel, Edwin A. *The Haunted Heroes of Eugene O'Neill,* Harvard University Press, 1953.

Floyd, Virginia, Editor. *Eugene O'Neill: A World View,* Ungar, 1979.

Shaughnessy, Edward L., *Down the Nights and Down the Days: Eugene O'Neill's Catholic Sensibility,* University of Notre Dame Press, 1996.

Skinner, Richard Dana. *Eugene O'Neill: A Poet's Quest,* Longmans, 1935.

Wainscott, Ronald H. *Staging O'Neill: The Experimental Years, 1920-1934,* Yale University Press, 1988.

FURTHER READING

Day, Dorothy, *By Little and By Little: The Selected Writings of Dorothy Day,* Knopf, 1983.

Day was a friend of O'Neill's in the 1920s and they had a strong influence on each other. The woman who founded the Catholic Worker movement can be experienced through this collection of her writings over the years.

Egan, Leona Rust. *Provincetown As a Stage: Provincetown, the Provincetown Players, and the Discovery of Eugene O'Neill,* Parnassus Imprints, 1994.

This book recounts the story of the artistic life of Provincetown where O'Neill was nurtured and rose to prominence. This is a scholarly work that, at times, offers tidbits of gossip courtesy of some excerpts from Carlotta O'Neill, the playwright's last wife.

Moorton, Richard F., Jr. *Eugene O'Neill's Century: Centennial Views on America's Foremost Tragic Dramatist,* Greenwood Press, 1991.

With essays by thirteen writers, this book looks at specific plays and at special themes in O'Neill's work, including the concept of searching for a home.

The House of Bernarda Alba

FEDERICO GARCIA LORCA

1936

The House of Bernarda Alba is Federico Garcia Lorca's last play, written the year he was killed at the outbreak of the Spanish Civil War. The play, along with *Blood Wedding* and *Yerma,* forms a trilogy expressing what Lorca saw as the tragic life of Spanish women. These late works Dennis Klein in *Blood Wedding, Yerma, and The House of Bernarda Alba* called "the most accomplished and mature efforts of the finest Spanish playwright of the twentieth century." If *Blood Wedding* is a nuptial tragedy and *Yerma* the tragedy of barren women, *The House of Bernarda Alba* might be seen as the tragedy of virginity, of rural Spanish women who will never have the opportunity to choose a husband. It is also a play expressing the costs of repressing the freedom of others.

The House of Bernarda Alba finally had its stage premiere nearly a decade after Lorca's death. The play was produced in Buenos Aries in 1945, and was published the same year, in Argentina. The play later had important productions at the ANTA Theater, New York, in 1951 and the Crescent Theatre, Birmingham, England, in 1952. In 1960 it was adapted for American television and in 1963 produced at the Encore Theater in San Francisco. Given the repression of artistic expression in Spain during Franco's regime, it was not until 1964 that Lorca's last play was finally produced in his native country, at Madrid's Goya Theatre. *The House of Bernarda Alba* continues to be revived and read all over the world. Its setting is specific to the values

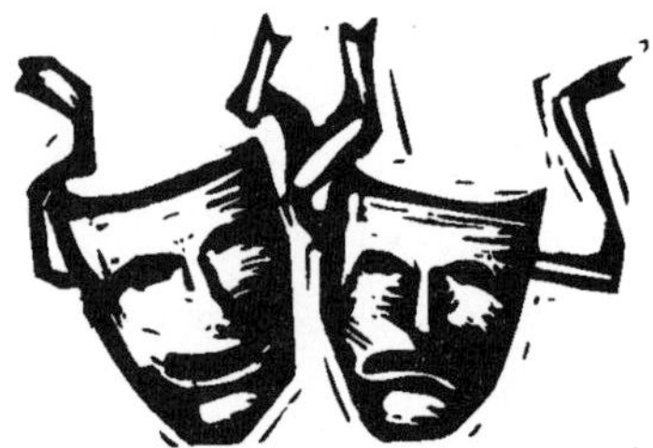

and customs of a rural Spanish people, but the play's appeal is universal rather than national. In the United States, the play has been enjoyed in both English and Spanish productions.

AUTHOR BIOGRAPHY

Federico Garcia Lorca was born June 5, 1898 in a village near Granada, Spain, the son of Federico Garcia Rodriguez, a liberal landowner, and Vicenta Lorca, a schoolteacher. (Although by Spanish custom his surname is properly Garcia Lorca, he is more commonly known by his mother's surname.) Lorca produced a body of work that is considered among the greatest in the Spanish language, and which has been enthusiastically embraced by audiences around the world. Although celebrated primarily for his writing about the Spanish countryside, Lorca did not wish to be labeled merely a poet of rural life. His writing is intellectual in its conception and symbolism, but nevertheless touches basic human emotions. Lorca felt acutely the suffering of oppressed people, but avoided direct involvement in politics. Hiding his homosexuality from the public, Lorca felt condemned to live as an outcast, and he frequently struggled with severe depression.

Lorca experienced traditional rural life growing up in the southern region of Andalusia, but was propelled into the modern world when his parents moved to the city of Granada in 1909. As an adolescent Lorca wrote plays which were enjoyed by his family and their servants, but his father tried to influence him to study law and pursue what he considered to be a more responsible career. Lorca attended university in Granada, and later in Madrid, but he was a poor student (although he eventually earned his law degree in 1923). At the same time, however, he was becoming known as a multitalented artist. Already skilled as a pianist and singer, Lorca wrote his first poems in 1915 and published his first book in 1918, the prose work *Impressions and Landscapes.* In 1920 his first play was produced; *The Butterfly's Evil Spell,* a highly personal allegory about the doomed love of a cockroach for a butterfly, was an artistic disaster. The setback was minor, however; throughout the 1920s Lorca achieved great success as a poet, writing about the traditional world of his childhood with a blend of traditional and contemporary techniques.

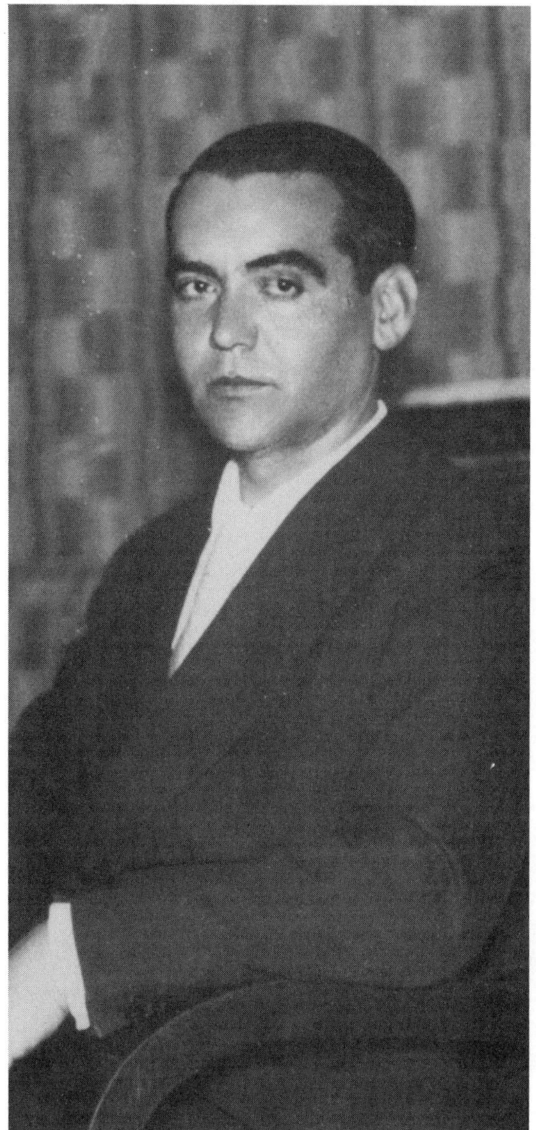

Federico Garcia Lorca

His collections from this period include *Poem of the Deep Song* and *Gypsy Ballads.*

Lorca continued to write for the theater, and in 1927 a production of his play *Mariana Pineda* was a success in Madrid. In 1929 Lorca traveled in the United States and Cuba, and from the experience of roaming the streets of foreign cities, he crafted the collection *Poet in New York.* Upon his return to Spain in 1930, his play *The Shoemaker's Prodigious Wife* was produced successfully. Other plays of note followed, including *Yerma* and *Blood Wedding.* Lorca also served as director and producer of plays for a state-sponsored traveling theater group,

La Barraca (''The Hut''). Lorca went on a short lecture tour of Argentina and Uruguay, and was greeted as a celebrity everywhere he went, even by other major writers like Chilean poet Pablo Neruda. Lorca wrote *The House of Bernarda Alba,* his last play, in 1936, and in July of the same year left Madrid for Granada. He was one of the earliest casualties of the Spanish civil war, executed by fascist rebels, his body thrown into an unmarked grave.

PLOT SUMMARY

Act I

The action opens in a ''very white room in Bernarda Alba's house.'' Bells toll for the funeral of Bernarda's second husband. The housekeeper La Poncia speaks with a maid about Bernarda and her family. La Poncia reports that one of the daughters, Magdalena, fainted during the funeral service. Magdalena is the only one who loved her father, La Poncia explains. Maria Josefa, Bernarda's mother, calls from within, where apparently she has been locked up against her will. La Poncia laments Bernarda's treatment of the servants, cursing her with the ''pain of the piercing nail.'' After La Poncia exits, a beggar woman and a little girl appear, but the maid drives them away. The servant hears the bells tolling and curses Bernarda's dead husband: ''You'll never again lift my skirts behind the corral door!'' The mourning women begin entering until the room is full. The servants now wail, putting on a show of grief for Antonio's passing. Bernarda and the five daughters enter, and Bernarda says a prayer for her dead husband.

The mourning women depart, and Bernarda curses what she sees as their hypocrisy: ''Go back to your houses and criticize everything you've seen!'' Bernarda explains to her daughters that they will mourn for eight years, during which ''not a breath of air will get in this house from the street.'' The grandmother calls again, and Bernarda orders a servant to let her out. Bernarda strikes Angustias, the oldest daughter, upon learning that she has been looking out the cracks in the door at the men departing the funeral. La Poncia comforts Angustias as Bernarda orders everyone but her maid out of the room. Bernarda questions La Poncia about the men Angustias was watching. La Poncia then expresses concern about the daughters, who are growing older and not finding husbands. Bernarda feels she's being protective: ''For a hundred miles around there's no one good enough to come near them.'' Bernarda leaves, ordering her servants to work.

Amelia and Martirio enter. They discuss Martirio's poor health, and the fact that their neighbor Adelaida did not attend the funeral (apparently because her boyfriend will not let her out in public). After speaking more about Adelaida's difficulties, Martirio concludes: ''It's better never to look at a man.'' Magdalena enters, deep in mourning. The three sisters discuss the talk of the town, that Pepe el Romano intends to ask their sister Angustias to marry him. Martirio and Amelia are happy about this news, but Magdalena is more cynical, feeling that Pepe is only interested in Angustias for her money. Adela enters, and hearing the news of Angustias's suitor first grows depressed, then defiant and angry. ''I'm thinking,'' she says, ''that this mourning has caught me at the worst moment of my life for me to bear it.'' Everyone exits at the announcement of Pepe's arrival. Bernarda and La Poncia enter, discussing the division of the inheritance. When Angustias enters, she is chastised by Bernarda for having her face powdered. Bernarda violently removes the powder and sends Angustias out. The other sisters enter, arguing about the inheritance. The grandmother, Maria Josefa, enters after escaping from her room. Yelling at the daughters, ''not a one of you is going to marry,'' Maria Josefa expresses a desire to return to her home town and be married herself. The act ends with everyone grabbing hold of Maria Josefa to subdue her again.

Act II

The daughters are seated with La Poncia, sewing. The betrothal of Angustias has brought out bitter jealousy between them. Angustias expresses a hope that she'll ''soon be out of this hell.'' She explains to her sisters how Pepe asked her to marry him. La Poncia contributes stories about her courtship, and the mood grows lighter. Magdalena goes to fetch Adela, and when they return, everyone questions the youngest daughter about what she did the night before. Adela resents this curiosity, and when she and La Poncia are left alone, she resists the maid's insinuations that she has feelings for Pepe. The housekeeper forces the issue, however, and warns Adela, ''if you like Pepe el Romano, keep it to yourself.'' Gradually the other daughters enter, showing off the lace that has just been delivered for Angustias's wedding sheets. A distant chorus is heard, the sound of men singing on their way to the wheat fields. La Poncia and some of the daughters go to watch the men from a window, leaving Amelia and Martirio alone. Martirio tells Amelia she thought she heard someone in the yard last night.

Angustias bursts in, furious that a picture of Pepe has been taken from beneath her pillow. The disturbance brings La Poncia and the other daughters, followed by Bernarda. She orders La Poncia to search the bedrooms. "This comes of not tying you up with shorter leashes," Bernarda fumes. La Poncia returns with the picture, which she found in Martirio's bed. While Martirio pleads that she only took the picture as a joke, Bernarda starts beating her. Further argument rages over Pepe. Bernarda, disgusted, sends the daughters away. La Poncia speaks her mind, warning her employer, "Something very grave is happening here." La Poncia insists that Bernarda has never given her daughters enough freedom. Martirio had at one time a suitor, whom Bernarda sent away because his father was a shepherd. To La Poncia this is an example of Bernarda putting on airs, and as a result, denying her daughter a chance to be married. La Poncia tries to convince Bernarda that Adela is Pepe's real sweetheart, the daughter he should be marrying. A servant enters, announcing there is a big crowd gathering in the street. Adela and Martirio are left alone, each accusing the other of trying to steal Pepe away from Angustias. Bernarda, the other daughters, and the servants enter, announcing that the crowd outside is calling for the death of a young woman who gave birth to an illegitimate child, and then in her shame, killed and buried it. Bernarda and her daughters join the cry, but Adela, holding her belly, cries out, "No! No!"

Act III

The act opens at night, in a room in Bernarda's house adjacent to the corral. The family and a guest, Prudencia, are eating. Prudencia tells Bernarda that her family is feuding, that her husband has never forgiven their daughter for an indiscretion. "A daughter who's disobedient," Bernarda says, "stops being a daughter and becomes an enemy." Everyone discusses Angustias's impending betrothal, and Prudencia admires the pearl engagement ring, though she comments that in her day, "pearls signified tears." The church bells toll, and Prudencia leaves to attend the service. Angustias goes off to bed because Pepe is not coming to visit her tonight. The daughters wonder why, and Bernarda explains he is away on a trip; Martirio, however, looks suggestively at Adela and mutters, "Ah!"

The daughters exit; La Poncia and Bernarda continue their discussion about the "very grave thing" which Bernarda insists is not happening in her house. Bernarda goes to bed, and the servants leave to investigate the sound of dogs barking in the yard. Maria Josefa passes through with a lamb in her arms, singing a lullaby. Adela passes through on her way out to the corral. Martirio enters by another door and is confronted by her grandmother. Encouraging Maria Josefa to return to bed, Martirio calls out for Adela. When she arrives, Martirio warns her, "Keep away from him." Adela is defiant: "You know better than I he doesn't love her." Martirio reluctantly admits this is the truth. Pepe whistles from the yard for Adela, who runs toward the door, but Martirio blocks her way. She calls for Bernarda, who enters quickly. Adela grabs Bernarda's cane and breaks it in two. La Poncia and some of the other daughters enter. Bernarda retrieves a gun, and shoots at Pepe waiting in the yard. Adela runs off after her lover, believing he has been shot. A thud is heard a moment later, and when La Poncia breaks open the door, she discovers that Adela has hanged herself. Bernarda orders Adela's body cut down, insisting, "My daughter died a virgin." The play ends with Bernarda stubbornly maintaining her illusion, ordering her daughters to be silent and defiant in the face of death.

CHARACTERS

Adela

Adela, age 20, is the youngest, most attractive, spirited, and rebellious of Bernarda's daughters. As Magdalena says of her, Adela "still has her illusions," and thus has difficulty submitting to the strong will of her mother, who keeps all the daughters under tight reign. As a form of rebellion, Adela puts on a green birthday dress and goes out in the yard shouting "Chickens, look at me!" She craves social interaction and cannot bear to be locked away from the world. She has a deep connection to nature, yearning to be free of the house and breathe the fresh air of the fields. As the conflict with her mother's will intensifies, Adela's defiance is symbolized in her breaking of the walking stick with which Bernarda has beaten her daughters. Ultimate-

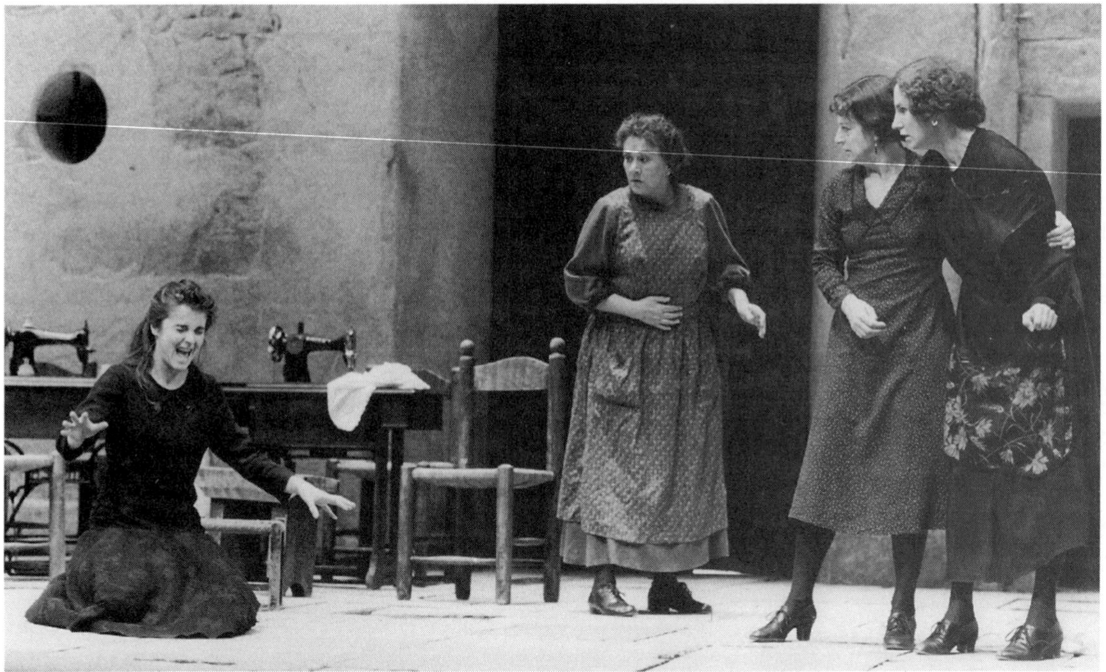

Adela (Amanda Root) reacts to the news regarding the illegitimate birth. Looking on are, left to right, La Poncia (Joan Plowright), Magdelena (Christine Edmonds), and Martirio (Deborah Findlay)

ly, Adela chooses death as a means of escape from an intolerable life when the only alternative she can envision—Pepe—is no longer available.

Bernarda Alba

At age 60, she feels out of place in the village, sure that everyone in the town despises her. She feels superior to her neighbors in social station, and will not allow her daughters to be courted by the men of the area, whom she generally finds inferior. She curses ''this village full of wells where you drink water always fearful it's been poisoned.'' Bernarda runs her house with an iron hand; La Poncia calls her a ''domineering old tyrant.'' Her husband, Antonio Maria Benavides, has recently died, and the family has gathered at her house for the funeral. Her domination of the family and servants intensifies the day of her husband's funeral. She is hard on her own daughters out of a sense of what is proper behavior for women in a period of mourning. She plans to keep the house shut up for eight years, and requires the daughters to cover their heads in mourning. She is a vicious and manipulative person who keeps a mental record of every scandal that involves her neighbors so she can use the information as a weapon against them. Bernarda seems unmoved by her daughter Adela's death, more concerned about the perceptions of her neighbors as she orders her daughters to uphold the lie that ''She, the youngest daughter of Bernarda Alba, died a virgin.''

Amelia

Of all the characters, Amelia, Bernarda's third youngest daughter at age 27, perhaps stands out the least as an individual. She is kindhearted and hates to hear her mother speak unkindly. She is concerned about Martirio's health even if Martirio is not. Like Martirio, she feels uncomfortable and embarrassed around men. Like Magdalena, she feels that being born a woman is life's worst punishment. Amelia seems to be afraid of almost everything; unlike Adela who seeks the truth, Amelia would rather close her eyes to it.

Angustias

The eldest daughter at age 39, Angustias is a half-sister to the others because she was born of Bernarda's first marriage. She is therefore the only one with any inheritance worth mentioning, and thus has a suitor, Pepe el Romano. Bernarda strikes her when she learns that Angustias has been looking out the cracks in the door at the men departing the funeral. Angustias knows that Pepe only wants her for her money, but is resigned to this fact. Near the conclusion of the play, Angustias stands her ground when a hysterical Adela orders her to tell Pepe that Adela will be his. She curses her sister: ''Thief! Disgrace of this house!''

First Servant

See Maid

La Poncia

She expresses bitterness about Bernarda's treatment of her and the other servants. (Bernarda must have everything perfect, and works her servants hard to get it.) La Poncia, who is 60 years old, is perhaps the most complex character in the play. A mediator, she is all things to all people without being a hypocrite. La Poncia is torn between debt to and hatred of Bernarda. Additionally, her sons work Bernarda's fields, so Bernarda controls the economic fate of the entire family. Nevertheless, La Poncia is extremely frank with her employer, which may be a privilege of age (Lorca is careful to indicate they are exactly the same age). La Poncia provides the daughters with friendly conversation, which they lack, and on occasion defends them to Bernarda. La Poncia persists in trying to make Bernarda recognize there are real problems brewing in the house.

Magdalena

Apparently the only daughter who truly loved her father, Magdalena, 30 years old, faints during his funeral. Realistic to the point of pessimism, she is convinced she is never going to get married. Like Martirio, she claims not to care if she lives or dies. She speaks out against hypocrisy when she hears it, and believes women should be strong and not tolerate poor treatment by men. She refuses to contribute a stitch to the making of clothes for the christening of Angustias's future first child. Her form of escape is a pleasant memory of the past.

Maid

Like the other servants in Bernarda's employ, her life consists of nothing more than cleaning the house until her fingers bleed, without ever earning Bernarda's approval. When the maid hears the bells tolling for Bernarda's dead husband, she curses him, ''You'll never again lift my skirts behind the corral door!'' She is 50 years old.

MEDIA ADAPTATIONS

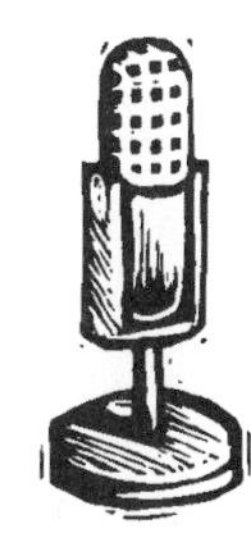

- *The House of Bernarda Alba* was produced on American television in 1960 for the ''Play of the Week'' series, translated and adapted by James Graham-Lujan and Richard O'Connell. Anne Revere starred as Bernarda Alba, with Eileen Heckart as La Poncia, and Suzanne Pleshette as Adela.
- In 1990, the play was adapted as a Spanish film, directed by Mario Camus (Gala).
- A British television production of the play premiered in 1992, directed by Nuria Espert and Stuart Burge (Channel 4).

Maria Josefa

Bernarda's mother, 80 years old, is the most poetic character in the play, identified closely with Adela (they share a desire to escape the house and be free). Maria Josefa is a voice of truth, painful to Bernarda who keeps her locked away. What she claims to want—marriage to a virile young man and lots of children—is irrational. But Maria Josefa is also very perceptive, more aware than Bernarda of the dire situation in the house. When she cradles the lamb she knows it is not a real baby, but accepts it as better than nothing.

Martirio

Martirio, Bernarda's second youngest daughter at 24, has been under the care of a doctor but does not express any hope of her condition improving. (Indeed, she takes her medicine more out of routine than any concern for health.) She is in many ways a younger picture of her mother, called ''a poisoned well'' by La Poncia. Martirio feels that God has made her weak and ugly and that all things considered, ''it's better never to look at a man.'' She hypocritically says having a boyfriend does not matter to her, but she is consumed by jealousy and sexual frustration. She steals the picture of Pepe el Romano so she can at least possess the image of a man. Martirio is the one daughter who reluctantly agrees that Pepe el Romano really loves Adela and not Angustias, to whom he is engaged. Still, she does all she can to keep Adela and Pepe apart.

Prudencia

One of Bernarda's few friends in the area. She is frustrated with her husband, who refuses to forgive their daughter for an incident long in the past. Prudencia is 50 years old.

THEMES

Beauty

Beauty—specifically the beauty of Adela, Bernarda's youngest daughter—is a source of conflict in the play. Beauty becomes corrupted, Lorca suggests, in an environment where people are not permitted to pursue their desires and passions. Pepe el Romano is passionate for Adela, but is bound by economic necessity to court Angustias instead. ''If he were coming because of Angustias' looks, for Angustias as a woman, I'd be glad too,'' Magdalena comments, ''but he's coming for her money. Even though Angustias is our sister, we're her family here and we know she's old and sickly, and always has been the least attractive one of us!'' The daughters are all in such a state of repressed isolation that they will resent both Angustias, for having a suitor, and the beautiful Adela, for possessing Pepe as a lover.

Fate and Chance

The characters' attempts to control their own lives bring them into contact with the inevitable and result in the tragedies that conclude not just *The House of Bernarda Alba,* but each of the plays in Lorca's trilogy. Destiny is intermingled with the repetition of the life cycle; what occurred in the past is often fated to occur again. For example, all the women in Adelaida's family suffered before her, and she is destined to suffer, too. (Martirio observes elsewhere in the play, ''History repeats itself. I can see that everything is a terrible repetition.'') In the scene with Prudencia, several symbols of bad luck appear (spilled salt and an engagement ring of pearls rather than diamonds). All the bad luck predicted in this scene comes to pass. Martirio comments, ''Luck comes to the one who least expects it.'' But good luck does not seem to come to anyone in Bernarda's house, whether they expect it or not. Adela, meanwhile, struggles against her fate and fails. The other sisters are resigned to their fate, lacking Adela's faith that she can control the course of her life.

Death

Each of the three plays in Lorca's trilogy ends with a significant death. Death is a mounting inevitability as the frustration of the characters grows more intense. Death comes to characters in situations with no hope, who are helpless victims of their destiny. Ultimately, Adela chooses death as a means of escape from an intolerable life when the only alternative she can envision—Pepe—is no longer available. Adela seems bound by fate not to survive, but Bernarda brings about tragedy through actions that have the opposite of their desired effect. In this, she appears more like a heroine of Greek tragedy, although she survives, perhaps to make the same mistakes again.

Freedom

The play is formed by Lorca's sense of social justice, warning society at large about the tragic cost of repressing any of its members. Adela's dilemma is Lorca's central concern. She has more to lose than the others in the dashing of her two hopes, men and freedom. Her optimism is irrational because of the isolation in which Bernarda keeps her and her sisters, and because she should be able to see from the society around her that men and freedom are mutually exclusive possibilities for a Spanish woman. But even servitude to a husband would likely provide Bernarda's daughters with more freedom than they have under her tyrannical authority. The land, which produces wealth, also serves as a metaphor for procreative power and other freedoms. The fields are a source of refreshment and escape for Bernarda's daughters. They see the men who work the land as free and independent, as having everything the women who are prisoners in the house do not have.

Honor

Honor is closely related in the play with themes such as status, money, and gossip. Bernarda feels she has a social position to maintain in the town; she won't let her daughters marry beneath this imagined station, and she won't give up her social airs. The tyranny of Bernarda is fueled by her own sense of honor and tradition. The desire to act honorably—to mourn her husband's death for eight years—ruins the lives of Bernarda's daughters. Bernarda's sense of honor is formed by her awareness of the judgmental opinions of her neighbors. However, she has only herself to blame for her fear of what the neighbors think because she has manipulated them by gossip in the past. Adelaida, for example (a character never seen), is afraid of Bernarda because the woman knows her sordid past, and throws it in Adelaida's face every chance she gets. Part of La Poncia's job is to keep Bernarda informed of what is going on in the town. When the neighbors awaken at the end of the play, however, it appears there will be no more controlling them (although Bernarda is desperately trying to keep up appearances).

Sex Roles

Lorca's primary identification was always with female characters, and all the plays in his late trilogy are about the plight of Spanish women. *The House of Bernarda Alba* bears the explicit subtitle "Drama about Women in the Towns of Spain," and there are more frustrated women in it than in any other Lorca play, perhaps than in any other modern play in the world theater. In Lorca's view, men and freedom are mutually exclusive for Spanish women. Although no male characters appear in the play, it is clear that the women's feelings of isolation are largely the consequences of men's actions and attitudes. In depicting sexual frustration, Lorca maintains the masculine mystique by keeping Pepe from appearing. Pepe acts only on instinct; his desires pit mother against daughter, sister against sister. Magdalena curses womanhood if it consists of nothing more than being bound by tradition. A woman has little control in achieving personal satisfaction and in determining the course of her own life, and therefore must often resort to desperate measures. The three plays of the trilogy dramatize tragic attempts by women to free themselves from impossible situations: the Bride runs off with Leonardo in *Blood Wedding,* Yerma kills her husband, and Adela kills herself.

Wealth and Poverty

Angustias suffers because she knows Pepe is only marrying her for her money, that even when they are together his thoughts are far from her. Land is the source of wealth throughout the three plays of the trilogy, and wealth creates stature. When Bernarda judges the men of the area as unfit for her daughters, she does so not on their individual merits, but because as shepherds and laborers they are all beneath her economic ideal. In such circumstances, wealth controls fate. Not only does Pepe become engaged to Angustias because of it, but the play is rich with other symbolic battles over money. Prudencia's family, for example, is torn apart by a struggle over money: a disputed inheritance.

TOPICS FOR FURTHER STUDY

- Following Adela's suicide, do you think Bernarda will continue to maintain such tight control over her surviving daughters? Do you think she will be successful at keeping the circumstances of Adela's death a secret from the town? Explain.
- Research the social status of women in Spain in the 1930s. Based on historical records, how successful does Lorca seem to have been at depicting the issues faced by women of this time?
- Examine the ways in which La Poncia serves as a mediator for the various conflicts in Bernarda's house. Why is she ultimately unsuccessful in preventing the tragic outcome of the play?
- Research the impact of Francisco Franco's regime on Spanish culture. Why do you think *The House of Bernarda Alba* did not premiere in Spain until 1964?
- Research Lorca's poetic and dramatic technique in the last years of his life. Why was he so adamant about achieving a more realistic style in *The House of Bernarda Alba* (so much so that he described the play as a "photographic document")?

STYLE

Realism and Surrealism

Lorca was a great experimenter with poetic and dramatic form, and was certainly influenced by the variety of new artistic forms developed in his day. Although the term surrealism is specific to the work of a handful of artists at a particular time, it is often used to describe a variety of techniques that seek to express the human subconscious directly, rather than revealing it through external actions, as is the case in realist drama. In writing his last play, Lorca worked against such a technique, trying to reach a more ''objective'' tragedy by stripping away the overtly poetic elements that had characterized his style before this. His friend Adolfo Salazar noted that as Lorca finished reading each scene he would exclaim, ''Not a drop of poetry! Reality! Realism!'' *The House of Bernarda Alba* lacks the stylized elements of the other two plays in the trilogy, but never approaches unadulterated realism. Lorca asserted that the play was a ''photographic record,'' suggesting an attempt to capture rural Spanish life in a naturalistic manner. The language of the play is carefully shaped to expose elements of character, however; it is poetic without overtly sounding like poetry. Similarly, while the play's settings appear naturalistic, evocative of a real house in the Spanish countryside, they are also stylized, with the white walls evoking purity but also the sterility and monotony of life in Bernarda's house.

Classical Tragedy

As Dennis Klein noted, Lorca wanted his theater to ''capture the drama of contemporary life and inspire passion as classical drama did,'' Lorca stated that his purpose in writing his tragic trilogy was to follow the Aristotelian canon for tragedy. He departed widely from this goal, however. *The House of Bernarda Alba* moves closer to the structure of classical tragedy than the other two plays, but still differs significantly. Lorca is true to the spirit of classical tragedy without rigorously applying the rules, such as the unities of time, place, and action. The breaking of the unities is consistent with the history of the Spanish theater, and indeed Lorca's drama was rooted as much in the traditions of the Spanish Golden Age, and those of European puppet farce, as in classical precedent. The plays of Lorca's trilogy are all structured as dramatic crescendos with a key event around which the rest of the action revolves. In this respect *The House of Bernarda Alba* has a classical structure. The play is also reminiscent of Greek tragedy in its focus on a household or lineage, its powerful sense of fatalism, and the cathartic quality of the final scenes. Additionally, Lorca did make subtle use of the classical technique of the chorus that comments on the action of the play. Each of the plays in the trilogy has a chorus; in *The House of Bernarda Alba* the function of the chorus is served both by the neighbors in act one, and the other daughters besides Adela.

Dramatic Structure

Eliminating most of the details of telling a story, Lorca designed his plays to be skeletal so he could concentrate on other theatrical elements. *The House of Bernarda Alba* is episodic in structure, and almost perfectly circular. The play starts with Bernarda returning from one funeral and ends with her arranging another. She appears to have learned nothing from the experience of losing her youngest daughter, for she exerts the same repressive control against which Adela rebelled with such tragic results. With the repetition of Bernarda's ''Silence!'' the command has an authoritarian ring at the beginning of the play, but a hollow one at the conclusion.

Folklore

Known primarily for his works about peasants and gypsies, Lorca drew extensively on his familiarity with rural Spanish life. Edward Honig observes that ''Lorca was rebelling against the realistic middle-class drama, which in Spain had succeeded in shutting off from the stage the rich atmosphere of folk speech and imagination.'' Lorca's work succeeds as a blend of surrealistic imagery and popular folklore. Lorca achieved a very personal style by relating with a modern sensibility and a variety of techniques his understanding of a folk world. Folk elements are crucial to a play like *The House of Bernarda Alba,* but Lorca does not romanticize rural life as did many of his contemporaries.

Among folk elements, the lullabies of Andalusia were especially important to Lorca; he once gave a lengthy lecture on these songs. Singing is employed throughout the trilogy, although the other two plays employ more poetry than does *The House of Bernarda Alba.* Maria Josefa's lullaby to the lamb, for example, allows her to express her maternal instincts and her feelings about her daughter.

Poetic Devices

Lorca is usually treated as a poet who happened to turn to theatre because he found lyric poetry inadequate. His brother argues against this interpretation, explaining how theatre and theatricality were important to Lorca as a child, and thus throughout his entire life. ''I would say that, just as someone called him 'poet by the grace of God,' he was dramatist by the same grace. . . . We need to say, then, that his dramatic expression was as pressing in him as the need for lyric expression.'' While writing *The House of Bernarda Alba* Lorca was intent on keeping it free of poetry, to eliminate the special effects and metaphorical characters that he used in the other two plays. Yet the touch of the poet is present; there is poetry even if there is no verse.

Symbolic elements such as one associates with poetic verse abound in the play. The characters are all fully realized individuals, with specific names, a transition from the allegorical characters of Lorca's other plays. Yet the characters also function symbolically through the use of onomastic imagery (attributing character traits through the names). Angustias suggests anguish, for example; Martirio, martyrdom; and Prudencia, prudence. Water is another important symbol for Lorca, suggesting sexual potency. Bernarda's daughters drink water not just to quench their thirst but to lessen their sexual frustration. At the same time, however, water can come down in torrents; the trouble in Bernarda's house is referred to metaphorically as a storm. Weather in general is symbolic; the heat suggesting intense sexual frustration. Since the men are outside, they are cooler on the patio (i.e., they do not suffer from sexual repression). By using these and other symbolic images (animals are especially important referents), Lorca retains a poetic quality to his writing in this otherwise prosaic play.

HISTORICAL CONTEXT

Spain at the time of Lorca's youth was experiencing a lengthy crisis of confidence spurred by the country's defeat by the United States in the War of 1898, during which Spain lost its remaining colonies. Political life was torn between a desire on one hand to strengthen traditional values and revive past glory, and the need on the other to move progressively forward, to foster intellectual inquiry and learn from the example of modernized nations. The split between these positions grew more acute in the 1930s. Lorca resisted efforts to recruit him for the communist party, but at the same time his social conscience caused him to be outspoken in his criticism of Spanish conservatives.

In 1936 civil war broke out as conservative army officers under General Francisco Franco revolted against the liberal Spanish government. Lorca was living in Madrid at the time and decided to wait out the conflict at his parents' home in Granada. His decision turned out to be disastrous, as Granada was filled with coup sympathizers, and quickly fell to rebel forces. Many liberal politicians and intellectuals in the area were executed, including Lorca. In the years of civil conflict which followed (in many ways a prelude to the war that was soon to rock all of Europe), the attention of the world was focused on Spain. Men and women of many nations traveled there to fight against fascism in international brigades. Franco's forces were victorious, however, and by 1939 he controlled all of Spain. Franco's regime never accepted responsibility for Lorca's death, but Lorca remained a forbidden subject for years.

Franco's victory stalled the flowering of the arts in Spain, which had been ongoing for several decades. Previously, Spain's Golden Age in the sixteenth and seventeenth centuries was the highpoint of its creativity in the theatre and the other arts. Pedro Calderon de la Barca, Felix Lope de Vega, and others created a dramatic canon that has stood as a standard for centuries. Lorca was born in the year of, but too young to be a part of, the literary Generation of 1898, which examined Spain's past and the problems that caused the country to fall from international power. Lorca was part of the second Spanish literary movement of the twentieth century, the Generation of 1927, an erudite group using cerebral imagery and believing in a code of Art for Art's sake.

Lorca's generation challenged audiences with its daring techniques and often controversial subject matter. This was a period of artistic liberation and the development of new artistic forms. Surrealism and Dadaism exerted influence over a number of arts, inspiring works that sought through imagery to pierce the human subconscious. Spain at the time was moved by the films of Luis Bunuel, and the painting of Salvador Dali and Pablo Picasso. Lorca's work is similarly sophisticated and shares a complex awareness of human psychology. While other artistic innovators appealed primarily to the intellect, however, Lorca was concerned with addressing basic human emotions and needs. Lorca championed the plight of the Andalusian gypsies, who were accorded the worst possible social position in the region. He was also passionate about the injustices done to Spanish women: the personal stigma associated with not being married, and a woman's inability to marry the man she loves.

The House of Bernarda Alba finally had its stage premiere nearly a decade after Lorca's death. It was produced in Buenos Aries in 1945, near the end of World War II, during which Argentina had maintained an uneasy neutrality. The play was published the same year, also in Argentina. Given the repression of artistic expression during Franco's

COMPARE & CONTRAST

- **1936:** The values and traditions of rural society remain strong in Spain, despite the influence of various modernizing forces.

  Today: While rural communities survive, in Spain and elsewhere traditional ways of life have largely disappeared. As populations migrate to urban areas to seek work, television and other media bring urban issues back to rural areas in ways that were not possible before.

- **1936:** The rights of women are highly circumscribed, and their economic dependence upon men holds them in traditionally subordinate gender roles.

  Today: Women, in Spain and elsewhere, have achieved important rights but many still continue to struggle against perceptions of their ''proper'' role in society, which often does not include success in a professional realm.

- **1936:** Spain is in the throes of a civil conflict brought about by economic inequalities which are felt more acutely in a depressed economy.

  Today: Spain has diversified and strengthened its economy to some extent, but the country continues to struggle with high levels of unemployment and is one of the poorest member nations of the European Union. Assassinations and other actions by rebel groups like the ETA in the Basque region suggest that many social and political issues remain unresolved.

- **1936:** Lorca is arrested and executed by rebels who support General Francisco Franco's fascist coup. Lorca and his works will be a forbidden subject in Spain for years to come.

  Today: Since Franco's death in 1975, Lorca is understood and appreciated on his own terms. He is openly admired in his homeland as one of the century's greatest poets, a status he never lost elsewhere.

- **1936:** Believing in a communist ideal of shared ownership of the land and other resources, brigades of Spanish Republicans and international sympathizers fight passionately against Franco's military forces.

  Today: Since the breakup of the Soviet Union and the effectiveness of the American embargo against Cuba, communism is widely viewed as a failed political experiment. Support for the concept of shared ownership is not considered a valid political position in the United States.

regime, it was not until 1964 that Lorca's last play was finally produced in his native Spain, at Madrid's Goya Theatre.

CRITICAL OVERVIEW

By the time of his death, Lorca was widely considered one of the greatest poets of the modern era, perhaps of all time. Since *The House of Bernarda Alba* differs from Lorca's other works in his attempt to employ a more realistic style, critics have differed in their assessment of the play's value in Lorca's canon. Most have found it a work of real theatrical power, demonstrating Lorca's versatility as a writer. A minority, however, have suggested that the work pales in comparison to Lorca's more lyric poetry and drama.

Lorca's assassination was a shocking tragedy not only to his Spanish audience, but to lovers of his writing all over the world. Some critics were particularly indignant about the circumstances surrounding Lorca's death. ''Lorca was assassinated, and his books burned,'' wrote William Rose Benet in a 1937 review of Lorca's *Lament for the Death of a Bullfighter,* ''but his burning words live on in the present book, beyond the reach of the bloody ape [i.e., Franco].'' Benet praised the ''fierceness'' in Lorca's poetry, calling some of his images ''striking and beautiful.'' Eulogizing Lorca a year after ''his criminal and stupid murder,'' Rolfe Humphries praised Lorca's versatility and his ability ''to write both simply and subtly at the same time.'' While dwelling on the lasting value of Lorca's poems, Humphries also praised Lorca as a total artist, saying that ''in achieving a synthesis of all that . . . he had received from the world of dance and painting, music and theater, he abandoned nothing of value, and was able to work his erudition down into the substance of his art.'' The American poet William Carlos Williams observed in the *Kenyon Review* that Lorca ''belonged to the people and when they were attacked he was attacked by the same forces.'' Williams praised the reality and immediacy of Lorca's verse, his skill at ''invoking the mind to start awake.''

At the time of Lorca's death, Humphries and other critics have noted, Lorca's work was not widely available in English. This fact has certainly been remedied in subsequent decades, but translation of Lorca's writing continues to be a tricky issue. Some critics have claimed that qualities of Lorca's style, especially his feel for the sound of language, are impossible to capture in translation. These critics suggest that the strength of Lorca's plays, meanwhile, is limited to their language. Others, however, have pointed out the quality of Lorca's stagecraft, suggesting the plays remain dramatically viable in translation. (This is especially true for a prose work like *The House of Bernarda Alba.*) There is merit to both perspectives, and unsurprisingly, while Lorca's plays are respected by the English-speaking public, they retain their greatest impact in their original language.

The House of Bernarda Alba finally premiered in Argentina nearly a decade after Lorca's death. Critics there hailed the work, comparing Lorca's drama to the works of the great Golden Age playwrights of Spain. A reviewer in *La Nation* identified Lorca's work with that of Calderon de la Barca, who also focuses intensely on issues of honor. This same critic, according to Dennis Klein, observed that in the present play, Lorca as strong realist dominates over Lorca the poet. Another critic, writing in the publication *Blanco y Negro,* traced patterns throughout the trilogy of plays about the lives of Spanish women. While praising both *Blood Wedding* and *Yerma,* this critic, according to Dennis Klein, concluded that ''the tragic inspiration of Garcia Lorca reaches its summit in this work.''

Not all critics have been as enthusiastic about Lorca's last play, however. Reviewing the 1960 production for the American television series ''The Play of the Week,'' John P. Shanley noted in the *New York Times* that Lorca's ''talent for poetic imagery'' was demonstrated in selections from his poetry read as an afterpiece to the telecast. The play itself, however, Shanley thought was ''better dismissed as an experimental diversion of limited appeal.'' While the play ''abounds with sounds of grief and anguish'' in a manner suggestive of the later works of Tennessee Williams, it ''lacks the range and compassion of Mr. Williams' better efforts.'' Edwin Honig commented in his 1963 study of Lorca that ''the personal dilemma . . . prevents Lorca's folk dramas as well as his other plays from rising so often out of pathos to real tragedy.'' Other American critics have found much wider appeal in Lorca's last play. Reviewing a production by the Actors' Workshop of San Francisco, Stanley Eichelbaum, as quoted by Dennis Klein, wrote that the play was ''superbly atmospheric to the eye and gloriously affecting to the ear.''

The House of Bernarda Alba has continued to be produced and read extensively, both in Spanish and in translation. Literary critics, meanwhile, have found much of interest in the complex themes of the play. Given the transition in Lorca's style at the time he wrote *The House of Bernarda Alba* (moving to a more prosaic and realistic style of drama), many critics have sought to contextualize the play in terms of Lorca's poetry. Warren Carrier, for example, concludes that *The House of Bernarda Alba* ''is so stark as prose, it is so essential in language and feeling, it stares so directly into the heart of the characters, that it may be said to be more poetic than many of the more patently poetic plays.'' In *The Contemporary Theatre: The Signigicant Playwrights of Our Time,* Allan Lewis shows himself to be among critics who have focused on the elements of folklore both in *The House of Bernarda Alba* and other plays of Lorca. Lewis observed, ''Lorca's plays are a tribal theatre of primitive power, ancient in form but shaped by a sophisticated modern mind.'' John Gilmour in *Religion in the Rural Tragedies* has surveyed the importance of religion and religious imagery in the three plays of Lorca's trilogy. ''Lorca's principal characters,'' Gilmour commented, ''are tormented souls who, despite their strict Catholic upbringing and proud sense of honour, are incapable of displaying the Christian virtues of love and forgiveness.'' Of course, given the theme of Lorca's last plays, many critics have studied his complex portrayal of gender roles in Andalusian society. Julianne Burton in *Women in Hispanic Literature: Icons and Fallen Idols* has grounded Lorca's rural trilogy in a social and historical context, suggesting that his depiction of the lives of Spanish women demonstrates "Lorca's commitment to a more egalitarian, humane, and personally fulfilling society."

CRITICISM

Christopher G. Busiel

Intertwined with other complex images and themes, Bernarda's house serves on a number of levels as the central image in The House of Bernarda Alba.

In order to arrive at an understanding of the complex images and themes in Federico Garcia Lorca's last play, *The House of Bernarda Alba,* one must start with the title. Lorca did not call his play *Bernarda Alba,* or even *The Family of Bernarda Alba.* (The latter would have been especially appropriate given that, like many of the great tragedies of classical Greece, the play focuses on a lineage and the impact of characters' actions on subsequent generations.) The title, *The House of Bernarda Alba,* draws attention both to Bernarda's "house" in the sense of her household or lineage, and to the physical space of the house itself, which serves as the central image of the play.

From his experience directing a production of the play, Eric Bentley discovered the paramount importance of the house, observing the significant role of windows and doors that serve as both barriers and bridges. The symbolism of what is inside the house and what is outside could not be more important to the themes of the play. To the daughters, the outside represents freedom and possibility, as well as romantic and sexual fulfillment. Throughout the play the daughters run repeatedly to the windows to observe the outside world: the crowd departing the funeral, the men going to work in the fields, and the arrivals and departures of Pepe el Romano. Bernarda upbraids Angustias for looking out through the cracks of the back door, becoming so angry that she strikes her daughter. To Bernarda, the outside of the house represents only negative possibility: corruption from which she wants to protect her daughters, and prying neighbors from whom she wants to keep her secrets.

The house is a self-contained society which Bernarda rules with an iron hand. "To Bernarda's way of thinking," wrote Dennis Klein in *Blood Wedding, Yerma, and The House of Bernarda Alba,* "virginity is decency and sex corruption." Therefore, it is understandable that when Adela commits suicide, Bernarda's first thought is to make the world believe her daughter died a virgin. Bernarda's rule also means that sexual activity always takes place outside the house: Pepe and Adela meet in the corral, and the maid speaks of Bernarda's husband lifting her skirts behind the corral. The story of Paca la Roseta, who spends a night with some local men deep in an olive grove, is to Bernarda a perfect example of the corruption which runs rampant outside her domestic space. The displacement of sexual activity to the outside is reflected in the symbolism of the weather. The daughters suffer in the heat of a house which is shut up tight for a period of mourning, during which, Bernarda explains, "not a breath of air will get in this house from the street. We'll act as if we'd sealed up the doors and windows with bricks." The heat in the house thus serves as a symbol for the sexual frustration of the daughters. The men of the town, meanwhile, are of course free to move about outside. They are cooler on the patio and in the fields, suggesting symbolically that they do not suffer from sexual repression.

The heat inside may be what causes Angustias to describe Bernarda's house as hell, and the ongoing torment of all the characters within it suggests the accuracy of her metaphoric description. (Interestingly, in her desperation at the end of the play, Angustias reverses herself and adopts her mother's proud rhetoric, cursing Adela: "Disgrace of this house!") Bernarda's house is also referred to as a house of war, again reminiscent of the lineages of Greek tragedy. Hell is perhaps the strongest lingering image of the house, but other locations of confinement are suggested throughout the play. In his study of the religious imagery in Lorca's trilogy, John Gilmour in *Religion in the Rural Tragedies* refers to Bernarda's house as "convent-like," observing that Lorca uses the funeral in the first act to establish an important theme for the remainder of the play. "A theatre audience," Gilmour wrote, "could not fail to be struck by the sheer number of women, all in mourning, filling the stage, and by their slow, processional entry in a hundred pairs. It is as though they were members of a religious house filing into chapel for their communal worship." If the house does function as a convent, it is only in the sense of deprivation and without, it seems, any

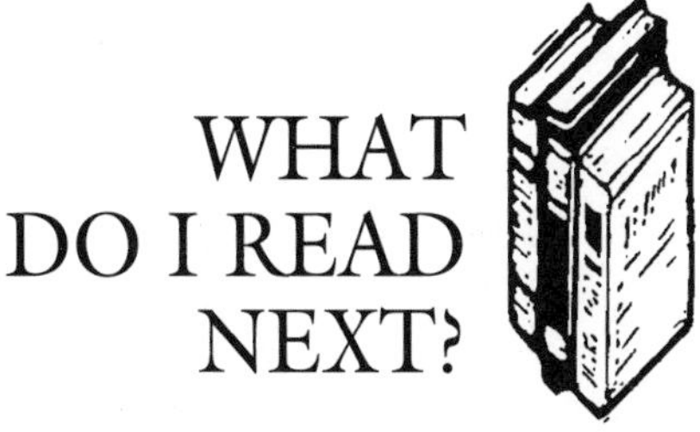

WHAT DO I READ NEXT?

- *Blood Wedding* (1932) is the first play of Lorca's tragic trilogy about life in rural Spain. It concerns a man and a woman who are passionately attracted to each other but enter loveless marriages out of a sense of duty to their relatives. At the woman's wedding feast, the lovers elope. The play uses many more poetic and allegorical devices than *The House of Bernarda Alba.*
- *Yerma* (1934) is the second play of the trilogy. Yerma is a woman who dutifully allows relatives to arrange her wedding. When she discovers her husband does not want children, she is torn between her desire for a baby and her belief in the sanctity of marriage. Her frustration grows uncontrollable, with tragic results.
- *The Poetical Works of Federico Garcia Lorca* (Farrar, Strauss & Giroux, 1991). Students may be interested in reading some of Lorca's more lyrical works about rural Spain, such as the poems originally included in the collections *Gypsy Ballads* and *Poem of the Deep Song.*
- *Life Is a Dream.* The most famous play by Pedro Calderon de la Barca, a seventeenth-century playwright whose works, together with those of the older Lope de Vega, dominated Spain's Golden Age. Like Lorca, Calderon saw life in terms of a symbolic formula, and he was concerned with the traditional Spanish respect for honor. This play examines the conflict between free will and predestination.
- *The Spanish Labyrinth: An Account of the Social and Political Background of the Civil War* by Gerald Brenan. (Cambridge UP, 1974) is a rigorous study of Spanish history from 1874 to 1936. Ian Gibson's *The Assassination of Federico Garcia Lorca* (W.H. Allen, 1979) provides a comprehensive examination of the political and other circumstances surrounding Lorca's death.

---

genuine religious devotion. Bernarda raises a compelling point of contrast when she chastises La Poncia: ''How you'd like to see me and my daughters on our way to a whorehouse!''

La Poncia highlights the dominant sense of confinement in the house when she comments to Bernarda: ''Your daughters act and are as though stuck in a cupboard.'' If larger than a cupboard, the house does function extremely well as a prison. Maria Josefa is most explicitly a prisoner, for Bernarda keeps her locked in a room and relies on the assistance of family and servants to keep her there. Bernarda also imprisons her daughters, saying to them at one point, ''I have five chains for you, and this house my father built.'' The house, the audience knows, has extremely thick walls and bars on the windows through which, for example, Angustias watches Pepe depart. When Adela defies Bernarda near the conclusion of the play, she highlights her mother's role as warden, saying: ''There'll be an end to prison voices here.'' While it is Bernarda's mother, daughters, and servants who are most explicitly imprisoned in the house, the play suggests that Bernarda is herself a prisoner. Although she commands power over others, she is so confined by her own sense of honor and proper appearance that she cannot act any more freely than the rest.

In the settings of each of the three acts of *The House of Bernarda Alba,* there is a symbolic penetration deeper and deeper into the house, which reflects the gradual exposing of the family's secrets. The first act is set in a room near the entrance hall, appropriate for the public nature of the funeral and the visitation of neighbors, which Bernarda must endure. In the second act, the setting moves to a more intimate room near the bedrooms, bringing the audience deeper into the hearts and motives of the various characters. The final act moves to a room adjacent to the corral, which is the site of sexual liaison and the symbolic source of conflict in the play. Bernarda's desire to keep the secrets of the

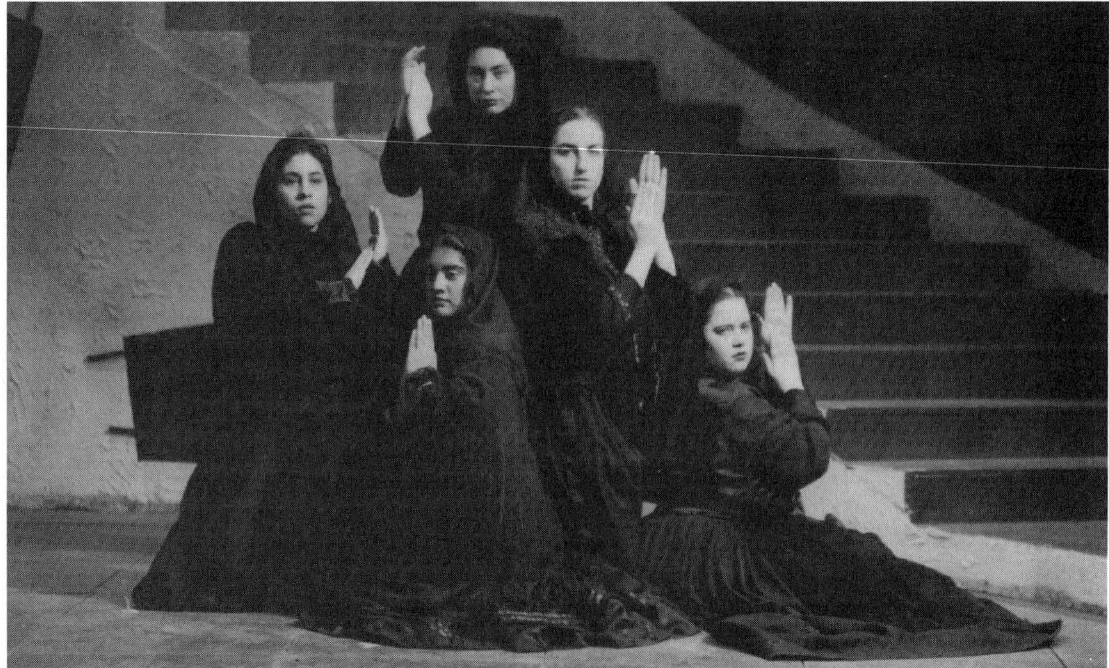

The women of Bernarda's house in a production staged at Case Western Reserve University

family deep within the house may prove impossible now that the neighbors have awakened. With her desperate cry of "Silence!" Bernarda can merely, as the old saying has it, close the barn door after the horse is out.

Lorca described the structure of the play as a "photographic document," and the imagery of the house supports this theme. Photographs in Lorca's day were of course in black and white, and the stark whiteness of the house's walls is contrasted perfectly with the black mourning clothes of the women in the first act. The uniform whiteness of the walls suggests a sense of purity which Bernarda would like to maintain. The color also suggests a whitewash of hypocrisy, which dominates the household, as well as the sterility and monotony of life for Bernarda's daughters in the house. The stark black and white patterns of the play are modified later when the walls appear tinged with blue, suggesting evening. (Ironically, it is in the dark cover of night rather than in stark light of day that the secrets of the family are "brought to light.") The blue tones suggest the doubt that now tinges the purity and decency which had previously prevailed. The green dress of Adela is the only other color which appears in the play, contrasting the white walls of the house not only in hue but also in theme, for the color is symbolically associated with nature, hope, jealousy, sex.

Bernarda's house thus functions as a central symbol in Lorca's final play, in the use of color and other elements of scenic design, in metaphoric references to prisons and convents, and in providing a physical structure to the layers of secrecy within which Bernarda wraps her family life. Since theater is an art form based on the physicality of performance, it is fitting that a great modern work of drama like *The House of Bernarda Alba* should make use of a setting that is both visually striking and serves so well to develop the images and themes contained in the play.

Source: Christopher G. Busiel, for *Drama for Students*, Gale, 1998.

Morris Freedman

Freedman elaborates on the theme of passion in Lorca's dramatic work, examining the conflict between individual character's emotions and the morals of the society portrayed.

With Lorca we enter an altogether different landscape in the modern drama, the landscape of passion. His three great tragedies—*Blood Wedding, Yerma, The House of Bernarda Alba*—are stripped nearly bare of the details of setting and time, that sense of locale we need for Ibsen, Wilde, Shaw, or O'Casey. Yet we do not leave the area of reality, as we do with some of Strindberg and of Pirandello. Lorca empties his drama of nearly all forces but passion. Even his settings always seem nearly barren, simply all whites or all blacks, so that only the colors emerge that are evoked by the action and the characters. The motivation and energy for plot are in passion; the definition of character is through passion. There is no "thought," no "idea" of any significance.

Lorca is preeminently the playwright of passion in the modern theater although we can find elements of Lorca in Williams, Osborne, O'Neill, and Genet; but in each of these there is a significant admixture of other thematic material. Lorca's passion is not related to a program, as in D. H. Lawrence, or in Williams, or in Genet. Lorca's "blood consciousness" is a consciousness of what is, already; of what must be observed, acknowledged, assimilated, lived with, understood, and, finally, even forgiven. Lorca's passion is rooted in an established social context. The tragedy in his plays comes from the tension between passion, which is necessarily always entirely individual and personal and whimsical, and the society in which the individuals move, which defines them and also gives a particular value and shading to passion and its manifestations. In Lorca, the conflict is between passion and honor, where passion is the mark of the personal (willful and private and powerful in its needs) and honor that of the social (rigid and public and equally powerful in its rules and taboos, the denial of needs). . . .

In *The House of Bernarda Alba,* we have what amounts to a nunnery and all that implies of the suppression of passion: nunneries are refuges from the usual passion of the world. Bernarda Alba is sadistically compulsive about order, pathological about cleanliness. As in *Yerma,* in which the two old maids spend all their time keeping their house spotless, so the barrenness, immaculateness of Bernarda Alba's establishment are related to sterility; her house is not merely a denial of passion but a denigration of it. Bernarda, loudly: "Magdalena, don't cry. If you want to cry, get under your bed."

We remember that in *Blood Wedding,* Leonardo lives a "disordered" life: he cannot hold down a job, he is hot-tempered and impatient, he comes from a line of murderers. He is thematically equated with a wild stallion. But none of this is pejorative, merely descriptive; Leonardo is of that world where violence alone is heroic. The Bridegroom represents order, cleanliness, and wealth. Bernarda Alba is rich and viciously opposed to irregular emotions: "Hot coals in the place where she sinned," she screams horribly about the local girl who has given herself to a number of men. As we hear the threat of the galloping stallion in *Blood Wedding,* threatening the orderly arrangement of events, so one hears the hoofbeats of the caged animal in *Bernarda Alba,* a tattoo of threatening disaster again.

> "THE TITLE, *THE HOUSE OF BERNARDA ALBA,* DRAWS ATTENTION BOTH TO BERNARDA'S 'HOUSE' IN THE SENSE OF HER HOUSEHOLD OR LINEAGE, AND TO THE PHYSICAL SPACE OF THE HOUSE ITSELF, WHICH SERVES AS THE CENTRAL IMAGE OF THE PLAY."

Bernarda Alba is an extreme distillation of social honor; she exemplifies a passion that has gone too far in excluding the mortally impulsive, irrational, emotional, self-indulgent. It has become in its extremity antipassion. When one daughter says, "I should be happy, but I'm not," Bernarda Alba replies, "It's all the same." (Of course, it's not all the same, not even for Bernarda, as her frenzy to undo things at the end of the play testifies.) In effect, Bernarda is a Satanic spirit, living in an atmosphere of death, perversion, and denial. The play starts with a funeral and ends with a suicide; between we have sadism, insanity, onanism. There are black curtains on the windows. Sexual passions are outside this territory: the stallion drumming in his stall; the village escapades. No men appear on stage. The setting is on the edge of action. The only action that occasionally can burst out in Bernarda Alba's house is the poultrylike squabbling of the sisters, a parody of life.

In *The House of Bernarda Alba,* then, we get an extended examination of the pathology of social

"LORCA IS PREEMINENTLY THE PLAYWRIGHT OF PASSION IN THE MODERN THEATER."

passion, of an honor that is contemptuous of the individually human, that is, finally, self-defeating. Bernarda Alba did bear five children, but we are to gather that this was in the cause of social honor, that whatever private passion she might have begun with has attenuated into nothingness, been distorted into self-hatred. She hates her daughters. Bernarda Alba's passion is exercised in the extinguishing of passion: the sadist can only have definition through the masochist, his diametrical opposite. As the play opens, we see Bernarda Alba finally retiring into the "ideal" existence, waiting primly for death, her social duties done, indifferent to the suppressed but smoldering vitality of the unattached daughters. Bernarda Alba fears and hates sex in any form, for sex means only life.

The conclusion of *Bernarda Alba* crystallizes earlier thematic hints and motifs. Adela hangs herself on learning, mistakenly, that her lover has been killed. In a veritable hysteria, Bernarda Alba shrieks that Adela died a virgin, forbids tears except in private, and calls for silence, silence, silence, as the curtain descends. Cleanliness, purity, silence, defining marks of death itself, envelope Bernarda Alba's house. "Death must be looked at face to face," she pronounces as Adela's body is cut down. . . .

Bernarda Alba climaxes this trilogy of the tragedy of passion by seeming to assert that it is "honor," passion perverted by a sense of the social that excludes the human, which somehow survives and even triumphs, however abominably, over the personal passion. We may thus read these tragedies as concluding on a pessimistic note: the world of Bernarda Alba is one in which human impulses may not range freely, must be constrained, even expunged, even at the risk of the ugliest consequences, of perversions of passion and of life, including madness, self-stimulation, torture, suicide. But the very extremity of this view suggests its own rebuttal; Bernarda Alba's mode cannot sustain itself except by a restlessly conscious, eternally remorseless exercise of death-dealing. Even as Bernarda Alba is hysterically improvising her sterile stagecraft for the future, managing the appearance of Adela's suicide ("Take her to another room and dress her as though she were a virgin"), arranging to face death daily, another daughter, Martirio, mutters: "A thousand times happy she, who had him." The personal, physical passion continues to assert its independent power. Honor may finally turn to antipassion, as in Bernarda Alba, certainly with its own power, but the primal force is personal passion.

Lorca's tragedy, then, resides in the domain of passion: passion destroys itself and its possessors, the personal can ultimately only come in conflict with the social, the social enlarges itself into vengeance or into death-serving sterility. Life and fulfillment may reside in passion alone, but precariously, never without risk, not casually. Humans cannot truly be alive without passion, but with passion they must wage a running, alert, and subtle battle with those guerilla forces intent on its destruction. It is the classic opposition between life and death itself; and death, of course, as Freud not least has sadly indicated, is an expression, a wish, of life itself. But to celebrate passion is to celebrate life, living, feeling, reaching, erring: vitality, vivacity, whimsicality, impulsiveness, energy of every sort. There is a final rightness about Lorca's characters who strive toward goals that define them as they live, as there is about Oedipus, and to fail is simply—and greatly—to be human.

Source: Morris Freedman, "The Morality of Passion: Lorca's Three Tragedies" in his *The Moral Impulse: Modern Drama from Ibsen to the Present,* Southern Illinois University Press, 1967, pp. 89–98.

Richard Watts, Jr.

In this review of an English language production of Lorca's play by the American National Theatre and Academy, Watts offers a positive critique of the material while finding the translation somewhat lacking.

Federico Garcia Lorca, the Spanish playwright who was murdered by his country's Fascists in 1936, is a figure of international literary importance, and the American National Theatre and Academy was fulfilling one of its proper functions when it offered his most famous drama, *The House of Bernarda Alba,* as the fourth item in its subscription season at the ANTA Playhouse last night. It must be added, however, that the production provided additional evidence that the theatre of Spain does not fit any too snugly into the American stage and presents barriers that it is not easy to cross.

The House of Bernarda Alba is a somber and brooding tragedy about a family of girls ruled over by a grim and tyrannical matriarch who seeks to suppress their natural instincts in the interest of her own stern social code. With the father dead, the mother drives the young women into a lengthy period of mourning in which they are to be cut off completely from association with men, with the not altogether surprising result that they are filled with bitterness, hatred and general unrest and the youngest of them commits suicide after it had been discovered that she was having a secret love affair with the eldest daughter's fiance.

The conflict between natural instincts and the forces that try to suppress them seems to be one of the dramatist's favorite themes, and there is no denying that, in *The House of Bernarda Alba,* he goes about his story with a single-minded intensity that is capable of engendering considerable dramatic power. Although on the English-speaking stage there appears to be a certain artificiality in the theatrical style of Garcia Lorca, it is still evident that he is a playwright of authentic tragic force. There are moments in the play that are highly impressive in their concentrated emotion.

The mood of ominous impending doom that hangs over the unhappy household of savage old Bernarda is captured in both the writing and the production with effective skill and presents the most successfull feature of the drama. But the tragedy itself, it seems to me, is made less moving and believable than its materials should make it through a kind of artificial stylization that may be eloquent and hauntingly lyric in the original Spanish but is a little flat and unpersuasive in its English translation. The final effect, which might have been devastating, is somehow far from overwhelming.

For me, one of the troubles with the play's effectiveness is the acting of Katina Paxinou as the matriarch. I have now seen Miss Paxinou on the stage in *Hedda Gabler* and on the screen in *For Whom the Bell Tolls* and *Mourning Becomes Electra,* and I must confess that her art continues to escape me. There is something about her highly mannered style that seems to me grotesque and extravagant, rather than powerful and moving, and this struck me as being all the more noticeable last night because that style happened to be contrasted with the less ornate playing of the other members of the cast.

" IN *THE HOUSE OF BERNARDA ALBA,* GARCIA LORCA GOES ABOUT HIS STORY WITH A SINGLE-MINDED INTENSITY THAT IS CAPABLE OF ENGENDERING CONSIDERABLE DRAMATIC POWER."

Such interesting young actresses as Ruth Ford, Helen Craig, Mary Welch and Kim Stanley are prominent in the all-woman cast, and they all play skillfully, but I couldn't escape the feeling that they were in a different play from the one in which Miss Paxinou was appearing. The set and the costumes by Stewart Chaney and the direction by Boris Tumarin are of help in creating the mood that is the most successful feature of *The House of Bernarda Alba,* and I certainly agree that the tragedy was worth doing. But I am also sure that Garcia Lorca must have been a finer playwright than he seems in the American theatre.

Source: Richard Watts, Jr., "The Grim House of Bernarda Alba" in the *New York Post,* January 8, 1951.

SOURCES

Bentley, Eric. "The Poet in Dublin" in *In Search of Theatre,* Knopf (New York City), 1953.

Benet, William Rose. "Singing Spain" in the *Saturday Review,* October 2, 1937, p. 18.

Blanco-Gonzalez, Manuel, "Lorca: The Tragic Trilogy" in *Drama Critique,* September 2, 1966, pp. 91-97.

Burton, Julianne. "The Greatest Punishment: Female and Male in Lorca's Tragedies" in *Women in Hispanic Literature: Icons and Fallen Idols,* edited by Beth Miller, University of California Press (Berkeley), 1983, pp. 259-79.

Carrier, Warren. "Poetry in the Drama of Lorca" in *Drama Survey,* February 3, 1963, pp. 297-304.

Cobb, Carl. "Federico Garcia Lorca" in *Twayne's World Author Series,* Volume 23, Twayne (New York City), 1967.

Garcia Lorca, Francisco. Prologue to *Three Tragedies by Federico Garcia Lorca,* New Directions Publishing Corporation (New York City), 1955, pp. 1-29.

Gilmour, John. "The Cross of Pain and Death: Religion in the Rural Tragedies" in *Lorca: Poet and Playwright,* edited by Robert Havard, St. Martin's Press (New York City), 1992, pp. 133-55.

Honig, Edwin. *Garcia Lorca,* New Directions (Norfolk, CT), 1963.

Humphries, Rolfe. "The Life and Death of Garcia Lorca" in the *Nation,* September 18, 1937, pp. 293-94.

Lewis, Allan. "The Folklore Theatre—Garcia Lorca" in *The Contemporary Theatre: The Significant Playwrights of Our Time,* Crown (New York City), 1971, pp. 242-58.

Shanley, John P. "Garcia Lorca Work on 'Play of the Week'" in *New York Times,* June 7, 1960.

Williams, William Carlos. "Federico Garcia Lorca" in *Selected Essays of William Carlos Williams,* Random House (New York City), 1954, pp. 219-30.

FURTHER READING

Colecchia, Francesca, Editor. *Garcia Lorca: A Selectively Annotated Bibliography of Criticism,* Garland (New York City), 1979; *Garcia Lorca: An Annotated Primary Bibliography* Garland, 1982.

Extensive bibliographies with many useful listings for researchers. One volume covers scholarship on Lorca's plays, the other Lorca's works in Spanish and in translation.

Klein, Dennis A. *Blood Wedding, Yerma, and The House of Bernarda Alba: Garcia Lorca's Tragic Trilogy,* G.K. Hall & Co. (Boston), 1991.

The first full-length critical study devoted to Lorca's tragic trilogy, which the author calls "the most accomplished and mature efforts of the finest Spanish playwright of the twentieth century." Klein works through the original Spanish texts (providing quotations in his own English translations), examining the trilogy both in the larger context of Lorca's career as a poet, playwright, director, and visual artist, and in the social context of Spain in Lorca's era.

Lima, Robert. *The Theater of Garcia Lorca,* Las Americas (New York City), 1963.

A critical study surveying all the plays of Lorca's available in print at the time of its publication.

Londre, Felicia Hardison. *Federico Garcia Lorca,* Ungar (New York City), 1984.

Examines Lorca's artistry by emphasizing a synthesis of approach to his poetry, drama, music, visual art, and stage direction. Includes a full chapter devoted to what Lorca called his "unperformable plays." *The House of Bernarda Alba* is treated in detail, pp. 172-180, and discussed elsewhere in the work.

Newton, Candelas. *Understanding Federico Garcia Lorca,* University of South Carolina Press (Columbia), 1995.

Newton provides her audience with an understanding of the Andalusian region where he was born, as a basis for appreciating his writing. She establishes connections between Lorca's works to illustrate the variety of approaches that Lorca employed. Contains an annotated bibliography and other resources for the student researcher.

Twentieth Century Literary Criticism, Vols. 1, 7, 49, Gale (Detroit), 1978, 1982, 1994.

This resource compiles selections of criticism; it is an excellent beginning point for a research paper about Lorca. The selections in these three volumes span Lorca's entire career. Also see Volume 2 of Gale's *Drama Criticism.* For an overview of Lorca's life, see the entry on him in Volume 108 of the *Dictionary of Literary Biography.*

The Importance of Being Earnest

OSCAR WILDE

1895

Oscar Wilde's most successful play, *The Importance of Being Earnest* became an instant hit when it opened in London, England, in February, 1895, running for eighty-six performances. The play has remained popular with audiences ever since, vying with Wilde's 1890 novel *The Portrait of Dorian Gray* as his most recognized work. The play proves vexing to critics, though, for it resists categorization, seeming to some merely a flimsy plot which serves as an excuse for Wilde's witty epigrams (terse, often paradoxical, sayings or catch-phrases). To others it is a penetratingly humorous and insightful social comedy.

When *Earnest* opened, Wilde was already familiar to readers for *Dorian Gray,* as well as for collections of fairy tales, stories, and literary criticism. Theatre-goers knew him for his earlier dramatic works, including three previous successes, *Lady Windermere's Fan* (1892), *A Women of No Importance* (1893), and *An Ideal Husband* (1895), as well as for his more controversial play, *Salome* (1896), which was banned in Britain for its racy (by nineteenth century standards) sexual content.

The Importance of Being Earnest has been favorably compared with William Shakespeare's comedy *Twelfth Night* and Restoration plays like Richard Brinsley Sheridan's *School for Scandal* and Oliver Goldsmith's *She Stoops to Conquer.* While it is generally acknowledged that Wilde's play owes a debt to these works, critics have contended that the

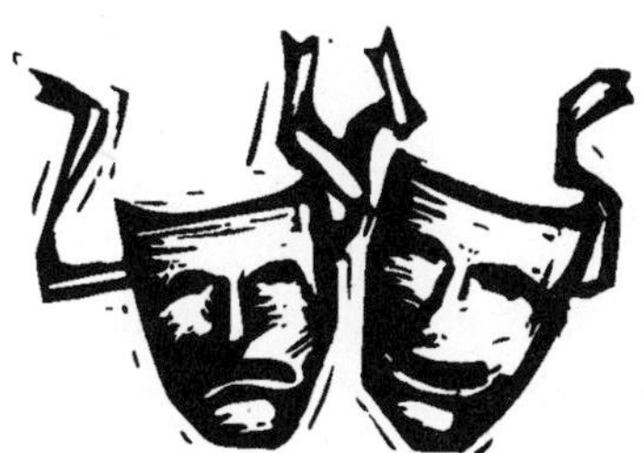

playwright captures something unique about his era, reworking the late Victorian melodramas and stage romances to present a farcical, highly satiric work—though audiences generally appraise the play as simply great fun.

Tragically, as *The Importance of Being Earnest,* his fourth and most successful play, received acclaim in London, Wilde himself became embroiled in the legal actions against his homosexuality that would end his career and lead to imprisonment, bankruptcy, divorce, and exile.

AUTHOR BIOGRAPHY

Oscar (Fingal O'Flahertie Wills) Wilde was born on October 15 (though some sources cite October 16), 1854 (some sources cite 1856) in Dublin, Ireland, where he would spend his youth. His father was a celebrated eye and ear surgeon who was knighted by Queen Victoria for founding a hospital and writing an influential medical textbook. Wilde's mother, Jane Francesca Elgee Wilde, came to be called "Speranza," writing poems, stories, essays, and folklore meant to give hope to advocates of rights for women and Ireland.

Wilde won prizes in the classics at Portora Royal School in Ulster, and his continued success in classic studies at Dublin's Trinity College won him a scholarship to attend Magdalen College, Oxford, where he earned a B.A. In 1878, the undergraduate Wilde won the Newdigate Prize for his poem "Ravenna."

While at Oxford, the ideas of Walter Pater and John Ruskin shaped Wilde's thinking about art. He became known for flamboyance in dress (his trademark became wearing a green carnation in his lapel), collecting peacock feathers, and blue china; he came to personify the term "Dandy" used to describe men who paid excessive attention to their appearance. He also became a spokesman for Aestheticism, a belief in the supreme importance of "Art for Art's sake," without regard for its practical, ethical, or social purpose. ("The object of Art is not simple truth but complex beauty," Wilde wrote later in his 1889 essay "The Decay of Lying.") Following publication of the first volume of his *Poems* in 1881, which included "The Harlot's House" and "Impression du Matin," Wilde spent ten months giving 125 lectures throughout the United States. The Aesthetics movement and Wilde were satirized in the magazine *Punch* and in W. S. Gilbert's *Patience* (1881).

After the disappointing reception of his first play, *Vera,* in 1883, Wilde returned to Britain to spend eighteen months lecturing on "Impressions of America." In 1884, he married Constance Lloyd and began working as a reviewer and editor. *The Happy Prince and Other Tales,* a volume of fairy tales originally written for his sons appeared in 1888, followed two years later by Wilde's novel, *The Picture of Dorian Gray.*

Success eluded Wilde's second play, *The Duchess of Padua* (1891), but his subsequent theatrical efforts received increasing acclaim: *Lady Windermere's Fan* in 1892, *A Women of No Importance* in 1893, *An Ideal Husband* in 1895, and, that same year, his greatest theatrical success, *The Importance of Being Earnest.*

While in Paris, Wilde wrote *Salome* in French, but the play was refused a license for performance in England, though the 1896 Paris production starred noted actress Sara Bernhardt. An English translation of *Salome* appeared in 1894 with illustrations by famed illustrator Aubrey Beardsley and the play provided the libretto for Richard Strauss's successful 1905 opera of the same name.

Social criticism of Wilde's openly homosexual behavior (though married with children, he professed a deep passion for young men) led to the end of his career. Wilde's relationship with Lord Alfred Douglas led Douglas's father, the Marquess of Queensberry, to publicly accuse Wilde of sodomy. Encouraged by Lord Alfred, Wilde sued the Marquess for slander, losing his suit when the Marquess offered evidence of Wilde's homosexuality. Wilde refused the advice of friends to flee to the Continent and in subsequent trials was convicted of "public indecency" and sentenced to two years of hard labor. With the scandal, Wilde's plays ceased production.

Two major works written in prison were published following Wilde's release. *De Profundus* appeared in 1905, offering an apologetic confession of Wilde's conduct, while *The Ballad of Reading Gaol,* published initially in 1898, indicts England's prison system and tells of his experiences there. Upon his release, Wilde, divorced and bankrupt, adopted the name Sebastian Melmouth and moved to Paris, France, where he died in 1900.

Wilde's literary reputation enjoyed a considerable resurgence in the years following his death. He is now regarded as one of modern literature's major figures. His skill and diversity within multiple genres has earned him respect as a poet, novelist, essayist, and playwright. His works are still widely studied and his plays enjoy frequent revivals.

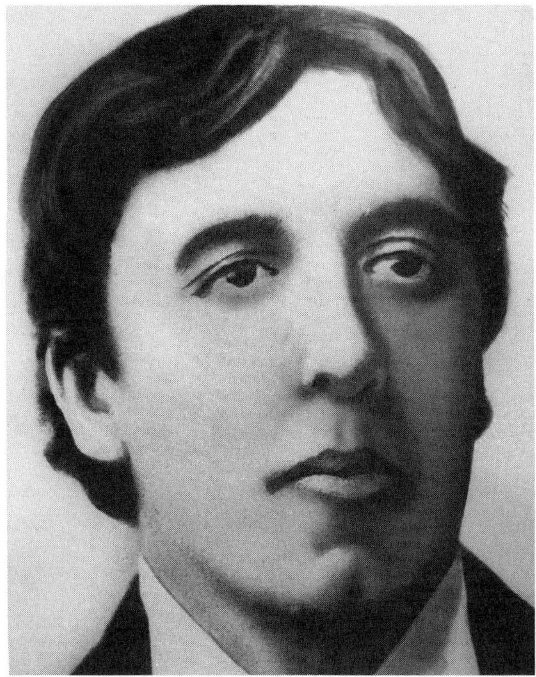

Oscar Wilde

PLOT SUMMARY

Act One

The play opens in the fashionable London residence of Algernon Moncrieff. His friend Jack (who goes by the name "Earnest") Worthing arrives, revealing his intention to propose matrimony to Algernon's cousin Gwendolen Fairfax. In the course of their conversation, Jack admits that he is the ward to a young woman, Cecily Cardew. Also, he admits to leading a double life, stating that his "name is Earnest in town and Jack in the country." In the country, he pretends to have a brother in London named Earnest whose wicked ways necessitate frequent trips to the city to rescue him.

Algernon's aunt Lady Augusta Bracknell arrives with his cousin Gwendolen Fairfax. While Algernon and his aunt discuss the music for her next party, Jack—claiming his name is Earnest—confesses his love for Gwendolen and proposes marriage. She is delighted, because her "ideal has always been to love someone of the name Earnest." When the lovers tell Lady Bracknell their news, she responds frostily, forbidding marriage outright after learning that while Jack has an occupation—he smokes—and money, he has no lineage to boast of—in fact, he has no knowledge of his real family at all. He was discovered as an infant, abandoned in a handbag in Victoria Station.

Because Cecily seems too interested in Jack's imaginary brother, Earnest, Jack decides to "kill" him. Gwendolen informs Jack that while Lady Bracknell forbids their marriage and that she "may marry someone else, and marry often," she will retain her "eternal devotion" to him.

Act Two

July in the garden of Jack's Manor House in Hertfordshire. Miss Prism, Cecily's governess, chides her for not attending to her German lesson, as Jack has requested. Prism informs Cecily that when younger, she had written a novel. The Rector, Canon Frederick Chasuble enters, suggesting that a stroll in the garden may cure Miss Prism's headache. She feels fine but a headache develops soon after his suggestion, and they walk off together.

Algernon arrives, and, finding Cecily alone, introduces himself as Jack's "wicked" city brother, Earnest. Cecily and Algernon (as Earnest) walk off. Prism and Chasuble return as Jack shows up unexpectedly. Hoping to end his double-life, Jack informs them that his brother Earnest has died in Paris of a "severe chill." They console him, until Cecily enters with Earnest (Algernon), who seems very much alive. Jack is bewildered, but Cecily, thinking Jack's coolness is resentment at his brother's dissipated lifestyle, insists that the "brothers" mend their relationship.

Left alone, Algernon proposes to Cecily, only to discover that—according to Cecily—they have already been engaged for three months. It seems that since Cecily heard from Jack about his wicked brother, Earnest, she fell in love with him. She entered in her diary their entire romance, complete with proposal, acceptance, break-up, and reconciliation.

Gwendolen arrives and chats with Cecily, until both women realize they are engaged to a man named Earnest. When Algernon and Jack return, their true identities—and the fact that neither of them is actually named Earnest—are revealed. As the scene ends, both men admit to having arranged for Chasuble to re-christen them with the name Earnest.

Act Three

Later the same day at the Manor house, Gwendolen and Cecily prepare to forgive the men, though they are disappointed that neither is named Earnest. Lady Bracknell arrives, in pursuit of Gwendolen. She learns from Jack that his ward Cecily is quite wealthy and therefore a desirable match for her nephew Algernon. When she hears of Miss Prism, Lady Bracknell recognizes her as a former family servant. Prism and Lady Bracknell's infant nephew had disappeared at the same time under mysterious circumstances.

Miss Prism confesses that she had left the house with her novel manuscript in one hand and the baby in the other. In her confusion, however, she had put the book in the baby carriage and the baby in the handbag at the train station. The baby, Jack, turns out to be Lady Bracknell's lost nephew and Algernon's older brother. Lady Bracknell now gives her permission for Algernon to wed Cecily, but Jack, as Cecily's guardian, refuses his permission unless Lady Bracknell consents to his marriage to Gwendolen. She does, and as the act closes, they learn that Jack was named after his father, General Earnest John Moncrieff—Earnest for short.

CHARACTERS

Algy

See Algernon Moncrieff

Lady Augusta Bracknell

Algernon's aunt and the sister of Jack's mother. She opposes Jack's marriage with her daughter Gwendolen, though relents when she learns that Jack is actually her nephew. More accurately, she wants Algernon to be able to marry the very wealthy Cecily, but that match cannot take place without Jack's permission, which he refuses to give unless Lady Bracknell approves his marriage with Gwendolen. Overall, she is realistic, hard-nosed, and an upholder of convention—though not entirely conventional herself.

Cecily Cardew

Jack's pretty, young ward, whom Algernon woos but who remains determined to marry a man named Earnest. Not quite as naive as she may appear, Cecily keeps a diary, which "is simply a very young girl's record of her own thoughts and impressions and consequently meant for publication." Tutored by Miss Prism, Cecily fails to attend to her studies and marries Algernon at the play's conclusion.

Canon Frederick Chasuble

Canon Chasuble is the rather foolish, pedantic Rector attracted to Miss Prism. Both Jack and Algernon ask Chasuble to christen them Earnest, though no christening actually takes place. As Cecily says, "He has never written a single book, so you can imagine how much he knows."

Earnest

See John Worthing

Gwendolen Fairfax

Algernon's cousin, with whom Jack—as Earnest—is in love and to whom he proposes marriage. She accepts, believing him to be Algy's friend Earnest. As she explains to Jack, her "ideal has always been to love someone of the name Earnest. There is something in that name that inspires absolute confidence." Her mother, Lady Augusta Bracknell, initially forbids their marriage, because while Jack seems an otherwise eligible bachelor, he cannot identify his parents, as he was found abandoned in a handbag. The play's end, however, establishes Jack's identity; Lady Bracknell grants permission, and the lovers are united.

Lane

The self-deprecating butler who serves Algernon in his London residence.

Merriman

The servant at Jack's country manor house in Hertfordshire.

Algernon Moncrieff

Jack (Earnest) Worthing's friend, Lady Bracknell's nephew, and Gwendolen's cousin. In order to free himself from unwanted social and family responsibilities, Algy has invented an invalid friend, Bunbury, whose ailing health frequently—and conveniently—requires Algernon's attention, enabling him to skip dinners with boring guests and tiresome relatives.

Ostentatiously cynical and constantly hungry, Algernon pretends to be Jack's brother Earnest and visits Jack's ward Cecily Cardew. He falls in love with her and proposes matrimony. Jack refuses his permission for Algernon to marry Cecily unless Lady Bracknell gives her permission for Jack to marry Gwendolen, which, at the play's end, she does. The mystery of Jack's parentage reveals that Jack and Algy are actually brothers.

Miss Laetitia Prism

Cecily's absent-minded governess who is wooed by Chasuble. Formerly, while working for Lady Bracknell, she wrote a novel then lost Jack in the railway station. She ''deposited the manuscript in the bassinet, and placed the baby in the handbag,'' which was lost in the cloak room of Victoria Station.

John Worthing

John ''Jack'' Worthing (Earnest) begins the play of unknown parentage, an orphaned infant found in a handbag in a cloak room at London's Victoria Station. Discovered and raised by Thomas Cardew, Jack becomes guardian of Cardew's granddaughter, Cecily. Though he calls himself Jack in the country, he identifies himself as Earnest when in the city. In order to excuse himself when he leaves for the city, he tells Cecily that he must get his wicked citified brother, Earnest, out of various scrapes. In time, Cecily becomes infatuated with this imaginary brother Earnest. By the play's end, it is revealed that Miss Prism had left Jack at the station, that Lady Bracknell's sister Mrs. Moncrieff is his mother, and that Jack is Algy's elder brother. Also, significantly, Jack, who has been named after his father General Earnest John Moncrieff, actually *is* named Earnest.

MEDIA ADAPTATIONS

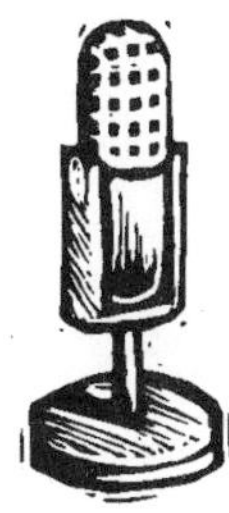

- Universal International Films released a film adaptation of *The Importance of Being Earnest* in 1953. Directed by Anthony Asquith, the film stars Michael Redgrave as Jack/Earnest. It is available on video from Paramount.

THEMES

Morals and Morality

Much of *The Importance of Being Earnest*'s comedy stems from the ways various characters flaunt the moral strictures of the day, without ever behaving beyond the pale of acceptable society. The use of the social lie is pervasive, sometimes carried to great lengths as when Algernon goes ''Bunburying'' or Jack invents his rakish brother Earnest so that he may escape to the city. Another example is Miss Prism's sudden headache when the opportunity to go walking (and possibly indulge in some form of sexual activity) with Canon Chasuble presents itself.

Love and Passion

One of Wilde's satiric targets is romantic and sentimental love, which he ridicules by having the women fall in love with a man because of his name rather than more personal attributes. Wilde carries parody of romantic love to an extreme in the relationship between Algernon and Cecily, for she has fallen in love with him—and in fact charted their entire relationship—before ever meeting him. She writes of their love in her diary, noting the ups and downs of their affair, including authoring love letters to and from herself.

Culture Clash

The play's action is divided between the city and the country, London and the pastoral county of Hertfordshire. Traditionally, locations like these symbolize different attitudes toward life, contrasting, for example, the corruption of urban living with the simple bucolic pleasures of rural farm life. As Jack says, ''when one is in town one amuses oneself. When one is in the country one amuses other people. It is excessively boring.'' Wilde's symbolism does not adhere rigidly to audience expectations, however. Though Jack is more sedate while in the country and more festive when in London, Cecily is far from the innocent she appears (and pretends to be around her guardian). Her handling of her ''affair'' with Algernon/Earnest shows her to be as competent in romance as any city woman. The

TOPICS FOR FURTHER STUDY

- Wilde's play revolves around the necessity of telling lies in order to keep polite society polite. Is such dishonesty really necessary? What would the world be like if everyone were absolutely honest? What would happen to you if you were honest for one week?
- Many psychologists, sociologists, and literary scholars consider Oscar Wilde's trial as the moment which marks the birth of the modern homosexual identity. Read an account of Wilde's trial or his novel *The Portrait of Dorian Gray* and consider the social and aesthetic issues which surround sexual identity.
- In many ways, Wilde's play is a send up of gender roles and a travesty of romantic idealism. Are love and marriage really as simple—or complicated—as they seem in *Earnest?* How should men and women behave toward each other? What do people really want in relationships? What makes for a successful or unsuccessful marriage?
- In *Earnest,* people in the country behave—or at least, are expected to behave—differently from their counterparts in the city. Are the stereotypes of city and country life still with us? Identify those stereotypes and consider how population growth, shifting demographics, and urbanization have affected the ways we think about rural and urban life.
- Critics have commented on the "triviality" of Wilde's play—that is, it's celebration of the superficial at the expense of earnest seriousness. As an advocate of the Aesthetic movement, though, Wilde might agree with those characters in *Earnest* who value form over content. Consider the ways Wilde's play critiques contemporary Victorian values.

trait is seen again when Gwendolen visits. During their tiff over just who gets Earnest (who they believe to be one man), Cecily holds her own and then some against her sophisticated city guest.

Language and Meaning

Those familiar with semiotic theory (signs and symbols) will notice the ways various characters in the play obsess over the signifier. The best example is the desire of both Gwendolen and Cecily to love men named Earnest. They see something mystical in the processing of naming and assume some connection between the word (the signifier) and the person (the signified), that one who is named Earnest will naturally behave earnestly.

Freedom

Both Jack and Algernon struggle to remain free of the restrictions of Victorian convention. Jack does so by maintaining a double identity, being Jack in the country and Earnest in the city. Algernon achieves similar results by inventing an invalid named Bunbury who constantly requires his attentions. This similarity in Algernon and Jack's behavior also offers a clue to the men's true relationship as brothers (further duality is indicated by their respective attractions to very similar women, Gwendolen and Cecily).

STYLE

Romantic Comedy

Most commonly seen in Shakespeare's romance plays like *As You Like It* or *A Midsummer Night's Dream,* the plot of a typical romantic comedy involves an idealized pair of lovers who the circumstances of daily life or social convention seem destined to keep apart. Along the way, the lovers escape their troubles, at least for a while, entering an ideal world (like the Garden of Eden) where conflicts resolve and the lovers ultimately come together. The plots of such comedies contain pairs of characters and conclude happily, often exhibiting poetic justice, with the good rewarded and the evil punished.

While *The Importance of Being Earnest* certainly fits this description, it is a play that is appraised beyond simple romantic comedy. In fact, part of the play's wide and lasting appeal is that it so competently fits into any number of comedy genres, including comedies of manners, farces, and parodies.

Comedy of Manners

Generally set in sophisticated society, this type of intellectual comedy privileges witty dialogue over plot, though social intrigue involving the problems of lovers—faithful and unfaithful—can be complicated. The comedy arises from the critique of the fashions, manners, and behavior of elevated society. While often featuring standard characters such as fools, fops, conniving servants, and jealous husbands, the action itself is largely realistic. At least one character, like the audience, accurately comprehends the foolish nature of the people and their situations. In addition to Restoration Comedies like William Congreve's *The Way of the World,* other examples would be Goldsmith's *She Stoops to Conquer,* Sheridan's *School for Scandal,* and Noel Coward's *Private Lives.*

Farce

This type of low comedy relies on physical gags, coarse wit, and generally broad humor. Laughter arises as exaggerated characters, sometimes caricatures of social types, extricate themselves from improbable situations. Farce occasionally involves disguise or the confusion of gender roles. Algernon's indulgence with food and his short attention span qualify him as a farcical character, as does Miss Prism's bumbling mix-up with her novel and the infant Jack.

Parody

A work which, for comic or satiric effect, imitates another, familiar, usually serious work, mocking the recognizable trademarks of an individual author, style, or genre. Successful parody assumes an informed audience, with knowledge of the parodied target. For example, one of the most parodied works today is the "Mona Lisa" painting which shows up in cartoons, advertisements, and fine art. In *Earnest,* Wilde parodies, among other things, love at first sight by having his characters fall in love before they ever see each other.

HISTORICAL CONTEXT

As the nineteenth century drew to a close, England witnessed a cultural and artistic turn against the values of Queen Victoria's reign (1837-1901). These earlier virtues, such as self-help and respectability, were widely touted during the boom years of the 1860s and 1870s. However, people were less able to help themselves and raise their social standing in the late 1870s, when farming practices underwent a change which affected society as a whole.

Wheat-fields were converted to cattle pastures on a sweeping scale, and farmers suffered. While farmers were struggling, industrialists were profiting from their factories which employed workers at cheap wages. Factory owners and other businessmen formed the new middle class in England, and as they rose on the social ladder, they desired to imitate the aristocracy by owning houses in the countryside and becoming patrons of art.

As people began questioning the values of the mid-nineteenth century, artists responded in their own way by reacting against the mass-produced goods which were made possible by the Industrial Revolution and technological advances. Artists such as William Morris desired a return to simpler times when handmade furniture, for example, was valued for its craftsmanship. Morris despised the mass-produced objects which filled the Victorian home, fearing that traditional crafts such as woodworking and bookbinding would be lost in an era that overlooked the beauty of handmade objects in favor of high quantity. The term "Arts and Crafts," coined in 1888, refers to Morris's revival of traditional crafts, which he considered to be equal to any form of so-called "high art."

Morris argued that in earlier times, such as the Middle Ages (of which he held a decidedly romantic view), art was all around, in everyday life, in the form of beautifully worked tapestries, furniture, and books, which were not just admired as art objects but had a practical function as well.

COMPARE & CONTRAST

- **1800s:** Theatre is one of the most popular forms of mass entertainment. The number of theatres built in England doubles between 1850 and 1860, and on a given night in London alone, 150,000 people attend the theatre.

  Today: While theatre remains an important force in contemporary culture, many more people watch television and films.

- **1800s:** Women in England cannot vote or control their own property until a series of Married Women's Property Acts (1870-1908). Though the first college offering advanced education to women is founded in London in 1848, by the 1890s, women can take degrees at twelve British universities, and study, though not take degrees, at Oxford and Cambridge.

  Today: British women, like their American counterparts, vote, control their own property, and have all the same legal rights as men, including the right to advanced degrees in education.

- **1800s:** During the Victorian period, travel by rail makes business and vacation travel possible. Trains bring city and country closer together, expediting mail service and supplying rural areas with London newspapers and magazines.

  Today: Few people in American travel by rail; most drive cars or fly.

- **1800s:** Britain has a far-flung imperial empire, with colonies around the globe.

  Today: Most of Britain's colonies have achieved their independence, though they continue to be affiliated with the former empire as members of the British Commonwealth.

Another way in which artists reacted against earlier Victorian values was by challenging the view that art had to be didactic or morally instructive. The leading critic of the time, John Ruskin, had earlier written that art's highest purpose was to instruct and enlighten. Ruskin was shocked when he saw a sketchy, impressionistic painting by James Abbot McNeill Whistler which had paint spattered on it; he claimed that Whistler had ''flung a pot of paint in the public's face.'' Whistler sued Ruskin for libel, winning the case and bringing the debate over the purpose of art into the public.

Supporters of Whistler approved of ''art for art's sake,'' meaning that paintings like Whistler's need not have a purpose other than to be aesthetically pleasing. Even if it was pleasing to see paint spattered on the canvas. The public could now decide for themselves what was ''good'' art; they did not need to rely on the views of critics like Ruskin to instruct them in the meaning of a painting.

This new movement in art came to be known as Aestheticism, as art could now be appreciated on purely aesthetic terms. Wilde followed Whistler as the chief spokesperson for the movement, writing and lecturing on the beauty of art for art's sake and became known for his own desire to have life imitate art, not the other way around. Aesthetes such as Wilde were mocked in the popular British magazine *Punch* as foppish, unrealistic individuals who strove to live up to the beauty of their home furnishings.

CRITICAL OVERVIEW

Two major issues predominate much of *The Importance of Being Earnest*'s criticism. First, while audiences from the play's opening have warmly received it, Wilde's contemporaries questioned its seeming amorality. Playwright George Bernard Shaw (*Major Barbara*), after seeing the original London production, attacked the play's ''real degeneracy'' in an article reprinted in *Oscar Wilde: A Collection of Critical Essays.* Shaw described Wilde's repartee as ''hateful'' and ''sinister.'' A second and related concern arises about *Earnest*'s dramatic structure, which exhibits elements of the farce, comedy of manners, and parody. Critics often disagree as to how the play should be categorized.

On the play's morality, critical opinion remains divided. In his book *Oscar Wilde,* Edouard Roditi, for example, believed that Wilde's comedy never rises above ''the incomplete or the trivial.'' Because none of the characters see through the others or critique their values, Roditi believed the play lacks an ethical point of view. Eric Bentley, in *The Playwright As Thinker,* raised similar issues, concluding that because of its ''ridiculous action,'' the play fails to ''break . . . into bitter criticism'' of serious issues.

For Otto Reinert, writing in *College English,* Wilde's comedy results in ''an exposure both of hypocrisy and of the unnatural convention that necessitates hypocrisy.'' As a consequence, ''bunburying,'' the reliance on white lies that keeps polite society polite, ''gives the plot moral significance.'' For example, when Lady Bracknell criticizes Algernon for caring for his imaginary friend, Bunbury, who should decide ''whether he was going to live or to die,'' she voices the conventional belief that ''illness in others is always faked [and] . . . consequently sympathy with invalids is faked also.''

Though Lady Bracknell respects convention, Reinert wrote, ''she has no illusions about the reality her professed convention is supposed to conceal.'' She assumes that both Algernon and Bunbury are ''bunburying,'' and her behavior ''exposes the polite cynicism that negates all values save personal convenience and salon decorum.''

Nor is Lady Bracknell immune from her own lapses in earnestness. Stating her disapproval of mercenary marriages, she admits, ''When I married Lord Bracknell I had no fortune of any kind.'' That is, though she opposes marrying for money, she had no money when she married a wealthy lord. For her, according to Reinert, this position ''is neither cynical nor funny. It represents . . . [a] compromise between practical hardheadedness and conventional morality.''

Overall, the play does not endorse social dishonesty, for while the plot ridicules respectability, ''it also repudiates Bunburyism.'' Wilde's use of ''paradoxical morality'' serves as a critique of ''the problem of manners,'' for ''Bunburying Algernon, in escaping the hypocrisy of convention, becomes a hypocrite himself by pretending to be somebody he is not.'' Wilde sees that Victorian respectability forces people to lead ''double lives, one respectable, one frivolous, neither earnest.''

The second critical issue concerns the play's categorization. Reinert unapologetically describes the play as a farce ''that represents the reality that Victorian convention pretends to ignore.'' The characters themselves are not being ironic, i.e. saying one thing and meaning another. They actually mean what they say. For example, Algernon despairs of attending Lady Bracknell's dinner party because she will sit him beside ''Mary Farquhar, who always flirts with her own husband.'' As Reinert wrote, ''Algernon is indignant with a woman who spoils the fun of extramarital flirtation and who parades her virtue. He is shocked at convention. And his tone implies that he is elevating break of convention into a moral norm,'' that is, making the unconventional conventional.

Characters like Algernon, who resemble those in works by Alexander Pope (*The Rape of the Lock*) and Jonathan Swift (*Gulliver's Travels*), ''derive their ideals for conduct from the actual practice of their societies, their standards are the standards of common corruption, they are literal-minded victims of their environments, realists with a vengeance.''

For Richard Foster, writing in *College English,* Wilde's comedy works through parody, by transforming ''stock comedic techniques, plot devices, and characters.'' Foster defended the play against charges that it is merely farce, because farce ''depends for its effects upon extremely simplified characters tangling themselves up in incongruous situations,'' as in Shakespeare's *The Comedy of Errors* or Goldsmith's *She Stoops to Conquer.* Instead, ''the comedy of *Earnest* subsists, for the most part, not in action or situation but in dialogue'' which is too witty and intellectual ''to be described simply as a farce.''

Nor is *Earnest* actually a comedy of manners, according to Foster, though it does use verbal wit to expose and ridicule ''the vanities, the hypocrisies, and the idleness of the upper classes.'' After all, a

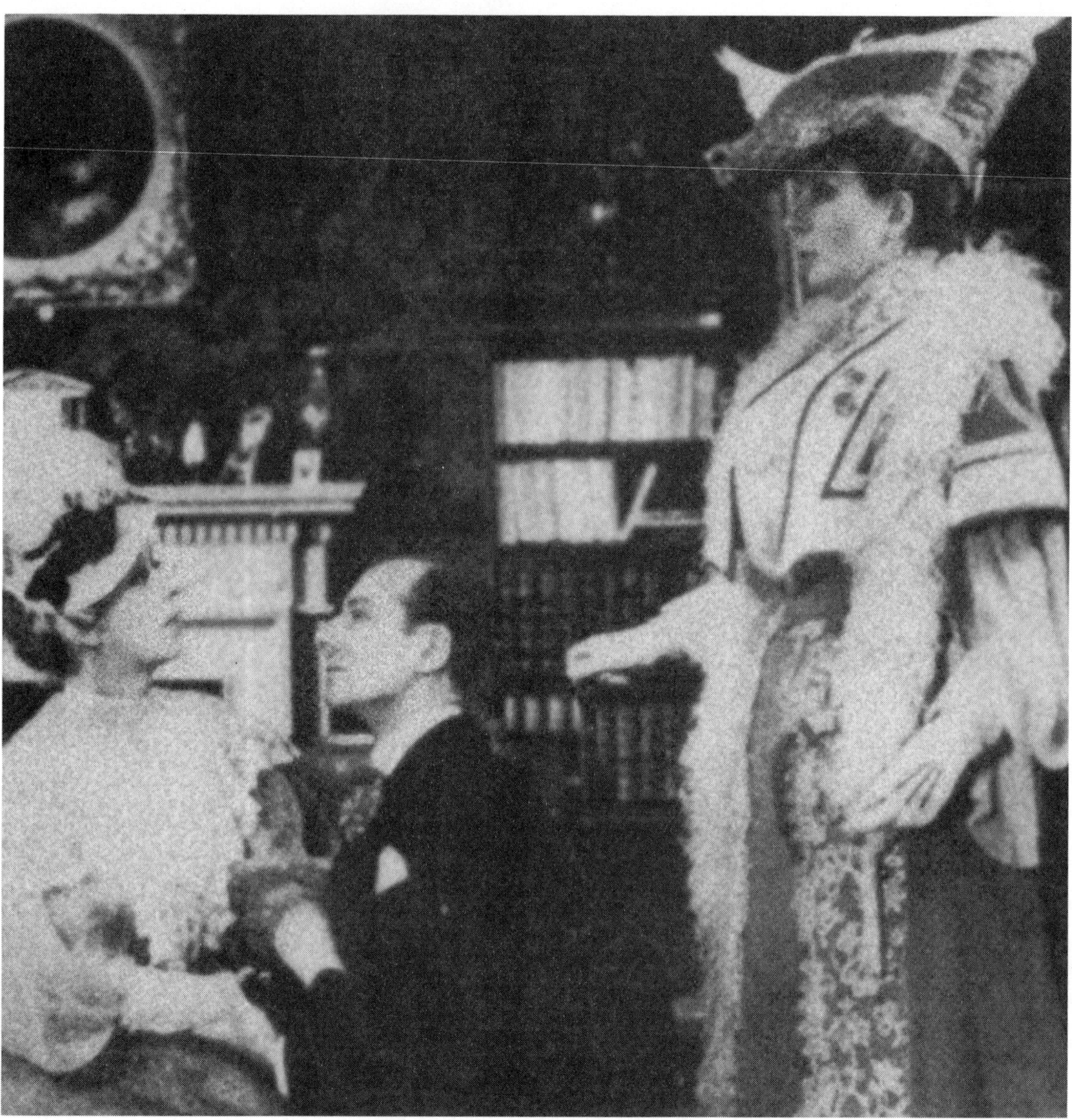

John Worthing (John Gielgud, who also directed the production) woos the hand of Gwendolen (Gwen Frangeon-Davies) as Lady Bracknell (Edith Evans) observes. This production of The Importance of Being Earnest *was staged at the Globe Theatre in 1939*

''comedy of manners is fundamentally realistic,'' requiring the audience to see the stage world as real or possible, if exaggerated. To assist in this recognition, some characters and the audience recognize the fools. In a comedy of manners, folly is recognized by some characters and the audience, while in *Earnest,* according to Rosemary Pountney in *The International Dictionary of Theatre,* Wilde creates ''a world of deliberately reversed values'' in which the wicked are charming and the good, boring.

Rather than a farce or comedy of manners, then, Foster saw Wilde using familiar plot devices and characters to satirize Victorian society. Jack's relationship with Gwendolen evidences a stock problem of lovers prevented from marriage by class differences. Wilde's solution: establishing the true patrimony of Jack, the railway station infant. Another commonplace of romantic literature is love at first sight, but in *Earnest,* Cecily has fallen in love with Algernon before first sight, solely because she believes his name to be Earnest. And while Algernon is cynical, there is evidence that his cynicism is superficial, for immediately on meeting Cecily, "Algernon is engaged to be married and reconciled to getting christened."

Cecily, seemingly sheltered and innocent, suggests it would be hypocritical for Algernon to actually be good while presenting to be wicked. "The moral of Wilde's parody: the rake is a fake, girlish innocence is the bait of a monstrous mantrap, the wages of sin in matrimony." What some critics identify as dramatic problems, then, are perceived by others as the play's strengths. "Nothing in the play," wrote Foster, "is quite what it seems. . . . The play's 'flaws'—the contrivances of plot, the convenience of its coincidences, and the neatness of its resolution—are," according to Foster, "of course, its whole point."

CRITICISM

Arnold Schmidt

Schmidt holds a Ph.D. from Vanderbilt University and specializes in literature and drama. In this essay, he examines Wilde's play in the context of Victorian concepts of "earnestness."

To modern theatre audiences, the title of Oscar Wilde's most popular play, *The Importance of Being Earnest,* seems a clever play on words. After all, the plot hinges on the telling of little—and not so little—white lies, while the title suggests that honesty (earnestness) will be the rule of the day. The title also implies a connection between the name and the concept, between a person named Earnest and that person being earnest. The narrative action does not bear out this assumption but rather its opposite. Audiences who saw the play when it opened in London in 1895 would have brought to it more complex associations with "earnestness," a word which historians, sociologists, and literary critics alike see as, at least in part, typifying the Victorian mindset.

The word "earnest" has three related meanings: to be eager or zealous; to be sincere, serious, and determined; and to be important, not trivial. During Queen Victoria's more than half-century reign, tremendous economic, social, and political changes rocked Great Britain. These were caused by earnest actions and their consequences required, indeed demanded, earnest responses. The Agricultural Revolution dislocated rural populations, forcing people to leave the countryside for cities. There, those people became workers in the factories created by the Industrial Revolution. While, over the long term, the British nation as a whole benefited from these changes, individuals often suffered greatly.

Even the wealthy were not immune to the changing economy's negative impact on land values. In *The Importance of Being Earnest,* this becomes clear when Lady Bracknell inquires into the finances of Jack Worthing, Gwendolen's choice for a husband. When Jack indicates that he has suitable income, she is pleased it comes from stock rather than land, for the declining value of "land . . . gives one position, and prevents one from keeping it up."

By the mid-nineteenth century, discussions concerning issues of economic disparity came to be known as the "two Englands" debate. People considered what would happen to Britain if economic trends continued to enrich the few while the majority of the population worked long hours in dangerous factories, underpaid and living in squalor.

Writers and intellectuals as well as evangelicals and politicians earnestly engaged in this debate. Poets and novelists such as Elizabeth Barrett, Charles Dickens, and Elizabeth Gaskell, created literary works which portrayed the lives of the underprivileged. Writings such as these ultimately contributed to changing public attitudes—and more importantly—public policy toward practices like child labor and public executions. Reforms in hospitals and orphanages, prisons and workhouses, schools and factories can all be traced to debates initiated or fueled by writers. The earnestness of all these reformers—artistic, intellectual, religious, and political—improved the quality of the life in Victorian Britain.

Earnestness did not characterize only those who addressed social evils, however, but also those whose activities created social problems in the first place. The farmers, investors, and manufacturers whose actions dislocated rural populations and resulted in the squalor of factory towns like Manchester, were also "earnest" about their actions. They believed they were improving the quality of peoples' lives and, in some ways, they were.

Overall, the country produced more abundant, cheaper food and better quality, affordable mass produced goods like clothing. Indeed, historian Asa

- William Congreve's comedy *The Way of the World* (1700), like *The Importance of Being Earnest,* features romance, mix-ups, and high comedy, though of a broader and bawdier variety.
- Wilde's novel *The Portrait of Dorian Gray* has elements of gothicism and melodrama. It tells the story of a corrupt young man who never ages, instead, his portrait ages as he should.
- Noel Coward's plays *Private Lives* (1930) and *Blithe Spirit* (1941) have much of the polish and wit of Wilde's writing. Coward was particularly noted for his skill with the comedy of manners.

Briggs termed the middle of the nineteenth century ''The Age of Improvement'' (a phrase he employed as the title of his book on the subject), because of the rising living conditions but also because of the concern to improve the quality of life, to ensure that each generation lived better than the last.

Like British farmers and industrialists, British colonial administrators also justified the nation's imperial ambitions because they ''improved'' the lives of ''uncivilized'' peoples, giving them Christianity, British cultural values, and higher living standards. This attitude came to be know as, in author Rudyard Kipling's words, ''the white man's burden.''

Many of those enriching themselves in this way would acknowledge that their actions caused suffering as well as benefits. They justified their actions based on the utilitarianism of thinkers like John Stewart Mill. Utilitarians determine the rightness of an action by asking if certain actions produce the most good for the most people. If people in general benefited, the suffering of a few specific people could be tolerated as the price paid for progress. While this approach may seem callous and self-serving, these thinkers and tycoons were also ''earnest'' in their actions.

Yet the characters in Wilde's play are not earnest in this sense. Their actions satirize popular notions of the idle rich but also poke fun at Utilitarianism as well. When Jack admits to Lady Bracknell that he smokes, she replies that ''a man should have an occupation.'' Later, Algernon admits that he doesn't ''mind hard work where there is no definite object of any kind.'' Jack and Algernon have no real occupations or professions; their purposelessness critiques the ''earnest'' nature of Utilitarian activities.

Now we can see that Wilde's use of ''earnestness'' is more complex than it may first appear to modern audiences. Indeed, his play offers rather biting, if understated, criticism of the institutions and values that had, by the end of the nineteenth century, made Britain the world's greatest colonial power. Ironically, it is exactly the earnestness exhibited by Britain's exploitative class, industrial, and colonial systems that enables the life of leisure enjoyed by the play's main characters. When asked about his politics, Jack replies, ''Well, I am afraid I really have none,'' though the Liberal Unionist party with which he identifies supports the continued colonial status of Ireland.

Britain's colonial system comes up again when Algernon jokes about sending Jack to Australia, emigration then being a common way to prevent excess population from causing unemployment and lower wages. Investment in stocks—the source of Jack's wealth—provided economic support for Britain's expanding economy, and by the play's end, we learn that his father served as a general in colonial India, a common road to personal enrichment during the Victorian age.

The rich are not the only targets of Wilde's wit, for the playwright satirizes earnestness and reformers of all kinds, in morality, education, women's rights, and marriage.

Reformers religious and secular alike expended much energy on improving the morals of the working classes, particularly in regard to family life, procreation, and child-rearing. In this regard reformers often emphasized the importance of the positive example to be set by upper class behavior. The servant Lane tells Algernon he had "only been married once. That was in consequence of a misunderstanding between myself and a young person." Algernon turns the reformers' ideas on their heads, observing "Lane's views on marriage seem somewhat lax. Really if the lower orders don't set us a good example, what on earth is the use of them." The comedy comes by satirizing the serious ideas of earnest critics of the class system (particularly communist thinkers such as Karl Marx), who wondered exactly what the purpose of the wealthy might be. Finally, Miss Prism's conversation about christening the poor reveals an underlying anxiety about the sexuality and population growth of the working classes.

Earnest reformers engaged in the public debate about education, which expected to "improve" the middle and working classes and enhance the "culture," as Matthew Arnold wrote, of the country in general. One forum for popular education, begun during the eighteenth century, was public lectures, and Wilde satirizes the earnest, if misdirected, efforts of educational societies whose talks have titles like "Society for the Prevention of Discontent among the Upper Orders" and a "Lecture by the University Extension Scheme on the Influence of a Permanent Income on Thought."

Wilde also satirizes the ineffectiveness of the education for the privileged in the scenes between Miss Prism and her reluctant student Cecily. More generally, though, Lady Bracknell proclaims: "The whole theory of modern education is radically unsound. Fortunately in England, at any rate, education produces no effect whatsoever. If it did, it would prove a serious danger to the upper classes and probably lead to acts of violence." Lady Bracknell links education of the poor with social unrest, fearing that the educated masses might forget their place and reject hierarchical class structure.

The independence and audacity of Wilde's female characters reflects the changing status of Victorian women, part of a public debate known as "The Women Question." It was only with the passage of a series of Married Women's Property Acts (1870-1908) that women could hold property in their own names. The opinions of Queen Victoria herself, who opposed women's suffrage but advocated women's education, including college, exemplified the ambiguous situation of women in England during this period.

"TO MANY, WILDE'S *THE IMPORTANCE OF BEING EARNEST* MAY SEEM A WORK OF 'SURFACE' AND 'STYLE,' BUT FURTHER EXAMINATION SHOWS IT TO HAVE DEPTH AND SUBSTANCE AS WELL AS HUMOR."

Cecily and Gwendolen discuss changing gender roles in their conversation about male domesticity, indicating their belief that "home seems to me to be the proper sphere for the man." Marriage, however, remained most women's primary goal and occupation. Arranged marriages had been on the decline since the late-eighteenth century but were not unknown among the Victorian era's upper classes. This may have made economic sense, but it did not always create domestic harmony. Consider Algernon's lament about the low quality of champagne in the homes of married men and his belief in the necessity of adultery, "for in marriage, three is company and two is none." Both comments highlight the lack of companionship resulting from marriage without compatibility and love, suggesting that the Victorian husband requires alcohol and a mistress to be happy.

Wilde describes the situation for married women in equally depressing terms. When Lady Bracknell tells of her visit with the recently widowed Lady Harbury, Algernon remarks that he's heard that "her hair has turned quite gold from grief." The audience anticipates the cliched response, that her hair turned gray or white from sorrow, but Wilde turns the phrase around.

Why might her hair have turned gold instead? Like many Victorian women, Lady Harbury seems to have been trapped in a loveless marriage, the kind Lady Bracknell proposes to arrange for Gwendolen. Now that Lady Harbury's husband is dead, she is finally free to become who and do what she wants. She feels younger, more attractive and changes her hair color. While the joke requires that we associate aging and grief, Wilde turns that around, associating widowhood instead with gold hair and joy. Algernon's statement could also be an indication of the new wealth and independence Lady Harbury gained in inheriting her husband's money. The simple turn of a phrase communicates a complex reality, in this case, about economic, social, and sexual politics.

The status of the nineteenth century's educated women remained grim, however, with few occupational outlets other than teaching. Miss Prism, Cecily's governess, combines two common female occupations, teaching and novel writing, another activity at which women flourished (and for which they were criticized). Prism's confusion between a baby and a manuscript pokes fun at changing ideas about parenthood and child-rearing. The misplaced baby symbolizes what critics saw as a confusion of gender roles, when women entered the traditionally masculine world of the mind. The plight of orphaned baby Jack illustrates the destabilization of family ties, which in his case are sequentially lost, invented, changed, and discovered.

As Lady Bracknell says, ''we live, I regret to say, in an age of surfaces,'' a position echoed by her daughter's comment that ''in matters of grave importance, style, not sincerity is the vital thing.'' To many, Wilde's *The Importance of Being Earnest* may seem a work of ''surface'' and ''style,'' but further examination shows it to have depth and substance as well as humor.

Source: Arnold Schmidt, for *Drama for Students,* Gale, 1998.

Brooks Atkinson

In a review that was originally published on March 4, 1947, Atkinson offers words of praise for a production of Wilde's play starring John Geilgud.

Owing to unavoidable circumstances, this department cannot solemnly swear that John Gielgud's performance of *The Importance of Being Earnest* is immeasurably superior to the original performance in 1895. Even Mr. Gielgud, wise though he is, cannot know that from personal observation. But traditions grow slowly, and it is highly unlikely that the original actors blessed Oscar Wilde's comedy with the knowing perfection that Mr. Gielgud and his colleagues are bestowing on it.

Having played *The Importance* triumphantly in London, Mr. Gielgud has now brought it across the Atlantic with no appreciable seachange—not, let it be said, with the entire original cast, but with superb players of artificial comedy, and they all set it meticulously on the stage of the Royale last evening. By the accuracy and uniformity of their style in acting, directing and setting they transmute a somewhat mechanical comedy into a theatre masterpiece.

Even when it was new, to judge by the records, ''The Importance of Being Earnest'' seemed mechanically contrived in plot and dialogue. It was a bit like Gilbert without the Sullivan music. Especially in the central parts of the second act the brilliance of the wit today shines with an effort as though Wilde were puffing a little.

That might be a point worth dwelling upon in a performance less stylized than Mr. Gielgud's. But he has approached it as if it were a score to be played for its own sake as artificial comedy without laying emphasis on the plot and without speaking the lines like jokes or deliberate rejoinders. Absurdly self-conscious, dry and arrogant, Mr. Gielgud and his associates are marvelously entertaining. In the purest meaning of the word they are ''playing'' Oscar Wilde. Nothing here is seriously intended except the manner of the comedy.

Notice how all the actors hold their heads high as though they were elevating themselves above vulgarity. Notice how they greet each other with dainty touches of the fingers, avoiding at all costs the heartiness of a handshake. The lines of dialogue are written elaborately; each word is carefully chosen for its satiric value; by modern standards, some of the lines are long. But notice how disdainfully these actors speak them. Instead of hammering away at the jokes, they speak dryly in an insufferable fashion, as perhaps Oscar Wilde spoke when he, too, had a large, admiring audience at some fashionable reception.

As John Worthing, who has invented a dissolute brother, Mr. Gielgud plays with an ascetic arrogance that is enormously witty quite apart from the dialogue. No play could ever match the sustained perfection of his stylized acting. But this is no exercise in star-casting. For Mr. Gielgud has surrounded himself with actors who have mastered the same attitudes. As the overbearing Lady Bracknell,

Margaret Rutherford is tremendously skillful—the speaking, the walking and the wearing of costumes all gathered up into one impression of insufferability.

Pamela Brown plays Gwendolen with the same icy condescension. As the more rustic Cecily, Jane Baxter is lovely and full of merriment in a more humane style. Jean Cadell is playing the spinster Schoolma'm with an acidulously sweet and nervous virtue. Robert Flemyng's Algernon Moncrieff is an excellent foil for Mr. Gielgud's John Worthing. Without rubbing the edge off the style, Mr. Moncrieff gets a dash of well-bred revelry into his acting. As the bachelor's servant, Richard Wordsworth is also immensely expert; and John Kidd is delightfully dull and fatuous as the rector.

Especially for the two interiors Motley's settings are models of period decor; they can be played against without staring the acting out of countenance or overwhelming the performance with color. The costumes, which presumably Motley has also designed, convey the character of the parts and the satire of the comedy without sacrificing beauty. What Motley has accomplished completes Mr. Gielgud's design for artificial comedy. Like the play, it is inhuman. It sacrifices personality to style—detached, egotistical, condescending, arid, satirical and marvelously enjoyable.

Source: Brooks Atkinson, review of *The Importance of Being Earnest* (1947) in *On Stage: Selected Theater Reviews from the New York Times, 1920–70,* edited by Bernard Beckerman and Howard Siegman, Arno Press, 1973, p. 277.

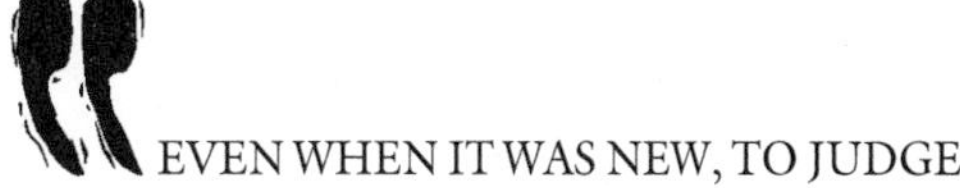

EVEN WHEN IT WAS NEW, TO JUDGE BY THE RECORDS, *THE IMPORTANCE OF BEING EARNEST* SEEMED MECHANICALLY CONTRIVED IN PLOT AND DIALOGUE. IT WAS A BIT LIKE GILBERT WITHOUT THE SULLIVAN MUSIC."

Max Beerbohm

In this chapter from his book, Beerbohm appraises The Importance of Being Earnest, *finding it to be that rare play that stands the test of time and continues to appeal to audiences of numerous generations.*

Of a play representing actual life there can be, I think, no test more severe than its revival after seven or eight years of abeyance. For that period is enough to make it untrue to the surface of the present, yet not enough to enable us to unswitch it from the present. How seldom is the test passed! There is a better chance, naturally, for plays that weave life into fantastic forms; but even for them not a very good chance; for the fashion in fantasy itself changes. Fashions form a cycle, and we, steadily moving in that cycle, are farther from whatever fashion we have just passed than from any other. The things which once pleased our grandfathers are tolerable in comparison with the things which once pleased us. If in the lumber of the latter we find something that still pleases us, pleases us as much as ever it did, then, surely, we may preen ourselves on the possession of a classic, and congratulate posterity. Last week, at the St. James', was revived "The Importance of Being Earnest," after an abeyance of exactly seven years—those seven years which, according to scientists, change every molecule in the human body, leaving nothing of what was there before. And yet to me the play came out fresh and exquisite as ever, and over the whole house almost every line was sending ripples of laughter—cumulative ripples that became waves, and receded only for fear of drowning the next line. In kind the play always was unlike any other, and in its kind it still seems perfect. I do not wonder that now the critics boldly call it a classic, and predict immortality. And (timorous though I am apt to be in prophecy) I join gladly in their chorus.

A classic must be guarded jealously. Nothing should be added to, or detracted from, a classic. In the revival at the St. James', I noted several faults of textual omission. When Lady Bracknell is told by Mr. Worthing that he was originally found in a handbag in the cloak room of Victoria Station, she echoes "The cloak-room at Victoria Station?" "Yes," he replies; "the Brighton Line." "The line is immaterial," she rejoins; "Mr. Worthing, I confess I am somewhat bewildered," &c. &c. Now, in the present revival "the line is immaterial" is omitted. Perhaps Mr. Alexander regarded it as an

> "*THE IMPORTANCE OF BEING EARNEST* ALWAYS WAS UNLIKE ANY OTHER, AND IN ITS KIND IT STILL SEEMS PERFECT. I DO NOT WONDER THAT NOW THE CRITICS BOLDLY CALL IT A CLASSIC, AND PREDICT IMMORTALITY."

immaterial line. So it is, as far as the plot is concerned. But it is not the less deliciously funny. To skip it is inexcusable. Again, Mr. Wilde was a master in selection of words, and his words must not be amended. ''Cecily,'' says Miss Prism, ''you will read your Political Economy in my absence. The chapter on the Fall of the Rupee you may omit. It is somewhat too sensational.'' For ''sensational'' Miss Laverton substitutes ''exciting''—a very poor substitute for that mot juste. Thus may the edge of magnificent absurdity be blunted. In the last act, again, Miss Laverton killed a vital point by inaccuracy. In the whole play there is no more delicious speech than Miss Prism's rhapsody over the restored hand-bag. This is a speech quintessential of the whole play's spirit. ''It seems to be mine,'' says Miss Prism calmly. ''Yes here is the injury it received through the upsetting of a Gower Street omnibus in younger and happier days. There is the stain on the lining caused by the explosion of a temperance beverage—an incident that occurred at Leamington. And here, on the lock, are my initials. I had forgotten that in an extravagant moment I had had them placed there. The bag is undoubtedly mine. I am delighted to have it so unexpectedly restored to me. It has been a great inconvenience being without it all these years.'' The overturning of a Gower Street omnibus in younger and happier days! Miss Laverton omitted ''and happier''. What a point to miss! Moreover, she gabbled the whole speech, paying no heed to those well-balanced cadences whose dignity contributes so much to the fun—without whose dignity, indeed, the fun evaporates. In such a play as this good acting is peculiarly important. It is, also, peculiarly difficult to obtain. The play is unique in kind, and thus most of the mimes, having trained themselves for ordinary purposes, are bewildered in approaching it.

Before we try to define how it should be acted, let us try to define its character. In scheme, of course, it is a hackneyed farce—the story of a young man coming up to London ''on the spree,'' and of another young man going down conversely to the country, and of the complications that ensue. In treatment, also, it is farcical, in so far as some of the fun depends on absurd ''situations,'' ''stage-business,'' and so forth. Thus one might assume that the best way to act it would be to rattle through it. That were a gross error. For, despite the scheme of the play, the fun depends mainly on what the characters say, rather than on what they do. They speak a kind of beautiful nonsense—the language of high comedy, twisted into fantasy. Throughout the dialogue is the horse-play of a distinguished intellect and a distinguished imagination—a horse-play among words and ideas, conducted with poetic dignity. What differentiates this farce from any other, and makes it funnier than any other, is the humorous contrast between its style and matter. To preserve its style fully, the dialogue must be spoken with grave unction. The sound and the sense of the words must be taken seriously, treated beautifully. If mimes rattle through the play and anyhow, they manage to obscure much of its style, and much, therefore, of its fun. They lower it towards the plane of ordinary farce. This was what the mimes of the St. James' were doing on the first night. The play triumphed not by their help but in their despite. I must except Miss Lilian Braithwaite, who acted in precisely the right key of grace and dignity. She alone, in seeming to take her part quite seriously, showed that she had realised the full extent of its fun. Miss Margaret Halstan acted prettily, but in the direction of burlesque. By displaying a sense of humour she betrayed its limitations. Mr. Lyall Swete played the part of Doctor Chasuble as though it were a minutely realistic character study of a typical country clergyman. Instead of taking the part seriously for what it is, he tried to make it a serious part. He slurred over all the majestic utterances of the Canon, as though he feared that if he spoke them with proper unction he would be accused of forgetting that he was no longer in the Benson Company. I sighed for Mr. Henry Kemble, who ''created'' the part. I sighed, also, for the late Miss Rose Leclerq, who ''created'' the part of Lady Bracknell. Miss M. Talbot plays it in the conventional stage-dowager fashion. Miss Leclerq but no! I will not sink without a struggle into that period when a man begins to bore young people by raving to them about the mimes whom they never saw. Both Mr. George Alexander and Mr. Graham Browne rattled through their parts. Even in the second act, when not only the situation, but also the necessity for letting the audience realise the situation, demands that John Worthing should make the slowest of entries, Mr. Alexander came bustling on at break-neck speed. I wish he would reconsider his theory of the play, call some rehearsals, and have his curtain rung up not at 8.45 but at 8.15. He may argue that this would not be worth his while, as "Paolo and Francesca" is to be produced so soon. I hope he is not going to have "Paolo and Francesca" rattled through. The effect on it would be quite as bad as on *The Importance of Being Earnest*—though not, I assure him, worse.

Source: Max Beerbohm, review of *The Importance of Being Earnest* in his *Around Theatres Volume 1,* Knopf, 1930, pp. 240–43.

SOURCES

Beckson, Karl. "Oscar Wilde" in *Concise Dictionary of British Literary Biography,* Volume 4: *Victorian Writers, 1832-1890,* Gale, 1991, pp. 340-55.

Bentley, Eric. *The Playwright As Thinker,* Reynal & Hitchcock, 1946.

Foster, Richard. "Wilde As Parodist: A Second Look at 'The Importance of Being Earnest'" in *College English,* Vol. 18, no. 1, October, 1956, pp. 18-23.

Pountney, Rosemary. "The Importance of Being Earnest" in *The International Dictionary of Theatre,* Volume 1: *Plays,* edited by Mark Hawkins-Dady, St. James Press, 1992.

Reinert, Otto. "Satiric Strategy in 'The Importance of Being Earnest'" in *College English,* Vol. 18, no. 1, October, 1956, pp. 14-18.

Roditi, Edourd. *Oscar Wilde,* New Directions, 1986.

FURTHER READING

Beckson, Karl, Editor. *Oscar Wilde: The Critical Heritage,* Routlege, 1970.

Focusing on the years 1881 to 1927, this book offers particular insight into Wilde's theatrical writings.

Briggs, Asa. *The Age of Improvement,* Longman, 1988.

A readable, comprehensive history of the mid-Victorian years in England. Useful for understanding the nineteenth century generally, including social history.

Ellmann, Richard. *Oscar Wilde,* 1988.

This is the standard literary biography of Wilde, providing a wealth of detail about his personal life as well as insight into the composition of his works.

Ellmann, Richard, Editor. *Oscar Wilde: A Collection of Critical Essays,* Prentice-Hall, 1969.

Most helpful for exploring the thinking about Wilde by his contemporaries such as W. B. Yeats and George Bernard Shaw.

Hobsbawm, Eric.*The Age of Capital, 1848-1875,* McKay, 1975.

Although this history concentrates on the middle of the nineteenth century, Hobsbawm usefully situates the roots of social trends that would influence British society in the 1890s.

Holland, Vyvyan B. *Oscar Wilde: A Pictorial Biography,* Viking, 1961.

Holland is Wilde's son. While this book contains a brief biography, the highlights are the fine photographs of Wilde and many of the people in his life, public and private.

Iphigenia in Taurus

EURIPIDES

c. 414 B.C.

To a modern audience, there is very little dramatic intensity in *Iphigenia in Taurus.* Those who hunger for action, deep emotion, or sharp irony may find this straightforward play ''boring.'' *Iphigenia in Taurus* seems a strange combination of tragedy and romance because although tragic conditions precede the events of the play and tragic events *nearly* happen, no one dies or ends in misfortune in this play. The misfortunes plaguing both Orestes and Iphigenia already exist before the play begins and by the end they are freed of their problems with little effort. The characters talk about past or potential traumas, then neatly dismiss or avoid them. All of the dangerous action occurs offstage or outside of the events of the play itself. Thus, in addition to its traditional classification as a tragedy, *Iphigenia in Taurus* has been called a ''romantic melodrama.''

But the play does meet Artistotle's definition of a work that releases pity and fear through exciting and then resolving these emotions (as a tragedy should). The prolonged scene wherein Orestes and Pylades refuse to reveal their identities to Iphigenia and she fails to reveal her own, allows a build up of pity and fear that are released when Iphigenia pronounces her brother's name. This moment of recognition constitutes one element that Aristotle considered key to tragedy: a reversal of situation and recognition.

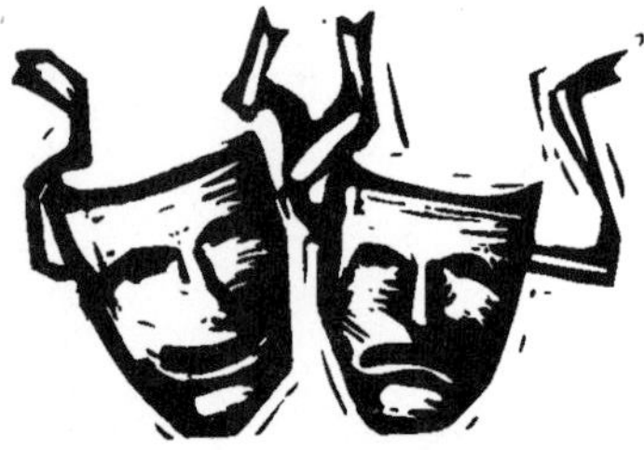

Iphigenia in Taurus lacks the heightened sense of drama often associated with tragedies, yet it is not unworthy of study, for it opens up a window to the ancient Hellenic mind, which enjoyed the quiet contemplation of the ironies of expectation versus fulfillment. It is a play that explores the mirror image of what is commonly called tragedy: not the descent of a tragic figure but the rise from tragic fate by characters who sidestep human sacrifice and still achieve ritual purification. In that respect, *Iphigenia in Taurus* is a kind of ancient Greek "escape" literature.

AUTHOR BIOGRAPHY

As far as historians can tell, Euripides was born in the Greek city-state of Athens around 484 B.C. to parents affluent enough to provide their son a good education and a library of philosophical works. He received training in athletics and won prizes in athletic competitions. Euripides also served briefly in the army, an obligation of Athenian youths. He then became a scholar and moved among the rich intellectual environment of the Sophist thinkers, although he always maintained his independence from them. Euripides knew the philosopher Anaxagoras, who speculated that energy from tiny "atoms" of matter drove the universe, not the gods; he socialized with the Sophist Protagoras, who ostensibly read his radical treatise, *Concerning the Gods* in Euripides's home; and he was a friend and contemporary of the great playwright Socrates (*Electra*), who frequently attended his plays.

While such a life seems rich and fulfilling, Euripides's halcyon pleasures did not last: during his life the philosophical mood of Athens swung from free-thinking optimism to a kind of fascist conservatism, wherein Anaxagoras barely escaped with his life, Protagoras died trying to escape, and Socrates was executed a few years after Euripides's death. Politically, Athens underwent a number of major changes as well. When Euripides was in his early twenties, the democrats, led by Pericles, seized power in a bloody coup. Pericles's rule would usher in the Golden Age of Athens, but this period would meet its cataclysmic demise at the end of the Peloponnesian Wars, which coincided with the final years of Euripides's life.

These extremes of political and philosophical moods contributed to the pessimism and uncertainty of Euripides's dramatic tragedies. In his lifetime Euripides won few prizes for his work (only four wins at the Dionysia play festival compared to Sophocles's twenty-four). Perhaps this lack of recognition led the aging Euripides to withdraw from the world to live in a cave on Salamis. At the advanced age of seventy, he left his beloved Athens, which was collapsing in the final throes of the Peloponnesian Wars, for Macedonia, to help the Macedonian king establish a cultural center there to rival Athens. He died there in 406 B. C.

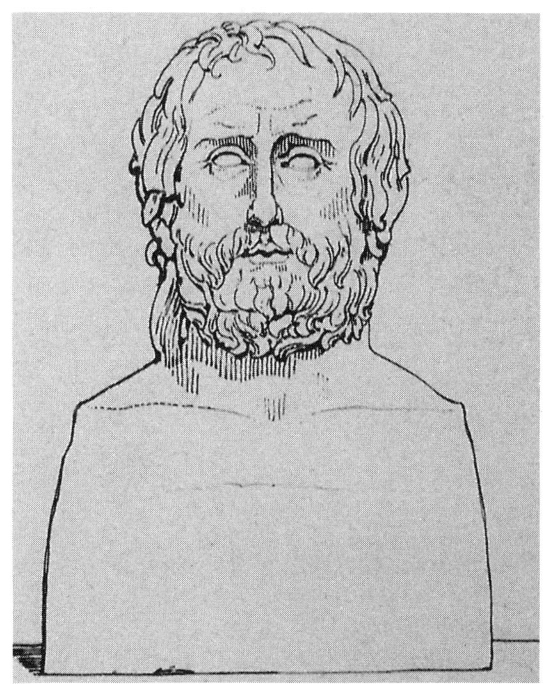

A bust of Euripides

There are historical references to ninety plays by Euripides; of these, only nineteen have survived to the modern era, although eighty of the titles are known. The best-known of Euripides's work include *Medea* (431 B.C.), *Iphigenia in Taurus* (c. 414 B.C.), *Orestes* (408 B.C.), and *Bacchae* (produced posthumously, c. 406 B.C.). After Euripides's death, his plays were carried from Athens to Alexandria, then to Rome, and finally to the Byzantine Empire. One measure of his renown is that Aristophanes dedicated three plays to burlesquing him. The extant versions of Euripides's plays probably stem from Byzantine texts. Over the ages, the original plays were most likely corrupted as they were copied and recopied and as various performers embellished the scripts, yet the unique essence of Euripides's style has survived.

The playwright's characters have more psychological depth than those of his dramatic predecessors, Aeschylus and Sophocles. Euripides broke with traditional Greek theater in his examinations of realistic humans and *their* motivations—as opposed to characters manipulated by the will of the gods. He also challenged preconceptions regarding plot, heroes and heroines, and use of stock characters, yet he mostly confined himself to the form and structure of traditional tragedies. He explored the plight of women in seven plays and he challenged religious thought through his radical ideas about the gods and society. Some called Euripides an atheist, but he did not reject religion—he merely had the courage to challenge and denounce its shortcomings.

PLOT SUMMARY

Act I

Iphigenia in Taurus takes place in a temple to the goddess Artemis along the shore of Taurus. It opens with a prologue spoken by one of the main characters, Iphigenia. In Euripidean prologues, the events preceding the story are recounted and the upcoming action foretold. Iphigenia explains why she was yet alive after ostensibly being sacrificed by her father, Agamemnon, who offered his child in order to dispel storms preventing his fleet from departing for an important battle.

Artemis, the virgin goddess of childbirth, had once extracted from Agamemnon the promise to sacrifice the loveliest creature born in a twelve-month period. His wife Clytemnestra had borne Iphigenia, and Artemis demanded her blood. Agamemnon contrived a false pretext for stealing his daughter, asking Clytemestra to prepare the child to wed Achilles. But once on the altar of sacrifice, Artemis snatched the young maiden away, placing a deer in her place to fool the humans. Artemis magically transported Iphigenia to Taurus, a ''barbarian'' land and made her a priestess in her temple. Ironically, Iphigenia often prepares her fellow Hellenes for sacrifice upon the shrine.

Iphigenia further relates a strange dream she had the previous night, in which an earthquake crumbled her father's house and left only one column standing. This column wore brown hair and Iphigenia weeped over it and prepared it for the deadly ritual of Artemis's temple. Iphigenia interprets her dream to mean that her brother, Orestes, has died and that she cannot properly bury him. She retreats into the temple to pour libations for him.

As she departs, Orestes and his friend Pylades enter from the ocean shore. He and Pylades have been sent by the oracle of Phoebus in retribution for avenging his father's death by killing his mother, Clytemestra (who killed Agamemnon because he sacrificed Iphigenia). Phoebus, the sister of Artemis, has ordered Orestes to steal her statue from Artemis's temple and give it to Athens. Only by this act of courage will Orestes be freed from the furies who have pursued him since he killed his mother. The two friends discuss how they can accomplish their mission and decide to hide in the caves of the sea cliffs until nightfall.

The chorus enters and sings of Artemis's temple and rituals. These are the girls who assist Iphigenia in her ritual preparations, and she shares with them her interpretation of her dream. They echo her mourning chant and then draw her attention to some herdsmen approaching the temple. The herdsmen explain to Iphigenia that while driving their cattle to the seashore to wash them, they saw two young Hellene men in one of the sea caves. They decided to capture the two to sacrifice to Artemis, according to their local custom. Then one of the strangers began to babble like a madman about ''fiends from Hades'' attacking him (this is the work of the furies that torment Orestes). Orestes slays some of the cattle, thinking they are the furies, and the herdsmen respond by stoning the two and taking them as prisoners to the king. The king ordered the prisoners sent to Iphigenia for purification and then sacrifice. Iphigenia commands the men brought before her; the ''loss'' of her brother makes her eager to sacrifice these two strangers.

Iphigenia once again recalls the horror of her aborted sacrifice, this time mentioning poignant details that create empathy with the audience, as she addresses the chorus. She ends by saying she believes the gods could not have caused her pain—that men blame the gods for their own evil actions. The chorus support her prayer to return to her home in Athens. In appraising the two approaching Hellenes, the chorus indirectly reminds the audience that human sacrifice is not allowed by Hellenic law.

Iphigenia has the prisoners unbound while she interrogates them about their identity and the events back in Athens. Out of pride, Orestes refuses to tell his name. He even recounts the story of murdering Clytemestra as though another committed the act and speaks of himself in third person. There are moments when the audience understands the dramatic irony of comments such as Iphigenia's wish that her own brother might be as noble as the man standing before her and Orestes's wish that his sister might be the one to purify him before his sacrifice.

The pair earn Iphigenia's respect, so she devises a plan to let one of them go, as long as he carries a message back to her brother. When she leaves to get the letter, Orestes and Pylades remark on her knowledge of their city. It seems as though they might recognize who she is, but instead Pylades expresses concern that he will be accused of killing Orestes. Iphigenia returns and she and Pylades trade oaths that they will accomplish what they promise. Pylades will go free and deliver the letter.

To assure that Pylades cannot fail by losing the letter, she has him memorize it. It is during the recitation of the letter that the two men recognize Orestes's sister. Orestes turns in joy to Iphigenia, but the chorus accuses him of desecrating her holy robes. Iphigenia demands proof that he truly is his brother and is not merely trying to trick her so that he may go free. When he proves himself, Iphgenia bemoans the crimes she nearly committed.

After Iphigenia explains how it is that she is still alive, the three strategize an escape plan. They cannot kill the king because that would violate the "law of guest and host." Iphigenia devises a plan to pretend that they have desecrated the statue Orestes must steal. She will tell Thoas that she must cleanse it and the two prisoners in the sea. That will allow them to make a run for Orestes's ship. Iphigenia prays to Artemis for help, and the chorus sings encouragement.

King Thoas enters with his guards asking the whereabouts of Iphigenia. She enters with the statue and silences him with the news that "impurity" has violated it. He agrees to honor her desire to purify it, after hearing her say the prisoners are guilty of horrific deeds at home. Her demand for solitude during the purification does not make him suspicious because she asks him to purify the temple with fire while she is busy at the sea. Keeping onlookers away from the unholy statue, she makes her way to the sea with her two "prisoners." The chorus sings the story of Artemis and Phoebus, ending with a story about the unreliability of dream interpretation.

A messenger rushes up to tell King Thoas that the two prisoners have fled in their ship, along with Iphigenia. Despite the trio's successful getaway, the ship is in danger of grounding near shore. Thoas orders horsemen to capture them, but he is stopped by Athena, goddess of reason, who informs the king that Apollo wants Orestes to convey the holy image to Athens. Athena orders the end of human sacrifice and decrees that all accused will be given the benefit of a fair trial in which a majority vote will decide their fate—treatment that Orestes received when he was judged for Clytemnestra's murder. Thoas agrees, and Athena applauds his decision, saying that even the gods must end to Necessity.

CHARACTERS

Athena

The goddess Athena appears at the end of the play to order King Thoas not to pursue the fleeing Hellenes. She represents wisdom and the disciplined aspects (rather than the aggressive aspects) of war, and she announces that human sacrifice will no longer be practiced. She also announces that it will henceforth take a majority of votes to condemn a man for a crime. Finally she blesses the safe return of Orestes, Iphigenia, and Pylades. The goddess supports the interests of the Hellenes, not the Taurians.

Chorus

The chorus consists of female attendants to Iphigenia. These are captured Greek women who occupy a lower social status than Iphigenia. Their choral strophes comment upon and generalize the events of the play, transforming tragic events to moments of lyric beauty.

Herdsman

The herdsman is a messenger who supplies the part of the story concerning the capture of Orestes and Pylades by the Taurians. He is one of the men who discovers and surrounds the two strangers, and his own account of the fight shows the Hellenes better warriors than the barbarians, who fought with stones.

Iphigenia

Euripides was known for his striking portrayals of female characters, and Iphigenia is no exception, although she lacks the dramatic depth of his Medea and Electra. Iphigenia, haughty and proud, has for twenty years grimly led her countrymen to Artemis's sacrificial altar whenever the barbarian Taurians captured them in their land. Although she longs for her culture, she vehemently hates her countrymen for what they did to her. She loves only her siblings

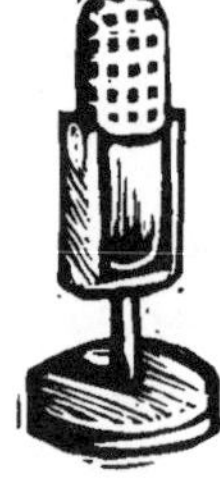

MEDIA ADAPTATIONS

- In 1779, Johann Wolfgang von Goethe created a prose version of *Iphigenia in Tauris* in five acts that closely follows Euripides's plot line.
- In 1779, Christoph Willibald Gluck produced an opera version of the play, called *Iphigenie en Tauride* that is still produced. A recording of the opera is available on compact disk from Phillips.

and laments that she cannot pour libations on Orestes's grave after misinterpreting a dream as an omen that he is dead. Discovering from the stranger Hellenes that he is alive brings her some respite from her misery, which quickly turns to elation when the stranger turns out to be Orestes. Her quick thinking and formidable bearing facilitate their escape. Iphigenia is daring, cool, and passionate.

Messenger

In a long descriptive monologue, this messenger informs Thoas that Iphigenia is not purifying her prisoners but escaping with them. The messenger threatens the chorus of captive Greek temple attendant that they will pay for having protected their mistress.

Orestes

Orestes lives under the curse of the Furies, who torment those who spill the blood of relatives. He has avenged his father's death by murdering his mother and has been acquitted of this crime by an Athenian jury; but he can find no peace until he satisfies the command of Apollo to retrieve the altar statue at the temple of Artemis in Taurus. Orestes is plagued with bouts of madness, caused, perhaps, by the Furies, perhaps by his own sense of guilt. Orestes shares a close friendship with Pylades, his sister Electra's husband. When Iphigenia offers to spare one of them, Orestes insists on sacrificing himself rather than to live at the expense of Pylade's life. Orestes ultimately accomplishes the task assigned him by Apollo and receives Athena's blessing, thus presumably ending his curse.

Pylades

Pylades epitomizes friendship, having accompanied Orestes on his dangerous mission, simply to keep his friend company. Pylades is married to Electra, Orestes's sister. When Iphigenia strikes a bargain to set free one of her prisoners, Pylades at first refuses, wanting to die with his friend. But he submits to Orestes's reasoning: that it is Orestes whom Apollo sent on this mission and that Pylades must not desert his wife.

Thoas

Thoas is king of Taurus. He is a barbarian (barbarian then meaning stranger, not savage) king, in the eyes of the Hellenes. He proves a rather unthreatening enemy to the Hellenes. Although he questions Iphigenia about her disposition of the prisoners, she easily deludes him. He submits to her order to purify the temple with fire while she goes to the ocean to purify the statue and prisoners. When he learns of Iphigenia's trickery, he commands his soldiers to follow the escapees but once again submits to the voice of reason, this time in the form of Athena.

THEMES

Sacrifice

The theme of sacrifice dominates the play *Iphigenia in Taurus.* Sacrifice holds a double bind over Iphigenia, in that she was to be sacrificed by her father as homage to Artemis, and was then ''rescued'' by that goddess, who made Iphigenia serve in her temple, preparing the ritual sacrifice of other Hellenes.

Although human sacrifice was not practiced during the fifth century B.C. in Greece, its symbolic stand-in, animal sacrifice, was integral to Greek religious culture. Animals to be slaughtered were reared with care, promenaded to the altar with dignity, and the sacrifice itself was an occasion of silent solemnity. Only young, beautiful animals were chosen for sacrifice. Their innocence made the offering more valuable and served to intensify the religious experience. Iphigenia was an innocent maiden who thought she was being prepared for a marriage when her father Agamemnon took her to the sacrificial altar. Her innocence would have been a poignant matter to a culture that regularly experienced the sacrifice of innocent creatures. Artemis snatches the young maiden away before she is destroyed.

A reversal of this event nearly happens to Orestes. He thinks he is about to be sacrificed but does not know that his blood relation, Iphigenia, would have led him to the altar, just as their father led Iphigenia. Iphigenia's duty is to prepare victims for sacrifice in the temple of Artemis, and the usual victims are her fellow Hellenes, whom she now passionately hates because of their cold-blooded intent to use her as a means to placate the gods. Thus she holds an office similar to her father's when he set out to sacrifice her. Her position as temple priestess is a tragic irony: she avoided sacrifice only to facilitate sacrificing others.

Interestingly enough, it is her office that enables her to escape her bondage to the Taurians. She has an aura of mystical power because of her priestess station, so she is able to tell Thoas to stay away from her and the defiled prisoners, allowing them space enough to escape. The reason behind both sacrificial necessities is war. Agamemnon chose to sacrifice his young daughter to appease Artemis, who held his ships in bay with a strong wind. The Taurians sacrifice Hellenes because of a current war between the two groups. The theme of sacrifice is further foretold in the dramatic irony that Iphigenia might actually sacrifice her own brother, whose death she thinks her dream has foretold.

Finally, it is under the ruse of preparing for the ritual sacrifice of Orestes and Pylades that Iphigenia and her cohorts escape. The Taurian king, Thoas, trusts this foreign temple priestess who has already killed so many Hellenes on Artemis's altar. Although human sacrifice looms large in this play, it never is actually committed. In each case, though, the question is raised whether this particular person should be sacrificed by the one preparing to do so. The Greeks, who were inclined to generalize from particulars, would see the larger question as whether or not human sacrifice should be committed at all. Athena cleary answers no, when she comes in at the end to explain that sacrificial offerings will henceforth require only a drop of human blood, not a whole human life.

TOPICS FOR FURTHER STUDY

- What political and social issues would have made the topic of human sacrifice pertinent to the fifth-century Athenian audience?
- Does this play corroborate a commonly held belief that the house of Atreus (Agamemnon's family) was unavoidably doomed? Explain your answer.
- What is the effect or role of Orestes's temporary madness upon the rest of the play? Why is this detail included?
- Does this play, in your opinion, effectively meet Artistotle's criteria for a tragedy, meaning that it purges the emotions of pity and fear through raising them? Does it effectively portray a change of fortune that is resolved in a recognition scene?

Mistaken Identity

The theme of mistaken identity, as it occurs in many of William Shakespeare's plays such *A Midsummer Night's Dream* and *Twelfth Night* in which two characters are mistaken for each other or purposely dress up to elude identification, is not common in Greek drama. The ancient Greeks were more familiar with human transformations to and from inanimate objects, as evidenced in the stories of Ovid's *Metamorphosis.* The mistaken identity of both Iphigenia and her brother, Orestes, constitutes the dramatic irony of *Iphigenia in Taurus.*

Characters mistake blood relatives for strangers. Iphigenia assumes that the man she will prepare for sacrifice could not possibly be her brother—because her dream has already told her that he has died. The irony consists in the possibility that she herself may kill him. At the same time, Orestes assumes that his sister died on the Athenian altar to Artemis, never expecting her to perform a like service upon him.

In any play of mistaken identity, the crisis resolves in a recognition scene. The artful recognition scene is painfully drawn out, as the characters approach and retreat without recognizing what the audience sees with agonizing clarity. To Athenian audiences, being in exile in a foreign land, suffering long absences, and nearly killing a blood relative resonated with the plight of citizens of a city at war with a sister Hellenic city. The irony and double-meanings within the lines would intensify their response to the play.

STYLE

Prologue

The prologue precedes the action of the play with a description of what will happen in the subsequent narrative. This may seem odd to modern theater-goers, who expect to experience surprise in watching a play. But the purpose of theater and therefore the purpose of the prologue was different in ancient Greek times. Fifth century Greek theater was closely aligned with solemn religious ceremony. The audience was attending a ritual performance that was a form of serious entertainment. The topic of the performance would be intimately familiar to all present. The prologue served not to introduce a novel situation but to hint at the subtle variations to a common theme this particular performance would explore. Both Euripides and Sophocles (in his *Electra*) explored the same material, yet each author brought his own subtleties to their respective dramas.

Before Euripides's time, the prologue was spoken, chanted, or sung by a chorus, but it had by now evolved into a speech presented by one of the players. Euripides's plays often begin with a single actor addressing the audience directly, recounting the story leading to the events about to be portrayed. *Iphigenia in Taurus* opens with a monologue by Iphigenia, saying simply, "I am Iphigenia" and then summarizing the pivotal event of her past, when her father tried to sacrifice her. (This event is the focus of another Euripides play, *Iphigenia at Aulis.*)

Chorus

Euripides made less use of the chorus than did his elder Sophocles, who demoted the chorus from a protagonist role to that of speaking spectator. Euripides reduced its role even further and employed it in a slightly different way. For Sophocles the chorus still served as a major character in the play; Euripides removed it from the action almost completely.

The chorus in Euripides's plays transforms the intense, personal emotions of the central characters into poignant statements about the situation in general. For example, after Iphigenia, Orestes, and Pylades depart from the temple on their way to the sea and freedom, the chorus sings of another brother and sister, Apollo and Artemis, in a moment when Apollo demands restitution of the gods for a wrong committed against him. Zeus applauds his pluck and restores reason to the earth. The story of Apollo foreshadows Athena's intervention on behalf of Orestes and Iphigenia. Euripides also demoted the chorus by giving it fewer songs and lines than did other poets; thereafter it disappeared completely from ancient Greek theater.

Deus ex Machina

The "deus ex machina," literally "god from a machine," was a common closing device in ancient Greek theater. Normally, a god would descend from the heavens to bring the action to a close. On the ancient Greek stage, the descent would have been accomplished by means of a large crane hoisting the actor playing the god. In Euripides's final scene, the goddess Athena appears from above the temple porch and prevents Thoas from pursuing the fleeing Hellenes. Athena informs Thoas that the gods ordered Orestes to steal the statue. She projects her voice to the fleeing Orestes as well, and she tells him to build a special temple to contain the statue, and to name the new temple after Taurus.

Furthermore, Athena hands down other laws, including the forbiddance of further human sacrifice. Instead a mere drop of human blood will now signify reverence to Artemis. Her closing words reinforce the rituals being celebrated by the Athenian audience.

HISTORICAL CONTEXT

The Peloponnesian Wars

The Peloponnesian War waged off and on for twenty seven years (431-404 B.C.), finally ending with the near total destruction of Athens by its economic rival Sparta. Pericles, for twenty years the

COMPARE & CONTRAST

- **5th century B.C.:** Greek tragic theater is produced in March for the ritual celebration of Dionysus, the god of wine. Everyone in the city attends the festival and the overall mood is festive though respectful and serious. Theater lies at the heart of Greek culture, integrated with religious ceremony and serving as a bond for the community.

  Today: Theater no longer has no ties to religion, although dramas for religious rituals are produced in some organized religions for important holidays. In the public theater, the sense of solemn ritual as experienced by the Athenians has no counterpart today. Theater is a form of entertainment that holds a rather peripheral status in modern society.

- **5th century B.C.:** The conflict between Sparta and Athens, the "super powers" of ancient Greece, has raged for ten years and a seven-year truce has just ended as *Iphigenia in Taurus* is first produced. The wars, which will ultimately last twenty-seven years, are devastating to Athens; Sparta plunders the city, destroys hundreds of valuable warships, and decimates Athenian population.

  Today: The United States has enjoyed over one hundred years of peace on its North American territory. Although its armed forces have engaged in wars in other countries, Americans and their way of life have enjoyed little threat from outsiders. The threat comes rather from within, from urban violence and from a slow erosion in moral values.

- **5th century B.C.:** Athenians value their democratic political and social system. Words have more power than weapons. Any citizen accused of a crime can defend *him*self (women did not share Athenian men's rights) before a jury. While slavery and other unsavory civil practices are common, the society is primarily democratic and free.

  Today: Democratic privileges extend to all citizens of the United States. Although inequalities still exist in practice, the American legal system guarantees citizens its rights and provides professional legal representation to those accused of crimes.

military general—the Greek equivalent of a president—of Athens, had engineered Athens rise to greatness through his superior oratory skill and his determination to build a true democracy through the education of Greek peoples. But he aggravated the rivalry between Athens and Sparta, sparking the Peloponnesian War, thus named because Sparta led the league of southern Greece called the Peloponnese.

The war waxed and waned between years of intense fighting, siege warfare, and periods of stalemate. Athens held the advantage at sea, while the Spartan army dominated land conflicts. Eventually, Sparta allied with Persia, obtaining needed funds to develop a naval force, and Athens, already weakened at sea, was undone. The political basis for the conflict lay in Sparta's adherence to oligarchy, which was threatened by the presence of Athen's democratic ideology. The psychological effect on Athenians of the decimation of its population and finances. The final, crushing blow came in admitting defeat to an enemy whose political philosophy was abhorrent to Athenians.

Greek Oracles and Omens

The importance of accurately interpreting dreams, omens, the ambiguous messages of oracles and the intentions of others certainly intensified during the long years of the Peloponnesian War. It was a time of deep superstitious belief. All humans experience the desire to foresee the future; during this time of crisis in Athenian life and culture, this desire became paramount.

The fifth-century historian Herodatus notes the profusion of oracles that flourished before and during the war. Archeologists have found leaden tablets listing questions as mundane as whether purchasing a piece of land would lead to prosperity as well as indications that some generals made no moves without the encouragement of an oracle or omen. Knowing this, political factions could and did manipulate the omens to sway decision-makers.

Iphigenia plays upon Thoas's superstitions in *Iphigenia in Taurus;* she convinces him that the two Hellenes are too impure to sacrifice, having committed the crime of matricide. Under the guise of purifying the statue and the intended sacrificial victims, she is able to lead them freely to the sea, first assuring that Thoas averts his eyes to avoid contamination. She also busies him with purifying the temple with fire. Even prisoners could gain a measure of control through the skillful manipulation of their conqueror's superstitions.

Greek Theater

Plays in fifth-century Athens were performed annually in honor of the Great Dionysia, a religious festival that took place on the *agora,* or marketplace. There was a wooden platform for the chorus and performers at the center of a bowl-shaped site that provided excellent natural acoustics for the audience. An altar to Dionysus lay at the center of the stage, a remnant of the fertility ritual that was the predecessor of the Dionysian festival. Players wore masks and chanted their lines, with little body movement. The festival also included a dramatic contest, where playwrights submitted and directed tetralogies consisting of tragedies and a satyr play, the latter a comic fertility rite.

CRITICAL OVERVIEW

Euripides wrote *Iphigenia in Taurus* before he wrote *Iphigenia in Aulis,* making *Aulis* a kind of ''prequel'' to *Taurus.* Euripides is one of a trio of great tragedians in fifth-century Greece: Euripides, Sophocles, and Aeschylus. Euripides was renowned during his lifetime, but he was not nearly as popular as either Sophocles or Aeschylus. Sophocles admired Euripides as a master playwright and honored the latter's death by having the participants in the subsequent Dionysian festival dress in mourning rather than in their usual festive costumes.

Philip Vellacott, a twentieth-century translator, explained in *Ironic Drama* that ''as a poet he was revered; in his function as a 'teacher of citizens' he was misunderstood.'' A century later, Euripides gained more notoriety, if not appreciation. During the fourth century B.C., his plays were more commonly produced and adapted than those of his fifth-century rivals. Aristophanes (448-380 B.C.) dedicated three whole plays to burlesquing—ridiculing—his style. This simple historical fact implies that Athenian audiences must have been familiar enough with Euripides's plays to make Aristophanes's jibes recognizable—Euripides's plays were an institution of drama during this period. While his theater was legendary, it was for his poetry and dramatic artistry for which Euripides was appreciated, not his ideas. Euripides was considered a fine poet with a misguided message. Aristotle (384-322 B.C.) used four of Euripides's works to illustrate various concepts of tragedy in his *Poetics,* wherein Aristotle defined the standards for drama. In that work he referred to Euripides as ''the most tragic of the poets'' who nevertheless had many ''faults.''

Euripides's skepticism was not condoned in the rather conservative fourth century. Greek culture was in decline, and as it declined even further, Euripides's plays were carried to Alexandria, and then to Rome, and the Byzantine culture. Plutarch (46-c. 120 A.D.) related three historical anecdotes of Hellenes who were allowed to escape their enemies by showing proficiency in reciting Euripidean poetry; this evidence corroborates Euripides's reputation, at least as a poet, in ancient Greece.

During the Middle Ages and Renaissance, the very aspect of Euripides's ideas that alarmed his contemporaries, his criticism of the pan-Hellenic gods, fueled an interest in his work by scholars, especially humanists such as Erasmus. Dante mentioned Euripides in his *Divine Comedy* and Ben Jonson used one of his plays as a model. Euripides's plays (along with those of Aeschylus and Sophocles) were required reading for the classical education valued during the Renaissance. In the seventeenth century Jean Racine adapted many of his plays and considered Euripides his master. John Milton (*Paradise Lost*) also expressed his admiration.

The eighteenth century lost interest in Euripides because his work was too innovative for the classical revival then in progress. Then Johann

Wolfgang von Goethe (*Faust*) paid him the ultimate Romantic period compliment by calling his work "sublime." Goethe created a new version of *Iphigenia in Taurus* that follows the original closely. It was of Euripides that Goethe wrote his oft-adapted expression: "Have all the nations of the world since his time produced one dramatist who was worthy to hand him his slippers?"

In the nineteenth century, Robert Browning made conspicuous allusions to certain plays by Euripides, and the Greek playwright was once more instated as a cornerstone of a good, classical education. Gilbert Murray's accessible translations in the early twentieth century made Euripides's work available to the larger public.

Twentieth-century literary criticism holds a reserved judgment regarding Euripides. Modern critics appreciate his championing of the underdog—slaves, women, the elderly, and children—and his lampooning of religious and secular hypocrisy. But he remains a shadowy figure whose actual political and religious beliefs are difficult to discern. Twentieth-century critics are more wary than earlier critics of associating ideas in an artist's works with his personal philosophy. The move toward New Criticism, with its emphasis on the text itself, has had a negative impact on Euripides's reputation in this century.

Under such assessments, Euripides, once again, does not measure up to Sophocles or Aeschylus. Furthermore, twentieth-century readers are accustomed to works of more dramatic intensity than *Iphigenia in Taurus,* which is considered a "romantic melodrama." Contemporary classical scholars find it interesting for its complex replication and reversal of certain paradigms found in the *Oresteia,* such as the near sacrifice of a blood relative. It seems unlikely that *Iphigenia in Taurus* will ever regain the popularity it enjoyed in its day, since its specificity to the status of the Hellenic state in the middle of the Peloponnesian Wars lies at the heart of the play.

CRITICISM

Carole Hamilton

Hamilton is an English teacher at Cary Academy, an innovative private school in Cary, North Carolina. In this essay she explores the multi-layered ironies of Iphigenia in Taurus *and suggests that to probe these layers sharpens the drama student's critical thinking skills.*

Because *Iphigenia in Taurus* is not as tragic or as compelling a story as such works as Sophocles's *Oedipus the King* or *Antigone,* (or even Euripides's own *Medea*), it is not produced as often on the modern stage or studied in the classroom as frequently. This play, written by a septuagenarian Euripides, pales in comparison to the violent action films of today's cinema, a genre of entertainment familiar to most students. *Iphigenia in Taurus* does not carry the legitimizing title of tragedy; it is often more accurately labeled a melodrama or romance. It has also frequently been dismissed as ancient Greek "escape" literature.

In a 1974 article for *Classical Journal,* R. Caldwell compared the play to a "pleasant day-dream" because "the danger is quite unreal, the escape is quite fantastic, the gods are clearly literary inventions. We are invited to indulge our fantasies, to subject repression to a process of catharsis, precisely because the work of art assures us, by its tone, that the dangers of such a task are not to be taken seriously." Yet despite these judgements, this play has much to offer contemporary viewers. The world of television and cinema is filled with sensationalism—violence, profanity, exaggerated special effects. Subtle works such as *Iphigenia in Taurus* can be a thought-provoking antidote to such mind-numbing sensationalism, offering an invitation to the art of active thinking while viewing.

Iphigenia in Taurus is filled with subtle ironies. It has been said that the ability to detect irony is a sign of mental aptitude, but this aptitude requires practice if it is to be developed to its full potential. To perceive irony the viewer must follow closely the unraveling of the plot, yet also remain aloof enough from the action to compare what is seen with his or her own experience and to make judgements accordingly. This means that the viewer cannot subsume critical thinking to emotional involvement or passively submit to the ideas presented in the play. Euripides knew this, and he portrayed the foolishness of accepting things at face value. Both Iphigenia and Orestes model the negative consequences of submitting passively to one's anticipated fate: they each assume the other is dead and only begin to use their own thinking capacities

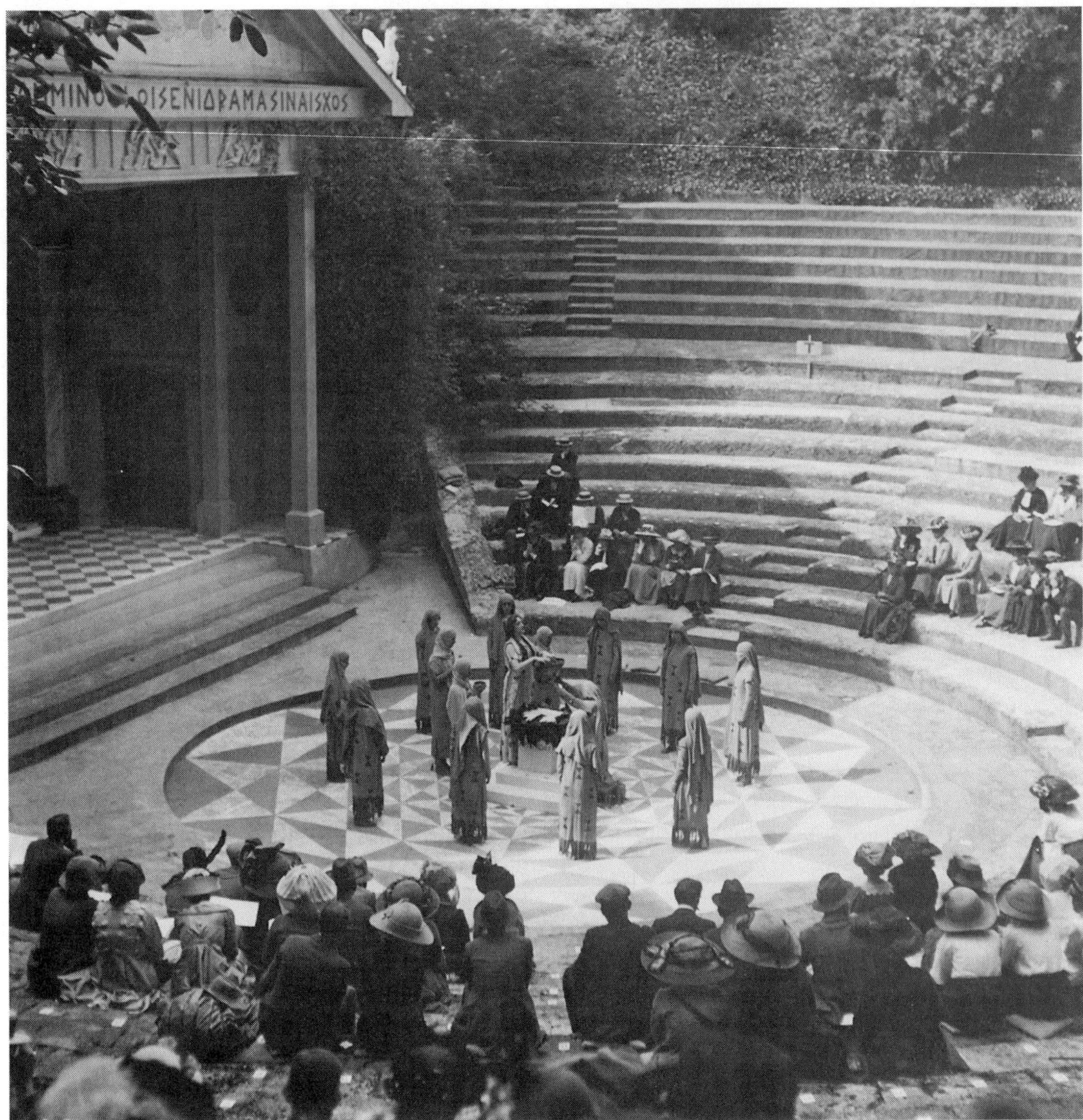

Iphigenia in Taurus *is staged at the Greek Theatre at Bradfield College in Berkshire. The theater is modeled after the traditional structure of Athenian theaters*

fully when they find each other alive and begin to work out a plan of escape.

Irony is a reversal of expectations, a difference between appearances or perception and reality. One can express irony through tone of voice, saying one thing and meaning another, such as when Shakespeare's Antony repeatedly states that ''Brutus is an honorable man'' in *Julius Caesar* when it is clear from his inflection and body language that he thinks the exact opposite. Dramatic irony consists of situations that the characters themselves accept at face value but which the audience understands in a different, usually opposite, way. *Iphigenia in Taurus* abounds in moments of dramatic irony where the audiences perceives a truth to which the characters are blinded, for various reasons.

Euripides's characters misread situations, such as when Iphigenia misinterprets her dream of one column still standing in the House of Atreus as an indication of Orestes's death, rather than considering the possibility that the standing column may mean her brother is alive. Orestes, in a moment of madness, stabs wildly at cattle which he misperceives as the Furies. At these times as well as in

WHAT DO I READ NEXT?

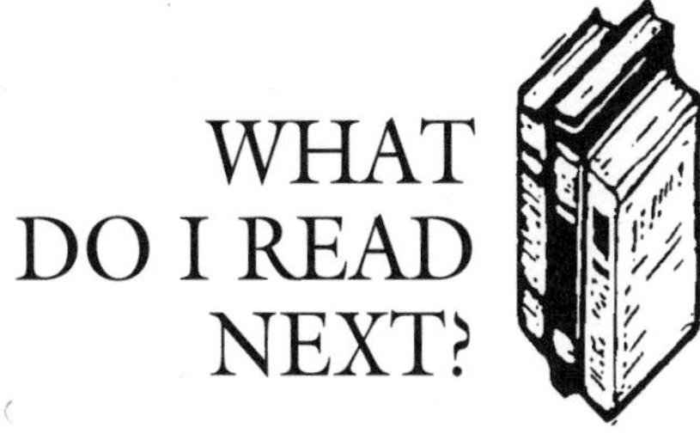

- The myth of the family of Atreus was portrayed by each of the three great dramatists of the Golden Age of Athens: Euripides, Sophocles, and Aeschylus. Euripides's play *Iphigenia in Aulis* recounts the moving story of Agamemnon's attempt to sacrifice his daughter. Euripides's other extant plays on the House of Atreus are *Orestes* and *Electra.*
- Sophocles also wrote an *Electra* (c. 409 B.C.), although this play assumes Iphigenia's death and focuses on the plight of her sister, Electra, and brother, Orestes, exacting revenge against Clytemnestra.
- Aeschylus wrote a trilogy on the myth called the *Oresteia.* In the first of the trilogy, *Agamemnon,* Clytemnestra murders Agamemnon in vengeance for sacrificing their daughter. In the second play, *The Libation Bearers,* Orestes kills Clytemnestra to avenge his father, and in the final play, *The Eumenides,* Orestes is tried and acquitted in an Athenian court.

numerous verbal or situational oxymorons, the audience easily recognizes the true meaning that the characters themselves do not fathom or guess.

Iphigenia's oxymoron, a "just evil" aptly describes both the necessity and the criminality of Orestes's murder of his own mother. The phrase takes on added dimension for the audience who know that she is speaking of a crime designed to avenge her own sacrifice at the hands of her father, Agamemnon. When Iphigenia wishes that her brother might resemble the young man before her who chooses to die in place of his friend, the audience recognizes the irony that her wish is only too true, and that she will destroy her brother. When Orestes wishes that his sister, meaning Iphigenia, could pour his libations, the audience knows that this wish might also, tragically, be fulfilled.

In each case, it is important for the audience to infer the reasons that the character fails to perceive the reality behind appearances. At the first level, Iphigenia fails to recognize her brother simply because he has not yet told her his name; but at another level of perception, she has a disinclination to feel empathy for any Hellene, because her father's betrayal has embittered her heart. Orestes is likewise blinded by his overwhelming sense of guilt, which has driven him partly mad. Thus he is unwilling to reveal his true nature to the one person who would accept him.

In places, the irony is not so obvious, making it more difficult for the audience to infer the deeper meaning of the characters' actions. This deeper irony demands a perceptive viewer, reader, or listener to detect it. The irony resides in the "gap" that Euripides's translator Philip Vellacott, in his introduction to the play, explained "must exist in the work of every profound and creative dramatist between what he knows he has put into a scene and what he knows most of his audience will receive from it." Most of Euripides's Athenian audience would have noted the irony that when Iphigenia tells Thoas she must purify the altar statue, she deceives him with the very means that landed her in Taurus to begin with—the desire for purification through sacrifice. She manipulates the appearance of her actions, to make Thoas think that she intends to purify the altar and sacrifice another Hellene; instead she intends the opposite: to set free and purify the Hellene, not the Taurians, and to purge the temple of its altar, not purify it.

Likewise, an ironic reversal occurs when Orestes, asks Iphigenia to save him (by procuring the statue), whereas just moments before she was desperately attempting to contact him to come and save her: the tables have now turned. Recognizing an event in which the "tables are turned" is the province of the sophisticated audience. Athenian audiences were better prepared to notice these sub-

"IT IS IMPORTANT FOR THE AUDIENCE TO INFER THE REASONS THAT THE CHARACTER FAILS TO PERCEIVE THE REALITY BEHIND APPEARANCES."

tleties, having plenty of time to contemplate the play and being unused to the onslaught of violent and extravagant performances that daily bombard the modern audience. The twentieth-century student of Euripides will benefit greatly from slowing down to appreciate and contemplate this profound and quiet masterpiece. Insights always reward the careful study of a work of great literature, but with Euripides's *Iphigenia in Taurus,* such analysis is critical to understanding the play as Athenian audiences understood it.

A deeper level of irony detection lies in the correspondence between the events of the play and the social or political context of the audience. Here the modern viewer may feel hamstrung by the distance of almost fifteen hundred years and the paucity of information about Euripides's opinions regarding the issues of his day. However, human nature has changed very little over the centuries; much of what Euripides has to say is perfectly comprehensible to contemporary human thought.

Orestes, we recognize, has fallen under the cloud of fatalistic thinking: he assumes the herdsmen will defeat them on the shore and only raises his arm to avoid dying a coward. The towering walls of the Taurian temple so intimidate him that Pylades has to convince him not to run away. Both of these instances pit appearances against reality, and Orestes remains stuck on appearance. Orestes has succumbed to the belief that his fate lies in the hands of Apollo, that he cannot change it, and he blames the gods rather than taking responsibility for his own decisions.

Iphigenia is similarly afflicted: years of enforced service in the temple have clouded her thinking, causing her to misinterpret her dream as an omen that Orestes is dead. In her case, appearances do not make the same impression on her as they would on another Hellene. The audience would identify with the siblings' difficulties. An attitude of embittered fatalism had become the norm to the Athenians, who had suffered catastrophic losses during eighteen years of strife with Sparta (and were further decimated by a plague). The Athenians were beginning to realize that despite their philosophical superiority, they could lose the Pelloponnesian War. The parallels between the doomed House of Atreus and the besieged city of Athens would have been painfully apparent. As the chorus chants "blow after blow staggers the cursed city," the substitution of Athens for Argos would have been automatic.

Another of Euripides's ironic comments involves the efficacy of human sacrifice for purification purpose. Cedric Whitman in his 1974 book,*Euripides and the Full Circle of Myth,* explained that the goal of purification lies at the heart of this play. "All must be purified, Orestes of his madness, Iphigenia of her involvement in human sacrifice, and Artemis of a cult unworthy of a Hellenic deity." Iphigenia says that "The rites I celebrate are unfit for song." The happy ending restores three Hellenes to their land and exorcises the Furies from further tormenting Orestes, whom the Athenian court has acquitted of a justified homicide. Thus besides resolving the individual characters' misperceptions and terminating the curse upon the House of Atreus, the ending also confirms the Athenian urge to trust in themselves rather than succumb to the fatalism and despondency of interpreting the omens of the gods. The ending is an exhortation communicated through the medium of irony to use the "double" vision of irony to see through appearances to the reality underneath.

Source: Carole Hamilton for *Drama for Students,* Gale, 1998.

Peter Walcot

In this essay, Walcot provides an overview of Euripides's play.

The *Iphigenia in Tauris* is the type of romantic melodrama with a happy ending characteristic of the later work of Euripides. Its setting is appropriately exotic: the forecourt of a temple of Artemis on the Taurian coast in the modern Crimea. The play tells how Iphigenia, the daughter of Agamemnon, is serving as a priestess of the Taurians, having been rescued when on the point of being sacrificed at Aulis by her father, who was leading the Greeks to Troy. Her brother Orestes and his friend Pylades come to the Crimea in search of a statue of Artemis which will release Orestes from his sufferings. A report that a pair of men has been captured is brought to Iphigenia whose responsibility it is to sacrifice arrivals from Greece on the altar of Artemis. When they meet, brother and sister fail to recognise one other, but a desire on the part of Iphigenia to have a letter smuggled back to Greece leads to a realisation that the two men are Iphigenia's own brother and his companion. Now reunited, they plot an escape to Greece together with the statue, but their plan is threatened by the arrival of King Thoas who, however, is persuaded that the statue must be cleansed in the sea. Once they reach the shore, escape is achieved, but only after a fight and a most opportune intervention by the goddess Athene. Throughout the play intense excitement is sustained by the seemingly endless twists and turns of a far from simple plot.

Iphigenia delivers a lengthy prologue of a type common in Euripides' plays. This does more than just impart basic information; it also reveals the pathos inherent in the woman's present plight. Furthermore, we learn of a dream which, ironically, is both optimistic (in depicting Iphigenia's restoration at home) and pessimistic (in seeming to anticipate the sacrifice of Orestes). It appears almost inevitable that as Iphigenia vanishes into the temple, Orestes and Pylades should take her place, busying themselves in careful examination of the blood-stained altar of Artemis. A reference to the goddess's statue and the instruction from Apollo to present it to Athens completes all we need to know in the way of information; Orestes' hesitation but Pylades' stern determination to fulfil their mission similarly complete our picture of the play's major characters.

The herdsman's account of the capture of Orestes and Pylades is certainly long, but any danger of tedium is eliminated by vivid description of an Orestes stricken by madness as he imagines himself pursued by a Fury and falls upon cattle in a belief that these too are Furies. The actual capture is almost hilarious as the herdsmen are scattered and then regroup and stone the young men into submission. The chorus finds a story so rich in detail astounding. And Iphigenia herself has another long speech in which, yet again, a heavy vein of irony is exploited: believing her brother dead Iphigenia declares her heart now to be hardened while, at the same time, delivering a pathetic account of how she came to Aulis ostensibly to be married, and then indulging in typical Euripidean philosophizing when she claims that it is men and not the gods who are evil.

" *IPHIGENIA IN TAURIS* IS THE TYPE OF ROMANTIC MELODRAMA WITH A HAPPY ENDING CHARACTERISTIC OF THE LATER WORK OF EURIPIDES."

The scene between Iphigenia and Orestes, who both talk vigorously but at cross-purposes, is a masterpiece of misunderstanding although it does reveal that Orestes is still alive. At every point it is expected that the full truth will come out, but it never does and our expectations are constantly frustrated. Euripides has a fondness for simple stage-props and one is then introduced: Iphigenia offers not to kill Orestes if he will carry a letter back to Argos for her, but Orestes proposes that Pylades performs the mission and proceeds to persuade his friend to do this in an exchange of an especial appeal to a Greek audience (deeply appreciative as it was of the art of rhetoric). But a complication is raised: what if Pylades' ship sinks and the letter lost but Pylades saved? The obvious solution to this dilemma is to tell Pylades the contents of the letter and this information, thus conveyed in such a way as not to strain credulity, identifies Iphigenia to the captives.

It is also quite natural that Iphigenia should delay the planning of their escape by seeking all the family news from Orestes. If Euripides drags out this episode at what initially appears inordinate length, it is done deliberately to heighten suspense. Less realistic, but again characteristic of Euripides, is the request for secrecy made to the chorus. But Thoas has still to be deceived, and Iphigenia's claim that the intended victims were unclean and so unfit for sacrifice and that Artemis's image must be purified illustrates, again surely to a Greek audience's considerable delight, its proponent's cleverness and superiority over a "barbarian." There remains one more drawn-out exposition: the messenger's description of the actual escape. In spite of their suspicions, the guards entrust the prisoners to Iphigenia; eventually they decide to investigate and find a Greek ship ready to depart and the two heroes climbing on board; both groups fight with fists in an attempt to secure Iphigenia and the Taurians are forced to fall back and use stones; the Greeks retaliate with arrows as Orestes carries his sister and statue safely aboard the ship which sails away but is then driven to the shore again by the wind. Thoas and his men make off to the shore, and it is at this point that Euripides plays his last card—the goddess Athene appears and orders Thoas to desist. The playwright has wrung an audience's every emotion and brought the most devious of plots to a happy conclusion. But Euripides adds a last detail with the obvious intention of pleasing his Athenian audience: Athene also orders the building of a sanctuary on the borders of Attica to house the statue of Artemis. The establishment of a local cult centre gives the play a special relevance to the original spectators and stresses the Athenian context of the drama.

Source: Peter Walcot, ''*Iphigenia in Taurus*'' in *The International Dictionary of Theatre I: Plays,* edited by Mark Hawkins-Dady, St. James Press, 1992, pp. 372–73.

Michael J. O'Brien

In this essay, O'Brien examines the plot of Euripides's play and compares its plot points to prevalent legends during the playwright's time. He argues that Euripides had a specific agenda in building his drama upon the history and legends of ancient Greece, although there are significant points at which the play differs from history.

The plot of *Iphigenia in Tauris* is usually thought to be Euripides' own invention. Its basic assumption can be found in Proclus' summary of the *Cypria,* viz. that a deer was substituted for Iphigenia during the sacrifice at Aulis and that she herself was removed to the land of the Tauri. Her later rescue by Orestes and Pylades, however, cannot be traced with probability to any work of art or literature earlier than Euripides' play. In this play, in which Orestes rccognizes and then saves the sister whom he had long thought dead, it is assumed that her replacement by a deer went unseen by those present at the sacrifice. The sequel which this assumption allowed Euripides to invent (if it was he who invented it) is original only in a limited sense, since it bears the imprint of several familiar story types. These types include the following: (1) the murder of a kinsman is narrowly averted by a recognition; (2) a reunion is followed by an intrigue; and (3) a maiden is rescued. Each is used elsewhere by Euripides. The first two, for example, are found in *Cresphontes,* the second in *Electra,* and the third in *Andromeda.* Correspondences of this sort, based on plot patterns, will naturally gain in interest if it can be shown that they throw light on a play's meaning or on the process that led to its creation. The student of dramatic plots, however, soon discovers that analogies between them are easy to draw and can be quickly multiplied. It is much harder to decide which analogies are genuinely enlightening. This study addresses that question as it applies to *I.T.* (*Iphigenia in Taurus*) and suggests certain criteria which may help to answer it for other plays as well.

The recurrence of patterns in tragic plots has been extensively discussed in recent decades, and it is now well understood how readily plots and their components can be classified and parallels drawn between them. Richmond Lattimore deals with this subject in a broad but enlightening way in a book which takes all of tragedy (and much else) for its subject. He shows that, since stories tend to crystallize in certain forms, these forms are encountered again and again in drama. T. B. L. Webster, in reviewing the evidence for Euripides' lost plays, also calls attention to recurrent plot elements but speaks as if these repetitions were the result of rapid composition and the pressure of time. Anne Burnett, in contrast, tabulates patterns in order to dwell on their variations, since she is convinced that Euripides' art lay partly in manipulating the educated expectations of an audience familiar with all the standard plot forms. She illustrates this theory by analysing seven Euripidean plays, one of which is *I.T.,* as combinatory adaptations of a limited set of six matrix plots. These three scholars write in English, but important work on plot forms had appeared earlier in German in such publications as Strohm's book on Euripides. It is sometimes alleged against such studies that they tend to confuse the tabulated results of scholarly analysis and generalization with the creative thoughts of poets and, at their worst, reduce the art of tragedy to the management of abstractions; furthermore, that these classifications too readily generate dubious norms of critical judgement. There is some truth in these charges. For all that, the practice of speaking of the tragic art in this way is well established; it is at least as old as Aristotle, who divides plots into the simple and the complex (which are said to be better), and whose other listings of typical plots and plot elements include a catalogue of recognition types in which these too are ranked by merit. Even he has not escaped the charge that his exercises in classification were 'slightly artificial'.

Whatever criticisms may be made against their excesses, these studies have undeniably advanced our understanding or traditional plot forms and shown to what degree tragic poets in the act of creation were constrained by precedent. But the kind and degree of attention that an audience was expected to pay to these recurrent forms is another matter. On this point Burnett at least has probably gone too far. She assumes that the typical spectator of a new tragedy was a man enthralled by its interplay of structural commonplace and constantly mindful of the formal precedents being followed or broken in the development of its plot. In questioning this view I do not mean to deny that audiences were often aware of broad similarities between stories and poets ready to turn this fact to account. Tragedy may sometimes appeal to this awareness by its use of generalizations. . . . Such generalization as occur, however, tend to carry an ethical or religious point, and the sum of them would not match very well the lists of plot types developed by modern scholars. This is to be expected: not every plot follows the lines of a maxim. Aside from examples like these, we should be wary of assuming that poets and audiences were preoccupied with general patterns or 'norms' of tragic action or that an awareness of deviations from these norms could have been a central element governing anyone's reaction to a play. The Greeks understood well enough that almost nothing in myth is unprecedented, but the most striking evidence for this in the plays is neither commonplace patterns nor general statements but the large number of passages where the legend being dramatized is compared with some other specific legend. In these passages what occupies the foreground and engages the attention is the concrete detail of the counterpart legend itself. These mythological paradigms or *exempla* may fill an entire stasimon or a mere single line of dialogue and may refer to the whole action of a play or a passing moment. Their use in tragedy is an inheritance from earlier poetry, where meaning is often clarified or emotion heightened through the well-known names and incidents of some legend not itself the main subject of a poem. Beyond these familiar facts, two less obvious points about *exempla* deserve particular notice. (1) Although in tragedy they are often linked to their contexts by some expression of comparison, at times there is no such link and their function as paradigms must be inferred. The latter is also true of some Pindaric myths used as *exempla,* if common interpretations of these are valid. (2) Although any analogy between a dramatized story and another legend will be based on similarity of form and will to that extent appeal to an awareness of pattern, the other legend may be chosen for its particular associations as much as for the general

"AS A TRAGEDY WITH A HAPPY ENDING, *IPHIGENIA IN TAURUS* CONTAINS MORE THAN IT MIGHT SEEM TO AT FIRST SIGHT: NOT ONLY A CHEERING SEQUEL TO THE ORESTES AND IPHIGENIA LEGENDS, BUT ALSO AN ALTERNATIVE HISTORY OF THE PELOPIDS, ONE THAT BEGINS AND ENDS WITH A TALE OF SUCCESS."

features which the two happen to share with many others. Whenever this is true, the relation of greatest interest will be one that joins specific legends, and the shared story pattern will be no more than one aspect of it.

This paper is meant to illustrate these last two points. It is a study of *I.T.* which finds analogies between its story and two other legends mentioned prominently in the play, the courtship of Pelops and Hippodameia and the sacrifice at Aulis. It will argue that the poet perceived a special relation between these legends and the action of his play and found means to convey this to the audience. In each case the relation is made perceptible through a shared pattern of action, but its affective power derives primarily from the blood tie which unites the principal agents of all three legends. Pattern repetition in this case is therefore the formal aspect of family history repeating itself, a subject of undeniable interest to fifth-century tragic poets. Since Euripides may actually have invented the story of Iphigenia's rescue, these related legends may also be the story's models. If that is so, his new sequel to Atreid history is fully organic. That assumption, however, will not be essential to the argument. It will be enough to show that these legends are present in *I.T.* as paradigms of the action, helping to colour and define it and foreshadowing its outcome. As I have argued elsewhere, Euripides made a similar use of the Tantalus myth in *Orestes;* therefore the technique displayed in *I.T.* is no isolated example.

Pelops' marriage contest is expressly referred to twice in *I.T.*, at the start of Iphigenia's first speech and at the climactic moment when she recognizes Orestes. . . .

For some reason, out of the long and complicated legend of the house of Atreus, Euripides has chosen to put at the beginning of his play an allusion to Pelops' successful contest with Oenomaus and his marriage to Hippodameia. The career of Tantalus is left out; he is mentioned only as Pelops' father. The gap in generations between Pelops and Iphigenia herself is bridged in steps as economical as the iambic metre allows. The family history is therefore effectively compressed into two events, the victory of Pelops and the sacrifice at Aulis. The latter will be narrated at length in the passage immediately following. Its great prominence in Iphigenia's opening speech requires no explanation, but it is not immediately apparent why she begins her speech, and the play, with Pelops.

At the beginning of the second episode. Orestes is brought into Iphigenia's presence, and after a long dialogue he realizes her identity. His identity, in turn, is revealed by Pylades, who addresses him by name in her presence at line 792; but 35 lines will pass before she accepts the fact that this is her brother. He first calls her 'dearest sister' (795) and attempts to embrace her. When the chorus (or Iphigenia herself, according to Monk's reattribution) rebukes him and she turns away, he invokes the name of Agamemnon (801). Another expression of disbelief follows. But by line 806 her interest seems aroused. . . .

His way of affirming his identity, as Pelops' descendant, is worth noting, though it cannot carry much weight by itself. Iphigenia now asks for evidence to support this claim. His reply, given in dialogue, is measured and orderly and designed to lead to a climax. First, what he has heard from Electra: that Atreus and Thyestes quarrelled over the golden lamb, and Iphigenia once wove this story on a tapestry; that the sun changed course, and she wove this too; that her mother gave her bathing water in preparation for what was supposed to be her marriage at Aulis; that before she was to be sacrificed she gave her mother locks of her hair as a relic. So much Orestes had from hearsay. . . .

[The] mention of the spear of Pelops, which Orestes saw hidden in Iphigenia's chamber, accomplishes the recognition and breaks down her reserve. [823 6]

These lines mark the end of an unusually prolonged and suspenseful recognition-scene and receive much emphasis from their position. Once again, as at the beginning of the play, what is said in 811–26 constitutes a selective review of family history: the quarrel of the brothers and the consequent reversal of the sun's course, the sacrifice at Aulis, and Pelops' victory. All three involve memories personal to Iphigenia, but in the first case and the last this connection is established by contrivance (the tapestry, the hidden spear). Why did Euripides choose these three episodes? It is the beginning of an answer to observe that only the third is a happy memory. The recognition, itself a triumphant moment in the stage action, is achieved through the memory of an ancestral victory. The other memories, all bitter, serve as preamble and contrast. They end with a line and a word designed to stand in the sharpest emotional opposition to what follows. . . (821).

Even this partial explanation of 811–26, which speaks only of the emotional development of the lines, involves difficulties. In most accounts, the outcome of Pelops' contest with Oenomaus was not an unreserved triumph. At *Orestes* 988ff. and 1548 a version is assumed in which Pelops won with the help of Myrtilus, Oenomaus' charioteer; his help is explained in other sources as the removal of the linch-pins of his master's chariot, which caused it to crash. Pelops later killed Myrtilus, and his dying curse became the source of endless troubles in the house. For this reason, at Sophocles' *Electra* 505 Pelops' ride is called 'a source of many sorrows'. But at least one notable literary version of the legend before Euripides, that of Pindar's *Olympian I,* left out Myrtilus and allowed Pelops to win with the help of winged horses provided by Poseidon. The presence of different versions in the tradition means that care is needed in deciding whether Myrtilus' trick and his later curse are meant to be assumed in *I.T.* The matter cannot be decided by saying that in the late fifth century they had become part of the standard version of the legend and could be presumed even when not explicitly mentioned. In a recent article, T. C. W. Stinton has discussed several tragedies in each of which important features or some legend in its standard version are purposefully ignored. He shows that suppression of such detail is one aspect of an author's freedom to adapt myth. Moreover, it hardly needs argument to say of the author of *Helen* that he was not bound to treat his myths consistently from play to play. We cannot simply fill in *I.T.* 823–6 with details drawn from *Orestes* 988ff. In Murray's Oxford text of *I.T.* the evidence on this point was blurred by a conjecture printed *exempli causa* in a corrupt choral passage at 192–3, one which introduced the killing of Myrtilus to the text. But Myrtilus is not otherwise to be found in the play; nor can any claim be made that he is required in order to explain how Oenomaus died. In accounts in which Oenomaus is killed in the crash of his chariot, Myrtilus is the agent of his death and to that extent indispensable. But at *I.T.* 825, as at Pindar, *O.* 1.88, Pelops is named as the one who kills him; in neither version is Myrtilus mentioned, and in neither can his presence be assumed. If he is absent from *I.T.*, then so is his curse, and the contest for the hand of Hippodameia need not be judged. . . . The troubles in the house may be thought of as beginning later, with the quarrel of Atreus and Thyestes, mentioned in the corrupt passage at 193–7 and again at 812ff. The career of Pelops himself will figure only as an example of good fortune. To say that much helps to justify an allusion to it in the very limited context of this moment of recognition, where good fortune again prevails.

Its appearance at the beginning of the play, however, as the point of departure for family history, may mean that it has a less limited relevance. To begin with what is most obvious, this play, like Euripides' summary version of the Pelops legend, ends happily. A review of the basic details of the legend reveals further analogies. The conditions imposed by Oenomaus upon anyone wishing to marry Hippodameia were that the suitor and his intended bride should ride off in a chariot, while Oenomaus, armed with a spear, rode in pursuit. Pelops won where others had lost and paid with their lives. Even in its barest outline, the legend implies a cruel Oenomaus. By the fifth century, he was being portrayed as a savage who cut off and exhibited the heads of unsuccessful suitors. This practice was attributed to him in Sophocles' *Oenomaus,* thought by some to have been an early production. One of the few fragments from that play is a reference to scalping 'in the Scythian fashion'. This is probably to be explained, in accordance with Herodotus 4.64, as an indignity like that practised by the Scythians upon the severed heads of slain enemies. In Sophocles' play, the impaled heads may have been part of the stage setting. Less is known about Euripides' *Oenomaus,* the fragments of which throw little light on how the legend was handled. Hyginus 84.3 appears to summarize a tragic scene in which Pelops is so frightened by the heads of Oenomaus' victims that he regrets having come to challenge him; his source is sometimes taken to be Euripides' play. Though individual authors certainly embellished the picture, the legend readily lent itself to the portrayal of Oenomaus as an ogre to be classed with several other mythical figures famous for outrages against strangers. Seen in this light, Pelops' successful courtship of Hippodameia was also her rescue from cruel and savage surroundings.

Calder and Sutton, in writing about Sophocles' *Oenomaus,* have noticed that in extant tragedy the closest parallels to the vanquished ogre-king of Oenomaus' type are Thoas of *I.T.* and Theoclymenus of *Helen.* They do not connect this fact with the references to Pelops and Oenomaus in *I.T.;* but Calder, in speaking of the probable display of skulls in the prologue of Sophocles' play, calls the similar spectacle at *I.T.* 74–5 an 'imitation' of it. This is a reference to Orestes' and Pylades' first sight of the temple of the Taurian Artemis and the altar stained with human blood; here Orestes immediately points out the 'spoils' attached under the cornice (74) and Pylades answers, 'Yes, first fruits of the foreigners who perished'. It seems almost certain that these words refer to a display or severed heads. This would tally with Herodotus 4.103, where the Taurians are said to sacrifice victims of shipwreck and fugitives from storms, then cut off and exhibit their heads. In other ways too, Euripides represents the king of the Taurians as the ruler of a barbarous country and a man personally willing to enforce its customary abuse of strangers. The parallel with Oenomaus, including the specific detail of line 74 with its probable reminiscence of Sophoclean staging, is clear. It is significant, however, only as part of a larger analogy that includes three of the play's characters. Iphigenia, like her ancestress Hippodameia, is held captive by a savage but finds a deliverer.

The name of her captor is Thoas. . . .

Wilamowitz, in *Analecta Euripidea,* cited this etymology as a mere display or sophistic erudition. If that is true, the charge is graver than it may seem, because Euripides, in attaching this name to Iphigenia's captor, has probably gone out of his way to create an opportunity for the etymology. If one sets aside the doubtful possibility that Sophocles' *Chryses* was both a sequel to the rescue of Iphigenia and an earlier play than *I.T.*, there is no evidence that Thoas was the name of a Taurian king in legend or fact before the date of *I.T.* Thoas the Lemnian, the son of Dionysus, who is known to Herodotus (6.138), is another man, even though he is identified with the Taurian by two late authors in defiance of mythical chronology. Euripides' character is 'a mere name', in Immisch's phrase, endowed with definable traits but with no place in any genealogy. Why this name should have been chosen for Orestes' adversary is not immediately clear, as Wilamowitz himself later pointed out. Significant names in Euripides, however, often make an important dramatic point. To take two other examples from prologues, Theonoe's 'godlike knowledge' gives her the power to ruin Helen and Menelaus, and the name of Dionysus declares the paternity that is the point at issue in *Bacchae.* Why is the king of the Taurians swift? Learned irrelevance is not the only possible answer. This is an escape play, and the threat which Thoas represents is that of a swift pursuer: at 1325–6 and 1422–34 he threatens to overtake the fugitives, and at 1435 he must be stopped by Athena. To that extent, his name fits: like Theonoe's name, it marks his function in the story. But even if it is strictly beyond proof that this is so by design, there should be little doubt about the nature of Thoas' role. As the pursuer, no less than as the warder of Iphigenia, he is the counterpart of Oenomaus, whose speed as a charioteer enabled him to run down and kill thirteen suitors with his spear. In both contests, the maiden flees with the young hero. Iphigenia rides in the ship with her brother; and, though the flight of Pelops is commonly described as a race with Oenomaus, it takes the form of a bride-theft. Hippodameia rides on Pelops' chariot; she does not wait at home for the outcome.

Analogies can be carried only so far, and there are important and obvious differences between the two stories: in *I.T.,* the maiden rescued is a sister, not a bride; the flight is by ship, not by chariot; and Iphigenia's captor is stopped by divine intervention, not killed. The first two arise from the intractable data of the Iphigenia legend. The killing of Thoas, on the other hand, is considered at 1020–3 and is expressly rejected by Iphigenia on moral grounds. . . . Here the desire to make a pointed ethical distinction between Iphigenia and Thoas, . . . has caused a departure from the pattern of the older story. In other respects the correspondences are striking; they constitute the main reason for thinking that the references to one story foreshadow the outcome of the other. The emphatic position of these references, at the beginning of the play and at its emotional climax, also argues for their significance; standing where they do, they claim attention. It is fair to ask why Euripides, who had other choices in each passage, chose them. The answer proposed here is that they are suitable in a play that dramatizes an escape from danger and from barbarism. Mythical allusion, elsewhere common in the form of paradigms of misforture, here foreshadows deliverance. *I.T.,* therefore, in adding an epilogue to Atreid history, has also reshaped that history into one circumscribed by two episodes of good fortune.

The pattern so far discussed accounts for only a part of the plot, viz. the arrival of Orestes and his escape with Iphigenia. It omits the near-sacrifice of Orestes. As Burnett has explained it, this is not a simple rescue story but one which has embedded in it a misdirected and interrupted vengeance plot. This is true, provided one accepts a broad definition of 'vengeance plot'; but the terms used, being general, may not be the most useful ones. They are appropriate if we think of the poet as manipulating 'structural commonplaces' and arousing in the audience its 'combined memories' of all other rescue plots and vengeance plots. But here again particular memories are the ones most obviously being aroused, and the structural analogy insisted upon in passage after passage links two stories, not many: the sacrifice of Orestes and the sacrifice of Iphigenia.

They are first associated in Iphigenia's opening monologue. This speech encompasses the allusion to Pelops (1–2), three transitional lines consisting largely of proper names (3–5), the sacrifice at Aulis (6–30), her life as priestess of Artemis (31–41), her recent dream (42–60), and her present intentions (61–6). The bulk of the speech is occupied by the sacrifice and the dream. The latter turns out to have taken the form of preparations for another sacrifice, that of Orestes, in which she plays the role of priestess. Her interpretation of it is wrong (that Orestes is already dead), but the dream itself is a true augury of her preparations to sacrifice him later in the play. Her speech, therefore, is largely occupied with her own apparent death, about which only she knows the truth (see line 8), and Orestes' apparent death, about which only she is deceived. Both deaths are cast in the form of sacrifices. Some parallelism of treatment is already discernible in all this.

It continues to be discernible in the parodos and kommos at 123ff. Here the two subjects recur, and there is more formal symmetry in the way they are balanced than in the earlier speech. If one omits the introductory lines before 143, the passage falls into three distinct parts, of which the first and last belong to Iphigenia (143–77, 203–35). The first is a lament for Orestes, with a brief reference to her own illusory sacrifice and death in the closing lines. The last is devoted to the same two subjects, but with their order and proportions reversed. The shorter chant of the chorus (179–202) which separates these is about the woes of the house, now reaching their final stage. As far as the corrupt text allows one to say, these begin with the quarrel of Atreus and Thyestes.

Up to this point, the correspondence between the two imagined deaths is merely something implicit in the poetic form. At 337–9 it becomes explicit, and it takes the special form of a claim that sacrifices of victims such as those now in hand can serve as retribution for the sacrifice at Aulis. The speaker is the herdsman who brings news of the capture of Orestes and Pylades. Iphigenia responds to this report in a speech (342–91) full of bitter reminiscence about her two sources of grief, the supposed death of Orestes and her own slaying, here spoken of without mention of her final rescue. The two captives, she says, will find her unsympathetic and fierce, as she never was before with Greeks (344–53). Her preferred victims would be Helen and Menelaus, whom she would gladly pay back by a re-enactment of Aulis. . . .

She does not speak of the sacrifice of two innocents now in prospect as a new Aulis; that would erase the moral distinction between her and the sanguinary Taurians, and this distinction will be consistently maintained in the play. But she does say that she has turned savage and that her victims will find her hostile. Euripides allows her no further comment in that vein, but her words seem designed to place her for a moment in the attitude of a vengeful killer about to balance her own sacrifice with the one to come. This attitude will not be maintained when the victims appear, but while it lasts it keeps alive the herdsman's notion of retributory correspondence.

The intended sacrifice is forestalled by the revelation of Orestes' identity. In the *amoibaion* which follows this recognition, it becomes clear that what happened at Aulis and what has just now happened here are linked both in Iphigenia's thoughts and in the design of the poet; this fact is reflected in the structure of the central section (850–72). Orestes begins this by stating a theme [at 850–1]. . . .

Of the many misfortunes that might have illustrated this statement, only two are mentioned, and the language used of these is chosen to reflect their essential similarity. Aulis comes first: the knife at the throat, the ruse of the betrothal to Achilles, the holy water. Then there is a transition to the attempted sacrifice of Orestes, which is linked with Aulis by a simple responsion of the idea 'reckless action committed against one's own kin'. . . . When she goes on to say that Orestes has barely escaped an unholy death . . . her language is not easily reconciled with her statement at 622–4 that she sprinkles holy water on the victims but others do the killing (cf. 40, 54). A possible explanation is that what she says here is meant to make her more clearly the counterpart of her father in the role he plays earlier in this same passage. A specific reminiscence may also be intended, since the verb she uses . . . is unparalleled in Euripides but is used by Aeschylus at *Ag.* 208 of the sacrifice of Iphigenia. At all events, this lyric exchange is so managed as to concentrate attention equally upon these two averted misfortunes while charting a pattern into which both will fit. It becomes clear that, in a sense she did not foresee, Iphigenia has performed the reenactment she envisaged at line 358. . . .

The re-enactment is closer than the imagined sacrifice of Menelaus and Helen because it too ends with the victim's escape from the knife. For Iphigenia this was a swift flight through the air; for Orestes the escape has just begun and will be less simple. Its completion will require the intrigue, the deception of Thoas, the flight to the ship, and Athena's intervention. In the development of this part of the tragedy, where a young man and woman flee before a savage pursuer, the paramount analogy is the flight of Pelops. But both of these myths in the background of the story, the sacrifice at Aulis and the flight of Pelops, end with an escape from death; to that extent both are mirrored in the conclusion of *I.T.* The connection with Aulis is made explicit at lines 1082–4; here Iphigenia asks Artemis to play once more the role she played at Aulis so that the present story will end as that one did. . . .

She asks Artemis to save them once again at 1398–1402, when the wave threatens to bring them back to shore. The active agents in her rescue, however, turn out to be three other gods: Athena, who stops the pursuit by Thoas; Poseidon, who stills the sea; and Apollo, by whose command Orestes is acting (1435–45). Iphigenia's repeated pleas do not cause any direct intervention by Artemis, though Artemis' acquiescence in the outcome can be assumed. Their principal effect, in reminding us of the goddess's more active role in the rescue at Aulis, is to keep alive the parallel between that former rescue and the more complicated present one, which began with the recognition and is now about to be completed.

Of the two legends reflected in the plot of *I.T.* the sacrifice at Aulis comes to the surface more often in the utterances of the characters. This is natural, since it is part of Iphigenia's own past, whereas the story of Pelops is a distant part of family tradition. Aulis means several things to Iphigenia: a betrayal of her hopes for marriage, a threat of death, an escape, and the beginning of exile. In the prologue of the play, the meaning she reads into her dream seems to put beyond remedy her separation from her family. In spite of her rescue at Aulis, the end result for her has not been happy, and it has left the need for another deliverance. In allowing his story to develop partly along the lines of that earlier averted sacrifice, Euripides has done more than fall into the familiar general pattern of kin-slaying averted by recognition; he has found a way to interweave two particular stories, in each of which Iphigenia has a role. While one story is acted out, the other emerges by reminiscence. Both arouse powerful emotions, and the lyric that follows the recognition is in equal measure about both. That dramatic moment is strengthened by the coincidence of theme which this interweaving allows: a brother has almost been killed by a sister as she once was by her father; brother and sister have until now each thought the other dead. Since each now knows the other's identity, their present emotions, like their past experiences, are matched and complementary. Earlier, while they were both still in ignorance, the recollection of Aulis was used to give the present story an ironic cast. For example, at 344ff., Iphigenia speaks of her harsh feelings towards the present victims; though these arise from the recent dream, her speech turns mainly on Aulis and the unfeeling treatment she suffered there from her father. We cannot fail to be made aware that at this moment her own actions are unwittingly moving in a pattern similar to his.

Unlike the sacrifice at Aulis, the courtship of Pelops and Hippodameia is no part of Iphigenia's personal experience and seems at first sight an unlikely cause of strong emotion in her or in Orestes. What sets it apart from the other legends of the house and gives it a claim to special relevance is the correspondence of form between its story and the plot of *I.T.*: both are escapes from a barbarous pursuer, and both end happily. Euripides, however, has also contrived a place for it in Iphigenia's life, in the form of the spear hidden in her chambers. Moreover, he has so placed the recollection of this token that it brings about the recognition and releases the strongest outburst of emotion in the play (822ff.). As far as anyone knows, the hidden spear is his own invention; as a means of recognition it stands well apart from the usual repertoire of necklaces, rings, scars, and articles of clothing. But if Euripides' purpose was to remind the audience of Pelops' victory over Oenomaus, nothing could have served better. The degree of artifice in all this should not be underestimated. A similar artifice, found at the start of the play, is that of beginning the family's history with the same victory, rather than earlier or later. In spite of their prominent positions, the two passages are short, and they are given little attention by modern scholars. Here the ancient spectator of *I.T.* undoubtedly had the advantage, since the legend of the contest with Oenomaus is known to have been a theme of sculpture, painting, and lyric in the fifth century and, it is likely, of at least one tragedy before *I.T.* In stating what that spectator was likely to be alert to we must therefore include the readily visible coincidences of plot line between one story and the other and at least one striking reminiscence of the Oenomaus legend in the staging of *I.T.* (72–5). Admittedly, the capacities of the ancient spectator to grasp and interpret such references are not well understood. The direct testimony about his knowledge of myths is inconclusive. It is clear, however, from tragic parodies in comedy and from the often fleeting allusions to myth in tragedy itself that poets habitually wrote as if for a knowing audience; and the relevant issue is the practice of poets rather than the culture of spectators. The long tradition of the *exemplum* in epic, lyric, and drama had, in any case, familiarized both poet and audience with the use of mythological paradigms. By convention, any legend can become part of the presentation of any other legend if it resembles it in some way and if mythical chronology allows its use. . . . But poetic logic is not always explicit, and not every paradigm will have its function announced so clearly. Euripides does not have Iphigenia or Orestes say after *I.T.* 826 that their fates have been similar, though by that point the similarity should be clear to us, as it was to Polyidus the sophist; and Pelops' contest is mentioned only before the pattern it foreshadows is complete.

My argument has been about a single Euripidean tragedy but may point the way to more general conclusions about recurrent plot patterns in Euripides. Among the many echoes of previous stories which these patterns bring into a play, some may be more important than others. . . . Some plots, admittedly, may lend themselves to nothing more than formal analysis, couched in general terms. Even here, we might keep in mind that our ability to interpret allusions and recognize particular analogies is limited by the loss to us of most of the literature known to Euripides. In deciding whether any of the many possible prototypes of an action has special significance, we should take into account Euripides' interest in the continuity of family history, a topic now given much less than its due. Euripidean characters and choruses, like those of Aeschylus and Sophocles, often mention family history and sometimes do so as an explanation or a model for the events being dramatized. These references are frequently dismissed as mere undigested relics of the tradition, since Euripides, unlike Aeschylus, is thought to be more interested in the inner life of his characters than in the actions of their ancestors. He is, of course; but there is no need to think of these interests as mutually exclusive or to judge Euripides incapable of combining them. It is clear, for example, that many of his characters retain a strong sense of their origins. Whenever they present their own experiences as the latest episodes of family history they call attention to family continuity and solidarity. One effect of this is to give added significance to any present crisis or success. Iphigenia's dream is threatening because it seems to mark the end of the house as well as the death of her brother. When she sees that she has misread it, both the house and her brother are in sight of rescue. The recurrence within that rescue of old patterns of action is a reminder of the continuity of the house and of the involvement of its fortunes in the outcome of the play. As a tragedy with a happy ending, *I.T.* contains more than it might seem to at first sight: not only a cheering sequel to the Orestes and Iphigenia legends, but also an alternative history of the Pelopids, one that begins and ends with a tale of success.

Source: Michael J. O'Brien, ''Pelopid History and the Plot of *Iphigenia in Taurus,*'' in *Classical Quarterly,* Volume 38, no. i, 1988, pp. 98–115.

SOURCES

Barlow, Shirley A. *The Imagery of Euripides,* Bristol Classical Press, 1971.

Caldwell, R. ''Tragedy Romanticized: The *Iphigenia Taurica*'' in *Classical Journal,* Vol. 70, 1974, pp. 23-40.

Decharme, Paul. *Euripides and the Spirit of His Dramas,* Kennikat Press, 1968.

Dodds, E. R. ''Euripides the Irrationalist'' in the *Classical Review,* Vol. 43, 1929, pp.97-104.

Dodds, E. R. *The Greeks and the Irrational,* University of California Press, 1951.

Faas, Ekbert. *Tragedy and After,* McGill-Queens University Press, 1984.

Grube, G. M. A. *The Drama of Euripides,* Methuen, 1961.

Halleran, Michael. *The Stagecraft in Euripides,* Barnes & Noble, 1985.

Hopper, R. J. *The Early Greeks,* Barnes & Noble, 1976.

Kerford, G. B. *The Sophistic Movement,* Cambridge, 1981.

Kott, Jan. *The Eating of the Gods: An Interpretation of Greek Tragedy,* Random House, 1970.

Melchinger, Siegfried. *Euripides,* Frederick Ungar, 1973.

Michelini, Ann Norris. *Euripides and the Tragic Tradition,* University of Wisconsin Press, 1987.

Nilsson, Martin P. *Greek Folk Religion,* University of Pennsylvania Press, 1961.

Rankin, H. D. *Sophists, Socratics and Cynics,* Canberra, 1983.

Segal, Erich, Editor. *Oxford Readings in Greek Tragedy,* Oxford University Press, 1983.

Vellacott, Phillip. ''Introduction'' in *The Bacchae and Other Plays,* translated by Vellacott, Penguin, 1973.

Vellacott, Phillip. *Ironic Drama,* Cambridge University Press, 1975.

Verrall, Arthur Woollgar. *Euripides the Rationalist: A Study in the History of Art and Religion,* Russell & Russell, 1967.

Whitman, Cedric. H. *Euripides and the Full Circle of Myth,* Harvard University Press, 1974.

FURTHER READING

Bieber, Margaret. *The Greek and Roman Theatre,* 1961.
A thorough description of the function and form of theatrical performances in ancient Greece and Rome.

Kitto, H. D. F. *The Greeks* Penguin Books, 1991.
This work describes the daily life, religion, philosophy, and political world of the Greeks, written in a conversational style with excerpts of famous speeches woven into the narrative to give a better sense of the Greek mind.

Lucas, F. L. *Euripides and His Influence,* Marshall Jones, 1923.
Lucas describes some of the innovations of Euripides's plays and how his work influenced later generations of writers.

Murray, Gilbert. *Euripides and His Age,* Oxford University Press, 1955.

A landmark work describing the historical context of Euripides's Athens, including the Peloponnesian War and the rise of the Sophists. Murray describes the function of such dramatic elements as the prologue, chorus, and messenger, and explains Euripides's unique use of them.

I, Too, Speak of the Rose

EMILIO CARBALLIDO

1965

Carballido's *I, Too, Speak of the Rose* is considered by many to be his greatest play and has become a masterpiece of the Mexican theatre. This play was first published in 1965 in *Revista de Belles Artes.* In 1966, it was first seen on stage at the Teatro Jimenez Rueda in Mexico City.

This one-act play was translated into English and published first in *Drama and Theatre* in 1969. The translation was by William D. Oliver. The play was produced in English in 1972 at San Fernando State College in Northridge, California, in a translation by Myrna Winer. This version of the play had the title *I Also Speak About the Rose.* This work received a couple of awards—the best play award in Mexico in 1967 and the Heraldo Prize.

I, Too, Speak of the Rose was also translated into French and produced in 1974. It received good reviews. It was also produced on French television.

Carballido's work has been influenced especially by playwrights such as Jean Anouilh, Tennessee Williams, and Arthur Miller. Like much of Carballido's work, *I, Too, Speak of the Rose* employs realistic elements but has clearly an expressionistic bent to it. The play uses at times very poetic language and employs the metaphor of the rose throughout. On another level, it, like much of Latin American theater, has a social agenda and explores the state of poverty and criticizes the varied responses society offers to the problem. On a

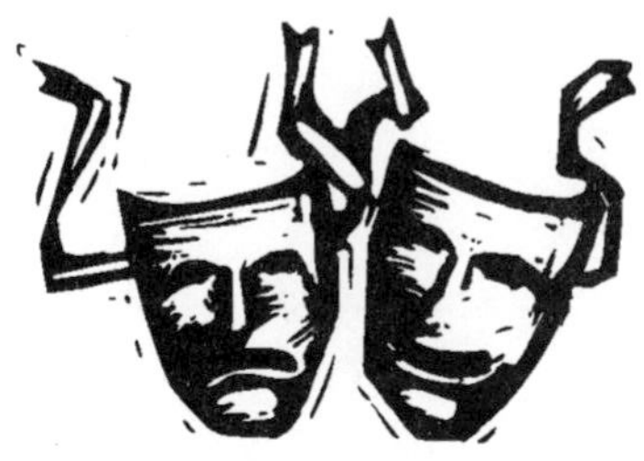

deeper level, the play explores questions about the nature of reality.

AUTHOR BIOGRAPHY

Emilio Carballido was born May 22, 1925, in Cordoba, Veracruz, Mexico. At the age of one, he moved to Mexico City with his mother. His father was a railroad man, and although he lived mostly with his mother, Carballido spent time with his father in 1939, living in a more rural environment, and occasionally traveling on the train with his father.

He started to write when he was young, but began to write most earnestly when he was twenty-one. Within a couple of years he had several produced and published plays under his belt.

When he turned twenty-five, he became a father, had his first commercial production of a play, and was sent to study in New York on a Rockefeller fellowship.

Carballido pursued an academic career, working as assistant director of the School of Theater at the University of Veracruz, and later as professor at the National University in Mexico City.

Carballido has been a prolific writer, producing a large body of dramatic works, including more than thirty-three one-act plays, more than five full-length plays, more than fifty screenplays, short stories, and novels. His dramatic works have regularly been honored with awards. Some of his awards include Centro Mexicano de Escritores fellowship, Universidad Nacional Autonoma de Mexico, Festival Regional of the Instituto Nacional de Bellas Artes, Instituto Internacional de Teatro, Ruiz de Alarcon Prize, and the Asociation de Criticos y Cronistas prize.

Carballido has spent time in the United States as a visiting professor at Rutgers University, the University of Pittsburgh, and the University of California. Some of the major influences on his writing have been Jean Giraudoux, Arthur Miller, Jean Anouilh, Sor Juana, and Ines de la Cruz.

Although not identified with a specific school of dramatic writing, Carballido is considered an important voice in Mexican theater and as part of an important movement in the theater towards neo realism. His work has been performed extensively in Mexico, and has also been produced in the United States, Spain, Germany, Switzerland, Belgium, Israel, Columbia, Venezuela, and Cuba.

PLOT SUMMARY

The play is set in Mexico City in the 1960s, with the focus on two poor young people who accidentally derail a train, and then have to face the consequences of punishment and everyone's varying perceptions of their deed. The play is broken up into twenty-one short scenes, opening with a spotlight on the Medium. She has a long poetic monologue in which she sees her heart as a sea anemone and claims she stores part of everything she's seen in herself. She says she receives information about events that will happen.

The next scene starts in the dark with the sound of a train crash, and a Newsboy hawks his papers with news about a train derailment. The play then shifts to a city scene with two young people, Tona and Polo, struggling to fish coins out of a telephone booth so they can buy candy. They tell a man who wants to use the booth that the phone is broken and eventually succeed at getting a coin but then gamble it away with Tona's bus fare on a bet with the candy vendor. Polo finds another coin and they buy candy. Tona asks Polo why he isn't going to school. He says it's because he doesn't have shoes and will not have money to get any for another week or so. They are joined by an older friend, Maximino, who clearly is watching out for them. He complains that his motorcycle isn't working but he is going to fix it at the garage where he works. Tona inspects his wallet and begs a picture from him which he signs. She says she will put it on her mirror. She makes fun of the photo of his girlfriend, saying she's cross-eyed.

The next scene finds Tona and Polo in a dump along with a scavenger who begs money so he can buy a drink. Tona gives him all their money. They find things like an old engine, thorny flowers, and a tub that would be good for planting flowers. They discover the tub is filled with concrete and put it on the tracks in the path of an approaching train to try and break out the concrete.

The Newsboy appears again, announcing that the train disaster was caused by delinquent children.

The Medium makes her second appearance, where she talks about dogs, cats, hens, and eggs. She also marvels at the wisdom of butterflies, bees, and snakes.

While the Newsboy again sells his papers, a lady and gentleman discuss the train derailment and the poverty that caused these children to be so barbaric.

The scene changes to a schoolroom where a teacher lectures about the evils of delinquency, using their classmate Polo as an example. In another scene, two university students discuss the train derailment. They are envious of the inspired action and the children's courage, thinking the action a premeditated one against the establishment.

Maximino gets a call at the garage where he is working. He asks his boss if he can have a little time off to go get Tona and Polo out of jail. His boss wonders about why they were playing around a train.

At the scene of the train derailment, a scavenger packs a large sack with goods from the derailed train. Several poor people come and gather food while wondering if this is stealing or not. They send for other family members to help them cart off as much as they can.

The Medium again appears to tell of a dream that two brothers had in two different cities. The dream instructed each brother to go to the other brother's house. They meet in the middle of the trip but are confused about where they are to fulfill the demands of the dream, so they stop where they are and build a little church and an altar where they pray and dance.

The Newsboy reappears, expanding the story, claiming that the damage from the train derailment is over a half million pesos.

In the next scene, Tona's mother and sister talk as her mother prepares to visit Tona in jail. They comment on her photo in the paper. Polo's mother visits him in jail, and moans over his imprisonment and berates him for being so stupid, not to have run from arrest. Their absent fathers are blamed for the children's delinquency.

The Newsboy again announces the news declaring that ''schizoid children'' have induced a public trauma.

The next two scenes are different interpretations of the event that happened. The first is presented by a Freudian psychologist who interprets all of the children's actions and the world before and at the time of the wreck, as having sexual significance. He sees the incidents as connected with repressed libido, or sexual energy.

A second professor, who is a Marxist economist, analyzes the experience based on class and economic factors. The children represent the lowest and poorest part of society. The action of the children, in his interpretation, is the natural result of years of oppression.

Maximino visits Tona in prison. Of course he wants to understand why she did it, but she is most interested in her picture in the paper and whether he will carry it in his wallet. He counsels her to avoid the other women in jail, whom she has found quite interesting. She asks him to carry only her photo in his wallet, not his cross-eyed girlfriend's. He agrees.

The scavengers appear again in the next scene at the dump. They are celebrating their abundance—the things they have scavenged from the train wreck. Some of the items they have traded for food and drink, including tequila, so they are becoming quite happy.

Lights come up on Maximino calling his girlfriend from the garage, trying to explain what he has been doing. He ends up calling her a cross-eyed bitch.

The next scene focuses on an Announcer with a rose to examine. He seems like the host of some kind of game show, with questions to answer. He asks his audience what he has and then goes into a monologue about a rose, wondering what it becomes when the petals drop. He goes further to examine a rose fiber and then asks of these three images—the whole rose, the rose petal, and the rose fiber—which is the true image? Which one is the real rose?

The Newsboy again comes and promises that the paper offers the total truth of the train crash. The Medium appears briefly. She explains the derailment, seeing the children as becoming part of all that surrounded them, and in the process, unearthing truth. Tona and Polo join the scene and dance ecstatically. And as the Medium replays the incident, with a view much different than the two professors, she shows the future—Polo owning his own garage and Tona marrying Maximino. The play ends with a sort of chant that links Tona, Polo, Maximino, and the Medium, and looks at the reality of a unity among them, ''a single beating heart.''

CHARACTERS

Announcer

Acting as a master of ceremonies, he energetically gives a lengthy monologue about the rose, the rose petal, and the rose fiber, and then poses questions to an unseen audience about what is the real rose.

Candy Vendor

He is selling candies and has no problem with gambling with Polo and Tona and taking away their money when he wins a coin toss.

Female Student

She is also a university student and is slightly envious of the action taken by the two children and the impact it had.

First Female Scavenger

She banters with the male scavengers, after having helped collect some of the food from the derailed train. She worries, though, whether they will be discovered by the police and blamed for stealing. She parties later with the other scavengers at the dump.

First Male Scavenger

He begs money from Tona to buy a drink. Later he discovers the food in the derailed train car and takes some. He runs off to share the good news of this plenty with others of his friends and family. Later he and his friends have a celebration with food and drink they bartered with goods from the derailed train.

First Professor

He is rather pompous and fastidious and imposes his own ideas on a current event, deciding what was really motivating Tona and Polo. He is a Freudian psychologist and interprets all of their actions based on this approach to understanding human behavior.

Gentleman

He sees the item in the news and criticizes the children as barbaric.

Maximino Gonzalez

He's a young man of nearly twenty-three who works in a garage. He has befriended Tona and Polo and looks out for them, even giving them money when they need it. He has an old motorcycle that isn't running but that he's going to fix. He defends his girlfriend's looks when Tona criticizes her but eventually turns against her, charmed and attracted by Tona's adoration of him. He is kind and caring and worries about the negative influences Tona is experiencing in jail.

Lady

She obviously likes sensationalism in the news. She thinks the poor are criminal, and that they are born that way without hope.

Male Student

A university student, he reads about the train derailment in the newspaper and declares it ''wild.''

The Medium

Dressed first in peasant garb, the Medium appears only four times in the play, and with each appearance her clothing becomes lighter and brighter and is finally all white. She is otherworldly and talks of things that seem unrelated to the central action of the play. She starts with a monologue about being a part of everything she sees and then comments on knowledge. She next appears with some old scientific illustrations and discusses animals in very poetic terms, including a warning about gold fish and a praise of butterflies. Later she relates a dream that two brothers had and the action it precipitated—a seemingly unconnected story. In the conclusion of the play she draws a totally different conclusion to the action in the play—a conclusion that connects the trains of thought she has laced throughout the work.

Newsboy

He starts out running on stage with his newspapers and calling out the news of the day. He is seen or sometimes just heard between a number of scenes later in the play, each time offering a different slant on the story of the train derailment. Throughout the play his newspaper changes, ending up with ancient parchment written in hieroglyphics when he offers the truth.

Paca

She is Tona's sister. She wants to visit her sister but is enlisted to babysit her younger sisters while her mother visits Tona instead. She seems a little amused about the event and the newspaper coverage and sends her sister a pin that she likes.

Don Pepe

He is a Spaniard, the owner of the garage where Maximino works. He appears kind and understanding when he allows Maximino to go visit his newly imprisoned friends.

Polo

Like Tona, Polo is an average school child. He is fourteen years old. His truancy from school is based in his shame and embarrassment about his poverty. He doesn't have shoes to wear and he knows the teacher will inspect the students for polished shoes. Although he is poor, he is resourceful and knows how to find money, or fish it out of phone booths. But he is easily relieved of his money when presented with an opportunity to gamble and hopefully win much more. This happens a couple of times but he accepts it gracefully since he had nothing in the beginning. He, like Tona, isn't particularly bad, just unsupervised with too much time on his hands. His putting the cement filled tub on the rails was not premeditated, and his lack of fear and unwillingness to run when the accident occurred illustrate his purity of heart.

Polo's Mother

She visit's him in jail and what she's concerned about is whether she'll lose her job because of her son's notoriety. She berates him for being as bad as his no-good father but then sinks to criticizing herself for spoiling him.

A Poor Boy

He discovers the overturned opened car from the derailed train and wants to steal from it. He goes to get sacks to carry the food.

A Poor Girl

She is scared that she and the boy will get caught taking things from the train but is assured that there is no one watching them, so she makes off with some food and gets help.

A Poor Man

He is certain that taking things from the abandoned train is stealing but is willing to help the poor woman with her sacks. He really doesn't care if it's stealing or not, because it's needed food—corn and beans.

A Poor Woman

She is guilt-stricken and tries to rationalize that this isn't stealing since there is no guard at the train. She does not let her guilt keep her from loading up sacks and carting them off. She decides to tell other family members about this abundance.

Second Female Scavenger

She joins the other scavengers around the fire at the dump, enjoying what they have to eat and drink.

Second Male Scavenger

He is in the scavenger party at the dump and finds time to flirt with the female scavengers while enjoying their plenty.

Second Professor

This professor is less precise in his dress and demeanor but has a view of the world which colors his interpretation of the train derailment. He sees everything through his Marxist economist rose-colored glasses and sees all of the children's actions as evidence of their social consciences and as a significant political protest.

Teacher

She is an unsympathetic and harsh character who uses the train derailment to try and get appropriate behavior from her class.

Tona

A poor Mexican schoolgirl of twelve, she has little parental supervision and little money but plenty of time to hang out with her friend. She easily skips school, and although the press immediately labels her and her friend as delinquents, she is really just an ordinary girl who wants to have friends and play. Her friendship with Polo is not without problems—they bicker back and forth and blame each other when something doesn't go as expected. But she has a good heart and is very willing to share her bus fare to buy something for them both. She is generous also when giving money to one of the scavengers. She has a crush on Maximino and the feeling comes out in criticism of his motorcycle and his girlfriend. She begs a photo of him and wants him to sign it so she can put it on her mirror. Later she is pleased to see he is carrying her photo from the newspaper. She is impressed with the cell mates she has, who seem a lot more real and interesting than the people she meets normally.

Tona's Mother

She is poor and trying to raise her children by herself. She is somewhat bewildered about what has happened and struggles to get time to go to see her daughter in prison. She doesn't trust the prison guards or the system and is worried about Tona missing school.

Woman Peddler

She is selling food and prepares jicama with chile for the children.

THEMES

Social Criticism

Social criticism is often embedded in or clearly on the surface of Latin American theater. *I, Too, Speak of the Rose* does this by making a commentary on the social conditions of the times (1965) as well as questioning the solutions to the problems.

Although the play commences with a Medium, who throughout the play presents a broader, other–worldly point of view, it is soon clear that the play focuses on the lives of the disadvantaged. Tona and Polo are representative children in Mexico City who are clearly lacking in parental supervision and in financial resources. When Tona asks Polo why he isn't in school that day, he responds that it is because of his lack of shoes. He will have to go to school barefoot and stand in line when the teacher inspects each student to check if his shoes are polished. He says, "I'll be damned if I am going to polish my feet."

So Tona and Polo work to find money just to buy candy. As Carballido proceeds with the play, he clearly paints a picture of the lowest level of society. These young people may be denied an education because of their poverty.

There are other glimpses of the plight of the poor in the play. The scavengers at the dump, and those taking advantage of the derailed train, show a bottom rung of the socioeconomic structure that could not survive without the castoffs.

More of this is shown when the mothers of the children deal with the reality of this offense. Tona's mother is worried whether there will be consequences for her taking time off from work to go visit her daughter in jail. In the same way, Polo's mother worries for her job. Will she be fired because of what her son has done?

The scavengers demonstrate some concern for right and wrong and question whether emptying the derailed train car is really stealing. They decide ultimately that it isn't, and then the goods on the car are redistributed. Carballido looks at the derailment of the railroad car from many different angles and examines the social significance of each of them. The Newsboy shouts throughout about the varying views of this event. And although he makes some criticism about poverty and how the poor are treated, Carballido is not totally one-sided in his view. In fact, he almost pokes fun at the Marxist professor interpreting the incident as a political event and that the innocent action of these two young people was a major political statement. He most clearly raises questions about the lack of power and control and the state of the poor in Mexico, but he also does not rely on one system to answer or solve the problem. This play represents a question more than an answer.

He attacks the school system that would willingly exclude students just because they don't have enough money for school. He takes issue with teachers that are without sympathy. Also in the line of his criticism are university professors who will bend events to support their views. He notes the situation of single mothers who are struggling to raise children without support. And he also alludes to the effect of Yankee imperialism.

Truth

Truth is not singular, Carballido tries to tell the audience in *I, Too, Speak of the Rose*. In fact, there are many sides to truth. Truth is explained as a kaleidoscope, as the audience is shown ever shifting interpretations and understandings of one singular event. As the lines between truth and non truth are blurred, so the lines between reality and fantasy. Carballido enters the minds of key players in this incident and shows the inner thoughts of these characters, or what could have been the inner thoughts.

The reader or audience member is left without a firm foundation, wondering about the correct interpretation of the event. Eventually the conclusion may be that the many views of the incident show that there are many truths to consider. The Announcer points out a rose, then a lone petal of a rose, and then a microscopic view of rose fiber. Which is the real rose, he asks. Which is the correct view? The viewer is left with this enigmatic question, and perhaps with an answer that all views are truth in some way, just as all of the views of the rose really are the rose.

STYLE

Monologues

Carballido begins *I, Too, Speak of the Rose* with a lengthy monologue by the Medium, which sets the tone for the rest of this one-act play. The action is often stopped and explanation is made of what is happening, or commentary is heard on the significance of it. This approach goes back to the Greek theater, when the action of the play occurred offstage. Often it was the Chorus that explained what had happened and at times the importance of it, before the main characters responded to the news and anguished over outcomes.

Monologues are found in Shakespeare's work often, like Hamlet's gloomy monologues or Macbeth's tortured ones. With these, the audience finds out more of what is happening within the mind of the character. A contemporary example of the use of monologue is found in Tennessee William's *Glass Menagerie* when Tom Wingfield engages in lengthy monologues as he introduces the audience to his memory, which becomes the present action of the play.

Within Carballido's play, monologues stop the action of the play, and in fact break the illusion that the theater creates—the illusion that the audience is in the space and time in which the action is supposed to occur and that the actions and characters are real. The character of the Medium seems to exist outside of the play, or outside of what might be called the frame of the play. She at times seems to be talking about different things than the main body of the play because other scenes and commentary speak directly of the train derailment. She doesn't speak of it directly but is more philosophical or spiritual in her reflections. When she appears, the audience is reminded that it is watching a play, that this is not real, it is only a representation of something. Monologues are used for the discussions by the two professors, as well as the Announcer. The Newsboy is woven throughout and has brief monologues where he is ostensibly selling his wares, but for the purposes of the playwright, announces a shift of perception of the event of the train derailment. Monologues wound together with other dialogue create a mosaic effect and further support Carballido's attempt to get the viewer to question reality and the nature of truth.

Nonconventional Style

Carballido's work often balances between realism and fantasy. He makes quick scene changes using changed lighting or blackouts to mark the change. The scenes are short and these short bursts that are punctuated by blackouts create almost a sense of images being flashed on a screen. The play presents the longest scene near the beginning, with a very realistic look at the life of the children and what was happening that afternoon for them in Mexico City.

TOPICS FOR FURTHER STUDY

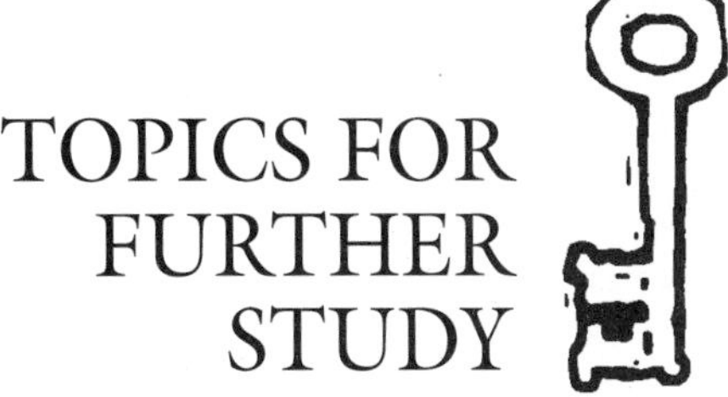

- Research the beating of Rodney King by Los Angeles police officers. Although there was undeniable evidence, a videotape, that the police officers did beat him, still they were acquitted. Discuss the possible different interpretations of the videotape that are possible.
- Compare and contrast this play with Peter Weiss's *Marat/Sade*. Which play makes a stronger social commentary and why do you think that?
- Investigate the work of two philosophers who discuss the nature of reality and truth. Try to distill their ideas in a couple of sentences. How does this compare with the message found in this play?
- Investigate the economic situation in Mexico at this time. How does this compare to the economic situation in 1965? Have improved trade agreements with the United States helped Mexico's economy?

The scenes switch to things that might have happened, so the viewer sees the response of academics whose ideas are then played on as if in a fantasy. So the Freudian psychologist presents a view of the repressed sexuality in these young people and places words in their mouths. The audience views his fantasy. Then the Marxist takes the very same scene and rewrites the script. The action is the same but the words are different. And again it is a fantasy. He is imagining what they might have been saying.

The scene with the announcer and his three views of the rose is clearly a scene from the imagination, juxtaposed with the realistic scenes of Tona and Polo in prison.

Some people have wanted to place labels on his work, but Carballido has resisted that. Although he avoids in this play a traditional theatrical structure, he is not easily pegged. The scenes where the children are replaying the events leading up to the derailment are certainly in the imagination or a sort of fantasy of the professors interpreting the action. But then the playwright pulls the play back to some very realistic scenes, keeping the viewer on edge.

HISTORICAL CONTEXT

It was the best of times; it was the worst of times. Just like Charles Dickens's description of the French Revolution, so too were the 1960s in the United States. The Democratic-controlled government made bold strides towards trying to deal with poverty and racism. The year 1965 was the year when the term "The Great Society" was coined and large appropriations were made to provide for programs to help the poor. And although concerned on paper with poverty at home, the U.S. government discouraged companies from selling wheat to the Soviet Union, which had experienced a devastating crop failure, by mandating that half of sales would have to be shipped in U.S. owned vessels. This would make the wheat significantly more expensive. Civil Rights legislation that had been passed was supported by concerned citizenry confronting racists and segregationist practices, forcing the government to deal with it. Sometimes, however, these protests took very violent turns resulting in the death of civil rights workers. At other times race riots in cities left lives lost and property destroyed.

But while the U.S. government was making attempts to better things for the poor within U.S. boundaries, it was at the same time engaging in a growing military action in southeast Asia, an initiative that was uninvited and was denounced by some countries as being clearly imperialistic. This war in Vietnam was not without opposition in the United States as well as in other parts of the world, with much of the protest coming from students and from the arts community. The Civil Rights movement and the anti-war movement grew throughout the 1960s, creating a sense that some sort of revolution could happen within the borders of the United States, not just in less stable countries like those South of the border.

I, Too, Speak of the Rose creates a view of life on the lower levels of society in that tumultuous decade in the country right to the South. And while Timothy Leary was pushing psychedelic drugs meant to alter reality, the play is questioning what people perceive and what reality is. In popular culture, the rock group The Rolling Stones had major success with the song "I Can't Get No Satisfaction." The Grateful Dead started in San Francisco and was soon connected with both psychedelic drugs and psychedelic colors. Other popular singing groups included the Beatles, Simon and Garfunkel, Sonny and Cher, Bob Dylan, and Big Brother and the Holding Company with Janis Joplin. The message behind much of the music was either a criticism of society, or an attempt to escape it.

CRITICAL OVERVIEW

Theater in Latin America is known to be a force for social change and so is often looked at not as entertainment but as a vehicle to make a statement. Carballido's work fits well within this tradition. His work is what can be called socially engaged.

Eugene Skinner in *Dramatists in Revolt: The New Latin America Theater* commented on *I, Too, Speak of the Rose* and labeled this work a masterpiece. "It delineates the repressive effects of ideologies and institutions through popular satire and alternating scenes of commentary and representation." For Skinner this play seems a complete work and shows what theater should do. Margaret Sayers Peden in *Emilio Carballido* agreed with Skinner on

COMPARE & CONTRAST

- **1965:** The military action in Vietnam escalates with major U.S. bombing missions on North Vietnamese targets and a doubling of draft calls. This is a war that is looked on by many outsiders as an imperialistic action and based mostly on economic interests in the United States. Antiwar rallies attract crowds in major cities and on college campuses. Most of the antiwar support comes from the young.

  Today: The Near East is the most potentially explosive section of the world, with Iraqi dictator Saddam Hussein regularly acting in a threatening manner and the United States trading threats sometimes accompanied by bombing missions. Although the Gulf War of the early 1990s sparked antiwar protest, there is little response to any aggressive military actions.

- **1965:** Martin Luther King, Jr., and more than 700 civil rights demonstrators are arrested for protesting Alabama state regulations for voter registration in Selma. This sparks further violence in the South and serves as a landmark in the civil rights struggle.

  Today: While the Civil Rights movement has made great advances, there is still a great deal of prejudice and injustice toward minorities in America.

- **1965:** Harvard psychology professor Timothy Leary, then 44, publishes *The Psychedelic Reader,* advising readers to use drugs and ''turn on, tune in, drop out.''

  Today: Drug use continues to be popular with many people. The emphasis, however, seems to be on the ''turn on,'' with fewer users actually employing drugs as a spiritual path. Drug use in the 1990s is often recreational. Yet it too frequently is symptomatic of social and economic malaise, with many people turning to drugs to escape the harshness of their reality.

- **1965:** The International Society for Krishna Consciousness is founded in New York by Swami Prabhupada. Followers can be seen with shaved heads and saffron robes chanting ''Hare Krishna.'' The way to enlightenment is through an ascetic life of devotion and spreading the truth, not through drugs.

  Today: Religious and spiritual cults have taken a dark turn. Many such organizations are accused of kidnapping and brainwashing their members. Other groups, such as the Branch Davidians, Heaven's Gate, and Aum Shinri Kyo (''supreme truth''), have turned to violence and mass suicide.

- **1965:** The National Endowment for the Arts (NEA) and the Humanities (NEH) is founded and funded by the Congress. The organizations are meant to encourage and support the growth of the arts and of individual artists as a way to preserve and endorse culture.

  Today: The NEA and the NEH struggle each year for Congressional funding. Both agencies have been under siege by right-wing Republican groups which have been offended by the work of some artists who have received grants.

---

the significance of this play. She said it was ''the most important one-act play written by Carballido, and one of his best plays of any length.''

In the *Latin American Theatre Review* Sandra Messinger Cypess said ''Carballido's one-act play has one of the most provocative titles of the many suggestive works'' by this playwright. Diana Taylor in the *International Dictionary of Theatre: Plays* saw this work as being about discourse, or the nature of discourse. ''Discourses not only stem from differing traditions and create their own realities, but they also vie for explanatory power and authority.'' She saw this work as making a statement about a lessened importance of a eurocentric (white European) society as represented by the idea and talk of the professors. What emerges is another way of seeing things, or many ways of seeing things, which may be rooted in an oral culture, not one based on writing.

Jacqueline Eyring Bixler in the *Latin American Theatre Review* commented on later works by Carballido that gave evidence of characteristics which were consistent throughout his body of work. She mentioned two patterns of audience participation, that of fusion and that of fission. This latter, the fission, ''produces an opposition or fission of impressions, which leads to a final fusion of concept. The pattern of fission, which is the one that characterizes Carballido's theatre, is naturally the more challenging for the audience, who is left to close the fissure, or bridge the conceptual gap.'' She saw this as allowing the audience to have a moment of seeing discovery. For her, this was participatory theatre, because the audience adds to the meaning of the piece, as they make the connection conceptually between the different levels of reality that exist in the play.

From the very beginning of his career Carballido attempted to mix fantasy and realism. According to George Woodyard in the *Encyclopedia of Latin American History and Culture,* he has done that in new ways in *I, Too, Speak of the Rose.* At the same time he has been involved with experimental works ''in his search for ways to express a Mexican reality deeply rooted in tradition.''

In the play, Tona reflects on the star and its connection with the ancient primitive hunter and the artwork he produced on the walls of his cave. Skinner sees this as a statement the playwright makes about the real function of art. ''The artist produces an image that persists long after the event or person represented ceases to exist. The sole function of the artist is to affirm . . . the existence of his contemporaries as a complex web of creative potential.'' Peden, who has written extensively about Carballido's works, saw his most important contribution as being the personal blend of humor and fantasy in a realistic framework. These ''create plays that transcend the specifically realistic and restrictively Mexican to achieve a theater that can be called modern, contemporary, and universal.'' At the same time, she said, the plays stay rooted in Mexican tradition.

Carballido himself is very conscious of the interrelationship of content and form. ''Content and form are exact equivalents one separates for purposes of analyses, for practical reasons, but the idea that they may be separated is fallacious; it would be like separating the heart from the rest of the bodily organs.'' He has done much experimenting and Peden labeled him the greatest innovator in form in the theater since Sor Juana.

He allows his audience or readers to make some conclusions. Emmaunuel Carballo has called him a ''demonstrative'' rather than a ''directive'' writer. The characters that he creates have a certain amount of freedom or autonomy but they see things with the playwright's judgments or biases.

Though critics talk about his realistic work, the playwright does not see it in that way. ''The majority of the things I do are not realistic; these days a minimum of my work is of that style. Many pieces have narrators, or have no set, or work through a series of expressionistic or didactic or surrealistic motivations.'' Peden praised his social satiricism and keen social criticisms. ''Carballido has changed the course of Mexican theatre.'' Critics seem to agree that both in style and content Carballido has contributed significantly to the literature of his country.

CRITICISM

Etta Worthington

Worthington is a playwright and a teacher. In this essay she examines the use of metaphor in Carballido's play and how it enriches his message

The poetic imagery in *I, Too, Speak of the Rose* creates a rich tapestry as a background to the social criticism on the surface of the play, which makes the work much richer than just a political tract. Eugene Skinner in *Dramatists in Revolt: The New Latin American Theater* says that *I, Too, Speak of the Rose* ''further elaborates the concept of human existence as a complex web of interrelationships through a fusion of realistic and poetic techniques.''

This is clear from the very beginning when one is greeted with the Medium, a woman who wears simple peasant garb but speaks in poetic language. She weaves a teasing web of language, comparing knowledge to a heart that beats and distributes its currents into various canals. She compares her heart to a timid knock on the door, to a chick trying to get out of its cell, and then to a sea anemone. She sees herself and her memory as a collector of all things,

- First published in Spanish as *El Norte* in 1959, this novel by Carballido is the story of a woman growing old and her young lover, who discovers how alone he really is in the world. It was published in English in 1968 as *The Norther,* translated by Margaret Sayers Peden.
- The famous Mexican muralist Diego Rivera died in 1959, but he was a contemporary of Carballido. *My Art, My Life: An Autobiography* is a 1991 reprint of this work released in 1960. Rivera's work chronicles the struggles and triumphs of the workers, and evidence a strong leftist orientation.
- The work of Mexican novelist Carlos Fuentes is known internationally. Although he is also a playwright and a critic, his fiction has won him the most acclaim. *Burnt Water* is a translation of twelve of his stories written from 1954 and published in English in 1980.
- Many call Mexican poet Octavio Paz the foremost poet in Latin America. His work *Selected Poems*, published in 1979, gives an interesting overview of his work. He was at times a diplomat as well, and although a socialistic in his leanings, he was quite critical of the leftist movement.
- *The Golden Thread and Others* is a collection of nine of Carballido's plays translated by Margaret Sayers Peden. Published in 1979, the play *The Intermediate Zone* may be most similar stylistically to *I, Too, Speak of the Rose.*

---

and as a collector, she assimilates everything into herself, or is assimilated.

When she next appears in the play, she comes with a book full of animal and plant images and she ruminates about many. She thinks about man and his sense of property. Then she considers other animals. There is the cat who offers sacrifices—captured mice—and who also connects with the mysteries of the universe. There is the hen, the producer of eggs. There are snakes, gold fish, butterflies, bees. And the images she produces brings us back to the core thing—knowledge. What bees know. What she knows.

She reappears later to relate a seemingly disconnected story of two dreamers and their similar dreams. This seems like a parable that spins our minds off onto other tangents. But at the end of the play, she takes her metaphors and tries to explain. "Now I'm going to explain the accident," she says. They children are gaining enlightenment. They are becoming everything around them. "they understand . . . they see."

She ends the play and her explanation of the significance of the event by pointing out how all human beings are connected. She goes back to a metaphor she began with, the heart. "Let us listen to the beating in each and every hand of the mystery of our single heart." "Through these references, Carballido proposes a mystical definition of knowledge; he intimates that knowledge posses qualities of beat and diffusion, and that these qualities originate in the pulsing center of the universe, the human heart," writes Margaret Sayers Peden in *Emilio Carballido.*

There is more than just the Medium's' poetic language in this work. At the core of the play is the metaphor of the rose. This image is not brought out too often, but it is very strong when it appears. The first encounter is, of course, the rose in the title. One is expecting to experience the rose since one has been warned it is coming. It is, says Peden, "an extended metaphor concerning the nature of reality."

The rose first appears in the dump where Tona and Polo are looking for something of value to scavenge. Tona finds an engine and some flowers. There is no explanation of the kind of flower, but she admits to being pricked by the flowers, and so the thorny stem of a rose comes to mind. It is an

"THE POETIC IMAGERY IN *I, TOO, SPEAK OF THE ROSE* CREATES A RICH TAPESTRY AS A BACKGROUND TO THE SOCIAL CRITICISM ON THE SURFACE OF THE PLAY, WHICH MAKES THE WORK MUCH RICHER THAN JUST A POLITICAL TRACT."

image of a perfect rose, a symbol of love and beauty, in the midst of a garbage dump. This juxtaposition of images is shocking and jarring. But this juxtaposition is part of the message of the play, the plain and simple beauty in the context of unpleasant situations. This is the reality to which Peden refers.

The idea of the rose is mentioned by the first professor, who examines the complexity of self and likens this to the rose, that unfolds its petals. He is searching for the core, the root, which for him is in the sometimes repressed and unexpressed sexuality of the individual.

The image of the rose is again brought into the play when the scavengers are together and one man sings to a woman a little song calling her a rose of the few. It is a song about making love and the images of love are rather common and base and sung to another scavenger in a makeshift shelter at the dump. Here the image of the rose is common and banal.

The rose comes up again with the announcer. Suddenly the viewer is put in almost a game show environment, where one must compete for prizes, and three images are shown: the rose in total, a rose petal, and a microscopic view of the fiber of a rose. The question then is posed: which is the real rose? Pursing the imagery of the rose and what it represents, one must then ponder this symbol of love and beauty and wonder at the evidence. Is life perfect and complete like the whole rose—is this the real picture, is this the real truth? Or is it the petal, the small dropped leaf that makes one think of the total flower, a part that has some of the smell and texture of the whole, and which one can close his eyes and imagine. Is this the moment in life when one experiences love and beauty—is this segment of the whole the true picture of the rose? Or is it the small fiber of the rose, like a fragment of human life, the beauty and love that at a daily microscopic level, without grandeur, without sweet smell, and without perfect construction, makes up real life? The relationship of Polo and Tona seems evidence of that rose fiber. It is a simple and at times painful thing. But it is, as much as any grander expression, something that is real and of value.

The action of the play focuses on a train derailment, the events that lead up to it and the results of the derailment. Although this event doesn't call attention to itself in the play as a metaphor, it is another core metaphor that runs throughout the work.

What does the derailment represent, or what is derailed? A derailment clearly is an abrupt halt to something that was on a rail, that was certain to happen. What is derailed? Many things. The lives of the children are derailed. Their regular life of going to school and playing has come to a jarring halt as they are faced with the enormity of the consequences of their actions. They will never be the same. Perhaps, in a way, this represents when their childhood is derailed. But at the end one has a bit of hope when the Medium gives a glimpse into the futures of Polo and Tona. Although their childhood and innocence have been derailed, their lives as adults are not without hope. Perhaps, in fact, the derailment is necessary for them to get onto another rail and take the trip towards adulthood.

More can be thought of as derailed in this work. There is a certain redistribution of goods that takes place when the train is derailed and the cars filled with food are off the track with their doors open. Something that seems sinister and bad contains something good as the poor rob the coffers of those better endowed with wealth and create a little bit more of life. This is a revolution on a small scale. So the derailment can represent a sort of revolution with the rebalancing effect that occurs in the economy.

Much of Mexican and Latin American theater attempts to make social criticism significant. This is certainly true for *I, Too, Speak of the Rose.* One can sense Carballido's biting and sarcastic criticism throughout the play. He aims his sights at many targets. He points to the school system, one without sympathy, that unfairly discourages the poorest from participating. Higher education also is criticized. The professors use their lecterns to impose their singular view of the world on the students.

Unfortunately their view severely distorts the truth of the actual event, and thus the viewer starts to question knowledge and existing systems of knowledge as we know them. Carballido even asks the audience to question the source of news as represented by the newsboy whose presentation of the news goes through a significant metamorphosis.

Although viewers will grasp Carballido's social criticism, they will stay much longer with the work, toying with the metaphors, with the poetic language, and questioning the nature of knowledge and reality. They will go with him to a deeper place where he questions not just social structures and politics but the very nature of knowledge and reality, and ultimately truth.

Source: Etta Worthington, for *Drama for Students,* Gale, 1998.

Diana Taylor

In this article, Taylor provides an overview of I, Too, Speak of the Rose.

I, Too, Speak of the Rose (Yo también hablo de la rosa) is a play set in modern Mexico City. Throughout the play only one thing happens—two lower-class children, Tona and Polo, derail a freight train carrying food and go to jail for an unspecified (though we assume brief) period of time. The rest of the play's 21 scenes focus on the process and politics of interpretation. For the police, the incident is a criminal offense. For the scavangers picking up the food, the strewn bounty is a miracle of good fortune. The mothers blame their children's vagrancy on the absent father. The school teacher refers to Tona and Polo as truants. For the university students reading the newspaper, the event is an anarchistic, brilliant act. The bourgeois couple, reading the same paper, refer to the children as ''little savages, that's what they are. All of them. They're all a bunch of savages.'' A Freudian psychologist expounds on the repressed libidinal component to the act. The Marxist economist interprets the destruction as the logical outburst of an oppressed class. What does the derailment mean? Whose interpretation or discourse gains authority?

While many perspectives are introduced in the play, not all of them are equal. The Intermediaria (Medium), an indigenous, or ''mestizo,'' peasant woman, dominates the play. She appears four times, linking the episodic scenes together by telling stories that indirectly elucidate the incident involv-

"CARBALLIDO'S HUMOROUS PLAY DOES NOT CONDEMN OR ENDORSE ANY ONE PERSPECTIVE. RATHER, IT SHOWS ALL OF THEM AS CO-EXISTING SIMULTANEOUSLY WITHIN A HIGHLY COMPLEX SOCIETY."

ing the two children. Interestingly, however, her perspective is not valorized as correct, but as indispensible in illuminating Mexico's racial and cultural mestizage. Carballido does not suggest that she knows more than the professors, but that her source of knowledge differs from theirs. She begins the play claiming ''I know many things!'' As she narrates what she knows—herbs, faces, crowds, the texture of rocks, books, pages, illusions, roads, events—we come to understand that her knowledge represents a mode of perception different in kind and origin from the ''scientific,'' objective knowledge posited by the eurocentric professors. Her epistemological framework is primarily of an oral tradition, conserved by memory, and passed on by word of mouth: ''I also retain memories, memories which once belonged to my grandmother, my mother or my friends . . . many which they, in turn, heard from friends and old, old people.'' Her orality is both a *product of* and a *producer of* a network of communication, and establishes her central position in it as much as literacy shapes the professors. The philosophic schools which shape the professors' perception, and the literacy maintaining it, do not, by and large, form the traditions within which most Mexicans have lived, and to different degrees still continue to live. In a country like Mexico, characterized by the co-existence of literary and primary oral cultures, consciousness changes according to how people receive and store information and knowledge.

The most immediate distinction between the oral and literary cultures we see in the play lies in the relationship between knower and known. The Intermediaria's knowledge cannot be called ''objective''—it is not empirically verifiable or in any way outside or disconnected from herself as knower.

Unlike the professors with their methodological and causal framework, she does not aspire to the Cartesian ideal of objectification. From her first line in her first speech, the Intermediaria approaches knowledge reflexively, comparing it to her heart which, with its ''canals that flow back and forth'' connects her with the rest of the world. As the fluidity of her speech shows, her way of knowing is anything but isolating or reductive—each idea opens a way to another, defying the possibility of any conclusion. The Intermediaria's role demonstrates the supreme importance of the speaker in an oral culture. In contrast, the professors' way of knowing is shown as eccentric in that they stand outside and removed from the source of their knowledge and information which now, in the literate society, lies in books and newspapers. Their physical presence is gratuitous; they only read or speak what has already been prepared in writing. They maintain a marginal, alienated position in both the acquisition and transmission of their knowledge. Alienation, then, is not an existential given, but a product of the knower/known relationship. The separation between knower/known changes, reduces and fragments human experience. Ironically, then, while literacy allows us to know more as well as more accurately, with greater abstraction and sophistication, it simultaneously widens the gap between knower and known.

Carballido's humorous play does not condemn or endorse any one perspective. Rather, it shows all of them as co-existing simultaneously within a highly complex society. If he condemns any position whatsoever it is only the folly of those who maintain that there *is* only one correct interpretation. His ludicrous characters (such as the Announcer of the game show in which the audience is asked to identify the one ''authentic'' image of a rose), illustrate not only the fallacy, but the potentially inquisitorial violence, of imposing any one view at the expense of others. There is only one valid response, the Announcer asserts; the rest ''should be stricken from the books so that they will be forgotten forever. And any person who divulges them should be pursued by law. All those who believe in these false images should be supressed and isolated!''

I, Too, Speak of the Rose is a discourse about the nature of discourse. Discourses not only stem from differing traditions and create their own realities, but they also vie for explanatory power and authority. Historically, western theories have displaced Mexican and Latin American worldviews. In this play Carballido moves the marginalized experience to the very center of inquiry. This re-centering constitutes an important, liberating act for, by the same move, the eurocentric view (the professors) receeds, seen to be reduced in importance. Changing the relationship between the marginal and the dominant can change history, for as Hayden White points out in *Tropics of Discourse,* histories ''are not only about events but also about the possible set of relationships that those events can be demonstrated to figure.''

I, Too, Speak of the Rose is then a theatrical collage of many conflicting views of an accident and proposes a method of inquiry into the politics of perception and interpretation. Like the rose of the title, which Carballido depicts as a complicated and interconnected entity inextricable from (and inconceivable without) its multiple parts—stalk, petals, and fibers—the play too is made up of numerous, yet irreducible, interpretations.

Source: Diana Taylor, ''*I, Too, Speak of the Rose,*'' in *The International Dictionary of Theatre I: Plays,* edited by Mark Hawkins-Dady, St. James Press, 1992, pp. 353–54.

Eugene R. Skinner

In this excerpt, Skinner delineates much of the action in Carballido's play, offering his interpretation of the major events and the play's themes and symbols.

Yo también hablo de la rosa (I Too Speak of the Rose) synthesizes earlier thematic concerns and technical achievements of Carballido. This one-act masterpiece further elaborates the concept of human existence as a complex web of interrelationships through a fusion of realistic and poetic techniques, as in *La hebra de oro.* Also, it delineates the repressive effects of ideologies and institutions through popular satire and alternating scenes of commentary and representation, as in *Silencio, pollos pelones, ya les van a echar su maíz.* Finally, it succeeds in realizing both an explicit statement on the function of the theater and an exemplary model of total theater.

The action occurs in Mexico City during the present, and the central realistic event is the derailment of a freight train by two adolescents, Tona and Polo. The technique and structure of the play focus the spectator's attention on the process of interpretation rather than on the event itself. There are eighteen basic scenes with twenty-nine characters portrayed by thirteen actors. Transitions are fluid and rapid, effected by lighting and the commentary of the Medium and the Newsboy.

The initial scene establishes a nonrealistic atmosphere. A spot comes up on the Medium, dressed in peasant costume. In her monologue, she conjures up an image of her heart. The heart, like the rose of the play's title, symbolizes human existence, complex and fragile, but also precise and powerful. The Medium herself is an objectification of the social function of theater. In the final lines of her monologue, she outlines the following process: events are perceived and images formulated, and the latter are then communicated and contemplated. The artist provides a representation of the people and their surroundings, an image that is physical and integral as opposed to the abstract and fragmentary analyses employed by scientists and politicians to manipulate reality. With each appearance the Medium's costume becomes increasingly lighter in color until the pure white of the final scene. This externalizes the process of clarification through which art succeeds in transcending the chaos of diverse partial visions in a total concrete image.

During a blackout following the monologue, the event is first presented sensorially: the sound of the derailment, silence, lightning flashes; then the Newsboy: "Get your papers now! Delinquents derail a train!" Although apparently a neutral medium for the news, he varies his salespitch according to the version he is vending. The Medium, however, remains constant in her refusal to offer a limited fragmentary interpretation.

Scene 2 provides a realistic representation and employs a linear progression: street scene, derailment, effects of the derailment. The behavior of the young truants is spontaneous. They steal some coins from a public telephone, and then they decide to buy some candy. Their encounters with the Candy Vendor, the Old Woman selling *jícama,* and the young mechanic Maximino develop a contrast between human relationships motivated by self-interest and, in the latter case, mutual respect. Later, at the dump, Tona and Polo give their remaining coins to a Scavenger. Objects that they find, scrap iron and flowers, are seen as gifts for their friend Maxi. In an unpremeditated gesture, they roll a metal tub filled with concrete onto the train tracks. The brief tableau (din of the crash, lightning, Tona and Polo awed by the wreck) suggests the import of the change effected by their actions.

"THIS ONE-ACT MASTERPIECE FURTHER ELABORATES THE CONCEPT OF HUMAN EXISTENCE AS A COMPLEX WEB OF INTERRELATIONSHIPS THROUGH A FUSION OF REALISTIC AND POETIC TECHNIQUES."

In scene 3 the Medium reads from a Bestiary. Diverse interpretations of human existence are illustrated by animal images. They range from the canine guardian of physical integrity and property rights, the cat watching over man's spiritual integrity, the hen, fish, butterfly, and snake, to the bee that knows "*all* about solar energy and light. Things we don't suspect!" The latter most closely approaches the dramatist's concept of man as an intricate web of interrelationships based upon cosmic energy.

The next five scenes provide brief interpretations of and reactions to the derailment. Commenting upon the newspaper report, a Gentleman identifies poverty as the cause of delinquency. A Lady agrees: "Oh, yes, their poverty's something awful. But they didn't say anything about the trunk murder, huh?" Even if the cause is identified, there is no active response, only the passive consumption of journalistic sensationalism. The Teacher uses the newspaper to illustrate the "dangers of idleness." She, too, refuses to accept any responsibility or attempt to alleviate the problem. Two University Students react with greater sympathy, revealing perhaps a desire to rebel against society. All three responses, however, contrast with that of Maxi. Informed by phone that his friends have been arrested, he immediately requests that his employer give him money and time off so that he can go to the aid of the adolescents. Scene 8 shifts to the dump where the Scavengers and others reap the fruits of the wreck, carrying off sacks of food.

Scene 9 returns to the Medium. She narrates a story that is enacted by two dancers. Living in different towns, they both receive the same command in a dream: to dance and pray *together* at the sanctuary near the house of their brother. They meet in mid-route and, confused by the ambiguous dream, celebrate the rite at the place of their encounter. Each returns home, feeling he has only half-fulfilled the command. The anecdote reflects the image of human existence presented by the play. Man has no foreknowledge of the consequences of his actions. Therefore, primary emphasis is placed upon the process: contradictions should be faced and choices made in a spirit of solidarity with others.

The next seven scenes supply additional interpretations, and the basic opposition is human-vs.-inhuman response. First, we see Tona's mother preparing food and clothing to take to her daughter, and then Polo's mother visits him in prison. Both mothers are confused and vacillate in assigning blame. However, they do reveal a human maternal concern for their children's welfare and establish an obvious contrast with the two following scenes, which employ more elaborate distancing techniques. Both are introduced by the Newsboy: first, he hawks a Freudian analysis holding up papers covered with Rorschachlike ink blots and, later, a Marxist interpretation carrying papers printed in red on black. Each scene includes a narrator (Professor One, Professor Two) who comments upon his version as it is presented by Tona and Polo. The result is the satire of two opposing overrationalizations: the first exaggerating the repression of the libido in the individual, the second stressing the exploitation of the proletariat under capitalism. The three following scenes underscore the inhumanity of the preceding ones by focusing upon the mutual bond of love. Maxi visits Tona in prison. He had come to free his two friends by paying their fines. This is impossible because the derailment has resulted in a half-million-peso "crime." That the real crime is poverty is implied by Tona's expression of solidarity with her fellow inmates, who have violated society's laws in order to live. Tona and Maxi embrace as he vows to carry only Tona's picture in his wallet. What had begun as idol worship on her part and friendship on his part ends in love. A scene at the dump develops a similar bond on the collective level. Here, it assumes a more popular and realistic form, as four Scavengers (two male, two female) celebrate around a fire with food, drink, and song. The earthy language of the songs contrasts strongly with the dehumanizing terminology of analysis employed by the two Professors. The scene concludes with the same gesture as the preceding one: the two couples embrace. Scene 16 returns to the Tona-Maxi plot. On the telephone at the garage, he breaks his engagement with his previous girlfriend and thus prepares the way for his future union with Tona.

Scene 17 restates the theses of the two Professors, adds a third, and requires the audience to make a choice. The Announcer illustrates the theses with three projected images and offers a magnificent prize to those who select the correct interpretation. In addition to the Freudian and Marxist rationalizations (rose petal and rose respectively), we have the weblike fiber of a rose petal seen under a microscope. This is the Medium's image, "primal matter" that is also "energy." The latter thesis destroys the former: there is no rose, no petal, only "a fusion of miraculous fictions. . . . Without the least possibility of rational explanation."

In the transition to the final scene, the Newsboy carries parchmentlike papers imprinted with magical signs and offers *all* the news. This introduces the Medium, now dressed in white, who gives her version. The previous representations by Tona and Polo, commented upon by the two Professors, were basically satires of exaggerated rationalizations, whereas the final scene achieves the total physical effect of ritual. The street scene included by the Professors is eliminated and dramatic intensity heightened as the Medium narrows the focus to the dump, where the change effected by the derailment occurs. As Tona and Polo enter, she explains: "They are changing into all that surrounds them." Their dance harmonizes with and evokes the creative potential of the cosmos. The flowers respond as a Feminine Chorus in a liturgy: "I have strength . . . / I have promise . . ." The dump itself begins to glow from within, and the Medium adds: "With rhythms such as these we summon and arouse fertility." After the derailment, all the characters in the play embrace, kiss, dance, at first chaotically and finally in a chain, with precise and complex movements. A change from sterility to fertility occurs on all levels: Tona and Polo pass from adolescents to adults (she marries Maxi, he gets his own garage), the situation of the poor shifts temporarily from lack to abundance, and the cosmos itself participates in this realization of creative potential.

Now, instead of commenting upon the representation, the Medium addresses a question to the characters:

> *Medium. (Asking in the manner of a teacher)* —And now, what about that light from that star—extinguished for so many years?
>
> *Tona.* —. . . It kept flowing into the telescope . . . but all it meant to say . . . all it meant to reveal . . . was the

humble existence of the hairy hunter, who was drawn by his friend, the painter, on the walls of an African cave.

This exchange provides, within the play, a statement on the function of art. The artist produces an image that persists long after the event or person represented ceases to exist. The sole function of the artist is to affirm, through an integral objectification, the existence of his contemporaries as a complex web of creative potential. Thus, the web becomes an image not of entrapment but of liberation, transcending, through a complex yet precise physical representation, the limits imposed by analytical rationalizations of human existence. The play itself is an exemplary realization of this concept of drama.

Source: Eugene R. Skinner, "The Theater of Emilio Carballido" in *Dramatists in Revolt: The New Latin American Theater,* edited by Leon F. Lyday and George W. Woodyard, University of Texas Press, 1976, pp. 19–36

SOURCES

Bixler, Jacqueline Eyring. "A Theatre of Contradictions: The Recent Works of Emilio Carballido" in *Latin American Theatre Review,* spring, 1985, pp. 57-66.

Cypess, Sandra Messinger, "I, Too, Speak: Female' Discourse in Carballido's Plays" in *Latin American Theatre Review,* fall, 1984, pp 45-50.

Jones, Willis, Knapp. *Behind Spanish American Footlights,* University of Texas Press, 1966.

Peden, Margaret Sayers. *Emilio Carballido,* Twayne Publishers, 1980.

Skinner, Eugene R. "The Theater of Emilio Carballido: Spinning a Web" in *Dramatists in Revolt: The New Latin American Theater,* edited by Leon F. Lyday and George W. Woodyard, University of Texas Press, 1976, pp. 19-36.

Taylor, Diane. "I, Too, Speak of the Rose" in *International Dictionary of Theatre:* Volume 1: *Plays,* edited by Mark Hawkins-Dady, St. James Press, 1992, pp. 353-54.

Woodyard, George. "Emilio Carballido" in *Encyclopedia of Latin American History and Culture,* Simon & Schuster, 1996, p. 550.

FURTHER READING

Bixler, Jacqueline Eyring. *Convention and Transgression: The Theatre of Emilio Carballido,* Bucknell University Press, 1997.

This book is a newly published one with extensive criticism and interpretation of all the writings of Carballido, including his plays.

Camin, Hector Anguilar, and Lorenzo Meyer. *In the Shadow of the Mexican Revolution: Contemporary Mexican History, 1910-1989,* translated by Luis Alberto Fierro, University of Texas Press, 1993.

This provides a good look at Mexican history in the twentieth century, with an examination of the economic situation and its impact on the poor.

Taylor, Kathy. *The New Narrative of Mexico: Sub-versions of History in Mexican History,* Bucknell University Press, 1994.

This author present an up-to-date look at Mexican fiction in the twentieth century, combining both history and criticism of the works.

Versenyi, Adam. *The Theatre in Latin America: Religion, Politics, and Culture from Cortes to the 1980s,* Cambridge University Press, 1993.

By exploring the history of Latin American theater, the author shows how the theatre has been a force for social change and has combined religious and political concerns.

Look Back in Anger

JOHN OSBORNE

1956

On May 8, 1956, *Look Back in Anger* opened at the Royal Court Theatre as the third production of the newly formed English Stage Company. The English Stage Company had been founded in 1955 to promote the production of new plays by contemporary authors that might not find production in the commercial West End theatre (London's equivalent of Broadway in New York City). West End theatre provided quality acting and high standards of production, but very little drama that related to life in contemporary England. Most plays of the time were generally innocuous light comedies, thrillers, and foreign imports—fourteen American shows in 1955 alone. Osborne had submitted copies of *Look Back in Anger* to every agent in London and to many West End producers and had been rejected by all. When the script arrived at the Royal Court, the Artistic Director George Devine and his young assistant director Tony Richardson knew it was exactly what they were looking for. *Look Back in Anger* was viewed as a play that would, as Devine later put it, "blow a hole in the old theatre."

Critical reception was strongly mixed: some detested the play and the central character, but most recognized Osborne as an important new talent and the play as emotionally powerful. They also recognized the play as one that fervently spoke of the concerns of the young in post-war England. Although the first production of *Look Back in Anger* was not initially financially successful, after an excerpt was shown on BBC the box office was

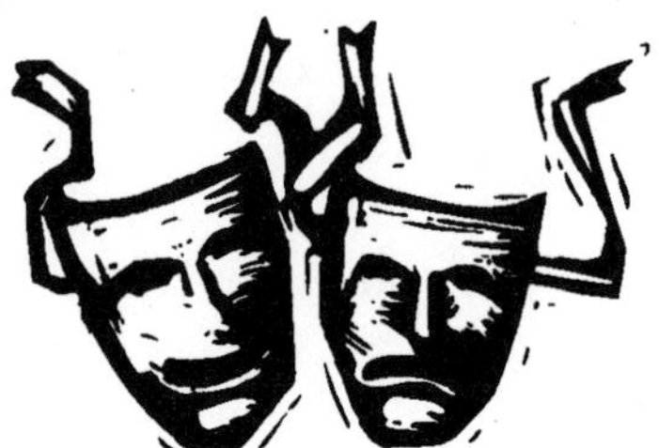

overwhelmed. Osborne was publicized as the ''Angry Young Man'' and the success of *Look Back in Anger* opened the doors to other young writers who dealt with contemporary problems.

AUTHOR BIOGRAPHY

John James Osborne was born on December 12, 1929, in Fulham, South West London. His father, Thomas Godfry Osborne, was then a commercial artist and copywriter; his mother, Nellie Beatrice Grove Osborne, worked as a barmaid in pubs most of her life. Much of Osborne's childhood was spent in near poverty, and he suffered from frequent extended illnesses. He was deeply affected by his father's death from tuberculosis in 1941 and also remembered vividly the air raids and general excitement of war. Osborne attended state schools until the age of twelve when he was awarded a scholarship to attend a minor private school, St. Michael's College, in Barnstaple, Devon. He was expelled at the age of sixteen after the headmaster slapped Osborne's face and Osborne hit him back. After spending some time at home, he took a series of jobs writing copy for various trade journals. He became interested in theatre while working as a tutor for children touring with a repertory company. After an education inspector found him to be uncertified as a teacher, Osborne was relieved of those duties but invited to stay with the company as assistant stage manager and eventually as an actor. He made his stage debut in March, 1948, in Sheffield and for the next seven years made the rounds of provincial repertory theatres as an actor.

Osborne's playwriting career began while he was still an actor. He wrote five plays before the production of *Look Back in Anger* made him an overnight success. *The Devil Inside Him,* coauthored with Stella Linden, was produced in Huddersfield in 1950; *Personal Enemy,* coauthored with Anthony Creighton, was produced in Harrogate in 1955; and *Epitaph for George Dillon,* also written with Creighton, was later produced in 1958 by the English Stage Company and has been published. The real breakthrough came when *Look Back in Anger* was staged in 1956 as the third production of the newly formed English Stage Company at the Royal Court Theatre. *Look Back in Anger* was the first play Osborne had written alone. He had submitted copies of the script to every agent in London and to many West End producers and had been rejected by all. After the success of *Look Back in Anger,* Osborne continued to have a highly successful career as playwright. His next play, *The Entertainer,* was written with Laurence Olivier in mind for the central character, Archie Rice. It was produced by the English Stage Company in April 1957 with Olivier giving what has been widely considered to be one of his finest performances. Both *Look Back in Anger* and *The Entertainer* were adapted for film. Following *The Entertainer,* Osborne continued to have a productive career, writing seventeen more stage plays, eleven plays for television, five screen plays (including *Tom Jones,* for which he received an Academy Award), and four books, including two volumes of autobiography.

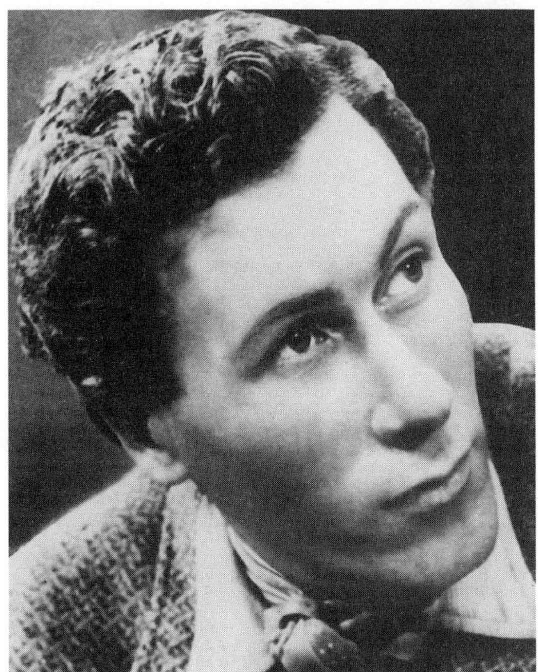

John Osborne in the 1950s

Osborne was married five times: to actress Pamela Lane from 1951 to 1957; to Mary Ure, who played Alison in *Look Back in Anger,* from 1957 to 1962; to Penelope Gilliatt, film and later drama critic for *The Observer,* from 1963 to 1967; to actress Jill Bennett from 1968 to 1977; and to journalist Helen Dawson beginning in 1978. He died of heart failure on December 24, 1994.

PLOT SUMMARY

Act I

The plot of *Look Back in Anger* is driven almost entirely by the tirades of Jimmy Porter rather than outside forces. The play is set in a one-room attic apartment in the Midlands of England. This large room is the home of Jimmy Porter, his wife Alison, and his partner and friend Cliff Lewis, who has a separate bedroom across the hall.

The play opens with Alison at the ironing board and Jimmy and Cliff in easy chairs reading the Sunday papers. Jimmy complains that half the book review he is reading in his ''posh'' paper is in French. He asks Alison if that makes her feel ignorant and she replies that she wasn't listening to the question. Immediately one of the main themes is introduced, Jimmy's railing against the inertia of Alison and the inertia of the whole middle-class of England. Jimmy teases Cliff about being uneducated and ignorant and Cliff good naturedly agrees with him. Jimmy says that Alison hasn't had a thought for years and she agrees. Jimmy is depressed by their Sunday routine and says their youth is slipping away. He says, ''Let's pretend that we're human beings and that we're actually alive.'' Cliff complains about the smoke from Jimmy's pipe. When Alison says she has gotten used to it, Jimmy says she would get used to anything in a few minutes. He then rails about the fact that ''Nobody thinks, nobody cares. No beliefs no convictions and no enthusiasms.'' He says that England has lost her soul, that it is dreary living in ''the American Age.'' There is talk of the candy stall that Jimmy and Cliff own and operate in an outdoor market. Jimmy talks about Alison's brother Nigel, whom he has dubbed ''the chinless wonder from Sandhurst,'' and who is a Member of Parliament. Jimmy resents Nigel and all that he stands for, including the fact that he will succeed in the world because of his social class and the schools he has attended in spite of his stupidity and insensitivity. He then turns on Alison, calling her ''the Lady Pusillanimous.'' Jimmy tries to listen to a concert on the radio and complains at the noise made by Alison's ironing and Cliff's rustling of the newspaper. He then harangues against women in general, Alison, and even Mrs. Drury, their landlady. Cliff and Jimmy then playfully wrestle and accidentally push over Alison and the ironing board. Alison has burnt her arm and finally tells Jimmy to get out. Cliff ministers to Alison's burn and calms her. She tells him that she is pregnant. She is afraid to tell Jimmy lest he think she planned it. Cliff holds Alison and Jimmy enters. There is teasing and play as Jimmy reestablishes himself. Cliff goes out for cigarettes. Jimmy tells Alison that he wants her; they play a private and affectionate game of ''squirrels and bears'' and Alison is about to tell him of her pregnancy when Cliff returns to say Helena Charles, an actress friend of Alison, is on the phone downstairs. When Alison returns she says she has invited Helena to stay with them during her engagement at the local theatre and Jimmy launches his most shocking diatribe yet. He tells Alison that if she were to have a child and if that child would die, then she might suffer enough to become a human being. The act ends with Jimmy saying of Alison, ''She'll go on sleeping and devouring until there is nothing left of me.''

Act II, scene 1

It is evening two weeks later. Helena and Alison are getting ready to go to church. Jimmy is in Cliff's room practicing jazz on his trumpet. Jimmy's friend Hugh and Hugh's working-class mother, who provided the money needed to start the candy business, are discussed. Alison talks of being cut off from the kind of people she had always known. She still hasn't told Jimmy she is pregnant. After Cliff and Jimmy enter, Jimmy launches into another attack on the Establishment in general and Alison's mother in particular. He then tells of keeping his father company as he lay dying for months and says he ''learnt at an early age what it was to be angry—angry and helpless.'' Jimmy is called to the phone. Helena tells Alison that she has telegraphed Alison's father to come and take her home. Jimmy returns and says Hugh's mother has had a stroke and he will go to London to be with her. He tells Alison he needs her to go with him. She leaves with Helena.

Act II, scene 2

It is the following evening and Colonel Redfern, Alison's father, is visiting. Redfern is bemused by the modern England; he spent his whole career, from 1913 to 1947, in the colonial service in India. He sees some right on Jimmy's side and was horrified by his wife's brutal attempts to prevent Alison from marrying Jimmy. He says he and Alison are much alike in that they both ''like to sit on a fence. It is rather comfortable.'' Alison tries to explain why she married Jimmy: "I'd lived a happy, uncomplicated life and suddenly this—this spiritual barbarian—throws down a gauntlet at me." Helena comes in followed shortly by Cliff. Helena will stay one more night so she can attend an audition nearby. Alison asks Cliff to give a letter to Jimmy and he refuses. Alison and her father leave, followed shortly by Cliff. Helena lies down on the bed and looks at the toy bear. Jimmy crashes in. He reads Alison's letter and berates her for being polite and "wet" instead of emotionally honest. Helena tells him Alison is pregnant and Jimmy says he doesn't care. He has watched Hugh's mother die and has no pity for Alison. He turns on Helena calling her an "evil-minded little virgin." She slaps his face; then, as he cries in despair, she kisses him passionately.

Act III, scene 1

It is early Sunday evening several months later. Jimmy and Cliff are sprawled in their armchairs reading the Sunday newspapers and Helena is at the ironing board. All seems very relaxed. They talk about a newspaper article and Jimmy starts in on religion and politics. They then go into a vaudeville routine and Helena joins in. Jimmy and Cliff do a song and dance and end with playful wrestling. Cliff's shirt gets dirty and Helena leaves to wash it. Cliff says he is going to move out and give up the candy stall. He says he might find a woman of his own. When Helena returns with his shirt, Cliff hangs it over the gas fire in his room. Helena tells Jimmy that she loves him and has always wanted him. The door opens and Alison enters, looking ill and obviously thin. Jimmy exits and leaves the two women looking at each other.

Act III, scene 2

It is moments later. There is the sound of Jimmy's trumpet from across the hall. Alison has suffered a miscarriage. She says she doesn't know why she came, that she doesn't want to cause a breach between Helena and Jimmy. Helena says that it is all over between her and Jimmy, that she realizes that what she has been doing is wrong, and she can't live with that. She calls Jimmy in and tells him she is going to leave, and she does. Alison says she will go. Jimmy berates her for not sending flowers to the funeral. Then he softens and talks of the old bear going through the forest of life alone. He remembers their first meeting and says, "I may be a lost cause, but I thought if you loved me, it needn't matter." Alison cries and says she has found strength in the humility of not having been able to protect her unborn child. She is in the mud now, groveling. Jimmy gently comforts her. They enter into their game of bear and squirrel in what is apparently a loving reconciliation.

CHARACTERS

Helena Charles

Helena is Alison's friend, a very proper middle-class woman. She is an actress who comes to stay with the Porters while she performs in a play at the local theatre. Jimmy has long despised her, as he considers her a member of the Establishment. When she contacts Alison's father and asks him to take Alison home, Helena seems genuinely concerned about Alison. However, she seduces Jimmy and replaces Alison in the household. When Alison returns, Helena realizes that her affair with Jimmy is wrong and decides to leave.

Cliff Lewis

Cliff is Jimmy's friend and partner in the candy stall business and shares the Porters' flat, although he has his own bedroom across the hall. Cliff is a poorly educated, working class man of Welsh heritage. He is warm, loving, and humorous. He genuinely loves Alison but adjusts when she leaves and Helena moves in. Cliff's first allegiance is to Jimmy. Nevertheless, ultimately he decides to go out on his own.

Alison Porter

Alison has been married to Jimmy for three years. She comes from the solid upper-middle-class Establishment. Her father was a colonel in the colonial Service and the family lived very comfortably in India until 1947. Her brother Nigel attended Sandhurst, the British equivalent of West Point, and is a Member of Parliament. She married Jimmy partly as a rebellion against the proper, predictable, stultifying precepts of her class. However, she has been molded by her upbringing and it is her "fence

MEDIA ADAPTATIONS

- *Look Back in Anger* was adapted in 1958 as a film by John Osborne and Nigel Kneale. It was produced by Woodfall Films, a company formed by John Osborne and Tony Richardson. It was directed by Tony Richardson and starred Richard Burton and Claire Bloom. Available on video.
- A second film as made in 1980, directed by Lindsay Anderson (a former artistic director of the Royal Court Theatre). It starred Malcolm McDowell and Lisa Banes. Available on video.
- The 1989 revival directed by Judi Dench for a very limited run in Belfast was filmed for Thames Television. The television version was directed by David Jones and starred Kenneth Branagh and Emma Thompson. Available on video.

sitting,'' her lack of total emotional commitment, that provokes Jimmy's attacks. Alison is warm and open with Cliff without ever harboring a sexual attraction to him. When Helena takes charge and arranges for Alison to leave Jimmy, Alison does not protest and does indeed return to her parents, their values, and the security they offer. Alison is drawn back to Jimmy at the end after she has suffered the pain and loss brought by the miscarriage of her child.

Jimmy Porter

Jimmy Porter is a character of immense psychological complexity and interest. He dominates the play through the power of his anger and language. He unleashes his invective on what he calls the Establishment (those ''born'' to power and privilege), the church as part of the Establishment, and his loved ones. Osborne describes him as ''a disconcerting mixture of sincerity and cheerful malice, of tenderness and freebooting cruelty; restless, importunate, full of pride, a combination which alienates the sensitive and insensitive alike.'' Critic Harold Ferrar assessed him as a man of decency and charity who is ''one of life's beautiful losers,'' while critic Michael Coveney called him ''a lovable monster with the gift of the gab and a talent for resentment.'' Although Jimmy has graduated from a university—albeit one with no prestige—he works with Cliff as owner/proprietor of a candy stall in an outdoor market. In spite of his tendency to sometimes cruelly insult Cliff, Jimmy genuinely likes him. His assaults on Alison are nasty and sometimes savage. He seems to be trying to force her to have a genuine response, something coming from her that is not colored by her class and upbringing. He says she is not real because she has not suffered real pain and degradation. When she leaves he is hurt but quickly adjusts. Jimmy has hated Helena for the same reasons he hated Alison, namely her social class and ''proper'' upbringing. While Jimmy apparently hates Alison's mother, he seems to like Colonel Redfern because he can feel sorry for him.

Colonel Redfern

Colonel Redfern, Alison's father, is a retired army officer who served in India from 1913 to 1947. During that time he seldom spent any time in England. He represents the values and beliefs of another period, a time of British Empire. His values are those of duty, honor, and loyalty to one's country and one's class. His world ended with the independence of India. He is a reasonable man somewhat bemused by the post-World War II England. He does not approve of Jimmy, but he does find things to admire in him and even agrees with Jimmy in some instances. He does not hesitate to help Alison and does not attempt to control her.

THEMES

Alienation and Loneliness

Jimmy Porter spoke for a large segment of the British population in 1956 when he ranted about his alienation from a society in which he was denied any meaningful role. Although he was educated at a ''white-tile'' university, a reference to the newest and least prestigious universities in the United Kingdom, the real power and opportunities were reserved for the children of the Establishment, those born to privilege, family connections, and entree to the "right" schools. Part of the "code" of the Establishment was the "stiff upper lip," that reticence to show or even to feel strong emotions. Jimmy's alienation from Alison comes precisely because he cannot break through her "cool," her unwillingness to feel deeply even during sexual intercourse with her husband. He berates her in a coarse attempt to get her to strike out at him, to stop "sitting on the fence" and make a full commitment to her real emotions; he wants to force her to feel and to have vital life. He calls her "Lady Pusillanimous" because he sees her as too cowardly to commit to anything. Jimmy is anxious to give a great deal and is deeply angry because no one seems interested enough to take from him, including his wife. He says, "My heart is so full, I feel ill—and she wants peace!"

Anger and Hatred

Jimmy Porter operates out of a deep well of anger. His anger is directed at those he loves because they refuse to have strong feelings, at a society that did not fulfill promises of opportunity, and at those who smugly assume their places in the social and power structure and who do not care for others. He lashes out in anger because of his deeply felt helplessness. When he was ten years old he watched his idealist father dying for a year from wounds received fighting for democracy in the Spanish Civil War, his father talking for hours, "pouring out all that was left of his life to one bewildered little boy." He says, "You see, I learnt at an early age what it was to be angry—angry and helpless. And I can never forget it."

Apathy and Passivity

Although Alison is the direct target of Jimmy's invective, her apathy and passivity are merely the immediate representation of the attitudes that Jimmy sees as undermining the whole of society. It is the complacent blandness of society that infuriates Jimmy. When speaking of Alison's brother Nigel, he says, "You've never heard so many well-bred commonplaces coming from beneath the same bowler hat." The Church, too, comes under attack in part because it has lost relevance to contemporary life. For Helena it spells a safe habit, one that defines right and wrong for her—although she seems perfectly willing to ignore its strictures against adultery when it suits her. Jimmy sees the Church as providing an easy escape from facing the pain of living in the here and now—and thus precluding any real redemption. Of course, Jimmy has also slipped into a world of sameness as illustrated by the three Sunday evenings spent reading the newspapers and even the direct replacement of Alison at the ironing board with Helena. Deadly habit is portrayed as insidious.

TOPICS FOR FURTHER STUDY

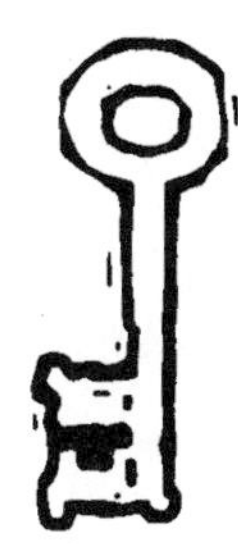

- Research the "Welfare State" programs and policies in post-World War II England. Why would these not satisfy someone like Jimmy Porter?
- Compare August Strindberg's *The Father* or *Dance of Death* and Henrik Ibsen's *A Doll's House* with *Look Back in Anger* for both style and content.
- Research the decline of the British Empire. How would that decline affect England itself and people as different as Jimmy Porter and Colonel Redfern?
- Is Jimmy Porter an "angry young man" with a purpose, or is he merely a tiresome, cruel whiner?
- Does rock music of the 1960s and 1970s contain any of the themes of *Look Back in Anger?* Does the rock music of today contain any of those themes?

Class Conflict

Jimmy comes from the working class and although some of his mother's relatives are "pretty posh," Cliff tells Alison that Jimmy hates them as much as he hates her family. It is the class system, with its built-in preferential treatment for those at the top and exclusion from all power for those at the bottom, that makes Jimmy's existence seem so meaningless. He has a university degree, but it is not from the "right" university. It is Nigel, the "straight-backed, chinless wonder" who went to Sandhurst, who is stupid and insensitive to the needs of others, who has no beliefs of his own, who is already a Member of Parliament, who will "make it to the top." Alison's father, Colonel Redfern, is not shown unsympathetically, but her mother is portrayed as a class-conscious monster who used every tactic she could to prevent Alison from marrying Jimmy. The only person for whom Jimmy's love is apparent is Hugh's working-class mother. Jimmy likes Cliff because, as Cliff himself says, "I'm common."

Identity Crisis

While Jimmy harangues everyone around him to open themselves to honest feeling, he is trapped in his own problems of social identity. He doesn't seem to fit in anywhere. As Colonel Redfern points out, operating a sweet-stall seems an odd occupation for an educated young man. Jimmy sees suffering the pain of life as the only way to find, or "earn," one's true identity. Alison does finally suffer the immeasurable loss of her unborn child and comes back to Jimmy, who seems to embrace her. Helena discovers that she can be happy only if she lives according to her perceived principles of right and wrong. Colonel Redfern is caught out of his time. The England he left as a young army officer no longer exists. Jimmy calls him "just one of those sturdy old plants left over from the Edwardian Wilderness that can't understand why the sun isn't shining anymore," and the Colonel agrees. Cliff does seem to have a strong sense of who he is, accepts that, and will move on with his life.

Sexism

A contemporary reading of *Look Back in Anger* contains inherent assumptions of sexism. Jimmy Porter seems to many to be a misogamist and Alison a mere cipher struggling to view the world through Jimmy's eyes.

STYLE

Setting

The play takes place in the Porters' one-room flat, a fairly large attic room. The furniture is simple and rather old: a double bed, dressing table, book shelves, chest of drawers, dining table, and three chairs, two shabby leather arm chairs. The drab setting of the play emphasizes the contrast between the idealistic Jimmy and the dull reality of the world surrounding him.

Plot

The construction of *Look Back in Anger* is that of an old-fashioned well-made play in the tradition of Henrik Ibsen, August Strindberg, Tennessee Williams, or most of Osborne's contemporary commercial playwrights. There is one plot developed over three acts (the expected number in 1956), and the basic plot device is ancient: misalliance in marriage compounded by a love triangle. There is some exposition that has been characterized as clumsy, such as when Jimmy tells Alison, to whom he has been married three years, how his business had been financed. Some plot devices stand out as the author's contrivances, such as Cliff's exit in Act I to buy cigarettes, and his unconvincing reasons for returning a couple of minutes later just as Alison is about to tell Jimmy that she is pregnant; the telephone call from Helena prepares for the Act I curtain and a phone call saying Hugh's mother is dying prepares the Act II, Scene 1 curtain. The end of Act II, Scene 2, with the two women left looking at each other, has been viewed as artificial. Osborne's innovations were not in form but rather in character, language, and passion which, for the most part mask the clumsy mechanics when the play is being acted.

Imagery

Two sound images from off-stage are used very effectively in *Look Back in Anger:* the church bells and Jimmy's jazz trumpet. The church bells invade the small living space and serve as a reminder of the power of the established church, and also that it doesn't care at all for their domestic peace. The jazz trumpet allows Jimmy's presence to dominate the stage even when he is not there, and it also serves as his anti-Establishment "raspberry."

Language

Osborne's use of language is basically in the realistic tradition. The characters' speech and rhythms reflect their class and education. Helena is very proper and conventional and so is her speech. Cliff is humble, Colonel Redfern is calm and reflective, Alison is proper and non-judgmental and non-committal. Jimmy Porter, though, broke with tradition. Working class characters were not new to the English stage, but previously they had been comic figures who were usually inarticulate, or even angry figures who were inarticulate and thus held back by their class and lack of language skills and could thus be pitied. Jimmy is extremely articulate and self-confident. Whatever one thinks of Jimmy, it is not going to be pity. His passion is overwhelming and he has the language to overwhelm others with that passion. His language is not polite, though one suspects it would be a great deal *more* impolite if theatre censorship had not been in effect when it was written. Jimmy can also be very humorous and even poetic, as when he describes Colonel Redfern as a "sturdy old plant left over from the Edwardian Wilderness." Indeed, the powerful use of language seems almost to be a second form of structure for the whole play, one that covers various other faults.

HISTORICAL CONTEXT

By 1956 the British Empire had been shrinking for decades. With the granting of independence to India in 1947 after Gandhi's thirty years of struggle and the loss of African colonies and the near independence of the Commonwealth nations such as Canada, Australia, and New Zealand, the British Empire was all but gone. The Suez crises in 1956, in which Egypt refused to renew the British-owned Suez Canal Company's concession and which resulted in a disastrous and humiliating intervention by England, simply emphasized the lack of power wielded by Britain in the Post World War II world.

There had also been incursions into the power structure since early Victorian times, with the ruling classes resisting every inch of the way. In 1945, the Labour Party won an impressive victory over the Tories, thus turning the war-time hero Winston Churchill out of office. This was a mandate for the welfare state and the end of the class system. Prosperity for all was the hope of the people. Nationalized medicine became a reality and a social welfare system was constructed. In the words of Harold Ferrar, "an era of affluence was predicted, and a meritocracy that would supersede the reign of old school ties." The new "red-brick" universities were built and greatly expanded educational opportunities, but the old power structure did not simply hand over the reins of control. Price controls and other austerity measures were imposed. By 1951 it was apparent that the land of milk-and-honey had not arrived. Winston Churchill was again voted into office.

The Church of England, too, was out of contact with the daily lives of most Englishmen. The Church is not simply a spiritual leader but also owner of vast properties and thus a member of the landholding class. The Church is attacked by Osborne when he has Jimmy quote the fictional Bishop of Bromley as saying that he is upset because someone has suggested that he supports the rich against the poor. He denies class distinctions and says, "The idea has been persistently and wickedly fostered by—the working classes!"

The international scene was also fraught with dangers. The Berlin crisis in 1948-1949 clearly pointed out that the peace following World War II was fragile. The Boer and Irish risings and the Palestine question further reminded the English that this new hard-won peace was not going to be easy or complete. Everyone lived under threat of instantaneous annihilation from the A-bomb. Jimmy says, "If the big bang does come, and we all get killed off, it won't be in aid of the old-fashioned, grand design. It'll just be for the Brave New-nothing-very-much-thank-you. About as pointless and inglorious as stepping in front of a bus." Less than two weeks after *Look Back in Anger* opened the first airborne hydrogen bomb was exploded. In October, 1956, England's first full scale use of nuclear fuel to produce electricity went into effect at Calder Hall. The facility also manufactured plutonium for military use in developing their own H-bomb. That same year there were uprisings in Hungary and Poland and the Soviet Union put them down with military force.

In the United States following World War II there was a period of general and unprecedented prosperity. However, opportunity was "deferred" for some, especially blacks, the rural poor, and women. Movements to challenge the status quo of exclusion were beginning. Reverend Martin Luther King, Jr., organized a boycott of Montgomery, Alabama, public transportation as a protest against

COMPARE & CONTRAST

- **1956:** The welfare state was in place in England with public ownership of the main public utilities, such as the telephone, gas, and electric production, national health was in place, and a national welfare system that provided at least minimal economic security for nearly the whole population.

  Today: The public utilities have been privatized, and there have been broad reductions in public programs, including national health.

- **1956:** The European Common Market was still an idea and movement across national boundaries was strictly controlled.

  Today: The European Common Market is firmly in place, Europe is on the brink of having a common currency, and borders between countries are practically open.

- **1956:** The Cold War between blocks of nations led by two superpowers was in full effect and nuclear annihilation was felt as a constant possibility.

  Today: With the collapse of the Soviet Union the Cold War was effectively won by the West and the threat of nuclear annihilation reduced; however, there are more nations with nuclear weapons ability and the threat of annihilation is still real if not popularly perceived as such.

- **1956:** Rock and roll music was just starting in the United States and was hardly known in England.

  Today: Rock and roll music has gone through many stages, with many of the most influential strains originating in England, and is the popular music of youth, as well as a powerful means of rebellion.

- **1956:** Radio and television was provided by the state-financed British Broadcasting Corporation, which produced most of what was broadcast.

  Today: Commercial radio and television compete with the BBC, satellite transmission and home satellite reception provide an immense choice of popular fare, and the major centers of production are in the United States.

- **1956:** The newly-founded English Stage Company at the Royal Court Theatre provided the only major outlet for contemporary relevant drama of doubtful commercial value in London

  Today: The Royal National Theatre and the Royal Shakespeare Company both provide major outlets for relevant contemporary drama, and there are dozens of ''fringe'' theatres—the equivalent of New York's Off Broadway and Off Off Broadway—that produce new plays.

discrimination. The Supreme Court had issued an historic desegregation ruling in 1954 and in 1956 a bloc of Southern Congressmen issued a manifest pledging to use ''all lawful means'' to upset that ruling.

Among the best selling books in 1956 was the nonfiction *The Organization Man* by William Hollingsworth Whyte, Jr., who argued that a new collective ethic has arisen from the bureaucratization of society. ''Belongingness'' rather than personal fulfillment has become the ultimate need of the individual, said Whyte.

My Fair Lady opened in New York. The musical is based on George Bernard Shaw's *Pygmalion* in which a working-class Cockney flower girl who, after learning the language and manners of upper-class society, is able to ''pass'' as one of them.

London theatre at the time has been described as ''a vast desert;'' ''only interested in innocuous little plays which would provide a vehicle for a star to achieve a long and tedious run;'' ''fairly frivolous.'' The Arts Council of Great Britain had been formed after World War II to support the arts nationwide, but it had severely limited funds. London theatre in 1955 was commercial theatre. The most decisive success on every level was Enid Bagnold's glittering and artificial high comedy-mystery *The Chalk Garden,* a play that could have been written any time since Oscar Wilde. Terence Rattigan was represented with his plays *The Deep Blue Sea* and *Separate Tables.* Most plays were light comedies, farces, and mysteries—including Agatha Christie's *The Mouse Trap,* which has continued to enjoy successful productions. The musicals included the contemporary *Salad Days* and *The Boyfriend,* frothy pieces set in what seemed to be an idealized Edwardian England. There were fourteen American shows of one kind of another and six imports from Paris playing in the West End. London theatre remained a middle-class, middle-aged theatre. The fare was dictated by the public and that particular public liked what was given to them. They wanted something ''safe.''

CRITICAL OVERVIEW

Look Back in Anger has been recognized as a bombshell that blew up the old British theatre. However, when *Look Back in Anger* opened as the third play in the repertory of the English Stage Company at the Royal Court Theatre (a company that had been founded the year before precisely to stimulate new writing that would have contemporary relevance), it was not an immediate success. The critical reaction was mixed, but many of the critics, whether or not they liked the play, acknowledged its merits and those of its young author. Cecil Wilson in the *Daily Mail* assessed Jimmy Porter as a ''young neurotic who lives like a pig,'' whose ''bitterness produces a fine flow of savage talk, but is basically a bore because its reasons are never explained.'' But Wilson also said that the English Stage Company ''have not discovered a masterpiece, but they *have* discovered a dramatist of outstanding promise, a man who can write with searing passion but happens in this case to have lavished it on the wrong play.'' John Barker, critic for the *Daily Express,* asserted that *Look Back in Anger* ''is intense, angry, feverish, undisciplined. It is even crazy. But it is young, young, young.'' Milton Shulman of the *Evening Standard* attacked the play, saying: ''It aims at being a despairing cry but achieves only the stature of a self-pitying snivel.'' Nevertheless, Shulman admitted that ''Mr. Osborne has a dazzling aptitude for provoking and stimulating dialogue, and he draws characters with firm convincing strokes.'' Philip Hope-Wallace of the *Manchester Guardian* responded negatively to the play as well, calling it ''a strongly felt but rather muddled first drama,'' but conceded that ''they have got a potential playwright at last, all the same.'' Harold Hobson of the *Sunday Times* provided a positive assessment of the play and wrote of Osborne: ''Though the blinkers still obscure his vision, he is a writer of outstanding promise.'' The critic for the *New Statesman and Nation* maintained that although *Look Back in Anger* was ''not a perfect play,'' ''it is a most exciting one, abounding with life and vitality. . . . If you are young, it will speak for you. If you are middle-aged, it will tell you what the young are feeling.'' But it was Kenneth Tynan of the *Observer* who created the most excitement with what is perhaps the most famous review in contemporary theatre. Tynan remarked: ''That the play needs changes I do not deny: it is twenty minutes too long, and not even Mr. Haigh's bravura could blind me to the painful whimsy of the final reconciliation. I agree that *Look Back in Anger* is likely to remain a minority taste. What matters, however, is the size of the minority. I estimate it at roughly 6,733,000, which is the number of people in this country between the ages of twenty and thirty. And this figure will doubtless be swelled by refugees from other age-groups who are curious to know precisely what the contemporary young pup is thinking and feeling. . . . It is the best young play of its decade.''

In spite of the tremendous critical excitement it generated, *Look Back in Anger* was not financially successful during its first run. Part of the problem was thought to be the fact that rotating repertory—a practice new to 1950s London—was confusing to audiences who were unable to determine when any particular play was being performed. It was decided in August to cancel the other plays and run *Look Back in Anger* alone for eleven weeks, but even then the ticket sales failed to meet expenses. A twenty-five minute excerpt from the play was broadcast by BBC on October 16, and following that the play sold out for its run and a three-week run in another theatre. A production of *Look Back in Anger* then toured England. It received the *Evening Standard Award* as best new play of 1956.

Look Back in Anger opened at the Lyceum Theatre on Broadway October 1, 1957, with the original cast and received very strong reviews. It ran for 407 performances, had a second Broadway production beginning in November, 1958, and toured the United States and Canada. It received the New

York Drama Critics Circle Award as the best foreign play of 1957. It then played all over the world. It continues to be produced, both by professional and amateur theatre groups.

That *Look Back in Anger* still has the power to move audiences was shown by Judi Dench's 1989 revival of the play in Belfast, Northern Ireland, which starred Kenneth Branagh. Maureen Paton, in the *Daily Express,* commented: "This devastating study of a disintegrating marriage has never dated since it changed British theatre back in 1956." Damian Smyth, in the *Independent,* declared: "At the point when Jimmy prescribes for Alison's lack of authenticity that she should have a child and that it should die, when he doesn't know she is already pregnant by him, there went up an instinctive gasp of shock. That's not bad after 33 years, and it is a testimony to the strength of this production in a city not unaccustomed to shock." Michael Billington, critic for the *Guardian,* asserted that "Good plays change their meaning with time; and it is a measure of the quality of John Osborne's *Look Back in Anger* that it now seems a very different work to the one staged at the Royal Court in 1956." Although to Billington the play "seemed less an incendiary social drama than [a Eugene] O'Neill-like exploration of personal pain," he went on to note that "what is slightly chilling is to realise how topical many of Osborne's ideas remain."

CRITICISM

Terry W. Browne

Browne holds a Ph.D. in theatre and is the author of the book Playwrights' Theatre, *which is a study of the company that first produced* Look Back in Anger. *In this essay he discusses elements that made Osborne's play important when it was first produced and why it remains a dynamic play today.*

When *Look Back in Anger* opened in 1956 it brought a new force to the English theatre. It was written in the prevailing form of a three-act well-made realistic play, a form that had existed for at least eighty years. The fact that the play was somewhat clumsy in its construction and needed editing was not lost on the critics, even those who championed the play as a major breakthrough in English drama and a new hope for English theatre. Not only that, but *Look Back in Anger* has received many revivals and has continued to speak to audiences, to hold their attention, and even to shock them. Although the form was not innovative, this clearly is no ordinary play.

The subject matter of twentieth-century English theatre until 1956 had been polite, perhaps witty, and even elegant and glittering in the use of language; however, it did not speak to the concerns of the nation, either young or old. It was a theatre of diversion, a theatre careful not to upset the illusions of its middle-class audience, a theatre that had lost all relevance to life as it was in fact being lived in post-World War II England. John Osborne changed that. As Kenneth Tynan said in the *Observer* on December 19, 1959: "Good taste, reticence and middle-class understatement were convicted of hypocrisy and jettisoned on the spot." They were not jettisoned in polite, or even comedic, political or social analysis; they were jettisoned by an articulate, educated, furious young man who pointed out what his contemporary world was really like. It was not the world of egalitarianism and idealism that had been envisioned by the socialist intellectuals. It was a dreary world in which, as Jimmy says, "There aren't any good, brave causes left."

In spite of the broadening of opportunities for university education, the old power structure based on "the old boy" network of school and family connections was still very much in place. The old power structure was cynical and bent on its own perpetuation. The Church of England was as much a part of the Establishment as the politicians and also seemed out of touch with the everyday realities of the people. For Jimmy, and for Osborne, the answers provided by the Church were a simple bromide that prevented people from looking at their lives and their society honestly. The "Bishop of Bromley" who is quoted by Jimmy may be a fictional person, but his call for Christians to help develop the H-Bomb was not fictional. John Osborne found a form that captured the unformed mood and discontent of the audience in 1956 England and gave it voice. Once the British Broadcasting Company (BBC) had shown a twenty-five minute segment of the play, that broad audience responded with letters asking to see the whole play.

It is not enough simply to point out that people, especially young people, are discontent. The theatre must bring that reality to life in a memorable way. Jimmy Porter is a magnificent character, and the power of his invective is certainly memorable.

John Osborne said many times that his aim was not to analyze and write about social ills but rather to

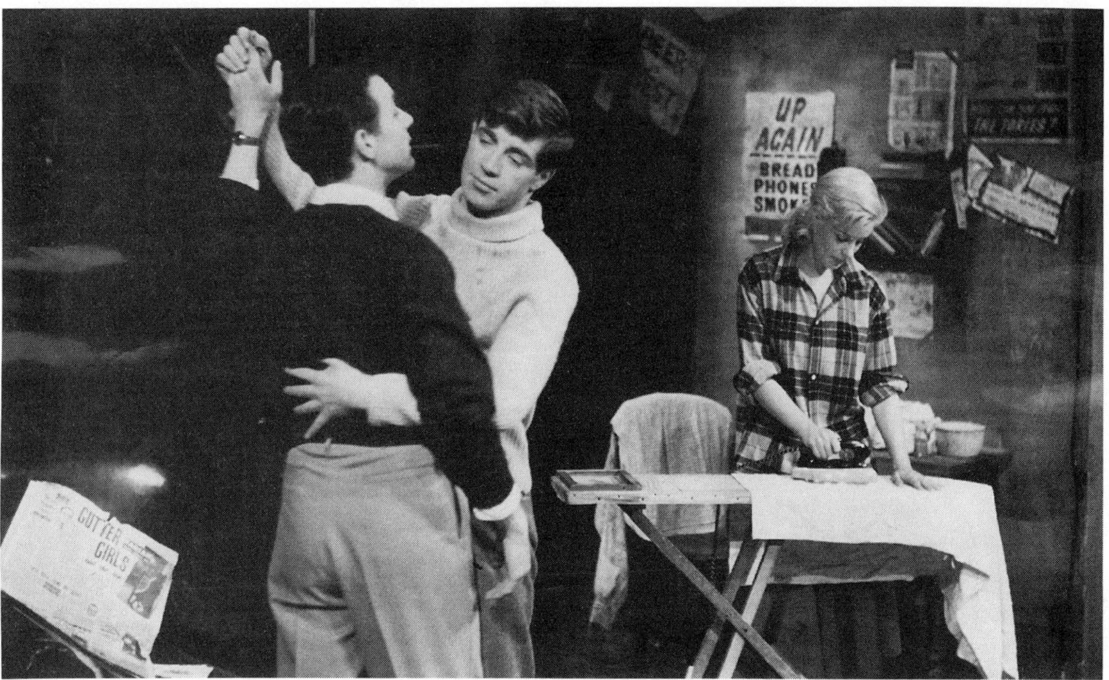

A 1956 production of Look Back in Anger. *Jimmy Porter (Kenneth Haigh) dances with Cliff (Alan Bates) while Jimmy's wife, Alison, irons*

make people *feel.* Jimmy Porter is not a political activist: he is a man living day-to-day in a world in which feelings and imaginative response to others has been deadened by convention. Jimmy's attacks are not against abstract ideas. He realizes what this world of dead ideas and moribund custom is doing to him and to those he loves. It is his desire to awaken them to feelings, to being truly and vibrantly alive, that drives Jimmy Porter. *Look Back in Anger* is a deeply felt drama of personal relationships, and it is because of that personal element that the play remains not only valid but also vivid to audiences today.

Jimmy's main conflict is with Alison. While the marriage is a misalliance, it is not just that of a Colonel's daughter marrying the rough-hewn commoner; it is the misalliance of someone who is alive and suffering to one who shuts off all suffering and sensitivity to the suffering of others to avoid the pain of life. They have been married for three years and their own routine has become deadening.

Jimmy's first direct attack on Alison comes barely a minute into the play when he says, "She hasn't had a thought in years! Have you?" Shortly after, he says, "All this time I have been married to this woman, this monument of non-attachment," and calls her "The Lady Pusillanimous." Alison's cool remoteness extends even to their lovemaking. Jimmy says, "Do you know I have never known the great pleasure of lovemaking when I didn't desire it myself. . . . She has the passion of a python." He wants to awaken her to life, with all its pain. That his passion and despair lead him to excess is undeniable: he wishes her to have a child and to have that child die. He says, "If only I could watch you face that. I wonder if you might even become a recognizable human being yourself." He later says he wants to watch her grovel in the mud. "I want to stand up in your tears, and splash about in them, and sing."

To be alive is to feel pain. Certainly, the notion that suffering validates human existence is an idea that runs through world drama from the time of Sophocles. Moreover, Jimmy recognizes that Alison's lack of emotional commitment to anything is draining him of his own zest for life. He tells of Alison's mother doing all she could to prevent the marriage, "All so that I shouldn't carry off her daughter on that old charger of mine, all tricked out and caparisoned in discredited passions and ideals! The old grey mare actually once led the charge against the old order—well, she certainly ain't what

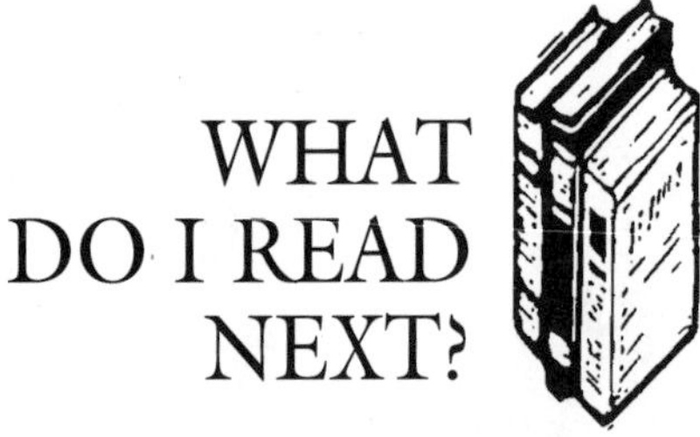

- *The Entertainer* is Osborne's second play, produced by The English Stage Company in 1957. Osborne offers the outdated and dying English music hall and the main character, second-rate performer Archie Rice, as a metaphor for England.
- *Luther* is Osborne's psychological study of Martin Luther as a private man, rather than as a public religious figure and instigator of the Protestant Reformation.
- *Inadmissible Evidence* is the product of a more mature artistic mind and evidenced that Osborne could successfully break traditional dramaturgical rules. It picks up Osborne's chronicle of the state of contemporary England where *Look Back in Anger* left off.
- *A Better Class of Person* is Osborne's autobiography up to the production of *Look Back in Anger.*
- *Almost a Gentleman* is Osborne's second volume of autobiography and begins with his fame as a playwright that followed the production of *Look Back in Anger.*
- *Roots* is a play by Arnold Wesker produced by the English Stage Company. It deals with a young woman of the rural working class finding her own voice and is an example of the many plays dealing realistically with contemporary England that followed *Look Back in Anger.*
- *Plays for Public Places* are short plays written by Howard Brenton in 1971 which deal with England from a generation after the time of *Look Back in Anger.*
- *A Doll's House* by Henrik Ibsen is a realistic play written in 1879 that focuses on a marriage in which a wife is seen as a possession and finally asserts her selfhood and independence. It also deals with the stultifying effects of social conventions and strictures.
- *The Father,* written by August Strindberg in 1887, is a realistic play which deals with extreme marital stress which results in the husband's mental instability.

she used to be. It was all she could do to carry me, but your weight was too much for her. She just dropped dead on the way.'' Jimmy is fighting for his love and for his own inner life. He needs to break down Alison's neutrality.

It was Jimmy's vibrant life that attracted Alison to him in the first place. In Act II, scene 1, she describes to Helena the time she first met Jimmy: ''Everything about him seemed to burn, his face, the edges of his hair glistened and seemed to spring off his head, and his eyes were so blue and filled with the sun.'' In Act II, scene 2, she also shows insight when she tells her father why she married Jimmy: ''I'd lived a happy, uncomplicated life, and suddenly, this—this spiritual barbarian—throws down the gauntlet at me. Perhaps only another woman could understand what a challenge like that means. . . .''

Alison does suffer the loss of her unborn child and she does return to Jimmy richer in the humility and pain of living. At the end of the play they have entered into their game of ''bears and squirrels,'' which Alison explained earlier was a place where ''[w]e could become little furry creatures with little furry brains. Full of dumb, uncomplicated affection for each other. A silly symphony for people who couldn't bear the pain of being human beings any longer.'' It seems doubtful that such a withdrawal from the world is likely to last, and it is likely that Osborne recognized the irony of the ending of the play when he wrote it. Jimmy's anger is deep and it is not new or brought on by current circumstances, either in his domestic life or society at large.

At the age of ten, Jimmy watched his idealistic father dying for twelve months, and ''I was the only one who cared!'' He says, ''You see, I learnt at an early age what it was to be angry—angry and helpless. And I can never forget it.'' Jimmy's source of pain and anger seem to come from the same source as that of John Osborne who, at an early age, watched his own father die of tuberculosis.

''Good plays change their meaning with time,'' said critic Michael Billington in the *Guardian* after seeing the 1989 revival of *Look Back in Anger.* It is a measure of its worth that even forty-two years after it premiered, the play still rings true and excites as the emphasis moves from the social comment to the personal angst that was propelling it from the first.

Source: Terry W. Browne, for *Drama for Students,* Gale, 1998.

Brooks Atkinson

In this review that was originally published on October 2, 1957, Atkinson cheers Osborne's play as ''the most vivid British play of the decade.'' The critic lauds Look Back in Anger *for its courage to challenge complacency and the common perceptions regarding everyday life.*

"TO BE ALIVE IS TO FEEL PAIN. CERTAINLY, THE NOTION THAT SUFFERING VALIDATES HUMAN EXISTENCE IS AN IDEA THAT RUNS THROUGH WORLD DRAMA FROM THE TIME OF SOPHOCLES."

To see *Look Back in Anger* at the Lyceum, where it opened last evening, is to agree with the British who saw the original performance. John Osborne has written the most vivid British play of the decade.

Since we have had angry young men writing bitter plays for a quarter of a century, *Look Back in Anger* will not be the landmark here that it is already in London. But Mr. Osborne is a fiery writer with a sharp point of view and a sense of theatre. Under the direction of Tony Richardson, five British actors give his savage morality drama the blessing of a brilliant performance.

Mr. Osborne is in blind revolt against the England of his time. In a squalid attic somewhere in the Midlands three young people are railing against the world. They are Jimmy Porter, a tornado of venomous phrases; his wife, who is crushed by the barrenness of their life and the wildness of her husband's vocabulary, and Cliff Lewis, an unattached young man who is the friend of both.

Being in a state of rebellion, neither Mr. Osborne nor his chief character has a program or a reasonable approach to life. From any civilized point of view, they are both impossible. But Mr. Osborne has one great asset. He can write. The words come bursting out of him in a flood of satire and invective. They are cruel; they are unfair, and they leave nothing but desolation as they sweep along.

But they are vibrant and colorful; they sting the secondary characters in the play, to say nothing of the audience. You know that something is going on in the theatre, and that the British drama has for once said a long farewell to the drawing-room, the bookshelves, the fireplace and the stairway. If Mr. Osborne is disgusted with England today, he is also disgusted with the pallor of British drama.

Not that he does not have trouble with the form. After inveighing against everyone and his wife for two acts with a certain malevolent though tolerable logic, he switches to the craft of writing a play. At the curtain of the second act Helena, a girl who despises Jimmy and is despised by him and who has persuaded his wife to go back home to escape further torture, becomes his mistress, and takes over where the beaten wife leaves off. When the curtain goes up on the third act Helena is at the ironing-board, as the wife was in the first act. Everything has been turned upside down.

This is a bit too pat. During the first scene of the third act, Mr. Osborne finds himself more preoccupied with the job of keeping a play in motion than with hurling words at the world. But in the last scene he is in control again. He is hack in top form—twisting and turning, sulking and groaning, turning civil morality inside out and doing other things he hadn't oughter. He is not the man for temperate statements.

If *Look Back in Anger* recovers its stride in the last scene, it is partly because the performance has so much pressure and passion. The acting is superb; it makes its points accurately with no waste motion. As Jimmy, Kenneth Haigh absorbs Mr. Osborne's furious literary style in an enormously skillful per-

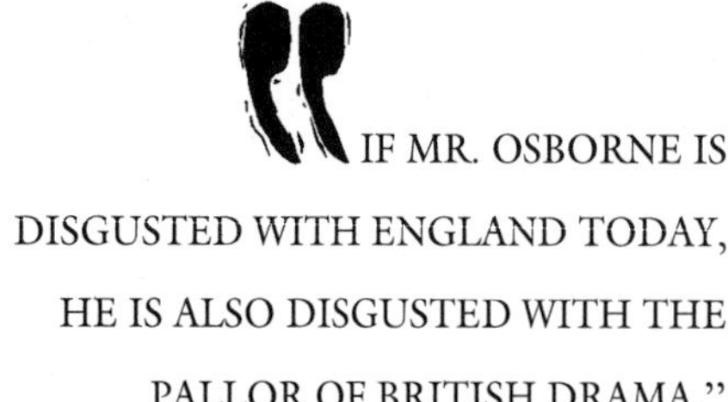

IF MR. OSBORNE IS DISGUSTED WITH ENGLAND TODAY, HE IS ALSO DISGUSTED WITH THE PALLOR OF BRITISH DRAMA."

formance that expresses undertones of despair and frustration and gives the character a basis in humanity. This wild man is no impostor.

As the tormented wife, Mary Ure succeeds in retaining the pride of an intelligent young woman by filling her silences with unspoken vitality, by being alive and by glowing with youth in every sequence. Alan Bates gives a vigorous performance in a more fluid style as the mutual friend. Vivienne Drummond plays the more ambiguous part of the intruding female with charm and guile.

Everything occurs inside a cheerless, slatternly attic room well designed by Alan Tagg. Miserable though it is, it is sturdy enough to withstand Mr. Osborne's thunderbolts. With the lightning that goes with them, they shake quite a lot of complacency out of the theatre.

Source: Brooks Atkinson, review of *Look Back in Anger* (1957) in *On Stage: Selected Reviews from the New York Times, 1920–1970,* edited by Bernard Beckerman and Howard Siegman, Arno Press, 1973 , pp. 388–89.

Harold Clurman

In this review of a 1957 New York production of Osborne's play, Clurman examines the motivations for Jimmy Porter's anger—which spring from sources that the critic feels are not immediately evident to American viewers. While generally laudatory, Clurman feels that the playwright's talents have been overstated but that his talent clearly promises that greatness in the future.

John Osborne, an actor still in his twenties, wrote a play two or three years ago, *Look Back In Anger* (Lyceum), which has also knocked at the door—this time at the door of British drama. The knock reverberated momentously through the English theatre, and its echo, slightly muted by its ocean passage, may now be heard on our Broadway shore.

I saw the play at its opening in London, where it was received by the leading critics with an excited gratitude which astonished as much as it pleased me. What the play represented to its English audience was the first resounding expression in the theatre not only of troubled youth but of the tensions within large segments of the middle class in England today. The play is contemporary in a way in which Rattigan on the one hand or Eliot and Fry on the other are not.

The play brings before us two young men of working-class origin in the English midlands who have a candy stand concession in a local cinema. One of them—Jimmy Porter—has had a university education and acts as a self-appointed protector to his Welsh buddy, an uncomplicated person happily free of metaphysical anguish.

Jimmy is married to a pretty girl whom he feels he almost had to steal away from her family, the kind of family whose strength and graces were grounded on England's 1914 Empire. Jimmy not only resents his wife's family and all the institutions that bred them because they led to nothing but the dust and ashes of 1945; he also berates her for having lost the stamina presumed to be characteristic of her background, without having replaced it with any new values of her own—even romantically negative ones like his.

A fourth character, a young actress, represents that middle class which obstinately holds on to its customary traditions, and there is also the wan figure of Jimmy's father-in-law, bewildered and impotent in an England he no longer recognizes.

Jimmy Porter then is the angry one. What is he angry about? It is a little difficult at first for an American to understand. The English understand, not because it is ever explicitly stated, but because the jitters which wrack Jimmy, though out of proportion to the facts within the play, are in the very air the Englishman breathes. Jimmy, "risen" from the working class, is now provided with an intellect which only shows him that everything that might have justified pride in the old England—its opportunity, adventure, material well-being—has disappeared without being replaced by anything but a lacklustre security. He has been promoted into a moral and social vacuum. He fumes, rages, nags at a world which promised much and has led to a dreary plain where there is no fibre or substance, but only fear of scientific destruction and the minor comforts of "American" mechanics. His wife comments to the effect that "my father is sad because everything has changed, Jimmy is sad because nothing has.'' In the meantime Jimmy seeks solace and blows defiance through the symbolic jazz of his trumpet, while his working-class pal, though he adores Jimmy and his wife, wisely leaves the emotionally messy premises.

Immanent reality plus a gift for stinging and witty rhetoric are what give the play its importance. It is not realism of the Odets or Williams kind nor yet poetry, although it has some kinship to both. It adds up to a theatrical stylization of ideas about reality in which a perceptive journalism is made to flash on the stage by a talent for histrionic gesture and vivid elocution. While the end product possesses a certain nervous force and genuineness of feeling it is also sentimental, for it still lacks the quality of an experience digested, controlled or wholly understood.

Someone asked me if I didn't believe the play might achieve greater dimensions if American actors were to play it in a manner now associated with the generation influenced by the Group Theatre. The question reveals a misunderstanding of the play's nature. It calls for the verbal brio and discreet indication of feeling which it receives from the uniformly excellent, attractive English cast—Kenneth Haigh, Mary Ure, Allan Bates, Vivienne Drummond.

Jimmy Porter, ''deepened'' in another vein, would prove an intolerable nuisance, a self-pitying, verbose, sadistic jackanapes. He is a sign, not a character. We accept him because in the final count he is more amusing than real. We can look beyond him and the flimsy structure of the fable in which he is involved and surmise some of the living sources in the civilization from which he issues.

That John Osborne is attached and attuned to those sources is the virtue and hope of his talent. It may take ten years for him to achieve what most people have declared he already has.

Source: Harold Clurman, review of *Look Back in Anger* in the *Nation,* Volume 185, no. 12, October 19, 1957, p. 272.

"IMMANENT REALITY PLUS A GIFT FOR STINGING AND WITTY RHETORIC ARE WHAT GIVE *LOOK BACK IN ANGER* ITS IMPORTANCE."

SOURCES

Athanason, Arthur Nicholas. ''John Osborne,'' in *Concise Dictionary of British Literary Biography,* Volume 7: *Writers After World War II, 1945-1960,* Gale, 1992, pp. 231-54.

Barker, John. A review of *Look Back in Anger* in *Daily Express,* May 9, 1956.

Billington, Michael. A review of *Look Back in Anger* in *Guardian,* June 8, 1989.

Carter, Alan. *John Osborne,* Oliver & Boyd, 1969, pp. 1-4, 22.

Coveney, Michael. A review of *Look Back in Anger* in *Financial Times,* June 13, 1989.

Elsom, John. *Post-War British Theatre,* Routledge & Kegan Paul, 1976, pp. 72-87.

Elsom, John. *Post-War British Theatre Criticism,* Routledge & Kegan Paul, 1981, pp. 74-80.

Ferrar, Harold. *John Osborne,* Columbia University Press, 1973, pp. 3-12, 46.

Hobson, Harold. A review of *Look Back in Anger* in *Sunday Times,* May 13, 1956.

Hope-Wallace, Philip. A review of *Look Back in Anger* in *Manchester Guardian,* May 10, 1956.

Osborne, John. *Look Back in Anger,* Penguin, 1982.

Page, Malcolm. *File on Osborne,* Methuen, 1988, pp. 11-17.

Paton, Maureen. A review of *Look Back in Anger* in *Daily Express,* June 8, 1989.

Shulman, Milton. A review of *Look Back in Anger* in *Evening Standard,* May 9, 1956.

Smyth, Damian. A review of *Look Back in Anger* in *Independent,* June 10, 1989.

Tynan, Kenneth. A review of *Look Back in Anger* in *Observer,* May, 13, 1956.

Wilson, Cecil. A review of *Look Back in Anger* in *Daily Mail,* May 9, 1956.

FURTHER READING

Browne, Terry W. *Playwrights' Theatre; The English Stage Company at the Royal Court,* Pitman, 1975.

This book details the first production of *Look Back in Anger* and gives a broad view of theatre conditions, including censorship, both before and after the production.

Rusinko, Susan. *British Drama, 1950 to The Present,* Twayne, 1989.

This book offers a concise view of developments in British both leading up to and after *Look Back in Anger.*

Taylor, John Russell. *The Angry Theatre,* Hill and Wang, 1969.

Taylor deals with the movement in theatre from the production of *Look Back in Anger* to 1968 and examines playwrights who were encouraged and influenced by Osborne.

Trussler, Simon. *The Cambridge Illustrated History of British Theatre,* Cambridge University Press, 1994.

An illustrated volume that places the period of *Look Back in Anger* in a broad context of theatre. It also includes pictures of the Royal Court Theatre and productions of *Look Back in Anger.*

Miss Julie

AUGUST STRINDBERG

1888

First published in 1888, August Strindberg's *Miss Julie* shocked early reviewers with its frank portrayal of sexuality. Although it was privately produced in Copenhagen, Denmark, in 1889, the play was banned throughout much of Europe and was not produced in Sweden, Strindberg's native country, until 1906. Britain's ban on public performances of the play was not lifted until 1939. Notoriety is often the best publicity, however, and the play soon gained an underground popularity in both Europe and America; mainstream acceptance and success came a bit slower, but by the early twentieth century the play was considered an important facet of modern drama.

The root of contention over the play stemmed from its frank portrayal of sex. Not only does *Miss Julie* contain a sexual encounter between a lower-class servant and an upper-class aristocrat (in itself outrageous for the times), the play clearly describes the sex act as something apart from the concept of love. The idea of intercourse based completely on lust was scandalous to late-nineteenth century thinking and enough to provoke censure. And it was nothing more than the idea of sex without love that caused the trouble: the act is only referred to in the play, not actually depicted on stage.

Strindberg's drama focuses on the downfall of the aristocratic Miss Julie, a misfit in her society (the author refers to her in his preface as a ''man-hating half-woman''). Julie rebels against the re-

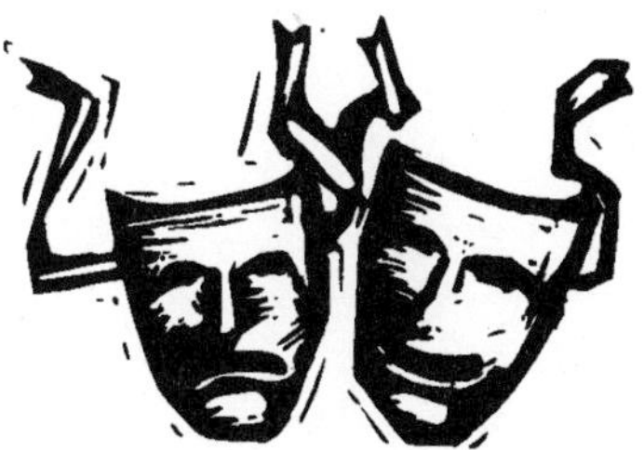

strictions placed on her as a woman and as a member of the upper-class. From the beginning of the play, her behavior is shown to alienate her peer class and shock the servants. She displays a blatant disregard for class and gender conventions, at one moment claiming that class differences should not exist and the next demanding proper treatment as a woman of aristocracy. Her antics result in her social downfall, a loss of respect from her servants, and, ultimately, her suicide.

Miss Julie is widely regarded as the most important drama to come out of the literary movement known as naturalism. The movement was based largely on the theory of social Darwinism, which proposed that individuals fight for position in society much as animals fight for their survival in the wild, and that, in humans (as in animals) only the fittest can survive (this theory is known as ''Natural Selection'' and was first proposed by Charles Darwin). As a naturalistic drama, *Miss Julie* focuses on Julie and Jean's struggle for survival in their society. Strindberg claimed that the basis for the plot of *Miss Julie* was a true story he had heard of a young noblewoman who had had sexual relations with a servant, although that young woman did not commit suicide. Strindberg lived in a time in which gender and class roles were becoming more fluid, and the play reflects the conflicts that are inevitable in a society struggling with change.

Today *Miss Julie* is regarded as remarkable for the same reason early critics and censors found it so shocking: it is the first play in which sex is separated from love. Strindberg's portrayal of the strength of sexual desire (and the often calamitous situations that result when one surrenders to such desires) strongly influenced later playwrights, most notably Tennessee Williams (*Cat on a Hot Tin Roof*). Although the play's importance was not widely recognized during Strindberg's lifetime, its place in modern drama, particularly as an example of naturalism, is now virtually undisputed.

AUTHOR BIOGRAPHY

Strindberg was born Johan August Strindberg on January 22, 1849, in Riddarholm, Stockholm, Sweden. His father was a middle-class merchant, his mother a former servant. He suffered through an emotionally difficult childhood; when he was four his father went bankrupt, and when he was thirteen his mother died. A year after her death, his father married the family housekeeper.

As Strindberg grew older, he struggled to choose a profession. He worked as an elementary school teacher, studied medicine and philosophy, worked as a journalist, and had an appointment in the Swedish Royal Library, cataloguing holdings in the Chinese section. He also made two unsuccessful attempts at becoming an actor. It was during the first of these attempts that Strindberg began writing plays and, in 1870, his first two plays, *The Freethinker* and *In Rome,* were produced. His early plays were poorly received, however, and it was not until 1881 that a reworked version of an earlier play, *Major Olof,* brought him some success.

In 1894, Strindberg's first collection of short stories was published. Frankly sexual in nature and critical of the upper classes, the book was considered immoral by many, and Strindberg was eventually put on trial for blasphemy. Although he was finally acquitted, the episode made him realize that the government could take away his freedom of expression. He nonetheless continued to explore sexuality as well as class issues in subsequent writings. In addition to working in other genres, Strindberg continued to write plays, gaining more success with his naturalistic dramas, the most well known of which are *The Father* (1887) and *Miss Julie* (1888).

In 1897, Strindberg briefly quit writing in order to pursue scientific experiments, particularly in alchemy, the attempt to turn less valuable metals into gold. He also became interested in mysticism and the occult. In 1896, he began developing psychotic symptoms, experiencing obsessions and hallucinations. Putting himself under a doctor's care, he eventually recovered and began writing again. After this experience, however, he developed a new interest in the reality of the psyche, particularly dreams. He began to write his ''dream plays,'' surrealistic pieces such as *A Dream Play* (1902) and *The Ghost Sonata.*

Strindberg's personal life mirrored his professional career, with many ups and downs. In 1877, he married Siri von Essen, a divorced actress. This union ended in divorce in 1891. Strindberg would marry and divorce two more times. He fathered a total of six children: Karin, Greta, and Hans from his first marriage (a daughter also died in infancy); Kerstin from his second marriage; and Anne-Marie from his third.

In addition to his writing, Strindberg was active in other artistic areas. He founded the Scandinavian Experimental Theatre in Copenhagen, Denmark, in 1888, and founded the Intimate Theatre in 1907. Strindberg remained active throughout his adult life, continuing to write until his death from stomach cancer on May 14, 1912. Today he is regarded as one of the most important of modern dramatists.

PLOT SUMMARY

Miss Julie opens with Jean, a valet, and Kristine, a cook, in the kitchen of the Count, their master. The two begin to talk about Miss Julie, the Count's daughter. Jean says she is crazy, dancing with the servants at a Midsummer's Eve celebration when she should be visiting relatives with her father. Kristine remarks that Julie has always been crazy but has gotten worse since breaking off her engagement with her fiance. Jean reveals that he once saw Julie ''training'' her fiance as one would train a dog, making him jump over her riding crop and hitting him with it after each jump until he finally took the riding crop from her, struck her with it, and broke it into pieces. According to Jean, Julie, like her late mother, acts in some ways like an aristocrat and in others like a commoner.

Julie enters and asks Jean to dance with her. At first he declines, noting that he has already promised this dance to Kristine, but Julie finally persuades him. The two go offstage together, leaving Kristine working in the kitchen. When Julie and Jean return, they engage in conversation while Kristine sleeps at the table. Jean reveals to Julie his aristocratic tastes—he drinks wine, speaks French, and uses the language of the upper classes. In contrast Julie chooses to drink beer instead of wine, saying she prefers it.

Julie wants to dance with Jean again, but Jean warns her that she is talked about because of her familiarity with the male servants. Kristine goes to bed, leaving Julie and Jean alone and, in the ensuing conversation, Julie alternates between urging Jean to treat her as an equal and ordering him around. Jean reveals that he was in love with Julie when they were both children and that to him her father's garden was the Garden of Eden, while Julie herself symbolized the hopelessness of his ascension to a higher class. As they are speaking, a crowd of servants comes to the door, singing a vulgar song about Julie and Jean. The servants are about to enter

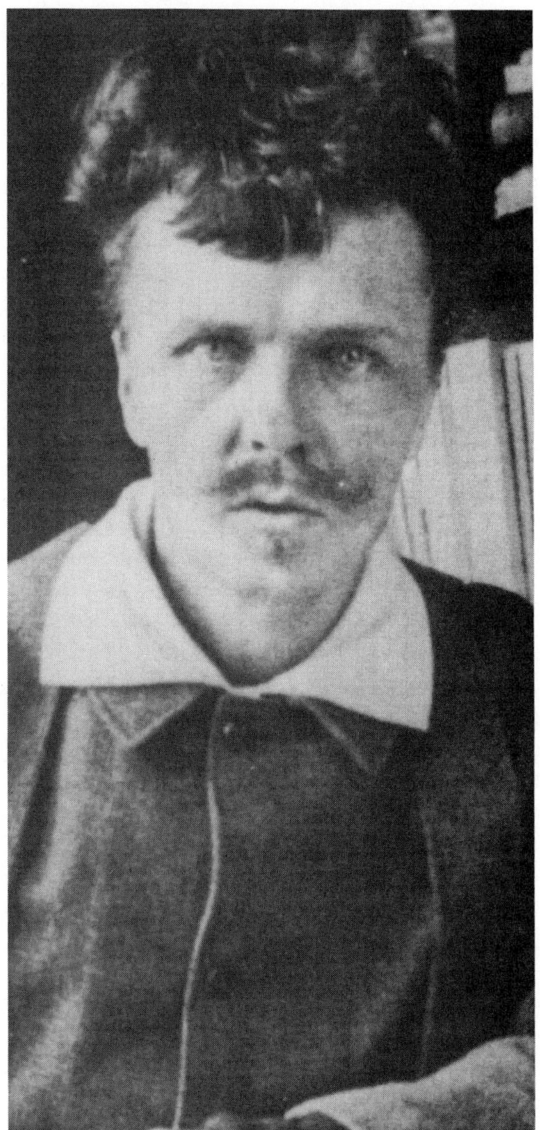

August Strindberg in 1886

the kitchen, and Jean tells Julie that, in order to safeguard her reputation, the two of them must hide and that the only possible place for them to go is his room. Julie and Jean leave the kitchen and the servants enter, continuing their singing. When the servants are gone, Julie and Jean return; it is clear that they have had sexual intercourse in Jean's room.

With both of their reputation endangered by their tryst, Jean says that the two of them must leave together, perhaps go to Switzerland to open a hotel. Julie, trying to create a romantic relationship from their purely carnal encounter, asks him to say he loves her and tells him to call her Julie rather than

Miss Julie. Jean refuses, saying that such familiarity is only possible in the future, when his ambition leads him to great heights—perhaps to becoming a count in Rumania, where titles can be purchased. He begins to speak harshly to Julie, saying he needs money to leave. When Julie says that she has no money, Jean says that they will have to stay. Julie expresses alarm at the prospect of the servants laughing at her for taking Jean as a lover. Jean calls her a whore, saying her actions are below those of a female servant, who would never throw herself at a man as Julie has.

Later, Jean softens in his attitude toward Julie. They return to the idea of running away together. Julie tells Jean about her family history. She relates her mother's belief in women's equality to men, beliefs which resulted in Julie being raised as a boy in order to show that women could be as good as men. Julie's mother also insisted that, on the estate, male servants take on the tasks of women and female servants do the work of men, a policy that resulted in financial ruin. Finally Julie's father took control, but a suspicious fire, later revealed to be started by Julie's mother, burned the house and other buildings. The family then faced poverty, but Julie's mother was able to secure a loan from a brick manufacturer, later discovered to be her lover. The "loan" was actually money that belonged to Julie's family in the first place. From her mother, Julie learned to hate all men. Despite such hatred, she is still sexually attracted to men and a victim to her passions.

Although Julie says she hates Jean, she wants the two of them to leave together. Jean says that the only solution is for Julie to go away alone. She says she will go if he will come with her. When he refuses, Julie, unable to make a decision, asks him for an order. He now tells her to go and dress for their trip, that the two of them will leave together. Julie leaves the room and, shortly afterwards, Kristine enters. Guessing what has happened, Kristine is disgusted with Julie and no longer respects her. Kristine leaves and Julie enters the room, carrying a bird cage. Jean agrees to leave with her but says they cannot take the bird; Julie agrees to let him kill it. When he decapitates the bird, Julie screams that she hates him and that she will tell her father everything.

Jean leaves, Kristine returns, and Julie begs her for assistance, suggesting that all three of them go to Switzerland, attempting to paint a beautiful picture of their future. Kristine is not interested, and she leaves for church, cutting off Julie and Jean's chance for escape when she remarks that she will tell the groomsman not to let any of the horses go. Julie asks Jean what to do. He tells her that she should commit suicide. The bell rings, and the two realize that the Count has returned. Jean becomes subservient at the sound of the bell, but he hands Julie the razor and tells her to go the barn. She walks out, carrying the razor.

CHARACTERS

Jean

Jean is the ambitious valet who engages in sexual relations with Julie. Although he is a servant, he longs for a higher social position. He tells Julie of his desire to open a hotel and become a count like her father. In his discussion with her, he reveals a taste for fine food and good wine as well as a dream of climbing a tree, a symbol of his desire to move up in the world. It is clear, however, that his actions will keep him a servant for life. He has become engaged to Kristine, the cook, further cementing his place in the lower classes and, when he and Miss Julie sleep together, he is primarily concerned with the fact that, because of his actions, he may lose his position as a servant—the very station he says he wants so desperately to leave.

Although Jean freely insults Julie after their sexual encounter, apparently no longer seeing himself as her inferior, when Kristine insults Julie, Jean tells her she must be respectful towards her mistress. Although Jean is brave enough to steal wine from his master, when the Count returns, ringing for his boots and coffee, Jean immediately returns to subservience, leading the audience to doubt that his ambitions will ever turn into reality.

Miss Julie

Miss Julie is the play's main character. She does not understand her place in society as an aristocrat or as a woman; her confusion and lack of understanding is the primary focus of the play. When the audience first sees her, she has been dancing with the servants at their Midsummer's Eve festivities when it would be more appropriate for her to be visiting relatives with her father, the Count. During the course of the play, she spends most of her time with Jean, her father's valet. In her conversations with Jean, Julie alternates between giving him commands and trying to convince him to treat her as an equal. In order that the other servants will not see her with Jean, however, she hides with him in his room. While they are locked in together, the two engage in sexual intercourse.

Julie not only rebels against her place as an aristocrat, but—having given in to animal passion, to sex without love—she has revealed a confused gender identity as well. Respectable women at this time did not engage in such behavior. Julie also reveals that her mother raised her as a boy, which contributes to her gender confusion. At the end of the play, although Julie is ashamed of her actions, she has really learned nothing. As in the beginning, she still alternates between seeing herself as an aristocrat and as an equal of the servants. At the end of the play, she commands Jean to order her to commit suicide.

Kristine

Engaged to Jean, Kristine is the Count's cook. Unlike Jean and Julie, she recognizes her place in society and stays within what she considers proper bounds. Traditional in every way, she is also extremely religious. Julie's actions appall Kristine from the beginning, but when she discovers that Julie has slept with Jean, Kristine says she can no longer work for people who have no sense of decency. She does not show such anger at Jean, however, and tells him that, in fact, his indiscretion with Julie is not as bad as if he had committed a similar act with a fellow servant. In Kristine's view, it is only Julie who has completely debased herself and is so deserving of disdain. Kristine cuts off Julie and Jean's only possibility of escape when she announces that she will tell the groom not to let any of the horses out, thus revealing that her loyalty is to her master, the Count.

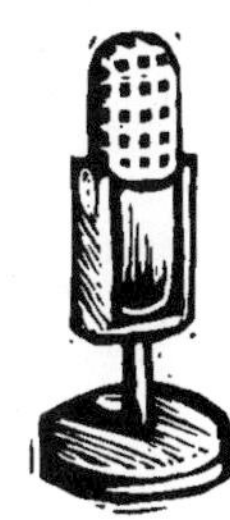

MEDIA ADAPTATIONS

- *Miss Julie* was made into the 1951 Swedish film *Froken Julie,* directed by Alf Sjoberg.
- A television version of *Miss Julie* was produced by the British Broadcasting Corporation (BBC) in 1965. The program was directed by Alan Bridges and stars Stephanie Bidmean, Ian Hendry, and Gunnel Lindblom.
- In 1972, John Glenister and Robin Phillips directed another version of *Miss Julie.* This adaptation stars Helen Mirren, Donal McCann, and Heather Canning.

THEMES

Gender Roles

Miss Julie's confusion over her sexual identity ultimately leads to her ruin. For Strindberg, men and women have specific roles in society; in the play's preface he describes Julie as a ''man-hating half-woman.'' Julie's problems stem from her heritage as well as the way she was reared. Her mother did not bring Julie up according to accepted standards regarding women's roles; she also believed—incorrectly, Strindberg implies—that men and women are equal. She refused to conform to traditional female roles. At first, she would not marry Julie's father, although she had sexual relations with him, was the mother of his child, and was essentially mistress of his household. In this position, she forced the servants into ''unnatural'' occupations, with men assigned to traditionally female tasks while women did the work of men. The result was financial ruin. In keeping with this philosophy, Julie was raised as a boy, expected to match or exceed the role of a male child. She was forced to wear boys' clothes, engage in physical chores such as caring for horses, and even go hunting.

In addition to forcing male traits on her daughter, Julie's mother also taught her to despise all men. Julie says she only became engaged so she could make her fiance her slave, and it is clear that this is what she did, even to the point of making her betrothed jump over her riding crop while whipping him like an animal. When Jean kills Julie's greenfinch, Julie's rage at men is nakedly revealed. ''I'd like to see your whole sex swimming in a sea of blood,'' she tells him. The situation is complicated, however, by the fact that Julie despises women as well and blames her father for bringing her up to revile her own sex. Complicating matters is Julie's sexual desire, which forces her to adopt female behavior she abhors and seduce the men she hates. The result, Julie says, is that she is neither fully male nor fully female but has become ''half-woman,

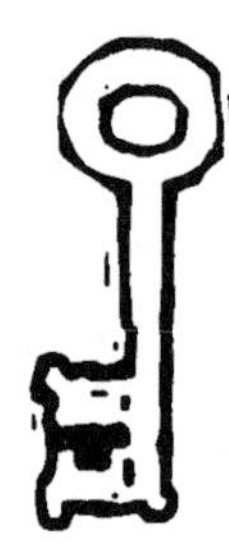

TOPICS FOR FURTHER STUDY

- Compare Miss Julie to Edna in Kate Chopin's novel *The Awakening*. How do both women respond to the restrictions of their societies? How does Edna's suicide differ from Julie's? Could the authors' genders be an influence in the differences between these two works?
- Although the Count affects the action of *Miss Julie,* he never appears onstage. Discuss the Count's importance to the play. What might be the purpose of his remaining an offstage presence? How would the play be different if he appeared onstage?
- Compare *Miss Julie* to the Ibsen plays *A Doll's House* and *Hedda Gabler.* How does Strindberg's apparent view of the changing roles of women in his society differ from Ibsen's?
- Compare and contrast Jean and Miss Julie's characters. How do they differ in their dissatisfaction with their class positions? Why is Jean able to live while Julie sees no option but suicide?
- Research the theory of social Darwinism. How do the fates of the characters in *Miss Julie* reflect Strindberg's belief in this theory?

half-man,'' an unnatural role in which, according to Strindberg, she can never find happiness.''

Class Conflict

Much of the action of *Miss Julie* focuses on the conflict between the upper and lower classes. Both Julie and Jean are dissatisfied with their class positions. Julie, the aristocrat, relates a recurring dream in which she is high atop a pillar yet longs to come down to the ground. Jean, the servant, also has a recurring dream: he conversely sees himself struggling to climb a tree in order to obtain the golden eggs at the top. Julie, although she is mistress of the house, attends the servants' party, participating in their revelry rather than visiting relatives with her father. Jean, on the other hand, has aristocratic pretensions. He is fussy about his food and drink, speaks in cultured tones, and plans to escape his role as a servant, open his own hotel, and become a count like his employer.

In spite of their desires, however, Strindberg's characters are destined to remain in the class to which they were born. Julie is, at heart, an aristocrat and Jean, despite his refined playacting, has the soul of a servant. While she longs to belong to their common class, Julie also snobbishly states that she honors her servants with her presence at their dance; she alternates between entreating Jean to treat her as an equal and ordering him about. Jean speaks of his ambitions, but, after his sexual encounter with Julie, he desperately searches for a way to keep his lowly position and tells Kristine she must respect her mistress. When the Count returns and rings for his boots and coffee, Jean reverts to a state of complete subservience. As far as these characters are concerned, Strindberg believes that there is no escaping class destiny.

Sexuality

In *Miss Julie,* sex is divorced from love—a fact that caused Strindberg and his play a good deal of trouble when it first appeared. Although there is mild flirtation between Julie and Jean at the beginning of the play, there is no sense that their subsequent sexual encounter arises from unrequited passion or love, especially as it occurs while the other servants sing what Jean describes as ''a dirty song'' about himself and Julie. In addition, when the two emerge from Jean's room, Jean confesses that his previous story of romantic longing for her as a child was merely a lie invented to seduce her. When he saw her as a child, he later reveals, he had ''the same dirty thoughts all boys have.'' Julie is horrified by this revelation. She asks Jean to say he loves her, but her desperate attempt to introduce romance into their relationship is forced, an attempt to convince herself that she has not been disgraced in her surrender to carnal desire.

Strindberg makes it clear, though, that Julie's sexual act with Jean is not romantic but unbridled lust. Jean says he has never seen a woman throw herself at a man as Julie has, that such sexual baseness exists only in animals and in whores. Julie says that, although she despises men, she cannot control herself ''when the weakness comes, when passion burns.'' Julie's sexuality ultimately contributes to her downfall. Not only do her passions drive her to sex with a lower-class man—an act that will forever sully her reputation—they force her to intimately interact with the male sex she so despises, behavior that will further damage her conflicted personality. Julie's sexual encounter with Jean causes a breakdown of both her external and internal status: she is disgraced in the eyes of others and has dealt an irreparable injury to her already precarious self-esteem.

STYLE

Allusion

An allusion is a reference to another literary work. In *Miss Julie,* the name of Julie's dog, Diana, is an allusion to the Roman goddess of hunting. According to her legend, when a man caught sight of her bathing, Diana unleashed her hounds to tear him to pieces. The goddess Diana's rejection of men mirrors Julie's. Another allusion is found in the subject of the church sermon Kristine will attend, the beheading of John the Baptist. According to the Biblical story, John the Baptist was beheaded by the Palestinian ruler King Herod Antipas, who was tricked into killing the disciple of Jesus Christ by his wife, Herodias, and daughter, Salome. John the Baptist's death is reflected in the death of Julie's bird as well as in the death of Julie herself.

Foreshadowing

In foreshadowing, words, symbols, or an event suggest a future incident. Julie's dog Diana's sexual encounter with the gatekeeper's dog, an encounter that horrifies Julie, foreshadows her own sexual act with Jean—as well as her subsequent shame and horror following the act. The beheading of Julie's bird by Jean foreshadows Julie's own death.

The Unities

The three classical unities, unity of time, unity of place, and unity of action, are a Renaissance-era interpretation of the rules of ancient Greek drama (as they are described in Aristotle's *Poetics*). Unity of time dictates that the action of a drama occur within a twenty-four hour period. In order to conform to unity of place, the action of a play must take place in either a single location or locations that are close to one another; one cannot, for instance, set one scene in Paris while another is set in Rome. Unity of action means that all of the incidents of a drama must follow each other logically. In writing *Miss Julie,* Strindberg strictly adhered to the classical unities.

Structure

The structure of *Miss Julie* differs from contemporary late-nineteenth century drama in that Strindberg, believing that the intermissions between acts interrupted an audience's concentration, chose to write a shorter play. He conceived *Miss Julie* as a one-act rather than the traditional three-act play so that the audience could experience his drama in a single sitting. Nevertheless, the play's structure reflects the traditional structure in that it has three distinct parts. Instead of being divided by an intermission, the first and second acts occur on either side of the mime, in which Kristine appears alone onstage. The second and third parts are separated by the servants' ballet, which occurs onstage while Jean and Julie are alone (having sex) in Jean's room.

Symbol

A symbol represents something outside of itself. In *Miss Julie,* the Count's boots and bell symbolize his offstage presence as well as his continuing power over Julie and Jean. When Jean hears the Count's bell, his dreams of social mobility evaporate, and he once again becomes a lackey. Likewise, Jean and Julie's respective dreams are symbols of their desire to escape their reality.

Naturalism

Naturalism is a literary movement that began in France in the mid-1800s. The French writer Emile Zola (the *Rougon-Macquart* series of novels) is considered the most influential in defining the principles of the movement. Naturalists were influenced by the theory of social Darwinism, in which the human struggle for social survival mirrored the struggle of animals for physical survival (survival of the fittest). In Naturalism, humans are controlled by social and biological factors, heredity, and environment, rather than by their own strength of will and character. *Miss Julie* is widely considered to be the most important naturalistic drama.

HISTORICAL CONTEXT

In 1859, less than thirty years before Strindberg wrote *Miss Julie,* Charles Darwin published *The*

COMPARE & CONTRAST

- **1888:** Although published in 1859, Charles Darwin's *The Origin of Species* is still the focus of controversy as religious people feel threatened by Darwin's findings and the resulting conception of human beings as animals.

  Today: Darwin's theories are widely accepted, and most people consider humans to be, biologically, animals. Few religious people consider their beliefs shaken by evolution.

- **1888:** The role of women is rapidly changing as women gain more equality with men under the law. Husbands, however, retain legal rights over their wives and the proper position of married women is widely debated.

  Today: European and American women have close to complete legal equality with men, but many believe much progress remains to be made. In some third-world countries there is still great inequality between the sexes.

- **1888:** Social Darwinism gains importance as a theory as people see the concept of the survival of the fittest at work in society.

  Today: Circumstances beyond individual control and genetics are now seen as having a great impact in determining who will gain status and wealth. Acceptance of the theory of social Darwinism has greatly declined.

- **1888:** Social reforms in Sweden are in the process of increasing the rights of workers, who are demanding higher wages and shorter workdays. In Sweden, workers are kept from voting by a law that requires a minimum income of those who vote.

  Today: The position of workers throughout the world has greatly improved. Due to a government welfare system, all Swedes have a relatively high standard of living.

Origin of Species, a book that revolutionized scientific thought on the subjects of evolution and environmental adaptation. Darwin identified a process he called natural selection. According to this theory, the earth cannot support all organisms that develop and so these life forms must compete with one another for environmental resources such as food and living space. The tendency for the hardier species to prevail and propagate while the weaker species die off is what Darwin termed the survival of the fittest.

Darwin's ideas were extremely controversial at this time. Previously, people believed that God had created each species individually. Further, Darwin's theories indicated that humans evolved from lower life forms—more specifically lower primates such as apes. To many, this idea was sacrilegious (as they believed God had created humans in his image, as fully-evolved creatures), a repudiation of God, and a threat to religion. Although some pious individuals accepted Darwin's theories, believing evolution occurred under God's guidance, others found their beliefs challenged. After all, if humans descended from other species, then there was little to separate man from beast.

In spite of such objections, acceptance of Darwin's theories grew. And while Darwin's ideas applied to biology, the concept of survival of the fittest began to influence other disciplines as well. Most notable was the development of social Darwinism, a concept that came to prominence in the late-1800s. Social Darwinists saw natural selection occurring within the social as well as biological realm; the concept was used to explain disparities—why some rose to aristocracy while others languished in the lower-classes—in social status. Those who were wealthy or had accomplished much had done so because they were better adapted to compete for scarce social resources. Those who were poor and had achieved little were in their positions because of their own nature. The concept of social Darwinism became important to the Naturalist literary movement from which *Miss Julie* arose. In Strindberg's play, the concept of social Darwinism can be seen in the fall of Julie, who is clearly unfit for a superior position and cannot survive. Jean's ability to rise, while questionable, is presented more optimistically; he is stronger and consequently more likely to improve his position in society.

The social position of the lower-class was improving at the time Strindberg's work appeared. Workers in Sweden began to strike for higher wages and shorter workdays. In 1881, a law was passed to limit child labor in factories, but it was not until 1909 that all adult males in Sweden were given the right to vote. The possibility of social mobility was becoming greater at this time as well. In his preface to *Miss Julie,* Strindberg, himself the child of a servant, wrote of "the old . . . nobility giving way to a new nobility of nerve and intellect."

The position of women in society was also an important issue at this time. It was only in 1845 that women in Sweden were given the right to own property. In 1846 women were also given the right to hold certain specific jobs, such as teaching, and finally, in 1862, the right to vote. In the 1870s, women were let into the universities for the first time, although they were not allowed to study theology or law. In general, women were gradually becoming, at least in the eyes of the law, more independent and closer in equality with men.

Strindberg himself showed mixed feelings about the changing roles of women. In many ways he sympathized with women, but while Norwegian playwright Henrik Ibsen created Nora, the heroine of *A Doll's House* who walked out on her husband and children to meet her own needs, Strindberg placed more importance on the sanctity of marriage and spoke in his preface to *Miss Julie* about the rise of the "man-hating half-woman." A general opposition to feminism is also apparent in *Miss Julie.*

CRITICAL OVERVIEW

With its frank portrayal of sexuality, *Miss Julie* has been a controversial play since its inception—even before it was produced onstage. Initially, Strindberg was only able to get the play published, and reviews of this published version were largely negative. Michael Meyer, in his biography *Strindberg,* quoted a number of early critics. The play was called "a filthy bundle of rags which one hardly wishes to touch even with tongs" as well as "a heap of ordure . . . [with] language that is scarcely used except in nests of vice and debauchery." One critic cited in Meyer's book prophesied that the play "will surely nowhere find a public that could endure to see it." Another said that, in order to write *Miss Julie,* Strindberg "must . . . have been troubled by some affectation of the brain which rendered him . . . not wholly normal."

Production of the play was initially banned by censors, but Strindberg, who opened his own experimental theater company in order to produce the play, was able to have *Miss Julie* shown privately in Copenhagen in 1889. In the next few years, the play was banned in various European countries, and it was not until 1906 that *Miss Julie* was performed publicly in Sweden. While the play gradually began to receive more frequent productions, it continued to be perceived as shocking. As Margery Morgan noted in her book *August Strindberg,* as late as 1912 one critic called the play "the most repellent and brutal play we have ever had to sit through." In spite of repeated censure and harsh criticism, however, the importance of *Miss Julie* was gradually recognized. According to Meyer, after seeing a production of the play, playwright George Bernard Shaw (*Major Barbara*) wrote of Strindberg as "that very remarkable genius who was left by Ibsen's death at the head of the Scandinavian drama."

Miss Julie is no longer considered shocking because of its sexuality, and critics have turned instead to viewing the play largely through the lens of psychology, a fledgling science in Strindberg's time. In *Gradiva,* Harry Jarv wrote that the pre-Freudian psychological theories of the 1880s focused on the elements of a personality but "did not produce a synthesis," a whole integrated personality. Jarv noted that other literary critics have found fault with Julie's lack of cohesiveness as a character. Jarv, however, pointed out the multitude of motivations Strindberg gives for Julie's actions in the preface and remarked that, in his understanding of personality, Strindberg was actually ahead of his time. According to the critic, "the master psychologist Strindberg has managed, in Julie and Jean, to give form to the exceedingly complicated functional units of human personalities." Jarv also suggested that Strindberg drew upon elements of his own psychology in developing Julie. "Like Julie," Jarv wrote, "Strindberg had personally felt drawn to a life of the instincts, but at the same time he has perceived it as something shameful." Jarv's article focused on Strindberg's own battles with madness as well. As is often the case in Strindberg criticism, Jarv analyzed the play by offering an analysis of its author.

Writing at the same time as Jarv, Martin Lamm, in his book *August Strindberg,* also saw Julie as a psychological study. Lamm called her a "psychological enigma." According to Lamm, Strindberg's lengthy list of the "causes" of Julie's fall were an answer to Georg Brandes, who considered Julie's suicide "psychologically unbelievable." Lamm noted that there is no simple single-theory psychological explanation for the suicide. "Strindberg's intention," he wrote, "was to go beyond simple explanations for answers and to present the multiplicity of conscious and unconscious motivations upon which actions are based."

Like Lamm, Harry G. Carlson, in his 1982 book *Strindberg and the Poetry of Myth,* also focused on the complexity of Julie's personality, calling her downfall "the [result] of the awesome power of nature's twin forces, heredity and environment." In addition, however, Carlson pointed out that Julie and Jean's dreams are also a window into the psychology of their characters. However, Carlson went beyond psychology, suggesting that "a mythic destiny had long ago designed and determined the characters' fate." For Carlson, Strindberg's psychological play also has mythical overtones.

Lesley Ferris, in her 1989 study *Acting Women: Images of Women in Theatre,* also showed an interest in the psychology of Julie, but saw that psychology from a feminist perspective. Ferris focused on Strindberg's characterization of Julie as a "half-woman," androgynous because of her upbringing. Julie, according to Ferris, has absorbed the patriarchal concept of what women should be but cannot assume the role patriarchy assigns her. Consequently she does not have "access to an autonomous self." Like earlier critics Ferris believed that Julie has no integrated personality, in essence no self, and this is what leads to her downfall.

Current psychological examinations of Julie and Jean reflect late-twentieth century thought and its emphasis on psychology as surely as the earliest critiques reflected common views on propriety in Strindberg's time. As times continue to change, further viewpoints will lead to a greater understanding of *Miss Julie.*

CRITICISM

Clare Cross

Cross is a Ph.D. candidate specializing in modern and contemporary drama. In this essay she discusses Miss Julie's inability to live within the gender and class roles imposed on her by society.

In his preface to *Miss Julie,* Strindberg refers to Julie as a "man-hating half woman," and indeed, the playwright draws her as such—though it should be pointed out that Julie despises not only men but women as well. Nonetheless, psychologically—considered within the context of her time—Julie is neither wholly male nor wholly female, and she cannot find a place for herself within the social confines of either gender role. In addition, Julie, though an aristocrat by birth, does not fit in with either the upper classes or with the lower. Although she lives in a time during which rigid divisions in class and gender were softening, nineteenth-century Sweden was still a highly structured society with clearly defined class and gender roles. Because Julie cannot distinctly identify with male or female, master or servant, there is no place for her in this world. It is this fact that finally leads to her suicide.

From the beginning of the play, well before she even sets foot on stage, Julie's class and gender confusion become clear as the servants Jean and Kristine discuss their mistress's idiosyncrasies. Julie's inability to act within the bounds of acceptable female behavior is illustrated by an act Strindberg makes so extreme that it becomes ludicrous: Julie "training" her fiance by having him jump over her riding crop and striking him each jump. Clearly, Julie desires power over men to a point that is pathological.

Strindberg provides further evidence of Julie's lack of class identity. On one hand, Kristine reveals Julie's extreme anger over her dog's sexual encounter with the gatekeeper's dog, an act that foreshadows Julie's own indiscretion with Jean. On the other hand, Julie has chosen to stay at home and dance with her servants when it would be more appropriate for her to be visiting relatives with her father.

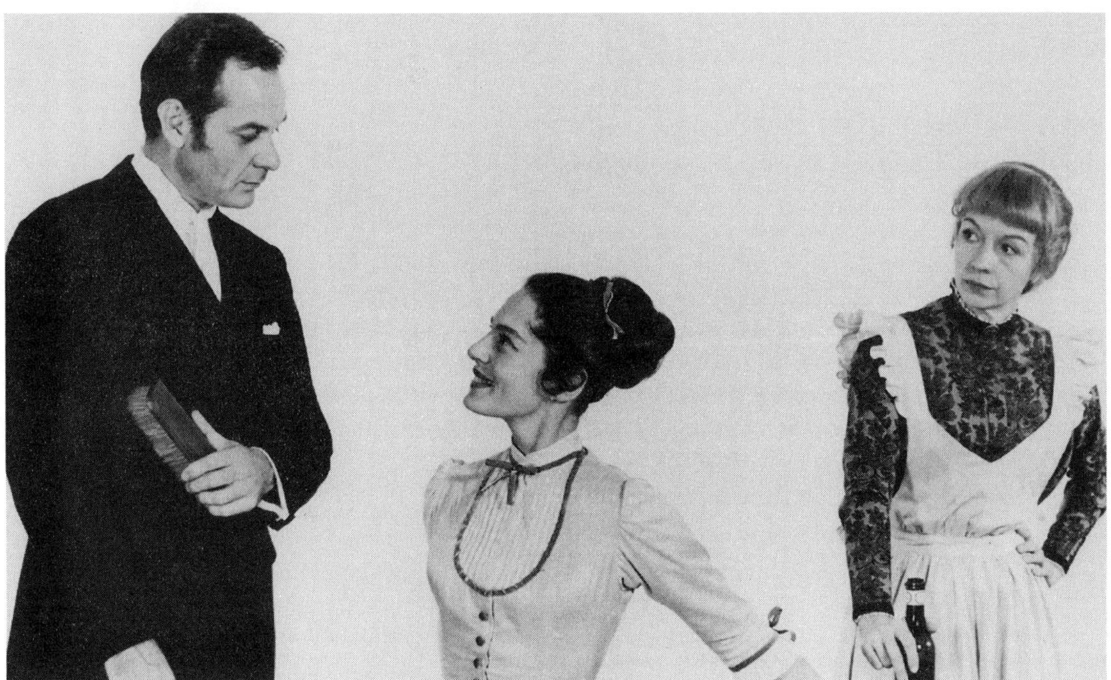

Jean (James Daly) talks to Miss Julie (Veronica Linford) while Kristine looks on disapprovingly

''Miss Julie,'' Jean says, ''has too much pride about some things and not enough about others.'' Jean reveals that Julie's mother was the same way. As he recalls, ''the cuffs of her blouse were dirty, but she had to have her coat of arms on her cufflinks.'' Like her mother, Julie is unrefined, even less refined than her own servants. Jean remarks that Julie ''pulled the gamekeeper away from Anna and made him dance with her.'' Such an act is unheard of in the world of the servants. ''*We* wouldn't behave like that,'' Jean says.

Julie's inconsistency in matters of class is revealed again when she appears onstage for the first time. When Jean points out that, by dancing with him, she risks losing the respect of her servants, she replies, ''As mistress of the house, I honor your dance with my presence!'' Yet when Jean says he will act ''as [she] orders,'' Julie replies, ''don't take it as an order! On a night like this, we're all just ordinary people having fun, so we'll forget about rank'' As much as Julie tries to force a sense of social equality, Strindberg makes it clear that she also demands the respect her position dictates.

In her book *Acting Women: Images of Women in Theatre,* Lesley Ferris pointed out that Kristine, the cook, acts as a counterpoint to Julie. As Ferris wrote, Kristine ''clearly knows her place as a woman and a member of the lower class—waiting on Jean, the footman, and enjoying this subservient position.'' When Jean asks Kristine if she is angry at him for dancing with Julie when he had promised to dance with her, Kristine tells him, ''I know my place.'' Jean responds, ''You're a sensible girl . . . and you'd make a good wife,'' a statement that plays up the contrast between Kristine and Julie, who is not sensible and would never make a good wife. Shortly after Julie and Jean return from their dancing, Kristine does the sensible thing; she goes to bed. In contrast, Julie stays up with Jean, telling him the story of a recurring dream, in which she is up in a tower and wants only to come down, clearly a reference to her discomfort with her position in society.

As Jean tries to point out to Julie, she is a woman and the mistress of the house, and she tremendously endangers her reputation by drinking alone with him in the kitchen: Julie, however, will not accept (at least initially) the fact that she cannot simply act as she pleases. Even when the other servants arrive and begin to sing the song of the swineherd and the princess, Julie believes they sing

WHAT DO I READ NEXT?

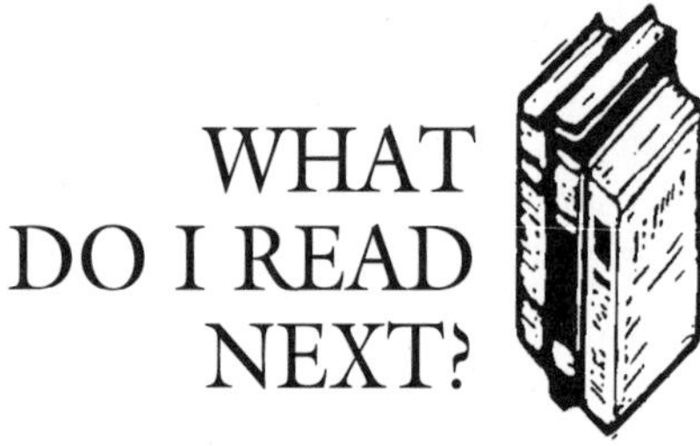

- *A Doll's House,* a play by Henrik Ibsen first produced in 1879, considers the place of the heroine, Nora, as a woman in her culture. Strindberg expressed a strong dislike of this play's portrayal of gender roles. *Miss Julie* is widely believed to be Strindberg's answer to *A Doll's House.*
- *Hedda Gabler,* an 1890 play also written by Ibsen, is the story of a woman who, like Miss Julie, cannot live within the confines of her society's gender roles. The play is regarded by some to be Ibsen's answer to *Miss Julie.*
- *A Streetcar Named Desire,* a 1947 play by Tennessee Williams, is considered to be strongly influenced by *Miss Julie.* This play focuses on Blanche DuBois, a southern belle who has seen better times, and Blanche's relationship with her sister's husband, Stanley Kowalski. Sexual desire as well as class and gender roles are important issues in this drama.
- *The Awakening,* an 1899 novel by Kate Chopin, tells the story of Edna Pontellier, who also rejects society and its conventions. Like Julie, Edna commits suicide. Chopin, however, presents a view of a troubled woman very different from that of Strindberg.
- *The Father,* Strindberg's 1887 play, is another naturalistic drama that is concerned with the difficulties of relationships between men and women.

---

out of love for her; she cannot see the gulf between herself and the workers. Finally persuaded that she has invited the disrespect of her servants, Julie hides with Jean in his room, another clear violation of her proper role. Her downfall becomes complete when she willingly has sex with Jean; at this point, her reputation is damaged beyond repair.

After their sexual encounter, Jean and Julie initially seem to believe that they can rectify the situation by fleeing to Switzerland, a place where no one knows them and their class differences will not matter. At this point, Julie, having acted with the sexual freedom reserved for men, now reverts to a traditionally female viewpoint; she wants to turn their purely carnal encounter into an expression of love. Jean, however, will not go along with her romantic fantasy. In addition, the sexual encounter has made them, in a sense, more equal; at least Jean is now able to openly express disdain for Julie. He tells her that her actions make her lower than her servants, calls her a whore, and, fearing no reproach, reveals that he has stolen wine from her father's cellar as well. At this point, Julie no longer wishes to play at social equality, and she attempts to regain her superior position. Insulted by Jean, she commands him, "You lackey, you menial, stand up when I speak to you!" He responds in kind: "Menial's strumpet, lackey's whore, shut up and get out of here!" This exchange brings Julie to realize the consequences of taking liberties with her socially-prescribed role; the respect that she feels is her due—and which she desperately needs for her self-esteem—has been erased.

At this point in the play, Strindberg chooses to provide the audience with some explanation for Julie's inability to accept her gender and class roles. Strindberg shows Julie as the product of heredity and environment, and his explanation for Julie's gender and class confusion even predates her birth, extending back to the character of her mother. Earlier Jean revealed that Julie's mother tried to act as both master and servant, that she insisted that her dirty cuffs be adorned with cufflinks bearing her coat of arms. After her sexual encounter with Jean and the ensuing arguments, Julie reveals to Jean more of her background. She describes her mother as "a commoner—very humble background." Because her father is a gentlemen, genetically, Julie truly is a hybrid of the upper and lower classes. Environment, however, has also played a strong part in bringing Julie to her present position. Her mother was "brought up believing in social equality, women's rights, and all that." Julie herself was reared according to her mother's bizarre ideas about gender equality.

As when he described Julie's "training" of her fiance, Strindberg once again presents a situation so extreme that it becomes ridiculous. Not only did Julie's mother believe women to be equal to men; she actually forced complete changes in gender roles. Male servants were assigned tasks normally reserved for women and women did the work of men. As a child, Julie was not simply freed from the conventional roles of women; she was forced to take on the activities and even the clothing of men. Julie was not brought up to see men as equals but to hate men and to want to make them her slaves. In addition, Julie complains that her father "brought me up to despise my own sex, making me half woman, half man." Because Julie hates women as well as men, she cannot help but hate herself and is doomed to confusion and misery. Because she is an aristocrat who cannot fully take on the role required by her class, there is no place where she belongs.

Up until the end, Julie's sense of gender and class identity remains ambiguous. For a time she is able to convince herself that she can escape her society by going to Switzerland with Jean, again trying to see their relationship as that of equals, but when Jean kills her greenfinch (her pet bird), her hatred of his sex and class resurfaces. Her words are remarkable for their violence: "I'd like to see your whole sex swimming in a sea of blood . . . I think I could drink from your skull! I'd like to bathe my feet in your open chest and eat your heart roasted whole!" In addition to this expression of hatred for men, Julie again reveals her sense of social superiority in her diatribe against Jean: "By the way, what is your family name?. . . I was to be Mrs. Bootblack—or Madame Pigsty. —You dog, who wears my collar, you lackey." Again, however, Julie changes her attitude. Retaining a sense of ambiguity in matters of class superiority, she essentially orders Jean to tell her to commit suicide, seemingly taking the roles of both master and slave.

John Ward offered a somewhat different interpretation in his book *The Social and Religious Plays of Strindberg:* "In a sense, Julie decides to kill herself; Jean merely says the words. If anyone is controlled or conditioned, it is Jean by the bell, not Julie who . . . makes her own decision." In her book *The Greatest Fire: A Study of August Strindberg,*

"BECAUSE JULIE CANNOT DISTINCTLY IDENTIFY WITH MALE OR FEMALE, MASTER OR SERVANT, THERE IS NO PLACE FOR HER IN THIS WORLD. IT IS THIS FACT THAT FINALLY LEADS TO HER SUICIDE."

Birgitta Steene expressed a similar opinion. During the course of the play, Steene pointed out, Jean and Julie exchange roles. At times Julie acts as the master but at other times assumes the position of servant. According to Steene, however, Julie shows her superiority to Jean in her act of suicide. As she wrote: "While Julie walks to her death holding her head high, Jean cringes in fear before the count's bell. The servant is victorious as a male, but he remains a servant. The aristocrat is defeated sexually and socially, but she dies nobly."

It is common in the study of literature to romanticize suicide. In reality, however, the nobility of Julie's suicide is questionable and problematic. Ferris denied that Julie even makes a choice at all. "Miss Julie makes no decision here," she wrote, "except the joint decision with Jean that they have 'no choice.' . . . there *is* no option, no choice in this world where the hierarchy of gender and class reigns supreme. Ferris went on to say that "Miss Julie is Strindberg's 'battle of the sexes' personified; her selfhood, whose existence she denies, manifest itself in a psychotic struggle between her male and female halves." One could add that Julie also engages in such a struggle between her aristocratic and common halves. For Ferris, Julie's suicide is not a noble act, but the only way out for one, neither male nor female, neither master nor servant, whose divided identity "gives her no willful action to an autonomous self." Having at best a divided identity, Julie sees self-destruction as her only option.

Source: Clare Cross, for *Drama for Students,* Gale, 1998.

Freddy Rokem

Citing the playwright's background as a photographer and filmmaker, Rokem explains the stage-

craft techniques employed by Strindberg in writing Miss Julie.

Strindberg succeeded in arriving at theatrical effects that resemble the way a photograph "cuts out" a piece of reality: not a symmetrical joining of one wall to the other walls in the house—the basic fourth-wall technique of the realistic theater—but rather an asymmetrical cutting-out. Furthermore, Strindberg used cinematographic techniques resembling zoom, montage, and cut, which are highly significant from the strictly technical point of view and for the meaning of the plays. Historically, photography and movies were making great strides at the time and were art forms to which he himself—as photographer and as movie writer—gave considerable attention and interest. During Strindberg's lifetime, both *The Father* and *Miss Julie* were filmed as silent movies by the director Anna Hofman-Uddgren and her husband, Gustaf Uddgren, writer and friend of Strindberg, but only *The Father* has been preserved.

Strindberg thus developed dramatic theatrical techniques that, like the movie camera, can bring the viewer very close to the depicted action and, at the same time, can quite easily change the point of view or direction of observing an event or succession of events. The disappearance or near disappearance of the static focal point is largely the result of the introduction of these different photographic and cinematographic techniques. When the characters, the action, and the fictional world are continuously presented, either from partial angles or from constantly changing ones, it is often impossible for the spectator to determine where the focal point is or what the central experiences are in the characters' world. This in turn is a reflection of the constant and usually fruitless search of the characters for such focal points in their own lives.

Whereas Hedda Gabler's lack of will to continue living was based on her refusal to bear offspring within the confines of married life, Miss Julie's despair primarily reflects her unwillingness merely to exist. Of course, there are external reasons for her suicide, and Strindberg has taken great care both in the play and in the preface almost to overdetermine her final act of despair. Nevertheless, as several critics have pointed out, there are no clear and obvious causal connections between her suicide and the motives presented. Instead, this final act of despair is triggered by an irrational leap into the complete unknown, as she herself says "ecstatically" (according to Strindberg's stage direction) in the final scene when she commands Jean, the servant, to command her, the mistress, to commit suicide: "I am already asleep—the whole room stands as if in smoke for me . . . and you look like an iron stove . . . that resembles a man dressed in black with a top hat—and your eyes glow like coal when the fire is extinguished—and your face is a white patch like the ashes." These complex images within images resemble links in a chain, and they illustrate the constant movement or flux of the despairing speaker's mind. For Miss Julie there is no fixed point in reality, no focal point, except her will to die, to reach out for a nothingness.

In Strindberg's description of the set in the beginning of *Miss Julie,* he carefully specifies how the diagonal back wall cuts across the stage from left to right, opening up in the vaulted entry toward the garden. This vault however, is only partially visible. The oven and the table are also only partially visible because they are situated exactly on the borderline between the stage and the offstage areas. The side walls and the ceiling of the kitchen are marked by draperies and tormentors. Except for the garden entry, there are no doors or windows. As the play reveals, the kitchen is connected only to the private bedrooms of the servants Jean and Kristin; there is no direct access to the upper floor where the count and his daughter, Julie, live except through the pipe-telephone.

In his preface to the play, Strindberg explained: "I have borrowed from the impressionistic paintings the idea of the asymmetrical, the truncated, and I believe that thereby, the bringing forth of the illusion has been gained; since by not seeing the whole room and all the furnishings, there is room for imagination, i.e., fantasy is put in motion and it completes what is seen." Here Strindberg describes the imaginative force of this basically metonymic set. But rather than following the custom in realistic theater of showing the *whole* room as part of a house that in turn is part of the fictional world of the play, Strindberg very consciously exposes only *part* of the room. He claims it should be completed in the imagination of the audience. As Evert Sprinchorn comments: "The incompleteness of the impressionist composition drew the artist and the viewer into closer personal contact, placing the viewer in the scene and compelling him to identify with the artist at a particular moment."

The audience comes closer not only to the artist through this view of the kitchen from its interior but also, by force of the diagonal arrangements of the set, to the characters inside the kitchen. This is because the fourth wall, on which the realistic theater was originally based, has been moved to an undefined spot somewhere in the auditorium, the spectators are in the same room as the dramatic characters. It is also important to note that, to achieve this effect, Strindberg also removed the side walls from the stage, thus preventing the creation of any kind of symmetrical room that the spectator could comfortably watch from the outside. Furthermore, the audience is not guided regarding the symmetries, directions, or focal points in the set itself, which the traditional theater strongly emphasized. The only area that is separated from the kitchen is the garden, visible through the vaulted entry, with its fountain and, significantly enough, its statue of Eros. Thus, the physical point of view of the audience in relationship to the stage is ambiguous.

"IN STRINDBERG'S FICTIONAL WORLDS THERE IS DEFINITELY AN AWARENESS OF PAST ACTIONS, THAT IS OF GUILT, BUT IT EXISTS AS A PRIVATE LIMBO IN THE SUBJECTIVE CONSCIOUSNESS OF THE INDIVIDUAL CHARACTERS AND THUS CANNOT BE PROJECTED ONTO THE OBJECTIVE OUTSIDE WORLD."

What is presented is a "photograph" of the kitchen taken from its interior, drawing the audience's attention to different points inside or outside as the play's action develops. The set of *Miss Julie* can, furthermore, be seen as a photograph because while the spectators get a close view from the inside of the kitchen, they also experience an objective perception of it and the events taking place there through the frame of the proscenium arch. The comparison between Strindberg's scenic technique in *Miss Julie* and the photograph is compelling because of the very strong tension between intimacy and closeness on the one hand and objectivity and distance on the other; this sort of tension has often been observed to be one of the major characteristics not only of the play but also of photography, as the practice of documenting and preserving large numbers of slices of reality. The photograph also "cuts" into a certain space from its inside, never showing walls as parallel (unless it is a very big space photographed from the outside), at the same time it freezes the attention of the viewer upon the specific moment. In photography the focus is on the present (tense), which is "perfected" into a "has been" through the small fraction of a second when the shutter is opened. Barthes even goes so far as to call this moment in photography an epiphany.

This is also what happens in *Miss Julie* when the attention of the audience is continuously taken from one temporary focal point to the next by force of the gradual development of the action. Our eyes and attention move from the food Jean is smelling to the wine he is tasting, to Miss Julie's handkerchief, to Kristin's fond folding and smelling of the handkerchief when Jean and Miss Julie are at the dance and so on. In *Miss Julie* these material objects force the characters to confront one another and to interact. They are not objects primarily belonging to or binding the characters to the distant past toward which they try to reach out in their present sufferings—as are the visual focal points in Ibsen's plays or even the samovars and pieces of old furniture in Chekhov's plays. The objects in *Miss Julie* are first and foremost immersed in the present, forcing the characters to take a stance and their present struggles to be closely observed by the audience.

In *Miss Julie* the past and the future have been transformed into fantasy, so the only reality for the characters is the present. Because Jean and Miss Julie are forced to act solely on the basis of the immediate stimuli causing their interaction, and because the kitchen has been cut off diagonally leaving no visually defined borders on- or off-stage, it is impossible to locate any constant focal points, either outside or inside the fictional world of the play and the subjective consciousness of the characters. This "narrative" technique achieves both a very close and subjective view of the characters and a seemingly objective and exact picture of them. The temporal retrospection has also been diminished because Jean and Miss Julie are not as disturbed by irrational factors belonging to a guilt-ridden past as, for example, the Ibsen heroes are. Strindberg's characters are motivated primarily by their present desires.

This of course does not mean that there are no expository references to the past in *Miss Julie,* on the contrary, there are a large number of references to specific events in the lives of the characters preceding the opening of the scenic action. The play, in fact, begins with a series of such references, all told by Jean to Kristin. Thus, we learn that Miss Julie is "mad again tonight" (inferring that it is not the first time this has happened), as represented by the way she is dancing with Jean. And to give her behavior some perspective (just before her entrance), Jean relates to Kristin how Miss Julie's fiancé broke their engagement because of the degradations he had to suffer, jumping over her whip as well as being beaten by it. These events are, however, never corroborated by other characters in the play. Miss Julie's subsequent behavior does to some extent affirm Jean's story, but we can never be completely sure.

What is specific to Strindberg's plays is not the omission of the past—which absurdist drama emphasizes—but rather a lack of certainty regarding the reliability of what the characters say about that past. And since in many of Strindberg's plays there is no source of verification other than the private memory of the character speaking, the past takes on a quite subjective quality. Miss Julie gives *her* version of *her* past and Jean relates *his,* and the possible unreliability of these memories is confirmed when Jean changes his story of how he as a child watched her in the garden. (pp. 112–15)

The major outcome of past actions, guilt, is objectified in Ibsen's plays. That is the reason why it can be given a specific geographical location in the outside world, which becomes the "focus" (in all respects) for it. In Strindberg's fictional worlds there is definitely an awareness of past actions, that is of guilt, but it exists as a private limbo in the subjective consciousness of the individual characters and thus cannot be projected onto the objective outside world. That is why in Strindberg's plays there is either no visual focus or a constantly moving one.

In *Miss Julie* the two principal characters continuously try to turn their respective opponents into the focal point onto which their own guilt and related feelings of inadequacy and general frustration can be projected. That is one of the major reasons for their sexual union and the distrust and even hatred to which it leads. Just how fickle those focal points are, however, can also be seen as in Miss Julie's last desperate attempt to find some kind of support in Jean for her step into the unknown realm of death. Jean's face has become a white spot, resembling to Miss Julie the ashes of a fire because the light of the sun—which is rising at this point in the play—is illuminating him. Again the present situation becomes the point of departure for her wishes. And when Miss Julie wants to die, her wish is thus focused on Jean's illuminated face. In *Ghosts* Ibsen used the same images (the fire and the sun) at the end of the last two acts as objective focal points. Strindberg has compressed these images into one speech in which they are projected onto Jean by the fantasy of Miss Julie's subjective consciousness. Ibsen gives a "scientific" explanation of Oswald's madness for which the sunset is a circumstantial parallel, whereas Strindberg lets the sunset motivate the outburst of Julie's death wish, as expressed from within. Thus the preparations for the introduction of expressionism, wherein everything is projection, had already been made in Strindberg's pre-Inferno plays.

Source: Freddy Rokem, "The Camera and the Aesthetics of Repetition: Strindberg's Use of Space and Scenography in *Miss Julie, A Dream Play,* and *The Ghost Sonata*" in *Strindberg's Dramaturgy,* edited by Goran Stockenstrom, University of Minnesota Press, 1988, pp. 107–28.

Wolcott Gibbs

Calling Strindberg's drama "more a pathological curiosity than a clear and moving play," Gibbs nevertheless offers a positive appraisal of this 1956 production.

Miss Julie is something, and with bells on, as the pretty saying goes. The heroine's mind is the battleground for a hundred warring impulses, inherited from a family of distinguished peculiarity, and her behavior, to put it very mildly, is bizarre. She is an incurable aristocrat who hates the idea of class distinctions, a passionate woman (the performance at the Phoenix suggests nymphomania, but I doubt if that was the author's intention) who has a horror of men, an idealist ceaselessly, corrupted by her senses. It is apparently Strindberg's contention that no tragedy has a single, pat explanation, and Julie's ultimate suicide, coming as the climax of her grotesque affair with her father's valet, surely bears this out. She is a figure of infinite complexity, but whether she is pitiful, ludicrous, or simply incredible is quite another point. It is my opinion that a perpetual shifting back and forth between love and hatred for the same things—an emotional confusion nearly indistinguishable from lunacy—is too difficult a conception for the stage, and that *Miss Julie* is more a pathological curiosity than a clear and moving play. If I'm mistaken—and it should be noted that *Miss Julie* has been performed regularly since1888— the blame can be laid partly to Viveca Lindfors' rather lurid rendering of the title role at the Phoenix. It has always been my aim to keep vulgarity as far as possible out of these essays, but I am almost forced to note that Miss Lindfors gives it the old Ophelia, with darker rumblings from Medea here and there. She is abetted by James Daly and Ruth Ford, the second of whom, incidentally, stars in the curtain-raiser, also by Strindberg, a sort of one-woman filibuster called "The Stronger."

Source: Wolcott Gibbs, "Two Crazy, Mixed-up Kids" in the *New Yorker,* Volume XXXII, no. 2, March 3, 1956, pp. 63–64.

SOURCES

Carlson, Harry G. *Strindberg and the Poetry of Myth,* University of California Press, 1982, pp. 61-64.

Ferris, Lesley. *Acting Women: Images of Women in Theatre,* New York University Press, 1989, pp. 121-24.

Jarv, Harry. "Strindberg's 'Characterless' *Miss Julie* in *Gradiva,* Vol. 1, 1977, pp. 197-206.

Lamm, Martin. *August Strindberg,* translated and edited by Harry G. Carlson, Benjamin Bloom, 1971, pp. 216-17.

Meyer, Michael. *Strindberg: A Biography,* Secker & Warburg, 1985, pp. 203-04, 515.

Steene, Birgitta. *The Greatest Fire: A Study of August Strindberg,* Southern Illinois University Press, 1973, p. 55.

Ward, John. *The Social and Religious Plays of Strindberg,* Athlone, 1980, p. 62.

FURTHER READING

Ferris, Lesley. *Acting Women: Images of Women in Theatre,* New York University Press, 1989.

This book is a good basic introduction to the depiction of female characters in drama from the Greeks to the present.

Hawkins, Mike. *Social Darwinism in European and American Thought: 1860-1945. Nature As Model and Nature As Threat,* Cambridge University Press, 1997.

This book provides a basic introduction to the theory and history of social Darwinism, particularly as it was perceived during Strindberg's time.

Morgan, Margery. *August Strindberg,* Macmillan, 1985.

This book provides a brief biography of Strindberg and an introduction to his works.

Sprinchorn, Evert. *Strindberg As Dramatist,* Yale University Press, 1982.

Dividing his work into periods, this book integrates a study of Strindberg's development as a dramatist, including biographical information and criticism of his plays.

Murder in the Cathedral

T. S. ELIOT

1935

In 1163, a quarrel began between the British King Henry II and the Archbishop of Canterbury, Thomas Becket. The men had been good friends, but each felt that his interests should be of primary concern to the nation and that the other should acquiesce to his demands. Becket fled to France in 1164 in order to rally support from the Catholic French for his cause and also sought an audience with the Pope. After being officially (although not personally) reconciled with the King, Becket returned to England in 1170, only to be murdered as he prayed in Canterbury Cathedral by four of Henry's Knights. Three years later, he was canonized and pilgrims—Henry among them—have made their way to his tomb ever since.

The allure of such a story for a dramatist is obvious: there is a great conflict between human and divine power, a strong central character and a number of complicated spiritual issues to be found in his death. In 1935, T. S. Eliot answered this ''calling'' to compose a play for that year's Canterbury Festival; the result was a work that revitalized verse drama—a form that had not been widely employed for almost three hundred years. Critics praised Eliot's use of verse and ability to invest a past historical event with modern issues and themes, such as the ways in which lay persons react to the intrusion of the supernatural in their daily lives. In part because it is a religious drama which appeared long after such plays were popular, *Murder in the Cathedral* is still performed, studied, and regarded

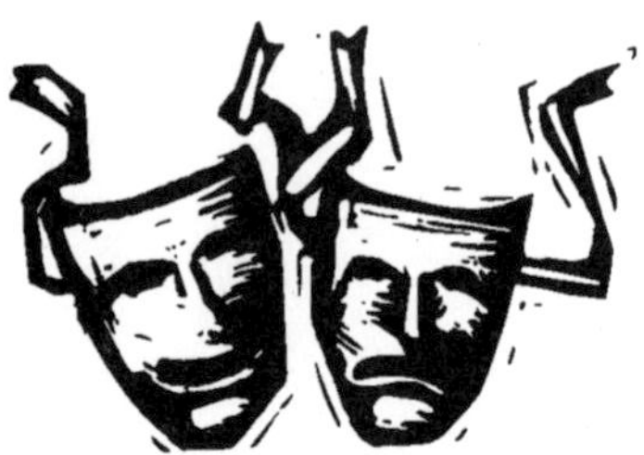

as one of Eliot's major works, a testament to his skill as a poet and dramatist.

AUTHOR BIOGRAPHY

T. S. Eliot was born in St. Louis, Missouri, on September 26, 1888, into a family that stressed the importance of education and tradition. His paternal grandfather had moved to St. Louis from Boston and founded Washington University; the young Eliot entered Harvard University in 1906 to study French literature and philosophy (he received a baccalaureate degree in 1909 and a master's degree in 1910). In 1910, Eliot attended the Sorbonne and studied under the philosopher Henri Bergson; he later studied at Oxford and completed his dissertation on philosopher F. H. Bradley in 1916, when he was living in London with his first wife, Vivien Haigh-Wood.

During this phase of his life, Eliot was befriended by the American poet Ezra Pound, who helped him shape and publish his poetry, specifically *''The Love Song of J. Alfred Prufrock''* which first appeared in the journal *Poetry.* 1917 saw the publication of Eliot's first volume of verse, *Prufrock and Other Observations* which was greeted with enthusiasm by its readers. Eliot's success, however, was not enough to relive the stress he felt from his failing marriage; he suffered an emotional breakdown and sought treatment at a sanitorium in Switzerland. It was there that he completed the first draft of what is regarded as his best—and most difficult to interpret—work, *The Waste Land.* Upon returning to London, Eliot edited the poem (at Pound's request) and published it in the American journal the *Dial.* More and more readers began paying attention to Eliot's new verse forms, which reflected the angst and desperation of people who had just lived through the terror and chaos of World War I.

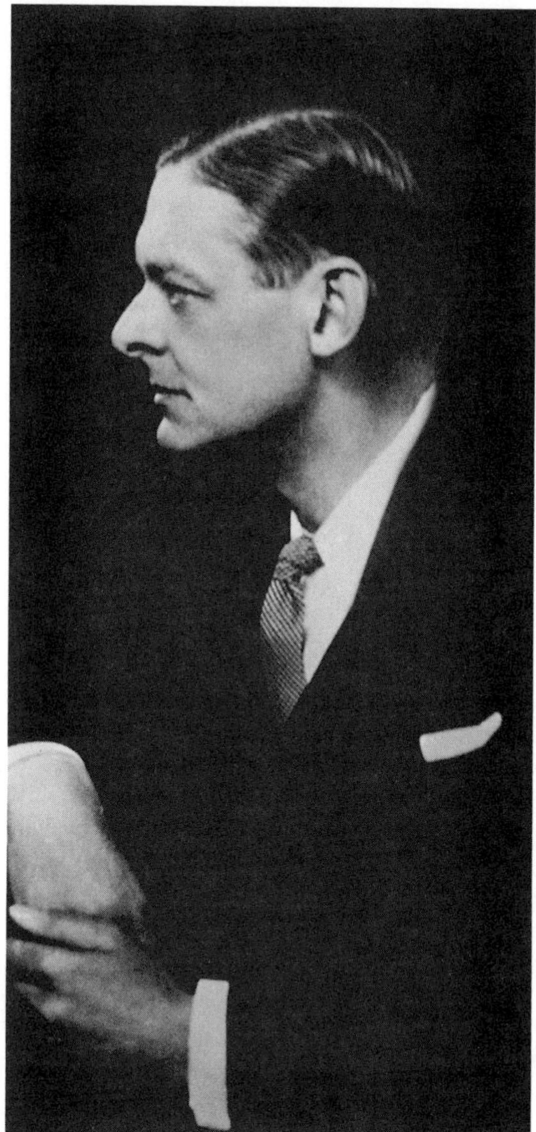

T. S. Eliot

Eliot renewed himself personally as he had the world of poetry: in 1927, he became a British subject and a confirmed member of the Anglican church. During this same year, he stated his controversial creed of conservatism, describing himself as ''Anglo-Catholic in religion, royalist in politics and classicist in literature.'' In 1930, another of his important poems, *Ash Wednesday,* was published, and in 1932 Eliot returned to the United States to become the Charles Eliot Norton Professor at Harvard. He was almost completely estranged from his wife and remained in the United States to lecture at various universities. In 1934 his first play, *Sweeney Agonistes,* was produced, followed the same year by his second drama, *The Rock.* However, it was 1935's *Murder in the Cathedral* that drew as much attention to Eliot's playwriting as his poetry. His next play, *The Family Reunion,* was produced in 1939, followed in 1943 by the poem *Four Quartets.* Vivien died in 1947 and in 1948 Eliot received the Nobel Prize in Literature and the Order of Merit by George VI. His next play, *The Cocktail Party,* was produced in 1949 and proved to be a critical and commercial success. Two other plays followed: *The Confidential Clerk* (1953) and *The Elder Statesman*

(1958). During his playwriting career, Eliot continued to write verse, essays, and volumes of criticism. He was remarried in 1957, this time to Valerie Fletcher, to whom he remained married until his death in 1965. He is buried in Westminster Abbey.

PLOT SUMMARY

Part One

The action of *Murder in the Cathedral* occurs in and around Canterbury Cathedral; Part One takes place on December 2, 1170, the day that Archbishop Thomas Becket returned to England and twenty-seven days before his murder by four knights of King Henry II. When the play begins, a Chorus comprised of the Women of Canterbury huddle outside the cathedral, certain that something is about to happen but unable to articulate any details: ''Some presage of an act / Which our eyes are compelled to witness, has forced our feet / Towards the cathedral.'' They then describe their lives to the audience and these descriptions mark them as common people who fear any threat of change: ''We try to keep our households in order,'' they explain, but ''Some malady is coming upon us.'' Ultimately, they decide that ''For us, the poor, there is no action, / But only to wait and witness.''

Three Priests enter and briefly discuss a major issue of the play: the differences between temporal (i.e., worldly) and spiritual power. The Third Priest claims that, ''King rules or barons rule'' and that politicians ''have but one law, to seize the power and keep it.'' The First Priest hopes that the Chorus has not become too jaded and hopes that they will realize that they have a ''friend'' in ''their Father in God.'' (Clearly, the populace and their religious leaders are living in spiritually trying times.)

A Messenger then arrives and informs them that their archbishop, Thomas Becket, is returning to England after a seven-year absence. Due to a feud with the King, in part over the degree to which the church would assert its power in the British government, Thomas has been exiled to foreign shores and has been seeking support for his ideas in Catholic France. The Priests' reactions to this news varies: The First Priest comments on Thomas's pride, which makes him ''fear for the Archbishop'' and ''fear for the Church''; the Second Priest looks towards his superior's return in the hope that ''He will tell us what we are to do, he will give us our orders, instruct us''; the Third Priest dismisses the very act of predicting what will happen, for, as he says, ''who knows the end of good or evil?'' Instead, he thinks they must simply ''let the wheel turn.''

The Chorus expresses its terror at the thought of Thomas's return: although they have endured previous hardships, they are unprepared ''To stand to the doom of the house, the doom on the Archbishop, the doom on the world.'' They are merely ''small folk drawn into the pattern of fate'' and beg the still-absent Thomas to ''leave us, leave us, leave sullen Dover and set sail for France.''

After the Chorus is scolded by the Second Priest for their ''croaking like frogs,'' Thomas enters, calling for ''Peace'' and telling the Priests that the Women of Canterbury ''speak better than they know, and beyond your understanding.'' He explains how he managed to arrive safely in Canterbury and remarks that ''the hungry hawk'' may still strike at any moment. However, he explains that ''End will be simple, sudden, God-given'' and that ''All things prepare the event.'' His faith in the divine will is thus asserted.

Thomas is then visited by four Tempters, symbolic characters who approach and attempt to lure Thomas away from his devotion to the Church. The First Tempter offers Thomas the glory of his past friendship with the King. The Second Tempter offers political power in the form of Thomas's former position at Court: the Chancellorship. The Third Tempter tells him to ''fight for liberty'' and end ''the tyrannous jurisdiction / Of king's court over bishop's court, / Of king's court over baron's court.'' All three Tempters are easily dismissed by Thomas, who asks, ''Shall I, who keep the keys / Of heaven and hell, supreme alone in England, / Who bind and loose, with power from the Pope, / Descend to desire a punier power?'' Proclaiming that he ''has good cause to trust none but God alone,'' Thomas refutes all of their enticements with assertions of his faith in God's will.

The Fourth Tempter, however, approaches Thomas from a different angle. Advising Thomas to ''Fare forward to the end'' and ''think of glory after death,'' this Tempter argues that ''Saint and Martyr rule from the tomb'' and that Thomas should ''Think of pilgrims, standing in line / Before the glittering jeweled shrine.'' Allowing himself to be martyred will, the Tempter promises, eventually see his enemies ''in timeless torment.'' Without martyrdom, Thomas will be only a footnote to future scholars who ''Will only try to find the historical fact.''

Unlike the first three Tempters, whose offerings are easily mocked and spurned by Thomas, this Tempter causes the Archbishop to experience a crisis of conscience: he asks, "Who are you, tempting me with my own desires?" and asserts that the Tempter offers only "Dreams to damnation" since the very act of courting one's fame through martyrdom is an act of "sinful pride."

After a short passage in which the three Priests and Chorus express their paranoia, fear of "a new terror" and the thought of being abandoned by God, Thomas announces his decision to remain in Canterbury. "Now is my way clear, now is the meaning plain," he begins, explaining that "The last temptation is the greatest treason: / To do the right thing for the wrong reason." In other words, allowing himself to be martyred is the "right thing" to do—as long as he does not do so for "the wrong reason"—a desire for fame and retribution. Acknowledging to the Priests and Chorus that "What yet remains to show you of my history / Will seem to most of you at best futility, / Senseless self-slaughter of a lunatic, / Arrogant passion of a fanatic," Thomas concludes, "I shall no longer act or suffer, to the sword's end" and invokes his "good angel" to "hover over the swords' points." The Archbishop will allow himself to be martyred only if it is the will of God, for he will not act in order to hasten his own murder. His own pride must not seduce him into presuming that he can know the mind of God.

Interlude

This short scene depicts Thomas preaching in the cathedral on Christmas morning, 1170. In his sermon, Thomas explores the meaning of a number of paradoxes inherent in the celebration of Christmas, the first being that, since Christ died to redeem the sins of the world, "we celebrate at once the Birth of Our Lord and His Passion and Death upon the Cross." A similar paradox is then explored in the meaning of the word "peace" as Christ used it when he said to his followers, "My peace I leave with you"; after describing the afflicted lives of the disciples (who suffered "torture, imprisonment, disappointment" and "martyrdom") Thomas concludes that Christ's peace is "not as the world gives"—in the form of, for example, an end to war—but as spiritual solace.

His final paradox lies in the nature of martyrdom: "we both rejoice and mourn at the death of martyrs," he explains, for the "sins of the world" have killed an innocent person who will, nonetheless, be "numbered among the Saints in Heaven." Thomas expands upon this idea by asking his listeners to remember that martyrdom "is never the design of man," for "the true martyr is he who has become the instrument of God, who has lost his will in the will of God, and who no longer desires anything for himself, not even the glory of being a martyr." Obviously considering his own possible martyrdom, Thomas's definition both instructs his listeners and allows him to once again consider his possible fate. "I do not think I will ever preach to you again," Thomas remarks in closing, noting that "in a short time you may have another martyr."

Part Two

Four days have passed since Thomas's sermon in the cathedral, but the Chorus is still fearful and awaiting a sign from God in the form of a cleansing Spring. As Part One saw the entrance of the four Tempters, this Part features four Knights, who enter the Archbishop's Hall, telling the three Priests that they have "urgent business" from the King that they must share with Thomas. Impatient and anxious, the Knights bully the Priests until Thomas appears, remarking, "However certain our expectation, / The moment foreseen may be unexpected / When it arrives." The Knights charge Thomas with being "in revolt against the King" since he "sowed strife abroad" and "reviled / The King to the King of France, to the Pope, / Raising up against him false opinions."

After they level other charges and demand that he absolve those bishops that he had previously excommunicated, Thomas refuses, explaining, "It is not Becket who pronounces doom, / But the Law of Christ's Church." He exits and the Knights follow, leaving the Chorus to describe the odd harbingers of evil that they have recently witnessed in the natural world. Thomas reenters to comfort the Chorus, telling them that "These things had to come and you had to accept them." The Priests, however, refuse such advice and drag Thomas into the cathedral while he protests, "all things / Proceed to a joyful consummation."

The scene then shifts inside the cathedral, where the Priests are barring the doors while Thomas insists, "I will not have the Church of Christ, / This sanctuary, turned into a fortress." "The Church will protect her own," he states, but the Priests argue that the Knights are "maddened beasts." Thomas persists, however, and commands the Priests to open the door. The Knights enter ("slightly tipsy" as Eliot notes in the stage direction), searching for ''Becket the faithless priest.'' After refusing to recant any of his former convictions or renounce any of his former actions, Thomas prays: ''Now to Almighty God . . . I commend my cause and that of the Church.'' The Knights then begin to kill him, during which the Chorus laments the curse being placed on their land and their lives. After their cry of ''Clean the air! clean the sky! wash the wind!'' Thomas is finally dead.

It is at this moment that Eliot surprises everyone in the audience by having the four Knights directly address them: ''We know that you may be disposed to judge unfavorably of our action,'' the first Knight explains, adding, ''Nevertheless, I appeal to your sense of honor. You are Englishmen, and therefore will not judge anybody without hearing both sides of the case.'' The other three Knights then take turns justifying their actions, stressing the fact that they acted in a ''perfectly disinterested'' manner and that Thomas was not the ''under dog'' as he was presented in the play. Ultimately, they ask the audience to ''render a verdict of Suicide while of Unsound Mind.'' When they exit, the Priests discuss the murder's meaning and eventually leave the Chorus to proclaim to God that ''the blood of Thy martyrs and saints / Shall enrich the earth, shall create the holy places.'' Finally, they beg forgiveness of God for doubting his ''blessing'' and petition their new Heavenly patron: ''Blessed Thomas, pray for us.''

CHARACTERS

Thomas Becket

Thomas Becket is the Archbishop of Canterbury and hero of the play. When the play opens, the viewer learns that he has not been in England for the last seven years because of a power struggle with King Henry II, who wants the church to serve the state. His return from France provokes a variety of reactions from the Chorus, the Priests, and the four Knights who serve the King; as the play progresses, Thomas responds to a number of these reactions with the calm, measured voice of one who believes ''there is higher than I or the King.''

Although he is repeatedly tempted away from his desire to lead his people and threatened with death by the four Knights, Thomas becomes convinced that only ''The fool, fixed in his folly, may think / He can turn the wheel on which he turns'' and places the question of whether or not he will be martyred into the hands of God. He accepts his martyrdom as part of a larger pattern that he, with his human limitations, cannot fully understand.

Richard Brito (Fourth Knight)

See The Four Knights

Chorus

Similar to those found in ancient Greek drama, the Chorus in *Murder in the Cathedral* serves as a mediator between the play and the audience. Composed of women of Canterbury, this group originally fears the unknown act that their ''eyes are compelled to witness'' and begs Thomas to return to France; they have accepted their common and often miserable lives (where ''King rules or barons rule'') and do not wish to ''stand on the doom'' of their church. At the play's conclusion, however, they have been enlightened to the fact that there is a higher power at work in the world other than that found in politics and they sing praises to the wisdom of God: ''We thank thee for Thy mercies of blood, for Thy redemption by blood,'' they proclaim, for ''the blood of Thy martyrs and saints shall enrich the earth, shall create holy places.''

Sir Hugh de Morville (Second Knight)

See The Four Knights

Baron William de Traci (Third Knight)

See The Four Knights

The Four Knights

Sent by King Henry to kill Thomas, the Four Knights parallel the Four Tempters of Part One. While the Tempters offer intellectual and spiritual trickery, the Knights threaten Thomas with physical violence, ultimately following through on their threat when they kill him near the end of the play. When they arrive at the cathedral and demand that Thomas acquiesce to the King's demands, he refuses. They murder him and then ''present their case'' to the audience in the form of a mock inquest in which they assert their blamelessness in the entire affair. Although their names are mentioned during their speeches to the audience, the Knights are not as different from each other as are the Three Priests.

The Four Tempters

During Part One, Thomas is visited by four Tempters who promise him a number of rewards in return for recanting his former judgments against the King and his minions. The First Tempter tells him that ''Friendship is more than biting Time can sever'' and asks Thomas to befriend the King (as he did once before) so that there will be ''Fluting in the meadow'' and ''Singing at nightfall.'' The Second Tempter suggests that Thomas should reclaim the Chancellorship (from which he resigned after his feud with King Henry); doing so would, the Tempter assures him, let Thomas ''set down the great'' and ''protect the poor.'' The Third Tempter, dubbing himself ''A country-keeping Lord who minds his own business,'' attempts to seduce Thomas into representing the barons at court in order to ''fight a good stroke / At once, for England and for Rome, / Ending the tyrannous jurisdiction'' of Henry's reign.

All three Tempters are easily deflated by Thomas, who is unaffected by their empty promises: ''Shall I,'' he asks, ''who ruled like an eagle over doves, / Now take the shape of a wolf among wolves?'' The Fourth Tempter, however, is more difficult for Thomas to dismiss, since he tempts him with his ''own desires'' of becoming a saint and martyred leader of his people. Eventually, the Fourth Tempter teaches Thomas about the degree to which his own pride stands between him and the will of God.

The Messenger

The Messenger arrives in Part One to announce to the Priests that Thomas is returning to Canterbury. He peppers his news with his own thoughts on Thomas, remarking that ''He is at one with the Pope'' and that his new ''peace'' with the King is, at best, a ''patched-up affair.''

The Three Priests

As a unit, the three Priests provide a context for Thomas's religious speculations and offer the audience different opinions of him before he enters the play. Throughout *Murder in the Cathedral,* the Priests express their desire to help Thomas guide his people and remain safely in Canterbury. Although they may seem interchangeable by virtue of their names (''First Priest,'' ''Second Priest,'' and ''Third Priest''), they are distinguished at times by Eliot according to the way in which they approach the danger of Thomas's return. The First Priest, for example, is uneasy and remarks, ''I fear for the Archbishop, I fear for the Church,'' before concluding that Thomas's troubles began when he wished for ''subjection to God alone.''

MEDIA ADAPTATIONS

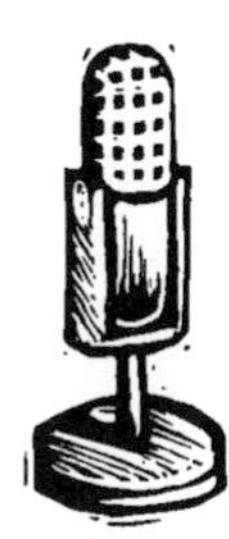

- *Murder in the Cathedral* was adapted as a British film in 1952, directed by George Hoellering. Paul Rodgers and Leo McKern are featured in the cast and Eliot provided the voice of the Fourth Tempter.
- A recording of the 1953 Old Vic cast performing the play was recorded by Angel Records.
- A recording of the play, starring Paul Scofield, was produced in 1968. It is available through Caedmon Recordings.

The Second Priest, less world-weary than the First, voices the hope that Thomas will dispel ''dismay and doubt,'' for ''He will tell us what we are to do, he will give us our orders, instruct us.'' The Third Priest expresses neither the doubts of the First nor the optimism of the Second; his only certainty is that fate will unwind as it must: ''For good or ill, let the wheel turn,'' he remarks, ''For who knows the end of good or evil?'' These differences, however, fade in Part Two, when the Priests act as a group in order to convince Thomas to flee the cathedral.

Reginald Fitz Urse (First Knight)

See The Four Knights

THEMES

Flesh vs. Spirit

Throughout *Murder in the Cathedral,* Thomas is warned about the danger of his remaining in Canterbury and the threat of danger from his enemies, who seek to please King Henry by murdering him. Before he enters, the Chorus begs, ''O Thomas return, Archbishop; return, return to France,'' for he comes ''bringing death into Canterbury''; when he does arrive, Thomas tells them and the three Priests that none should fear his possible death, for ''the hungry hawk / Will only soar and hover'' until there

TOPICS FOR FURTHER STUDY

- Research the historical Thomas Becket and his reasons for quarreling with King Henry II. To what degree does Eliot's version of these events accord with that found in historical sources?
- The British poet Alfred, Lord Tennyson also composed a verse play on the life of Thomas Becket, *Becket* (1884). Read Tennyson's version of Becket's martyrdom and compare and contrast it with Eliot's. How, for example, does each poet present Becket's decision to remain in the cathedral when threatened by the knights?
- Renaissance artists frequently painted saints in symbolic settings. Locate some paintings of Becket and explain the ways in which their artists have manipulated color, light, and form in order to present their subject. What aspects of Becket's personality do they wish to stress?
- Eliot admired the morality play *Everyman* (1500) for its versification, i.e., for its author's use of sound and meter in creating certain effects. Compare the nature of *Everyman*'s verse to Eliot's: are there any patterns of rhythm or sound that can be found in both works? Why would Eliot appropriate the patterns he did?
- In Part Two of the play, several musical cues are mentioned, such as ''*a* Dies Irae *is sung in Latin by a choir in the distance.*'' Look in an encyclopedia of music to learn what a Dies Irae is and how it and the other types of songs mentioned by Eliot are used in the Catholic Mass. Then explain why Eliot would use them in his play: how do certain types of hymns suit certain dramatic situations?

is an ''End'' that will be ''simple, sudden, God-given.'' The very fact of his return suggests Thomas's refusal to fear death and belief that God will decide whether he will live or die: as he tells the Priests, ''All things prepare the event.''

Thomas's disregard for earthly pleasures and power is heightened during his conversations with the first three Tempters. When the First Tempter offers him ''wit and wine and wisdom'' if he will only ''Be easy'' in his condemnation of King Henry, Thomas calls his temptations a mere ''springtime fancy'' belonging to ''seasons of the past.'' When the next Tempter urges him to take up again the Chancellorship and ''guide the state again,'' Thomas argues that ''what was once exaltation / Would now only mean descent'' to a ''punier power,'' since, as an Archbishop, he is able to ''keep the keys / Of heaven and hell.'' ''To condemn kings, not serve among their servants,'' he explains, is his ''open office.''

Clearly, Thomas is not interested in any form of temporal power. The Third Tempter attempts to appeal to Thomas's political and religious faith, stating that Thomas could help the barons fight for the ''liberty'' of England and Rome; still dismissive of man's law, however, Thomas asserts that if he ''break'' the tyranny of the King, he must not do so for promises of power but must ''break myself alone.'' The fact that Thomas is able to so easily refuse these Tempters reflects his desire to serve divine—rather than human—law; this also accounts for his turmoil when facing the Fourth Tempter, who questions Thomas's desire to become a martyr for purely spiritual (as opposed to temporal) reasons. Once Thomas considers his own heart and concludes that he must not be tricked by his own pride into coveting his martyrdom, he is assured that even if he is killed, his ''good Angel, whom God appoints'' will ''hover over the swords' points.''

Thomas's unshaken devotion to his spiritual life is seen throughout the Interlude and Part Two. When preaching to his congregation on Christmas Day, he tells them that martyrdom is ''never the design of man,'' for ''the true martyr is he who has become the instrument of God'' and ''who no longer desires anything for himself.'' He then bluntly acknowledges his acceptance of his possible fate by saying, ''I do not think I shall ever preach to you again'' and ''it is possible that in a short time you may have another martyr.''

In Part Two, when faced with the menace of the four Knights, Thomas refuses to flee (as the Priests beg him to do), since he is ''not in danger: only nearer to death.'' Believing that ''all things / Proceed to a joyful consummation,'' Thomas orders a Priest who has bolted the Cathedral door to open it. He then proclaims, ''I give my life / To the Law of God above the Law of Man.'' As the Knights kill him, Thomas does not beg for any mercy or postponement; instead, he begins a prayer in which he ''commends [his] cause and that of the Church'' to ''Almighty God.'' Although tempted with physical pleasures and threatened with physical violence, Thomas remains true to what he sees as the ''pattern'' of God's will in his life.

Obedience

Closely allied with the theme of flesh vs. spirit is that of obedience, an issue of the play that is seen in Thomas's unflagging devotion to God. The very nature of the argument between Thomas and King Henry, occurring before the play begins, is centered on this issue: Henry wants Thomas to obey his (and thus the state's) commands, but Thomas is a man described by the First Priest as one ''Loathing power given by temporal devolution, / Wishing subjection to God alone.'' Convinced that God is his only judge and ruler with any authority, Thomas mocks those who view themselves as sources of power in a worldly sense: ''Only / The fool, fixed in his folly, may think / He can turn the wheel on which he turns.'' Another example of Thomas's belief in the power of divine law is found in his rebuttal of the Second Tempter, who offers him his previous power as Chancellor:

> Temporal power, to build a good world, To keep order, as the world knows order. Those who put their faith in worldly order Not controlled by the Order of God, In confident ignorance, but arrest disorder, Make it fast, breed fatal disease, Degrade what they exalt.

Here, Thomas asserts that the only order is that found in the will of God and that any attempt to stray from one's obedience to it can only result in the ''fatal disease'' of chaos. Only God can provide any sort of harmony between one's temporal and spiritual lives and Thomas chooses to remain in the ''confident ignorance'' of one who does not know—but who nevertheless trusts—the force of Providence.

While Thomas's refusal to flee the cathedral certainly proves his obedience to God, it is in an earlier conversation that Eliot dramatizes the conflicting forces within Thomas that solicit his obedience. After speaking to the Fourth Tempter, who asks, ''What can compare with the glory of Saints / Swelling forever in presence of God?'' Thomas must examine his own conscience to determine whether or not his pride is encouraging him to (as the Tempter commands), ''Seek the way of martyrdom.'' Thomas's problem lies not in dying, but in determining if he is doing so out of an obedience to his pride or his God. Eventually, he reaches the enlightenment for which he searches:

> Now is my way clear, now is the meaning plain: Temptation shall not come in this kind again. The last temptation is the greatest treason: To do the right deed for the wrong reason.

Thomas has learned that the ''right deed'' (martyrdom) must not be performed for the ''wrong reason'': his self-interest. To allow his desire for glory to interfere with the will of God—which is, ultimately, what will determine his fate—would be like ''treason'' in its attempt to subvert the authority of an all-powerful ruler. Only by remaining obedient to God can he ever hope to ''do the right deed'' and become a martyr for his church and his people. He will remain God's obedient servant, living in ''confident ignorance'' of God's eternal plan.

STYLE

Tragedy

''Tragedy'' as a dramatic form is usually defined as the story of a noble individual who struggles against himself or his fate in the face of almost certain defeat. Perhaps the ideal example of tragedy is Sophocles's *Oedipus the King* (5th century BC) in which Oedipus, the King of Thebes, attempts to cleanse his city against an evil that is plaguing it, only to learn that this evil is found in himself. Eliot's play does employ several classical tragic conventions, such as the use of a Chorus to comment on the action, the characters' speech written in verse, and a plot which culminates in the hero's death.

Thomas is a tragic figure in his larger-than-life passion and search for what can be done to solve the problem with which he is faced. Unlike many tragic heroes, however, Thomas's character harbors no ''flaw'' or (as Hamlet called it) ''mole of nature'': he is not blind to his fate (like Oedipus), he is not the slave of passion (like Othello) and he is not a man destroyed by the promises of his own imagination (like Willy Loman).

Instead, Thomas is steadfast and assured; even when he questions his own motives for seeking martyrdom, he summons enough strength in himself to determine that he will allow himself to be the ''instrument'' of God. While Thomas is eventually killed, something more wonderful than terrible occurs when the Chorus finally understands the will of God and praises Him for His wisdom and power. Unlike Hamlet, who dies amongst a litter of corpses and evokes the audience's pity and fear, Thomas dies as he describes Christ as having done: bringing the ''peace'' of God to the world. *Murder in the Cathedral* makes use of the tragic form, but the tragic outcome is to be found in its *physical* plot only—the spiritual life of its hero is stronger than death.

Setting

Murder in the Cathedral was written especially for performance at the 1935 Canterbury Festival and was performed in the Chapter House of the cathedral, only fifty yards away from the very spot on which Becket was killed. Aside from its being written for the Festival, Eliot must have had other artistic aims in having it be performed in a non-traditional theater space.

Foremost among these is the fact that anyone in the original audience would be conscious of the fact that he was not in a theater as he viewed the play; instead, he was in a place resonant with the history of the play's protagonist. The effect of such a setting is obvious: by having the action take place in the Chapter House, Eliot stressed the relationship between the past and present. While the action of the play occurs in 1170, a 1935 audience member would become more aware of the fact that the play's issues are as contemporary as its audience. As the cathedral still stands, so are the issues explored by the play still relevant to modern life.

Rhetoric and Oratory

There are only two sections in the play in which characters do not speak in verse: Thomas's sermon on Christmas Day and the ''apologies'' by the Knights to the audience. Both of these sections feature a speaker (or speakers) attempting to manipulate language in order to convince their listeners of a certain point (rhetoric) and trying to deliver the words in a way that gives them the greatest impact (oratory). In Thomas's sermon, he attempts to engage the congregation in the same mental processes which he himself has been experiencing, specifically, to consider the paradoxical nature of martyrdom. To do so, he offers a number of paradoxes for them to consider, such as the idea that ''at the same moment we rejoice'' at the birth of Christ, we do so because we know that he would eventually ''offer again to God His Body and Blood in sacrifice.''

He similarly attempts to convince his followers that God creates martyrs upon a similar paradoxical principle: ''We mourn, for the sins of the world that has martyred them; we rejoice, that another soul is numbered among the Saints in Heaven, for the glory of God and the salvation of men.'' Because he suspects that his people will soon ''have yet another martyr,'' Thomas wishes to convince them to consider the reasons for—and bounties of—martyrdom, which they do at the very end of the play.

When directly addressing the audience, however, the Four Knights prove themselves to be more adept at cliched political hustling than sincere attempts at public speaking. The First Knight attempts to ingratiate himself to the audience by addressing its members as ''Englishmen'' who ''believe in fair play'' and will certainly ''not judge anybody without hearing both sides of the case.'' The Third Knight stresses the point that the four of them ''have been perfectly disinterested'' in the murder; they are not lackeys of the King, but ''four plain Englishmen who put our country first.'' The Second Knight promises that, while defending their actions, he will ''appeal not to your emotions but to your reason,'' since ''You are hard-headed, sensible people . . . and not to be taken in by emotional clap-trap.''

Again the viewer sees another example of a Knight attempting to ingratiate himself to the audience through hollow rhetoric and flattery. Following this lead, the Fourth Knight then employs the language of pseudo-psychology in an attempt to offer a ''logical'' and ''scientific'' view of Thomas's actions: he calls him ''a monster of egoism'' and explains that ''This egoism grew upon him, until it at last became an undoubted mania,'' as found in the ''unimpeachable evidence'' that the Fourth Knight has gathered. He concludes his speech (and the Knights' presentation of their ''case'') with the aplomb of a trial lawyer: ''I think, with these facts before you, you will unhesitatingly render a verdict of Suicide while of Unsound Mind. It is the only charitable verdict you can give, upon one who was, after all, a great man.''

Despite these attempts at sounding logical (''with these facts before you''), proclaiming their confidence in the audience's judgment (''you will unhesitatingly render'' a ''charitable verdict''), use of jargon (''Suicide while of Unsound Mind'') and attempt to seem dispassionate and logical about the murder (''who was, after all, a great man''), the Fourth Knight, like his companions, stands as an example of one who uses language to defend his temporal action and fulfill a political agenda—unlike Thomas, who uses his rhetorical skills to help his listeners understand the will of God.

HISTORICAL CONTEXT

World War I and Modernism

The ravages of World War I (1914-1918) brought about the deaths of millions of soldiers and civilians and caused many artists and intellectuals to question the values and assumptions of their worlds and the permanence of civilization. The growth of Modernism, a literary and artistic movement, attested to this newfound refusal to apply old-world values to contemporary life. Writers such as Ezra Pound (1885-1972), Wyndham Lewis (1882-1957), Virginia Woolf (1882-1941), James Joyce (1882-1941) and Eliot himself attempted to create new forms of prose, drama, and verse which they thought would reflect what they saw as the often fragmented and hollow nature of their world.

As William Butler Yeats's 1920 poem ''The Second Coming'' explains, ''Things fall apart; the center cannot hold; / Mere anarchy is loosed upon the world.'' Eliot's long, bitter and complicated poem, *''The Waste Land''* (1922) is regarded as one of the most perfect examples of modernist attitudes in verse. Other notable modernist works include Joyce's *A Portrait of the Artist as a Young Man* (1916) whose protagonist rejects the previous generation's religious and patriotic faith and Samuel Beckett's *Waiting for Godot* (1952), a play without any apparent plot concerning two tramps seeking a meaning to their lives which is never bestowed upon them.

Ironically, it was only after many of his own groundbreaking experiments in literary form that Eliot composed *Murder in the Cathedral,* which has more in common with the drama of the Middle Ages than it does with modernist, experimental pieces. However, the very use of such an antiquated form assists Eliot in exploring one of his chief ideas, specifically, that the values of Becket—who believes in a ''pattern'' of life that culminates in a meaningful act—are exactly what is lacking in the chaos of modern experience. Seen in this light, *Murder in the Cathedral is* modern in its attitudes and longing for a ''center'' that will ''hold'' the world together—something which many writers could not locate in modern life.

Drama between the Wars

Drama in both Europe and the United States flourished between the wars and playwrights offered audiences a number of experimental plays that now stand as landmarks in the attempt to revolutionize the dramatic form. Foremost among these was the American playwright Eugene O'Neill (1888-1953), who wrote a number of plays that accomplished this goal, among them *Desire under the Elms* (1924) which used Freudian psychology to explore a New England infanticide, *The Great God Brown* (1926) in which the actors use masks to present their ''personalities'' to each other, *Strange Interlude* (1928) a long play where characters frequently ''step outside of themselves'' to reveal their thoughts directly to the audience and *Mourning Becomes Electra* (1931), a trilogy of plays in which O'Neill appropriates the Orestes myth into the era of Civil War America.

Another notable dramatic revisionist was Luigi Pirandello (1867-1936), whose *Six Characters in Search of an Author* (1921) follows the exploits of six roughly-drawn fictional characters as they attempt to describe their existence to a group of rehearsing actors.

Eliot's chief contribution to the rethinking of dramatic forms was his use of verse. While the verse play found its greatest practitioner in William Shakespeare (1564-1616), the use of verse on stage had dwindled over time. As a poet, Eliot was able to successfully employ verse as dramatic language while still allowing his characters to speak in a ''realistic'' fashion. In his 1951 book *On Poetry and Poets,* Eliot explained that the problem with many nineteenth-century verse plays was ''their limitation to a strict blank verse [lines of ten syllables with alternating stresses] which, after extensive use for non-dramatic poetry, had lost the flexibility which blank verse is to have if it is to give the effect of conversation.''

COMPARE & CONTRAST

- **1170:** King Henry II and Archbishop Thomas Becket begin to quarrel over the growing strength of the Catholic Church, marking the first hints of an anti-Catholic sentiment lasting until the Catholic Emancipation Act of 1829, which permitted Roman Catholics to sit in Parliament and hold almost any public office.

  1935: Belfast is ravaged by anti-Catholic riots. Northern Ireland expels Catholic families and Catholics in the Irish Free State retaliate.

  Today: Although their British counterparts generally live in peace, tensions between Irish Catholics and Protestants are still seen in the number of bombings and acts of terrorism in Northern Ireland. British Prime Minister Tony Blair holds talks with Irish representatives in an effort to end these and other problems, collectively referred to as the ''troubles.''

- **12th-14th Centuries:** ''Miracle'' and ''Morality'' plays grow in popularity. These plays present the lives of Christ or the saints in dramatic form, often performed in a church as part of religious holidays or festivals.

  1935: Eliot's *Murder in the Cathedral* is written for the year's Canterbury Festival and is performed in the Chapter House of the cathedral. Eliot's play makes use of conventions and ''stock'' characters similar to those found in medieval morality plays.

  Today: While morality plays are not common commercial fare, long-respected titles such as *Everyman* are frequently studied and revived. Many churches perform ''passion plays''—morality plays based on the crucifixion and resurrection of Christ—as part of their Easter celebrations.

- **1170:** The feud between King Henry II and Thomas Becket—who defended the political rights of the church without any compromise—marks one of the first times in European history where the church and state are fiercely opposed to each other's workings.

  1935: In the most notorious attempt of a government to control the religious practices of its people, the Nazi Party congress, meeting at Nuremberg, deprives Jews of German citizenship and makes intercourse between ''Aryans'' and Jews punishable by death.

  Today: While the separation between church and state is taken for granted by Americans, the debate can still be seen in battles over school curricula, such as school districts prohibiting the teaching of Darwin's theory of evolution because it conflicts with the Creationist views found in the Bible or groups protesting the Pledge of Allegiance's use of the phrase, ''One nation, under God.''

Therefore, the versification in *Murder in the Cathedral* avoids any set metrical pattern which, as Eliot said, ''helped to distinguish the versification from that of the nineteenth century.'' The use of verse was a crucial decision for Eliot, who defended it (in his 1928 *''Dialogue on Dramatic Poetry''*) with the remark, ''The tendency . . . of prose drama is to emphasize the ephemeral and superficial; if we want to get at the permanent and universal we need to express ourselves in verse.'' While verse plays are still not as popular as those written in prose, Eliot's work did renew audiences' interest in this dramatic form.

CRITICAL OVERVIEW

Since the publication of his first book of verse, *Prufrock and Other Observations* in 1917 and *The Waste Land* in 1922, Eliot has been regarded as an important, if not crucial, figure in twentieth-century literature. When *Murder in the Cathedral* premiered on June 15, 1935, Eliot found yet another of his works greeted with enthusiastic and glowing reviews. Writing in the *London Mercury* in July of that year, poet Edwin Muir called it a ''unified work, and one of great beauty.'' The *Christian Century*'s Edward Shillito praised the play's force, stating (in the October 2, 1935 issue), ''Not since [George Bernard Shaw's] *Saint Joan* has there been any play on the English stage in which such tremendous issues as this have been treated with such mastery of thought, as well as dramatic power.'' Echoing the thoughts of many other critics, the American poet Mark Van Doren, in the October 9, 1935 issue of *The Nation,* stated that ''Mr. Eliot has written no better poem than this.''

Many critics were particularly impressed by Eliot's ability to compose a play almost entirely in verse and to make its sound as interesting as its subject. Writing for the July 11, 1935 edition of *New English Weekly,* James Laughlin stated that the play proves Eliot to be ''still a great master of metric'' and continued his praise with, ''Mr. Eliot has been to school and knows his language-tones and sound-lengths as few others do. . . . The craftsmanship of the verse is so unostentatious that you must look closely to see all the richness of detail.''

Frederick A. Pottle concurred with this judgment, writing (in the December, 1935, *Yale Review*) that the play ''shows Eliot's curious and inexhaustible resourcefulness in both rhymed and unrhymed'' verse. Such admiration for Eliot's ''resourcefulness'' with the intricacies of poetic language was also found in I. M. Parson's review for the *Spectator* (June 28, 1935): ''Its main quality is bound up inexorably with the written word, which cannot be paraphrased. And if one were to start quoting it would be hard to know where to begin or where to stop. For the play is a dramatic poem, and has an imaginative quality which does not lend itself to brief quotation.''

Perhaps the strongest endorsement for Eliot's use of the verse-play form was found in a review by the poet Conrad Aiken (writing in the July 13, 1935 *New Yorker* under the pseudonym Samuel Jeake, Jr.), who called the play ''a turning point in English drama'' because, while watching it, ''One's feeling was that here at last was the English language literally being *used,* itself becoming the stuff of drama, turning alive with its own natural poetry.''

While most reviews and essays on *Murder in the Cathedral* laud Eliot's ability to suit his verse to his subject, not everyone has been impressed. John Crowe Ransom, writing in the 1935-36 *Southern Review,* called the play ''a drama that starts religious but reverts, declines, very distinctly towards snappiness.'' F. O. Matthiessen, in the December, 1938, *Harvard Advocate,* faulted the play's ''relative lack of density'' when compared to *The Waste Land* and remarked that ''the life represented is lacking something in immediacy and urgency.''

And unlike those critics quoted above who praised Eliot's versification, Denis Donoghue, in his book *The Third Voice: Modern British and American Verse Drama* (1959), states that ''the text evades, rather than solves, the problems of dramatic verse'' and that the play's overall structure is marred by the absence of any ''unity of drama and metaphor.'' Harold Bloom (in the introduction to his anthology, *Modern Critical Interpretations of Murder in the Cathedral*) faults what he sees as the play's evasion of its central issue: ''How can you represent, dramatically, a potential saint's refusal to yield to his own lust for martyrdom? Eliot did not know how to solve that dilemma, and evaded it, with some skill.''

Criticism this harsh, however, is not as abundant as that which favors Eliot's daring in (as the June 13, 1935 *Time Literary Supplement* called it) moving drama ''farther from the theatre'' in order to ''come nearer to the church.'' Regardless of any one critic's censure or praise, the play still evokes commentary and interest due to the fact that, as described by Peter Ackroyd in his 1984 biography *T. S. Eliot,* ''The play is typical of Eliot's work in the sense that it is concerned with a figure, not unconnected with the author himself, who has some special awareness of which others are deprived and yet whose great strengths are allied with serious weaknesses.''

CRITICISM

Daniel Moran,

Moran is an educator specializing in literature and drama. In this essay, he examines the ways in which Eliot's play explores the processes an individual must undergo if he is to give his life for his faith and how such a gift affects the martyr's world.

In Eliot's *''The Love Song of J. Alfred Prufrock''* (1917) he presents a man on the verge of an emo-

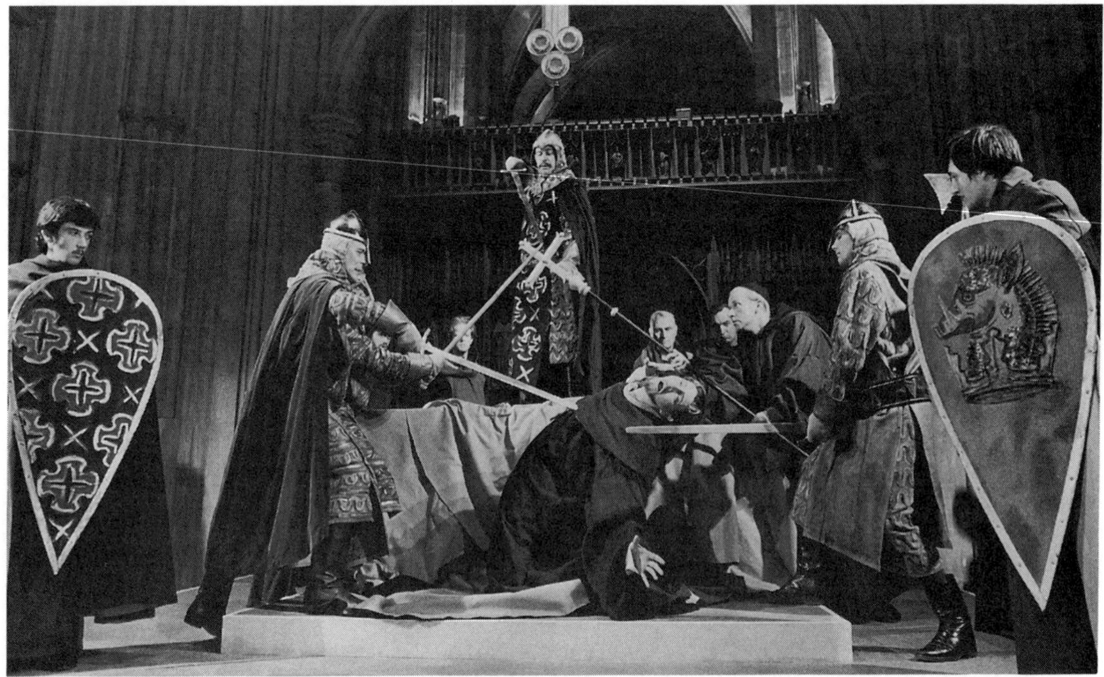

A production of Murder in the Cathedral *depicting the death of Thomas Becket (John Westbrook)*

tional crisis who finds that his fear of humiliation and of committing a social *faux pas* prevent him from revealing to a woman the depth of his love for her. "There will be time," he remarks, "For a hundred indecisions, / And for a hundred visions and revisions," since he knows that he will change his mind a hundred times before doing anything so brave. He asks, "Do I dare / Disturb the universe" with his desire to be frank; since he is "no prophet—and here's no great matter," since he is "not Prince Hamlet, nor was meant to be," he sees himself as insignificant, "an attendant lord, one that will do / To swell a progress, start a scene or two." Terrified of acting, yet dissatisfied with the results of inaction, fearful of revealing himself, yet dying to "say just what I mean," Prufrock stands in sharp contrast to a later Eliot hero, Thomas Becket, as seen in *Murder in the Cathedral* (1935).

Becket is a man who *does* "dare / Disturb the universe" with his arrival in Canterbury and refusal to concede to King Henry's demands; he needs no time for a "hundred indecisions" since he sees that the path chosen for him by God is clear. He is "like a prophet" and Prince Hamlet in that he serves the aims of a supreme, supernatural figure and sees himself as one faced with a task that can only culminate in his own death; unlike Hamlet, however, this knowledge causes him no great suffering of mind. While Prufrock's fear of rejection inhibits him from taking action, Thomas's determination to serve God prevents him from seeking asylum in a world governed by human law. Throughout the play, Eliot explores the ways in which Thomas's lack of "Prufrockian" fear allows him to answer his calling from God and how one who accepts such a call must do so at the expense of any and all temporal comforts. Rejecting this world in favor of the next may seem to Henry's Knights like the ultimate faux pas, but in doing so, Thomas renews his own spiritual life as well as the spiritual lives of the common people and the very world that martyrs him.

Eliot's original title for the play was *Fear in the Way,* and it is evident from the opening Choral ode that fear is a constant in the world of the play. The "poor women" huddle near the cathedral not for spiritual comfort but because "Some presage of an act / Which our eyes are compelled to witness, has forced our feet / Toward the cathedral. We are forced to bear witness." Already God is at work, "compelling" the women (and the audience) to attend to the drama at hand. Unlike the audience,

WHAT DO I READ NEXT?

- The sixteenth-century morality play *Everyman* (1500) was admired by Eliot for its versification, which he imitated in his play. A reader of *Murder in the Cathedral* will also immediately note the ways in which Eliot appropriated this play's use of symbolic characters (such as Death, Kindred, and Beauty) as the Three Tempters in his own work.
- John Milton's *Samson Agonistes* (1671) is, like Eliot's play, a religious drama in verse. The play examines the captivity of Samson (the Biblical hero) among the Philistines and his desire to strengthen his faith in God.
- Barry Unsworth's 1995 novel *Morality Play* offers a look at the performers of such medieval dramatic fare and raises questions similar to those found in Eliot's play, specifically, the ways in which the law of man—as opposed to the law of God—can be corrupted and suited to the desires of those in power.
- Sophocles's *Antigone,* a tragedy written in the 5th century B.C., is very much like *Murder in the Cathedral* in its exploration of a conflict between human and divine law. The play also features a Chorus much like that found in Eliot's play.
- Eliot's verse, particularly *''The Love Song of J. Alfred Prufrock,'' ''Journey of the Magi''* and *The Waste Land* shares many themes found in *Murder in the Cathedral,* such as individual spiritual decay, the desire to be led by a higher authority than man and fear of the unknown.

---

who by virtue of its position is intrigued, the women are terrified of any change in their lives: although they have ''suffered various oppression'' such as ''various scandals,'' ''taxes,'' and ''private terrors,'' they have ''Succeeded in avoiding notice, / Living and partly living.''

While a viewer might think that the intrusion of God into their lives would be welcomed as a form of deliverance from the ''poverty and license'' they describe, the women wish to maintain the status quo, which may be rife with ''minor injustice'' but which is also predictable and, more importantly, *understandable.* To be called by God to do anything—even to ''witness''—is too terrifying a task, especially when they learn that their Archbishop is returning:

> O Thomas our Lord, leave us and leave us be, in our humble and tarnished frame of existence, leave us; do not ask us To stand to the doom on the house, the doom on the Archbishop, the doom on the world. Archbishop, secure and assured of your fate, unaffrayed among the shades, do you realise what you ask, do you realize what it means To the small folk drawn into the pattern of fate, the small folk who live among small things, The strain on the brain of the small folk who stand to the doom of the house, the doom of their lord, the doom of the world?

The Chorus has accepted the world's indifference to them and all of its concomitant troubles and wishes to ''live among small things'' rather than answer the call of God, who will obviously make greater demands. Only through Thomas's death (which is his own answer to *his* calling) will they come to understand the greatness and glory of God.

As if God were presenting the Chorus with an example of one who rejects the very fears they vocalize, Thomas enters the play as one who knows he may die but who accepts this as part of a larger scheme. He tells the Chorus and the Three Priests that there is an ''eternal action, an eternal patience / To which all must consent'' and that the ''End will be simple, sudden, God-given.'' Already he is prepared to die for his return—but if he already knows this, why would Eliot write the play? In his *The Third Voice: Modern British and American Drama,* Denis Donoghue argues that an audience's knowledge of Thomas's death eliminates the dramatic force that his death may have. However, he seems to be missing the point that Eliot can use an

"BECKET IS A MAN WHO *DOES* 'DARE / DISTURB THE UNIVERSE' WITH HIS ARRIVAL IN CANTERBURY AND REFUSAL TO CONCEDE TO KING HENRY'S DEMANDS; HE NEEDS NO TIME FOR A 'HUNDRED INDECISIONS' SINCE HE SEES THAT THE PATH CHOSEN FOR HIM BY GOD IS CLEAR."

audience's knowledge of Thomas's impending death as a way to refocus its attention. The viewer then becomes more attuned to the issue of *how* Thomas will meet his death instead of whether or not this death will occur—and how Thomas struggles with the weight of martyrdom is Eliot's subject here.

Because a viewer knows Thomas will die, his thoughts on death and martyrdom take on an added significance, like when Henry Fonda's character in John Ford's film *Young Mr. Lincoln* walks into the sunset with "The Battle Hymn of the Republic" playing on the soundtrack. As Thomas explains to the Priests, "Heavier the interval than the consummation." The mental and spiritual processes *leading* to an acceptance of martyrdom and the means by which an individual gives himself completely to his faith are Eliot's concern here, and by having the audience know the end of the play before it begins (a function of its title), he is able to prod the viewer into becoming interested in the same things as himself.

Thomas's interaction with the Four Tempters allows Eliot to dramatize these very processes of denial and self-examination that a martyr must undergo if he is to remain true to his calling. The First, Second, and Third Tempters are easily spurned by Thomas, who knows that their promises of temporal power and comfort are "puny" when compared to those offered by God: "Shall I," he asks, "who ruled like an eagle over doves, / Now take the shape of a wolf among wolves?" Rejecting their insinuations that he can set right the world and its temporal problems, Thomas remarks, "Only / The fool, fixed in his folly, may think / He can turn the wheel on which he turns." Like Hamlet, Thomas believes "There's a divinity that shapes our ends" and will (again like Hamlet) "Let be," making the rejection of the Three Tempters a matter of course.

The Fourth Tempter, however, challenges Thomas on a much different—and more difficult—level. The strict meter of his verse attests to his potential bewitching of the future martyr:

> As you do not know me, I do not need a name, And, as you know me, that is why I come. You know me, but have never seen my face. To meet before was never time or place.

These figures have never met before because the "time or place" were not ripe with such a spiritual crisis, and it is the crisis of self-examination that this Tempter forces on Thomas. The Tempter asks, "But what is pleasure, Kingly rule" compared to "general grasp of spiritual power" and tells him that "Saint and Martyr rule from the tomb"; Thomas should "think of pilgrims, standing in line / Before the glittering jeweled shrine" and "Seek the way of martyrdom." If he refuses, he will become a footnote and "men shall declare that there was no mystery / About this man who played a certain part in history." As Thomas admits, the Fourth Tempter has exposed his "own desires"; like Prufrock, who imagines himself "pinned and wriggling on the wall" with a "magic lantern" throwing his "nerves in patterns on a screen," Thomas must now discern his own motives in seeking martyrdom:

> Is there no way, in my soul's sickness, Does not lead to damnation in pride? I well know that these temptations Mean present vanity and future torment. Can sinful pride be driven out Only by more sinful? Can I neither act nor suffer Without perdition?

The Tempter's answer to this question is an almost word-for-word recitation of Thomas's opening speech to the Chorus:

> You know and do not know, what it is to act or suffer. You know and do not know, that action is suffering, And the suffering action. Neither does the agent suffer Nor the patient act. But both are fixed In an eternal action, an eternal patience To which all must consent that it may be willed And which all must suffer that they may will it, That the pattern may subsist, that the wheel may turn and still Be forever still.

For what reason does the Fourth Tempter answer Thomas with his own words? The answer becomes more clear if the audience considers this Tempter—like his three counterparts—as not an external figure but a part of Thomas himself. Finding no allure in physical pleasure and certainly no use (after his split with the King) for temporal government, Thomas can reject these ideas quite easily. This part of himself, however—the part of his soul that *does,* to some ambiguous degree, covet fame and glory—is more difficult to resist. If he is to be martyred, he must look deep within himself, listening to his own voice, in order to be sure that he is not the slave of vanity. Seen in this light, the Fourth Tempter is unlike Satan, who tempted Christ, but like a mirror into which Thomas must gaze if he is to know himself. The Forth Tempter is a counselor more than an enemy.

Because of the Fourth Tempter's "friendly advice," Thomas is able to determine that "The last temptation is the greatest treason: / To do the right deed for the wrong reason." But what has Thomas decided? To let himself be killed? This is decided by him before the play even begins. To reject martyrdom? This is never an issue or possibility; Thomas wants to know if he seeks the "right thing" for the "wrong reason" of his own pride, not whether or not martyrdom itself is "right" or "wrong." What Thomas learns here *from his own words being thrown back at him* is that "action is suffering."

It is worthwhile to pause here and consider the implications of these words. For Thomas, who earlier in the play says that the women "know and do not know, what it is to act or suffer," to "act" would entail *inaction,* i.e., not protesting his death by sword when it finds him. To "suffer" would entail physical suffering (in his time of dying) but the word also carries the more important sense of "to allow" or "to be the object of some action." *This* is the key to Thomas's decision: he will "act" (through inaction) not because of his own pride, but by allowing himself to "suffer" the presence and workings of God. Only by seeking a martyrdom grounded in spiritual obedience (rather than temporal fame) will Thomas remain undefiled and avoid the "damnation in pride" that he fears. He now "knows" that "action is suffering" but "does not know" the actual experience of it yet. When this time does come, however, he will "no longer act or suffer, to the sword's end," obeying temporal commands and threats, but will instead "act and suffer" to obey the will of God.

Thomas's newfound enlightenment is offered to his congregation when he preaches to them on Christmas Day. Besides providing a dramatic fulcrum to the two halves of his play, the sermon allows Eliot to demonstrate the depth of Thomas's understanding of the nature of martyrdom. Christmas is, of course, the birthday of the ultimate martyr and Thomas uses this fact as a way to present the paradoxes inherent in martyrdom. For example, he speaks of the fact that they rejoice in the birth of one who died for their sins, explaining that "only in our Christian mysteries" can they "rejoice and mourn at once for the same reason." He also addresses the meaning of the word "peace" in Christ's statement to His apostles, "My peace I leave with you, my peace I give unto you," concluding that Christ "gave to His disciples peace, but not peace as the world gives."

A viewer can see the extent to which Thomas's sermon here is self-reflexive, since he too will soon find spiritual—rather than physical—peace. A final example of how the sermon reveals the working-through of the mysteries in Thomas's mind is found in his discussion of God's "first martyr, the blessed Stephen." Thomas states that "by no means" is it an "accident" that "the day of the first martyr follows immediately the day of the birth of Christ," so urging the congregation to ponder the "pattern" of God's will as he has done. He concludes by indirectly asserting his own triumph over the thoughts presented to him by the Fourth Tempter, saying, "Still less is a Christian martyrdom the effect of a man's will to become a Saint, as a man by willing and contriving may become a ruler of men."

The true martyr has "lost his will in the will of God" and does not even desire "the glory of being a martyr." Knowing that he is balanced on the knife's edge of divinity, Thomas pleads with the people to adopt his course of allowing God's will to work in their lives and to "suffer" His presence in Canterbury.

Part Two of the play presents the martyrdom that Thomas awaits. As Part One examines the processes involved in the individual's acceptance of martyrdom, Part Two examines the ways in which others may view and consider the same. The nervous First and Second Priests speak of the possibility of God acting through Thomas "To-day," but the Third Priest knows that such anticipation is pointless:

> What is the day that we know that we hope for or fear for? Every day is the day we should fear from or hope from. One moment Weighs like another. Only in retrospection, selection, We say, that was the day. The critical moment That is always now, and here. Even now, in sordid particulars The eternal design may appear.

Time is the mother of meaning (an issue raised in Eliot's poem *"Journey of the Magi"*) and the Third Priest is now certain, like Thomas, that the "critical moment" may arise even in "sordid particulars." As if to respond to this statement, the

Four Knights enter the play, much like Thomas's perfectly timed entrance in Part One. God's will is now hard at work, a fact acknowledged by Thomas when he enters and states, ''However certain our expectation / The moment foreseen may be unexpected / When it arrives.'' The Four Knights, however, have no interest in any discussion of ''the pattern'' or ''the wheel'' and demand that Thomas recant his former judgments to appease ''The King's Justice'' and ''the King's majesty.'' Thomas's refusal to do so reveals the extent to which he has (as he stated in his sermon), ''lost his will in the will of God'': it is not ''Becket who pronounces doom,'' he explains, ''But the Law of Christ's Church.'' Theory has been converted into practice and no threat can weaken Thomas's resolve: he is ''not in danger'' but ''only nearer to death.''

The Chorus's reaction to Thomas's fearlessness marks their gradual understanding of what they were ''compelled to witness'' in the opening of the play. Stating that they have seen ''subtle forebodings'' of the ''death-bringers'' in such natural signs as ''The horn of the beetle, the scale of the viper'' and the smell of ''incense in the latrine,'' the women beg Thomas for forgiveness for voicing their original fears. Thomas's cult of personality is growing stronger with each moment he remains alive. Naturally, Thomas forgives them with the command ''Peace'' and explains, ''Human kind cannot bear very much reality,'' an insight that is proven by the actions of the Four Knights and the previous lamentations of the Chorus: to Thomas, the only ''reality'' is that of God's will—all else is the vanity of temporal power and ''toiling in the household.''

The Priests, however, are still fearful and plead with Thomas to hide in the cloister. Thomas refuses, stating, ''I have therefore only to make perfect my will.'' It is at this point that Eliot again highlights the mental process of martyrdom by making Thomas's actions here slightly ambiguous and hinting—but only hinting—at his previously rejected desire for fame. Thomas commands the Priests to ''Unbar the doors! Throw open the doors!'' because he ''will not have the house of prayer'' turned ''into a fortress'': ''The Church shall protect her own, in her own way, not / As oak and stone.'' This train of thought is in perfect keeping with Thomas's earlier rejection of human law in favor of God's. When the Priests still insist on his hiding, however, Thomas flies into a rage less easily explained by a desire to remain solely an ''instrument'' of God:

> I give my life To the Law of God above the Law of Man. Unbar the door! unbar the door! We are not to triumph by fighting, by stratagem, or by resistance, Not to fight with beasts as men. We have fought the beast And have conquered. We have only to conquer Now, by suffering. This is the easier victory. Now is the triumph of the Cross, now Open the door! I command it. OPEN THE DOOR!

Thomas's logic here posits that only by self-sacrifice (''I give my life'') and allowing God to work his will through the Knights (''suffering'') will God's will be made complete. But why must God work today? At this moment? (Recall the Third Priest's explanation of how only ''retrospection'' yields meaning.) Thomas never considers this point and Eliot never addresses it, making this rallying of the Priests' faith one of the most ambiguous moments in the play. A viewer could easily understand this speech to imply that Thomas fears his *not* being martyred and that there are still some remnants of worldly pride clinging to his vestments.

While this may be a more cynical way to read the play, the point nonetheless seems valid—but only if that same viewer forgets a simple fact about Thomas: for all his wisdom and strength, *he is still a man* and still subject to the same apprehensions and doubts as everybody else. It is not surprising, then, that the very human Thomas fears the Knights will be prohibited from entering, for he has already completed a grueling process by which he has prepared himself for martyrdom. ''For my Lord I am ready to die,'' he states, ''That His Church may have peace and liberty.'' His resolve is stronger than any audience's doubts.

Thomas is killed onstage, so that the audience—like the Chorus—will be appalled by the event which God and Eliot have forced them to ''witness.'' The women long for a time when the land was free from the ''filth'' they ''cannot clean,'' found in the murdering Knights:

> A rain of blood has blinded my eyes. Where is England? Where is Kent? Where is Canterbury? O far far far far in the past; and I wander in a land of barren boughs: if I break them, they bleed; I wander in a land of dry stones: if I touch them, they bleed. How can I ever return, to the soft quiet seasons?

Although they are terrified by the murder of their Archbishop, the women still do not understand that God's will is at work here: ''We did not wish anything to happen,'' they cry, since their usual hardships ''marked a limit to our suffering.'' Only later will they ''know what it is to act and suffer.''

As they finish their ode and Becket dies, Eliot engages the viewer in the greatest surprise of the play: the Four Knights' direct address to the audience. In *On Poetry and Poets,* Eliot describes this device as "a kind of trick" added to "shock the audience out of their complacency," and the mock-inquest performed by the Knights serves several purposes in the total design of the play. First, the viewer sees the trivial nature of temporal power in The Second, Third, and Fourth Knights' sycophantic praise of the First Knight: "I am not anything like such an experienced speaker as my old friend Reginald Fitz Urse," states the Third Knight, while the Second Knight praises Fitz Urse for making his point "very well" and the Fourth Knight remarks that their "leader, Reginald Fitz Urse," has "spoken very much to the point."

The hollow rhetoric of the Knights, with their appeals to the "hard-hearted, sensible" people in the audience, heighten the sincerity and honesty that Thomas has displayed throughout the play. More importantly, the Knights' defense "shocks" the audience into understanding the degree to which the issues of the play are still relevant to modern life, as when the Second Knight explains,

> No one regrets the necessity for violence more than we do. Unhappily, there are times when violence is the only way in which social justice may be secured. At another time, you would condemn an Archbishop by vote of Parliament and execute him formally as a traitor, and no one would have to bear the burden of being called murderer. And at a later time still, even such temperate measures as these would become unnecessary. But, if you have now arrived at a just subordination of the pretensions of the Church to the welfare of the State, remember that it is we who took the first step. We have been instrumental in bringing about the state of affairs that you approve. We have served your interests; we merit your applause; and if there is any guilt whatever in the matter, you must share it with us.

The Second Knight looks forward to a future in which the Church's "pretensions" are subordinate to the State—a world very much like that of contemporary Western societies. But this is not a "message" play and Eliot is too clever to allow all the previous action to congeal into a tidy set of remarks. Instead, the Second Knight raises the question of how much the Church—or spirituality in general—affects the political lives of a nation's citizenry and the extent to which those who put their faith in temporal power (like Henry and his Knights) will go to ensure that the State is always in charge.

In *The Plays of T .S. Eliot* (1960), David E. Jones calls the Knights' apology "the temptation of the audience," and the Second Knight's remarks may seem tempting to one who wishes for no spiritual stake in the life of a nation. But who could be tempted by these "slightly tipsy" assassins with their fawning over earthly leaders and vocabulary of psychobabble ("render a verdict of Suicide while of Unsound Mind") that they use to cloud the issues? At most, they are like the first three Tempters in Part One: easily dismissable. Eliot has included their prose defense in order to show the gulf between men of politics and men of God—a contest in which Eliot never avoids revealing the side for whom he is rooting.

As a final way to illustrate the Knights' lack of understanding and as a way to illustrate the effect that Thomas's martyrdom has had on his world, Eliot closes the play with a Choral ode in which the women "Praise Thee, O God, for Thy glory" and describe their new understanding of the "pattern" and the "wheel":

> For all things exist only as seen by Thee, only as known by Thee, all things exist Only in Thy light, and Thy glory is declared even in that which denies Thee; the darkness declares the glory of light. Those who deny Thee could not deny, if Thou didst not exist; and their denial is never complete, for if it were so, they would not exist.

The Knights' sophistry or twentieth century cynicism are no match for devotion of this depth. The Chorus has moved millions of spiritual miles since the beginning of the play: where they formerly asked God to let them "perish in quiet," they now beg Him to forgive them for their former blindness. They describe their former selves as "the men and women who shut the door" and sat "by the fire"—seeking physical comfort—instead of as those who "fear the blessing of God." Any previous arguments raised about the depth of Thomas's devotion and spurning of pride are put to rest here, for the Chorus has been served by its Archbishop, regardless of the motives he may have had:

> We now acknowledge our trespass, our weakness, our fault; we acknowledge That the sin of the world is upon our heads; that the blood of the martyrs and the agony of the saints Is upon our heads. Lord, have mercy on us. Christ, have mercy on us. Lord, have mercy on us. Blessed Thomas, pray for us.

The women now fully "know that action is suffering" and will allow God's will to work through them. They have moved from Prufrockian doubts to Beckettian certainty and find solace in the presence of a Being that many moderns may be missing. Whether the modern age will produce more Beckets to assuage the doubts of the Prufrocks remains to be seen, but, as Hamlet says and Becket enacts, ''The readiness is all.''

Source: Daniel Moran, for *Drama for Students,* Gale, 1998.

Patricia Mosco Holloway

In this review, Holloway examines why Eliot composed his chorus entirely of women. The critic theorizes that, like many martyrs, women represent birth, new life, and renewal. She cites several examples of language and imagery that support this assertion.

When Carole M. Beckett observes that ''the dramatic function of the women of the Chorus (in *Murder in the Cathedral*] is to comment upon the events which they witness,'' she, like others, skirts the perplexing critical question of why the chorus is composed solely of women. What, in the design of the play, would necessitate an all female chorus?

The second priest in the play sees little use for the chorus of women:

> You are foolish, immodest and babbling women. . . . You go on croaking like frogs in the treetops: But frogs at least can be cooked and eaten.

These women, however, do perform a vital function: they expand our understanding of martyrdom through a metaphor of birth. The female chorus reminds us that both women and martyrs give birth to new life. For a woman, it is the life of her child; for a martyr, it is the life of his belief. In the play, the women's chorus shows us how before giving birth, a martyr, like an expectant mother, must wait and suffer.

To introduce his metaphor of birth, Eliot first shows us that both the women in the chorus and the martyr are waiting. The women open the play waiting ''close by the cathedral'' where they acknowledge they ''are forced to bear witness.'' As it turns out, they will bear witness to the birth of a martyr. At this point in the play, even though they are not consciously aware of waiting, intuitively they are expectant; they wait and wait. In fact, they repeat the word ''wait'' eleven times in just this first passage. This repetition, as well as words such as ''bear'' and ''barren,'' suggests a metaphor of birth. Similarly, Thomas' diction also points to a birth metaphor when he notes soon after he enters the play:

> Heavier the interval than the consummation. All things prepare the event.

Like the expectant women, he too is waiting for the birth of the martyr. Ironically, that birth will come only with the ''event'' of his death.

The women in the chorus, however, do not refer literally to Thomas' death. Instead, they speak metaphorically about an imminent, ominous birth:

> the air is heavy and thick. Thick and heavy the sky. And the earth presses up against our feet. . . . The earth is heaving to parturition of issue of hell.

The image of a round earth pressing up and the words ''heavy'' and ''thick'' suggest the physical appearance of women about to give birth. The word ''parturition'' itself literally depicts the act of childbirth. Later in the play, the women will repeat the image of a ''heaving earth'' as they again convey the metaphor of birth: ''I have felt the heaving of earth at nightfall, restless, absurd.''

Both the women and Thomas await the ''absurd'' birth described by the chorus, and as they wait, they suffer. The women agonize when they realize they await the death of Thomas. They fear the birth of which they speak because it will be a ''parturition . . . of hell''—the hell of their suffering when they experience the physical loss of their beloved Thomas. Like the expectant women, Thomas, too, suffers as he awaits his delivery. He suffers not only mentally through the temptations to his pride and power, but also physically through the pain of his death—the death that will deliver him into his heavenly birth.

Eliot uses the symbol of blood to link the suffering of the martyr and the suffering of the women. Just before he sheds his own blood, Thomas notes:

> I am . . . ready to suffer with my blood This is the sign of the Church always The sign of blood.

Blood is not only a sign for martyrdom, it is also a sign for motherhood. The shedding of Thomas' blood frightens the women, who would naturally associate it with the pain of childbearing, and their first reaction is to rid themselves of this sign of suffering:

> Clean the air! clean the sky! wash the wind! take stone from stone and wash them.

They echo the birth metaphor a last time when, in the same speech, they refer to themselves as wandering ''in a land of *barren* boughs.''

If, as seems to be the case, Eliot wants to show the similarities between giving birth and the making of a martyr, then a chorus composed of women makes sense not only thematically, but also structurally. After all, it is women who know best how to wait, suffer, and give birth.

Source: Patricia Mosco Holloway, review of *Murder in the Cathedral* in the *Explicator,* Volume 43, no. 2, Winter, 1985, pp. 35–36.

William J. McGill

McGill explicates the role of the chorus in Eliot's play, discussing how their choral speeches enhance the poet/playwright's language and the overall tone of the drama. The critic dissects several of the speeches to prove his point.

In staging T. S. Eliot's poetic drama *Murder in the Cathedral,* one of the principal technical and artistic-interpretive problems involves the presentation of the choral speeches. Textually they appear as odes with no specific instructions to indicate differentiation of voices. But the first staging of the play set the precedent for assigning parts within the choral odes to individual voices or varying ensembles. The decision is in part a musical one, involving an assessment of the voices available and an orchestration of those voices to produce a pattern of sound that enhances the aural effect of the language. Obviously, however, the arrangement of voices must also relate to the thematic development of the odes as well. We cannot separate sound and meaning. Thus, while the individual director has some freedom in designating parts of the choral speeches, the poetry itself places strictures on that freedom. What I seek to do here is to provide a reading of the choral odes which identifies the principal thematic and dramatic voices in them.

The choral ode which opens the play serves as prelude not only to the drama which follows, but also to the varying functions of the chorus and to the different voices which articulate aspects of those functions. The initial stanza is a full-voiced statement of the entire chorus speaking as "the poor women of Canterbury" and outlining their roles as harbingers of some danger which they cannot comprehend and which they can neither impede nor hasten, and as reluctant witnesses to whatever consequences that danger may bring. "Some presage of an act / Which our eyes are compelled to witness, has forced our feet / Towards the cathedral. We are forced to bear witness."

The second stanza takes up the theme of helpless waiting in a somber, yet strong, mellifluous voice (hereafter the first voice). The decline of "golden October" into winter, but not yet the wondrous winter of fresh snow and crystalline frost, rather the dead season of stubbled, muddy fields, sets the image of time suspended while "... The

"IF, AS SEEMS TO BE THE CASE, ELIOT WANTS TO SHOW THE SIMILARITIES BETWEEN GIVING BIRTH AND THE MAKING OF A MARTYR, THEN A CHORUS COMPOSED OF WOMEN MAKES SENSE NOT ONLY THEMATICALLY, BUT ALSO STRUCTURALLY."

New Year waits, destiny waits for the coming." In the chill of that mordant time the poor laborer from the fields seeks refuge before the fire, yet even in that refuge is not free: "and who shall / Stretch out his hand to the fire, and deny his master? who shall be warm / By the fire, and deny his master?"

The question points up the reluctance with which the women are drawn to their witness. The long third stanza opens with a querulous, almost whining voice which gives substance to that reluctance. Recognizing that the Archbishop Thomas had always been a gracious master, this second voice nonetheless regrets the possibility of his return. For the poor, what difference does it make who rules so long as things are quiet for them?—"we are left to our own devices, / And we are content if we are left alone." Left alone, they go about their business, keeping their households in order, trying to accumulate what they can, working their bit of land, "... Preferring to pass unobserved," leading colorless lives. But that hope diminishes. A third voice, dark and husky, Cassandra-like, dispels it with a vision to match the voice: "... Winter shall come bringing death from the sea, / Ruinous spring shall beat at our doors, / Root and shoot shall eat our eyes and our ears. ..." The full chorus now returns, and in the wake of this sequence of voices, the women are more fearful, more pessimistic. They have absorbed the qualities of the separate voices and their sense of premonition sharpens: "Some malady is coming upon us. We wait, we wait, / And the saints and martyrs wait, for those who shall be martyrs and saints." As before, the first voice intervenes to give resonance to the choral cry, while also developing its particular motif—all that happens depends on destiny which "waits in the hand

> "FROM THE EXISTENCE OF EVIL COMES THE POSSIBILITY OF GOOD, AND FROM THE VIOLENT DEATH OF THE ARCHBISHOP COMES A NEW SAINT, ANOTHER SAINT FOR CANTERBURY, A SOURCE OF SOLACE AND COMFORT TO THE POOR."

of God, shaping the still unshapen. . . . '' Confronted by that forceful affirmation of their own helplessness, the women conclude: ''For us, the poor, there is no action, / But only to wait and to witness.''

In the opening ode, then, we have three distinct voices standing out from the general chorus, each stressing a particular dimension of the choral function. The first with its recurrent appeal to destiny emphasizes that the women are but passive witnesses; the second with its recitation of the mundane preoccupations of the poor emphasizes that they are drawn unwillingly to fulfill the role of witness; and the third with its darksome, surreal vision emphasizes the fatalism, the pessimism of their witness. The reiteration of these voices develops the tone and consciousness of the full choral voice toward the final revelation.

Thus, in the second choral ode which occurs following the arrival of the messenger who announces the return of Thomas to England, an interchange between the second and third voices impels the women to a sorrowful plea to Thomas to go back to France. The third voice opens with a vivid invocation of the evil that is in the air and an intimation of its consequences: ''You come with applause, you come with rejoicing, but you come bringing death into Canterbury: / A doom on the house, a doom on yourself, a doom on the world.'' Then the plaintive second voice breaks in with a long recitation which, in effect, expands by specifics its earlier theme, though now in a more fretful, less certain fashion: ''We do not wish anything to happen. / Seven years we have lived quietly, / Succeeded in avoiding notice, / Living and partly living.'' That refrain persists, a recognition that the life of the poor, even when they succeed in avoiding notice, is tenuous and drab. The voice finally takes on some of the darksome quality of the others: ''We have all had our private terrors, / Our particular shadows, our secret fears.'' The third voice picks up this admission and intensifies it: ''But now a great fear is upon us, a fear not of one but of many. . . .'' That fear is a vivid intimation of the doom foretold in the opening stanza of this ode, and indeed it concludes with the refrain, ''the doom on the house, the doom on the Archbishop, the doom on the world.'' This ''dialogue'' closes with the full voice of the chorus which now echoes the rhetoric of the third voice in a petition, partly a whimper, partly a prayer: ''do you realise what you ask, do you realise what it means / To the small folk drawn into the pattern of fate. . . . / O Thomas, Archbishop, leave us, leave us, leave sullen Dover, and set sail for France.''

The third voice returns in a brief speech which follows the appearance of the four tempters. The premonitory sense now assumes graphic physical form—a sickly smell, a dark green cloud, the earth heaving, sticky dew—engaging all the senses. Then the full chorus joins the priests and the tempters in an alternating sequence which, with mounting anxiety, reports the omens and portents that now multiply.

A choral ode follows. The second voice opens, now readier to admit the drabness and sorrow of the life of the poor which seems more partly living than living. A wiser streak of fatalism has diluted the querulous tone of this voice. The third voice follows, and the physical details of the portents become even more distinct, more surrealistic: ''. . . The forms take shape in the dark air: / Puss-purr of leopard, footfall of padding bear, / Palm-pat of nodding ape, square hyaena waiting / For laughter, laughter, laughter. The Lords of Hell are here''. With the atmosphere now charged with premonition, a sense of foreboding in every voice, the poor women of Canterbury cry out, ''O Thomas Archbishop, save us, save us, save yourself that we may be saved; / Destroy yourself and we are destroyed.'' They have now realized, driven by the consciousness of fate and of their helplessness and of the impending violence, that they cannot be mere witnesses. However reluctant they are to watch, they must; however much they yearn to plow their fields, to tend their hearths, to let the princes and nobles rule, they know that the very act of witnessing draws them into the maelstrom.

The increasing anxiety of the poor women of Canterbury, which develops toward the final unison cry of fear that concludes part one, begins part two of the drama unabated, the interlude of Becket's Christmas sermon having done nothing to alleviate it. The full choral voice poses a series of questions which reiterates the pattern of part one, moving from mere anticipation (''Does the bird sing in the South?'') to anxious expectation (''What signs of a bitter spring?''). Hopefulness rapidly gives way to despair as, in response to each question, the resonant first voice consistently replies in gloomy tones, invoking the sense of destiny. This exchange concludes with a long rhetorical question that reaches the level of pain that tormented the last choral speech of the first part. This dialogue then is a reprise of the chorus's developing consciousness.

Having set the tone for part two, the chorus withdraws into the role of silent witness to the first encounter between Thomas and the four knights. When the knights depart with the threat to return armed, the dark and despairing third voice takes up the burden of the chorus in a long and gruesome ode. The shift from psychic to physical portents which characterized that voice earlier culminates here in orgiastic horror. The ''savour of putrid flesh . . .'', ''Smooth creatures still living . . .'', ''Corruption in the dish . . .'' are no longer signs beheld but immediate experiences, horrors not merely seen but ingested. The ''death-bringers'' are here. Thomas's refusal to heed the cathedral priests' harried pleas to escape brings death itself into full view: ''. . . The white flat face of Death, God's silent servant, / And behind the face of death the Judgement / And behind the Judgement the Void, more horrid than active shapes of hell; / Emptiness, absence, separation from God. . . .''

And so death comes to Thomas. As the knights murder him, the full chorus screams in agony, ''Clear the air! Clean the sky! wash the wind! take stone from stone and wash them!'' In frenzied succession the three distinct voices declare the maturation of their motifs. The first voice declares the desecration of England, of life itself, in blood: ''Can I look again at the day and its common things, and see them all smeared with blood, through a curtain of falling blood?'' The working out of destiny changes forever the world. The second voice, now perhaps older and wiser, yet retains its plaintive edge: the poor have known private catastrophe, have known suffering: ''Every horror had its definition, / Every sorrow had a kind of end: / In life there is not time to grieve long. / But this,. . . this is out of time, / An instant eternity of evil and wrong.'' And the third voice proclaims the final agony and helplessness of the poor: ''We are soiled by a filth that we cannot clean, united to supernatural vermin, / It is not we alone, it is not the house, it is not the city that is defiled, / But the world that is wholly foul.'' Again, the agonized full cry of the chorus: ''Clear the air! clean the sky! wash the wind!''

But man's avowal of helplessness and despair, calling from the depths, opens the way to the movement of God's grace. From the existence of evil comes the possibility of good, and from the violent death of the Archbishop comes a new saint, another saint for Canterbury, a source of solace and comfort to the poor. The concluding choral ode, delivered in procession while a choir sings a Latin Te Deum in the distance, is itself a Te Deum, a hymn of praise to God from those who, having watched, waited, and suffered, now celebrate the rebirth of hope through the martyr's blood. The ode is antiphonal with the strong vibrant first voice, now proclaiming like a celebrant the joy of God's destiny, while the full chorus responds, the interchange mounting in vigor and intensity until the concluding Kyrie.

Source: William J. McGill, ''Voices in the Cathedral: The Chorus in Eliot's *Murder in the Cathedral,*'' in *Modern Drama,* Volume XXXIII, no. 3, September, 1980, pp. 292–96.

SOURCES

Ackroyd, Peter. *T. S. Eliot: A Life,* Simon and Schuster, 1984, p. 227.

Bloom, Harold. Introduction to *Twentieth Century Interpretations of* Murder in the Cathedral, Chelsea House, 1988, pp. 1-4.

Donoghue, Denis. *The Third Voice: Modern British and American Verse Drama,* Princeton University Press, 1959, p. 83.

Eliot, T. S. ''Dialogue on Dramatic Poetry'' in *Selected Essays,* Faber and Faber, 1951, p. 46.

Eliot, T. S. *Murder in the Cathedral,* Harcourt Brace, 1935.

Eliot, T. S. ''Poetry and Drama'' in *On Poetry and Poets,* Faber and Faber, 1957, pp. 79-81.

Jeake, Samuel, Jr. [pseudonym for Conrad Aiken]. ''London Letter'' in the *New Yorker,* July 13, 1935, pp. 61-3.

Jones, David E. *The Plays of T. S. Eliot,* University of Toronto Press, p. 61.

Laughlin, James. ''Mr. Eliot on Holy Ground'' in *New English Weekly,* July 11, 1935, pp. 250-51.

Matthiessen, F. O. ''For an Unwritten Chapter'' in *Harvard Advocate,* December, 1938, pp. 22-24.

''Mr. Eliot's New Play'' in the *Times Literary Supplement,* June 13, 1935, p. 376.

Muir, Edwin. ''New Literature'' in the *London Mercury,* July, 1935, pp. 281-83.

Parsons, I. M. ''Poetry, Drama and Satire'' in *Spectator,* June 28, 1935, p. 1112.

Pottle, Frederick A. ''Drama of Action'' in *Yale Review,* December, 1935, pp. 426-29.

Ransom, John Crowe. ''Autumn of Poetry'' in *Southern Review,* 1935-36, pp. 619-23.

Shillito, Edward. Review of *Murder in the Cathedral* in *Christian Century,* October 2, 1935, pp. 1249-50.

Van Doren, Mark. ''The Holy Blisful Martir'' in the *Nation,* October 9, 1935, p. 417.

Yeats, William Butler. ''The Second Coming'' in *The Norton Anthology of English Literature,* Volume 2, W. W. Norton and Company, 1986, p. 1948.

FURTHER READING

Ackroyd, Peter. *T. S. Eliot: A Life,* Simon and Schuster, 1984, p. 227.

Although Ackroyd's book is an unauthorized biography, it does offer a general study of Eliot's growth as a poet and dramatist.

Eliot, T. S. *Selected Poems,* Harcourt Brace, 1964.

This is a compact edition of Eliot's verse, containing such famous poems as ''The Love Song of J. Alfred Prufrock,'' ''The Hollow Men,'' and ''The Waste Land.'' Reading these poems will give a student of *Murder in the Cathedral* a glimpse at how similar thematic concerns are explored in different forms.

Grant, Michael, Editor. *T. S. Eliot: The Critical Heritage,* Routledge & Kegan Paul, 1982, pp. 313-34.

This book collects a number of reviews of the original Canterbury Festival production of the play.

Hinchcliffe, Arnold P. *T. S. Eliot: Plays. A Casebook,* Macmillan, 1985.

This book contains a long introductory collection of essays titled ''Eliot's Aims and Achievements'' and then devotes a chapter to each play. There are many excerpts in this book by Eliot himself.

Malamud, Randy. *T. S. Eliot's Drama: A Research and Production Sourcebook,* Greenwood Press, 1992.

This is an invaluable book for any student of Eliot's plays. It contains a long introduction exploring Eliot's aims in writing verse drama, chapters on the production history of each play and a full annotated bibliography.

Plenty

DAVID HARE

1978

On April 7, 1978, *Plenty* was performed for the first time at London's Lyttelton Theatre. Its author, David Hare, directed this production starring Kate Nelligan as the play's protagonist, Susan Traherne. *Plenty* is one of Hare's most successful plays and the work with which he is most closely identified. Despite being one of the playwright's more popular works, the critical reception to *Plenty* was initially mixed. The play received a rather cool reception in England during its initial production, yet met with great approval in its U.S. debut in 1980 (the play's 1985 film adaptation was also greeted more favorably in America). The work's American popularity and the reluctance of British critics to embrace *Plenty* are at odds with both the author and the play's pedigree: Hare is an Englishman and *Plenty*—like the bulk of his work—is primarily set in England and deals with distinctly British themes. Like many literary works, however, time has shown Hare's play to be a valuable part of British (and worldwide) drama; the work gained new respect in the 1980s and 1990s—thanks largely to the successful movie adaptation.

As with the majority of his work, Hare's *Plenty* is noted for its well-defined characters, incisive dialogue, cinematic staging techniques, and a concern for social/political issues (Hare is an active socialist). The character of Susan is often cited as a prime example of the playwright's facility with strong female characters: in *Dreams and Deconstructions: Alternative Theatre in Britain,*

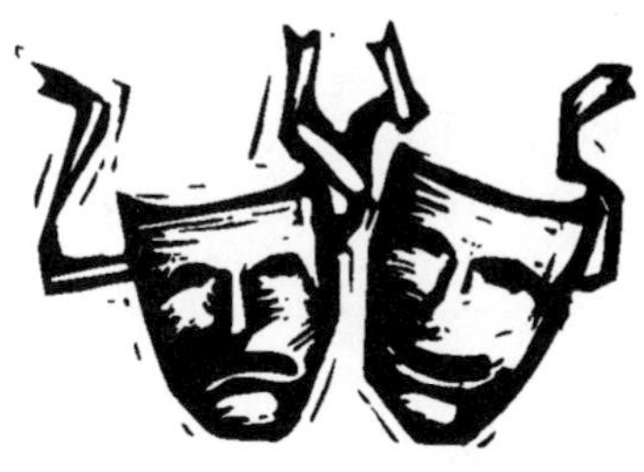

Steve Grant noted that Traherne is Hare's "most colossal role to date." Susan is a woman conflicted by the triumphs of her past and the mundane nature of her present circumstances. *Plenty* does not follow a linear chronology but rather shifts back and forth through Susan's adult life. In this manner Hare illustrates not only how one's youthful dreams are rarely realized but how a character's personal life can affect the outside world. This conflict of personal versus private life is often seen as one of the play's central themes. Audiences have been attracted to *Plenty* for this reason as well as for the play's unique characters, unconventional structure, and its bittersweet examination of lost youth and dreams.

AUTHOR BIOGRAPHY

David Hare was born to Clifford Theodore and Agnes Gilmour Hare on June 5, 1947. He was born in St. Leonard's which is located in Sussex, England. His father was a sailor and when he was five, his family moved to the small coastal town of Bexhill-on-Sea. Hare began his career as a playwright, director, and filmmaker while attending Jesus College in Cambridge where he earned his M.A. in English with honors in 1968. Prior to attending university, Hare was educated at Lancing College in West Sussex on a scholarship. In 1968 he founded and subsequently directed a traveling company called the Portable Theatre with which he was associated until 1971. Throughout his career, Hare has served as a resident dramatist, literary manager, and director of other reputable theatre companies, including the Royal Court Theatre in London.

In 1970 he married Margaret Mathieson, who at that time was his theatrical agent. Hare and Mathieson had three children, Joe, Lewis, and Darcy. After ten years of marriage, the couple divorced. Hare married for the second time, in 1992, to Nicole Farhi.

By 1998, Hare had close to thirty published plays, essays, and films as well as several unpublished works to his credit. His writing is noted for its political orientation and its focus on British themes. According to Mel Gussow in a *New York Times Magazine* article, Hare often treats such concerns "as the collapse of the English empire, the debilitating effects of the class system, the myths of patriotism, [and] the loss of personal freedom." Hare is also known for creating politically and morally ambiguous plays, despite his rather clear-cut leftist politics. His first published play, *How Brophy Made Good* was first produced in Brighton, England, at Brighton Combination Theatre in 1969 and was subsequently published in *Gambit* in 1970.

Hare did not begin to receive public attention until he produced *Slag* in April of 1970; however, since then he has been honored for his works on numerous occasions. In 1975 he became the first dramatist to win the presitigious John Llewellyn Rhys Prize and in 1983 *Plenty* received the New York Critics Circle Award for best foreign play. Hare is perhaps best known for *Plenty,* which achieved a high profile when it was made into a film starring Meryl Streep. Despite the fact that Hare's work has received severe criticism at times, he has still developed a fine literary reputation. As Joan Fitzpatrick Dean noted in her book *David Hare,* "Hare has earned an impressive reputation not only as a prolific writer but also as a theater and film director, theater founder, and literary manager." Hare's work is considered to have made an important contribution to his nation's body of contemporary literature.

PLOT SUMMARY

Scene 1

The play opens on Easter Sunday in Knightsbridge, England. The year is 1962. In this opening scene Susan Traherne gives her house to her friend of fifteen years, Alice Park. Alice intends to use the house as a home for unmarried mothers. Susan's husband, Raymond Brock, lies on the floor naked, bloodied (though unharmed), and full of Scotch and the drug Nembutal; he does not move throughout the scene. Susan leaves her husband at the end of the scene. She does not, however, take any of his possessions.

Scene 2

Scene 2 flashes back to the year 1943. The location is occupied France, where Susan works for the English government as part of the resistance efforts against Germany in World War II. In this scene, Susan awaits a shipment of explosives and guns to be parachuted down to her. Hearing a plane and thinking the drop is early, Susan flashes a beam of light only to find another English agent, Lazar, who is bailing out of his failing plane. Susan helps him parachute to safety. The two discuss the irony that the more successful they are at diverting the Germans from their military goals, the longer the war seems to continue. While they wait, the shipment drop arrives and it is taken by a Frenchman. Susan and Lazar argue with the man as to whom the supplies belong. Eventually, and by gun point, Susan and Lazar retrieve the shipment of arms from the Frenchman. Susan breaks down and confesses that she is not an agent, only a courier, and that she is afraid to die.

Scene 3

Scene 3 takes place in Brussels in June, 1947. After traveling with Susan in Europe, Mr. Tony Radley, a friend who served in the war with Susan as a wireless operator, drops dead in their hotel lobby. Susan approaches the British Embassy for assistance, pretending to be Tony's wife. After Sir Leonard Darwin, the British Ambassador, leaves the room, Susan asks Raymond Brock, then the Third Secretary, to call Tony's wife to explain how he died. Susan and Raymond discuss whether Raymond should tell the widow that Tony was traveling with Susan. Susan discloses that her relationship with Tony was not unphysical, but she claims nonetheless that it was innocent. Brock decides to lie to Tony's wife. Darwin returns and he and Susan discuss what the Ambassador perceives to be the great rebuilding of Europe in the postwar period.

Scene 4

Scene 4 is set in Pimlico (a suburb of London) in September, 1947. In a conversation with Alice, Susan repeatedly states how much she needs change and that she would like to move on. Susan also discusses her dissatisfaction with her job and her boss, who she believes is making sexual overtures towards her. Susan makes Raymond, now her lover, an omelette while Alice tells him about a new book she is writing. Susan also tells Alice that Brock thinks that Sir Leonard Darwin, his boss, is "a joke." Towards the end of the scene Susan recalls the war and her involvement with Lazar. She says she often wonders where he is. Susan tells Brock that she would like to try a winter apart. He leaves for Brussels, where he is now posted, without responding to her suggestion. Instead, he says goodbye and gives her a kiss.

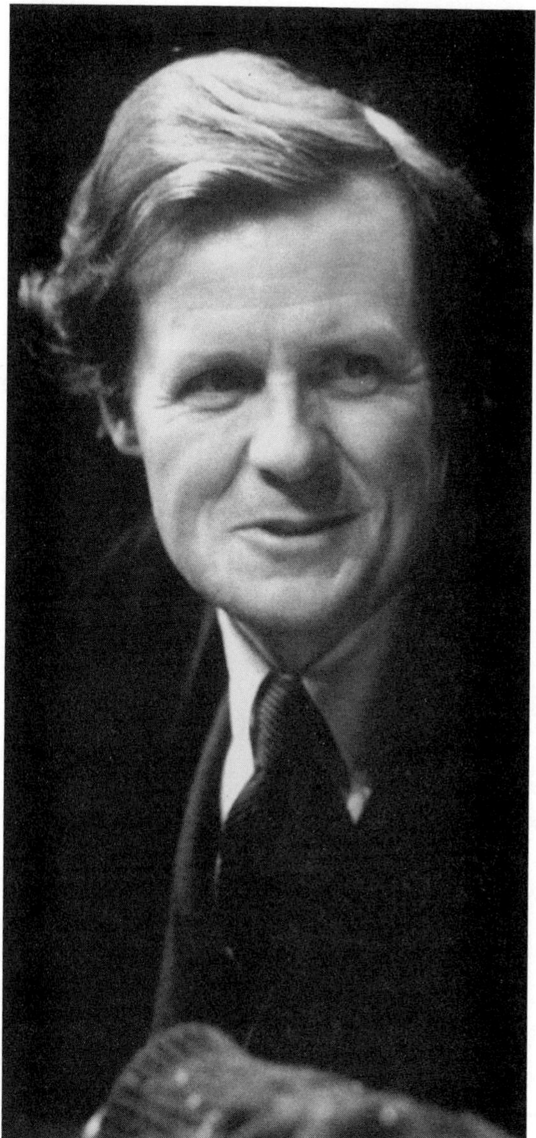

David Hare

Scene 5

This scene takes place in the London suburb of Temple in May, 1951. Susan meets Mick, a friend of Alice's from the East End and asks him to father her child. She says she would prefer to do it alone but that having someone she barely knows participate is her second choice. Mick agrees to Susan's plan.

Scene 6

The action returns to Pimlico in December, 1952. Susan complains about her job in advertising

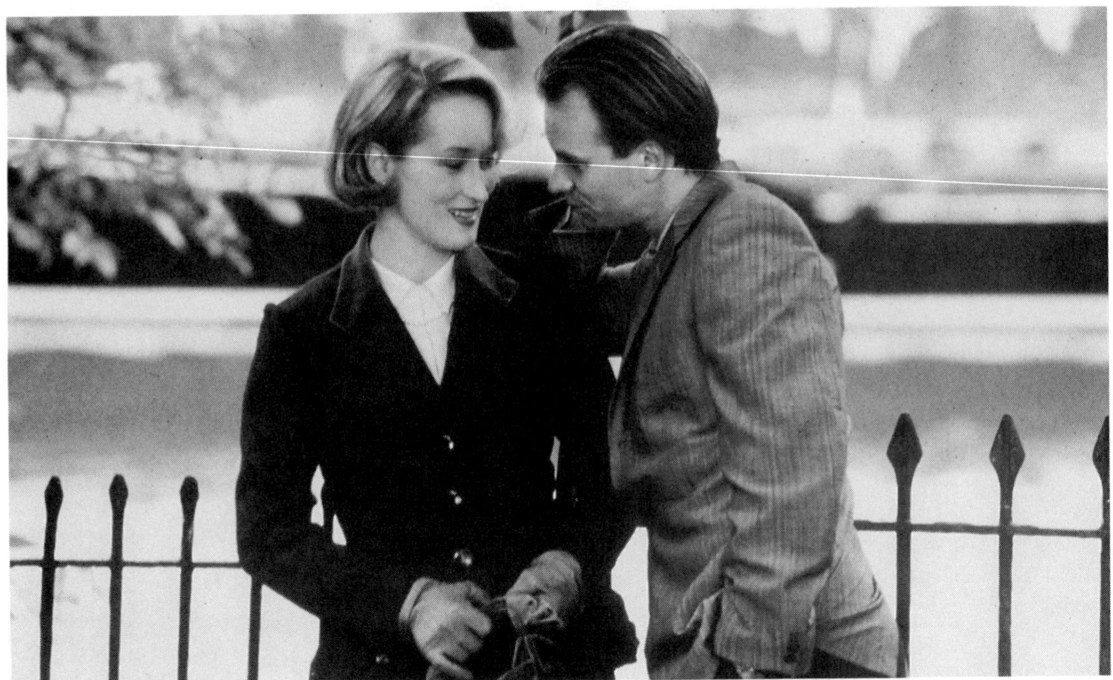

Susan (Meryl Streep) meets with Mick (Sting) in the film adaptation of Hare's play

and the dishonesty and stupidity that the position requires. Alice paints a nude of her friend Louise from Liverpool for the New Year's Arts Ball. Mick shows up and he and Susan have a heated discussion about their inability to conceive a child after a year and a half of trying. Susan takes out her gun and shoots it just above Mick's head.

Scene 7

It is October, 1956, in Knightsbridge. Susan and Brock have a dinner party. Their guests include the Third Secretary to the Burmese embassy, M. Aung; his wife, Madame Aung; Alice; and Brock's superior, Sir Leonard Darwin. Susan offends Darwin by making a scene about the English involvement in the Suez Canal fiasco (a conflict that arose over the control of the vital shipping passage. England eventually lost its claim on the canal). M. Aung spends most of his time kissing up to Darwin.

Alone, Brock and Darwin discuss Susan's previous bouts with mental illness. Darwin discloses that he believes that the Israeli/Egyptian war was fabricated so that the English would have an excuse for seizing the canal. Susan has what seems to be a breakdown and the guests leave. At the end of the scene Brock announces that Darwin will resign, and Susan celebrates that change is on the horizon.

Scene 8

Set in Knightsbridge in July, 1961, Scene 8 introduces Alice's student Dorcas Frey. Susan, Brock, Alice, and Dorcas have just come from Darwin's funeral. Susan explains that she and Brock have been posted in Iran. She also notes that not many people attended Darwin's funeral because he publicly revealed his negative thoughts about the Suez Canal incident. Dorcas asks to borrow money from Susan for an abortion. Alice tells Brock that Dorcas needs the money for a hand operation. Susan says that she would like to remain in England; she and Brock do not return to Iran.

Scene 9

The scene shifts to Whitehall, England, in January, 1962. In the first part of this scene, an unnamed BBC (British Broadcasting Company) radio reporter interviews Susan about her wartime efforts as one of the few female intelligence agents—and, at seventeen, one of the youngest to serve.

Later, Susan talks with Sir Andrew Charleson, the Chief Clerk in charge of personnel decisions, about her husband's career. She requests that he be given a more respectable post. Charleson comments that Brock's performance has always been quite mediocre. Susan tells Charleson that she will shoot herself in six days unless Charleson promotes Brock. She leaves after Charleson and Begley, another diplomat, try to detain her.

Scene 10

It is Easter, 1962, in Knightsbridge. This scene precedes the first scene in the play in which Alice returns to find Brock drunk, drugged, naked, and bloodied. Brock, who no longer works for the Foreign Service, tells Alice that he has told Susan that morning that they ought to sell the house. Brock now works in insurance. Susan is in a frenzy collecting all of the objects around the house. She suggests that Alice use the house to help her work with unmarried mothers. Brock asks Alice to get the Nembutal to sedate Susan and threatens to call the doctor to have Susan admitted to a mental hospital. Susan disregards his threat and suggests that Alice leave for a while so that she and Brock can discuss their problems.

Scene 11

Scene 11 takes place in Blackpool, England, in June of 1962. Susan has had sex with Lazar, with whom she was recently reunited. In bed, Lazar tells Susan that he found her because he heard her on the radio interview. Susan confides that she has not always been well; Lazar confesses that he has sold out to suburbia, marrying and taking a job in a corporate bureaucracy. Susan rolls a cigarette with marijuana and falls to the bed, waking to ask Lazar his real name as he leaves. "Lazar," he says, stating his codename. He departs.

Scene 12

The final scene takes place in France. It is August, 1944, and the Resistance has succeeded in liberating the occupied portions of France. Susan appears on a beautiful hillside talking with a Frenchman about the splendor of the day; she is radiant and happy, obviously joyous that her contributions aided in the Resistance's success. She is about to join the village party. The Frenchman complains about his life while Susan, somewhat oblivious to his comments, expresses optimism about the English improving the world. She agrees to have soup with the Frenchman and his wife. Looking out across the lush countryside, Susan pauses, stating: "There will be days and days and days like this."

CHARACTERS

Madame Aung

Madame Aung accompanies her husband to Susan and Raymond's dinner party in 1956. She is characterized by Hare as "small, tidy and bright." Her only action in the play is to begin to tell the story of an Ingmar Bergman film she recently viewed. She mistakenly states that Bergman is Norwegian and Darwin firmly corrects her by mentioning that the famed director is in fact Swedish.

Monsieur Aung

Monsieur (often abbreviated as M.) Aung is the First Secretary of the Burmese Embassy whom Susan and Raymond entertain in their Knightsbridge home in October of 1956. The stage directions describe M. Aung as "almost permanently smiling—short [and] dogmatic." Aung acts quite flattered to be in the presence of Sir Leonard Darwin and is overtly complimentary and deferential to him throughout Scene 7.

Raymond Brock

Susan first meets Brock when she approaches him at the British Embassy in Brussels, Belgium, in 1947 after her friend Tony dies in a hotel. Hare describes Brock as "an ingenuous figure, not yet thirty, with a small moustache and a natural energy he finds hard to contain in the proper manner." Brock becomes Susan's husband after taking her out of a mental hospital somewhere between December, 1952, and October, 1956. He does not seem bothered by dishonesty when it suits his purpose or coincides with his beliefs. He lies for Susan so that Tony Radley's wife does not find out that her husband was traveling with another woman. Later, Brock seems unruffled by the fact that Darwin was lied to about the Suez Canal episode. Brock is described by his superior, Sir Andrew Charleson, as an unexemplory employee; however, his patience with Susan and her various mental challenges throughout the years suggests a certain level of

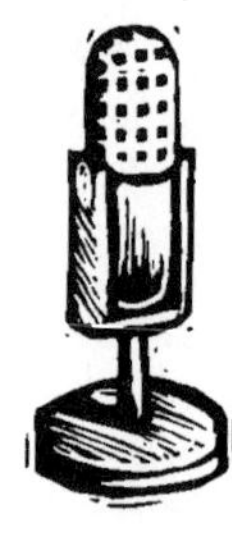

MEDIA ADAPTATIONS

- *Plenty,* was made into a film by Twentieth Century-Fox in 1985. Hare wrote the script and Fred Schepisi directed the film. The drama starred Meryl Streep as Susan, Tracy Ullman as Alice, Sting as Mick, Charles Dance as Raymond, and John Gielgud as Sir Leonard Darwin.

integrity. In the later years of *Plenty*'s chronology, Brock has lost his career in the foreign service and is working in the insurance industry. He is introduced in the first scene (what is, chronologically, his last scene in the play's non-linear sequence of events), naked, drunk, drugged, and unconscious, with his wife preparing to leave him.

Sir Andrew Charleson

Charleson is the Chief Clerk in charge of personnel matters for the Foreign Service. Susan discusses Brock's career with him following the couple's return from Iran. Charleson can be read as a condescending character in that he treats his assistant with little respect. Hare characterizes Charleson as a man in his early fifties with "far more edge" than Darwin. Perhaps by edge, Hare means to say that Charleson is direct and to the point. He tells Susan quite frankly that her husband has been tested and although he has risen beyond one challenge, he is honestly a rather average man in terms of his performance in the Foreign Service.

Sir Leonard Darwin

Darwin serves as a superior to Brock in the Foreign Service. He is a tactful and patriotic diplomat. He has faith in the reconstruction of Europe following World War II and does not take Europe's greatness for granted. He is an upstanding man who believes in his country until he is deceived about England's role in the Suez Canal incident. This deception provokes his resignation from the Foreign Service.

Darwin takes a moral stand that counters what would have been the appropriate diplomatic reaction, which is to support his country without question—despite his feelings of betrayal. As a result of his resignation—and, overall, his comittment to the truth regardless of decorum and expectations—Darwin is shunned by society, as evidenced by the small turnout at his funeral. While Susan claims to be motivated by truth, it is Darwin who represents genuine honesty in Hare's play.

Dorcas Frey

She is Alice's seventeen-year-old history student from Kensington Academy, where Alice begins to teach during the play. Dorcas attends Sir Leonard Darwin's funeral as Alice's guest. Having had sex with one of Alice's friends in an effort to acquire drugs, Dorcas becomes pregnant. After Darwin's funeral, Dorcas asks to borrow money from Susan in order to get an abortion, although she claims to need the money for a hand operation.

Lazar

Lazar is the man Susan accidentally meets while she waits for a shipment of guns and explosives during the war one evening. He is an agent for England and Lazar is only his code name (his real name is never revealed). Susan often wonders about Lazar in the years following the war. He tracks her down in England nineteen years after their first meeting in France. They have sex in a cheap hotel, and he tries to tell Susan about his life after the war. He feels that he has sold out in some fashion because he works in the corporate world and has a wife and a home in suburbia. Despite wanting to reveal something of his life following the war, Lazar ultimately hides his true identity from Susan. He leaves her, stoned on marijuana, without telling her his real name (he tells her the name she has always known: Lazar). Lazar's absence throughout most of the play as well as his shadowed identity code him as a mystery man. In a way, he represents all that has been elusive in Susan's life; it is the enigma that surrounds him—and the possibility that he possesses that which would make her life whole—that maintains Susan's interest for so many years.

Mick

Mick is a friend of Alice's who Susan approaches to father her child. He is a friendly younger man who still lives with his mother. He is from a lower class than Susan and thus does not spend time in the same social circles as she and Brock. Mick agrees to father the child and the two spend eighteen months trying; however, they are never successful. Mick winds up feeling quite horrible and used by the experience. He would like to continue to be involved with Susan yet the two agree not to see each other any longer. Mick later confronts Susan despite their agreement; however, she wants nothing to do with him and shoots her gun above his head. Later, Susan tells Lazar that Brock paid Mick to appease him after the incident.

Alice Park

Alice is Susan's self-proclaimed Bohemian friend. Susan meets Alice in 1947 and stays in touch with her until the play's end in 1962. Alice leads a rather carefree existence, sleeping with married men, doing drugs, working inconsistently, and crashing at Susan's home on occasion. Alice encourages Susan to break free from the things that Susan believes restrain her: Brock and her job. Alice seems to enjoy the drama that such action would present. Alice seemingly dislikes England as well as its social expectations. Throughout the course of the play she resists these expectations and helps those whose lives run counter to the country's dominant cultural expectations—as evidenced by her plans to use Susan and Brock's home as a kind of halfway house for expecting unwed mothers.

Susan Traherne

Susan Traherne is the rather complicated protagonist of the play. She is both volatile and passionate, as exemplified by her unpredictable outbursts and her lingering feelings for Lazar. Susan suffers from mental instability that manifests itself in her brutal and unabashed honesty. She serves in World War II as a courier for the English in France, and after the war she is disillusioned, constantly confronting the boredom and inanity of her subsequent jobs. She has trouble adjusting to postwar England and seems lost in her admiration of the past; through her memory and the mundane quality of her present life, her years with British intelligence have acheived an idealized (an unrealistic) perfection. She thinks longingly of the war and her love affair with Lazar.

Susan finds herself alone at the end of the play. She goes from serving a country in a war on foreign soil to being ostracized by that country by the end of the play's chronology. In the beginning, Susan willingly accepts this outsider status. In the end, her status as someone who is alienated can be seen as self-inflicted or as a punishment that others (perhaps unjustly) impose upon her (like other points in the play, Hare leaves this issue ambiguous). Although Susan is characterized as mentally unstable, she claims her actions are motivated by a desire for change and truth—bolstered by her willingness to say that which others will not. Despite her declarations of allegiance to the truth, Susan comes to represent something else entirely: unfulfilled hopes and ambitions. Like her native country, Susan reaches her apex in the victory of World War II; in subsequent years she and England will both fail to sustain their dreams of empire and influence.

THEMES

Duty and Responsibility

Much of the themes of duty and responsibility in *Plenty* revolve around social expectations and patriotic obligations. Susan fulfills her patriotic duty to England by serving in the resistance efforts during the war. Likewise, Brock, Darwin, Begley, Charleson, and M. Aung's service in diplomatic positions reflects their patriotic responsibility to represent their countries. Both Mick and Brock attempt to meet the traditional social responsibilities of men in that Mick tries to father a child with Susan and become involved with her while Brock later cares for Susan financially and emotionally as her husband. Interestingly, many of the characters in this play can be described as failures in these respects.

Although Susan feels that she is helping France curtail Germany's encroachment during the war, the Frenchman that she and Lazar encounter in the first scene tells them that the English are not welcome in France. From the Frenchman's perception, Susan and Lazar are fulfilling duties that are not necessarily required of them. After the war Susan fails to adhere to the unspoken civil responsibility of following social protocol. Instead of being quiet and acquiescent (as women were expected to do), Susan is often verbose and brash. Susan and Alice (who

TOPICS FOR FURTHER STUDY

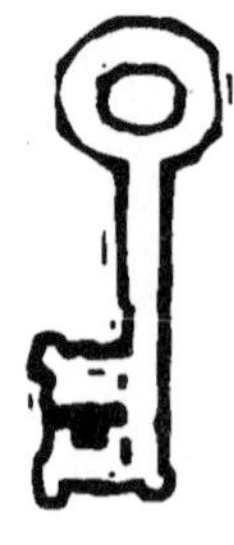

- Research the role of women in World War II. What did women contribute to resisting German dictator Adolf Hitler's forces in Europe or more specifically in France during the war?
- In Scene 4, the announcer discusses the BBC series, "Musicians and Disease" after mentioning that Vorichef died "in an extreme state of senile dementia." Do you think that Susan suffers from dementia or any other psychological disease? If so, where can you locate evidence in her behavior that she is or is not rational and mentally stable?
- Compare and contrast Alice's perceptions about the world around her with those of Susan. In what ways are the two women similar and in what ways are they different?
- How might Susan define love. Does she care most for Lazar, Brock, or perhaps Mick? Discuss her motivation to be with each of these three men.
- Research the Suez Canal incident. Do you believe that Darwin should have resigned from his post based upon your findings?

adheres to social mores even less than Susan) seem almost unpatriotic in their dislike for their nation, its policies and conventions. Susan also refuses to let Mick assume the responsibilities that being a lover, father, or even a friend would entail—despite his apparent willingness to be all of the these things to her.

Darwin relinquishes his duties in the foreign service in order to be honest with himself and others about what he perceives really happened over the Suez Canal. By abandoning the socially acceptable diplomatic role, Darwin refuses to take responsibility for the lies of his country. Ironically his honesty codes him as unpatriotic in that he does not unconditionally support England. For different reasons Brock fails to meet his professional responsibilities in the eyes of the foreign service. He does not advance through the ranks because he fails to excel in his duties. At the play's conclusion, he is working in the insurance industry. Ironically insurance protects people when and if they are unable to care for themselves. Thus it seems that while on the surface this play focuses on the ways in which the characters meet their duties and responsibilities, it also turns this notion upside down by exposing the ways in which they fail themselves and others as well.

Sanity vs. Insanity

Another central theme of *Plenty* revolves around the question of Susan's state of mind. Towards the end of the play Susan admits to Lazar that she has "not always been well"; however, just after this admission she also tells him that her clarity of mind is something that she controls. This scene suggests that, as Susan says, she simply "likes to lose control" at times. While "losing control" may have been an asset during her daring wartime work, it is a less desirable trait in England's staid postwar society.

In an earlier scene Brock denies that Susan is mad by suggesting that she simply "feels strongly." After Darwin's pressing however, Brock admits that Susan does have a history of mental illness. Brock actually admitted Susan to a mental institution after the shooting incident with Mick. Despite the apparent proof that Susan is mentally disturbed, the scenes which betray this instability are also marked by Susan's willingness to speak what she believes to be true. Some critics have suggested that, with the character of Susan, Hare intertwines truth and madness. As far as his protagonist is concerned, the truth and insanity are mutually dependent traits; her mental instability fuels her need to expose the truth.

Truth and Lies

The question of honesty permeates this play and most of its characters. Susan exemplifies someone who is willing to speak her mind despite the fact that what she says may be inappropriate and offensive. Despite her devotion to the truth, Susan is not above deception. In fact, her work in France was based on duplicity. Likewise, she does not intercede with the truth regarding the money she loans to Dorcas Frey. Alice tells Brock that the funds are for a hand operation while Susan knows—but does not betray—the truth: that Dorcas needs the money for an abortion.

Brock is another character who lies throughout the play. He lies to Tony Radley's widow about Tony traveling alone at the time of his death—although this lie does serve to protect both Radley's reputation and his widow's feelings. Later, Brock seems to not understand Darwin's consternation regarding the lies that surround England's role in the Suez Canal incident. Although the play does not explicitly incriminate M. Aung as a liar, his exaggerated deference seems insincere. His wife, though perhaps not a liar, does convey false information when she tells the dinner guests that Ingmar Bergman is Norwegian when in fact he is Swedish. Darwin, who is associated with truth throughout the play, corrects this false information. Later Darwin resigns because he is unable to live with the lie that continued diplomatic service might require. He feels betrayed and takes the higher moral ground. Darwin's morality is apparently respected by few of his peers, as evidenced by the small turnout at his funeral.

Hare seems to be criticizing the social practice of rewarding those who advance by any means necessary. While the characters who manipulate the truth are often successful, they are hardly respectable people. Although Susan is, for the most part, devoted to truth, her motivation is in part driven by bitterness over the lost hopes and dreams of her adventurous youth. Her obsession with exposing the truth also reveals her mental problems and may eventually lead her to imprisonment in an institution. Darwin, perhaps the most honest character in the play, is rewarded for his integrity with vilification. It's interesting to note that he shares the surname of Charles Darwin (author of the ground breaking *Origin of the Species*), the British naturalist known for advancing the theory of evolution. Darwin the scientist was frequently attacked for challenging preconceived notions regarding man's origins.

STYLE

Setting

Plenty takes place in the European countries of England, France, and Belgium. The twelve scenes occur in seven different cities or towns during eight different years ranging from November of 1943 up through June of 1962. The setting of this play is significant because it is far from unified. Not only does the action skip from location to location, but it also travels back and forth through close to nineteen years as well. Instead of highlighting the ways in which many things change over time, the skipping through the years exposes what remains constant in the lives of the characters, namely Susan's dissatisfaction.

The setting for Scene 1 and Scene 10 is particularly significant because it takes place on Easter. During these scenes, Susan prepares to and eventually does leave Brock. Because Easter symbolically recalls Jesus Christ's resurrection, Susan's leaving can perhaps be read as a rebirth of sorts. Hare concludes the play with an almost dream-like scene in which a radiant, young Susan celebrates the Resistance's victory in France. The audience's last impression of her is as a confident, optimistic young woman. Yet this scene evokes bittersweet emotions with the knowledge that Susan's life will never again be this rich or fulfilling.

Allusion

Hare employs several political allusions within his play. An allusion is a reference to a person, place, or event with which the reader/viewer is supposed to be familiar (likewise, a literary allusion makes reference to a written work with which familiarity is assumed). An example of a more overt allusion occurs in Scene 7 when Susan brings up the Suez Canal. Critics such as Ted Whitehead, who wrote for the *Spectator* in 1978, somewhat sarcastically criticized Hare because such allusions "may mean more to those for whom Suez still rings a bell." Whether one is familiar with the event or not, its inclusion in the text should prompt an investigation about the event, for knowing the history behind the canal will only further one's level of understanding regarding Hare's intent. The playwright's allusions highlight his refusal to spoon-feed his audiences with a neatly packaged message.

Ambiguity

Ambiguity is one of the more central literary devices Hare employs in *Plenty*. He intended ambiguity. He gives examples of this intention in his foreword to *Plenty*. Hare says of Susan, "in Scene

Four you may feel that the way she gets rid of her boyfriend is stylish, and almost exemplary in its lack of hurtfulness; or you may feel it is crude and dishonest.'' By not clearly defining a character's actions or motivations, Hare provokes thought in his readers and viewers. He intends to show that there are often many ways of perceiving a situation or person. Some may see Susan as heroic while others may find her crazy and unpredictable. The manner in which Hare portrays her makes it possible to view the character in both of these lights.

Unconventional

Convention in literature pertains to certain expected approaches and traditions associated with particular genres. Hare breaks with traditional approaches to drama and thus his work can be considered unconventional. In particular, *Plenty*'s plot is considered a departure from standard dramatic narrative. Hare's plot does not follow a linear development that progresses from a beginning through a middle to an end. Instead, the plot is broken up and begins at the end. Scene 2 is really the first of the chronology and Scene 12 is the second in the chronology. Although Scene 3 through Scene 11 follow in a linear fashion, they are separated by many years. In addition the setting for these scenes span the globe, taking place in different countries and cities throughout Europe. Rather than adhering to the unities of theater (place, time, and action as defined by Aristotle's *Poetics*), Hare jumbles the events of Susan's life to illustrate his themes; while time does not unfold in a typical fashion, the play's structure allows the playwright to build a ''linear'' concept of thematic unity.

Plenty is also considered unconventional in its liberal use of cinematic techniques such as flashbacks, quick scene changes that approximate film editing styles, and concise dialogue. While the play earned its share of criticism for appropriating such methods (many theater critics looked down on film as a bastardization of traditional drama), it also made *Plenty* appealing to a generation of theater goers who had become familiar with cinematic vocabulary.

Symbolism

One of the most blatant symbols in *Plenty* is Susan's gun. According to Joan Fitzpatrick Dean in *David Hare,* Susan's gun symbolizes her ''destructive powers that are intended to exact respect and submission.'' Often guns suggest a certain phallic presence in literature. Read in this way, Susan's gun could also be understood to symbolize the ways in which she controls, manipulates, and destroys the men in her life.

Hare also employs symbolism by linking Darwin (through the character's name) to noted scientist Charles Darwin, who, like the diplomat, sought to spread the truth despite harsh criticism. On a larger scale, the character of Susan can be seen to symbolize the unfulfilled promise of England in the postwar era. Like Susan at the end of World War II, the British empire is strong and confident, believing that it has the power to change the world for the better. Susan's disillusionment and growing unhappiness mirror the dissolution of the British empire and the country's increasing hardships with unemployment and domestic unrest.

HISTORICAL CONTEXT

England in 1978

England is one of the countries that comprise the United Kingdom along with Scotland, Wales, and Northern Ireland. In 1978, the year of *Plenty*'s debut, Prime Minister James Callaghan and Queen Elizabeth II presided over the United Kingdom, whose population at the time was approximately 55,780,000 people.

British Arts and Literature in the 1970s

According to Arthur Marwick in *British Society since 1945,* ''British art merged anonymously into the major international trends'' and thus did not necessarily advance a ''distinctively national or personal genius.'' Marwick identified ''super realism'' as one of the international trends with which British art blended. He included political works that emphasize feminism and homosexuality in this group. For dramatists, poets, and musicians, he noted that ''innovation tended to be at the unspectacular.'' Despite such derogatory comments, Marwick did—contrarily—suggest that in the 1970s ''the National Theatre at last entered into its magnificent new

COMPARE & CONTRAST

- **1940s:** During World War II, Great Britain envisions that it will be able to provide for the development of its colonies abroad. On February 20, 1947, Great Britain announces its intention to relinquish governing power over India. By 1948, the British colonies of India, Pakistan, Ceylon, and Burma have gained independence. These events indicate the downsizing of the British Empire.

  Today: The majority of England's colonies have achieved independence. The British Empire as a world power is no more.

- **1940s:** Retail sales decline in 1943 because citizens are urged to purchase items such as clothing and furniture on a need only basis. Expenditures on luxury items are low as a result. Other items are restricted such as coal.

  1978: Britain enjoys a booming economy in 1978 with many of its leading indicators up from previous years.

  Today: According to the *Economist,* in 1997 Britain experienced economic growth for "a fifth straight year" despite a more recent slow down.

- **1947:** Britain and Egypt attempt to negotiate a renewal of the Anglo-Egyptian Treaty of 1936 which granted Britain the right to post defense troops in the Suez Canal region to protect their interest in the route's security. Negotiations break down despite Britain's voluntary evacuation of the area.

  1956: President Nasser of Egypt nationalizes the Suez Canal in July and in October, after making an ultimatum that Egypt and Israel withdraw from the area, Britain and France invade the Canal Zone. Egypt sinks forty ships and effectively blocks the Canal in retaliation. By November British, French and Israeli troops withdraw from the area.

  Today: The Middle East continues to be a site of extensive political conflict.

architectural complex and thereafter continued to present a range of plays which could by no stretch of the words be deemed conservative or unimaginative."

Also during this period, novelists such as Angela Carter and Fay Weldon advanced feminist concerns while playwrights such as Hare addressed issues that directly affected women in postwar society. Marwick called the rise of women novelists and feminism as a literary theme "the most significant development in the indigenous novel"for the 1970s.

Economy

By the close of 1978, the British economy had not enjoyed a better year since 1973. Most of the leading indicators were up, including total output, export volume, spending power, earnings, and retail sales. The government aided this trend by reducing taxes during the summer of 1978. As a result of a strong pound (the basic unit of currency in England), the country experienced less expensive imports. In addition inflation was brought to a celebrated low of 7.4% in June of 1978.

Although 1978 signaled improvement in many areas, the mid- to late-1970s were a harkening back to the Depression of the 1930s according to Marwick in *British Society since 1945.* The author stated that this period was marked by "a general sense of a worsening economy and declining living standards . . . and the break up of the optimistic consensus which had carried Britain through the difficult post-war years into the affluence of the sixties."

Politics

According to *Encyclopedia Britannica's Book of the Year* for 1979, one of the principal successes of 1978 was Prime Minister Callaghan's ability to run the nation despite "a hung Parliament, a divided Labour Party, and Trades Union Congress opposition to his principle policies." Ironically, in 1978, opinion polls rated Margaret Thatcher less popular than James Callaghan. This suggests that the Labour Party enjoyed a higher approval rating than Thatcher's Conservative Party despite the fact that Thatcher assumed the Prime Ministership in 1979.

Foreign Relations

Callaghan's visit to India marked a major foreign relations event in 1978. Prior to this visit, a British Prime Minister had not visited India since 1971. The general concerns for the year involved increasing international trade and decreasing Soviet influence in Cuba and Africa. Britain's colonies continue to agitate for independence. Colonial Prime Minister Ian Smith signed an agreement that allowed the African nation of Zimbabwe's black majority to assume sovereignty by year's end.

Class

During the 1970s, Britain's society continued to confirm the endurance of its class-conscious system. The decade, however, was also a time of class mobility. Marwick noted that "Margaret Thatcher herself is a symbol of the educational opportunity and upward mobility offered by the British System." Marwick referred to the Prime Minister's "lower-middle-class" beginnings in contrast to her future distinction as the British head of state as an example of the possibility of social mobility afforded to British citizens during this era.

CRITICAL OVERVIEW

Plenty has most certainly not gone without its share of unfavorable criticism despite the fact that it is one of Hare's best-known plays. Prior to *Plenty*'s debut at the Lyttelton Theatre, Hare's plays had not been performed at Britain's National Theatre and following some of the rather scathing reviews from his critical contemporaries it may seem shocking that Hare has risen to such artistic acclaim—despite the mixed critical reaction his plays have received, he has continued to be popular with audiences.

It is perhaps Hare's often shocking and pointed commentary about England that elicited such a response from his nation's critics. After the release of the film adaptation in 1985, Gavin Millar wrote in *Sight and Sound,* "no one with any serious hopes for contemporary British writing can ignore him, yet what the devil is the chap saying about us?" Ted Whitehead, writing for the *Spectator* soon after *Plenty*'s first performance in April of 1978, had answered this question years earlier by detailing Hare's work as "a cry of disgust with Britain—with the wet, the cold, the flu, the flood, the loveless English—and with the horror of sexual repression, the futility of sexual freedom, the corruption of wealth, the lie of good behavior, the decay of belief, the deceit of advertising, the bureaucracy and the indignity of death."

Whitehead touched on the elements within the play which may have offended Britain's critics. He further noted that the play was somewhat confusing because of the inclusion of "some sketchy minor characters" such as Dorcas Frey and the Aungs. Their inclusion, along with the "hurtling forward, or backward and forward, gives the feeling of hectic development that never quite becomes organic growth" according to the critic. Whitehead was not alone in his confusion about *Plenty.* Bernard Levin wrote in the *Sunday Times* in April, 1978, "what does the author want us to think, to feel? What is he saying? What does he believe about his characters and their predicament? There is no telling, and it is no use searching the title for clues, either, for it has less discernible connection with the contents than in any play since *Twelfth Night.*"

Of the film version, George Perry echoed Levin's dismay in his November, 1985, article for the *Sunday Times.* He noted that "*Plenty,* albeit well dressed, entertaining, and cleverly written, is ultimately so shallow it might as well have been called Empty." While there seemed to be a consensus of confusion surrounding *Plenty,* which many critics viewed as the playwright's fault, one critic suggested that perhaps the viewers of Hare's work were themselves responsible for coming up empty. Writing for *London Magazine,* Colin Ludlow commented that the critical conclusion "that [*Plenty*] lacks substance and has nothing to say" results from "pure laziness" on the part of the critics. Further, Ludlow noted that his peers' inability to understand the play also highlights the way in which "Hare refuses to prescribe cures for the problems he highlights."

In a two-page "Note on Performance" published with *Plenty,* Hare confirms his intent to not answer the questions he poses. He wrote, "ambiguity is central to the idea of the play. The audience is asked to make its own mind up about each of the actions. In the act of judging, the audience learns something about its own values.'' Hare's work continued to frustrate, disappoint, and challenge critics both in England and in the United States, where he produced the play in 1982 prior to making the film version; however in general, *Plenty* was received much better abroad than at home.

In his introduction to his work *The History Plays,* which includes *Plenty,* Hare partially attributes this relative acceptance to the fact that Americans were ''not afraid to look English society in the eye, to see Suez as criminal and the Foreign Office as absurd. They also seemed less frightened of a strong woman.'' Despite the criticism Hare has received about the political content of his work, he has often been praised for his wit even by his most skeptical critics. In the same *Spectator* article of 1978, Whitehead applauded the playwright's ''glacially witty dialogue.''

Much to Hare's credit, he has been congratulated not only for his mastery of his craft but for his effect on audiences as well. After noting the intentional ambiguity of *Plenty,* Ludlow made the comment that ''the power of his [Hare's] work is to provoke thoughts and disturb complacency.'' He follows this with the appraisal that ''certainly the study of suffering and waste in *Plenty* does no less than that.'' While critics may have initially chafed at Hare's forthright commentary in *Plenty,* time has shown the play to be a significant contribution to both British and world drama. As Joan Fitzpatrick Dean noted in *David Hare,* ''*Plenty* deserves to be Hare's best-known work, not only because it is among his finest plays but because it epitomizes his themes and character types. Like many of his works of the 1970s, *Plenty* deals with specifically British experiences and personalities.''

CRITICISM

D. L. Kellett

Kellett is a professional writer with a specialty in drama. The following essay explores the theme of ambiguity in David Hare's Plenty.

The extent to which readers are able to understand or discern an author's intended meaning is often a topic of literary debate. Some authors refuse to discuss the meaning of their works and thus it is not possible to know for certain whether critical interpretations of their writings are accurate. Doris Sommer's article ''Resisting the Heat: Mench, Morrison, and Incompetent Readers'' in *Cultures of United States Imperialism,* expanded this debate even further. Sommer argued that readers may not necessarily be capable of accurately interpreting a work's meaning because ''some books resist the competent reader.''

Sommer noted that writers like Guatemala's Rigoberta Mench and the United States's Toni Morrison may intentionally prevent readers from pinning down an author's meaning. Sommer's article raises the point that authors go to varying lengths to either help or hinder interpretation of their work. In addition, she noted a critical distinction between ambiguity and what she calls resistance. She stated that ''ambiguity, unlike the resistance that interests me here, has been for some time a consecrated and flattering theme for professional readers. It blunts interpretive efforts and therefore invites more labor.''

David Hare's works combine resistance and ambiguity. In the introduction to *The Early Plays: Slag, Great Exhibition, Teeth 'n' Smiles,* Hare states, ''as you can't control people's reactions to your plays, your duty is also not to reduce people's reactions, not to give them easy handles with which they can pigeon-hole you, and come to comfortable terms with what you are saying.'' In the ''Note on Performance'' that precedes *Plenty,* Hare goes further. He says of *Plenty,* ''I planned a play in twelve scenes, in which there would be twelve dramatic actions. Each of these actions is intended to be ambiguous, and it is up to the audience to decide what they feel about each event.''

Taken as a whole, Hare's *Plenty* may seem rather overwhelming—in fact it has confounded many critics over the years. Taken piece by piece, however, the play may be more readily accessible. In the ''Note on Performance,'' Hare states that he intends for his audiences, or presumably his readers, to judge his characters and plots in order to arrive at conclusions about the work as a whole. One impediment to judging quickly, however, is the presence of ambiguity in Hare's writing. Thus prior to judging, one must explore the nature of *Plenty*'s ambiguities in further detail.

One of the greatest obscurities in *Plenty* surrounds the characterization of Susan Traherne. Should she be detested, admired, or pitied? Is she selfish, inspired, or crazy? Can she be detested, admired, and pitied because she *is* selfish, inspired, and crazy? These questions are not easily answered;

WHAT DO I READ NEXT?

- *Paris by Night* is another of Hare's works. It was first published in 1988, and was written expressly for film. The story is about an English woman attending a political conference in Paris who must confront her limits and her understanding of herself.
- The television play *Licking Hitler* (1978) was written by Hare at the same time he was working on *Plenty.* It takes place during World War II and, like *Plenty,* explores the themes of honesty and dishonesty in the public and private realms.
- Sefton Delmar's *Black Boomerang*(1962) was used by Hare as a factual source for *Licking Hitler.* In this autobiographical work, Delmar details his direct involvement in the black propaganda efforts of Britain during World War II.
- *Hedda Gabler* (1890), a play by Norwegian dramatist Henrik Ibsen, is the story of a strong female protagonist. The title character, Hedda, struggles with the world in which she lives much like Susan in Hare's *Plenty*—she also possesses destructive tendencies and an explosive personality. Ibsen and Hare are both known for addressing political and personal problems in their works.
- Chinua Achebe's *Things Fall Apart* (1959) examines England's role as a colonial power in Nigeria. The novel traces the empire's influence on an African tribal village.

---

however, they seem to be the very judgments that Hares insists his readers make. In *David Hare,* Joan Fitzpatrick Dean remarked that ''there is a fundamental ambiguity in Hare's presentation of Susan. On the one hand she is frustrated, trapped, and unfulfilled; on the other, she is selfish, insatiable, and unreasonable.''

Scene 7 is the pinnacle scene of Susan's frustration with the polite inanity of the British diplomatic world. Her barbs towards Darwin, who to that point had epitomized the acquiescence and silence Susan detests about diplomacy, reflect her deep dissatisfaction with Britain's social mores. In a heated moment she declares, ''I would stop, I would stop, I would stop . . . talking if I ever heard anyone else say anything worth . . . stopping talking for.'' But does Susan's outburst reflect a warranted frustration or simply the ranting of a self-centered unstable idealist who wishes to control the present and who cannot let go of the past? Susan's dealings with Mick suggest the latter.

In asking Mick to father a child for her, Susan exposes an intolerance for allowing other people into her private world. She is absorbed in her own wishes and would be more than happy to ''do the whole damn thing'' alone. After Mick and Susan's attempts fail, she reveals that she does not care for Mick's feelings. The Susan presented in Scene 6 is cold, calculated, and self-absorbed. She does not demonstrate compassion for Mick, who feels used, but rather she is preoccupied with the work she must do on her newest ad campaign. In the end, Mick concludes that ''she is actually mad,'' yet is she not just frustrated by his love for her?

Hare suggests that the answers to these questions betray the values of the one who judges, thus what does it imply to say that Susan is frustrated or Susan is a raving lunatic or Susan is selfish? Better yet, what does Hare evoke by wanting his readers to categorize Susan as one thing or another? To see Susan as a frustrated and trapped woman places the reader squarely within a camp that openly criticizes British culture; however, labeling her as crazy may indeed do the same. Susan's madness may account for the lack of perfect British decorum in her behavior, yet it does not necessarily diminish the impact of what she says.

Whether she is frustrated or crazy, Susan's honesty still reveals social criticism. The reader who is willing to label her as frustrated shows his or her willingness to be overtly critical, while the reader who prefers to call her crazy can be shielded from implicating him/herself in such criticism. In the end then, the ambiguity surrounding Susan Traherne ferrets out those folks who value honesty above decorum or those who value diplomacy above forthrightness.

Hare weaves ambiguity throughout *Plenty* not only through his characterization of Susan but within each scene as well. As he clearly states in his "Note on Performance," he intended each action to be ambiguous. One of the ambiguities raised in Scene 2 concerns the British presence in France. Angry about losing the guns and explosives from an armed Lazar, the Frenchman declares, "Nobody ask you. Nobody ask you to come." In French he adds, "you are not welcome here." The implicit "you" of the Frenchman's statement is not simply Susan and Lazar but the British in general.

In this scene Hare suggests that despite their allegiance in resistance to Germany, England and France were perhaps not as united as one might think. What then are the rules of engagement by which Susan and Lazar must abide when France, a supposed ally, becomes adversarial? She says, "they [the Gaullists] just expect the English to die. They sit and watch us spitting blood in the streets." In a frightened state of dismay Susan questions, "what's the point of following the rules?" Susan's questioning contrasts sharply with the comment she makes earlier in the scene that, "it really is best if you always obey the rules." Scene 2 thus embodies two contradictions that leave the audience or reader somewhat mystified: allies stand in opposition to one another and rules are both to be followed and not to be followed.

Although Scene 2 does not include Alice, the themes it raises have metaphorical implications on Susan's relationship with her. In that Alice and Susan share a distaste for England, she and Susan seem alike. In *David Hare,* Dean suggested that although Alice and Susan share such distaste, "the contrast between them is at least as strong as their shared disdain for convention." Dean noted that Susan "admires Alice's freedom and independence," but she does not achieve the same in her own life. In Scene 6 Alice prompts Susan to leave her job and Brock, yet Susan convinces herself not to do either. Susan does not leave Brock for another ten years and continues to torment herself with unfulfilling occupational choices. As she sees it, she chooses instead to continue "living in hell."

"DESPITE THE READING THAT EACH VIEWER OF *PLENTY* MAY CHOOSE, THE INCLUSION OF OPTIONS MAKES HARE'S PLAY AN EXERCISE IN DECISION-MAKING."

Susan and Alice's relationship symbolizes the notion that within similarity, differences may exist. Alice most definitely does not believe that one must always obey the rules. Her sexually active Bohemian lifestyle flies in the face of such social conventions. Susan's rejection of the rules manifests itself only sporadically and thus she can ironically be seen as someone who in part obeys the social mores of her time. The action advanced in Scene 2 involves Lazar and Susan in 1944 in France, yet the ambiguities it evokes permeate the play throughout its entirety.

Because ambiguity plays such an integral role in Hare's work, one should not be surprised that his title also reflects this basic organizing principle. The title calls to mind Susan's postwar optimism. In the final scene, which chronologically precedes the majority of the other scenes in the play, Susan declares "there will be days and days and days like this." Susan's perception of what the day is like differs greatly from that of the Frenchman who seems downtrodden and pessimistic about the future and his own reality. Thus, the days that follow or—in the jumbled chronology of the play—have passed, can either be seen as Susan perceives them or as the Frenchman perceives them.

The scene's placement at the end of the play also has important significance. First, it calls attention to the fact that the days that follow it chronologically do not meet Susan's expectations; however, if one reads the final scene as a 1962 dream sequence induced by Susan's drug use, her words may express a valid hope for her future. The title, like this final scene, embodies two possible perceptions of the past and the future: one of plenty and one of lack. Again, Hare leaves this judgment for his readers and audiences to make. The irony afforded by the more pessimistic reading may seem a bit more appealing; however, the two readings play into Hare's use of ambiguity. Despite the reading

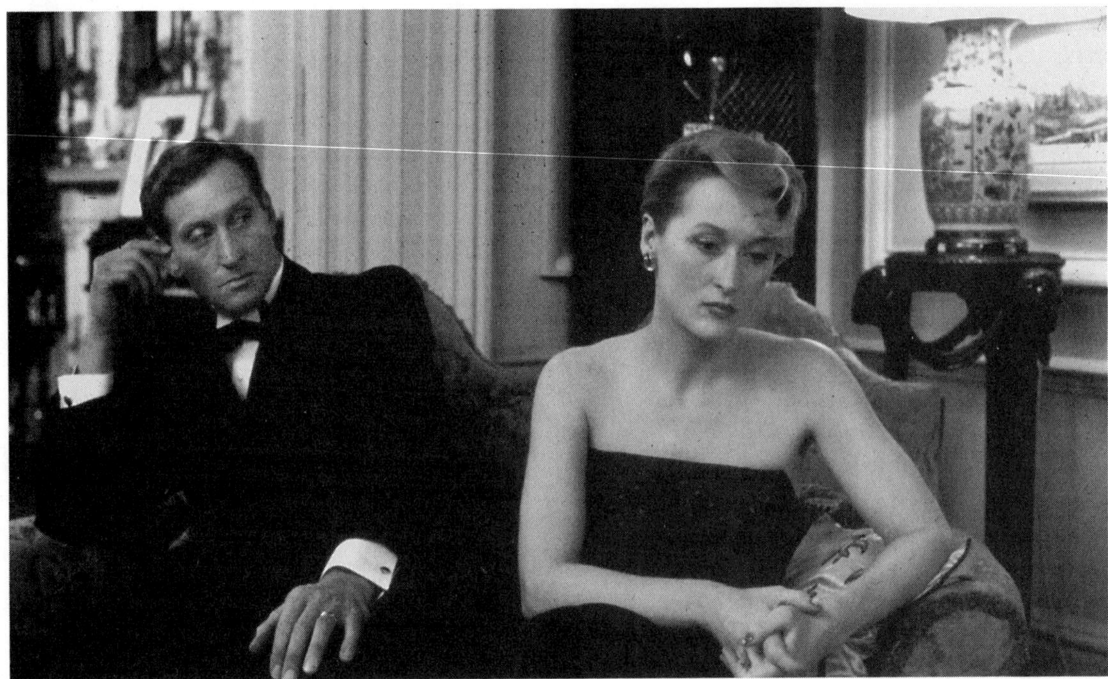

A scene from the 1985 film adaptation: Brock (Charles Dance) regards his unhappy wife, Susan

that each viewer of *Plenty* may choose, the inclusion of options makes Hare's play an exercise in decision-making.

As Colin Ludlow noted in an article for the *London Magazine,* ''the power of his [Hare's] work is to provoke thought and to disturb complacency.'' At the very least, Hare stirs his audience into debate. For this reason, I would argue that the title of ''Empty'' that George Perry suggested in his review of the play for the *Sunday Times* lacks the subtlety required of this wonderfully ambiguous play.

Source: D. L. Kellett, for *Drama for Students,* Gale, 1998.

Bert Cardullo

Cardullo examines the use of staging, particularly the elements of light and sound, as they pertain to the the character of Susan in Hare's work.

In Scenes 2 through 11 of David Hare's *Plenty* (1978), we hear sounds from the dark before the lights come up on the action. Those sounds are of a wireless (Scene 2); a small string orchestra (Scene 3); a string quartet (Scene 4); a brass band (Scene 5); Charlie Parker's saxophone (Scene 6); the music of the English composer Elgar (Scene 7); the voice of a priest (Scene 8); a radio interview (Scene 9); ''some stately orchestral chords: melodic, solemn'' (Scene 10); Elgar's music again (Scene 11). The lights come straight up on the action, without any sounds coming first from the dark, in Scene 1. In Scene 12, music is playing as ''the room [of Scene 11] scatters [and] we see a French hillside in high summer. The stage picture forms piece by piece. Green, yellow, brown. Trees. The fields stretch away. A high sun. A brilliant August day.''

Plenty, in the words of Robert Brustein,

> traces the career of a spirited Englishwoman from her youth as a courier [1943], aiding the French resistance against the Nazis, to her collapse, some fifteen years later [1956], into peacetime disillusionment—paralyzed by anomie, riddled with depression, rotting with despair and psychic rust. Hare's heroine, Susan Traherne, represents a particular example of a general condition, the personification of a hopeful, idealistic generation disaffected by a nation in moral collapse. It is Hare's conviction that World War II represented England's last heroic moment, after which it experienced a series of demoralizing deceptions and compromises, tied to the loss of empire. Ironically, this was a time of relative affluence, an era of peace and plenty.[*New Republic,* November 29, 1982]

The play begins in 1962 as Susan is about to leave her husband, Raymond Brock, whom she later says she married only because he had once been kind to her when she was in trouble (she had shot a man in a quarrel). The play begins, that is, with Susan's disillusionment and despair. We see that disillusionment and despair clearly from the start; there is no anticipatory moment of darkness and sound before Scene 1. There is such an anticipatory moment before Scene 2, and this scene itself is played in only "a small amount of light." Scene 2 is a flashback to Susan's days as a teenaged courier for the Resistance—a time of excitement, danger, mystery, and promise for her. There—we get not only "from the dark the sound of the wireless," but a whole scene played in semi-darkness: darkness is a metaphor, not for death, but for life lived at its highest pitch. Scene 11 is a flash forward to England in 1962, after Susan has left Brock and has been tracked down by Lazar, the parachutist whom she aided in Scene 2 and whom she hasn't seen since the war. Susan and Lazar are spending the night in a Blackpool hotel in a failed attempt to recapture the exhilaration and sense of purpose of 1943. The scene is played in semi-darkness, an ironic reproduction of the lighting of Scene 2.

Scenes 3 through 10 of *Plenty* chronicle Susan's life from 1947 to 1962. She meets Brock after the death in 1947 of Tony, a Resistance worker with whom she was carrying on a casual affair and whose sudden death of a heart attack can be seen as a mercy not afforded those who had to live through England's decline after World War II. She has an unhappy career as an advertising copywriter, where success is "simply a question of pitching my intelligence low enough"; she runs around with a bohemian crowd. Susan attempts to have a child by Mick, a man she barely knows: she wants a child, but not a husband; she likes sex, but she'd rather not know her sex partner very well, if at all. She marries Brock, whom she does not love. She shows signs of a mental imbalance that will never leave her.

Like Scene 2, Scenes 3 through 10 open with an anticipatory moment of darkness and sound; unlike Scene 2, these scenes present an increasingly sad reality exposed by light. Through light and sound, Hare repeats the outline of Susan's experience up to her leaving Brock eight times: the anticipation—the promise of darkness and sound—then the deflation—the disappointment of light and human bodies. Even though the sounds from the dark are usually meant to underline the mood of the scene to come (for instance, the music of a brass band before Susan's brassy request, made at a festival and fireworks site, that Mick father her child), still they have, occurring *before* not during the scene, an existence independent of it, an existence in darkness as pure, tantalizing sound. Scene 12, set in 1944 in newly liberated France, opens in light: even as we saw clearly Susan's disillusionment and despair in Scene 1, we see the past clearly now. We see it without illusions, with the knowledge about Susan and England that the play has given us, knowledge that Susan herself, for all her erratic behavior, achieved. The time is immediately after the liberation, and already the boredom and sluggishness of "peace and plenty" are setting in under a brilliant sun. Thus the "unnaturally gloomy" farmer whom Susan encounters speaks with "extreme disgust" of the ugly stretchmarks he sees on his wife's legs in bed, as if darkness with its attendant invitation or allure has completely deserted them, just as it will desert Susan.

"THROUGH LIGHT AND SOUND, HARE REPEATS THE OUTLINE OF SUSAN'S EXPERIENCE."

Source: Bert Cardullo, "Hare's *Plenty*" in the *Explicator,* Volume 43, no. 2, Winter, 1985, pp. 62–63.

Molly Haskell

Looking at two film versions of Hare's work, critic Haskell praises the author for his creation of strong female leads. She primarily focuses on the film adaptation of Plenty *starring Meryl Streep as Susan Traherne.*

First, Kate Nelligan, beautiful and sardonic as the larger-than-life and eternally dissatisfied heroine of David Hare's play *Plenty* (produced at New York City's Public Theater and transferred to Broadway several seasons ago). Then, Vanessa Redgrave, all natural radiance as a Yorkshire schoolteacher in *Wetherby,* Hare's first venture as filmmaker. And now, in the movie *Plenty,* Meryl Streep giving brilliantly muted and quite different shadings to the character of Susan Traherne. Together, they constitute a three-woman/one-man renaissance of great women's roles.

A male critic I know was so startled at the spectacle of these powerhouse heroines that he began looking for signs of misogyny in Hare. True, Jean Travers (Redgrave) sends her lover to his death . . . in a sense. And Susan Traherne is a man-eating tigress (though where Nelligan spit her men out for breakfast, Streep swallows them sadly). But there's more to it than that. All these women are too large to be contained by a label like misogyny—or veneration, for that matter.

In *Wetherby,* Travers is plagued by memories of the past, in particular the night her young fiancé went off to war . . . and died before he could get there. As her story unfolds in flashbacks (with Redgrave's daughter Joely Richardson playing Jean Travers as a young girl), we realize that she had only to say the word to keep her lover at home. That she didn't was partly, one suspects, because she refused to be responsible for another person's life decision; but more important, she had a duty to herself that marriage would have compromised. In the midst of his deliberately, tantalizingly cryptic narrative, Hare makes it quite clear that the kind of marriage she and her provincial young man were about to make would have ended forever her passionate desire for an education.

An abiding guilt mingled with the tremendous satisfactions of being a really good teacher—that's the life that Redgrave's glowingly attractive middle-aged "spinster" is content to live. Until the disruptive intrusion of a strange young man (Tim McInnerny) who kills himself in her presence, and an equally strange young woman (Suzanna Hamilton) who later appears on the schoolteacher's doorstep, Travers is as richly in tune with herself as she is with the old farmhouse that becomes the stage for unseemly melodrama.

Through the device of a psychological mystery that is never resolved, Hare gives us a richly atmospheric and slyly satirical study of a milieu, and the manners—ultra-British yet casually "country"—that maintain a smooth facade even as the underpinnings are about to crack.

For all its modernist, ellipses, *Wetherby* is a remarkably physical film, both in the sense of place it evokes, and the sensuality of the characters. The attraction between Redgrave and a stumblingly shrewd detective (Stuart Wilson), for example, provides one of the more erotically charged love scenes in recent cinema.

Susan Traherne, the heroine of *Plenty,* Hare's wittily scathing chronicle of postwar England, is also a woman nagged and imprisoned by the past, but in this case the past represents perfection. In France, during a night of lovemaking with a fellow Resistance worker, love and ideals came together. From that moment, life became a disillusioning descent.

In both play and film Traherne is a feverish idealist who, by her own admission, wants to change the world without knowing how. Her life is one long and increasingly reckless diatribe against what she considers the complacency of an England grown fat and conservative with postwar profits. But she is more (and less) than the scourge of the bourgeoisie. Sardonic and strong-minded, she rips apart the surface of life and shreds human beings as she does so. She works at jobs she despises; she takes a lower-class lover in order to get herself an illegitimate, and unconventional, child; she marries, without passion, a man in the diplomatic corps to whom she feels culturally superior. Finally, unable to find a niche or an outlet—and perhaps unable to face the wreckage of her life—she goes mad. Is she, finally, a lonely beacon of emancipation or an angel of destruction? More than a little of both, I should say.

Like Ibsen's Hedda Gabler before her, like Frances Farmer in the recent dramas of her life, she seems to lay claim to a feminist alibi: that of the woman too large and energetic for the options that society gives her. Yet, like Hedda, like Farmer, there is an arrogant, narcissistic fury that drives her to destroy rather than to nurture or create. She is smarter than everyone around her—yet she surrounds herself with people to whom she can condescend. Having done noble work in the Resistance, she dismisses an entire nation with the words, "People back in England seem a little childish."

"Don't you think," another character says to her, "you wear your suffering a little heavily?"

In adapting his own play, David Hare has barely changed a word, yet the whole feeling of the film is different. (The film is directed by Australian Fred Schepisi, who also directed the haunting "The Chant of Jimmie Blacksmith" about a scorned half-breed aborigine turned vengeful murderer of whites.) One of the beauties of the film version is that it takes the destructive side of Traherne's idealism into account without making us hate her. On the contrary, thanks to a more balanced cast and the genuine naivete Streep brings to the part, we like her more. As the diplomat husband, Charles Dance (Guy Perron in Masterpiece Theater's "The Jewel in the Crown") has more sex appeal and authority than Edward Herrmann had. Because Dance's Raymond Brock is clearly not a wimp, our sympathy is with him when he lashes out at Susan, but also with her for marrying him. Tracy Ullman as Susan's free-spirited friend and Sting as her anointed lover (both British rock stars turned actors) are sparkling, active presences that underline her own frustrated inertia.

These subsidiary characters, in raising all the objections that we feel and that Nelligan's dominance suppressed in the play, free us to sympathize more often with Susan Traherne, and feel her vulnerability. Nelligan, always in control, seemed too ironic, too shrewd, too blisteringly aware not to perceive the gap between her ideals and her actions. Streep, however, in her scenes with such elegant exemplars of tradition as John Gielgud as a British ambassador and Ian McKellen as a foreign service executive, seems more of a well-meaning innocent.

Under Schepisi's sometimes laborious direction—endless travelogue shots of the Dordogne and quaint French village life during the war—*Plenty* takes a while to get going. The phony, picture-postcard atmosphere of the early scenes infects Streep's performance. She seems forever out of place. But this quality of alienation suits her well as she matures, and grows ever more isolated from the people around her. Whether catatonic or lashing out in fury, she is tremendous in the bitterness and craziness of the later scenes. What makes these passages so moving is that Streep has managed to keep before us the shadow of the young woman Susan once was, who believed she could change the world. In a searing, deeply troubling yet exhilarating performance, Streep universalizes Susan. She challenges us to remember our own lost ideals, and to wonder if the world is any readier to receive the goadings of a fiercely independent woman.

Source: Molly Haskell, ''A One-Man Revival of Great Women's Roles'' in *Ms.*, Volume XIV, no. 4, October, 1985, pp. 19–20.

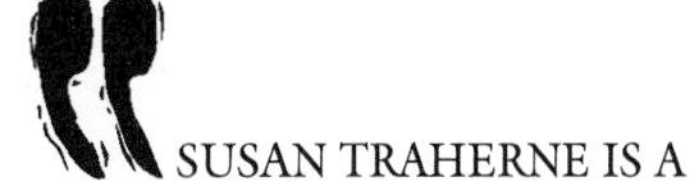

SUSAN TRAHERNE IS A WOMAN NAGGED AND IMPRISONED BY THE PAST, BUT IN THIS CASE THE PAST REPRESENTS PERFECTION.''

SOURCES

Craig, Sandy, Editor. *Dreams and Deconstructions: Alternative Theatre in Britain,* Amber Lane Press, 1980.

Economist, January 3, 1998, p. 52.

Gussow, Mel. Review of *Plenty* in the *New York Times Magazine,* September 29, 1985.

Hare, David. ''Note on Performance'' in *Plenty,* New American Library, 1983.

Hare, David. Introduction to *The History Plays,* Faber, 1978, p. 16.

Hile, Kevin S. ''David Hare'' in *Contemporary Authors, New Revision Series,* Vol. 39, Gale, 1992.

Levin, Bernard. Review of *Plenty* in the *Sunday Times,* April 16, 1978, pp. 37.

Ludlow, Colin. Review of *Plenty* in *London Magazine,* July, 1978, p. 78.

Marwick, Arthur. *British Society since 1945,* Penguin, 1982.

Millar, Gavin. ''The Habit of Lying'' in *Sight and Sound,* Autumn, 1985, p. 299.

Perry, George. ''Plenty of Nothing'' in the *Sunday Times,* November 24, 1985.

Sommer, Doris. ''Resisting the Heat: Mench, Morrison, and Incompetent Readers'' in *Cultures of United States Imperialism,* edited by Amy Kaplan and Donald E. Pense, Duke University Press, 1993, pp. 407-32.

Whitehead, Ted. ''North of the Suez'' in the *Spectator,* April 22, 1978, p. 26.

FURTHER READING

Bull, John. *New British Political Dramatists: Howard Brenton, David Hare, Trevor Griffiths, and David Edgar,* Macmillan, 1984.

This work explores Hare as well as other modern English playwrights. It dedicates a thorough, in-depth chapter to Hare and his work.

Childs, David. *Britain since 1945: A Political History,* Methuen, 1986.

Childs details post-World War II political issues up through 1985. The book focuses on domestic as well as foreign affairs.

Dean, Joan Fitzpatrick. *David Hare,* edited by Kinley E. Roby, Twayne, 1990.

This work offers information on the critical reception, themes, imagery, sources, settings and contexts of Hare's works.

Homden, Carol. *The Plays of David Hare,* Cambridge University Press, 1995.

Homden's work is a comprehensive resource about Hare's works and includes commentary about his 1993 trilogy which includes *Racing Demon, Murmuring Judges,* and *The Absence of War.*

Oliva, Judy Lee. *David Hare: Theatricalizing Politics,* UMI Research Press, 1990.

Oliva's work provides another comprehensive review of Hare's works and includes an interview with him from 1989. The appendix lists the sources for critical reviews of Hare's work.

Trussler, Simon, General Editor and Malcom Page, Compiler and Associate Editor. *File on Hare,* Methuen Drama, 1990.

This helpful short book provides summaries of many of Hare's works as well as quotations from Hare, his actors, and his critics about the works. The text includes nine pages about *Plenty* and additional bibliographic suggestions.

School for Scandal

RICHARD BRINSLEY SHERIDAN

1777

School for Scandal opened at the Drury Lane Theatre in London, England, in May of 1777. It was an enormous success. Reviews heralded the play as a ''real comedy'' that would supplant the sentimental dramas that had filled the stage in the previous years. While wildly popular in the eighteenth century, the play has not been as successful with contemporary audiences.

One significant problem is the anti-Semitism that runs throughout the play. Post-World War II audiences are understandably sensitive to the disparaging remarks made about moneylenders, who were often Jewish. That the character of Moses is portrayed as honest and concerned is depicted in the play as an aberration. When Sir Oliver is learning how to disguise himself as a moneylender, he is told that he must ask 100% interest because it is expected that he must behave as an ''unconscionable dog.''

But anti-Semitism is not the only problem with modern staging. By current standards, the play appears artificial in the characters' speech, dress, and motivations. A comedy about manners is not as interesting to twentieth century audiences because manners and the rules of society are far more permissive and wide-ranging than they were in the 1700s. When *School for Scandal* was revived on the London stage in 1990, the director stated that another problem with staging was the lack of any one strong character to drive the play.

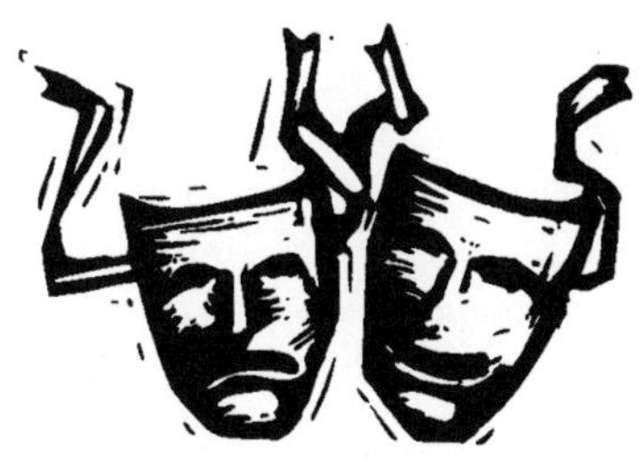

Perceptions regarding the nature of drama also play into contemporary perceptions of Sheridan's work. Peter Woods, who directed the 1990 revival, stated in an interview in *Sheridan Studies,* that "today's audience supposes itself to be watching ART. Sheridan's audience was looking at the funnies." Woods believed that audiences taking themselves and historical plays too seriously are what prevents Sheridan's comedy from being as successful today. Nevertheless, *School for Scandal* remains a standard for comedies of manner and is considered Sheridan's defining work.

AUTHOR BIOGRAPHY

Richard Brinsley Sheridan was born in Dublin, Ireland, and was christened on November 4, 1751. His father was an actor and author, a path that Sheridan himself would choose for his vocation. He was educated at Harrow School in London, England. After the family moved to Bath in 1770, Sheridan met and eloped with a young singer, Eliza Linley. Their marriage contract was invalid due to a lack of parental consent, however. Sheridan fought two duels on her behalf, nearly dying in the second, and finally, after three years, the couple's families withdrew their opposition and the pair were legally married in 1773.

Sheridan had begun to study the law the year before, and, in 1773, he entered as a barrister in the Middle Temple. When the law failed to provide him with adequate financial means, Sheridan turned his attention to writing drama. His first play, *The Rivals* was completed in a few weeks and opened in 1775 at the Covent Garden Theatre. The production closed the same day; Sheridan revised the work, shortening the structure and recasting his actors. The play reopened to great success only ten days later. A few months later his second work, *St. Patrick's Day,* opened. Sheridan next collaborated on an operatic play, *The Duenna,* with his father-in-law. Both of these works were popular with audiences.

After writing and producing three successful plays in 1775, Sheridan and some partners bought the Drury Lane Theatre in 1776, and he became its manager. In 1777, his play *A Trip to Scarborough* was presented at the Drury Lane, and, three months later, *School For Scandal* became his most popular play. In 1779, Sheridan became the sole owner of the theatre, and his last play for another twenty years, *The Critic,* opened to the same success as his earlier works.

Despite critical and popular success, Sheridan had accumulated a huge amount of debt. On the surface, he appeared a success. By his late twenties he was the owner of the most famous theatre in England and was a well-known, successful playwright, yet his finances were in ruins.

In 1780, Sheridan was elected to Parliament. By all reports, Sheridan was a brilliant orator, but he never achieved the kind of success he desired, due in part to British prejudices against his Irish birth. Sheridan's wife died in 1792; she had left him years earlier because of his drinking and infidelity. The same year, the Drury Lane Theatre was condemned and torn down. Sheridan went even further into debt but managed to rebuild the theatre. Three years after his wife's death, he married Hester Jane Ogle, the nineteen-year-old daughter of the Dean of Winchester. Sheridan wrote his last play, *Pizarro,* in 1799. The income from this last successful production only slightly reduced his mountain of debt. Finally, Sheridan was ousted from Drury Lane's management due to his mishandling of funds. When he lost his Parliament seat, he also lost protection against arrest for his debts. Sheridan was imprisoned several times for failure to pay his debts; his furniture was sold, and he was living in filth at the time of his death in 1816. Although he died in financial ruin and ignominy, the work that he produced for the stage in the years 1773-1779 earned Sheridan a place among the great writers of drama.

PLOT SUMMARY

Act I

School for Scandal opens with Lady Sneerwell and her henchman Snake plotting a means to break up the romance between Charles Surface and Maria. It is Snake's job to assist in disseminating the gossip that Lady Sneerwell creates, and when he asks why she wishes to destroy this romance, Lady Sneerwell reveals that she wants Charles for herself. Maria's hand would then go to Charles's brother, Joseph.

In the first act, the audience is introduced to the characters who surround Lady Sneerwell and their true nature is revealed. Gossip and slander fill their time; they consider the destruction of marriages and reputations as entertainment.

Maria is the exception in this group. She condemns their gossip and refuses to be persuaded that Charles is unworthy of her. Sir Peter and his servant, Rowley, arrive on stage at the change of scene. Sir Peter is openly questioning his wisdom in marrying such a young wife. He thought that by marrying an innocent country girl, his happiness would be assured. Instead, Sir Peter reveals to the audience that his wife spends too much time with her friends and too much money on dresses and extravagances. Rowley tells Sir Peter that Charles and Joseph's uncle, Sir Oliver, is returning to London after a long absence. The audience also learns that it is Rowley's opinion that Charles has more potential than Sir Peter recognizes.

Act II

The second act opens with an argument between Sir Peter and his wife, Lady Teazle, about the money she is spending. He focuses on her extravagant purchase of fresh flowers during the winter. She is not intimidated by his anger. When her husband reminds her of how he rescued her from a simple but poor life, Lady Teazle nearly admits that she would wish her husband dead as his next step toward rescuing her.

In the next scene, the gossips are busy slandering everyone they know as they prepare for a card game at Lady Sneerwell's. Lady Teazle joins them and in a few moments is joined by her husband. Maria is also there and is joined by Joseph who presses his suit for her attention. She is clearly annoyed and pleads with him to change the subject.

In the following scene, Sir Oliver has returned and is briefed by Rowley and Sir Peter regarding his nephews, Joseph and Charles. Rowley and Sir Peter differ in their appreciation of the two young men. Sir Oliver is determined to investigate and decide the nature of his nephews for himself.

Act III

Rowley, Sir Peter, and Sir Oliver are joined by the moneylender, Moses. Moses will take Sir Oliver to meet Charles under the guise of a moneylender, Mr. Premium. Moses coaches Sir Oliver in the behavior and manners of a moneylender, and the two depart for Charles's home. When Maria enters, Sir Peter takes the opportunity to chastise her for her rejection of Joseph, but Maria stands her ground, proclaiming her love for Charles.

The scene ends with a humorous exchange between Sir Peter and his wife. Although the two begin lovingly enough, the compliments soon turn to an argument as the two each claim that the other one is always at fault for their constant quarreling.

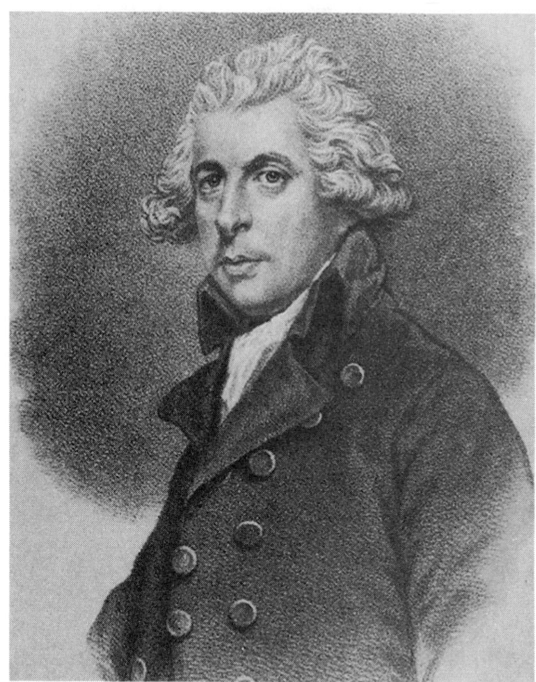

Richard Brinsley Sheridan

In the next scene, Moses and the disguised Sir Oliver arrive at Charles's home. Charles is happily at play gambling, singing, and drinking with his friends, but he is delighted to be visited by the moneylender, since Charles needs cash quite badly. Charles agrees to sell the family portraits to raise money. It is agreed that he will make a game of an auction to sell the pictures to Mr. Premium.

Act IV

During the auction, Sir Oliver buys all the portraits except his own, which Charles will not sell. He has a fondness for his uncle whom he has not seen in many years and refuses to part with the portrait. Sir Oliver is charmed and forgives Charles his faults. While still disguised, Sir Oliver gives Charles far more money than the agreed upon price and leaves with Moses. Charles immediately sends some of the money to a poor relation.

In the next scene, Lady Teazle has called upon Joseph. He has been attempting to seduce her, and, although she has resisted thus far, she has come to Joseph's home because she is tempted. When her husband is announced, Lady Teazle hides behind a

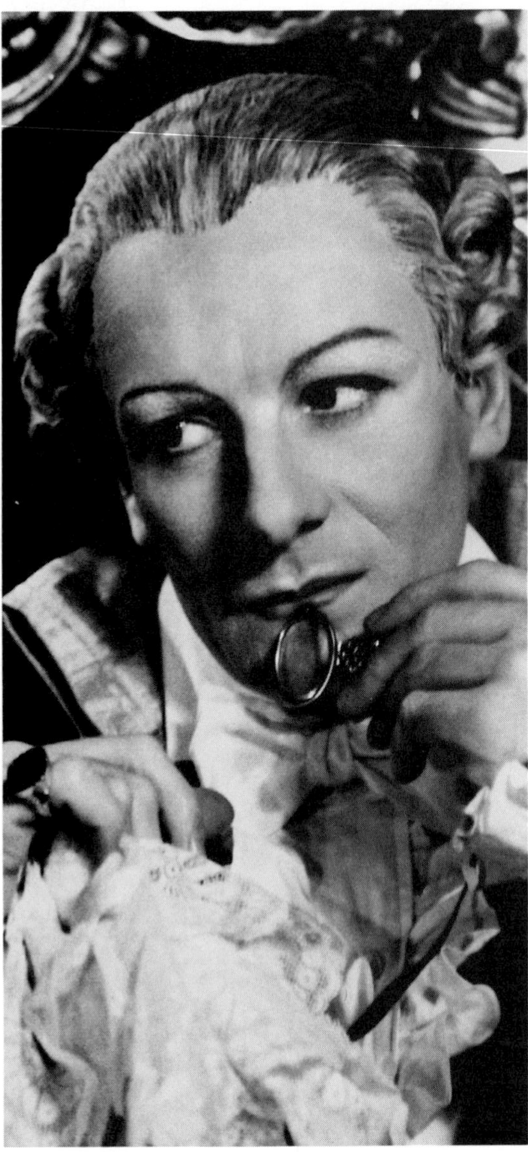

John Gielgud as Joseph Surface in a 1937 production staged at London's Queen Theatre

screen. Sir Peter has arrived to ask Joseph if his brother, Charles, is having an affair with Lady Teazle. Joseph is taken aback by the suggestion, and although he hedges a bit, finally states that he cannot think Charles guilty of such a thing.

At that moment Charles is announced, and Sir Peter asks to hide so that he might overhear Joseph ask Charles about Lady Teazle. When Sir Peter goes to hide behind the screen that conceals his wife, Joseph tells Sir Peter that his arrival had interrupted a rendezvous with a French milliner and the young woman is hiding behind the screen. Sir Peter hides in a closet just as Charles is ushered into the room.

In a few moments Joseph learns that Lady Sneerwell is arriving, and he leaves the room. Sir Peter, having heard Charles profess that he has no interest in Lady Teazle, reveals himself. When Charles pronounces Joseph too worried about his reputation to risk scandal, Sir Peter knocks down the screen, thinking that he will reveal a French milliner. Instead, his own wife is revealed hiding behind it.

Joseph rushes back into the room and attempts to create a story to explain everything. But Lady Teazle, who has overheard her husband's plans to honor her, is ashamed of her near betrayal and confesses everything to Sir Peter. Sir Peter declares Joseph a villain. The act ends.

Act V

Sir Oliver, unaware of the recent activities, arrives at Joseph's disguised as a poor relation. He asks Joseph for help but is turned quickly away. Rowley returns to tell Joseph that his Uncle, Sir Oliver, has returned to London and wishes to meet with both brothers.

The next scene opens with all of the gossips clamoring for more information about what really occurred between Sir Peter and his wife and Joseph. In a matter of moments, they have concocted a duel and a near fatal injury for the participants. They are interrupted when Sir Peter arrives and throws his wife's former friends outside. Lady Teazle resigns from the scandal club. In the library of Joseph's house, Sir Oliver arrives. Charles and Joseph recognize him from the disguised identities he assumed. Sir Oliver's true identity is revealed, but at that moment, Lady Sneerwell arrives for one last try at breaking up Maria and Charles.

Sneerwell fails when it is revealed that Snake has betrayed her to someone who would pay him a higher price. She leaves. Joseph follows her after it is made clear that everyone present now recognizes his hypocrisy. Sir Oliver and Sir Peter confer their blessings upon Maria and Charles.

CHARACTERS

Sir Benjamin Backbite

Backbite is a suitor to Marie. He is a gossip who will slander anyone, even those he does not know.

Lady Sneerwell admires Backbite's wit and poetry. Backbite is an especially malicious character whose rude behavior is encouraged in the company of his uncle, Lady Sneerwell, and Mrs. Candour.

Sir Harry Bumper

Toby is one of Charles's friends who spends his time drinking, gambling, and singing.

Mrs. Candour

Mrs. Candour is a good-natured and friendly gossip whose talkative nature makes her dangerous, since she spreads slander more effectively than Backbite or Crabtree.

Careless

Careless is one of Charles's friends. He plays auctioneer when the family pictures are sold to Mr. Premium.

Crabtree

Crabtree is Backbite's uncle and as big a gossip as his nephew.

Maria

Maria is Sir Peter's wealthy ward. She is in love with Charles and he is in love with her. Her nature is sweet, and she is very disturbed at the vicious gossip she encounters at social functions. Although Maria is considered a principle character, she has only a small role in the play.

Moses

Moses is the moneylender who has been lending money to Charles. He has tried to help Charles with his money problems and bring his spending under control. Moses is honest and helps Sir Oliver in his pretense as a moneylender.

Old Stanley

See Sir Oliver Surface

Mr. Premium

See Sir Oliver Surface

Rowley

Rowley is Sir Peter's servant and was formally a steward to Joseph and Charles's father. He recognizes that Charles is kind-hearted and good in spite of his problems managing money. Rowley has caught Snake at forgery and uses the information to force Snake to betray Mrs. Sneerwell. Rowley serves as go-between for Sir Oliver when he disguises himself to visit his nephews.

Snake

Snake works for Lady Sneerwell; he undertakes the actions that destroy reputations. He is indeed a snake, since his job is to slither around gaining and dispensing gossip. Snake willingly goes to the highest bidder and in the final scene admits that Rowley has paid him a greater fee to betray Lady Sneerwell.

Lady Sneerwell

Lady Sneerwell was the target of slander in her youth. She now directs her efforts at ruining the reputations of other women. She prides herself on her delicacy of scandal, which she manages with only a hint of a sneer (she "sneers well"). Slander is her primary source of pleasure. Lady Sneerwell is secretly infatuated with Charles, and that is the real reason she wants to break up his relationship with Maria. Lady Sneerwell plots with Joseph to secure Charles for herself and Maria for Joseph, but the plot blows up when Joseph is exposed to Sir Peter and when Maria refuses to consider Joseph as a suitor. She forges letters in a final attempt to further her plot but is revealed when her partner, Snake, sells his loyalty to a higher bidder.

Charles Surface

Charles is the protagonist of the play and the younger Surface brother. He is extravagant but good-natured. He is in love with Maria and wishes to marry her. Mrs. Sneerwell, however, wants him for herself. Charles sells his uncle, who is in dis-

MEDIA ADAPTATIONS

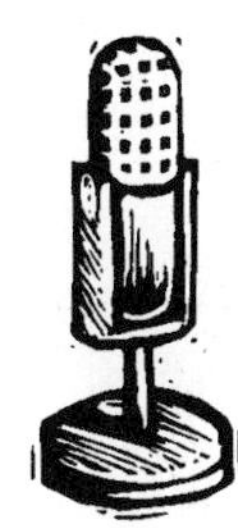

- *School for Scandal* was videotaped in 1965. The 100 minute-long black and white film, taped during a stage performance of the play, stars Joan Plowright and Felix Aylmer. The Hal Burton production is available from Video Yesteryear.

guise, the family portraits, since he, as usual, needs money. He wins his old uncle's heart when he refuses to sell his beloved uncle's portrait. Sir Oliver finds that Charles is honest and generous. In the final scene, Charles and Maria receive the endorsement and good wishes of her guardian, Sir Peter, and that of Sir Oliver.

Joseph Surface

The elder Surface brother, Joseph is amiable and well regarded. But he is a hypocrite, since he is courting the wealthy Maria behind his brother's back while also flirting with Lady Sneerwell and trying to seduce Mrs. Teazle. When Joseph refuses to help his disguised uncle, his true nature is revealed. He is artful, selfish, and malicious, but he has Sir Peter completely convinced of his merit and good name until Lady Teazle tells her husband that Joseph has attempted to seduce her. Joseph lacks the qualities of truth, gratitude, and charity.

Sir Oliver Surface

Sir Oliver is Charles and Joseph's rich uncle. He returns to England and attempts to test his nephews' character without revealing his identity. Sir Oliver assumes the identity of a moneylender, Mr. Premium, to test Charles's loyalty. Later, he assumes the identity of Old Stanley, a poor relation, to test Joseph. In the final scene he reveals his true identity to both brothers, and Joseph is disinherited while Charles is rewarded by his uncle for his honesty and generosity.

Lady Teazle

Lady Teazle is young and was educated in the country. But since her marriage and move to London, she has learned to dress well and to spend lavishly. She counts Lady Sneerwell among her friends and engages in flirtations with young men. She fights frequently with her husband, contradicts him, and flaunts his authority, but he continues to love her. When Lady Teazle engages in gossip with her friends, there is a noticeable meanness in her words. Yet her country upbringing makes her hesitate when she considers engaging in an affair with Joseph. When Lady Teazle overhears her husband's plan to settle an income on her, she realizes that he does love her and she quickly comes to her senses. She reveals to Sir Peter Joseph's attempts to seduce her. In the final scene, she resigns from the company of gossips and reaffirms her devotion to her husband.

Sir Peter Teazle

A neighbor of Lady Sneerwell, Sir Peter is also the guardian of Joseph and Charles Surface. Sir Peter was an older bachelor when he married his much younger wife six months before the start of the play. She is making his life miserable with her extravagances and her friends. But he loves his wife, although his friends sneer at him for letting her take advantage of him. Although Sir Peter has always favored Joseph (he even suspects Charles of trying to seduce Lady Teazle), Joseph's hypocritical nature is revealed when Lady Teazle confesses to her husband that Joseph was attempting to seduce her. Eventually, Sir Peter approves of the marriage of his ward, Maria, to Charles.

Toby

See Sir Harry Bumper

Trip

Trip is Charles's footman. He also needs to borrow money and seeks out the moneylenders when they come to see Charles.

THEMES

Honor

Initially honor seems to be in short supply in *School for Scandal:* The gossips are completely without honor; Lady Teazle is considering abandoning the lessons about honor that she learned growing up in the country; Joseph is ready to betray his brother to secure a wealthy wife; and Charles is hopelessly in debt to moneylenders. Even Sir Oliver, whose honor should be above question, is ready to assume a disguise to test his nephews' honor.

By the conclusion of the play, however, it is clear that only the gossips have no true honor. Lady Teazle realizes that she values her husband and that she has more honor than her friends had supposed. Charles, though foolish and intemperate with gambling and money, is honorable. He pays his debts, if slowly, and he is willing to help a poor relation without being asked. Sir Oliver's deception unmasks Joseph's hypocrisy. And the moneylender, Moses, is a man of so much honor that he assists Charles in managing his debts.

Morality

Sheridan asks his audience to question the morality of society in this play. Slandering one's

TOPICS FOR FURTHER STUDY

- Sheridan is a male writer who writes about marriage and women in *School for Scandal.* Research the role of women in London society. Do you think that Sheridan accurately portrays women? Is the marriage depicted in this play an accurate reflection of marriage in the late-eighteenth century?
- Sheridan's biography indicates that he made a lot of money from writing plays. Investigate playwriting and other theatre work as money-making ventures. How successful financially was acting? Or the writing of plays? Or owning a theatre?
- *School for Scandal* focuses on gossip and slander as a social disease. How serious a problem was slander in London society? In your research did you find that Sheridan was using slander as a symptom of a more serious social issue?
- The eighteenth century was a period during which the line between poverty and wealth became even more pronounced in England. Because of enclosure laws, more people, who had formerly made an adequate living in the country, were forced to move to London to look for employment. At the same time, gin bars proliferated, and public drunkenness became a serious problem. High unemployment and public drunkenness combined to created some serious issues in London. Research the effects of these two events. What new issues were created?
- Sheridan was one of the last playwrights to write a "comedy of manners." This genre of comedy became very popular after the Restoration but was waning when Sheridan began to write. Explore this genre and discuss the conventions that define a comedy of manners.

neighbors, acquaintances, and friends is an entertainment. There is no real interest in the truth—and even less consideration is given to the damage that such gossip causes.

In the early acts of *School for Scandal,* the subjects of such gossip are not known to the audience, who cannot determine the truth of Lady Sneerwell and Mrs. Candour's observations. But by the last act, it becomes clear that these gossips need absolutely no element of truth to fuel their stories. The felling of the screen in Joseph's library—and the confrontation that took place immediately after—are fresh in the audience's mind. This earlier scene serves as a nice contrast to the speculation and innuendo that engages the gossips. Although it is all comedy, it is comedy that teaches a lesson to the audience.

Sentiment

School for Scandal is generally regarded as a refutation of the sentimental drama that was prevalent on the London stage prior to and during Sheridan's era. Sentiment was much admired as a replacement for the debauchery of Restoration comedy, but it often proved bland and boring. Often the protagonists were pure to the point of generic blandness. In Sheridan's play, Joseph Surface is much admired for his sentiment. Conversely, his brother Charles is chastised because he is not the man of sentiment that his brother is: "He is a man of sentiment . . . there is nothing in the world so noble as a man of sentiment." That Joseph is really not at all noble or admirable makes Sir Peter's compliment more damning and more a mockery of this eighteenth-century convention.

Truth and Falsehood

Trying to determine the truth occupies much of Sheridan's play. Lady Sneerwell and Snake are engaged in deception and falsehood, and Joseph is willing to bend the truth to get what he wants. When Sir Oliver, disguised as old Stanley, approaches Joseph to ask for money, Joseph easily lies that he has no money. He even blames his brother, Charles, stating that Charles's free-spending has left Joseph without funds. Of course the gossips have no interest in the truth; their goal is to entertain one another with wild speculation. When compared to such exciting exaggerations as theirs, reality—and the truth—is boring.

Wealth

This is certainly a play about wealth. The poor in London were much too busy trying to find shelter and food to engage in such idle distractions as gossip or gaming. Wealth really sets the characters in this play apart from the rest of society. For instance, Sir Peter complains that his wife spends too much on silk dresses and fresh out-of-season flowers. Charles spends his money gaming and drinking with his friends, and the moneylenders are on their way to being wealthy, thanks to idle young men such as Charles. Maria is the object of Joseph's plotting only because she is wealthy, and Sir Oliver is primarily interested in the morals of his nephews because he plans to leave them him wealth.

STYLE

Act

A major division in a drama. In Greek plays the sections of the drama signified by the appearance of the chorus were usually divided into five acts. This is the formula for most serious drama from the Greeks to the Romans and to Elizabethan playwrights like William Shakespeare. The five acts denote the structure of dramatic action. They are exposition, complication, climax, falling action, and catastrophe. The five act structure was followed until the nineteenth century when Henrik Ibsen (*A Doll's House*) revolutionized dramatic structure by combining elements into fewer acts.

School for Scandal is a five act play. The exposition occurs in the first act when the audience learns of Lady Sneerwell and Joseph's plan to break up the romance between Charles and Maria; the audience also meets the gossips. By the end of Act II, the complication, the audience has met Sir Oliver and knows that he plans to test his nephews' morality. The climax occurs in the third act when Charles meets his uncle disguised as a moneylender and agrees to sell him the family portraits.

The conflict between Maria and her guardian, Sir Peter, is revealed when she refuses his request to allow Joseph to court her. There are several near misses as a series of visits, Lady Teazle and her husband, Charles, and Lady Sneerwell all arrive at Joseph's. As Lady Teazle and her husband each hide in separate areas and each peek to see what is occurring, the screen finally provides the falling action, and the catastrophe occurs in the last act when Sir Oliver's arrival restores order and Sir Peter is reconciled with Maria and Charles.

Plot

This term refers to the pattern of events. Generally plots should have a beginning, a middle, and a conclusion, but they may also be a series of episodes connected together. Basically, the plot provides the author with the means to explore primary themes. Students are often confused by the two terms; but themes explore ideas and plots simply relate what happens in a very obvious manner.

Thus the plot of *School for Scandal* is the story of how Joseph and Lady Sneerwell each try to lie their way to getting what they want, while its parallel plot is how Sir Oliver attempts to discover the truth about his nephews. But the themes are those of falsehood (in the form of malicious gossip), honesty, true love, and a rejection of sentiment as a virtue.

Setting

The time, place, and culture in which the action of the play takes place is called the setting. The elements of setting may include geographic location, physical or mental environments, prevailing cultural attitudes, or the historical time in which the action takes place. The location for Sheridan's play is London during the eighteenth century—more specifically, it is set in London's richer quarters. No exact time markers are provided, but the action takes place during a short period of time.

Character

A person in a dramatic work. The actions of each character are what constitute the story. Character can also include the idea of a particular individual's morality. Characters can range from simple stereotypical figures to more complex multi-faceted ones. Characters may also be defined by personality traits, such as the rogue or the damsel in distress. ''Characterization'' is the process of creating a lifelike person from an author's imagination. To accomplish this the author provides the character with personality traits that help define who he will be and how he will behave in a given situation.

School for Scandal provides two types of characters. There are traditional heroes and villains and a vulnerable young woman. But some characters are also defined by his or her name. Lady Sneerwell clearly does a good job of sneering contemptuously at everyone else. And Backbiter lives up to his name as well. Charles and Joseph's natures are revealed in their surname, Surface, indicating that they are somewhat superficial characters interested in appearances.

Genre

Genres are a way of categorizing literature. Genre is a French term that means "kind" or "type." Genre can refer to both the category of literature such as tragedy, comedy, epic, poetry, or pastoral. It can also include modern forms of literature such as drama novels or short stories. This term can also refer to types of literature such as mystery, science fiction, comedy, or romance.

School for Scandal is most frequently classified as a comedy of manners, although it has also been accurately described as social satire and anti-sentimental drama.

Comedy of Manners

"Comedy of manners" is a term applied to a type of play that provides a depiction of the very artificial manners and conventions of society. Characters are usually types and not individuals. Their names reflect their "type." The dialogue in these plays is witty and is of more interest to the audience than the plot, which serves more as an excuse to deliver humorous lines. The comedy of manners is associated most closely with the Restoration of the late-seventeenth century. But the illicit love affairs and lack of morality that defined the genre eventually resulted in their disappearing from the stage. Sheridan revived this genre in the late eighteenth century.

Satire

Satire attempts to blend social commentary with comedy and humor. Satire does not usually attack any individual but rather the institution he or she represents. The intent is to expose problems and create debate that will lead to a correction of the problem. In *School for Scandal,* Sheridan satirizes a society that is so shallow that gossip and slander—and the destruction of a reputation—are forms of entertainment.

HISTORICAL CONTEXT

Sheridan's England was a very different one than that of earlier British playwrights. The mid-seventeenth century had brought the German House of Hanover to the English throne. The first two King Georges spoke little English and had no interest in patronizing the arts. Royal patronage, which had supported so many writers in the past, ended. By the time George III became king in 1760, England was more concerned with colonization and reform than with supporting the arts.

While the British were cementing their control over Canada and India, the American colonists were proving themselves restless with Britain's rule. England had always seen itself as a military power; when the discontent in the colonies developed into the American Revolutionary War, which the British ultimately lost, George III took the news badly. But George III, who had always been popular with his subjects, was ill and at the mercy of his son who constantly plotted to seize the throne.

At the same time, the industrialization of England had resulted in an even sharper division between classes. Industrialization brought a great deal of wealth to England but little of it found its way to the working class or the poor. What the poor had, instead, was even less than before. With the Enclosure Act, the lower class were shifted from the country, losing a simple existence that permitted them to grow some of their food and trade for their needs.

With no where else to go, these displaced people moved into London. There was little shelter and even fewer jobs to greet them. But there was cheap gin, and public drunkenness became a serious problem. But there were also public executions to entertain the poor and prisons for those who could not pay their debts. For those with money, there was tobacco and opium. There were coffeehouses, where tea was served more frequently than coffee, and men met there to drink and talk and read the newspapers.

Women were usually excluded from these social activities, but they did make attempts at social integration and suffrage (the right to vote). Gambling was a proper occupation for gentlemen, as was the visiting of brothels. While paying a prostitute for sex or having a mistress was acceptable for men, the same behavior was not permitted for women.

COMPARE & CONTRAST

- **1777:** The Continental Congress votes to accept the services of the Marquis de Lafayette, who will command a division during the American Revolutionary War. Lafayette will assist the American Colonies, although he has been forbidden to do so by the king of France, Louis XVI. The French have secretly been supporting the American war effort for nearly two years.

  Today: The United States regards England as one of its closest allies and strongest supporters. The two countries frequently support one another in economic, military, and cultural efforts.

- **1777:** The victory at Saratoga is a turning point for the Revolutionary War. For the first time, the English realize that they can not beat the Americans. Parliament asks George III to back down and end the war. He refuses to consider the option.

  Today: The monarchy of England has little political power and could neither declare war nor sustain one in opposition to parliament.

- **1777:** Wolfgang Amadeus Mozart is composing music and his Concert No. 9 for Pianoforte and Orchestra in E flat major debuts in Salzburg. Europe remains a center for great music, with London better known for its theatre than its musical composers.

  Today: England has been an important force in popular music since the 1960s, delivering such influential groups as the Beatles, the Rolling Stones, and Led Zeppelin.

- **1777:** Disease is a major threat to living a long life. Ailments such as tuberculosis cripple and kill many people. George Washington obtains approval to have his troops inoculated against smallpox.

  Today: Advancements in medical technology have resulted in treatments, preventions, or cures for such diseases as tuberculosis and polio. Smallpox is considered to be completely eradicated, and vaccination is no longer required.

Ladies of the eighteenth century were to be chaste and early marriage was encouraged to ensure this; girls could wed at twelve years-of-age. Still, no such high standard interfered with men's behavior.

By the last half of the eighteenth century, drama had almost disappeared from the theatre. There were many great actors, but few playwrights were creating memorable work. There was little incentive for good writing. The playwright collected only the third, sixth, and sometimes (if the play lasted), ninth nights' profits. Theatre owners and actors, however, made a great deal of money. Still, theatre flourished, and several of London's more notable drama houses (including Sheridan's own Drury Lane Theatre) were established in the 1700s.

Surrounding the theatres were brothels, and this reflected the dual nature of the city. London was a complex city, and, in many ways, it reflected the chaos of the royal family. There were huge stores that imported the finest objects from around the world, and the city was crowded with artisans and street singers. The municipality tried to keep the streets cleaned and sewers were being built. But coal dust turned the buildings black and covered everything in its path. And on the edge of all this civility the slums existed. Sewage was dumped into the river Thames, and the poor made use with outside privies and slept in the doorways. Whole families shared one room—if they could afford it.

The city overflowed with life and vitality, but there were two distinct worlds present. One of the rigidly defined life of society, where social convention ruled behavior. This is the world of Sheridan's *School for Scandal.* The other world lay just outside the theatre's doors. Those dark, depressed, and often twisted lives would not be the subject of plays until the next century.

CRITICAL OVERVIEW

School for Scandal opened in May 1777 to enthusiastic audiences. Since it appeared at the end of the London theatre season, it played only twenty performances before the season closed, but Sheridan's play reappeared the following season for an additional forty-five performances. Since few plays enjoyed runs of more than fifteen performances, *School for Scandal* was, by prevailing standards, a success.

In the *Dictionary of Literary Biography,* Mark S. Auburn notéd that "the play engendered wildly enthusiastic support. Passing by the outer walls of Drury Lane just as the famous screen fell and the audience exploded in laughter and applause, a journalist of that day claimed to have run for his life in fear that the building was collapsing."

The reason for the play's success, stated Auburn, is "the witty repartee of fashionable society, the Cain-and-Abel motif, and the delightful recitation of the May-and-December theme." Richard C. Taylor, writing in *Sheridan Studies,* noted a different reason for the play's success. Taylor stated that critics overlooked the play's faults because they "recognized the topicality of Sheridan's moral concern and that Sheridan was targeting hypocrisy." Still, both Auburn and Taylor felt that *School for Scandal* was very popular with audiences and with reviewers. The audience appreciated the plot, especially since gossip had become an important feature in newspapers of the time (a foreshadowing of the gossip-frenzy that dominates many forms of multimedia information in the twentieth century).

But besides plot, Sheridan himself had ensured the play's success by opening it after a popular revival of William Congreve's comedies at Drury Lane. Sheridan eliminated some of the more offensive sexuality, and Congreve's work, which had been unpopular in recent years, received generally good reviews. When Sheridan opened *School for Scandal* immediately after showcasing three of Congreve's comedies, the critics quickly drew comparisons between the two dramatists. Suddenly Sheridan was the new comedic playwright of his generation, just as Congreve had been in his era.

Several critics, who made the intended connection between Congreve and Sheridan, pronounced Sheridan's work the superior while additionally congratulating him on resurrecting Congreve's reputation. In an examination of Sheridan's ties to Congreve, Eric Rump included several of the 1777 reviews of *School for Scandal* in an essay for *Sheridan Studies.* For instance, the reviewer for *The Gazetter* applauded Sheridan's "Manly sentiments, entirely divested of affectation, and which are conveyed to the heart through the purest channels of wit." But an even more important compliment follows when the same reviewer stated that Sheridan's work presents a real challenge to Congreve's "royal supremacy."

The reviewer for the London *Evening Post* celebrated *School for Scandal*'s "wit and fancy . . . decency and morals." Sheridan, stated the same reviewer, demonstrates that "the standard of *real comedy* is once more unfurled." Seven years later, the connection to Congreve was not forgotten; a critic for the *Universal Magazine* wrote that Sheridan's play "has indeed the beauties of Congreve's comedies, without their faults; its plot is deeply enough perplexed, without forcing one to labour to unravel it; its incidents sufficient without being too numerous; its wit pure; its situations truly dramatic."

School for Scandal has endured as a popular play worthy of revival. The work was produced in England in 1990, and while the language, dress, and behavior appear alien to modern audiences, the revival still found appreciative viewers. The 1990 London production's director, Peter Woods, stated in *Sheridan Studies* that the characters are difficult, since "Nobody's fond of anybody."

The play is more difficult to stage in the contemporary dramatic era because audiences are too far removed from the issues presented in the play. The falling screen is still considered funny, but the context is not as filled with tension. Adultery and divorce are simply not as scandalous to a twentieth-century audience. Whereas a 1777 London audience would be tense with anticipation that Lady Teazle might be discovered, with the falling screen providing an explosion of laughter and release, a modern audience might only appreciate the slapstick nature of the scene. Woods described *School for Scandal* as "an artificial comedy about an artificial society in an artificial city."

An additional reason for the difficulty in staging the play is the anti-Semitism in its references to moneylending. Contemporary audiences are not comfortable with this, said Taylor, and the sections cannot be cut without compromising an important part of the play. Still, many of the societal malignancies that Sheridan sought to criticize are just as prevalent in modern society as they were during the playwright's lifetime. Combined with its distinction as a model comedy of manners, these touchstones to contemporary life allow *School for Scandal* to be appreciated by generations of audiences.

CRITICISM

Sheri Metzger

In this essay, Metzger discusses the merits of viewing a production of School for Scandal *as opposed to merely reading the play. She also discusses the cultural problems—notably the anti-Semitism that is woven throughout the drama—that prevents a wider contemporary audience from embracing and fully appreciating Sheridan's work.*

I often tell my students that a play needs to be seen and heard to be properly appreciated. Reading a play requires an ability to visualize, and it is very difficult to manage this visualization without a careful scrutiny of the stage directions and some experience reading drama. This notion is especially true for Richard Brinsley Sheridan's, *School for Scandal,* which makes the reader *wish* for a fine production to view.

In the fourth act when Lady Teazle and Sir Peter are each peeking out of their respective hiding places, and Joseph is cautioning each to retreat, the reader can only imagine the fun occurring on stage. But when the screen falls later in that same act and Lady Teazle is exposed, this bit of slapstick demands to be seen. Mark S. Auburn related in *Sheridan Studies* that anyone passing by the theatre during that scene would have heard the riotous laughter of the audience that erupted from the theatre. This type of comedy was an early inspiration for the silly situation comedies that are a staple of television viewing; but if this play is so funny, why is it so infrequently staged?

Some critics suggest that the language is stilted or the subject matter not topical. When Peter Wood was interviewed about his 1990 production of *School for Scandal,* he expressed the opinion that the public might be developing a new appreciation for the rhythm and tone of language such as Sheridan's. And while it is true that the comedy of manners motif might be of less interest to twentieth-century audiences, it is certain that with tabloid journalism an especially hot topic on television and in mainstream newspapers, the public's interest in gossip, or in a play that satirizes gossip, should be apparent.

But if language and topic do not limit the play's reception, what other reasons might? One possibility is offered by Richard Taylor, who suggested in *Sheridan Studies* that the play's anti-Semitism may present a problem for audiences. Taylor asserted that "the anti-Semitism that runs through *School for Scandal* produces palpable discomfort in contemporary audiences, and no amount of directorial cutting easily eliminates it."

Anti-Semitism was a part of eighteenth-century English life. An act that would have permitted Jews to become naturalized citizens was repealed immediately when anti-Semitic street mobs loudly protested the law. When Moses is introduced in Act III of *School for Scandal,* his name is prefaced with the character descriptor "Honest." Since it was Moses who led the Jews from Egypt to their salvation during the Biblical Exodus, the audience should expect that this Moses will help Charles to his reward. But as important as his name is the qualifier that comes before it. Sheridan places great emphasis on "honest," using the word many times to describe Moses. The obvious inference is that Moses is an exception: moneylenders are stereotyped as dishonest.

The same is true for the overly used "friend" or "friendly." If descriptions of Moses must note his friendliness, then the point is made that most moneylenders are not their client's friends. Historically Jews have been identified with usury or moneylending, and in *School for Scandal,* Sheridan also identifies Jews as dishonest and unfriendly—proven by the fact that Moses's honesty and friendship are repeatedly inferred as anomalous to both his race and occupation.

In *School for Scandal,* to be a moneylender is to be a cheat. Sir Oliver is told that to be successful in his disguise, he must demand 50% interest. And if the subject seems especially desperate, then 100% interest would be appropriate. Thus, to be a successful moneylender, one must also be greedy, unfeeling, and unsympathetic. In Sheridan's play, Jews must even look different from other men. Sir Oliver asks if he shall be able to pass for a Jew. The response is that this moneylender is a broker—a step up socially, and since he is also a Christian, Sir Oliver's appearance will be satisfactory.

The text never explains what a Jew should look like, but Sir Oliver's "smart dress" is in keeping for a broker though not a moneylender. Sir Oliver is even told that moneylenders talk differently than other men. All of these points create an image of

- Sheridan's first play, *The Rivals,* written in 1775, is also a comedy that uses disguise and romance to probe social issues. A clever use of language is notable in this play, which, like *School for Scandal,* offers generational discord as a motif.
- Sheridan was often compared with William Congreve, whose *Way of the World* is considered to be one of his finest comedies. This comedy makes use of witty dialogue to demonstrate how foolish human nature can be.
- The French playwright, John Baptiste Poquelin Moliere, is often cited as an influence on Sheridan. *School for Wives,* was first presented in 1662. The play is a satire and makes use of mistaken identity and misunderstandings to help further its plot.
- Oliver Goldsmith's play, *She Stoops to Conquer,* presented in 1773, was also an attack against the sentimental comedy of the Restoration Age. Goldsmith is sometimes described as the only other successful playwright, besides Sheridan, to emerge in the latter part of the eighteenth century.
- *England in the Age of Hogarth,* written by Derek Jarrett and published in 1986, provides a glimpse of the social history of English in the years just before Sheridan began writing his plays.

Jews that sets them apart from other businessmen. The implication is that Jewish businessmen are different—in clothing, in speech, and in morality. While this depiction would have raised little concern in the last quarter of the eighteenth century, twentieth-century audiences have the example of the Holocaust. The realization that anti-Semitism is never harmless and never acceptable intrudes on the otherwise light-themed *School for Scandal.* It cannot and should not be forgotten, and since the scenes with Moses and the disguised Sir Oliver form an important section of the text, their deletion would be nearly impossible.

If its portrayal of moneylenders detracts from *School for Scandal,* Sheridan's glimpse at the morals and social manners of the period do offer much for an audience to appreciate. As Louis Kronenberger observed, this is a play with a ''sense of naughtiness''; this ''play is concerned with the *imputation* of sinning; of sin itself there is absolutely nothing. No one ever actually commits a sin. The actors only talk about sin.''

Of course, it could be argued that slander and gossip is in itself a sin, and Sheridan might have agreed; but for the audience, gossip is the subject of satire, and satire's result is laughter. All this talk about sin, accompanied by its absence, is a departure from Restoration theatre. The *comedy of manners* of the earlier century emphasized sexuality and sexual situations, and the writers relied on the titillation of the audience as a necessary component of comedy. But Sheridan's play offered a fresh voice. There is a mystery associated with what is hidden by shadow.

As Kronenberger noted, ''sin now seems far more wicked and important than it used to.'' All of this absence of sex might be as equally refreshing to modern audiences who have become jaded by the explicit sexuality portrayed in film and drama. When Kronenberger stated that with *School for Scandal,* ''we are back in an age when sex has become glamorous through being illicit,'' I am reminded of the popularity of Hollywood films of the 1930s and 1940s. The audience could anticipate a happy resolution. Romance ended in weddings, but only after one of the stars had resisted illicit temptation. This is also the happy ending of *School for Scandal.*

Although romance provides the play's happy ending, very little of the play is actually concerned with the romance that ends the play. Maria has a very small part, and there is little interaction on

"IN *SCHOOL FOR SCANDAL,* SHERIDAN CREATES A GENUINELY COMIC MOMENT WITH THE FALLING SCREEN; IT IS SINCERELY FUNNY BECAUSE THE AUDIENCE LIKES THESE TWO CHARACTERS."

stage between her and Charles, little to exemplify the devotion they profess for one another. The romance between Lady Teazle and Sir Peter is given greater emphasis. And although they are married, it is their discovery of romance that offers much entertainment for the audience.

Auburn related that Sheridan rejected the stock depiction of May-December romance. How to recreate a new approach to a familiar story was a challenge, and Auburn said that "in an early version [Sheridan] toyed with a harsh cuckolding story like Chaucer's "Miller's Tale" and Wycherley's *Country Wife* (1675), but in the final version he sought and achieved the amiable tone of Georgian comedy." The couple's happy resolution is based on an awareness of their love for one another. Lady Teazle's country origins, which led her to believe that Lady Sneerwell represented fashion, help remind the young bride of why she chose to marry. And Sir Peter, who had too often focused on his age, recognized that although he might be old enough to be Lady Teazle's father, he was, instead, her husband.

Sheridan's decision to soften the relationship between Lady Teazle and her husband was also noted by Rose Snider, who compared Sheridan's handling of May-December romance to that of Wycherely and Congreve. Snider stated that Sir Peter "reacts in a more gentlemanly fashion" than Wycherely or Congreve's similarly challenged husbands. Accordingly, "Sir Peter Teazle is a far pleasanter person than the earlier prototypes." Snider pointed out that the Teazles introduce some sentiment into the comedy; thus, Sheridan's play is more pleasant for the audience, as well.

Lady Teazle and Sir Peter are, as Aubrey de Selincourt noted, stock characters. The task for Sheridan was to make these familiar characters interesting. Sheridan does succeed, says de Selincourt, "with unsurpassed brilliance and precision." In *School for Scandal,* Sheridan creates a genuinely comic moment with the falling screen; it is sincerely funny because the audience likes these two characters. A cuckold husband and an unfaithful wife do not invite the audience's loyalty, but Sheridan creates two characters the audience can like. Their discovery of one another's value provides a more genuine appreciation of romance than the too brief framing of Maria and Charles's courtship.

Source: Sheri Metzger for *Drama for Students,* Gale, 1998.

Nancy Copeland

Copeland reviews a Stratford Festival production of Sheridan's play. While finding the text as theatrical and resilient as ever, the critic was less than impressed with the production.

As conceived by Robin Phillips, *The School for Scandal* displays a harsh and glittering world of exquisite beauty and viciousness, where sentimental sobriety—when genuine—is the only refuge from the savagery that lies in wait for vitality and virtue. Phillips has read the play as a piece of serious social criticism, with decidedly mixed results: his version of this classic comedy of manners is thought-provoking, visually stunning, but finally a failure.

Sheridan wittily exhibits the machinations of the hypocritical Joseph Surface, who joins with the malicious Lady Sneerwell in a campaign of slander originally designed to obtain his uncle Oliver's fortune and the hand of the wealthy Maria by the destruction of his brother Charles's reputation, but which eventually expands to threaten the marriage of Sir Peter and Lady Teazle. In his program note, Phillips emphasizes the importance of reputation in a mercantile society, where to lose respectability is literally to lose "credit." In such an environment, the power of Lady Sneerwell and her "scandalous college" of gossips is no laughing matter, and Phillips's production takes its tone from the seriousness of their crime. The characterizations are subdued, the comedy is underplayed: the audience is never allowed to forget that the events it is witnessing could end as easily in suffering as in happiness.

Flamboyant performances are therefore the rare exception in this *School.* As that victim of a May-September marriage, Sir Peter Teazle, William Hutt is a sober, tender husband, whose very irascibility is restrained. He is seen at his most characteristic in his Act III scene with his young wife, where his childlike delight in her affection succumbs with reluctance to her attacks, to be replaced by deeply felt hurt, rather than rage, when her wounding remarks struck home. His violent emotions are reserved for his ward Maria, whom he reduces to tears with his attempt to bully her into accepting Joseph as her husband. Douglas Campbell's excellent Sir Oliver is almost equally grave, although he is captivatingly comic during the debt-ridden Charles's private auction of the family portraits and in his encounter with the slanderers who gather at Sir Peter's door to gloat over Lady Teazle's apparent indiscretion with Joseph. Susan Wright's Mrs. Candour typifies the treatment of Sheridan's wit in this production, delivering her catalogue of scandal in a matter-of-fact tone that underlines the speech's audacity while it almost eradicates its humor. Only Richard Curnock and Keith Dinicol, as the arriviste gossips Crabtree and Sir Benjamin Backbite, are allowed to fully exploit the comedy of their roles, to the considerable delight of the audience.

Sheila McCarthy combines these two approaches to delineate this production's central action: the maturation of Lady Teazle. In her first scene McCarthy emphasizes the broad comedy of her role, playing a squeaky-voiced caricature of an empty-headed flirt as she tantalizes and torments her hapless spouse with her childlike longings for fashionable extravagancies. But in the course of her trials at the hands of Colm Feore's lascivious Joseph and the chorus of scandalmongers, she gradually adopts the subdued style of the more experienced characters, as the enthusiastic girl dwindles into the sedate—but safe—wife. The diminished Lady Teazle of the last act is the poignant symbol of the price to be paid for social security in Phillip's London.

This autumnal drama is played out most clearly in the visual aspect of the production. Michael Eagan's set is a vision of geometric opulence: a long, narrow thrust covered in white tile with a metallic border, terminated upstage by an enormous moveable three-tiered cage, in white and silver, that perfectly balances the proportions of the playing area. The spare luxury of the set is matched by an enormous silver rocking horse that appears, surrounded by a chorus of dancers and a fireworks display, in a spectacular *entr'acte* representing the temptations of fashionable London. Anne Curtis's equally lavish costumes provide an emblematic commentary on the action through a general movement from white and beige in the early scenes, punctuated dramatically by Lady Teazle's orange hair and gown and the complete blackness of Snake's costume, toward more sombre colors, as the circumstances of Charles and the Teazles became more precarious. Matters are at their darkest when the vultures descend on the house of the supposedly cuckolded Sir Peter dressed in deep brown and carrying black umbrellas. The arrival of Sir Oliver in fawn and Sir Peter in an oatmeal-colored coat prepared the way for the dénouement, in which the blacks and dark browns of the evil characters are ranged against the sensibly muted buffs and beiges of the virtuous. Maria arrives for her happy ending dressed in realistic beige and brown stripes, while the chastened Lady Teazle appears in very pale peach.

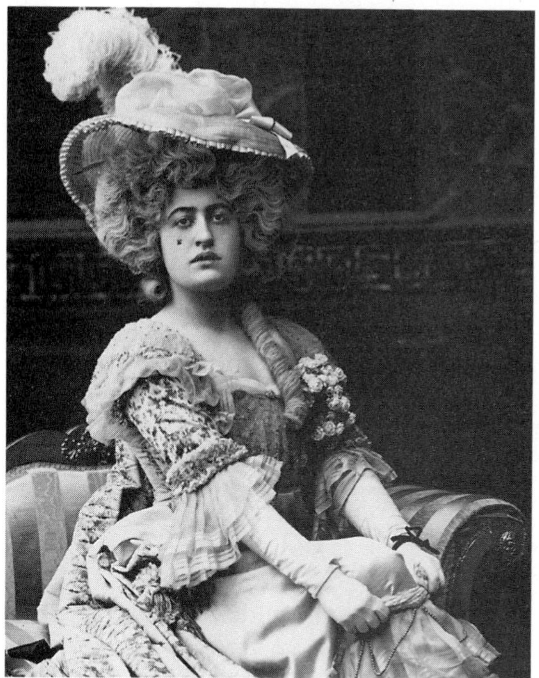

Constance Collier in an early-twentieth century production of School for Scandal

The emblematic quality of the costuming is echoed in Phillips's use of tableaux. The prologue is set against a spectacle of voyeurism: while Sir Peter describes the evils of slanderous newspaper paragraphs, upstage, inside the cage, Lady Teazle exhibits herself in a state of undress to a crowd of scandalized gawkers. Once again surrounded by an attendant crowd, she delivers the epilogue from the back of the silver rocking horse amid darkness and dry ice, the spotlit image of her wistful lament for her lost pleasures. The prologue tableau is preceded by a mysterious sound effect—a prop-driven airplane—but the use of sound is generally more

> "*THE SCHOOL FOR SCANDAL* DISPLAYS A HARSH AND GLITTERING WORLD OF EXQUISITE BEAUTY AND VICIOUSNESS, WHERE SENTIMENTAL SOBRIETY—WHEN GENUINE—IS THE ONLY REFUGE FROM THE SAVAGERY THAT LIES IN WAIT FOR VITALITY AND VIRTUE."

straightforward, indeed, prosaic: music underlines moment of turmoil and sentiment; Snake is accompanied by a synthesized rattle and hiss. Even the lighting design functions symbolically, reinforcing the theme of relentless social scrutiny by the frequent use of spotlights.

By taking Sheridan seriously, Phillips discovers in *The School for Scandal* a critique of urban consumerist culture that has unexpected resonance, but his approach is finally self-defeating. His reliance on schematic visual effects betrays the conflict between his interpretation and the text, which promulgates its ethics by means of blatantly theatrical comedy. In the service of his solemn interpretation, Phillips attacks the play's comic structure, retarding its rhythms, evading its comic builds, and eschewing its invitations to physical comedy and broad characterizations. Drained of comic energy, Phillips *Scandal* is ultimately a lackluster performance, despite its considerable intelligence and beauty, and, as such, a misrepresentation of Sheridan's work.

Source: Nancy Copeland, review of *The School for Scandal* in *Theatre Journal,* Volume 40, no. 3, October, 1988, pp. 420–21.

John Clifford

Clifford expresses disappointment at being denied the full pleasure of Sheridan's play. Complaining of poor technical values and a general lack of enthusiasm, the critic feels that the play deserves better attention.

To a writer a theatre like the Royal Lyceum is a magic box full of enticing possibilities—to all of which, almost invariably, you are denied access. To an Artistic Director, on the other hand, such a place must more often feel like a black hole—with row after row of empty seats that somehow, night after night, have got to be filled.

The theatre's understandable response to this has been to mount two classic comedies in repertory—a revival of their immensely successful production of *Tartuffe* in tandem with a new production of Sheridan's *School for Scandal.*

This opened recently to an almost uniformly hostile press, which the production did not really deserve. The Lyceum tends to open with a cheerful free preview and follow it with a press night that almost always falls flat; a strongly self-destructive process to which this in many respects perfectly acceptable show has also fallen victim.

Colin MacNeil's set is an elegant and serviceable rectangular box, fronted by a row of footlights, that neatly and effectively conjures up a feeling of the period; the cast are splendidly bewigged and crinolined; the show looks good, and by the end had enough basic buoyancy to it to ensure that the very special magic exerted by so beautifully structured a comedy would work on its audience.

The basic groundwork was all in place; the show's problems arose because somehow hardly anyone seemed to be working quite as hard or quite as sharply as they could.

One soon began to long, for instance, for a more elegant and imaginative solution to the problems of scene changing than the inevitably shame-faced lackeys embarassedly shoving bits of false bookshelf off and on the stage, or collapsing and re-erecting chinese screens; and particularly in the first half, when so much of the comedy depends on the words, one could often not stop longing for a cast more totally and incisively in command of the language. In fact it was hard, sometimes, to escape the feeling that most of them, given the chance, would probably have been happier doing something else.

The much stronger theatrical possibilities of the second half seemed to bring out much stronger and more lively performances. The cast's timing picked up, as did their capacity for inventiveness, and they began to approach the whole play with a delightfully infectious relish.

Garry Stewart, for instance, who had been looking wretchedly uncomfortable in wig and rouge as the foppish Benjamin Backbite, approached the part of the dissolute but good-hearted Charles with exactly the right kind of swagger; and Andrew Dallmeyer, who had produced a rather somnabulistically grotesque Crabtree, came into his own as the nameless but wonderfully malevolent lackey to Billy McElhaney's haplessly hypocritical Surface.

Sarah Collier's splendidly piratical Lady Sneerwell—complete with eye-patch—David McKail's pop-eyed and genial Sir Oliver, Gerda Stevenson's bubbly and charming Lady Teazle, all turned out consistent and skilfull performances which were a pleasure to watch. It all added up to a pleasant, entertaining, undemanding sort of evening, which did not quite do justice to the skills and talents of everyone concerned. With stronger direction, a greater sense of commitment and purposefulness, it could easily have added up to a very great deal more.

Source: John Clifford, review of *The School for Scandal* in *Plays and Players,* Number 407, August, 1987, pp. 33–34.

Anonymous

In this uncredited review, a 1963 production of School for Scandal *receives a favorable appraisal. The critic terms the play as ''iridescently enchanting, contagiously amusing.''*

The Shool for Scandal, by Richard Brinsley Sheridan, is a kind of dramatic harpsichord. It has surface vivacity rather than inner strength. It has elegance of style rather than profundity of substance. Thumped by realism's heavy hand, it would jangle and go mute; stroked with exquisite artifice, it enchants and amuses. The present import from Britain, top-starring Sir john Gielgud and Sir Ralph Richardson, is iridescently enchanting, contagiously amusing.

"*THE SHOOL FOR SCANDAL* IS A KIND OF DRAMATIC HARPSICHORD. IT HAS SURFACE VIVACITY RATHER THAN INNER STRENGTH. IT HAS ELEGANCE OF STYLE RATHER THAN PROFUNDITY OF SUBSTANCE."

Gielgud is Joseph Surface, the hypocrite as moral snob, a kind of holier-than-thou heel. Richardson is Sir Peter Teazle, a crusty, crestfallen bridegroom in his 50s, loving, but not loved by, young Lady Teazle (Geraldine McEwan), a predatory country kitten so sure of her city ways that her voice seems to be crunching canary-brittle. The ostensible question is: Will Lady Teazle cuckold Sir Peter with Joseph? But Sheridan is less concerned with virtue in peril than with vice masquerading as virtue. In the famously comic screen scene, when Lady Teazle is finally discovered by Sir Peter in Joseph's library, it is not her folly that is impugned and exposed but Joseph's bad character. All high comedy is a deliberately moral unmasking of moral pretense, the ultimate poseur being Society itself.

What Gielgud the director brings to *The School for Scandal* is a sense of how the play traps constancy of man's frivolity in its high-polish comic veneer. Gielgud the actor evokes an entire social structure with the delicate flourish of a snuffbox. Richardson *et al.* are similarly and superlatively good. The cast is sumptuously costumed, but its kingliest array is English speech, heard with the ringing clarity of fine crystal on a U.S. stage too long debased by caveman playwrights and actors who are masters of the grunt, the mumble and the slur.

Source: ''Elegantly on the Harpsichord'' in *Time,* Volume LXXXI, no. 5, February 1, 1963, p. 65.

SOURCES

Morrow, Laura. ''Television, Text, and Teleology in a *School for Scandal*'' in *Shakespeare on Film Newsletter,* Vol. 11, no. 2, 1987, p. 3.

Morwood, James and David Crane. ''On Producing Sheridan: A Conversation with Peter Wood'' in *Sheridan Studies,* edited by Morwood and Crane, Cambridge University Press, 1995, pp. 178-88.

Rump, Eric. ''Sheridan, Congreve and *School for Scandal*'' in *Sheridan Studies,* edited by James Morwood and David Crane, Cambridge University Press, 1995, pp. 58-70.

Snider, Rose. ''Richard B. Sheridan'' in *Satire in the Comedies of Congreve, Sheridan, Wilde, and Coward,* 1937, reprint by Phaeton Press, 1972, pp. 41-73.

Taylor, Richard. '''Future Retrospection': Rereading Sheridan's Reviewers'' in *Sheridan Studies,* edited by James

Morwood and David Crane, Cambridge University Press, 1995, pp. 47-57.

Wiesenthal, Christine. "Representation and Experimentation in the Major Comedies of Richard Brinsley Sheridan" in *Eighteenth-Century Studies,* Vol. 25, no. 3, 1992, pp. 309-30.

FURTHER READING

Auburn, Mark S. "Richard Brinsley Sheridan" in *Dictionary of Literary Biography,* Volume 89: *Restoration and Eighteenth-Century Dramatists,* edited by Paula R. Backscheider, Gale, 1989, pp. 298-322.

Auburn provides a general overview of Sheridan's plays and his life.

de Selincourt, Aubrey. "Sheridan" in *Six Great Playwrights: Sophocles, Shakespeare, Moliere, Sheridan, Ibsen, Shaw,* Hamish Hamilton, 1960, pp. 105-31.

This essay is an examination of the construction of several of Sheridan's plays, with a brief look at Sheridan's development of characters.

Hay, Douglas and Peter Linebaugh, Editors. *Albion's Fatal Tree: Crime and Society in Eighteenth-Century England,* Pantheon, 1975.

This book explores the legal problems that confronted the differences in class. The book includes a number of detailed studies.

Hogan, Robert. "Plot, Character, and Comic Language in Sheridan" in *Comedy from Shakespeare to Sheridan,* edited by A. R. Braunmiller and J. C. Bulman, University of Delaware Press, 1986, pp. 274-85.

Hogan compares Sheridan's use of plot and comedic language in *School for Scandal* and *The Rivals.*

Kronenberger, Louis. "*School for Scandal*" in *Restoration and Eighteenth-Century Comedy,* edited by Scott McMillin, W.W. Norton, 1973, pp. 558-63.

Kronenberger discusses the strengths and appeal of *School for Scandal.* He focuses on the themes and on the play's contrasts with Restoration comedy.

Jarrett, Derek. *England in the Age of Hogarth,* Hart-Davis, MacGibbon, 1974.

Derek presents a social history of the eighteenth century. The author uses diaries and letters to provide authenticity to his ideas.

Mikhail, E. H., Editor. *Sheridan: Interviews and Recollections,* St. Martin's Press, 1989.

Mikhail provides an interesting examination of the private Sheridan through the use of letters and recollections from the period to offer a different biography of Sheridan. The author has tried to use information that has not been previously printed in other biographies.

Porter, Roy. *English Society in the Eighteenth Century,* Penguin, 1982.

Porter tries to provide a comprehensive look at eighteenth-Century English life. He offers a number of small details on every aspect of English social life, from the small country town to London.

Stone, Lawrence. *The Family, Sex, and Marriage in England 1500-1800,* Penguin, 1977.

Stone's study of family life and the relationship between family, state, and law is easy to read and absorb. Stone includes examples to support this account of social history. This volume makes it easy to see the progression of family structure and values during 300 years of political and social transformation.

Six Characters in Search of an Author

LUIGI PIRANDELLO

1921

Six Characters in Search of an Author created Luigi Pirandello's international reputation in the 1920s and is still the play by which he is most widely identified.

With originality that was startling to his contemporaries, Pirandello introduced a striking and compelling dramatic situation that initially baffled but eventually dazzled audiences and critics alike. In what begins as a realistic play he introduces six figures who make the extraordinary claim that they are the incomplete but independent products of an artist's imagination—''characters'' the artist abandoned when he couldn't complete their story. These ''characters'' have arrived on the stage to find an author themselves, someone who will give them the fullness of literary life that their original author has denied them. Furthermore, these ''characters'' claim that they are more ''real'' than the actors who eventually want to portray them.

This concept was so startling it helped to incite a riot in the audience when the original production of the play was staged in Rome on May 10, 1921. Later that year, however, audiences and critics had assimilated the extraordinary idea and were enchanted by a remounted production in Milan. The play would then see successful productions in London and New York in February and October of 1922, in Paris in 1923, and in Berlin and Vienna in 1924. Pirandello's own theatre company, founded in 1925, then performed the play in Italian through-

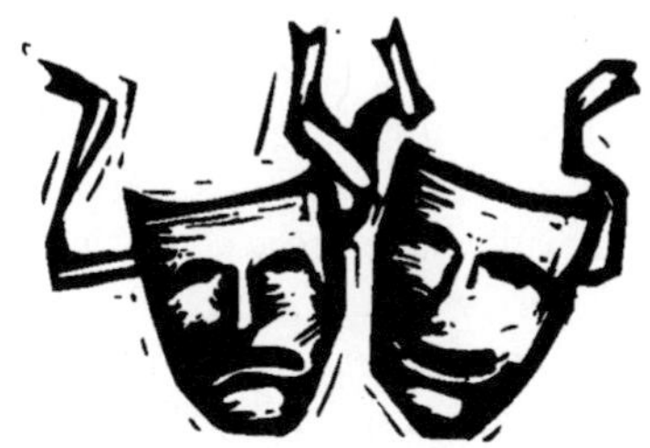

out the major cities of Europe and North and South America. As a result of this assault on the theatre world, Pirandello became one of the most respected and influential dramatists in the world by the end of the 1920s, and today *Six Characters in Search of an Author* is considered one of the most influential plays in the history of world literature.

AUTHOR BIOGRAPHY

Luigi Pirandello was born in Sicily (the large island near the ''toe'' of Italy) on June 28, 1867, to a wealthy father who owned sulphur mines. Though his father wanted him to pursue a business career, Pirandello preferred academics and by 1891 had earned a Ph.D. in linguistics, eventually spending many years of his life as a professor of Italian literature and language at a school for women in Rome.

In 1894 Pirandello's father arranged for his son to marry the daughter of his business partner, and Pirandello's resulting financial independence enabled him to live in Rome and pursue a writing career. Although he initially focused on poetry and short stories, Pirandello first achieved success as a writer in 1904 with the novel *The Late Mattia Pascal.* However, in 1903 floods in his father's sulphur mines had brought financial ruin to the Pirandellos and altered the playwright's life irrevocably. Pirandello's wife reacted to the catastrophe with an emotional breakdown from which she never recovered, spending the rest of her life in a condition of mental instability. His wife's condition made Pirandello's life miserable but also supplied him with the themes that would sustain the rest of his artistic career. Until he finally agreed to commit her to a mental institution in 1918, Pirandello was living with an insane wife who accused him of infidelity whenever he was out of her sight. This constant challenge to his sense of reality led Pirandello to investigate in his writings the question of personal identity and the relationship between madness and sanity and appearance and reality.

Pirandello became widely known in Italy as a poet, novelist, and short story writer, but around 1916, at the age of 49, he began writing more plays and when his famous themes appeared in his two dramatic masterpieces, *Six Characters in Search of an Author* (1921) and *Henry IV* (1922), Pirandello immediately became an international success, enabling him to create a theatrical troupe that performed his plays around the world. By the end of his life in 1936 Pirandello had written eight volumes of poems, seven novels, 250 short stories, and 44 plays. But it was mainly because of his internationally famous plays that Pirandello was awarded the Nobel Prize for literature in 1934, two years before his death from pneumonia in Rome on December 10, 1936. Pirandello has had a profound effect on twentieth-century drama and especially on what would be called the Theatre of the Absurd. Having given eloquent testimony to the issues of the relativity of truth, the instability of personal identity, and the nature of stage illusion, Pirandello remains one of the most influential dramatists of the twentieth century.

PLOT SUMMARY

Act I

When *Six Characters in Search of an Author* begins, the stage is being prepared for the daytime rehearsal of a play and several actors and actresses are milling about as the Producer enters and gets the rehearsal started. Suddenly the guard at the stage door enters and informs the Producer that six people have entered the theatre asking to see the person in charge. These six ''characters'' are a Father, a Mother, a 22-year-old Son, a Stepdaughter, an adolescent Boy, and young female Child. These ''characters'' claim that they are the incomplete creations of an author who couldn't finish the work for which they were conceived. They have come looking for someone who will take up their story and embody it in some way, helping them to complete their sense of themselves.

The Producer and his fellow company members are initially incredulous, convinced that these ''people'' have escaped from a mental institution. But the Father, speaking for the other characters, argues that they are just as ''real'' as the people getting ready to rehearse their play. Fictional characters, he maintains, are more ''alive'' because they cannot die as long as the works they live in are experienced by others. The Father explains that he and the other ''characters'' want to achieve their full life by completing the story that now only exists in fragments in the author's brain.

The Stepdaughter and Father begin to tell their ''story.'' The Father was married to the Mother but left her many years ago when she became attracted to a young assistant or secretary in his employ.

Though the Father was angered by his wife's feelings and sent his young assistant away, he grew impatient with his wife's melancholy and sent their son away, to be raised and educated in the country. He eventually turned his wife out and she sought her lover, bearing three more children by him before the man died two months before the play begins. These three children and the son from her marriage with the Father stand before the Producer and his theatrical troupe.

The Father's version of these events is variously contested both by the Mother and the Stepdaughter. The Father claims that he turned his wife out because of his concern for her and his natural son and that later he was genuinely concerned for his wife's new family. However, the Mother claims the Father forced her into the arms of the assistant because he was simply bored with her, and the Stepdaughter claims that the father stalked her sexually as she was growing up. They all agree that eventually the Father lost track of his stepchildren because the wife's lover took different jobs and moved repeatedly. When the lover died, the family fell into extreme financial need and the father happened upon his Stepdaughter in Madame Pace's brothel where the Stepdaughter was attempting to raise money to support the family.

Both the Father and Stepdaughter are anxious to play the scene in the brothel because both think the portrayal will demonstrate their version of that meeting. The daughter asserts that the father knew who she was and desired her incestuously while the father claims he did not know her and immediately refused the sexual union when he recognized her—even before the Mother discovered them in the room. After the incident, the Father took his wife and stepchildren home, where his natural son resented their implicit demands on his father.

The Producer and actors become intrigued by this story and are anxious to play it, putting aside their original skepticism about whether or not these ''people'' are ''real.'' The Producer requests the ''characters'' to come to his office to work out a scenario.

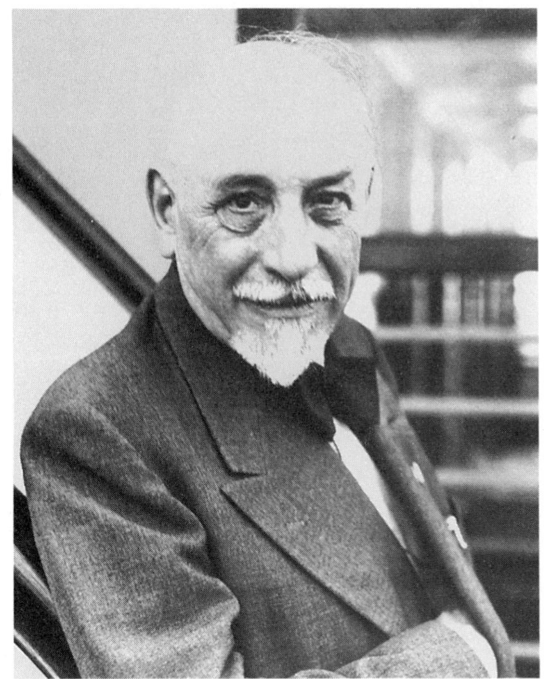

Luigi Pirandello

Act II

The Producer's plan is for the ''characters'' to act out their story, starting with the scene in Madame Pace's brothel, while the prompter takes down their dialogue in shorthand for the actors of the company to study and imitate. The ''characters'' suggest that they can act out the story more authentically, but the Producer insists on artistic autonomy and overrules their objections. It is soon discovered that Madame Pace is not available for the scene, but the Father entices her into being by recreating the hat rack in her brothel and she appears—much to the consternation of the acting company, who immediately consider it some kind of trick.

When they begin the scene in the brothel, the Producer is initially dissatisfied with Madame Pace's performance and the Mother disrupts the scene with her consternation over what's being acted out, but finally the Producer is pleased with what he sees and asks the actors to take over for the Father and Stepdaughter. However, the Stepdaughter cannot help but laugh when she sees how the actors represent their scene in such a different manner from the way she sees it herself. But when the Father and Stepdaughter resume the acting themselves, the Producer censors the scene by not permitting the Stepdaughter to use a line about disrobing. He explains that such suggestiveness would create a riot in the audience. The Stepdaughter accuses the Producer of collaborating with the Father to present the scene in a way that flatters him and misrepresents the truth of what the Father had done. The Stepdaughter asserts that to present the drama accurately the suffering Mother must be excused. But as

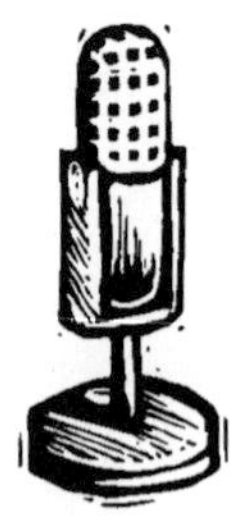

MEDIA ADAPTATIONS

- *Six Characters in Search of an Author* was presented in a full-length film version in 1992 by BBC Scotland, starring John Hurt as the Father, Brian Cox as the Producer, Tara Fitzgerald as the Stepdaughter, and Susan Fleetwood as the Mother. Adapted by Michael Hastings and produced by Simon Curtis, the film was directed by Bill Bryden. In 1996, the 110 minute film was released on videocassette with a teacher's guide.
- In 1987, sections of *Six Characters in Search of an Author* were represented in an episode on Pirandello for the BBC Channel 4 South Bank Show series called *The Modern World: Ten Great Writers.* This documentary recreated a day in the life of Pirandello's acting troupe as they brought *Six Characters in Search of an Author* to London in 1925. The show was written and adapted by Nigel Wattis and Gillian Greenwood and produced and directed by Nigel Wattis. Hosted by series editor Melvyn Bragg, the episode featured Jim Norton as Pirandello, Douglas Hodge as the Producer, Reginald Stewart as the Father, Sylvestra LeTouzel as the Stepdaughter, and Patricia Thorns as the Mother.
- A 59-minute videocassette version of *Six Characters in Search of an Author* was presented in 1978 as part of an educational television series called *Drama: Play, Performance, Perception,* hosted by Jose Ferrer. A co-production of Miami-Dade Community College, the BBC, and the British Open University, the episode was directed by John Selwyn Gilbert and included actors Charles Gray, Nigel Stock, and Mary Wimbush. The film was also distributed in 1978 by Insight Media and Films Inc. with actor Ossie Davis as guest commentator and additional direction by Andrew Martin. This version was re-released in 1992 as a 60 minute videocassette.
- A 48-minute audiovisual cassette version of the play was presented by the British Broadcasting Corporation in cooperation with the British Open University in 1976.
- A 58-minute VHS videocassette version of the play was produced in 1976 by Films for the Humanities (Princeton, New Jersey) in their History of Drama series as an example of Theatre of the Absurd. It was produced by Harold Mantell, directed by Ken Frankel, translated by David Calicchio, and narrated by Joseph Heller, with music by William Penn. The actors included Nikki Flacks, Ben Kapen, Gwendolyn Brown, Dimo Comdos, Bob Picardo, and Kathy Manning. In the same year this version was also released on two reels of 16 mm film with accompanying textbook, teacher's guides, and two filmstrips. The film was re-released in 1982 in Beta and VHS, in 1988 in VHS, and in 1988 in a 52-minute version.
- A commentary on the play by Alfred Brooks called ''Pirandello's Illusion Game'' was released on audiocassette in 1971 from the Center for Cassette Studies.
- A 38-minute commentary on the play on audiocassette by Paul D'Andrea was released in 1971 by Everett and Edwards out of Deland, Florida, in the Modern Drama Cassette Curriculum series. Another commentary by Robert James Nelson was released in 1973 as part of their World Literature Cassette Curriculum series.
- A production of *Six Characters in Search of an Author* appeared on BBC television on April 20, 1954 in a translation by Frederick May.

the Mother is explaining her torment, the final confrontation of the scene is actually played out, with the Mother entering the brothel to discover the Stepdaughter in the Father's arms. The Producer is pleased with the dramatic moment and declares that this will be the perfect time for the curtain to fall. A member of the stage crew, hearing this comment, mistakes it for an order and actually drops the curtain.

Act III

When the curtain rises again, the scene to be acted out is in the Father's house after the discovery at the brothel. The Producer is impatient with the suggestions given him by the "characters" about how to play the scene while the "characters" don't like references to stage "illusion," believing as they do that their lives are real. The Father points out to the Producer that the confidence the Producer has about the reality of his own personal identity is an illusion as well, that the key elements of his personality and identity change constantly while those of the "characters" stay constant. The Producer decides that regardless of what the "characters" want to propose, the next action will be played with everyone in the garden.

After considerable squabbling between the "characters" as to how the scene should be portrayed and after the revelation that the Little Boy has a revolver in his pocket, the Son reluctantly begins telling the story of what he saw when he rushed out of his room and went out to the garden. Behind the tree he saw the Little Boy "standing there with a mad look in his eyes . . . looking into the fountain at his little sister, floating there, drowned." Suddenly, a shot rings out on stage and the Mother runs over toward the Boy and several actors join her, discover the Boy's body, and carry him off. It appears to some actors that this "character" is actually dead, but other actors cry that it's only make-believe. The exasperated Producer exclaims that he has lost an entire day of rehearsal and the play ends with a tableaux of the "characters," first in shadow with the Little Girl and Little Boy missing, and then in a trio of Father, Mother, and Son with the Stepdaughter laughing maniacally and exiting the theatre.

CHARACTERS

Amalia

See The Mother

The Director

See The Producer

The Father

The Father is the leading spokesperson for the six "characters." He is the biological father of the 22 year-old son he had with the Mother, and he is the stepfather of the three children the Mother had during her relationship with the Father's secretary. In his "Preface" to *Six Characters in Search of an Author,* Pirandello describes the Father as "a man of about fifty, in black coat, light trousers, his eyebrows drawn into a painful frown, and in his eyes an expression mortified yet obstinate." The Father is mortified by his stepdaughter's charge that he has felt incestuous feelings for her since she was a child, stalking her when she was a schoolgirl, and attempting to buy her in Madame Pace's brothel. The Father insists that his concern for his family has always been genuine and that he was surprised to discover his stepdaughter at Madame Pace's establishment. The Father is determined to have their story told. According to Pirandello, the Father and Stepdaughter are the "most eager to live," the "most fully conscious of being characters," and the "most intensely alive" as the two of them "naturally come forward and direct and drag along the almost dead weight of the others."

The Little Boy

The Little Boy is 14 years old and the eldest son of the Mother from her relationship with the Father's secretary. The Little Boy is dressed in mourning black, like his mother and two sisters, in memory of the death of his natural father. He is timid, frightened, and despondent because in his short stay in the Father's house following the incident in Madame Pace's brothel he was intimidated by the Father's natural son. His elder sister, the Stepdaughter, also disdains the Little Boy because of his action at the end of their story. The Little Boy does not speak because he is a relatively undeveloped character from the author's mind, and in the "Preface" Pirandello lumps the Little Boy with his younger sister as "no more than onlookers taking part by their presence merely." At the end of the story, the Little Boy will shoot himself with a revolver when he sees his little sister drowned in the fountain behind his stepfather's house.

The Little Girl

About four years old, the youngest daughter of the Mother from her relationship with the Father's secretary, the Little Girl is dressed in white, with a black sash around her waist. For the same reason as with her brother, the Little Girl does not speak, and she will drown at the end of the story presented by the ''characters.''

The Mother

The wife of the Father and the mother of all four children (the eldest son by the Father and the other three by the lover who has just died). She is dressed in black with a widow's crepe veil, under which is a waxlike face and sad eyes that she generally keeps downcast. Her main goal is to reconcile with her 22-year-old ''legitimate'' son, to convince him that she did not leave him of her own volition. The Mother is deeply ashamed of the Father's experience with her eldest daughter in Madame Pace's brothel. According to Pirandello in the ''Preface,'' the Mother, ''entirely passive,'' stands out from all the others because ''she is not aware of being a character . . . not even for a single moment, detached from her 'part.''' She ''lives in a stream of feeling that never ceases, so that she cannot become conscious of her own life, that is to say, of her being a character.''

Other actors, actresses, and company members

The other members of the Producer's company are proud of their craft and initially contemptuous of the six ''characters'' but then become quite intrigued by their story and are anxious to portray it.

Madame Pace

The owner of the dress shop that doubles as a brothel, Madame Pace is old and fat and is dressed garishly and ludicrously in silk, wearing an outlandish wig and too much makeup. She speaks with a thick Spanish accent and is mysteriously summoned by the Father when she appears to be missing from the brothel scene between the Father and Stepdaughter. She is, essentially, the ''seventh'' of the ''characters.'' In the ''Preface'' Pirandello points out that as a creation of the moment Madame Pace is an example of Pirandello's ''imagination in the act of creating.''

The Producer

The Producer (or Director or Stage Manager, depending on the text and translation that is used) is the main voice for the theatrical company that is attempting an afternoon rehearsal for their current production when the six ''characters'' enter and request their own play to be done instead. The Producer initially attempts to dismiss these ''people'' as lunatics, intent on getting his own work done. Gradually, however, he becomes intrigued by the content of their story and comes to accept their ''reality'' without further questioning because he sees in their story the potential for a commercial success. An efficient and even violently gruff man, the Producer is also patient, flexible, and courageous, willing to go forward without a great deal of conventional understanding of where things are taking him. He is, however, comically inflexible in that he insists on modifying what the ''characters'' give him to fit the stage conventions to which he is accustomed.

Rosetta

See The Little Girl

The Son

The only biological child of both the Mother and Father, this tall 22- year-old man was separated from his mother at the age of two and was raised and educated in the country. When he finally returned to his father, the Son was distant and is now contemptuous of his father and hostile toward his adopted family. Pirandello describes him as one ''who stood apart from the others, seemingly locked within himself, as though holding the rest in utter scorn.''

The Stage Manager

See The Producer

The Stepdaughter

The Stepdaughter is 18 years old and the eldest child from the Mother's relationship with the Father's secretary. After her natural father died, the Stepdaughter was forced into Madame Pace's brothel in order to help the family survive, and it was at the brothel that she encountered her stepfather. Pirandello describes her as ''pert'' and ''bold'' and as one who ''moved about in a constant flutter of disdainful biting merriment at the expense of the older man [the Father].'' Desiring vengeance on the Father, the Stepdaughter is elegant, vibrant, beautiful, but also angry. She, too, is dressed in mourning black for her natural father, but shortly after she is introduced to the Producer and his company, she dances and sings a lively and suggestive song. The Stepdaughter dislikes the 22-year-old son because of his condescending attitude toward her and her ''illegitimate'' siblings, and she is also contemptuous of her 14 year-old brother because he permitted the Little Girl to drown and then ''stupidly'' shot himself. She is, however, tender toward her four-year-old sister. The Stepdaughter and the Father are the author's two most developed characters and thus dominate the play.

THEMES

Reality and Illusion

In the stage directions at the beginning of Act I of *Six Characters in Search of an Author,* Pirandello directs that as the audience enters the theatre the curtain should be up and the stage bare and in darkness, as it would be in the middle of the day, "so that from the beginning the audience will have the feeling of being present, not at a performance of a properly rehearsed play, but at a performance of a play that happens spontaneously." The set, then, is designed to blur the distinction between stage illusion and real life, making the play seem more realistic, but Pirandello has no intention of writing a realistic play. In fact, he ultimately wants to call attention as much as possible to the arbitrariness of this theatrical illusion and to challenge the audience's comfortable faith in their ability to discern reality both in and outside the theatre. Pirandello is concerned from the outset with the relationship between what people take for reality and what turns out to be illusion.

The audience has entered the theatre prepared to see an illusion of real life and to "willingly suspend their disbelief" in order to enjoy and profit from the fiction. In this way, human beings have long accustomed themselves to the illusion of reality on a stage, but in becoming so accustomed they have taken stage illusion for granted and in life they often take illusion for reality without realizing it. Furthermore, in life, as on stage, the arbitrariness of what is taken for reality is so pervasive as to bring into question one's very ability to distinguish at all between what is real and what is not.

When the action of the play officially begins, the audience knows they are watching actors pretending to be actors pretending to be characters in a rehearsal, but nothing can prepare an audience for the suspension of disbelief they are asked to make when the six "characters" arrive and claim that they are "real." The audience "knows" these are simply more actors, but the claim these "characters" make is so strange as to be compelling. Even before there are words on a page (not to mention rehearsals, actors, or a performance) these "characters" claim to have sprung to life merely because their author was thinking about them; they claim to have wrested themselves from his control and are seeking out these thespians to find a fuller expression of who they are. These claims understandably strain the credulity of the Producer and the members of his company, who perhaps speak for the audience when they say, "is this some kind of joke?" and "it's no use, I don't understand any more."

The "characters" insist to the end that they are "real" even though the audience "knows" they are actors, and this conflict between what is known and what is passed off as real is intensified by the actors' responses to crucial moments in the play. In Act I, for example, the Stepdaughter is summarizing the "story" of these "characters" when the Mother faints with shame and the actors exclaim, "is it real? Has she really fainted?" It is a question the audience would like to dismiss easily—"knowing" that everyone on stage is an actor—but this question is raised again even more dramatically at the end of the play when a real-sounding shot is fired and the Mother runs in the direction of her child with a genuine cry of terror. The actors crowd around "in general confusion," and the Producer moves to the middle of the group, asking the question that the audience, in spite of its certainty, is tempted to ask, "is he really wounded? Really wounded?" An actress says, "he's dead! The poor boy! He's dead! What a terrible thing!" and an actor responds, "What do you mean, dead! It's all make-believe. It's a sham! He's not dead. Don't you believe it!" A chorus of actor voices expresses the duality that Pirandello refuses to resolve: "Make-believe? It's real! Real! He's dead!" says one, and "No, he isn't. He's pretending! It's all make-believe" says another. The Father, of course, assures everyone that "it's reality!" and the Producer expresses a simple refusal to decide: "Make believe?! Reality?! Oh, go to hell the lot of you! Lights! Lights! Lights!"

Permanence and the Concept of Self

Pirandello was convinced that in real life much is taken for real which should not be. He had only to think of his insane wife's decades of groundless accusations to realize that what the mind takes to be true is often outrageously false. But if illusions are repeated often enough, believed long enough, and enough people take them to be real, illusions develop a compelling reality in the culture at large. Such,

TOPICS FOR FURTHER STUDY

- Read a biography of Pirandello to learn about the relationship Pirandello had with his mentally unstable wife. Then research the relationship between American author F. Scott Fitzgerald and his wife, Zelda, who had numerous emotional breakdowns after 1930 and was institutionalized several times, eventually dying in a fire in a mental hospital in Asheville, North Carolina, in 1948. Compare the two unstable marriages and their effects on the literary careers of the two authors.
- Read Pirandello's "Preface" to *Six Characters in Search of an Author* for his description of the genesis of his play. Then read interviews in such books as *In Their Own Words* (1988) and *The Playwright's Art* (1995) to see how contemporary playwrights respond to questions about how they initially discover their characters and stories. What conclusions can you make about the process of artistic creation?
- Research what psychologists say about the human concept of self and compare their generalizations with the observations that Pirandello presents in *Six Characters in Search of an Author*. Where does the concept of personal identity come from and why is it so important to the human psyche?
- Research the stage history of *Six Characters in Search of an Author* to see how various audiences and critics in different countries and times have responded to the play. How can expectations of the conventional and/or of the unconventional color an audience member's response to an artistic experience?
- Research the concepts of Relativity and the Uncertainty Principle in Physics, with especial attention to Albert Einstein and Werner Karl Heisenberg, and compare the scientific treatment of these issues with Pirandello's artistic treatment.

for example, is the commonly held belief in the permanence of a personal identity.

Most people believe that they exist as a relatively stable personality, that they are basically the same people throughout their lives. But Pirandello and the Father directly challenge this belief when the Father asks the Producer in Act III "do you really know who you are?" The Producer blubbers, "what? Who I am? I am me!" But the Father undermines this self-assurance by pointing out that on any particular day the Producer does not see himself in the same way he saw himself at another time in the past. All people can remember ideas that they don't have any more, illusions they once fervently believed in, or simply things that look different now from the way they once appeared to be. The Father leads the Producer to admit that "all these realities of today are going to seem tomorrow as if they had been an illusion," that "perhaps you ought to distrust your own sense of reality." Trapped by these observations, the Producer cries, "but everybody knows that [his reality] can change, don't they? It's always changing! Just like everybody else's!"

This question of a permanent personal identity is crucial to the Father because the Stepdaughter is trying to characterize him as a lecherous and even incestuous man. The Father knows that "we all, you see, think of ourselves as one single person: but it's not true: each of us is several different people, and all these people live inside us. With one person we seem like this and with another we seem very different. But we always have the illusion of being the same person for everybody and of always being the same person in everything we do. But it's not true! It's not true!" The psychological and physiological needs that led the Father to the brothel were a part of him he does not value; but other people, like his stepdaughter and former wife, choose to define him by this weak moment. "We realise then, [he says] that every part of us was not involved in what we'd been doing and that it would be a dreadful injustice of other people to judge us only by this one action as we dangle there, hanging in chains, fixed for all eternity, as if the whole of one's personality were summed up in that single, interrupted action.'' The Father regrets the incident at Madame Pace's brothel but asserts that a human being cannot be defined as a consistent personal identity. The reality is that a human being (from the real world at least) changes so drastically from day to day that he cannot be said to be the same person at any time in his life. A human being is perhaps different hour by hour and may end up being 100,000 essentially different people before his life has ended.

STYLE

The Play Within the Play

The most obvious device that Pirandello uses to convey his themes is to portray the action as a play within a play. The initial play within a play is relatively easy for the audience to handle—Pirandello's own *Rules of the Game* is being performed in rehearsal by a troupe of actors. Then the ''characters'' enter and they seem to embody a completely different play within the play. Furthermore, they insist on acting out the story that have brought to the rehearsal, which is done twice, once by themselves and again by the actors. And once the audience has more or less assimilated all of this, a seventh character, Madame Pace, is created on the spot, as if out of thin air. The effect is similar to that presented with nesting boxes, one inside another and another inside that until the audience gets so far away from their easy faith in their ability to distinguish between reality and illusion that they might throw up their hands like the Producer and simply say, ''Make believe?! Reality?! Oh, go to hell the lot of you! Lights! Lights! Lights!''

Throughout the production of *Six Characters in Search of an Author* the audience in fact experiences the difficulty of distinguishing between reality and illusion that constitutes Pirandello's main theme. And the Producer's company of actors in many ways speaks for the audience throughout—from the initial, derisive incredulity at the entrance of the ''characters'' to the ambivalent response at the end of the play. And a crucial moment in this process comes early in Act I, after the derisive laughter of the actors has died down somewhat, and the Father explains that ''we want to live, sir . . . only for a few moments—in you.'' In response, a young actor says, pointing to the Stepdaughter, ''I don't mind . . . so long as I get her.'' This comically libidinous response is ignored by everyone on stage, but it represents an important turning point in the minds of the actors in the company and in the minds of the audience as well. It embodies a playful, tentative acceptance of the illusion, a making do with what's available, an abandonment to the situation as it presents itself. In short, it represents the response to the mystery of life to which human beings obsessed with absolute certainty are ultimately reduced. One must simply get on with life and make the best of it, accepting the hopelessness of trying to draw fine distinctions between what is real and what is not.

Comedy

A less obvious device in the play is Pirandello's use of laughter to lighten the audience's confrontation with this frustrating collision of reality and illusion. The play is not easily seen as humorous on the page, but in production the humor can be rich and is certainly essential in order to reassure the audience that their inability to easily distinguish between reality and illusion is an inevitable but ultimately comic part of human existence.

The humor is most obvious in the frustrations of the acting troupe. Serious but self-important, they are comical in their inability to deal with anything they are too inflexible to understand. The Producer is admirable in the way he finally bends to the unusual situation and vaguely sees the emotional intensity that the ''characters'' have brought to him. But he is ultimately comical because he is hopelessly obsessed with stage conventions. He insists on trying to ''fit'' this phenomenon within the boundaries of what he's most familiar with and his efforts are comically doomed. In the Edward Storer translation of Pirandello's original text, the play ends with the Producer throwing up his hands and saying ''never in my life has such a thing happened to me.'' What often makes comedy rich is witnessing human beings forced into being resilient under the common, existential circumstance of confronting the ultimate mystery of the universe.

But the play also displays a grim kind of humor in the desperation of the ''characters,'' who stumble across this rehearsal looking for an ''author'' and end up settling for a director with decidedly commercial tastes. The Producer is not an author who can complete their story but someone who depends on a script that's finished. The best that he can do is to exemplify the incompleteness the "characters" have brought him; the worst he can do is to create more barriers to their sense of an accurate portrayal of their story, which he what he most comically does. The Father and Stepdaughter laugh when the actors portray them so differently from the way they see themselves, but the joke is ultimately on them.

At the very beginning of the play, the Producer is complaining of the obscurity of Pirandello's *Rules of the Game.* He is satirically instructing his leading actor that he must "be symbolic of the shells of the eggs you are beating." It is a very funny moment, given the actors' and Producer's frustration, as well as Pirandello's playful self-denigration. But it is also a moment filled with rich comic ambiguity because the Producer's dismissive explanation is quite seriously what Pirandello's play is all about: "[the eggs] are symbolic of the empty form of reason, without its content, blind instinct! You are reason and your wife is instinct: you are playing a game where you have been given parts and in which you are not just yourself but the puppet of yourself. Do you see? . . . Neither do I! Come on, let's get going; you wait till you see the end! You haven't seen anything yet!"

HISTORICAL CONTEXT

Surrealism

Pirandello's *Six Characters in Search of an Author* was a watershed in the history of drama because its form and content were so revolutionary. And to some extent Pirandello's play relates to a more systematic artistic revolution in the 1920s—Surrealism. As C.W.E. Bigsby has said, Surrealism "is essentially concerned with liberating the imagination and with expanding the definition of reality."

The Surrealists insisted that by freeing the mind from the limiting controls of rationality, logic, consciousness, or aesthetic conventions, an artist could reach a higher reality that would include the fantastic and the marvelous—qualities that had generally been considered antithetical to realism. Coined by French poet Guillaume Apollinaire and championed by French poet Andre Breton, the term was described in Breton's famous 1924 *Manifesto on Surrealism* as a resolution of two states of mind—dream and reality. Joined together, these two states of mind made a sort of absolute or sur-reality. When the movement made inroads in England, an attempt was made to substitute the phrase "superreality" but the alternate terminology never caught on.

Earlier movements like Cubism and Dada had prepared the way for the liberating spirit of Surrealism, and the general result of this liberation was a challenge to the dominance of the realistic movement, which had its roots in the 19th century and which still survives today as a very powerful standard in the popular arts. But the "avant-garde," of which Pirandello is now taken to be an important part, has always distrusted excessively powerful traditions and has continually sought to enlarge the scope of artistic possibilities.

In his book *Rococo to Cubism in Art and Literature,* art historian Wylie Sypher observed what he called a "cubist drama" in *Six Characters in Search of an Author,* claiming that "Pirandello 'destroys' drama much as the cubists destroyed conventional things. He will not accept as authentic 'real' people or the cliche of the theatre any more than the cubist accepts as authentic the 'real' object [or] the cliche of deep perspective." A more thorough discussion of Pirandello's affinity with the Surrealist movement comes from Anna Balakian, who recognized that "an affinity has often been seen between the theatre of Pirandello and the surrealist mode because both adhere to such notions as the 'absurd,' the unconventional, the iconoclastic, and the shocking to stir the receivers of the created work." But in examining closely the elements of the surrealist manifestos and Pirandello's plays, Balakian concluded that "Pirandello and the surrealists shared a moment in the history of the arts but followed parallel rather than converging paths in their spectacular irreverence for the traditional."

Italian Fascism

In 1921, as *Six Characters in Search of an Author* was creating an international celebrity of Pirandello, the Italian statesman Benito Mussolini was consolidating his power and rising toward the position he would hold through World War II as the fascist leader of Italy. An Italian nationalist, revolutionary, and socialist from his early years, Mussolini founded his own fascist party in 1919. Italy was suffering social upheaval as a result of World War I and Mussolini capitalized on the situation to raise support for armed fascist squads that attacked Mussolini's political opponents and killed hundreds of people. On May 15, 1921, five days after *Six Characters in Search of an Author* premiered in Rome, Mussolini and 35 other Fascists were elected

COMPARE & CONTRAST

- **1921:** Franklin Delano Roosevelt, 32nd President of the United States from 1933 to 1945, contracts the poliomyelitis that will cripple him for life and confine him to a wheelchair or require him to wear heavy braces to walk. Since the appearance of robust vitality was necessary for the presidential image, the reality of Roosevelt's paralysis was downplayed by the media and went largely ignored or undiscovered by the American public. Roosevelt became the only U.S. President to be re-elected three times.

  Today: Starting with the presidencies of Lyndon Baines Johnson and (especially) Richard Nixon, the media have become increasingly dedicated to examining the appearance of presidents and other political figures. However, Roosevelt's disability still remains a largely ignored part of his presidency. In 1997, a memorial statue of Roosevelt in Washington, D.C., created some controversy when—rather than obviously placing him in a wheelchair—the statue portrayed him as seated in an office chair with casters and with a large cloak draped over his legs that essentially obscured his disability.

- **1921:** Eight baseball players from the 1919 Chicago White Sox major league baseball team go to trial in June on charges of accepting bribes from gamblers to purposely lose the World Series against Cincinnati in 1919. Indicted in 1920, their trial in June and July of 1921 ended in an acquittal, but the presiding judge for the grand jury, Kenesaw Mountain Landis, had become the first Commissioner of major league baseball in 1921 and banned the players from baseball for life in spite of the court's verdict.

  Today: These eight members of the "Black Sox," including the great Shoeless Joe Jackson, are still considered ineligible for induction into baseball's Hall of Fame, the truth of their criminality having been decided by Judge Landis rather than by the process of the legal system. In what is perhaps a similarly contested process of judgment, the 7th Commissioner of major league baseball, A. Bartlett Giamatti, banned Cincinnati's Pete Rose from a place in the Hall of Fame in 1989, despite Rose's all-time major league record 4,256 hits, because Rose was accused of illegally betting on baseball games.

- **1921:** The futuristic drama of social satire, *R.U.R.,* (Rossum's Universal Robots), by Czechoslovakian playwright Karel Capek, opens in Prague. The robots are manufactured men and women who work without complaining. They are so difficult to distinguish from real people that one character decided the robots were capable of developing a soul. When robots around the world revolt against their masters, humanity is almost destroyed. The robots had finally begun to act precisely like human beings.

  Today: Though *R.U.R.* is not widely produced today, the term and concept it essentially created—"robot"—has now become an established part of our vocabulary and thought. The word "robot" was a translation from the Czech word for "forced labor" and while Rossum's robots were manufactured from artificial flesh and blood, Fritz Lang's popular 1926 film, *Metropolis,* used the term to describe a creature made of metal and that more mechanical concept of robot is what survives today. Today's widespread industrial use of robotics and the controversies over genetic engineering have perhaps given a new immediacy to Capek's drama.

to the Italian parliament and began their struggle for power from within the governmental structure. Already known to his followers as *il duce* (the leader), Mussolini organized squads of armed men at a Fascists' convention in Naples in October of 1922 and began his famous "march on Rome." Taking over the Italian government from his position as Prime Minister, Mussolini gradually consolidated his power and became virtual dictator by January of 1925.

Pirandello's connection with Mussolini and Italian Fascism is a complex and controversial part of Pirandello's life that is still being debated today. The connection with his art is roundabout but equally complex and controversial. In October of 1922, as Mussolini and his Blackshirts were marching on Rome, Pirandello's second masterpiece, *Henry IV,* was consolidating his rise to international recognition. Then, on June 10, 1924, Mussolini's men murdered a leading Socialist member of the Italian parliament named Giacomo Matteotti, arousing considerable public uneasiness and controversy. In September of 1924, Pirandello, now an international celebrity and an Italian literary hero, demonstrated his support of Mussolini by giving the fascist newspaper, *L'Impero,* a copy of a letter to Mussolini asking to join the Fascist party. Scholars still debate Pirandello's motives and the sincerity of his political commitment to Fascism, but the most significant ramification for the history of drama is that in the same year Pirandello and a group of his colleagues founded the Italian Arts Theatre company and Mussolini's political power helped Pirandello gain financial support for a theatre based in Rome. The company's first production was in May in Milan. As the company flourished Pirandello met actress Marta Abba, for whom most of his later plays were written, and his troupe began touring extensively throughout Italy, Europe, and North and South America. Thus, it was indirectly through Pirandello's involvement with Italian Fascism that his plays became so thoroughly disseminated around the world. Pirandello's theatre company collapsed in 1928 because of financial problems, but by that time his international reputation and dramatic impact were well-established.

CRITICAL OVERVIEW

The first production of *Six Characters in Search of an Author* at the Teatro Valle in Rome on May 10, 1921, astonished its unsuspecting audience. As Gaspare Giudice reported in his biography of Pirandello, ''things started to go badly from the first, when the spectators came into the theatre and realized that the curtain was raised and that there was no scenery.'' Some spectators considered this ''gratuitous exhibitionism,'' especially as it was yoked with stagehands and actors milling about as if they were not really in a play. The arrival of the ''characters'' was even more ''extraordinary'' and ''all this was enough to infuriate anyone who had gone to the theatre to spend a pleasant evening. The first catcalls were followed by shouts of disapproval, and, when the opponents of the play realized that they were in the majority, they started to shout in chorus, 'ma-ni-co-mio' ('madhouse') or 'bu-ffo-ne' ('buffoon').'' The production had its supporters, but their defense of Pirandello's play created even more confusion, and the audience members, actors, and critics ended up exchanging blows that even spread out into the street and into a general riot after the play had ended.

Cooler heads ultimately prevailed, led perhaps by the review the next day by Adriano Tilgher, who would later become one of the most important and influential critics of Pirandello's work. Tilgher pronounced that the production was ''a success imposed by a minority on a bewildered, confused public who were basically trying hard to understand.'' Tilgher concluded that ''from today, we can say that Pirandello is most certainly among the leading creators of a new spiritual environment, one of the most deserving precursors of tomorrow's genius if tomorrow ever comes.''

A few months later the production was remounted in Milan and because of the intervening publication of the text, audience and critics were prepared for the play's radical innovations of style and theme. Over the next three years, *Six Characters in Search of an Author* was produced successfully all over the world.

An especially important production of the play directed by Georges Pitoeff was mounted in Paris on April 10, 1923. The production had, according to Thomas Bishop, ''the effect of an earthquake.'' Most famous for Pitoeff's ingenious device of bringing the characters down onto the stage in an elevator, the production created ''characters'' who were deemed ''supra-terrestrial,'' and Germane Bree followed the famous French dramatist Jean Anouilh in saying that because of the influence that Pirandello had on generations of French dramatists ''the first performance of Pirandello in Paris still stands out as one of the most significant dates in the annals of the contemporary French stage.''

Another very important production of the play occurred in Berlin in December, 1924. Directed by the legendary Max Reinhardt, the characters were on stage from the beginning of the play but hidden from the audience until, as Olga Ragusa described it, ''a violet light made them appear out of the darkness like 'apparitions' or ghosts.'' The production was said in a review by Rudolph Pechel to have fully realized ''the magnitude and the possibilities of [Pirandello's] theme.'' According to Pechel, ''it was Max Reinhardt rather than Pirandello who was the poet of this performance'' because ''Reinhardt felt the potential of this piece and offered a master production of his art in which the audience became fully aware of all the horror of this gloomy world.'' According to Pechel, the ''characters'' were ''like departed souls in Hades yearning for life-giving blood.''

In 1925 Pirandello's own theatre company took the play to London as part of its world tour and the play was performed in Italian because the British censors had objected to the play's references to incest. A reviewer for the London *Times* maintained that in Italian ''the tragic personages are more tragic, the squalid personages more squalid, and the comic remnant more emphatically and volubly comic.'' He called it ''a new theatrical amusement. For it is certainly amusing to see characters disintegrated, as it were, on the stage before you, wondering how much of them is illusion and how much reality, and setting you pondering over these perplexing problems while enjoying at the same time the orthodox dramatic thrill.'' A reviewer for the *Manchester Guardian* simply proclaimed the production ''a dramatized version of a first-year course upon appearance and reality'' in which ''the author's strength lies not in any philosophical brilliance but in the practical cunning whereby he as made metaphysics actable.''

Between 1922 and 1927 productions of the play appeared throughout Europe, the United States, and even in Argentina and Japan, testing directors, audiences, and critics around the world. As a result of the many rich responses to his work, Pirandello fashioned a significantly revised version of his play in 1925 in which he suggested the use of masks for the ''characters'' and appended his famous ''Preface'' that reveals the genesis of the work and Pirandello's concept of its thematic elements. Today, the ''Preface'' remains an almost integral part of the play itself.

Important productions around the world continued throughout the decades following Pirandello's death, including a New York production in October, 1955, adapted and directed by Tyrone Guthrie and a three-act opera version that appeared in New York in 1959 with a libretto by Denis Johnston and a score by Hugo Weisgall. As Antonio Illiano reported, Pirandello's *Six Characters in Search of an Author* ''was like a bombshell that blew out the last and weary residues of the old realistic drama'' and today it is widely considered one of the most important and influential plays in the history of twentieth-century drama.

CRITICISM

Terry R. Nienhuis

Nienhuis is a Ph.D. specializing in modern and contemporary drama. In this essay he discusses the role that uncertainty plays in Pirandello's Six Characters in Search of an Author.

Pirandellian themes like the relativity of truth, the constantly changing nature of personal identity, or the difficulty of distinguishing between reality and illusion or between sanity and madness all have a common thread—they all point to uncertainty as a significant part of human experience. As John Gassner has observed, Pirandello was consistently ''expressing a conviction that nothing in life is certain except its uncertainty.''

In *Six Characters in Search of an Author* uncertainty begins with the introduction of the ''characters.'' The claim they make about their reality is obviously counter to fact (they are, of course, actors), but Pirandello makes their case so convincing that it is ultimately difficult for the audience to feel certain about what they know to be true. It is interesting to see how Pirandello does this.

First of all, Pirandello has encouraged the audience to adopt their customary willingness to suspend disbelief and accept the stage illusion as reality. As one-dimensional as the members of the theatrical troupe ultimately appear to be, the play seems to begin in a spirit of ultra-realism—with a stage hand nailing boards together (how mundane is the sound of a hammer meeting a nail), with a set that appears unprepared for a formal ''show,'' and with actors improvising their lines so as to sound as authentic as possible. Therefore, if the audience has taken these initial characters for real, what must they do with a group that claims they are even more real than the actors in the Producer's troupe? And the ''characters'' persist in their claim with such a vehemence that their claim becomes compelling.

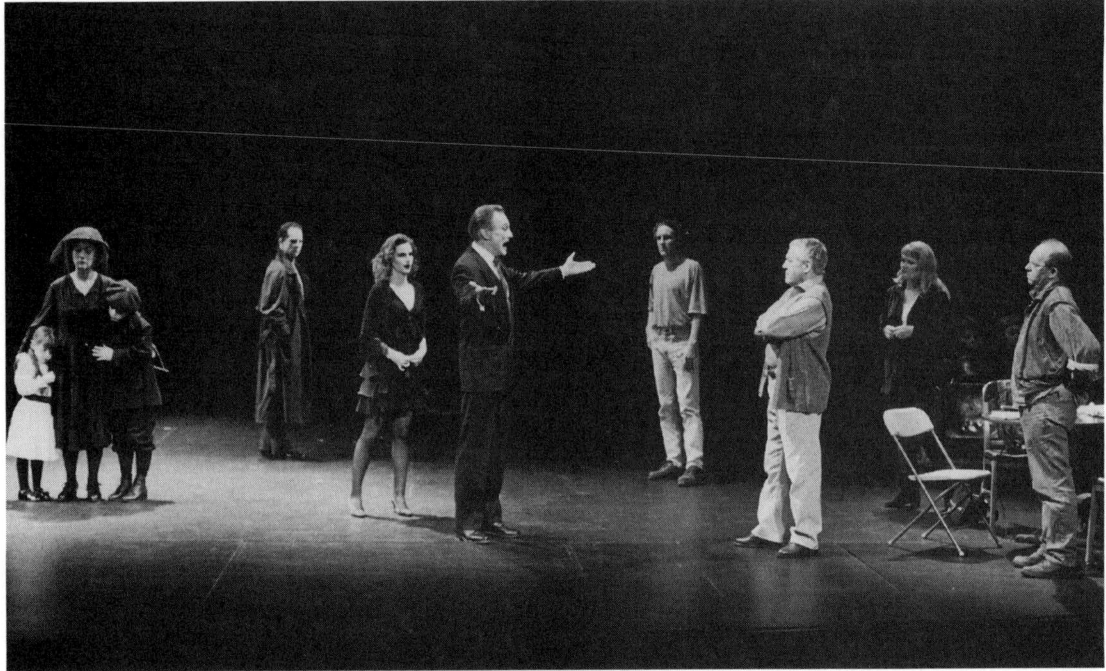

A scene from an American Repertory Theatre production of Pirandello's play directed by noted theater critic Robert Brustein

Contemporary jurisprudence demonstrates a similar phenomenon. No matter how certain a defendant's guilty conduct seems to be, if the person charged with a crime persists in claiming innocence an air of uncertainty eventually envelops the proceedings and significant numbers believe the defendant innocent.

In this way, the Mother is especially difficult for the audience to dismiss as "merely an actress" because she is so simple and direct in her assumption of "reality." As Pirandello says in his "Preface," the Mother "never doubts for a moment that she is already alive, nor does it ever occur to her to inquire in what respect and why she is alive. . . . she lives in a stream of feeling that never ceases." And perhaps her most powerful moment comes near the end of Act II when the Producer verbalizes a very common sense approach to her suffering. The Producer is willing to grant the Mother some kind of reality but points out that if her story has happened already she should not be surprised and distraught by its reoccurrence. But the Mother says, "No! It's happening now, as well: it's happening all the time. I'm not acting my suffering! Can't you understand that? I'm alive and here now but I can never forget that terrible moment of agony, that repeats itself endlessly and vividly in my mind." In spite of the collision with common sense that this assertion entails, intensity like this makes the fiction so compelling that the audience is forced to question its own certainty, if only subconsciously and only in a flashing moment. The genius of Pirandello is that he calls attention to the illusion and at the same time helps to perpetuate it, thereby demonstrating the awesome power that illusion has over the human mind and the inevitable state of uncertainty that must result.

An even more obvious contribution to the audience's sense of uncertainty is that Pirandello allows different versions of events to be presented but never suggests which might be more near the "truth." Under what circumstances, for instance, did the Mother leave with the Father's secretary? Did she leave of her own accord? Or was she forced to leave? What were the Father's feelings for his stepdaughter while the young girl was growing up? What actually happened in the brothel? The Father, Mother, and Stepdaughter all answer these questions differently but there is no adjudication. In fact, the resolution of the different versions is simply ignored and becomes moot as the play ends in the melodramatic drowning and suicide. And Pirandel-

WHAT DO I READ NEXT?

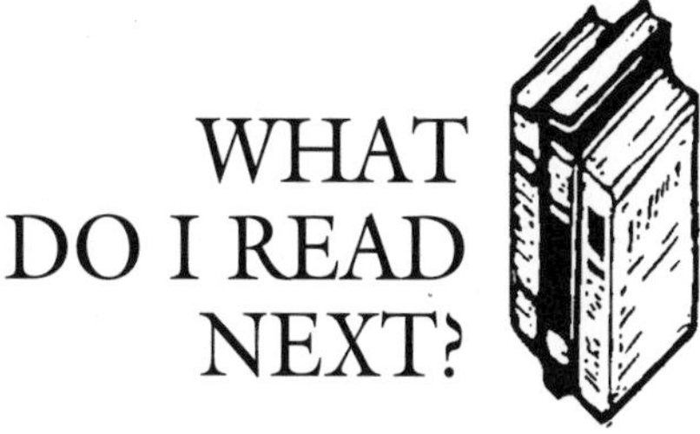

- Pirandello's second "masterpiece," *Henry IV* (1922), is another examination of human role-playing and the subtle differences between art and life, madness and sanity. An accident leaves a man thinking for years that he is the German Emperor Henry IV. One day in private the man regains his sanity but decides to continue playing the role of Emperor and is finally trapped in his assumed identity.
- Pirandello's *Right You Are (If You Think So)* (1917) has been called by many, including Eric Bentley, the "quintessential Pirandello." The situation in the story is told in three conflicting versions and the audience can never know which one to accept as true.
- Many of Pirandello's novels elaborate on themes developed in the major plays. In *The Late Mattia Pascal* (1904) the hero permits himself to be thought dead and assumes a false identity to escape his past but discovers that he cannot start a new life without his old self. In *One, None, and a Hundred Thousand* (1926) a man who realizes he cannot be known by the multiplicity of his many selves renounces life and becomes the inmate of a poorhouse.
- *R.U.R.* (Rossum's Universal Robots; 1922), by Czechoslovakian playwright Karel Capek, presents a slightly different kind of confrontation between human and non-human figures who closely resemble human beings.
- *No Exit* (1948), by French playwright Jean-Paul Sartre, takes place in Hell and focuses on the Pirandellian idea that we are the roles we play and that our personal identity is constructed by how others see us rather than by our own concept of ourselves.
- *The Rehearsal* (1950), by French playwright Jean Anouilh, presents a Pirandellian situation involving romance, role playing, and a play-within-a-play. A group of aristocrats meets in a villa and works out its romantic entanglements through their amateur production of a play.
- *Old Times* (1971), by British playwright Harold Pinter, frustrates the audience's desire for certainty when the memories of the three characters are quite contradictory and the audience cannot know whose version of the past is most accurate.
- *The Purple Rose of Cairo* (1985), a film by Woody Allen, is a modern, cinematic treatment of the Pirandellian idea that fictional characters can have a certain kind of reality that rivals the reality of human beings. A number of other Woody Allen films deal with similar Pirandellian situations, such as *Deconstructing Harry* (1997).

---

lo makes clear that the resolution would be impossible anyway because uncertainty is at the heart of language itself. In Act I the Father says, "we all have a world of things inside ourselves and each one of us has his own private world. How can we understand each other if the words I use have the sense and the value that I expect them to have, but whoever is listening to me inevitably thinks that those same words have a different sense and value, because of the private world he has inside himself too. We think we understand each other; but we never do. Look! All my pity, all my compassion for this woman (*Pointing to the Mother*) she sees as ferocious cruelty."

After one examines how Pirandello puts his audience into this condition of uncertainty, the next question is why does he choose to do this? In part, he creates uncertainty in his audience because he believes uncertainty is the natural condition that human beings must learn to live with. In his famous essay, "On Humor" (1908), Pirandello summed up this attitude toward human existence, asserting that "all phenomena either are illusory or their reason

"PIRANDELLIAN THEMES LIKE THE RELATIVITY OF TRUTH, THE CONSTANTLY CHANGING NATURE OF PERSONAL IDENTITY, OR THE DIFFICULTY OF DISTINGUISHING BETWEEN REALITY AND ILLUSION OR BETWEEN SANITY AND MADNESS ALL HAVE A COMMON THREAD—THEY ALL POINT TO UNCERTAINTY AS A SIGNIFICANT PART OF HUMAN EXPERIENCE."

escapes us inexplicably. Our knowledge of the world and of ourselves refuses to be given the objective value which we usually attempt to attribute to it. Reality is a continuously illusory construction.'' Consequently, the ''humorist,'' or artist, sees that ''the feeling of incongruity, of not knowing any more which side to take,'' is the feeling he or she must create in the audience. Illusions are the human attempt to create certainty where it doesn't really exist, and all fall prey to the temptation. Pirandello's art simply puts many of mankind's most common illusions on center stage to demonstrate their flimsy inadequacy and encourages the audience to recognize these illusions for what they are. Pirandello describes life as ''a continuous flow,'' with logic, reason, abstractions, ideals, and concepts acting as illusory constructs that attempt to fix this flux into a reality that can be stabilized and more certainly known. But Pirandello concludes that ''man doesn't have any absolute idea or knowledge of life, but only a variable feeling changing with the times, conditions, and luck.''

Umberto Mariani has asserted that the typical character in a Pirandellian work of art ''has lost the feeling of comforting stability'' and chafes under the ''tragic knowledge that he cannot achieve what he seeks and needs; a universe of certainties, an absolute that would allow him to affirm himself.'' Robert Brustein observed that ''[For Pirandello] objective reality has become virtually inaccessible, and all one can be sure of is the illusion-making faculty of the subjective mind.'' Brustein noted that ''man is occasionally aware of the illusionary nature of his concepts; but to be human is to desire form; anything formless fills man with dread and uncertainty.'' Aureliu Weiss has summarized all of this most abruptly, asserting that Pirandello simply ''derided human certainty and denounced the fragility of the truth.'' But Weiss has also brought this discussion of content back around to its ultimate focus on form. When everything seems uncertain, ''such a concept cannot be expressed through the traditional forms. It needs its own style. . . . What was needed to succeed in such an enterprise . . . was to strike an initial blow strong enough to shatter our certainty . . . to create an atmosphere where reality would become less concrete and where illusion could play freely and gently worm its way into the audience's consciousness. No longer sure of anything, the spectator would accept as normal the oscillation between reality and illusion.''

But Pirandello's obsession with uncertainty can also be accounted for by a basic understanding of the intellectual history of the Western world—which has witnessed a gradual erosion of certitude, from a relatively high degree of certainty in the Medieval world to the relatively high degree of uncertainty in the 20th century. Propelled, ironically, by the discoveries of science, this process has been developing for hundreds of years and has simply culminated in the implications of Darwin, Freud, and Einstein, among others. Anthony Caputi, in his *Pirandello and the Crisis of Modern Consciousness,* asserted that ''Pirandello began where Matthew Arnold began, with the conviction that the world was in disarray, that the system of beliefs that had provided coherence and continuity for centuries had broken down, and that the new sciences could yield little more than organized barbarism.'' What Caputi called ''the crisis of modern consciousness'' is ''that stage in which not just traditional ways of deriving coherence and value were lost but the capacity for deriving alternative coherences by way of the reason has been undermined as the reason itself has been subverted as an authority. As the idea gained ground that every mind is a relative instrument, subject not to the grand program for coherence provided by Christianity or, for that matter, by any other traditional orthodoxy, but subject to its own conditions, a new variability and a new insecurity were born. Not only did men and women not look to external sources for guides to value, they no longer looked to reason.''

As Renato Poggioli put it, "logic, or reason, according to the classics of philosophy, had always had a universal value, equally valid for each *individual of the human race.*" But "Pirandello does not believe in reason as an absolute and transcendent value." Reason for Pirandello is simply "a practical activity," a tool the mind uses as it needs to create and defend its illusions. Pirandello was the dramatist of consciousness, examining how the human mind apprehended the world, and he decided that humans could be certain of nothing that was produced from such a variety of mental platforms. The old standards of "reason" and "logic," thought to be constant guides implanted by God in the minds of all human beings, were dead, to be replaced by the disconcerting phenomenon of relativism. In a process of questioning that began most vigorously in the Renaissance, all that had been taken as certain for centuries was gradually re-examined until finally the process of consciousness itself fell under scrutiny and humans discovered that the workings of the mind delivered more tricks than dependable conclusions. As Caputi finally put it, Pirandello and "most of the artists and writers of the [twentieth] century" saw the human mind as "a frail, uncertain faculty capable of little more than self-deception."

John Gassner concluded that Pirandello's "work remains a monument to the questioning and self-tormenting human intellect which is at war . . . with its own limitations. Once the intellect has conquered problem after problem without solving the greatest question of all—namely, whether it is real itself rather than illusory—it reaches an impasse. Pirandello is the poet of that impasse. He is also the culmination of centuries of intellectual progress which have failed to make life basically more reasonable or satisfactory. He ends with a question mark." And Robert Brustein concluded by saying that "after Pirandello, no dramatist has been able to write with quite the same certainty as before."

Source: Terry R. Nienhuis, for *Drama for Students,* Gale, 1998.

Susan Bassnet

In this excerpt, Bassnet provides an overview of the play.

This is the play that established Pirandello's international reputation as a playwright. Already well-known in Italy as a prose writer, critic, and poet, he had begun to write for the theatre shortly before World War I, increasing his output rapidly after 1918. *Six Characters* caused a scandal when it first appeared, and the first night ended with a riot, due to the taboo subject-matter of the play: incestuous desire.

"THE INGENIOUS STRUCTURE OF THE PLAY CONTINUES TO RAISE IMPORTANT QUESTIONS ABOUT THE NATURE OF STAGE ILLUSION AND ITS RELATIONSHIP TO LIFE."

Six Characters is the first of three plays known as the "theatre-in-the-theatre" triology, because the action involves the attempted staging of a play within another play. A rehearsal of a Pirandello play is supposedly taking place in an Italian theatre, but is interrupted by the arrival of six people, who claim to be characters looking for a playwright to tell their story. That story then gradually unfolds, told principally by the Father and the Stepdaughter. At some point in the past, the Father and the Mother have separated, and the Mother has gone to live with another man by whom she has had children. She is accompanied on stage by the Son and by two smaller children, the Boy and the Little Girl. Relations between the characters are strained: the Stepdaughter detests the Son and the Boy, the Son has a grudge against the Mother, and the Father is an outsider altogether. The Father claims to have always loved the Mother and her children, but the Stepdaughter depicts him as a debauched elderly man who used to spy on her when she was a child.

In the second act, the Characters summon up a seventh person, Madame Pace, the owner of a seedy milliner's shop that serves as a brothel, where the Stepdaughter was working and where the Father met her when he came looking for a girl. The incestuous encounter between the Father and the Stepdaughter is interrupted by the Mother's cry. In the last act, the Mother tries to win over her sullen, resentful Son, but while her attention is distracted, the Little Girl drowns in a fountain and the Boy shoots himself. The Stepdaughter runs away and the Father, Mother, and Son are left, prisoners of their own despair. The boundary between fiction and reality has completely broken down, the Director and the other Actors are left bewildered by what has happened, and the play ends.

Pirandello uses ingenious devices to mark the passage from one act to another, and manages to preserve the shape of the well-made play while simultaneously deconstructing it as a form. The text of the play was modified considerably after the famous Pitoeff production in 1923, when the appearance of the Six Characters, one of the great moments of theatre magic, was heightened by having them arrive on stage in a huge elevator. In the preface that he added to the second version of the play, Pirandello explains the function of the Characters in relation to his own creative process. He was constantly concerned with the problem of the vital, moving process that constitutes life, in contrast to the rigid fixity of art, and *Six Characters* explores that duality. The Characters are fixed in their tragic story, unmovably, for as Pirandello says, they are created out of "unvarying fantasy." Ironically, although the Characters are fictitious, Pirandello argues that they appear more real than the Actors with their "changeable naturalness." Art, for Pirandello, can seem more real than life, and this is the paradox he seeks to expose.

What Pirandello does in *Six Characters* is to strip the play down to its bones, offering the audience the basic tools—the Actors, the Characters, a story—but leaving the final interpretation open. The play thus becomes an investigation of the processes of artistic creation; it is a play about playing that uses the device of play-making as its central, structural principle.

After the initial shock at the subject-matter of the play, *Six Characters* became a huge success, both in Italy and around the world. It has since come to be regarded as a classic experimental play that prefigured many later developments in the theatre. The work of Brecht and Piscator in exposing the theatricality of theatre finds its parallel in it, while the relativity of truth that means there is no single, straightforward solution to the story of the Six Characters, foreshadows the "Theatre of the Absurd."

Six Characters has remained one of Pirandello's most popular and best-known plays. It continues to be performed throughout the world and has been televised, filmed, and, (in 1959) turned into an opera. Although the subject-matter no longer causes feelings of outrage, the ingenious structure of the play continues to raise important questions about the nature of stage illusion and its relationship to life.

Source: Susan Bassnet, review of *Six Characters in Search of an Author* in *International Dictionary of Theatre 1: Plays,* edited by Mark Hawkins-Dady, St. James Press, 1992, pp. 747–48.

Martin Hoyle

Hoyle reviews a revival production of Pirandello's play. While he avers the classic status of the work, the critic has less-than-favorable impressions of the production.

If you think the critic's function is parasitic, wait till you hear Pirandello on actors. The writer's famed distinction between reality and illusion makes it plain, in *Six Characters* at least, that actors are as removed from the blood and sinew of real feeling as the recording angels of the centre stalls.

The mummer's endemic shallowness is underlined by Michael Rudman's new production at the Olivier. In the original, the theatre company that we meet in the throes of rehearsing another Pirandello play, *The Rules of the Game,* is not obtrusively characterized. Personalities are fleetingly illuminated by the odd detail. But the irrelevant waffle of Nicholas Wright's new version plunges, heaven help us, into a backstage comedy, as stereotype thespians swap banalities and Leslie Sands's old stager confuses Polonius with the Gravedigger. (Though still rooted in Twenties Italy, the company is preparing *Hamlet.*) It might be Rattigan's *Harlequinade.* On the lethargic second Press night this embarrassing attempt to individualise the boys and girls were hampered by the listless snail's pace and, from the smaller roles, a delivery of lines ('Shh—look!' 'What's going on?') that was little better than amateur—Paul Hastings' sympathetic and lively vignette as Horatio always excepted.

In an attempt, presumably, to anglicise and modernise the frame of emotional reference, if not the setting, Wright and Rudman flatly contradict the original at some points. The mysterious family, frozen forever in some ghastly tragedy, who interrupt the proceedings and beg to be dramatised, should enter normally but be noticeably 'different' (Pirandello suggested half-masks). Here they suddenly appear in a black-out to a clap of thunder, but are thereafter 'normal' to the point of triviality. Pirandello ends his play with the producer stumbling terrified through the darkened theatre at the final vision of those figures fixed in an eternity of anguish—like the still-living acquaintance whom Dante sighted in the Inferno: he lives and breathes and goes about his business but he is already in hell—and, to the mocking laughter of the

Stepdaughter who breaks the confines of stage, auditorium and building, we remember Petrushka's showman, appalled at the doll's ghost, at the spectacle of something created assuming an independent existence. At the Olivier the imperturbable Director (Robin Bailey, whose drily undercutting smoothness provides the evening's main pleasure) utters the character's last line, asking for more light, and settles down at his desk. And that's that.

Throughout, the supernatural is hinted at (though Italians, the Sicilian awe of the evil eye apart, are robustly disinclined to *feerie*) while formality is rendered dully prosaic. The result is J. B. Priestley crossed with Tom Stoppard: as it were, *The Real Inspector Hound Calls.*

Everything is emphatic, pedantic; and this affects the playing. Lesley Sharp, a powerful actress as we know from the Royal Court, makes a liberated, hectoring Stepdaughter. She suggests little horror at being pushed across the narrow divide between respectable poverty and the shame of prostitution. She, or the director, confuses intensity with earnestness. And she is lumbered with that modern semi-literate Americanism that someone at the NT should have blue-pencilled at rehearsal stage when announcing that she is 'nauseous'. No, Miss Sharp; your lines may be nauseous. You are nauseated.

Richard Pasco goes along with the prevalent mood by playing the lustful Stepfather as a verbose, almost professorial, droll. Barbara Jefford, as we were reminded by the Fellini film, *And the Ship Sails On,* has a potentially riveting star presence. By no means is she the cowed, illiterate little wife, perpetually bowed in shame (I wish I'd seen *her* Stepdaughter in the 1963 production). Ralph Fiennes carries off the almost unspeaking part of the cold Son with dignity and perceptible style; but Di Langford's dressmaker-procuress is colourless—why disregard Pirandello's detailed description of the bedizened, bewigged old madam?

I suspect Mr Rudman has been misled by the 'reality/illusion' duality of much of Pirandello's work, and has overlooked the fact that *Six Characters* is for the most part about different sorts of illusion. In an effort to draw distinctions in the wrong places, the production merely turns what, according to conventional wisdom, is a modern classic into a stilted museum-piece.

Source: Martin Hoyle, review of *Six Characters in Search of an Author* in *Plays and Players,* Number 404, May, 1987, pp. 16–17.

"PIRANDELLO'S FAMED DISTINCTION BETWEEN REALITY AND ILLUSION MAKES IT PLAIN, IN *SIX CHARACTERS* AT LEAST, THAT ACTORS ARE AS REMOVED FROM THE BLOOD AND SINEW OF REAL FEELING AS THE RECORDING ANGELS OF THE CENTRE STALLS."

SOURCES

Balakian, Anna. "Pirandello's *Six Characters* and Surrealism," in *A Companion to Pirandello Studies,* edited by John Louis DiGaetani, Greenwood Press, 1991, pp. 185-92.

Bentley, Eric. "Varieties of Comic Experience," in his *The Playwright as Thinker: A Study of Drama in Modern Times,* Reynal & Hitchcock, 1946, p. 178.

Bigsby, C. W. E. *Dada & Surrealism,* Methuen, 1972, p. 78.

Bishop, Thomas. *Pirandello and the French Theatre,* New York University Press, 1960, p. 5.

Bree, Germaine. "Foreword," in *Pirandello and the French Theatre,* by Thomas Bishop, p. xi.

Brustein, Robert. "Luigi Pirandello," in his *The Theatre of Revolt: An Approach to the Modern Drama,* Little, Brown, 1962, pp. 281-317.

Caputi, Anthony. *Pirandello and the Crisis of Modern Consciousness,* University of Illinois Press, 1988, pp. 1, 5, 10.

Gassner, John. "Latin Postscripts—Benavente and Pirandello," in his *Masters of the Modern Drama,* 3rd ed., Dover, 1954, pp. 424-45.

Guidice, Gaspare. *Pirandello: A Biography,* translated by Alastair Hamilton, Oxford, 1975.

Illiano, Antonio. "Pirandello's *Six Characters in Search of an Author:* A Comedy in the Making," in *Italica,* March, 1967, p. 1.

London *Times.* Review of *Six Characters in Search of an Author,* excerpted in *File on Pirandello,* compiled by Susan Bassnett, Methuen, 1989, pp. 44.

Manchester Guardian. Review of *Six Characters in Search of an Author,* excerpted in *File on Pirandello,* compiled by Susan Bassnett, Methuen, 1989, pp. 44-45.

Mariani, Umberto. "The 'Pirandellian' Character," in *Canadian Journal of Italian Studies,* Vol. 12, Nos. 38-39, 1989, pp. 1-9.

Pechel, Rudolph. Review of *Six Characters in Search of an Author,* excerpted in *File on Pirandello,* compiled by Susan Bassnett, Methuen, 1989, pp. 43-44.

Pirandello, Luigi. "On Humor," translated by Teresa Novel, in *The Tulane Drama Review,* Spring, 1966, pp. 46-59.

Pirandello, Luigi. "Pirandello Confesses . . . Why and How He Wrote *Six Characters in Search of an Author*" (a translation of Pirandello's "Preface" by Leo Ongley), in *The Virginia Quarterly Review,* April, 1925, pp. 36-52.

Poggioli, Renato. "Pirandello in Retrospect," in *Italian Quarterly,* Winter, 1958, pp. 19-47.

Ragusa, Olga. "Sei personaggi in cerca d'autore," in *Luigi Pirandello: An Approach to His Theatre,* Edinburgh University Press, 1980, p. 167.

Sypher, Wylie. "Cubist Drama," in *Rococo to Cubism in Art and Literature,* Random House, 1960, p. 294.

Tilgher, Adriano. Review of *Six Characters in Search of an Author,* excerpted in *File on Pirandello,* compiled by Susan Bassnett, Methuen, 1989, pp. 41-42.

Weiss, Aureliu. "The Remorseless Rush of Time," edited and translated by Simone Sanzenback, in *The Tulane Drama Review,* Spring, 1966, pp. 30-45.

Wurman, Richard Saul. *NYC Access,* 4th ed., Access Press, 1991, p. 144.

FURTHER READING

Bentley, Eric. "*Six Characters in Search of an Author,*" in *The Pirandello Commentaries,* Northwestern University Press, 1986, pp. 57-77.
An essay that interprets the Father as a schizophrenic.

Cambon, Glauco, ed. *Pirandello: A Collection of Critical Essays,* Prentice Hall, 1967.
A collection of fourteen essays, including excerpts from Adriano Tilgher's famous "Life Versus Form" and Robert Brustein's essay on Pirandello from his *The Theatre of Revolt.*

Charney, Maurice. "Shakespearean and Pirandellian: *Hamlet* and *Six Characters in Search of an Author,*" *Modern Drama,* September, 1981, pp. 323-29.
Compares Pirandello's play with Shakespeare's *Hamlet* and Tom Stoppard's *Rosencrantz and Guildenstern Are Dead,* finding remarkable similarities and crucial differences.

Clark, Hoover W. "Existentialism and Pirandello's *Sei Personaggi,* " *Italica,* September, 1966, pp. 276-84.
Examines Pirandello's play for elements that correspond to the main tenets of existentialist thought.

DiGaetani, John Louis. *A Companion to Pirandello Studies,* Greenwood Press, 1991.
A collection of critical essays that deal with philosophical issues, biographical and historical approaches, thematic interpretations, influence studies, feminist approaches, and non-theatrical works—with stage production histories and a thorough bibliography.

Guidice, Gaspare. *Pirandello: A Biography,* translated by Alastair Hamilton, Oxford, 1975.
The standard biography of Pirandello.

Pirandello, Luigi. "On Humor," translated by Teresa Novel, in *The Tulane Drama Review,* Spring, 1966, pp. 46-59.
Provides an understanding of what Pirandello was attempting to accomplish in *Six Characters in Search of an Author.*

Pirandello, Luigi. "Pirandello Confesses . . . ," in *The Virginia Quarterly Review,* April, 1925, pp. 36-52.
A translation of Pirandello's "Preface" to *Six Characters in Search of an Author.* Appended to Pirandello's revision of the play, the "Preface" offers a basis for understanding the genesis of the play and its themes.

The Skin of Our Teeth

THORNTON WILDER

1942

Thornton Wilder completed his sixth, and perhaps most ambitious, play, *The Skin of Our Teeth,* on January 1, 1942. After trial runs in New Haven, Connecticut, and Baltimore, Maryland, the play opened on Broadway at the Plymouth Theater on November 18, 1942. The production—directed by Elia Kazan and starring Tallulah Bankhead (Sabina), Frederic March (Mr. Antrobus), and Florence Eldridge (Mrs. Antrobus)—received positive reviews and ran for 355 performances. Audiences and critics applauded Wilder's unconventional drama about the history of humankind. Most reviewers agreed that the playwright had produced a work that would revitalize American theater; as Brooks Atkinson wrote in the *New York Times,* ''*The Skin of Our Teeth* stands head and shoulders above the monotonous plane of our moribund theater—an original, gay-hearted play that is now and again profoundly moving, as a genuine comedy should be.''

Disrupting traditional notions of linear time, Wilder's play tells the story of the twentieth-century American Antrobus family in three acts which recount such epochal events as the onset of the Ice Age, the start of Great Flood, and the end of the Napoleonic Wars. Ending exactly as it began, the play illustrates the cyclical nature of existence, celebrating humanity's resilience, inventiveness, and will to survive. Although the play offers an age-old message, it does so in an untraditional form, rejecting the conventions of naturalistic drama. Not only do the characters appear to be both middle-

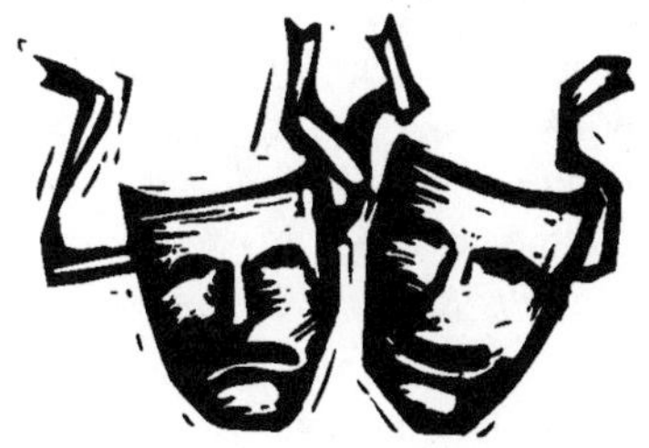

class Americans and allegorical figures, but they also repeatedly drop out of character and speak directly to the audience, breaking theatrical illusion and reminding viewers that they are watching a play. Combining modern theatrical experiments and timeless human themes, Wilder produced a work that would both challenge and entertain generations of Americans. Along with *Our Town* (1938), *The Skin of Our Teeth* is considered Wilder's theatrical masterpiece and an invaluable cornerstone of modern American drama.

AUTHOR BIOGRAPHY

Thornton Niven Wilder was born on April 17, 1897, in Madison, Wisconsin, the survivor of twin sons born to Isabella Thornton and Amos Parker Wilder. At the time of Wilder's birth, his father, a newspaperman with a Ph.D. in political science, was working as editor of the *Wisconsin State Journal.* A strict and religious man, Wilder's father exerted a forceful influence over his second child. The young Thornton often felt the pull between his mother's encouragement and his father's disapproval.

In 1906, the Wilder family moved to Hong Kong, where Amos assumed the diplomatic position of consul general. There, the nine-year-old Thornton went to a German school for six months before returning to the United States with his mother. In the following years, Thornton attended schools in California and China, eventually graduating from Berkeley High School in 1915. He then spent two years at Oberlin College in Ohio, transferred to Yale University, graduated from there in 1920, and spent the next academic year at the American Academy in Rome.

Back in America in 1921, Wilder settled into a job teaching French at the Lawrenceville School in New Jersey. On leave from Lawrenceville in 1925, Wilder entered the master's program in French at Princeton University. In that year, he revised his fictionalized account of his time in Italy which became his first novel, *The Cabala,* a work that earned favorable reviews when it appeared in 1926. That same year, critics greeted a production of Wilder's first play, an allegorical drama called *The Trumpet Shall Sound,* much less enthusiastically. But the next year, his second novel, *The Bridge of San Luis Rey,* would win the Pulitzer Prize for the best fiction work of 1927, allowing Wilder to resign his teaching position.

Wilder's career as a novelist and playwright would flourish in the succeeding decades. Two collections of one-act plays and two more novels were followed by a play destined to become an American classic, *Our Town* (1938), a drama about small-town life that would bring Wilder his second Pulitzer Prize. His thirteen later plays include: *The Merchant of Yonkers* (1938), a comedy he revised into *The Matchmaker* (1954) and which became the source for the popular musical *Hello, Dolly!* (1963); *The Skin of Our Teeth* (1942), which earned Wilder his third Pulitzer Prize; *Our Century* (1947), a short burlesque; and *The Alcestiad* (1955), a drama based on Greek playwright Euripides's *Alcestis.*

In his later years, Wilder continued to be honored. He received the Presidential Medal of Freedom (1963) and the National Medal for Literature (1965). His sixth novel, *The Eighth Day* (1967), earned a National Book Award. Two years after the publication of his final work, *Theophilis North* (1973), Wilder died on December 7, 1975, in Hamden, Connecticut, secure in his reputation as an innovative dramatist and important American literary figure.

PLOT SUMMARY

Act I

At the opening of *The Skin of Our Teeth,* images from a slide projector appear on the closed stage curtain. An Announcer narrates these pictures of "News Events of the World," telling the audience about events in both the theater (items left in the lost and found) and the world (a glacier is moving South over Vermont; Mr. George Antrobus has invented the wheel).

When the curtain rises, it reveals the living room of the Antrobus house in suburban Excelsior, New Jersey. Sabina, the sexy maid, gives an opening speech which parodies the clunky expositions that often begin traditional realistic plays: it is six o'clock and Mr. Antrobus is not yet home; it is so cold "dogs are sticking to the sidewalks"; and "the whole world is at sixes and sevens." But before the end of this speech, the actress playing Sabina drops her character and speaks in her own voice as Miss Somerset, complaining that she does not understand the play in which she is performing. After the stage manager sticks his head out to reprimand her, she picks up where she left off and is joined on stage by Mrs. Antrobus. The women discuss the weather, the fact Sabina has let the fire go out, Mrs. Antrobus's devotion to her ungrateful children, and Sabina's past affair with Mr. Antrobus. Their conversation is then interrupted by a baby dinosaur sticking his head in the window to say it is cold, followed by the entrance of a telegraph boy who delivers a message from Mr. Antrobus saying he will be late and instructing them to keep the children warm by burning ''everything but the Shakespeare.''

Before the telegraph boy departs, he helps Mrs. Antrobus re-light the fire. The dinosaur and a mammoth—who behave like family pets—have come into the house, and Mrs. Antrobus soon calls her children in as well. Yelling out the door, she orders her son, Henry, to put down a stone that he has picked up (and is contemplating throwing at something or someone). She yells at her daughter, Gladys, to put down her skirt (which she has raised to entice men). The ensuing conversation reveals that Henry—who, as Sabina told the audience earlier, killed his brother in an ''unfortunate accident''—was once called Cain. Soon, Mr. Antrobus returns home bearing his newly-invented wheel and offering humorous comments about his day. Before long he has to turn the animals outside in order to make room for the human refugees he has encountered on the way home—these wanderers include the poet Homer, the lawgiver Moses, a doctor, and a professor. In order to save these representatives of higher civilization—and themselves—the Antrobuses need to stoke the fire. Sabina, who, as Miss Somerset, had previously reassured the audience that in actuality ''the world's not coming to an end,'' now turns to the audience and tells them to help fuel the fire: ''Pass up your chairs everybody. Save the human race.''

Act II

Act II again opens with slide projections on the curtain: ''Time tables for trains leaving Pennsylvania Station for Atlantic City. Advertisements of Atlantic City hotels, drugstores, churches, rug merchants; fortune tellers, Bingo parlors.'' These are followed by the announcer's voice again narrating the ''News Events of the World.'' The news this time is that the hundred thousandth annual convention of the ''Ancient and Honorable Order of Mammals, Subdivision Humans'' is taking place in Atlantic City, New Jersey, and Mr. Antrobus has been elected president of the order.

The action begins with Mr. Antrobus giving a speech with the assistance of his wife, who whispers cues to him. He tells his listeners that ''the watchword for the future'' is ''Enjoy Yourselves.'' His wife, however, who steps up to speak next as president of the ''Women's Auxiliary Bed and Board Society,'' offers an alternate motto: ''Save the Family.'' Throughout the act we see the conveners following Mr. Antrobus's advice to seek enjoyment, while the president himself is tempted to sacrifice duty to pleasure and pursue an affair with Sabina, who now appears as Miss Lily Sabina Fairweather, Miss Atlantic City, 1942. During the seduction scene, Miss Somerset again drops her character, refusing to speak her lines because she believes they will offend a friend of hers in the audience. She does not ''think the theater is a place where people's feelings ought to be hurt.''

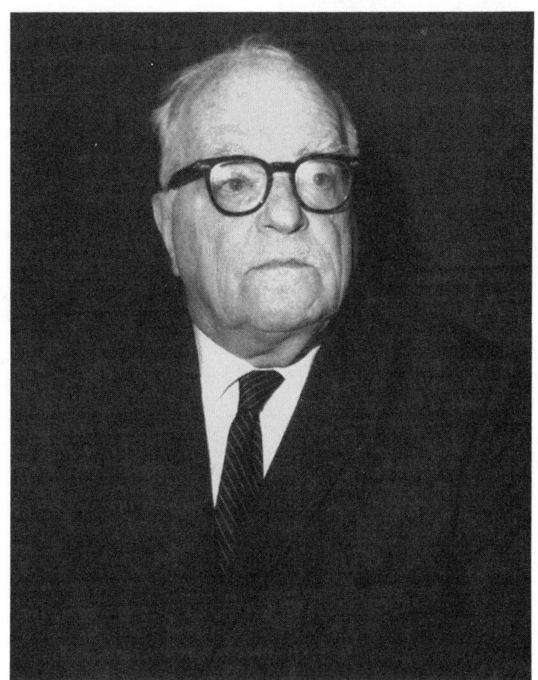

Thornton Wilder in 1968

Meanwhile, a fortune teller on the boardwalk offers advice to Sabina, and speaks words of warning to both the audience and the heedless conveneers. Mrs. Antrobus reprimands Gladys, who shows up in a sexually provocative outfit complete with red stockings, and Henry, who threatens a chair-pusher with his slingshot. As events on stage get more chaotic, a storm signal warns of a coming hurricane. At the end of the act, Mr. Antrobus is forced to abandon his plan to leave his wife for Sabina and instead must shepherd his family and two of every kind of animal onto a waiting ark.

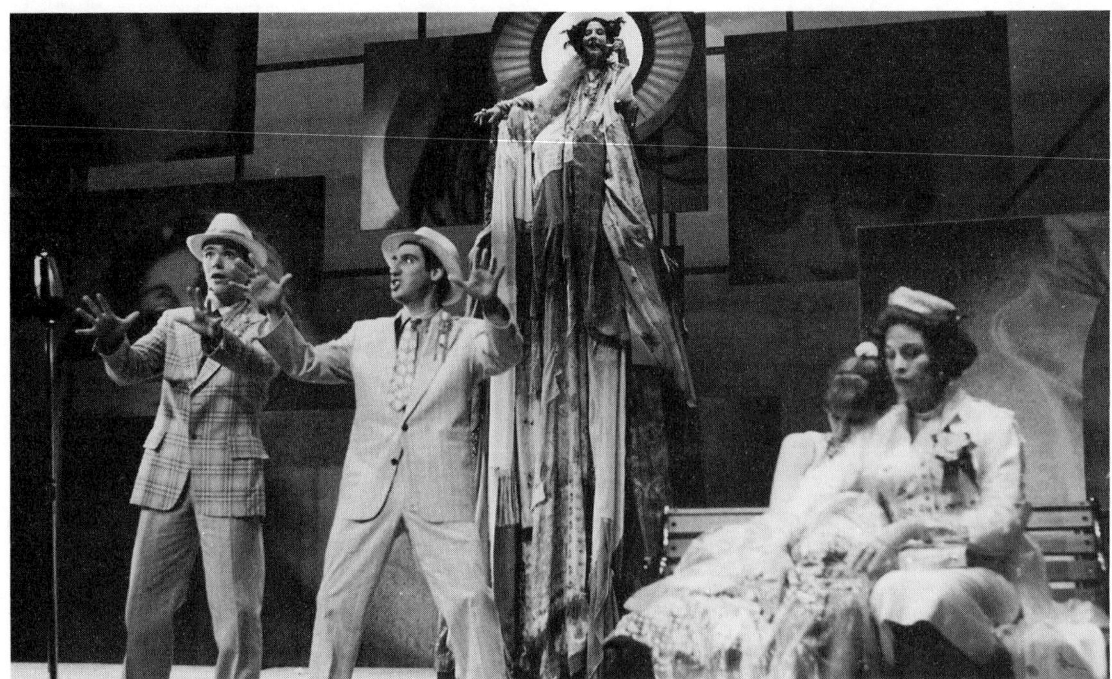

A scene from a Brandies University production depicting the Atlantic City convention of the ''Ancient and Honorable Order of Mammals, Subdivision Humans''

Act III

At the outset of Act III the curtain raises on a dark stage. The Antrobuses' Excelsior home is visible but the walls ''lean helter-skelter.'' The sound of a bugle is heard from off-stage and Sabina enters ''dressed as a Napoleonic camp follower.'' Ensuing dialogue makes it clear that a seven-year war has just come to an end.

Moments after Sabina enters, the stage manager interrupts the action to announce that several actors have fallen sick with food poisoning. He then asks the actor playing Mr. Antrobus to explain what is wrong. So Mr. Antrobus drops his character and tells the audience that the sick actors will be replaced by ''a number of splendid volunteers,'' including his own dresser and Miss Somerset's maid. He then asks those in the audience to ''just talk quietly among yourselves'' while the stage manager quickly takes the volunteers through their parts. After this ''rehearsal'' is through, the action resumes with Mrs. Antrobus and Gladys, who holds a baby in her arms, emerging from a trapdoor in the floor.

Not long after Mrs. Antrobus, Gladys, and Sabina are reunited, Henry and Mr. Antrobus return from battle. Mr. Antrobus has come to recognize that Henry is ''the enemy.'' Henry remains as angry as ever and swears to kill his father, but during their fight, Miss Somerset again drops character and warns them not to play the scene, ''You know what happened last night. Stop the play. Last night you almost strangled him.'' The actor playing Henry also steps out of character and confesses ''something comes over [him]'' when he plays the scene and the ''emptiness of being hated'' in his own life makes him want ''to strike and fight and kill.''

When the actors resume their parts, Sabina escorts Henry off stage while Mr. and Mrs. Antrobus begin a conversation in the living room which the women have put back in order. Mr. Antrobus explains he has momentarily lost ''the desire to begin again, to start building''; but his wife, hearing the cries of her grandchild, tells him matter-of-factly that he will ''have to get it back again.'' Sabina reenters in her outfit from Act I, ready to barter some beef-cubes in order to go to the movies. She knows she should have turned the cubes over to ''the Center downtown'' but in her opinion ''after anybody's gone through what we've gone through, they have a right to grab what they can find'' and she's just ''an ordinary girl'' who ''every now and then'' needs to ''go to the movies.''

Sabina's comments remind Mr. Antrobus of one of the three things that motivated him to keep going, "the voice of the people in their confusion and their need." This, along with the thought of his family and his books, reinvigorates him. He picks up a book and, as he looks into it, the "volunteers" from the earlier rehearsal come forward to recite passages from Spinoza, Plato, Aristotle, and the Bible. At the conclusion of these recitations, the stage goes momentarily black, then the lights come up on the exact scene of the play's opening with Sabina speaking the same opening lines before pausing to tell the audience, "This is where you came in. We have to go on for ages and ages yet. You go home. The end of the play isn't written yet. Mr. and Mrs. Antrobus! Their heads are full of plans and they're as confident as the first day they began—and they told me to tell you good night."

CHARACTERS

Announcer

The Announcer's voice narrates the slides and describes the "News Events of the World" at the beginning of Act I and Act II.

George Antrobus

Mr. Antrobus is the father of not only a typical suburban American family but also the entire human race. The play's central character, he possesses the virtues and flaws of both the biblical Adam and the American Everyman. The inventor of the wheel and the alphabet, he "comes of very old stock and has made his way up from next to nothing." In Act I, he is the hardworking and innovative businessman who loves his family and values his books and must preserve them all from the approaching Ice Age. In Act II, he is the President of the Order of Mammals who is tempted to leave his wife for a beauty contest winner, but with the onslaught of catastrophic rains, he returns to his family and loads them—along with his potential mistress and two of every kind of animal—onto a ship that will withstand the coming flood. And finally in Act III, he returns to his family after a seven-year war, ready to unearth his books and rebuild civilization.

Gladys Antrobus

The daughter of Mr. and Mrs. Antrobus, Gladys is constantly admonished to act like a lady, put down her dress, and not wear makeup or red stockings. Her mother reminds her that she should try to be as perfect as Mr. Antrobus thinks she is, and she does attempt to please her father by reciting lessons. But in Act III she appears with an apparently illegitimate baby which seems to be the result of her irrepressible sexuality.

Henry Antrobus

The son of Mr. and Mrs. Antrobus, Henry is introduced as "a real, clean-cut American boy" who killed his brother in "an unfortunate accident." Later dialogue reveals that the dead brother was named Abel and Henry—who has a red mark on his forehead—used to be called Cain. These references clearly remind the audience of the biblical story of the two brothers. Henry demonstrates his violent nature throughout the play. In Act I Sabina reports he has "killed the boy that lives next door"; in Act II he threatens people with his slingshot; in Act III he expresses his desire to kill his father. Although Mrs. Antrobus always loves her son despite his evil character, Mr. Antrobus acknowledges in Act III that Henry is "the enemy" who starts wars and disrupts peace.

Maggie Antrobus

Mrs. Antrobus is both the ideal suburban wife and the archetypal earth mother. She uncomplainingly endures nature's disasters, her husband's infidelities, and her children's disobedience, always facing each new crisis with energy and determination to survive. President of the Excelsior Mothers' club, "an excellent needlewoman" who "invented the apron," she "lives only for her children." Entirely defined by her domestic role, her motto is to "Save the Family," and in each Act of the play she manages to do just that.

Fred Bailey

The Captain of the Ushers, Fred is one of the backstage workers called forward in Act III to take the place of actors who have fallen sick with food poisoning.

Broadcast Official

In Act II, this man is trying, in the midst of chaotic activity, to get Mr. Antrobus to the microphone to give a broadcast to the conventions of the world.

Cain

See Henry Antrobus

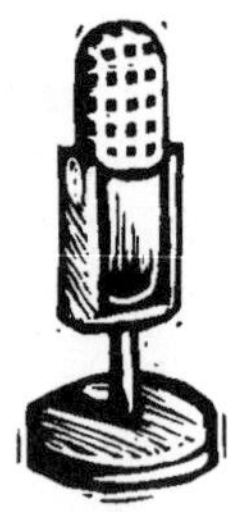

MEDIA ADAPTATIONS

- In 1950, Decca Records put out the American National Theater and Academy (ANTA) *Album of Stars: Great Moments of Great Plays* Volume I, which included sound recordings of selections from *The Skin of Our Teeth* performed by Frederic March, Florence Eldridge, and Alan Hewitt.
- On September 11, 1955, NBC televised a production of *The Skin of Our Teeth* starring Helen Hayes, Mary Martin, and George Abbott.
- Another production of *The Skin of Our Teeth,* starring Vivien Leigh, was televised live in London in March of 1959.
- In 1968, as the twelfth episode of its *One to One* television series, WETA-TV in Washington, D.C., aired ''Armchair Theater: *The Skin of Our Teeth*'' produced by Cherrill Anson and directed by David Powell. This episode, available on video, includes excerpts of the play performed by Jack Burn, Mary Lou Groom, Judy Margolis, and Ruth Mintz, followed by discussion.
- A video recording of the play, presented by the Kennedy Center and Xerox Corporation as part of the American Bicentennial Theater series in 1975, had a teleplay adapted by Douglas Scott and set design by Robert Kelsey.
- A sound recording of the play was produced by the Sydney A.B.C. company in 1979 as part of its World Theater series.
- As part of the ''American Playhouse'' series, PBS produced a live version of the play under the direction of Jack O'Brien in January, 1983.
- A production recorded on May 19, 1988 is available on video from Austin Peay State University in Clarksville, TN.
- The *Readings for the Blind* series (Southfield, Michigan, 1994) includes a sound recording of *Three Plays by Thornton Wilder.*

Chair Pushers

Wilder's stage directions for Act II, using the sort of stereotypical racial designations typical of the years preceding the Civil Rights movement, note that ''three roller chairs, pushed by melancholy Negroes, file by empty. Throughout the act they traverse the stage in both directions.''

Conveners

Six conveners—attendees of the Annual Convention of the Ancient and Honorable Order of Mammals—appear throughout Act II, walking on the Boardwalk. Determined to enjoy themselves, they do not heed the Fortune Teller's warnings about the coming rain. Engaged in drinking, gambling, and other sorts of revelry, they taunt Mr. Antrobus about being domesticated and tied to his family.

Dinosaur

The baby Dinosaur Dolly appears on the Antrobus's front lawn in Act I, is allowed in out of the cold, and behaves like a family pet. At the end of the Act when more room is needed for human refugees inside the house, Mr. Antrobus sends it and the Mammoth outside again, presumably to face extinction in the face of the oncoming ice age.

Doctor

The Doctor is the first refugee who comes into the Antrobus home in Act I.

Dolly

See Dinosaur

Esmerelda

See Fortune Teller

Miss Lily-Sabina Fairweather

See Sabina

Mr. Fitzpatrick

The stage manager who comes out front at several points to deal with problems, such as Miss Somerset's refusal to act certain scenes or the illness of other actors which necessitates their being replaced by volunteers.

Fortune Teller

The Atlantic City Fortune Teller who appears in Act II offers advice and words of wisdom to Sabina and other characters. The Fortune Teller also speaks directly to the audience, saying that it is easier to tell the future than to understand the past and that the Antrobuses are a reflection of those watching the play. Her comments point to the themes and concepts Wilder seeks to highlight.

Frederick

See Mammoth

Hester

The wardrobe mistress, Hester, is another backstage worker called forward in Act III to replace one of the actors who have fallen sick with food poisoning.

Homer

The second refugee, "a blind beggar with a guitar," who comes into the house in Act I. Homer is "an old man" and "particular friend" of Mr. Antrobus. His name and Mr. Antrobus's comment that it was this man who "really started off the A.B.C.'s," suggest to the audience that this is the poet Homer who authored the Greek epics the *Iliad* and the *Odyssey.*

Ivy

Miss Somerset's maid Ivy is one of the backstage workers called forward in Act III to take the place of actors who have fallen sick with food poisoning.

Lily Sabina

See Sabina

Mammoth

The Mammoth comes into the Antrobus home in Act I along with the Dinosaur. Both animals act like pets until Mr. Antrobus sends them outside at the end of the Act.

Judge Moses

The third refugee who enters the house in Act I, Judge Moses is an elderly Jewish man wearing a skull cap. The Judge's recitation in Hebrew, along with Mr. Antrobus's comment that this is the man "who makes all the laws," suggests that this is the biblical Moses who led the Jews out of Egypt and received the Ten Commandments from God in the Old Testament.

Muses

The three sisters—Miss E. Muse, Miss T. Muse, and Miss M. Muse—enter the Antrobus home in Act I along with the other refugees. Their name and relationship suggests they are the sister goddesses from Greek mythology who inspired song and poetry.

Sabina

The character of Sabina is described in the stage directions for Act I as "straw blonde" and "over-rouged"; she carries a feather-duster and plays the stock role from farce of the smart-mouthed maid. Her mercurial emotions, pessimism, and desire to have fun distinguish her from the unflinching, resilient, and pragmatic Antrobuses. The sexy Sabina—whose name variations are meant to remind the audience of the biblical stories of the Sabine women and Lilith (in biblical legend, Lilith was Adam's first wife who was supplanted by Eve)—is the opposite of the maternal Mrs. Antrobus. A house servant and Mr. Antrobus's former mistress in Act I, Sabina appears in Act II as the winner of an Atlantic City beauty contest who is determined to lure Mr. Antrobus away from his wife. She reappears in Act III as a returning camp follower whose numerous liaisons have left her wishing "never . . . to kiss another human being" again.

Not far into the first act, the actress playing Sabina, Miss Somerset, steps out of her role and addresses the audience in her own voice, revealing that she hates the play but has taken the part out of financial necessity. Miss Somerset will drop out of character several more times during the course of the play to express similar dissatisfactions. Her side comments, both as Sabina and Miss Somerset, provide much of the play's humor.

Miss Somerset

See Sabina

Mr. Tremayne

A dresser for the actor playing Mr. Antrobus, Mr. Tremayne is one of the backstage workers called forward in Act III to take the place of actors who have fallen sick with food poisoning.

Ushers

These two ushers rush down the theater aisles with chairs when Sabina calls out to the audience at the end of Act I, asking everyone to pass up their chairs for the fire to "save the human race."

THEMES

Absurdity

Much of the humor in *The Skin of Our Teeth* derives from Wilder's use of bizarre juxtapositions which place the characters in absurd situations and highlight the ludicrous aspects of seemingly ordinary events. Combining elements of twentieth-century suburban America with events from the historical and mythological past creates an odd world where a middle-class family can have a dinosaur and mammoth for pets, the Antrobuses can celebrate their 5,000th wedding anniversary, and the children can recite poems even though their father has only just invented the alphabet.

American Exceptionalism

By presenting his allegorical parents of the human race as a conventional American middle-class couple, Wilder reinforces Americans' belief in the exceptional nature of their country and its citizens. Mr. Antrobus's virtues of inventiveness, resilience, and diligence are those of the ideal American entrepreneur, and the family's continued ability to start from nothing and achieve greatness is the essence of the American dream. The play suggests the best human characteristics are also the best American qualities.

Illusion vs. Reality

While traditional realistic plays try to create a "real" world on the stage, encouraging viewers to forget that they are watching actors play roles in a fictional drama, Wilder constantly interrupts this sort of theatrical illusion to remind the audience that they are watching a drama. When actors step out of their roles and speak directly to the audience, they highlight the fact that this is a performance taking place on a stage, a fictional world that can be altered and adapted by the ordinary people who are putting it together. Wilder repeatedly reminds the audience of the realities of sets, actors, and scripts, disrupting the conventions of naturalistic theater.

Cycle of History

The Skin of Our Teeth emphasizes the repetitive nature of human history. The Antrobuses have faced disasters in the past, overcome more disasters during the course of the drama, and are ready to engage in further struggles at the performance's end. Wilder emphasizes the circular quality of the characters' lives, each act finds them starting over again. The play concludes with the exact same words and situation with which it began—another reminder that the cycle of history (and human existence) is on-going.

Family

Wilder's play both parodies and idealizes the image of the nuclear family. George and Maggie Antrobus are extreme examples of the masculine provider and the feminine caregiver. His enthusiasm for his inventions and books and her single-minded devotion to her children might be viewed as humorously exaggerated. Yet, their adherence to their stereotypical gender roles seems to contribute to the survival of the human race in each act, suggesting that the perpetuation of civilization depends upon the perpetuation of a traditional family structure in some form.

Good and Evil

The character of Henry, formerly known as Cain, emphasizes the constant presence of evil in

TOPICS FOR FURTHER STUDY

- Compare and contrast *The Skin of Our Teeth* with James Joyce's *Finnegan's Wake* (1939). Wilder acknowledged that Joyce's novel was an important influence and source for his play. What similarities in content and structure do you see between the two works? What significant thematic differences distinguish Wilder's world view from Joyce's?
- Research the political and cultural climate of post-World War II Germany. What issues and ideas confronting the German people during this time would account for their positive response to Wilder's *The Skin of Our Teeth?*
- Look up psychologist Carl Jung's definition of ''archetype.'' What archetypal images and figures appear in *The Skin of Our Teeth?* How does recognizing them as such influence viewer interpretation of the play?
- Compare and contrast *The Skin of Our Teeth* with a traditionally naturalistic play such as Henrik Ibsen's *A Doll's House* (1879) or Eugene O'Neill's *Long Day's Journey into Night* (1956). What staging techniques characterize each work? What theatrical conventions does Wilder's play break down?
- Read a book or view a film that portrays a post-apocalyptic world, for example, a novel such as Angela Carter's *Heroes and Villains* (1981) or Richard Matheson's short novel *I am Legend* (1954), or a movie like *The Road Warrior* (1982) or *The Day After* (1983). Then compare your chosen work's setting and characters to those of *The Skin of Our Teeth.* To what extent does this work share Wilder's cyclic vision and message about humanity's fortitude, adaptability, and duality? Do the two works present similar or contrasting views of the human condition?

the world. The angry and violent Henry is part of the human family—and appears in every act—suggesting that evil can never be left behind. Henry's fight with his father towards the end of the play illustrates the on-going struggle between good and evil. Wilder interrupts this fight, however, leaving it unresolved (as real world clashes between such forces often end). The play suggests that as humanity enters each new era, it always brings both its good and evil impulses along.

Human Condition

Wilder's characters exemplify basic human qualities and encounter basic human experiences. They illustrate the unchanging facts of the human condition. Representing in turn intelligence, maternal love, violence, lust, selfishness, and determination, the Antrobuses and Sabina endure work, betrayal, natural disaster, and war. In his depiction of them and their strangely timeless world, Wilder underscores the best and worst aspects of the human condition: humanity possesses the will and ability to survive and yet must repeatedly confront (and overcome) its own destructive tendencies.

STYLE

Allegory

An allegory is a narrative in which the characters and events can be read both literally and figuratively. In the case of *The Skin of Our Teeth,* the Antrobuses can be read as ordinary people (a middle-class American couple) and as allegorical figures (Adam and Eve, the progenitors of humankind). The action of the play can be viewed literally, as the experiences of a particular family, and allegorically, as the story of human history. Wilder, with both character names (such as Henry a.k.a. Cain and Sabina) and explicit comments, emphasizes the allegorical nature of his play.

Anti-Illusion Theater

Anti-Illusion theater was pioneered by German playwright Bertolt Brecht (*The Threepenny Opera*), who believed an audience should remain conscious of the physical realities of performance and not give into the illusion that events depicted on stage are real. Like Brecht and Italian dramatist Luigi Pirandello (*Six Characters in Search of an Author*), Wilder uses various techniques to break the theatrical illusion. Both by presenting actors who drop out of character, comment on their lines, and speak directly to the audience and by bringing ''backstage'' figures in front of the curtain, he calls attention to the efforts that go into producing a theatrical work, prompting viewers to think about how and why a story is told in a certain way. In so doing, Wilder engages in meta-theater, creating a play that comments on the process of creating a play. (Meta is a prefix placed before any creative work that is self-referential; metafiction is perhaps the best-known of this form, with the writings of John Barth exemplifying the genre.)

Characterization

Wilder does not try to present complex multifaceted characters in *The Skin of Our Teeth* but instead presents each person on stage as a generalized type. Every character is easily identified with an archetypal role—the mother/nurturer (Mrs. Antrobus), the temptress (Sabina), the provider (Mr. Antrobus)—and exhibits the personality traits traditionally associated with this role. These simple and flat characterizations, along with the technique of having actors interrupt the action and comment about the nature of the play, keeps the audience from identifying with the characters and destroys the illusion that the Antrobuses are ''real'' people. It is interesting to note, however, that even though the ''actors'' playing the roles in *The Skin of Our Teeth* do break character and address the audience—presenting themselves as real people—they themselves are characters created for the purpose of anti-illusion theatre. While Miss Somerset may seem a more tangible person than Sabina, she is in fact just another character created by Wilder. The playwright's purpose, however, is not to provide the actors with a forum to address the play process but to make the audience aware of the theatrical process they are viewing and provide a contrast to the broad character types.

Farce

Wilder's play employs many elements of farce—a comedic theatrical form characterized by broadly drawn characters, improbable situations, and physical humor. Sabina's character of the seductive, inefficient, wise-cracking maid is a stock figure in farce. Similarly, incongruous images such as a pet dinosaur curled up in front of the family fireplace, reflect staging characteristic of farce. Other farcical elements include Henry's violent tendencies (he is constantly warned against committing violent acts) and Gladys's nymphomania (in the first act her mother yells at her to lower her skirt, an action she presumably undertakes to attract men to have sex with her).

Juxtaposition

Throughout the play Wilder juxtaposes the modern and the ancient, the momentous and the insignificant, the serious and the silly. These ludicrously opposed images and ideas both produce humor and emphasize the simultaneous greatness and absurdity of humankind. A good example of this is found in Mr. Antrobus's qualities as an inventor and an educated man. The newsreel at the play's opening informs the audience that George Antrobus has just invented the wheel and the alphabet despite the obvious fact that the society in which he lives has already lived with archetypal inventions such as these for many years.

Wilder plays with audiences' notion of linear time by setting his play in past historical epochs and in 1940s New Jersey simultaneously. The three acts take place during the Ice Age, the Great Flood, and the Napoleonic Wars respectively, yet the characters dress and act like twentieth-century Americans. The play's notion of time is further complicated by the Antrobus's apparent agelessness (they have been married 5,000 years) as well as the repetitive cycle of events (at the end the play starts over where it began). This use of time emphasizes the play's message about humanity's ability to endure through the ages, while also contributing to Wilder's goal of reminding the audience of the non-reality of the staged events.

HISTORICAL CONTEXT

Wilder began writing *The Skin of Our Teeth* in 1940 at a time of great political and cultural change. As the 1930s drew to a close, Americans found themselves in an increasingly urban and secular world where market forces took precedence over moral ideals and psychology took the place of religion. The ideas of Sigmund Freud, a German psychologist who argued that the unconscious mind significantly impacted human behavior, greatly influenced the art of the era. Experimental movements in visual art, such as surrealism, reflected artists' attempts to move beyond traditional aesthetic standards they felt did not do justice to the imaginative resources of the human unconscious. Many writers and musicians engaged in similar experiments during the following decades, altering conventional forms so as to better express human consciousness and experience.

Although open to cultural influences from abroad, America had followed a policy of political isolationism throughout the 1930s. In Europe, Adolf Hitler's army attacked Poland in September of 1939, beginning World War II. The United States stayed out of the war even as the Germans continued their offensive, invading Norway, Denmark, and France in the spring and summer of 1940. As the situation worsened, President Franklin Roosevelt did encourage Congress to pass, in March of 1941, the American Lend-Lease Act which gave money and supplies to the Allied nations (England, France, and Russia) fighting against the Germans. But America did not officially enter the war until the Japanese air attack on the U.S. naval fleet at Pearl Harbor, Hawaii, on December 7, 1941. This event, followed by Germany's declaration of war against the United States days later on December 11, made further isolationism impossible.

When Wilder finished his play in January of 1942, the United States had joined the Allied forces and was engaged in a global war. Battles raged in Africa, Europe, and the Pacific with only four countries remaining neutral (Spain, Portugal, and Switzerland). In early 1942 things still looked bleak for the Allies, but three decisive battles that year would alter the course of the conflict. In February, the six-month-long battle for control of Stalingrad, Russia, finally ended with the Russian forces outlasting the demoralized German invaders. In June, the battle of Midway Island would leave the Japanese fleet permanently crippled. And in November, the British victory at the battle of El Alamein would turn the tide in Africa. Meanwhile, American forces were gradually gaining command of the Atlantic.

At home, Americans were closely following these military events and doing what they could to aid the war effort. Stateside industrial plants began to shift from producing commercial goods to producing war supplies; rubber and gasoline were rationed and families were encouraged to grow their own food in "Victory Gardens." Audiences who went to see the first production of *The Skin of Our Teeth,* although hardly suffering the hardship and starvation that afflicted the populations of Europe, still would have related to the images of war-induced sacrifice and destruction depicted in Wilder's play.

CRITICAL OVERVIEW

Since its premiere, *The Skin of Our Teeth* has maintained a solid critical reputation, earning consistent critical acclaim and winning over new generations of Americans with its frequent revivals.

The original Broadway production, which opened on November 18, 1942, prompted reviewers like the New York *Daily Telegraph*'s George Freedley to comment both that "Wilder certainly has the most vivid imagination in the theater today," and that the play is "a perfect piece of theater." Although a few critics complained that the work lacked substance and that Wilder's anti-illusion staging devices were awkward, such voices were distinctly in the minority.

The play did generate some controversy when two authors, Joseph Campbell and Henry Morton Robinson, published an article in the *Saturday Review of Literature* claiming that Wilder had plagiarized James Joyce's novel *Finnegan's Wake* (1939). Campbell and Robinson carefully pointed out the similarities in plot, theme, and presentation between the two works. Wilder, who freely admitted Joyce's influence on his play, did not directly answer the charges but merely encouraged critics to read both texts and judge for themselves. A small flurry of articles on the issue followed, some poked fun at Campbell and Robinson while most acknowledged that Wilder's use of Joyce's novel was no different

COMPARE & CONTRAST

- **1942:** German leader Adolf Hitler begins the methodical annihilation of millions of European Jews in what he calls the "final solution" and history will term the Holocaust. In July, Paris police, under the command of occupying German forces, gather 30,000 Jews and send them to German concentration camps, where all but thirty will die.

  Today: On September 30, 1997, Roman Catholic bishops in France offer the Church's first public apology to the Jewish people for its silence during the French participation in the Holocaust. Earlier in the year, the French medical association and the French police offer similar public apologies; while in Switzerland, the government finally responds to years of protests, creating a fund to reimburse survivors and relatives of Holocaust victims whose bank accounts and assets were kept by Swiss financial institutions after World War II.

- **1942:** German rocket engineer Wernher von Braun launches the first surface-to-surface guided missile.

  Today: Highly sophisticated guided missiles, as seen in the 1991 Persian Gulf War, play an important role in late-twentieth-century warfare. The United States military arsenal includes computer-guided missiles such as the Tomahawk cruise missile.

- **1942:** Congress establishes the Women's Auxiliary Army Corps (WAAC) and the Women Accepted for Voluntary Emergency Service (WAVES), bringing women into the United States armed services in an official, but limited, capacity.

  Today: Women are active in all branches of the American armed services. In the U.S. Army, for example, women make up 14% of the personnel. These 69,000 female soldiers, however, are still excluded from thousands of combat positions as well as the senior leadership roles attained through serving in combat jobs. Questions about women's equal participation in combat, as well as highly publicized reports of sexual misconduct and harassment on military bases during the late-1990s, continue to fuel debate about the role of women in the military.

- **1942:** The government asks Americans to grow vegetables in "Victory Gardens" to help alleviate war-time food shortages. Forty percent of U.S. vegetables will be grown in such gardens in 1942, but this percentage decreases in succeeding years as public interest wanes.

  Today: Agriculture in America is big business, and the United States possesses the world's largest food surplus. The United States exports double the amount of food it imports. While Americans still grow some of the food they eat, it is more of a leisure pursuit than an economic necessity.

- **1942:** Oxford University scholar Gilbert Murray founds the organization Oxfam to fight world famine. Millions of Europeans in German-occupied countries such as Greece, Poland, and Yugoslavia suffer from starvation as the war cuts off food supplies.

  Today: Oxfam International has grown into a confederation of ten Oxfam agencies that direct projects in more than one hundred countries. Oxfam America, founded in 1970, fights against global poverty, hunger, and social injustice in the United States as well as in countries such as North Korea, where over 100,000 people died of starvation in 1996.

---

than many other dramatists' creative use of their sources. Although this controversy may have prevented the New York drama critics from naming it the year's best play, *The Skin of Our Teeth* still won the Pulitzer Prize for drama in 1942 and ran for 355 performances.

In 1945, a London production starring Vivien Leigh and Laurence Olivier was also a success. Though the Soviet Union banned performances of Wilder's plays, other European countries responded favorably to *The Skin of Our Teeth;* performances in Amsterdam and Bavaria, as well as a 1946 London revival, were well-attended and positively reviewed. German theatergoers particularly loved the play, which offered hope for revitalization to a broken people. In years to come, the play would become even more highly regarded—and receive more critical attention—in German-speaking countries than in the United States.

By the 1950s, the play's reputation was solidly established. In 1952, Sheldon Cheney, in his survey of the history of theater *The Theatre: Three Thousand Years of Drama, Acting, and Stagecraft,* would pronounce *The Skin of Our Teeth* "the most notable event of the forties." Two years later Frank M. Whiting's *An Introduction to the Theater* would tell readers that "any survey of American playwriting must recognize the importance of Thornton Wilder." By 1956, several academic articles about *The Skin of Our Teeth* were published, and the work was discussed in three books on drama. Scholars continued to praise Wilder's theatrical technique and began to associate his work with Brechtian epic-theater. Critics also noted Wilder's influence on European absurdist drama.

In 1961, Rex Burbank published the first book entirely devoted to Wilder's work. Though this text would be followed by several other full-length studies in succeeding decades, and Wilder would continue to hold the status of a respected literary figure, his writings would not receive as much academic attention as some of the dramatists of the next generation like Arthur Miller (*The Crucible*) and Tennessee Williams (*Cat on a Hot Tin Roof*). Some critics attribute this relative neglect to the fact that Wilder's essential optimism and classical ideals were at odds with the late-twentieth century preference for the pessimistic worldview of modernist works influenced by romantic aesthetics.

Despite scholars' reserved responses, in the last half of the century live performances of *The Skin of Our Teeth* have continued to be popular. A 1955 revival at the National Theater in Washington, D.C.—starring Helen Hayes, Mary Martin, and George Abbot—earned critical raves. And although a national touring production of the play was less successful, the play again pleased critics when it was included as part of the American "Salute to France" in Paris. In 1961 the play once more went abroad as part of the Theatre Guild American Repertory Company's world tour and was embraced by audiences in countries as diverse as Chile, Greece, Trinidad, and Sweden. Americans again received the play favorably in a 1975 Kennedy Center production that was part of the national Bicentennial celebration, and more recently, a 1983 PBS "American Playhouse" production earned good reviews.

Throughout the 1990s, the play has remained a perennial favorite of high school, college, and community theater. In 1997, the centennial of Wilder's birth prompted numerous revivals of his plays, as well as the creation of an internet web page devoted to his life and writings. Today, *The Skin of Our Teeth* is not only performed frequently but also appears regularly in literature anthologies and on college course syllabi. It holds a place, alongside Wilder's *Our Town,* as one of the best examples of mid-twentieth-century American drama.

CRITICISM

Erika M. Kreger

Kreger is a Ph.D. candidate and instructor at the University of California, Davis. In this essay, she examines how Wilder joins innovative theatrical techniques, classic themes, and American optimism to create the mythic world of The Skin of Our Teeth.

The Skin of Our Teeth is a play full of paradoxes. When audiences first viewed Thornton Wilder's comedy in 1942, they were confronted by events which seemed to take place both in the distant past and the immediate present, characters who were both age-old allegorical figures and contemporary actors, and dialogue that was both irreverent and philosophical. Wilder's theatrical techniques were undeniably innovative for his time; he broke with the conventions of naturalistic theater that had guided previous generations of American playwrights. But perhaps the central irony of the play is that it uses these progressive techniques to present an extremely traditional message. In *The Skin of Our Teeth,* Wilder pairs modern form with classical content, disrupting viewers' assumptions about the nature of theater, while also reinforcing their beliefs about the nature of humanity.

- *The Bridge of San Luis Rey* (1927) is Wilder's Pulitzer Prize winning novel, a work made up of three connected stories detailing the experiences of several people killed by a collapsing bridge in eighteenth-century Peru.
- *The Making of Americans* (1925) is a novel by Wilder's good friend Gertrude Stein. This narrative about several generations of Stein's family uses her trademark techniques of simple language and repetition. Her goal was to create a sensation of a constant present, to begin again and again because "repeating is the whole of living and by repeating comes understanding." Stein's techniques greatly influenced Wilder.
- *Mother Courage and Her Children* (1941), is a drama by German playwright Bertolt Brecht. The narrative revolves around a seventeenth-century German canteen woman who is an allegorical figure representing the destructive forces of capitalism. The play exemplifies Brecht's ideas of epic-theater and the anti-illusion techniques which influenced Wilder.
- *Our Town* (1938) is Wilder's most famous work and possibly America's most-produced play. It depicts the daily existence of people in a small New Hampshire town, employing some of the same non-realistic theatrical techniques seen in *The Skin of Our Teeth.*
- *Six Characters in Search of an Author* (1921) is an experimental drama by Italian playwright Luigi Pirandello. This play challenged the tradition of naturalistic theater and greatly influenced Wilder's writing.
- *Watch on the Rhine* (1941) is a realistic play by Lillian Hellman that provides an interesting contrast to Wilder's work. This drama, about a couple fighting against Nazi ideas in the United States, deals explicitly with the political issues of its time.

Accustomed to plays which sought to create the illusion that events on stage were really happening, 1940s audiences were caught off guard by Wilder's disregard for such theatrical convention. They recognized, in the opening minutes of *The Skin of Our Teeth* when "Miss Somerset" stops speaking in the character of Sabina and starts complaining about her lines, that they were viewing a different kind of play. They were not used to actors breaking the proscenium barrier—the imaginary divide between the people on stage and the people in the audience—and asking the viewer to participate in events on stage by, for example, passing up their chairs at the end of Act I to fuel the fire that will "save the human race."

Wilder anticipated theatergoers' surprise, and knew, as he wrote in a journal entry for October 26, 1940, that "twenty years from now . . . audiences will be accustomed to such liberties and the impact of the method will no longer be so great" (published in *The Journals of Thornton Wilder, 1939-1961*). But in 1942, he felt American drama needed some shaking up. Theater, he explained in his 1957 preface to *Three Plays,* had "become a minor art," "an in consequential diversion." In the plays of the 1920s and '30s, "the tragic had no heat; the comic had no bite; the social criticism failed to indict us with responsibility." So Wilder decided to try a new approach; he began writing plays "that tried to capture not verisimilitude but reality."

Wilder's desire to present a different kind of reality on stage resulted in plays, like *The Skin of Our Teeth,* which can be classified as anti-illusion theater. Originating with European playwrights like Bertolt Brecht (*The Threepenny Opera*) and Luigi Pirandello (*Six Characters in Search of an Author*), this type of drama emphasizes the artificiality of performance while highlighting the actuality of performers. As Brecht explained the theory, in an essay collected in John Willett's anthology *Brecht on Theatre,* "the audience must not be able to think that it has been transported to the scene of the story but must be invited to take part" in the events on stage.

Anti-illusion dramatists, Thomas Adler explained in an essay in *Claudel Studies,* "write plays about plays . . . taking as their subjects the nature of the theatre and the act of going to the theatre and demanding that their audiences consciously think of themselves as an audience." (This self-referential technique is often referred to as meta-drama.) A play like Pirandello's *Six Characters in Search of An Author* (1921), in Adler's view, requires "absolutely no make-believe . . . in viewing it: the theatre is the theatre, the audience is the audience, the stage is the stage, the characters are the characters, and so forth." Although "ordinarily, we call a play realistic when what we see on stage presents . . . [a] convincing illusion that what we are seeing is a faithful representation of reality; and when we in the audience are separated from what is happening on stage by an imaginary fourth wall," Adler argued that this type of play is actually un-realistic because it asks audience to "make believe that [they] are *not* making believe." A play that breaks through the fourth wall actually emphasizes the true realities of performance: the fact of sitting in a theater watching a production put on by living people.

Wilder's use of anti-illusion techniques in *The Skin of Our Teeth* is both surprising and fun. Disrupting audience expectations might alienate or confuse theatergoers, but Wilder anticipates such resistance and cleverly uses the actors' asides to articulate and diffuse viewers' objections. Miss Somerset often speaks for the sort of theatergoer who does not want to tackle tough questions. She will express annoyance at the playwright's subject matter and then at other points exclaim: "Oh, I see what this part of the play means now!" Yet not entirely won over, she still refuses to ponder the big issues: "I'll say the lines, but I won't think about the play." Like the middle-class theatergoer who seeks escapist entertainment—the sort of person Wilder wanted to jolt out of their complacency—Miss Somerset thinks plays should be pleasant and predictable. She does not "think the theatre is a place where people's feelings ought to be hurt." Wilder is definitely poking fun at such timid responses to theater—but he is also giving the ordinary person a voice, a voice given some credence because it is associated with the most sympathetic and amusing figure in the play.

" WITH HIS DEPICTION OF THIS TYPICALLY SUBURBAN AND YET ARCHETYPICALLY MYTHIC FAMILY, WILDER TRANSFORMED THE AMERICAN THEATRICAL LANDSCAPE OF THE 1940S. HE WILL CERTAINLY BE REMEMBERED AS AN INNOVATOR IN TWENTIETH CENTURY DRAMA, THOUGH HE WOULD HAVE CLASSIFIED HIMSELF AS A TRADITIONALIST."

In addition to reassuring the audience and providing comic relief, Sabina/Somerset's out-of-character comments contribute to Wilder's goal of capturing the "reality" of theater. Early on, Somerset complains "I hate this play and every word in it," confessing she only took "this hateful job" out of necessity. Before viewers have a chance to connect with the character of the sexy maid Sabina, their attention shifts to the actress playing the part and the circumstances of her employment. Although Somerset's comment that "for two years I've sat up in my room living on a sandwich and a cup of tea a day waiting for better times in the theater" breaks the illusion that the woman speaking on stage is actually Sabina, it builds awareness of behind-the-scenes realities. Similarly, the "rehearsal" at the beginning of Act II brings backstage workers out front, emphasizing the labor that goes into producing a play. Other illusion-breaking moments—such as the Act III confession of the actor who plays Henry, who reveals he feels the same violent rage as his character—emphasize that hardship and passionate emotions are part of "real life" just as much as they are part of dramatic performance.

These moments in which the actors' and characters' experiences intersect illustrate Wilder's belief, expressed in his *Three Plays* preface, that theater "has one foot planted firmly in the particular, since each actor before us . . . is indubitably a living, breathing 'one'; yet it tends and strains to exhibit a general truth" as well. To get at this truth,

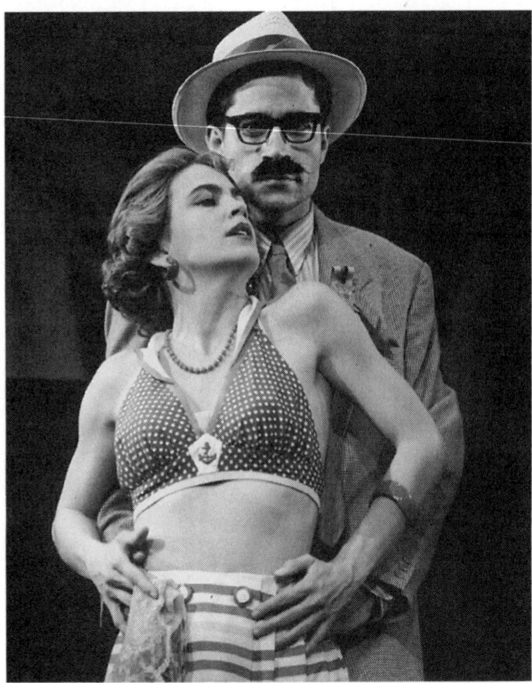

Mr. Antrobus is once again tempted by the charms of Sabina

Wilder emphasized general traits in his characterizations, another technique of anti-illusion theater. The play's characters are not psychologically developed and individualized but rather are broadly defined as common types, the sort of one-dimensional allegorical figures often found in myth. Despite their suburban setting, the main characters are presented as archetypes (age-old models of basic human roles such as the Great Mother, the Hero, the Fallen Woman). Each person on stage, when speaking in character, represents as essential human quality—intellect (Mr. Antrobus), nurture (Mrs. Antrobus), sexuality (Sabina and Gladys), violence (Henry)—and these qualities appear in every historical epoch.

Although such allegorical characterizations were a departure from the dramatic practices common in the era immediately preceding the composition of *The Skin of Our Teeth,* Wilder's approach to character was not new. He had, in fact, returned to very old ideas, reclaiming classical Greek dramatic forms. In his essay ''Some Thoughts on Playwriting'' (published in *Playwrights on Playwriting*), Wilder gave an example of the theatrical philosophy behind the staging of a classical play such as Euripides's *Medea* (c. 431 B.C.). In such plays, the actors wore large masks and spoke their lines loudly without significant inflection. ''For the Greeks,'' Wilder argued, ''there was no pretense that Medea was on the stage.'' They saw ''the mask, the costume, the mode of declamation'' as a ''series of signs which the spectator interpreted and reassembled in his own mind.'' These ancient viewers were active participants in the theatrical experience, assembling in their own minds the ideas and images presented on stage. Wilder wanted his twentieth century audiences to be just as active.

By the time Wilder began writing for the stage, modern drama had moved away from the staging techniques of Euripides and Sophocles (*Antigone*). In post-Sophoclean drama, as German writer Frederic Nietzsche explained it in *The Birth of Tragedy and the Genealogy of Morals,* ''the spectator ceases to be aware of the myth at all and comes to focus on the amazing lifelikeness of the characters and the artists power of imitation.'' But, as noted above, Wilder did not concern himself with this modern focus on ''lifelikeness'' and instead wished to regenerate awareness of the myth. He made his intent clear in an October 26, 1940, journal passage, complaining of the difficulties of his ''attempt to do a play in which the protagonist is a twenty-thousand-year-old man and whose heroine is a twenty-thousand-year-old woman and eight thousand years a wife.'' His ''challenge'' was to ''represent Man and Woman.'' And he believed that ''by shattering the ossified conventions of the well-made play [the] characters [would] emerge . . . as generalized beings.'' His ''favorite principle'' he wrote in another journal entry on October 29, 1940, was ''that the characters on the stage tend to figure as generalizations, that the stage burns and longs to express a timeless individualized Symbol.''

In addition to its symbolic characters, Wilder's play contains other elements of classical drama. Both the structure and content of the work emphasize the cycle of history often depicted in myth. Sabina's comment early in Act I emphasizes the cyclical nature of the Antrobuses' existence, as well as its ambivalence and uncertainty: ''Each new child that's born to the Antrobuses seems to them to be sufficient reason for the whole universe's being set in motion; and each new child that dies seems to have been spared a whole world of sorrow, and what the end of it will be is still very much open to question.'' Throughout the rest of the play, characters will frequently refer to the repetition in their lives—''always beginning again! Over and over again. Always beginning again.''—demonstrating how things circle around and return to the same place rather than progressing forward. Each Act finds the same characters having come through another disaster, essentially unchanged. The end of Act III finds Sabina exactly in the same place she was at the play's outset, speaking the same lines once more and only pausing briefly to tell the audience to go ahead and leave since the Antrobuses have to go on for ages and ages yet.''

Wilder's mythic vision, however, is less fatalistic than that of the classical works from which he drew inspiration. He did not want to portray humanity's helplessness in the face of adversity but rather wished to convince the audience of humanity's fortitude and strength. He wondered, in a December 2, 1941, journal entry, ''what does one offer the audience as explanation of man's endurance, aim, and consolation?'' He hoped his play would show that the representative man finds ''adequate direction and stimulation'' in ''the existence of his children,'' ''the inventive activity of his mind,'' and ''the ideas contained in the great books of his predecessors.'' His image of the persevering ordinary man reflected the optimistic ideals of American democracy. Although the ancient Greeks—as Winifred Dusenbury commented in *Modern Drama*—created ''no myth which symbolizes free men governing themselves.'' Two thousand years later, Americans have begun to write a ''mythology of the Common Man.'' A figure such as Mr. Antrobus, the inventive businessman and loving father, is an ordinary hero worthy of a democratic mythology. This Everyman—despite his flaws, failures, and crises of confidence—is a leader. His ingenuity ensures that his family—the human family—will get through more wars and more walls of ice and floods and earthquakes, even if they only make it through by the skin of their teeth. The play's concluding message, much like the optimistic outlook of other democratic American narratives, is that not only will people always come through such crises but they will learn something and start to get better.

The Antrobuses, the Fortune Teller informs the audience in Act II, are: ''Your hope. Your despair. Your selves.'' They represent the best and worst of humanity—and in Wilder's comic formulation perhaps offer a good deal more hope than despair. With his depiction of this typically suburban and yet archetypically mythic family, Wilder transformed the American theatrical landscape of the 1940s. He will certainly be remembered as an innovator in twentieth century drama, though he would have classified himself as a traditionalist, as he wrote in the preface to *Three Plays,* ''I am not an innovator but a rediscoverer of forgotten goods and I hope a remover of obtrusive bric-a-brac.''

Source: Erika M. Kreger, for *Drama for Students,* Gale, 1998.

Lewis Nichols

In this review of The Skin of Our Teeth, *which was originally published on November 19, 1942, Nichols offers a positive review of the original Broadway production of the play.*

A few seasons ago Thornton Wilder increased the stature of the theatre with *Our Town* and now that November again lies heavy over Broadway he has done it once more. For in *The Skin of Our Teeth,* which Michael Myerberg brought last evening to the Plymouth, he has written a comedy about man which is the best play the Forties have seen in many months, the best pure theatre.

Mr. Wilder is no pedantic philosopher, setting down the laws of the schoolmaster; when he is writing for the theatre he uses all of its arts. His story of man's constant struggle for survival, and his wonderment over why he so struggles, is presented with pathos and broad comedy, with gentle irony and sometimes a sly self-raillery. He does not believe the footlights should separate his players from his audience; his actors now and then step out of their characters to discuss the progress of the play, to comment on what it means or what it does not mean.

In *The Skin of Our Teeth* the scenery bounces up and down, the players carry on rehearsals, at one point there is a call to the audience to send along its chairs to keep the fire going against the advancing Ice Age. Everywhere in both the dialogue and the properties that surround it are a series of anachronisms, so beautifully blended as to make Excelsior, N. J., quite properly a hold-out against the Ice Age, and Atlantic City the point from which the ark took off against the flood.

The first act is Excelsior, and Mr. Antrobus—played by Fredric March—has had a considerable day in town: He has fixed up the alphabet by separating em from en, he has brought the multiplication table up to the hundreds, he has invented the wheel. But in August at Excelsior it is growing colder, so cold the ''dogs are sticking to the sidewalk,'' and obviously the ice is coming down from Vermont. The neighbors come in—Homer, Moses, others—and Mr. Antrobus and his wife, after wondering if it's all worth while, begin cramming

> "THORNTON WILDER HAS WRITTEN A COMEDY ABOUT MAN WHICH IS THE BEST PLAY THE FORTIES HAVE SEEN IN MANY MONTHS, THE BEST PURE THEATRE."

their children with knowledge, in the hope they will survive somehow and can build again on the other side.

The second act is Atlantic City, at the convention of the Ancient and Honorable Order of Mammals, Subdivision Humans, where Mr. Antrobus, pompous with power and tired of his wife, again almost falls to disaster. The third is at the end of the war—any war—when Mr. Antrobus is properly beaten, but finally decides to start off again. This time the things he sees as reasons are "the voice of the people in their confusion and need," his wife, children and home, knowledge. He goes on, having gotten by only by the skin of his teeth.

The cast Mr. Myerberg has assembled should always fill Mr. Wilder's plays. First, there is Tallulah Bankhead, in the role of Sabina, who is variously the Antrobus maid, the bathing beauty, the camp follower who has been off to the wars for seven years. Her role is the eternal Helen of Troy, Cleopatra, who wanders off on her own affairs when all is quiet, who comes home and helps out when the going is rough. Miss Bankhead is magnificent—breezy, hard, practical by turns. She can strut and posture in broad comedy, she can be calmly serene. It is she who steps out of character to discuss the play, marvelous interludes all of them.

As Mr. Antrobus, Mr. March is at first the roaring, blustering inventor and amasser of knowledge, bringing home his new wheel with a loud whoop; then the pontifical new president of the Mammals in convention assembled; finally the war-weary and discouraged soldier coming home from battle. Florence Eldridge is Mrs. Antrobus, the mother and home-builder, the steadying influence who, in the Atlantic City period, is out of place, too. Miss Eldridge can be either the steady housekeeper or a Helen Hokinson drawing. Each of the Marches has every reason to be proud of the other.

And there are others: Montgomery Clift, as Henry, the son, the Henry who used to be called Cain and has a scar on his forehead; and Frances Heflin, as Gladys, daughter of the Antrobuses. There also in Florence Reed as a cynical, surly, contemptuous fortune-teller, and Dickie Van Patten as a telegraph boy and E. G. Marshall as the stage manager, who grows more and more harassed as the evening goes on. Elia Kazan directed in the mood meant by Mr. Wilder, and Albert Johnson has provided the informal settings that tilt and slide as a perfect cover to the play.

As of last evening the theatre was looking up. Definitely.

Source: Lewis Nichols, review of *The Skin of Our Teeth* (1942) in *On Stage: Selected Theater Reviews from the New York Times, 1920–1970,* edited by Bernard Beckerman and Howard Siegman, Arno Press, 1973, pp. 242–243.

Peter Fleming

Terming Wilder's drama a "morality play" designed to make audiences think about the consequences of their lives, Fleming gives the work a favorable review. He singles out such high points as a "high degree of suspense" and the play's theme of the "invincibility of the human spirit"—factors which make The Skin of Our Teeth *"astonishingly successful" theatre.*

It is by the skin of our teeth, the author very plausibly asserts, that the human race escapes the consequences of its own proclivities for self-destruction. He calls his morality play "a history of mankind in comic strip," and though the history is allusive and surrealist the strip is undeniably comic. Nothing, in fact, could be less ponderous than Mr. Thornton Wilder's approach to his weighty theme. It is nevertheless truly philosophical.

Mr. and Mrs. Antrobus represent *Homo Sapiens* down the ages. They have a son and a daughter, and in the son germinate the seeds of what the Russians call "deviationism"—the itch first to break away from and then to overthrow the established order. The pert and lovely Sabina is their servant, feckless yet oddly faithful, shallow but percipient. Jabberwockian is the only word with which to describe the pattern of their vicissitudes. Some slight idea of the dramatist's technique may be conveyed by recalling that Moses and Homer are among refugees fleeing from the Ice Age who seek asylum in the Antrobus's New Jersey home, which already shelters a dinosaur and a mammoth. Nor is chronology the only convention which Mr. Thornton Wilder, with an engaging insouciance, defies. At frequent intervals the actors, and in particular Sabina, step outside the play and make their own adverse comments on it, so that a harassed stage-manager has to intervene to restore order. In short, the tactics of the Crazy Gang are employed in an attempt to solve the ultimate riddle of human destiny.

The result is astonishingly successful. One merit of the author's capricious (to put it mildly) methods is that they engender a very high degree of suspense; with no possible means of telling what is going to happen next on or, for that matter, off the stage, the audience has no choice but to remain alert and curious. But the play has solider virtues than this. Its theme is the invincibility of the human spirit, and despite the atmosphere of harlequinade there is something moving and noble in the spectacle of Mr. and Mrs. Antrobus, though conscious of their own follies and failings, and aware that each renewal of hope after a hard-won victory will be cheated by fresh disasters, refusing to admit defeat. The author takes every conceivable kind of risk—save only that of being pompous. Never was a message put across with less solemnity: and seldom with greater success.

The play unquestionably owes much to its producer, Mr. Laurence Olivier, who has imposed a tremendous pace on its zany symbolism. It is also deeply in debt to his wife, Miss Vivien Leigh, whose enchantingly detached Sabina is a very fine piece of comic acting. Mr. George Devine's rugged and impressive Antrobus is well matched by Miss Esther Somers's quiet but powerful portrait of his wife. I also liked very much poor Mr. Fitzpatrick, whoever he was; he does not appear on the programme, but he was frequently on the stage, composing with a dire embarrassment recurrent mutinies among the cast. *The Skin of our Teeth* is as topical as Mr. Molotov's liver, and is well worth going to see.

Source: Peter Fleming, review of *The Skin of Our Teeth* in the *Spectator,* Volume 177, no. 6169, September 20, 1946 , p. 287.

"THE AUTHOR TAKES EVERY CONCEIVABLE KIND OF RISK—SAVE ONLY THAT OF BEING POMPOUS. NEVER WAS A MESSAGE PUT ACROSS WITH LESS SOLEMNITY: AND SELDOM WITH GREATER SUCCESS."

James N. Vaughn

Vaughn reviews the original Broadway production of Wilder's play, finding the cast and production values to be of the highest quality. The critic feels, however, that the playwright's text does not achieve what his previous play, Our Town, *did in terms of enchanting an audience.*

Thornton Wilder in his new play has preached a sermon in a style joining asides like those of Saint Bernard with jarring juxtapositions like those of T. S. Eliot. Life, he wants to say, is struggle to discover truth, to build material conditions in the image of truth and above all to subdue natural forces and human anger, lust and unreason. Within himself and without, everyman meets such forces—inexhaustible supplies of arrogant energy blindly seeking his moral and material destruction. Working day and night they make moral and physical development a process ever balanced on the "razor edge of danger." Wilder says through this play that the unhuman irrational principles give us *in man* everything from bingo to war: everything sordid, dull, vulgar, carnal and murderous. In nature these principles develop a slow, unending series of frightful catastrophes from ice packs to hurricanes. Thus it has always been and so it will be always. Nevertheless we live, and rightly, with hope and faith because God has announced that our general conditions shall be permanently improved by thought, orderliness and the achievement of moral integrity.

The story is told of George Antrobus, his wife and two children. Antrobus, a kind of Adam, is the inventive, practical, home-building man. In the end he lives by thought and spirit despite momentary falls from grace. He is tried by nature, by lust and by the rebellion of his own son, but he survives because within him is an undying determination to begin anew the construction of the perfect world.

To preach his sermon Wilder has the advantage of the superlative talent of Fredric March and Florence Eldridge as Mr. and Mrs. Antrobus. Tallulah Bankhead supplies the comic touch and carnal intimations—with modest success, I should say. Florence Reed as the Fortune Teller charged with ominous passages regarding the unknowability of the human past is superb.

Had the play been placed in less capable hands it might have been a grotesque failure. It lacks enchantment. The device, freely employed, of bringing the audience into the play need not destroy continuity of audience feeling as Mr. Wilder in *Our Town* proved. But the same technique fails in the present play because it is too overt, too garish, too sensational in the literal sense. The reception of the audience was tepid.

Source: James N. Vaughn, review of *The Skin of Our Teeth* in *Commonweal,* Volume XXXVII, no. 7, December 4, 1942, pp. 175–76.

SOURCES

Adler, Thomas P. ''Theater Looking at Theater: A Self-Image of Post-World War II American Drama'' in *Claudel Studies,* Volume 9, number 1, 1982, pp. 31, 40.

Atkinson, Brooks. ''*The Skin of Our Teeth*—Thornton Wilder Writes a Wise and Frisky Comedy about People'' in the *New York Times,* November 22, 1942, section 8, p. 1.

Cheney, Sheldon. *The Theatre: Three Thousand Years of Drama, Acting, and Stagecraft,* Longmans, Green, 1952, p. 570.

Dusenbury, Winifred. ''Myth in American Drama between the Wars'' in *Modern Drama,* Volume 6, 1963, p. 298.

Freedley, George. ''The Stage Today'' in the *New York Morning Telegraph,* November 20, 1942, p. 2.

Nietzsche, Friedrich. *The Birth of Tragedy and the Genealogy of Morals,* Doubleday, 1956, p. 106.

Whiting, Frank M. *An Introduction to: The Theatre,* Harper & Brothers, 1954, p. 106.

Wilder, Thornton. *The Journals of Thornton Wilder, 1939-1961,* Yale University Press, 1985, pp. 22, 24, 37.

Wilder, Thornton. Preface to *Three Plays,* Harper & Row, 1957, pp. viii, xi-xiv.

Wilder, Thornton. ''Some Thoughts on Playwriting'' in *Playwrights on Playwriting,* edited by Toby Cole, Hill and Wang, 1960, p. 108.

Willett, John, Editor. *Brecht on Theatre,* Hill and Wang, 1964, p. 212.

FURTHER READING

Bigsby, C. W. E. *A Critical Introduction to Twentieth-Century American Drama: Volume One, 1900-1940,* Cambridge University Press, 1982.

A good overview of American theater before World War II, this discussion devotes a full chapter to Wilder.

Blank, Martin, Editor. *Critical Essays on Thornton Wilder,* G.K. Hall, 1996.

This is a good recent collection of articles on Wilder's work.

Harrison, Gilbert A. *The Enthusiast: A Life of Thornton Wilder,* Ticknor and Fields, 1983.

This biography, which makes use of Wilder's papers at the Yale University Beinecke Library, includes many excerpts from unpublished journals and notebooks that illuminate Wilder's troubled personal life.

Walsh, Claudette. *Thornton Wilder: A Reference Guide, 1926-1990,* G.K. Hall, 1993.

This comprehensive annotated bibliography of works by and about Wilder is an invaluable resource for anyone studying his writings.

The Threepenny Opera

BERTOLT BRECHT

1928

Bertolt Brecht's 1928 play *The Threepenny Opera* was his most financially successful play and the work with which he is most closely identified. The play is an early example of his ''epic theater,'' consisting of theatrical innovations designed to awaken audiences to social responsibility. Epic theater uses ''alienating'' devices, such as placards, asides to the audience, projected images, discordant music and lighting, and disconnected episodes to frustrate the viewer's expectations for simple entertainment. This ''theater of illusions'' (as anti-realists such as Brecht termed it) allowed the audience to comfortably and passively view a production without being changed by it. It was Brecht's intention to use drama to invoke social change, to shake his audiences out of their complacency and expect more from the theater than entertainment.

The disruptive capacity of Brecht's drama was designed to awaken the theater-goers critical mind and galvanize them into political awareness and action. *The Threepenny Opera,* which he produced with the aid of his secretary (and lover) Elisabeth Hauptmann (who had just translated John Gay's *The Beggar's Opera* [1728] into German) and composer Kurt Weill, is a satire of bourgeois society, containing many of the major elements of epic theater: placards announcing the ballad singers, discordant music, and a plot that frustrates expectations for romantic resolution. *The Threepenny Opera* is very closely based on Gay's eighteenth-century play, another social satire. Brecht and

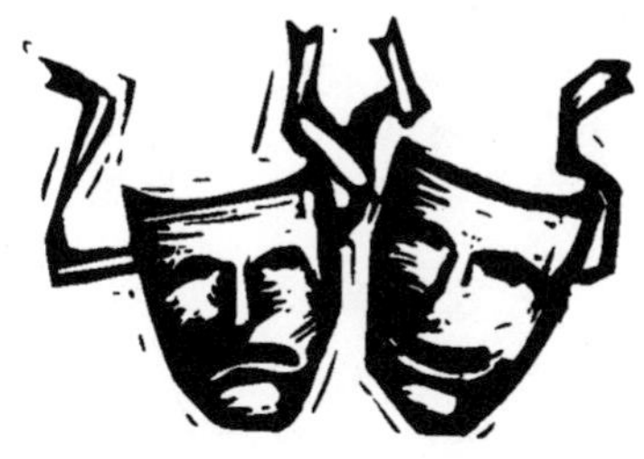

Hauptmann borrowed ballads from Francois Villon, and Weill turned them into darkly twisted cabaret songs for this version of the play.

Brecht also made some stylistic changes, transforming the protagonist, Macheath, into a morally ambiguous hero, emphasizing the parallels between Polly and Lucy, and creating the character of Sheriff Jackie Brown, a former army buddy of Macheath's who protects his friend's criminal activity in exchange for a percentage of his spoils. Brecht's play places blame on capitalist society for the criminal underworld that Gay presented merely as a mirror-image satire of eighteenth-century aristocracy. Weill's discordant mesh of jazz, folk, and avant-garde music adds to the play's popular appeal, which was the polar opposite of what Brecht wanted: he designed his ''epic theater'' to awaken the audience's critical judgement, not its empathy. Despite Brecht's designs, *The Threepenny Opera* has become one of the hallmarks of musical theater and his most popular play. While it is regarded in modern drama as a significant political work, it is equally revered for its unique music and darkly engaging characters.

AUTHOR BIOGRAPHY

Born Eugen Bertolt Friedrich Brecht on February 10, 1898, in Augsburg, Germany, Bertold Brecht is regarded as a founding father of modern theater and one of its most incisive voices. His innovative ideas would prove to have a profound effect on many genres of modern narrative, not the least of which are novels, short stories, and cinema. Brecht is considered a pioneer of socially conscious theater—especially in the subgenre of anti-reality theater, which sought to debunk the illusory techniques of realistic drama. His work reflects his commitment to his political beliefs. By the time he was a young adult he had firmly embraced the communist doctrines of Karl Marx, a German philosopher who authored the seminal texts *The Communist Manifesto* and *Das Kapital.*

Brecht began life as the intellectually rebellious son of a bourgeois (middle-class) paper factory director. His mother was Catholic, his father Protestant; Brecht disavowed any religious affiliation, and his first play, written when he was sixteen-years-old, exposes the conflicting lessons of the Bible—early evidence of his life—long effort to erode the infrastructure of complacency in his society. During World War I, he was unable to avoid conscription into the German army (by studying medicine) and so served as an orderly in an army hospital. The meaningless suffering he witnessed there embittered his already pessimistic worldview.

Always fascinated by dualities and cultural opposites, Brecht sought to expose the ridiculousness of either extreme, while never offering any kind of transcendent alternative, thus earning many critics' condemnation as a nihilist (one who believes that traditional values have no foundation in reality and that existence is pointless). Often his plays and poems depict situations that seem naturally aimed toward romantic conclusions yet avoid such easy resolutions. By the time he reached adulthood, Brecht had already established himself as a lady's man, often juggling wives, ex-wives, and lovers who lived within blocks of each other and bore his children—often at the same time.

One of Brecht's many significant others, Elisabeth Hauptmann, collaborated with him on his adaptation of John Gay's eighteenth-century play *The Beggar's Opera,* which he debuted in 1928 as *The Threepenny Opera.* The work featured music by renowned composer Kurt Weill and became one of the playwright's best-known dramas (thanks in large part to singer Bobby Darrin's popular cover of the play's song ''Mack the Knife''). Recent biographers speculate that Brecht ran a veritable writing sweatshop, using the talents of his harem of women, who stood little chance of literary success without his paternalistic shepherding or his political and intellectual inspiration.

Prior to the political ascension of Adolf Hitler's Nazi party in the 1930s, Brecht fled Germany and lived in exile in Europe and the United States. In 1947, he was unsuccessfully interrogated by the House Committee on Un-American Activities for his outspoken communist sympathies. He returned to Germany in 1948, where he established the Berlin Ensemble, a theatrical production troupe dedicated to political and artistic reform. In this latter period of his life, he produced what is regarded as some of his best work, including the plays *Mother Courage and Her Children* (1949) and *The*

Good Woman of Szechuan (1953). He died of coronary thrombosis on August 14, 1956, in the then-communist country of East Germany.

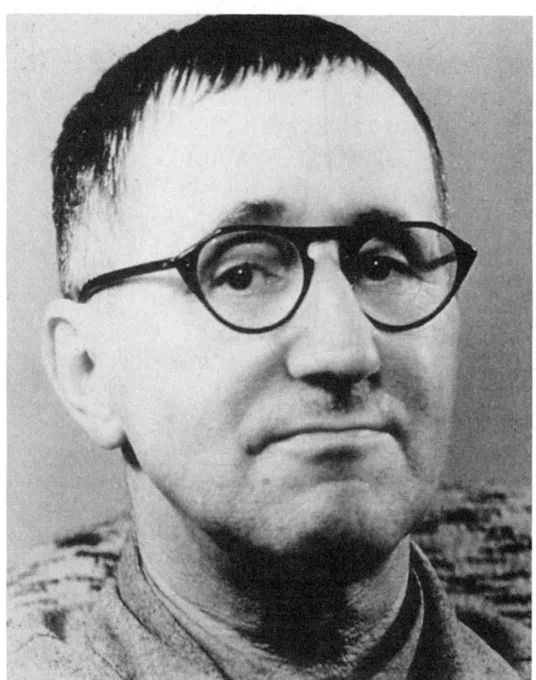

Bertolt Brecht

PLOT SUMMARY

Act I

The Prologue of *The Threepenny Opera* presents Fair Day in Soho (a suburb of London), where beggars, thieves, and whores ply their trades. A ballad singer steps forward to sing a macabre ditty about Mac the Knife. Peachum, proprietor of ''The Beggar's Friend Ltd.'' strolls back and forth across the stage with his wife and daughter. At the close of the song, Low-dive Jenny says that she sees Mac the Knife, who disappears into the crowd.

In Scene One, it is morning in the Peachum business emporium, where the proprietor outfits beggars for their swindling careers. The scene opens with Peachum singing his morning hymn to the glory of human betrayal and deception. Peachum appeals to the audience to consider the complexities of his business: raising human sympathy often necessitates counterfeit misery, because the public has become so jaded that it's donations diminish over time. He interprets the Biblical saying, ''Give and it shall be given unto you'' as meaning, provide new reasons to give to the poor.

A young man, Charles Filch (the word ''filch'' is slang for stealing), enters the shop. He reports that a beggar gang have beat him up for begging on their territory. Peachum offers him a district and an improved beggaring outfit in return for fifty percent of his take. Filch does not inspire Peachum's confidence because he succumbs too easily to pity; begging requires sterner stuff, less of a conscience. Mrs. Peachum enters and discusses the whereabouts of their daughter, Polly, with Peachum. The couple sing a brief satirical duet on love.

In Scene Two, beggar gang member Matthew (a.k.a. Matt of the Mint) enters a stable to ensure that it is empty. Macheath brings in Polly, dressed in a stolen wedding dress. Moments later large vans appear, containing luxurious—and certainly stolen—furniture and tableware for the wedding. The rest of the beggar gang also arrive. In a comedy of grotesque decorum, the gang critiques the wedding appointments while Polly and Macheath cling to the semblance of a dignified ceremony. Realizing that a wedding song is conventional, Macheath orders three of the boys, already considerably drunk, to sing one, to which they lamely comply.

Polly reciprocates with her own, rather hostile tune about a barmaid named Jenny, which Macheath pronounces art, wasted on trash. A Reverend, actually one of the gang, arrives to perform the ceremony. The party is nearly dispersed by the arrival of a special guest, Macheath's old army buddy, Jackie Brown, the High Sheriff of London. He and Macheath drink together and sing an old army tune, ''The Cannon Song.'' While Macheath makes maudlin comparisons to classical friendships such as Castor and Pollux and Hector and Andromache, Brown notices the wealth around him and grows pensive. Macheath has succeeded in life in a way that Brown has not. Before Brown leaves, Macheath confirms that Brown has kept his record clean at Scotland Yard. Finally, the gang displays the crowning glory of their stolen goods: a new bed. The scene closes with a cynical duet (''love will endure or not endure. . .'') between the newly ''married'' couple.

Scene Three takes place back at Peachum's place of business, where Polly sings a song to her parents revealing her new marriage. Her parents are appalled that she has married a notorious criminal. A group of beggars enter, one complaining about the poor quality of his false stump. Peachum grouses about the beggar's lack of professional deportment and then turns back to the problem of his daughter's bad marital match. Peachum lands upon a solution: turn Macheath into the police, get him hanged, and earn a forty-pound ransom at the same time. The family sings a trio on "The Insecurity of the Human Condition" containing the refrain "The world is poor and man's a shit." Then, Peachum exits to bribe Low-Dive Jenny to betray Macheath to the police.

Act Two

Scene Four (the scenes are numbered sequentially through the whole play) takes place in the stable, now Polly and Macheath's home. Polly begs Macheath to flee, because she has witnessed Brown succumbing to her father's threats; Macheath will be arrested. Macheath puts Polly in charge of the accounts and preps the gang for the upcoming coronation, a huge business opportunity for thieves and beggars. Macheath departs. In an Interlude, Mrs. Peachum and Low-Dive Jenny step in front of the curtain to sing "The Ballad of Sexual Obsession" after Celia bribes Jenny with ten shillings to reveal Macheath's whereabouts to the police.

Scene Five takes place at the whorehouse in Highgate. It is Thursday, the day Macheath normally visits but the proprietor and the whores don't expect him; they are ironing, playing cards, or washing. Macheath enters and cavalierly throws his warrant for arrest on the floor. Jenny offers to read his palm, predicting treacherousness at the hand of a woman whose name begins with "J." Macheath makes a joke of it, as Jenny slips out a side door. As Macheath sings "The Ballad of Immoral Earnings," Jenny can be seen beckoning to Constable Smith. She joins in a duet with Macheath, describing her battered life with him. As they end, Constable Smith takes Macheath away to the Old Bailey (the prison).

In Scene Six, Brown is wringing his hands at the Old Bailey, in fear that his buddy has been caught. Macheath enters, tied heavily in ropes and accompanied by six constables. Mac writes a check to Constable Smith in return for not applying handcuffs and sings "The Ballad of Good Living." One of Macheath's lovers, Lucy, enters, too enraged by jealousy to care about Macheath's fate. Polly then enters and the two women sing the "Jealousy Duet." Macheath denies that he has married Polly, accusing her of masquerading to get pity. Mrs. Peachum comes to drag Polly away. Now Lucy and Macheath make up, and he elicits her promise to help him escape. He does so, but talks her out of going with him.

Mr. Peachum arrives to enjoy the sight of his triumph over Macheath, only to find Brown sitting in his cell. Peachum convinces Brown to go after Macheath or imperil his reputation. The lawman departs. The curtain falls, and Macheath and Low-Dive Jenny appear to sing the duet, "What Keeps Mankind Alive?," the answers to which are: bestial acts and represssion.

Act Three

Scene Seven opens on the Peachum Emporium in preparation for their grand plan of disrupting the coronation ceremony with "a demonstration of human misery." This is a massive campaign: nearly fifteen-hundred men are preparing signs. The whores traipse in for their payoff, which Mrs. Peachum refuses to pay because Macheath has escaped. Jenny lets it slip that Macheath is with the whore Suky Tawdry, so Peachum sends word to the constables. Mrs. Peachum sings a stanza from "The Ballad of Sexual Obsession." Brown enters and threatens to arrest the lot of the beggars, but Peachum blackmails him by insisting that they are busy preparing a song for the coronation. The boys sing "The Song of the Insufficiency of Human Endeavor." As Brown disconsolately leaves to arrest Macheath, the curtain falls and Jenny sings a ballad about sexual urges.

Scene Eight takes place in the Old Bailey. Polly and Lucy compare notes on Macheath and befriend one another. Lucy hears a commotion and announces that Mac has been arrested again. Polly collapses, then changes into widows garb.

Scene Nine finds Macheath shackled and led by constables into his death cell. The police are worried that his hanging will draw a bigger crowd than the coronation. Smith is willing to help Macheath escape for one thousand pounds, but Macheath cannot get his hands on his money. Brown comes in to settle his accounts with Mac. Through all of this, visits from Lucy, Polly, Peachum, the gang, and the whores, Mac is notably casual about his impending doom. He sings a song asking forgiveness and proceeds to the gallows. Peachum presides, but his speech begins as a eulogy and ends as an announcement that Brown has arrived on horseback to save Mac. Brown announces that because of the coronation, Mac has been reprieved and raised to peerage. They cheer, sing, and the bells of Westminster ring.

CHARACTERS

Ballad Singer

The unnamed Ballad Singer serves as a kind of Greek chorus, commenting and explaining the play's action as it unfolds. He opens the story with a grotesquely playful tale of Mac the Knife, an actual historical character who murdered prostitutes in London. Although John Gay's *Beggar's Opera* (the source material for Brecht's work) included ballads about the thieves in his dramatic world, the songs were not as outrageous as those sung by Brecht's narrator—a credit to the musical talents of Brecht and his composer, Kurt Weil. Throughout *The Threepenny Opera,* the Ballad Singer punctuates the action with distastefully mordant commentaries on the seamy action of the play, sung to a discordant tune. He sings the play's best-known musical number ''Moritat'' (or ''Theme from the Threepenny Opera'')—more commonly known as ''Mac the Knife''—which was popularized by singer Bobby Darrin in 1959.

Sheriff Jackie Brown

Brown is the crooked High Sheriff who takes a portion of the beggars' earnings in return for tip-offs about planned police raids. He is a long-time friend of Macheath, having served with him as a soldier in India. Brown attends Polly and Mac's wedding and is taken aback by the wealth that surrounds his friend. When cornered by Peachum, who cites a list of Macheath's crimes, Brown is forced to send Constable Smith out to arrest his former pal. He is a weak-willed and greedy man who expresses sorrow upon seeing Macheath in jail at the Old Bailey but nevertheless accepts the money from Peachum. Finally, as Macheath stands at the gallows, Brown rides up on horseback with a reprieve.

Lucy Brown

Lucy is the Tiger Brown's daughter. Mac has been having an affair with Lucy, deceiving both his friend and Polly. Lucy appears to be pregnant—the father presumably Macheath—but she reveals to Polly that she has faked her pregnancy by stuffing a pillow under her dress. Lucy at first treats Polly with haughtiness but later agrees with Polly's assertion that Macheath loves her more. Lucy finally befriends her lover's wife.

Charles Filch

Filch comes innocently enough into Peachum's beggar's outfitting emporium, hoping to obtain Peachum's permission to beg on a certain street corner. Filch proves himself singularly unsuited for the career of begging, however, being naturally inclined to pity—he expresses guilt over accepting money from people.

The Gang

With fellows such as Bob-the-Saw, Crook-fingered Jake, Jimmy, Matthew (or Matt of the Mint), Ned, Robert, and Dreary Walt, the Gang consists of thieves, cutpurses, prostitutes, pimps, and beggars. All of them are supplied costumes for the trade of begging by Mr. Jonathan Jeremiah Peachum, and they forfeit a percentage of their earnings to Macheath, who uses the money as a pay-off to Sheriff Brown for protecting their racket. There is no honor among these thieves; all are ready to turn on their brothers if it will buy them an evening of food and pleasure. They give stolen gifts to Mac and Polly at their wedding.

Reverend Kimball

Kimball performs the impromptu wedding between Polly and Macheath. He is more than likely not a real priest, as he is also one of the thieving Gang.

Low-dive Jenny

Low-dive Jenny is a former lover of Mac's and now just one of the whores of the gang. Like the Biblical character of Judas (who deceived his leader Jesus Christ), Jenny betrays Macheath. She pretends to read Macheath's palm, hinting at a dismal future event, then she informs Constable Smith of the thief's whereabouts.

Mac the Knife

See Macheath

Macheath

A former war hero turned master thief, Macheath is the dark hero, the grotesque Christ figure of *The Threepenny Opera.* His name alludes to the murder-

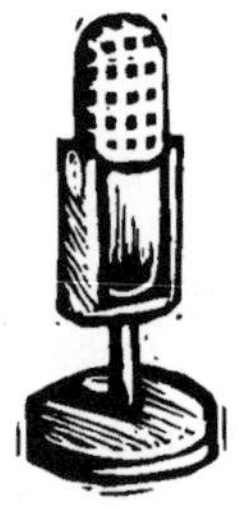

MEDIA ADAPTATIONS

- Brecht wrote *The Threepenny Opera* as a novel in 1934 (*Dreigroschenroman,* translated by Vesey and Isherwood as *A Penny for the Poor,* R. Hale, 1937; reprinted as *Threepenny Novel*, Grove, 1956); but it was his play that received the most attention. He revised the script for a 1931 film version to be more politically oriented than the original 1928 play script. The black and white German film (*Die Dreigroschenoper* with English subtitles), directed by G. W. Pabst and starring Antonin Artaud, is available on video from Embassy Home Entertainment.
- Metro-Goldwyn-Mayer (MGM) released a 1954 recording of Kurt Weil's music for *The Threepenny Opera.*
- Marc Blitzstein revived *The Threepenney Opera* in the 1950s and his revision of the ''Mack the Knife'' song became a worldwide hit for singer Bobby Darrin.
- A 1989 film version, alternatively titled *Mack the Knife,* was released by Columbia. Directed by Menahem Golan, the film features Raul Julia as Macheath and rock star Roger Daltrey (of the Who) as the Ballad Singer.

er Mac the Knife in Brecht's play; he was merely an underworld criminal and womanizer in Gay's *The Beggar's Opera.* His mother-in-law, Mrs. Peachum calls him a horse-thief and a highwayman (one who robs travelers). Much like Brecht, Macheath is also a womanizer who conducts simultaneous affairs with a variety of women; he plays the attentive husband to Polly while also pursuing an affair with his friend Tiger's daughter, Lucy.

Macheath is the kingpin of the beggar gang, a jaded criminal, and a slave to his ''sexual urges.'' He appears to pursue his lifestyle with little emotion or regret. He whistles nonchalantly when Polly reads him the list of charges the police have against him: ''You've killed two shopkeepers, more than thirty burglaries, twenty-three hold-ups, and God knows how many acts of arson, attempted murder, forgery, and perjury, all within eighteen months. In Winchester you seduced two sisters under the age of consent.'' Macheath's only response to the entire list of charges is that he thought the girls were twenty.

His father-in-law, Peachum, turns Macheath over to the police to rid his daughter (as well as his own business interests) of him. In the father's eyes, Macheath is not a desirable match. Despite facing a sentence of death for his crimes, Macheath is tough and practical, brusquely ordering Polly to watch over his interests. He accepts his fate like the soldier he once was, although he persists until the last minute in trying to bribe his way out of jail.

Celia Peachum

Polly's mother and Peachum's wife, Celia assists her husband at the emporium by bossing the beggars. She faints when she learns that Polly has married Macheath because she sees this as a good investment gone bad: In her mother's eyes, Polly had the potential to be a society lady and could have raised the family's status by marrying a wealthy man.

Jonathan Jeremiah Peachum

Peachum is the proprietor of ''The Beggar's Friend, Ltd.'' He runs the begging in London like an efficient business, outfitting the beggars, training them to perfect their methods (especially the art of swindling suckers), and assigning them districts in which to work. Peachum, like Fagin in Charles Dickens's *Oliver Twist,* takes a percentage of each of the Gang's earnings, slowly getting rich while his employees live hand-to-mouth. Peachum needs Polly around his business to attract customers with her good looks. This exploitation of his daughter's charms is disrupted when she falls in love with

Macheath, marrying the thief without her father's permission. True to his greedy and ruthless ways, Peachum solves the problem by selling Macheath out to the police.

Polly Peachum

Polly is the daughter of the beggar king, Jonathan Jeremiah Peachum. She is referred to by her father as ''a lump of sensuality''—a fact that he shamelessly exploits to increase his business. Polly marries her lover, Macheath, in a makeshift ceremony in a stable. During the proceedings, she learns that Macheath has also been sexually active with Lucy.

When Lucy and Polly meet they accuse each other ruining their respective relationships with Macheath. They sing a duet in which they trade lines berating each other. While Polly and Lucy are very similar characters, it is Polly who prevails in a sustained union with Macheath. While she does not like her husband's sexual promiscuity, she accepts it as a fundamental part of his nature.

Constable Smith

Smith is the police officer who arrests Macheath, though he accepts a bribe to leave the handcuffs off. He later offers to help Macheath escape for a one-thousand pound bribe.

Tiger

See Sheriff Jackie Brown

THEMES

Betrayal and Moral Corruption

Like the ''greatest story ever told,'' the story of Jesus, the protagonist of *The Threepenny Opera* is betrayed by a former intimate. But there the similarity ends, or rather, diverts to mirrored opposites. Macheath is not a savior like Christ but a moral corrupter, not a paragon of virtue but a fountainhead of sin, not the archetypal human ideal but a base man of bestial instinct. In contrast to Jesus, he marries the woman with whom he has been sleeping in a stable rather than being born of a chaste woman in a stable. The wedding gown and gifts are not humble attire and ritual offerings but stolen goods.

Despite these oppositions to one of the best-known symbols of purity, Macheath is not a completely evil figure. He has some appeal, especially to the whores and women of low virtue. He is gallant in his way, cuffing his gang members for not displaying enough gentility to his new bride; he has courage—or at least disdain for his fate; and he has a loyal friendship with his army buddy Jackie Brown. He has a roguish charm but his personality is presented not as a role model but as a warning against the seductive quality of such a dishonest life.

Nor is Macheath the only false idol in the play. Peachum is in the business of guiding beggars to larger profits falsely earned in the name of charity. He preys upon the generosity of the public, justifying his use of false wounds and artificial limbs with his own twist on the biblical homily ''Give and it shall be given unto you.'' Peachum argues that people are jaded and must be prodded to charity by ever newer and more ghastly representations of poverty. Yet the proprietor takes a whopping fifty percent of his beggars' earnings, betraying the very purpose of begging through his swindling.

Peachum also betrays his own daughter by having her new husband arrested. The whores are the chorus of this play, and they are as corrupt as the main characters. Low-dive Jenny (J as in Judas), a former lover of Macheath's, betrays him for a handful of money, which she is denied when Macheath escapes. In fact, Macheath has escaped due to the betrayal of the jail guard, whom the robber king has bribed. Furthermore, the whores know Macheath has escaped, and effectively are betraying Peachum when they demand payment for a job that was not satisfactorily completed. The list could go on, including Jackie Brown, who seesaws morally as he wrestles with remaining loyal to Macheath versus saving his own reputation and livelihood. The ubiquity of the corruption and betrayal in *The Threepenny Opera* goes beyond social criticism to a kind of macabre, black humor.

Art and Experience

The purpose of Brecht's plays (as they were originally staged by the author) was to create an experience that would force audiences out of their common perceptions of bourgeois theater (as merely a means of entertainment). His plays sought to instill a willingness to work for social change. Thus, ultimately, Brecht's plays were designed as tools of moral and social propaganda, yet they strangely lack what most propaganda, by definition, carries with it: a design for a utopian social paradise that social reform might achieve. Brecht's plays are largely pessimistic: they offer what biographer Martin

TOPICS FOR FURTHER STUDY

- Compare the plot of *The Threepenny Opera* with the plot of John Gay's 1728 *The Beggar's Opera.* Macheath is more villainous in Brecht's version, and Lockit (a Newgate prison chief in Gay's play) has transformed into Jackie Brown, a corrupt sheriff and old army buddy of Macheath's. Consider also the differences in language and staging. What is the significance of the changes Brecht made to Gay's work?
- The ''alienating effects'' of Brecht's staging have become standard fare in modern drama. Does this lessen their impact on contemporary audiences? Why or why not?
- Brecht was becoming a committed Marxist when he produced *The Threepenny Opera.* In his play, what evidence do you find of Marxist concepts such as dialectical materialism (that change occurs as problems are resolved through conflict), distrust in capitalism, and desire for a classless society?
- In the final scene, Brown enacts a ''deus ex machina'' ending by granting a pardon to Macheath at the last minute before his hanging. Such endings, where the hero is saved at the last minute, are common to drama, but seldom found in novels, short stories, or poems. Think of other deus ex machina endings and develop a theory of their significance in theatrical works.

Esslin chose as the subtitle to his book *Brecht,* a ''choice of evils'' rather than the choice between a right and a wrong way to live.

This aspect of Brecht's work has garnered much critical attention and warrants further contemplation. In *The Threepenny Opera,* the opera format—already stretching the viewer's sense of realism—is made even more alien through constant reminders of the artifice of the play. Placards announcing the events and songs, asides to the audience, and lyrics incongruent with the action disrupt and sully any positive sentiments being expressed. For example, when Brown and Macheath reminisce about their days in the army, the ditty they sing cynically celebrates the fate of all soldiers to be chopped into tartar (ground meat). When Peachum complains about his lot in life, he sings that God has humankind in a trap that is a ''load of crap.'' In both cases, what might be profound social commentary is turned into a sick joke. In places, Brecht does address seriously the social ills he wants his audience to face and be moved to change. But he does not offer answers or a rectifying course of action. Rather than offer pat solutions to complex social problems, Brecht forces the spectator to ponder these issues and arrive at their own remedy.

STYLE

Opera or Musical?

An opera is a play that contains music (instrumental and/or vocal) as well as dialogue, and the music is just as important to the piece as is the action and spoken words of the characters. The style of singing is known as *recitative,* which means that the sung words are slightly modified from normal speech, just enough to make them melodic. In operas, the characters sing in the recitative mode during the action of the drama, occasionally launching into a more definitive song, during which the action temporarily stops. It is not a true opera if the lines are spoken instead of sung.

In a musical, the players do not sing their lines but rather speak them normally. The players do, however, break into song and dance at certain points in the play. The action is punctuated by these musical interludes. In an opera, the songs are somewhat more integrated into the recitative singing in the rest of the drama (for the most part, the vocal activity in opera takes the form of singing). In addition, the artistry of an opera lies in the virtuoso singing performances of the performers, not in their qualities as actors or dancers. By contrast, the songs of a musical, while they may showcase the musical abilities of the actors and actresses, are not the *raison d'etre* (justification for existence) of the musical. The musical is a composite of song, dance, music, and drama in which each element contributes equally. In some cases (particularly cinematic musicals) one performer will record or ''dub'' the vocals while an actor (who may have no musical ability but can act) performs the speaking parts and lip-synchs to the pre-recorded singing. This practice would be unheard of in an opera, where the performance of the singers is paramount.

Following these guidelines, *The Threepenny Opera* is an opera in name only; its form of spoken *and* sung vocal parts defines it as a musical not a traditional opera. The musical was an American invention of the early twentieth century, a natural outgrowth of vaudeville, in which unrelated acts of singing, dance, jazz, juggling, mime, and stunts were performed. American musicals were pure entertainment. Jazz music and the ''cabaret'' style of entertainment were hugely popular in Germany during the 1920s. Brecht transformed the musical comedy and cabaret music into an instrument of satire, which is not unlike what John Gay did with opera when he wrote *The Beggar's Opera* in 1728.

Gay fused together a satire on Italian opera (the form which is most commonly identified with the definition of opera) and the common ballad that had been popular on London streets for many decades. Thus, his invention was called a *ballad opera.* The ballad opera took the music from familiar ballads and set new words to them, incorporating dozens into the fabric of a loose plot. Gay's work playfully ridicules the pretensions of society, aristocracy, and Italian opera. Brecht, on the other hand, intended his play to effect actual social change, but the extraordinary music by Kurt Weill led many viewers to perceive the work as entertainment.

Epic Theater

Epic theater (sometimes called ''open'' theater) was the unique invention of Brecht. He designed epic theater as a ''dialectical'' (educational) experience: to deviate from the theater's base goal of entertainment to turn the spectator into a judge. Brecht's drama is designed to stir the audience into action. He attempts to accomplish this by disrupting the viewer's passive stance toward the play in order to generate a mode of ''complex seeing,'' wherein the viewer follows the action, but also thinks about the construction of the play and the fabrication of its characters at the same time. Brecht wanted to develop the viewer's critical consciousness, the part of the observing mind that holds the drama at arm's length and judges not the action of the story but the reasons for presenting the characters.

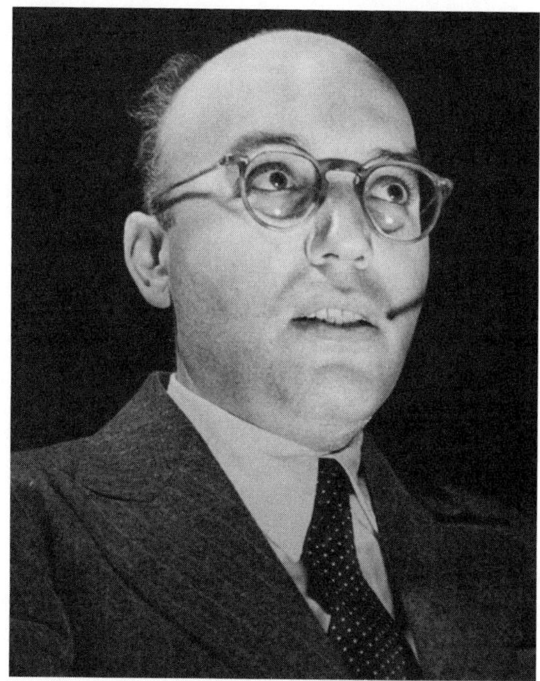

Kurt Weill, composer of The Threepenny Opera*'s unique music*

Brecht frustrates the viewer's usual passive stance toward the drama in a number of ways. One is through the performers' direct asides to the audience, where the character steps out of action momentarily to address the audience with his or her own observations about the proceedings. For example, Peachum asks the audience ''what's the use'' of touching Biblical sayings if people are going to become jaded by them. The songs also serve to disrupt a complacent reading of the story, because they amplify or deny the themes presented by the action. The song Macheath and Polly sing after their wedding is a stinging cynical commentary that taints any shred of romanticism in the couple's marriage ceremony when it says that ''love will endure or not endure / no matter where we are.''

Although Brecht's ideas about theater had a profound influence on later playwrights, his immediate effect on audiences was not as successful. Spectators sometimes developed empathy for his characters in spite of his ''alienating'' techniques.

This initial failure was due in large part to Weill's music, which many theatergoers found alluring; the intoxicating music often gave viewers the impression that the play's events were a fantasy and thus removed from their own world. Critics have also pointed to the characters' rakishly amusing behavior, the love story—albeit twisted—between Macheath and Polly, and Macheath's happy ending as reasons for audiences to misinterpret the play as light entertainment.

HISTORICAL CONTEXT

Germany After World War I

Just prior to World War I, Germany, more dramatically than any other country in Europe was undergoing a transformation from an agrarian economy to an urban, industrial economy. An abundance of wealth, generated by a more productive work force, contributed to a growing sense of national power. Thus Germany magnanimously offered unlimited aid to Austria-Hungary when it came into conflict with the Balkans, portions of which it was attempting to overtake. Out of this conflict arose World War I.

Germans believed that they had the manpower and the technological superiority to put a quick end to the conflict. They did not bargain, however, for the involvement of Germany's greatest European rivals, and after three years of bitter losses, Germany suffered utter defeat at the hands of the Allied forces (Russia, France, Great Britain, and towards the end of the war, the United States).

German leader Kaiser Wilhem II, after forcing the more politically astute Chancellor Bismarck to resign, had aggravated European politics to the point where Germany faced a hopeless two-front war against the countries (France and Russia) that enjoined its East and West borders. The arrogant sense of honor with which most Germans initially undertook the battle to back neighboring Austria-Hungary was completely overturned by the time that the German republic's representatives were forced to sign a humiliating treaty at Versailles, France, in 1919. This treaty was signed in the same Hall of Mirrors in the Palace at Versailles where Germany had in 1871 forced France to accept a humiliating treaty ending the Franco-Prussian War.

The financial demands (Germany was forced to pay $31 billion in war reparations), the emotional price of the 1919 Versailles Treaty, the decimation of the country's civilian and military population, and the crippling of its newly developed industrial machine seriously compromised Germany's ability to repay the war debt or to reestablish its economy until, in 1924, an American businessman arranged for the United States to loan money to the faltering republic. Thereafter the spiraling inflation of the immediate postwar years and accompanying sense of pessimism and bitterness at having lost the war, was quickly followed by a period of heady economic growth and hedonism constrained by a clinging and pervasive sense of shame. The sharp decline and sudden rebound of the economy only served to exacerbate existing class conflicts.

During Germany's involvement in the war, Brecht had avoided conscription for a time but finally had to serve as an orderly in an army hospital in 1916. His experience left an indelible cynicism about the effectiveness of armed combat. He found solace in the ideas of Karl Marx's 1848 *Communist Manifesto,* as did other German Social Democrats. This political party envisioned a classless society as a solution to the ills of capitalism and the remnants of feudalism inherent in Germany's political system. Brecht, along with other writers and artists of the period, produced *Expressionist* works that captured the revulsion of newly converted pacifists. While recognizing the moral obligation to effect social change, these artists also felt deeply the horrors of war, and the conflicting feelings were expressed in emotionally charged works of drama, literature, and perhaps most effectively, painting. Brecht's plays continued to explore the gut-wrenching choices that faced Germany as it proceeded toward the rise of the Third Reich (Adolf Hitler's Germany) and its second great defeat in World War II.

German Decadence

Out of the increasing hedonism that followed Germany's defeat in World War I sprung the cabaret culture, a nightclub scene that came to personify German decadence. Adopting a nihilist philosophy (one that posits that life is ultimately meaningless), young Germans would indulge in excessive drinking, carousing, and sex. Believing that an individual's actions made little difference whether a temperate or libertine lifestyle was followed, they indulged their every whimsy. Both in accordance with this philosophy and in reaction to it, a wealth of arts arose, notably the music of composers such as Kurt Weill and writers such as Brecht.

COMPARE & CONTRAST

- **1920s:** Germany transforms from pre-war optimism to a state of cynicism and violent class conflict in a matter of less than ten years. Political, economic, and social turmoil plunges Germans into a state of psychological shock, as evidenced in ''Black Expressionist'' art and in plays and literature expressing similar feelings of pessimism and bitterness.

  Today: The 1990 tumbling of the Berlin Wall (erected in 1961 to further defend the political demarcation between East Germany and West Germany following Hitler's defeat in World War II), marks a new era of unity for Germany.

- **1920s:** Class conflict exacerbated by the war and rampant inflation make the country ripe for the rise of Hitler's ''Third Reich'' and its promise of a new society.

  Today: Germany holds a strong position in the world economy as well as the respect of fellow members of the United Nations.

- **1920s:** Naturalist or Realist theater predominates in German drama. Brecht and others rebel against naturalism hoping to replace the ''theater of illusion'' with a theater for thinking and social change.

  Today: Like theater in the United States, Brecht's previously daring dramatic frameworks, characters addressing the audience directly, and open, symbolic rather than realistic staging and costumes are standard fare in German drama. While no longer shocking, these techniques are still effective ways of preventing theatergoers from viewing the production passively; modern theatergoers expect to be made to think.

Decadence would continue to influence German arts throughout the twentieth century. The concept pervades the literary works of such authors as Thomas Mann (*Buddenbrooks, Death in Venice*) and filmmakers such as Rainer Werner Fassbinder (*The Marriage of Maria Braun*) and Werner Herzog (*Aguirre, Wrath of God, Fitzcarraldo*).

CRITICAL OVERVIEW

A study of the critical reception of Brecht's plays must include references to his political and aesthetic ideology. More so than with most playwrights, it was Brecht's dynamic personality that generated his reputation. His charisma as a director and thinker made him the leader of a faithful group of artists and intellectuals.

Brecht had three opportunities with which to establish his notoriety under the adverse condition of being on the side of the wrong political party. In Germany prior to the Nazi takeover, he supported the Socialist Democrats; in the United States, he actively supported communism during the height of the McCarthy era (Senator Joseph McCarthy headed the hearings on Un-American Activities designed to root communism out of American society); upon his return to East Germany, he criticized the communists, once again embracing the ideals of a classless society as promoted by Socialist Democracy. Through all of this, Brecht's very peculiar form of drama elicited ever-widening circles of interest, first among the international intellectual elite, and then, slowly and inevitably, to a wider audience by way of his profound influence on other writers.

The Threepenny Opera opened at the Munich Schiffbauerdamm Theater on August 28, 1928. It ran there until Hitler banned it; early praise and the notoriety of the ban made Brecht an overnight success. The tunes were whistled on the street and a Threepenny Opera Bar opened in Berlin, featuring music exclusively from Brecht and Weill's work. In

1933 the play was produced at New York's Empire Theater, where it ran for a dismal twelve performances before closing. Audiences in the United States, beyond a small group of writers, artists, and avant-garde thinkers, would not recognize Brecht's genius for another thirty years.

Just as *The Threepenny Opera* was being produced in the main centers of culture across Europe (to considerable acclaim), Brecht was worrying about how he might survive at all, let alone write. He and a group of other writers persecuted by Hitler met frequently to decide where to go. By 1923, his works were on the Nazi ''burn'' list (Hitler frequently ordered any books that contradicted or undermined his philosophy to be destroyed), and his own safety was questionable. He fled to Vienna in 1933 and then to Denmark, where he published anti-fascist tracts. In 1939 he was forced once again to move, this time to Sweden and then almost immediately again to Finland, from where he obtained passage to the United States. Finland became an ally of Germany ten days after he left.

In 1941, after a long land trip across the Soviet Union, Brecht arrived in California, where he was virtually unknown. He proceeded to search for a market for his work, forming a circle of intellectual German refugees. He met Eric Bentley, then a graduate student of German who would later become a renowned drama critic. Bentley offered to translate his works; it was the beginning of a long and productive relationship. Actor Charles Laughton, himself quite an intellectual, also joined the playwright's coterie, and by 1943, Brecht's works were beginning to be produced in small but important avant-garde theaters. His work, however, earned no public acclaim and he had no Broadway productions during his lifetime, although several of his plays were big hits in New York during the 1960s.

Unfortunately for Brecht, the United States was going through a period of hysteria over the fear of communism. The House Committee on Un-American Activities subpoenaed Brecht in 1947. The committee was snowed by Brecht's charm and intellectualism. He affirmed that he had studied Karl Marx but only as a student of history, and he flatly denied his membership in the communist party. The committee let him go without further questioning. The result was a small leap in the popularity of his plays. In 1948 he returned to East Berlin and established there the Berliner Ensemble, which enjoyed the support of the intellectual elite in East Berlin and of audiences in the European cities where they visited.

In that troupe and in the work he did with his coterie of young German actors and writers, he left his indelible mark. Having left his country in exile, he had returned triumphant and remained so until he died in 1956. His political followers continued his penchant for attacking the establishment (now the communist regime in East Germany) after his death, while his literary successors still attribute their theatrical innovations to the ideas he planted with his own work.

CRITICISM

Carole Hamilton

Hamilton is an English teacher at Cary Academy, an innovative private school in Cary, North Carolina. In this essay she examines the social constructs of Brecht's revisions to The Beggar's Opera *and how these revisions played into his political ideals.*

When a writer revises and adapts an earlier work, as Bertolt Brecht did with John Gay's *The Beggar's Opera* (1728), they make revisions that are consistent with a particular aesthetic and ideology. These shifts are part and parcel of the thinking of that writer's age—an attempt to bring the older work into a contemporary frame and make it meaningful to modern audiences. For example, some late-twentieth-century adaptations of Shakespeare's *Hamlet* emphasize the tangled feelings between Hamlet and his mother Gertrude, indicating this age's acceptance of Freudian Oedipal concepts (sexual attraction between mother and son). Much of the criticism written on *The Threepenny Opera* has centered on Brecht's modifications to Gay's staging: the asides to the audience, the placards announcing events, the songs that belie the often somber action taking place, and the harsh white lighting (elements identified with ''epic theater''). However, Brecht also made small but significant changes to the storyline itself and these changes reveal his ideological leanings.

The Beggar's Opera is about Macheath, a small-time criminal who marries one of his mistresses while continuing his relationships with other women. Two of the women in his life, his wife, Polly, and lover Lucy, discover each other and vie for the right to claim him. As a way to rid himself of an unprofit-

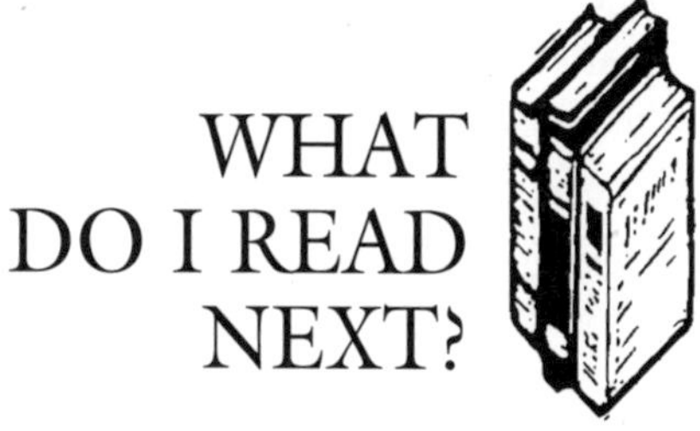

WHAT DO I READ NEXT?

- John Gay's 1728 comic opera, *The Beggar's Opera* was Brecht's source material and offers a good source for comparison. The differences between the two works illustrate the ideologies of the authors who produced them.
- Franz Kafka's *The Metamorphosis* and *The Trial* give an imaginative sense of the futility and nameless anxiety of the pre–World War I years in Europe. For a British perspective, T. S. Eliot's poem ''The Waste Land'' (1922) expresses a sense of spiritual vacuity, with imagery recalling the devastation of World War I.
- The 1972 film *Cabaret* directed by Bob Fosse and starring Liza Minnelli, Joel Grey, and Michael York presents a vivid and compelling picture of the hedonism, decadence, and spiritual longings of post–World War I Germany (circa 1931) in which Hitler began his ascent to power.
- Brecht had a profound influence on the literary artists who succeeded him. His epic theater gave rise to the ''theater of the absurd,'' which takes his idea of alienation to a new realm. In Samuel Beckett's 1952 *Waiting for Godot* (which Brecht had seen and to which he had planned to write another play in reply just before his death) four characters await salvation in the form of the arrival of Godot, who never appears; like Brecht, Beckett raises issues of expectation and fulfillment.
- Jean Genet's 1956 play *The Balcony* is another modernist play; it is about a brothel that transforms into a law court, battleground, and a slum, while the characters undergo similar transformations.
- Harold Pinter's 1957 drama *The Birthday Party* concerns the disruption of normal daily life by the bizarre and examines the sanctuaries that people build to protect themselves from reality. Pinter's fragmented and illogical plot causes theatergoers to question their assumptions of ''normality.''

---

able match (he had previously used his daughter's looks to attract customers to his business), Polly's father turns Macheath in to the police. After a couple of escapes, Macheath is led to the gallows but receives a last minute reprieve (and considerable rewards) just before he is hung.

Brecht's secretary (and one of the playwright's own lovers), Elisabeth Hauptmann, translated Gay's play into German for Brecht, who then added his inimitable stylistic changes. He transformed it into ''epic theater,'' but he changed more than the presentation. Gay's version makes no reference to Jack the Knife, does not include a wedding scene, has no counterpart to Sheriff Jackie Brown, and makes only one tiny reference to the coronation.

Jack the Knife was a nickname for the London serial killer more commonly known as Jack the Ripper. Jack targeted prostitutes and was never caught. The victims were each knifed in a characteristic style, with precise, surgical wounds that led many to suspect the murderer was a doctor or had medical training. The story of Jack the Knife has fascinated and horrified the world. Numerous theories have been proposed to reconcile his grisly methods with a psychological make-up and motive. By shortening Macheath's name to Mac and adding the words ''the knife,'' Brecht alludes to the famous serial killer and transforms Gay's protagonist.

As he is revised by Brecht, Macheath of *The Threepenny Opera* is already a more ruthless criminal than Gay's character. Yet the association with Jack the Ripper cloaks him with such an aura of dark menace that Gay's Macheath pales in comparison. In *The Beggar's Opera,* Macheath is a womanizer and a scoundrel but not a murderer. Both characters bribe their prison guard in hopes of escaping and

"*THE THREEPENNY OPERA* QUESTIONS THE SOCIAL LAWS THAT WERE LEADING GERMANS, INEVITABLY, TO A SECOND WORLD WAR."

both go gallantly to the gallows when recaptured. But Brecht's Macheath is cynical and jaded; murder and death are inescapable elements in his world, and he has learned to make peace with them. In *The Threepenny Opera,* he and his army buddy (now sheriff), Jackie Brown, sing a ditty about the inevitability of dying on the battlefield, of being chopped into human "tartar" by the enemy. They have seen the worst of war and they have made it into a joke. Mrs. Peachum says of Macheath, "There goes a man who's won his spurs in battle / The butcher, he. And all the others, cattle."

Macheath's attitude towards war has its roots in Brecht's personal military experience. He had done light duty as an army orderly during part of World War I, and he wrote poetry about the butchery of war. Macheath represents the macabre side of Brecht, who expresses his revulsion with war in grotesque poems that reek of forced machismo. His "The Legend of the Dead Soldier" tells of a corpse that is revived and re-enlisted with gruesome details—such as a canister of incense swinging over the marching cadaver to mask its putrid odor. Brecht's experience was by no means unique, nor was it extreme—anti-war feelings such as his were pervasive throughout Europe. In his version of *The Beggar's Opera,* Brecht has transformed Macheath into a member of the "lost generation" of the postwar years, like Brecht and his peers. The playwright revised the eighteenth-century play to address his era's prevailing state of mind: numbed and cynical.

When Macheath states his nihilistic case in the "Ballad of Good Living": "Suffering ennobles, but it can depress / The paths of glory lead but to the grave," he spoke for a large majority of the European audiences who first viewed the play. This nihilist philosophy justifies licentiousness; Macheath has a "live for today" attitude that closely resembles the decadent cabaret world of Germany in the 1920s. In fact, the lighting, staging, songs, and music all evoke the atmosphere of cabaret. No wonder that Brecht's early audiences loved the play instead of recognizing it as an admonishment to their bourgeois lifestyle.

Oddly enough, the connections to war and to Jack the Knife are made but not emphasized. In a way, Macheath is a lovable rogue whose vocation sometimes requires that he kill people, a career criminal who wants full credit for such acts as setting the Children's Hospital on fire. At the end of the play he is reprieved and given a high station, a manor, and a generous pension. He is not unlike those leaders who had actually profited by the war while Germany as a whole was devastated; men who were made heroes for their battleground butchery.

In Brecht's version of London's criminal underworld, Macheath marries Polly on stage, whereas Gay had this event occur offstage. The ceremony is made into a travesty of traditional marriage, with its stolen bridal gown, furniture, and food, all taking place in an abandoned stable. The stable element recalls Jesus Christ, who was born in such a humble setting. Macheath, however, tries to transform this setting into a palace, fooling himself that he is surrounded by luxury and becoming irritated by any notice of failure.

None of the furniture matches, and the thugs saw off the legs of a harpsichord to use as a table. The former owners were innocent victims of Macheath's bungling cohorts, who panicked while robbing the family and killed them. Polly cries, "Those poor people, all for a few sticks of furniture." In another twisted allusion to the Bible, Brecht has Macheath dragging stolen tables into his sanctuary (Christ overturned tables in the temple). In war-devastated Germany, the sight of valuable household items being sullied by the incompetence of thieves would have been especially distressing.

Jackie Brown is another intriguing revision implemented by Brecht. Brown, in some ways, is even more despicable than Macheath, for he has no redeeming charisma or sexual charm, and he equivocates endlessly over whether or not to turn in his friend Macheath. The shifting tides of German politics and power during these years must have unearthed many such creatures, who were more determined to be on the winning side—insuring their own survival at any cost—than to maintain their integrity. It is Brown who arrives on horseback to announce Macheath's gifts of a reprieve, elevation to peerage, castle, and a sizable annual pension

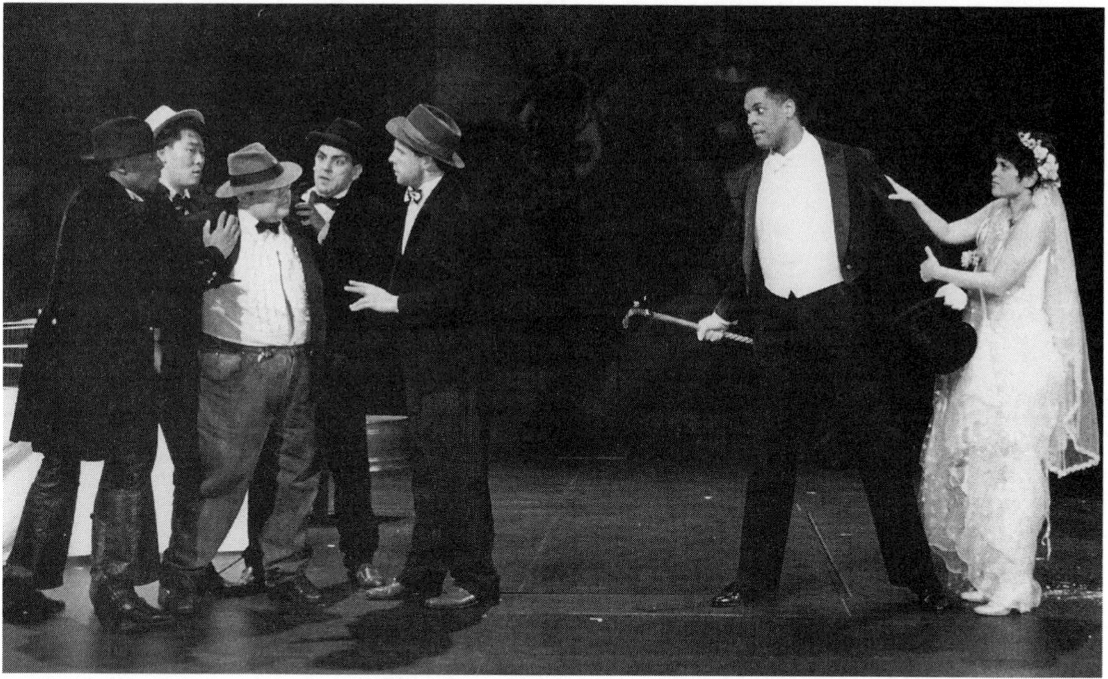

A scene from a 1995 American Repertory Theatre production depicting Macheath and Polly's wedding

from the Queen; with his questionable moral fiber, Brown is the instrument of authority and a symbol of a corrupt system.

The final telling variation from the Gay version involves the coronation ceremony. Brecht has Peachum plan a demonstration of "human misery" to coincide with the royal proceedings. John Gay would not have dreamed of having a character in his play put on such a demonstration—the eighteenth century did not have such a phenomenon. But demonstrations staged by political parties were standard fare in twentieth-century Germany. As the labor party factions evolved and disputed, marches and rallies were held to garner support. A group of beggars staging a demonstration would burlesque a common occurrence in postwar Germany, with its continuing contention between socialist democracy (which would become fascism) and communism. Brecht's comment upon this phenomenon seems to be that the political rallies are no more effective than a parade of "human misery" put on by the miserable themselves.

Brecht has been accused of failing to take a political stand in this play. Robert Brustein in his *The Theatre of Revolt* found *The Threepenny Opera* a complex of ambiguities that are never solved. The *deus ex machina* ("God from the machine") he finds especially obscure: "With the whole play inverted, and the whole world seen from its underside, even Brecht's positive affirmations seem to come out backwards." Yet the final lines literally bespeak an ironic or sarcastic solution: spare injustice from persecution. Brown spares the unjust Macheath from persecution by arriving on horseback to grant him a reprieve, and goes one step further by ennobling and enriching the criminal.

Brecht is saying that Brown's act, sanctioned by the highest authority in the land (the queen) makes no less sense than to allow any injustice to be tolerated. His ironic comment, along with the theatrical innovations of "epic theater" are designed to provoke the viewer to think; Brecht said that it "arouses his [sic] capacity for action, forces him to make decisions." Brecht believed that humans adapted to the social settings in which they lived, that "social being determines thought." Therefore, he adapted Gay's eighteenth-century play to better portray the social milieu that he was questioning. He set the play in London to provide a comfortable thinking distance, to avoid the politicization of his German audience's response. He wanted to appeal to his viewers' rational side (not the empathic response) so that they could revise themselves and their society.

The social elements that Brecht inserts into the play—a ruthless criminal (and possible serial killer), a wedding of thieves, an unjust reprieve—zero in on the very societal flaws he urged his audiences to correct. Brecht explained why he included certain social structures: "The epic theatre is chiefly interested in the attitudes which people adopt towards one another, wherever they are socio-historically significant (typical). It works out scenes where people adopt attitudes of such a sort that the social laws under which they are acting spring into sight." *The Threepenny Opera* questions the social laws that were leading Germans, inevitably, to a second World War.

Source: Carole Hamilton for *Drama for Students,* Gale, 1998.

Bernard F. Dukore

Dukore points out several Biblical references in The Threepenny Opera, *citing both obvious allusions and ones that are cloaked in metaphoric language. Of the latter, Dukore argues that there are numerous examples that compare the character Macheath to Jesus Christ.*

Several critics have quoted Brecht's statement that the work which made the greatest impression on him was the Bible. Although Martin Esslin discusses the biblical quality of Brecht's language, and although Von Thomas O. Brandt cites a number of biblical quotations in Brecht's plays (without, however, identifying their exact sources), Brecht's use of the Bible has, so far as I have been able to discover, been given only cursory notice. In this article, I should like to examine biblical references in *The Threepenny Opera.*

Brandt refers to *The Threepenny Opera's* "Bibelcollage"; his term is accurate. Following the Prologue, the play begins with the Bible-carrying Peachum singing a Morning Hymn and closes with a chorale that has a nagging resemblance to German Easter chorales. Not only are there such general biblical references as Judgment Day (Peachum's opening song, I,1) and basking in divine grace (first-act finale), but there are numerous specific references as well. For example, Peachum (first-act finale) sings of the desirability of "Being given bread to eat and not a stone," referring to *Matthew,* 7:9 ("Or what man is there of you, whom if his son ask bread, will he give him a stone?"). In I,1 there are such direct quotations as "It is more blessed to give than to receive" (*Acts,* 20:35) and "Give and it shall be given unto you" (*Luke,* 6:38). And the famous "whither thou goest, I will go" from *Ruth,* 1:16 is referred to three times: by Mr. and Mrs. Peachum in their song in I,1; by Polly when she introduces the duet with Macheath at the end of I,2; and by Polly when she tells her parents of the friendship between Macheath and Tiger Brown in I,3.

However, the major biblical references are those which relate Macheath to Jesus. Martin Esslin has called attention to the biblical parody in *Threepenny Opera,* citing the betrayal of Macheath on a Thursday. This is not the only point of resemblance. Like Jesus, Macheath may be called "a gluttonous man, and a winebibber, a friend of publicans and sinners" (*Luke,* 7:34). Very early in the play (I,1) a link between them is made obliquely. When Mrs. Peachum learns that the man who has been courting Polly, and whom Polly intends to marry, is Macheath, she exclaims, in a *double entendre* whose significance she does not realize, "For God's sake! Mackie the Knife! Jesus! Come, Lord Jesus, abide with us!" In the wedding scene too (I,2) there is a hint at this connection. The beginning of the "new life," as Polly calls it, between herself and Macheath, takes place in a stable. As soon as they enter he commands her to sit down on the crib ("Krippe," which can be translated not only as "crib" but also as "manger"). Then Macheath's gang bring gifts—stolen gifts, to be sure, but gifts nonetheless.

But the most significant parallels, as well as the most extended, concern the Crucifixion. Like Jesus, Macheath is betrayed on a Thursday. And he is betrayed by his own kind, his own people: Jenny and Brown. Jenny's treachery is explicitly related to that of Judas: "A female Judas has the money in her hand," Mrs. Peachum sings in III,1. Peachum resembles Caiaphas, for just as Peachum's business is in danger of being taken over by Macheath ("*He'd* have us in his clutches. I know he would! D'you think your daughter would be any better than you at keeping her mouth shut in bed?" says Peachum in I,1), so was Caiaphas' in danger of being superseded by Jesus', and Peachum hires Jenny to betray Macheath, as Caiaphas paid Judas to betray Jesus. Moreover, it is to be inferred that Tiger Brown carries the role of Peter, for he—in effect—denies his friendship with Macheath. This is made explicit when Macheath is brought to jail in II,3:

> BROWN (*after a long pause, under the fearful gaze of his former friend*). Mac, I didn't do it . . . I did everything I could . . . don't look at me like that, Mac . . . I can't bear it . . . Your silence is too terrible.

(*Shouts at a policeman.*) Don't pull him with that rope, you swine! Say something, Mac. Say something to your old friend . . . Give him a word in his dark . . . (*Rests his head against the wall and weeps.*) He doesn't think me worth even a word. (*Exit.*)

MACHEATH. That miserable Brown. That evil conscience incarnate. And such a creature is made commissioner of police. Lucky I didn't bawl him out. At first I thought of doing something of the sort. But then I thought a good, piercing, punishing stare would send the shivers down his back. The idea found its mark. I looked at him and he wept bitterly. That's a trick I got from the Bible.

The biblical passage to which Macheath refers in the last sentence may be *Luke,* 22:61–62.

And the Lord turned, and looked upon Peter. And Peter remembered the word of the Lord, how he had said to him, Before the cock crow, thou shalt deny me thrice.

And Peter went out, and wept bitterly.

Brown's request for a word for his dark (state? place?—he does not complete the sentence) recalls a number of biblical passages in which a godly word lightens darkness. There is the famous

In the beginning was the Word, and the Word was with God, and the Word was God.

. . .

In him was life; and the life was the light of men.

And the light shineth in darkness; and the darkness comprehended it not. [*John,* 1:1,4–5]

There is also, for example, "Christ shall give thee light" (*Ephesians,* 5:14), and the prophecy of Jesus is spoken of "as . . . a light that shineth in a dark place, until the day dawn, and the day star arise in your hearts" (2 *Peter,* 1:19).

In addition, Macheath, like Jesus, is to be executed on a Friday. The precise time is fixed: he is to be hanged at six o'clock (III,3). This was the hour when there came a darkness over the entire land that lasted until the ninth hour, at which time Jesus quoted the beginning of the twenty-second *Psalm,* "My God, my God, why hast thou forsaken me?" Macheath's cry as he is about to be killed (III, 3)—"Beware lest you go down as well as he!"—is reminiscent of "Remember the word that I say unto you, The servant is not greater than his lord. If they have persecuted me, they will also persecute you" (*John,* 15:20). Finally, there is a biblical parallel to the circumstances during which Macheath is released. Matthew tells us (27:15) that during the feast of Passover "the governor was wont to release unto the people a prisoner, whom they would." Macheath is pardoned by the Queen because it is Coronation Day.

"THERE IS NO VICARIOUS REDEMPTION, BRECHT IMPLIES. MACHEATH DOES NOT SAVE MANKIND BY HIS DEATH; HE DOES NOT PURCHASE REDEMPTION WITH HIS BLOOD. SALVATION—SOCIAL SALVATION—REMAINS TO BE ACHIEVED, PRESUMABLY BY THE AUDIENCE."

In *The Threepenny Opera* we have a satiric retelling of the Crucifixion in a manner which is in harmony with other satiric thrusts in this play. Brecht brings onstage many familiar elements. But he presents them through an unfamiliar angle of vision (thus making them appear strange—"alienating" them, as it were) and in so doing calls them into question. For example, Macheath's gang steal expensive furnishings and bring them to an empty stable (I,2). Brecht could have had the gang break into an unoccupied mansion for the wedding ceremony. However, by making the furnishings stolen goods, Brecht calls into question the manner by which their "legitimate" owners acquired them. Similarly, by presenting the prostitutes as not unlike the respectable bourgeoisie—the stage directions at the beginning of II,2 read: *A brothel in Wapping. An ordinary early evening. The girls, mostly in their underclothes, are ironing, playing draughts, washing themselves; a peaceful bourgeois idyll.*—he emphasizes by implication the prostitution underlying the business and domestic dealings of the bourgeoisie. And by having the crook Macheath confide to Polly that it is only a matter of weeks before he devotes himself exclusively to banking (II,1) he calls into question the morality of the legal business of banking. Occasionally, this practice of casting a critical light on traditional values and attitudes is made explicit, as when Macheath asks (III,3), "What is a picklock to a bank-share? What is the burglary of a bank to the founding of a bank? What is the murder of a man to the employment of a man?"

Relating the story of Macheath to the story of Jesus enables Brecht to use each to comment on the other. The actions of men under capitalism, Brecht appears to be saying, are direct reversals of the actions advocated by Jesus. We would all like to be good, Peachum sings in the first-act finale, but circumstances (presumably economic) prevent us. In III,1 he sings that man is not wicked enough for the (presumably capitalist) world we live in. And at the end of the play (III,3) he reminds us that if you kick a man he will not turn the other cheek but will kick you back. The immoral Macheath is therefore a more appropriate god than the humane Jesus, for while we pay lip service to the code of conduct of Jesus, we actually follow the actions and subscribe to the code of conduct of Macheath. In addition, there is the implication that Brecht is mocking the concept of salvation through divine grace. By making his Christ-figure a scoundrel, he is deriding Christianity. I think that Brecht would want us to infer that social regeneration must precede individual, religious regeneration.

However, Brecht is not simplistic. The biblical parallel does not make this play a simple anti-religious document. There is one essential difference between Macheath and Jesus: Macheath is released, not executed. Certain aspects of the story of Macheath may parallel that of Jesus, but Macheath's fate is—fittingly—the fate of Barrabas.

Macheath's knife, so to speak, cuts both ways. Brecht's mockery of religion is not a blanket condemnation of religious ideals. He may cast doubt on some biblical concepts, but he upholds others. Just as his *Verfremdungseffekt* does not banish emotion utterly but adds thought and detachment, so his Bible-chopping does not banish the Bible utterly. Brecht's vision appears to me to be essentially a Christian vision: he would like a world in which man could be good to his fellow man, and in which survival would not necessitate—as his characters state in the second-act finale that it presently does—cheating, exploiting, and forgetting one's humanity. However, such a world is not easily come by. When Brecht tells us, just before the arrival of the Mounted Messenger at the end of the play, that "in the whole of Christendom/There's nothing granted free to anyone," he is not making a cynically anti-Scriptural comment, but in fact the reverse, for the Bible offers numerous statements concerning the economics of redemption, *e.g.,* "Take heed therefore unto yourselves, and to all the flock, over the which the Holy Ghost hath made your overseers, to feed the church of God, which he hath purchased with his own blood" (*Acts,* 20:28) and "And almost all things are by the law purged with blood; and without shedding of blood is no remission" (*Hebrews,* 9:22). There is no vicarious redemption, Brecht implies. Macheath does not save mankind by his death; he does not purchase redemption with his blood. Salvation—social salvation—remains to be achieved, presumably by the audience.

Source: Bernard F. Dukore, "The Averted Crucifixion of Macheath," in *Drama Survey,* Volume 4, no. 1, Spring, 1965, pp. 51–56.

Harold Clurman

In this brief review, Clurman finds in The Threepenny Opera *an appeal that audiences can trace to historic events such as the Great Depression as well as more personal themes such as regret and loss.*

Kurt Weill's and Bert Brecht's *The Threepenny Opera* is a masterpiece; in its present production at the Theatre de Lys it very nearly misses fire. Such is the paradox of the theatre: the presentation is almost as much part of a play as the material itself.

The Threepenny Opera—called that because it is so oddly conceived that it might be a beggar's dream and so cheaply done that it might meet a beggar's budget—sums up a whole epoch and evokes a special state of mind. The epoch is not just the Berlin of 1919–1928; it is any epoch in which a lurid rascality combined with fierce contrasts of prosperity and poverty shapes the dominant tone of society. The state of mind is one of social impotence so close to despair that it expresses itself through a kind of jaded mockery which mingles a snarl with tears. Such in a way was the England of John Gay's *The Beggar's Opera* (1728), from which the Brecht "book" derives, and certainly the Germany which preceded Hitler. No wonder the one period produced Hogarth and the other George Grosz.

We do not live in such a time—though people who remember the depression days between 1930 and 1935 will appreciate the mood of *The Threepenny Opera* most readily—but it makes the mood irresistibly present and, strangely enough, induces us to take it to our hearts with a kind of pained affection. There is, despite the sharp sense of period that permeates it, a universal quality in *The Threepenny Opera.* It fosters a bitter sense of regret that we live so scabbily in relation to our dreams and also a kind of masochistic attachment to our wounds, as if they were all we have to show as evidence of our dreams.

This effect is achieved through Brecht's brilliant lyrics rendered with remarkable intuitive insight and witty skill in Marc Blitzstein's adaptation—and through the one score Weill composed which places him on the level of an Offenbach. What bite and tang, what insidious irony, in the clean thrusts of Brecht's verses; what economy and lightness in Weill's songs and orchestration! How poignant is the sullied lyricism of this work with its jeering bathos, its low-life romanticism, its sweetly poisonous nostalgia, its musical profanity, and its sudden hints of grandeur, godliness, and possible greatness! Here in contemporary terms and with a strange timelessness is the ambiguous, corrupt seduction of a submerged half-world akin to that which François Villon sang of long ago.

How disappointing, then, to have so unique a work—acclaimed practically everywhere since its première in 1928—reduced to a minor event by so ill-prepared a performance as the one we now see! Except for Lotte Lenya, who appeared in the original production, the cast ranges from the amateurish to the adequate. Lenya's nasally insinuating whore is superb for its incisiveness and triple-threat innuendo. But the fault is not the actors'—most of whom could do much better—but the director's. Everything seems labored and awkward instead of sprightly and bright. The miracle is that the inherent superiority of the material survives all hazards.

Source: Harold Clurman, "*The Threepenny Opera,*" in his *Lies like Truth: Theatre Reviews and Essays,* Macmillan, 1958 , pp. 113–15.

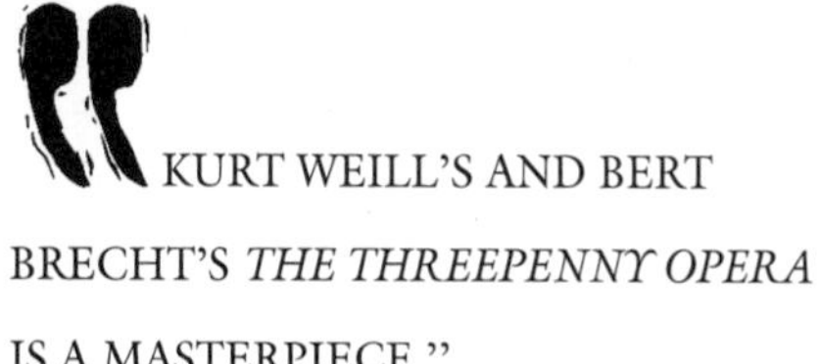

KURT WEILL'S AND BERT BRECHT'S *THE THREEPENNY OPERA* IS A MASTERPIECE."

SOURCES

Bartram, Graham, and Anthony Waine. *Brecht in Perspective,* Longman, 1982.

Bentley, Eric. *The Brecht Commentaries,* Grove, 1981.

Cook, Bruce. *Brecht in Exile,* Holt, 1983.

Esslin, Martin. *Brecht: The Man and His Work,* Anchor Books, 1960.

Esslin, Martin. *Bertold Brecht,* Columbia University Press, 1969.

Gray, Robert D. *Brecht the Dramatist,* Cambridge University Press, 1976.

Willett, John. *Brecht in Context: Comparative Approaches,* Methuen, 1984.

Williams, Raymond. *Drama from Ibsen to Brecht,* Hogarth Press, 1987.

Witt, Hubert. *Brecht: As They Knew Him,* International, 1974.

FURTHER READING

Bentley, Eric. *The Brecht Memoir,* PAJ Publications, 1985.

Bentley was Brecht's first English translator. In this book he chronicles his experiences working with the paradoxical playwright, generally concluding that despite Brecht's oddities and personal failings, he was a genius.

Brustein, Robert. *The Theatre of Revolt: An Approach to Modern Drama,* Little, Brown, 1962.

Brustein presents the thesis that modern theater consists of a rebellion against the classical norm wherein plays uphold a sense of community or communion. By contrast, the theater of revolt seeks not to reinforce community values to but to question and overturn them.

Esslin, Martin. *Brecht: A Choice of Evils,* Methuen, 1985.

Esslin has written three major treatments of Brecht. This one explains the dualities in his plays and in his nature, emphasizing that Brecht presented no transcendent utopia but exposed the evil in both sides of political and social issues.

Glossary of Literary Terms

A

Abstract: Used as a noun, the term refers to a short summary or outline of a longer work. As an adjective applied to writing or literary works, abstract refers to words or phrases that name things not knowable through the five senses. Examples of abstracts include the *Cliffs Notes* summaries of major literary works. Examples of abstract terms or concepts include ''idea,'' ''guilt'' ''honesty,'' and ''loyalty.''

Absurd, Theater of the: See *Theater of the Absurd*

Absurdism: See *Theater of the Absurd*

Act: A major section of a play. Acts are divided into varying numbers of shorter scenes. From ancient times to the nineteenth century plays were generally constructed of five acts, but modern works typically consist of one, two, or three acts. Examples of five-act plays include the works of Sophocles and Shakespeare, while the plays of Arthur Miller commonly have a three-act structure.

Acto: A one-act Chicano theater piece developed out of collective improvisation. *Actos* were performed by members of Luis Valdez's Teatro Campesino in California during the mid-1960s.

Aestheticism: A literary and artistic movement of the nineteenth century. Followers of the movement believed that art should not be mixed with social, political, or moral teaching. The statement ''art for art's sake'' is a good summary of aestheticism. The movement had its roots in France, but it gained widespread importance in England in the last half of the nineteenth century, where it helped change the Victorian practice of including moral lessons in literature. Oscar Wilde is one of the best-known ''aesthetes'' of the late nineteenth century.

Age of Johnson: The period in English literature between 1750 and 1798, named after the most prominent literary figure of the age, Samuel Johnson. Works written during this time are noted for their emphasis on ''sensibility,'' or emotional quality. These works formed a transition between the rational works of the Age of Reason, or Neoclassical period, and the emphasis on individual feelings and responses of the Romantic period. Significant writers during the Age of Johnson included the novelists Ann Radcliffe and Henry Mackenzie, dramatists Richard Sheridan and Oliver Goldsmith, and poets William Collins and Thomas Gray. Also known as Age of Sensibility

Age of Reason: See *Neoclassicism*

Age of Sensibility: See *Age of Johnson*

Alexandrine Meter: See *Meter*

Allegory: A narrative technique in which characters representing things or abstract ideas are used to convey a message or teach a lesson. Allegory is typically used to teach moral, ethical, or religious lessons but is sometimes used for satiric or political purposes. Examples of allegorical works include Edmund Spenser's *The Faerie Queene* and John Bunyan's *The Pilgrim's Progress.*

Allusion: A reference to a familiar literary or historical person or event, used to make an idea more easily understood. For example, describing someone as a ''Romeo'' makes an allusion to William Shakespeare's famous young lover in *Romeo and Juliet.*

Amerind Literature: The writing and oral traditions of Native Americans. Native American literature was originally passed on by word of mouth, so it consisted largely of stories and events that were easily memorized. Amerind prose is often rhythmic like poetry because it was recited to the beat of a ceremonial drum. Examples of Amerind literature include the autobiographical *Black Elk Speaks,* the works of N. Scott Momaday, James Welch, and Craig Lee Strete, and the poetry of Luci Tapahonso.

Analogy: A comparison of two things made to explain something unfamiliar through its similarities to something familiar, or to prove one point based on the acceptedness of another. Similes and metaphors are types of analogies. Analogies often take the form of an extended simile, as in William Blake's aphorism: ''As the caterpillar chooses the fairest leaves to lay her eggs on, so the priest lays his curse on the fairest joys.''

Angry Young Men: A group of British writers of the 1950s whose work expressed bitterness and disillusionment with society. Common to their work is an anti-hero who rebels against a corrupt social order and strives for personal integrity. The term has been used to describe Kingsley Amis, John Osborne, Colin Wilson, John Wain, and others.

Antagonist: The major character in a narrative or drama who works against the hero or protagonist. An example of an evil antagonist is Richard Lovelace in Samuel Richardson's *Clarissa,* while a virtuous antagonist is Macduff in William Shakespeare's *Macbeth.*

Anthropomorphism: The presentation of animals or objects in human shape or with human characteristics. The term is derived from the Greek word for ''human form.'' The fables of Aesop, the animated films of Walt Disney, and Richard Adams's *Watership Down* feature anthropomorphic characters.

Anti-hero: A central character in a work of literature who lacks traditional heroic qualities such as courage, physical prowess, and fortitude. Anti-heros typically distrust conventional values and are unable to commit themselves to any ideals. They generally feel helpless in a world over which they have no control. Anti-heroes usually accept, and often celebrate, their positions as social outcasts. A well-known anti-hero is Yossarian in Joseph Heller's novel *Catch-22.*

Antimasque: See *Masque*

Antithesis: The antithesis of something is its direct opposite. In literature, the use of antithesis as a figure of speech results in two statements that show a contrast through the balancing of two opposite ideas. Technically, it is the second portion of the statement that is defined as the ''antithesis''; the first portion is the ''thesis.'' An example of antithesis is found in the following portion of Abraham Lincoln's ''Gettysburg Address''; notice the opposition between the verbs ''remember'' and ''forget'' and the phrases ''what we say'' and ''what they did'': ''The world will little note nor long remember what we say here, but it can never forget what they did here.''

Apocrypha: Writings tentatively attributed to an author but not proven or universally accepted to be their works. The term was originally applied to certain books of the Bible that were not considered inspired and so were not included in the ''sacred canon.'' Geoffrey Chaucer, William Shakespeare, Thomas Kyd, Thomas Middleton, and John Marston all have apocrypha. Apocryphal books of the Bible include the Old Testament's Book of Enoch and New Testament's Gospel of Peter.

Apollonian and Dionysian: The two impulses believed to guide authors of dramatic tragedy. The Apollonian impulse is named after Apollo, the Greek god of light and beauty and the symbol of intellectual order. The Dionysian impulse is named after Dionysus, the Greek god of wine and the symbol of the unrestrained forces of nature. The Apollonian impulse is to create a rational, harmonious world, while the Dionysian is to express the irrational forces of personality. Friedrich Nietzche uses these terms in *The Birth of Tragedy* to designate contrasting elements in Greek tragedy.

Apostrophe: A statement, question, or request addressed to an inanimate object or concept or to a nonexistent or absent person. Requests for inspiration from the muses in poetry are examples of apostrophe, as is Marc Antony's address to Caesar's corpse in William Shakespeare's *Julius Caesar*: ''O, pardon me, thou bleeding piece of earth, That I am meek and gentle with these butchers!. . . Woe to the hand that shed this costly blood!. . . ''

Archetype: The word archetype is commonly used to describe an original pattern or model from which all other things of the same kind are made. This term was introduced to literary criticism from the psychology of Carl Jung. It expresses Jung's theory that behind every person's ''unconscious,'' or repressed memories of the past, lies the ''collective unconscious'' of the human race: memories of the countless typical experiences of our ancestors. These memories are said to prompt illogical associations that trigger powerful emotions in the reader. Often, the emotional process is primitive, even primordial. Archetypes are the literary images that grow out of the ''collective unconscious.'' They appear in literature as incidents and plots that repeat basic patterns of life. They may also appear as stereotyped characters. Examples of literary archetypes include themes such as birth and death and characters such as the Earth Mother.

Argument: The argument of a work is the author's subject matter or principal idea. Examples of defined ''argument'' portions of works include John Milton's *Arguments* to each of the books of *Paradise Lost* and the ''Argument'' to Robert Herrick's *Hesperides.*

Aristotelian Criticism: Specifically, the method of evaluating and analyzing tragedy formulated by the Greek philosopher Aristotle in his *Poetics.* More generally, the term indicates any form of criticism that follows Aristotle's views. Aristotelian criticism focuses on the form and logical structure of a work, apart from its historical or social context, in contrast to ''Platonic Criticism,'' which stresses the usefulness of art. Adherents of New Criticism including John Crowe Ransom and Cleanth Brooks utilize and value the basic ideas of Aristotelian criticism for textual analysis.

Art for Art's Sake: See *Aestheticism*

Aside: A comment made by a stage performer that is intended to be heard by the audience but supposedly not by other characters. Eugene O'Neill's *Strange Interlude* is an extended use of the aside in modern theater.

Audience: The people for whom a piece of literature is written. Authors usually write with a certain audience in mind, for example, children, members of a religious or ethnic group, or colleagues in a professional field. The term ''audience'' also applies to the people who gather to see or hear any performance, including plays, poetry readings, speeches, and concerts. Jane Austen's parody of the gothic novel, *Northanger Abbey,* was originally intended for (and also pokes fun at) an audience of young and avid female gothic novel readers.

Avant-garde: A French term meaning ''vanguard.'' It is used in literary criticism to describe new writing that rejects traditional approaches to literature in favor of innovations in style or content. Twentieth-century examples of the literary *avant-garde* include the Black Mountain School of poets, the Bloomsbury Group, and the Beat Movement.

B

Ballad: A short poem that tells a simple story and has a repeated refrain. Ballads were originally intended to be sung. Early ballads, known as folk ballads, were passed down through generations, so their authors are often unknown. Later ballads composed by known authors are called literary ballads. An example of an anonymous folk ballad is ''Edward,'' which dates from the Middle Ages. Samuel Taylor Coleridge's ''The Rime of the Ancient Mariner'' and John Keats's ''La Belle Dame sans Merci'' are examples of literary ballads.

Baroque: A term used in literary criticism to describe literature that is complex or ornate in style or diction. Baroque works typically express tension, anxiety, and violent emotion. The term ''Baroque Age'' designates a period in Western European literature beginning in the late sixteenth century and ending about one hundred years later. Works of this period often mirror the qualities of works more generally associated with the label ''baroque'' and sometimes feature elaborate conceits. Examples of Baroque works include John Lyly's *Euphues: The Anatomy of Wit,* Luis de Gongora's *Soledads,* and William Shakespeare's *As You Like It.*

Baroque Age: See *Baroque*

Baroque Period: See *Baroque*

Beat Generation: See *Beat Movement*

Beat Movement: A period featuring a group of American poets and novelists of the 1950s and 1960s—including Jack Kerouac, Allen Ginsberg, Gregory Corso, William S. Burroughs, and Lawrence Ferlinghetti—who rejected established social and literary values. Using such techniques as stream of consciousness writing and jazz-influenced free verse and focusing on unusual or abnormal states of mind—generated by religious ecstasy or the use of drugs—the Beat writers aimed to create works that were unconventional in both form and subject matter. Kerouac's *On the Road* is perhaps the best-known example of a Beat Generation novel, and Ginsberg's *Howl* is a famous collection of Beat poetry.

Black Aesthetic Movement: A period of artistic and literary development among African Americans in the 1960s and early 1970s. This was the first major African-American artistic movement since the Harlem Renaissance and was closely paralleled by the civil rights and black power movements. The black aesthetic writers attempted to produce works of art that would be meaningful to the black masses. Key figures in black aesthetics included one of its founders, poet and playwright Amiri Baraka, formerly known as LeRoi Jones; poet and essayist Haki R. Madhubuti, formerly Don L. Lee; poet and playwright Sonia Sanchez; and dramatist Ed Bullins. Works representative of the Black Aesthetic Movement include Amiri Baraka's play *Dutchman,* a 1964 Obie award-winner; *Black Fire: An Anthology of Afro-American Writing,* edited by Baraka and playwright Larry Neal and published in 1968; and Sonia Sanchez's poetry collection *We a BaddDDD People,* published in 1970. Also known as Black Arts Movement.

Black Arts Movement: See *Black Aesthetic Movement*

Black Comedy: See *Black Humor*

Black Humor: Writing that places grotesque elements side by side with humorous ones in an attempt to shock the reader, forcing him or her to laugh at the horrifying reality of a disordered world. Joseph Heller's novel *Catch-22* is considered a superb example of the use of black humor. Other well-known authors who use black humor include Kurt Vonnegut, Edward Albee, Eugene Ionesco, and Harold Pinter. Also known as Black Comedy.

Blank Verse: Loosely, any unrhymed poetry, but more generally, unrhymed iambic pentameter verse (composed of lines of five two-syllable feet with the first syllable accented, the second unaccented). Blank verse has been used by poets since the Renaissance for its flexibility and its graceful, dignified tone. John Milton's *Paradise Lost* is in blank verse, as are most of William Shakespeare's plays.

Bloomsbury Group: A group of English writers, artists, and intellectuals who held informal artistic and philosophical discussions in Bloomsbury, a district of London, from around 1907 to the early 1930s. The Bloomsbury Group held no uniform philosophical beliefs but did commonly express an aversion to moral prudery and a desire for greater social tolerance. At various times the circle included Virginia Woolf, E. M. Forster, Clive Bell, Lytton Strachey, and John Maynard Keynes.

Bon Mot: A French term meaning ''good word.'' A *bon mot* is a witty remark or clever observation. Charles Lamb and Oscar Wilde are celebrated for their witty *bon mots.* Two examples by Oscar Wilde stand out: (1) ''All women become their mothers. That is their tragedy. No man does. That's his.'' (2) ''A man cannot be too careful in the choice of his enemies.''

Breath Verse: See *Projective Verse*

Burlesque: Any literary work that uses exaggeration to make its subject appear ridiculous, either by treating a trivial subject with profound seriousness or by treating a dignified subject frivolously. The word ''burlesque'' may also be used as an adjective, as in ''burlesque show,'' to mean ''striptease act.'' Examples of literary burlesque include the comedies of Aristophanes, Miguel de Cervantes's *Don Quixote,*, Samuel Butler's poem ''Hudibras,'' and John Gay's play *The Beggar's Opera.*

C

Cadence: The natural rhythm of language caused by the alternation of accented and unaccented syllables. Much modern poetry—notably free verse—deliberately manipulates cadence to create complex rhythmic effects. James Macpherson's ''Ossian poems'' are richly cadenced, as is the poetry of the Symbolists, Walt Whitman, and Amy Lowell.

Caesura: A pause in a line of poetry, usually occurring near the middle. It typically corresponds to a break in the natural rhythm or sense of the line but is sometimes shifted to create special meanings or rhythmic effects. The opening line of Edgar Allan Poe's ''The Raven'' contains a caesura following ''dreary'': ''Once upon a midnight dreary, while I pondered weak and weary. . . .''

Canzone: A short Italian or Provencal lyric poem, commonly about love and often set to music. The *canzone* has no set form but typically contains five or six stanzas made up of seven to twenty lines of eleven syllables each. A shorter, five- to ten-line ''envoy,'' or concluding stanza, completes the poem. Masters of the *canzone* form include

Petrarch, Dante Alighieri, Torquato Tasso, and Guido Cavalcanti.

Carpe Diem: A Latin term meaning "seize the day." This is a traditional theme of poetry, especially lyrics. A *carpe diem* poem advises the reader or the person it addresses to live for today and enjoy the pleasures of the moment. Two celebrated *carpe diem* poems are Andrew Marvell's "To His Coy Mistress" and Robert Herrick's poem beginning "Gather ye rosebuds while ye may. . . ."

Catharsis: The release or purging of unwanted emotions— specifically fear and pity—brought about by exposure to art. The term was first used by the Greek philosopher Aristotle in his *Poetics* to refer to the desired effect of tragedy on spectators. A famous example of catharsis is realized in Sophocles' *Oedipus Rex,* when Oedipus discovers that his wife, Jacosta, is his own mother and that the stranger he killed on the road was his own father.

Celtic Renaissance: A period of Irish literary and cultural history at the end of the nineteenth century. Followers of the movement aimed to create a romantic vision of Celtic myth and legend. The most significant works of the Celtic Renaissance typically present a dreamy, unreal world, usually in reaction against the reality of contemporary problems. William Butler Yeats's *The Wanderings of Oisin* is among the most significant works of the Celtic Renaissance. Also known as Celtic Twilight.

Celtic Twilight: See *Celtic Renaissance*

Character: Broadly speaking, a person in a literary work. The actions of characters are what constitute the plot of a story, novel, or poem. There are numerous types of characters, ranging from simple, stereotypical figures to intricate, multifaceted ones. In the techniques of anthropomorphism and personification, animals—and even places or things—can assume aspects of character. "Characterization" is the process by which an author creates vivid, believable characters in a work of art. This may be done in a variety of ways, including (1) direct description of the character by the narrator; (2) the direct presentation of the speech, thoughts, or actions of the character; and (3) the responses of other characters to the character. The term "character" also refers to a form originated by the ancient Greek writer Theophrastus that later became popular in the seventeenth and eighteenth centuries. It is a short essay or sketch of a person who prominently displays a specific attribute or quality, such as miserliness or ambition. Notable characters in literature include Oedipus Rex, Don Quixote de la Mancha, Macbeth, Candide, Hester Prynne, Ebenezer Scrooge, Huckleberry Finn, Jay Gatsby, Scarlett O'Hara, James Bond, and Kunta Kinte.

Characterization: See *Character*

Chorus: In ancient Greek drama, a group of actors who commented on and interpreted the unfolding action on the stage. Initially the chorus was a major component of the presentation, but over time it became less significant, with its numbers reduced and its role eventually limited to commentary between acts. By the sixteenth century the chorus—if employed at all—was typically a single person who provided a prologue and an epilogue and occasionally appeared between acts to introduce or underscore an important event. The chorus in William Shakespeare's *Henry V* functions in this way. Modern dramas rarely feature a chorus, but T. S. Eliot's *Murder in the Cathedral* and Arthur Miller's *A View from the Bridge* are notable exceptions. The Stage Manager in Thornton Wilder's *Our Town* performs a role similar to that of the chorus.

Chronicle: A record of events presented in chronological order. Although the scope and level of detail provided varies greatly among the chronicles surviving from ancient times, some, such as the *Anglo-Saxon Chronicle,* feature vivid descriptions and a lively recounting of events. During the Elizabethan Age, many dramas— appropriately called "chronicle plays"—were based on material from chronicles. Many of William Shakespeare's dramas of English history as well as Christopher Marlowe's *Edward II* are based in part on Raphael Holinshead's *Chronicles of England, Scotland, and Ireland.*

Classical: In its strictest definition in literary criticism, classicism refers to works of ancient Greek or Roman literature. The term may also be used to describe a literary work of recognized importance (a "classic") from any time period or literature that exhibits the traits of classicism. Classical authors from ancient Greek and Roman times include Juvenal and Homer. Examples of later works and authors now described as classical include French literature of the seventeenth century, Western novels of the nineteenth century, and American fiction of the mid-nineteenth century such as that written by James Fenimore Cooper and Mark Twain.

Classicism: A term used in literary criticism to describe critical doctrines that have their roots in ancient Greek and Roman literature, philosophy, and art. Works associated with classicism typically exhibit restraint on the part of the author, unity of design and purpose, clarity, simplicity, logical organization, and respect for tradition. Examples of literary classicism include Cicero's prose, the dramas of Pierre Corneille and Jean Racine, the poetry of John Dryden and Alexander Pope, and the writings of J. W. von Goethe, G. E. Lessing, and T. S. Eliot.

Climax: The turning point in a narrative, the moment when the conflict is at its most intense. Typically, the structure of stories, novels, and plays is one of rising action, in which tension builds to the climax, followed by falling action, in which tension lessens as the story moves to its conclusion. The climax in James Fenimore Cooper's *The Last of the Mohicans* occurs when Magua and his captive Cora are pursued to the edge of a cliff by Uncas. Magua kills Uncas but is subsequently killed by Hawkeye.

Colloquialism: A word, phrase, or form of pronunciation that is acceptable in casual conversation but not in formal, written communication. It is considered more acceptable than slang. An example of colloquialism can be found in Rudyard Kipling's *Barrack-room Ballads:* When 'Omer smote 'is bloomin' lyre He'd 'eard men sing by land and sea; An' what he thought 'e might require 'E went an' took—the same as me!

Comedy: One of two major types of drama, the other being tragedy. Its aim is to amuse, and it typically ends happily. Comedy assumes many forms, such as farce and burlesque, and uses a variety of techniques, from parody to satire. In a restricted sense the term comedy refers only to dramatic presentations, but in general usage it is commonly applied to nondramatic works as well. Examples of comedies range from the plays of Aristophanes, Terrence, and Plautus, Dante Alighieri's *The Divine Comedy,* Francois Rabelais's *Pantagruel* and *Gargantua,* and some of Geoffrey Chaucer's tales and William Shakespeare's plays to Noel Coward's play *Private Lives* and James Thurber's short story "The Secret Life of Walter Mitty."

Comedy of Manners: A play about the manners and conventions of an aristocratic, highly sophisticated society. The characters are usually types rather than individualized personalities, and plot is less important than atmosphere. Such plays were an important aspect of late seventeenth-century English comedy. The comedy of manners was revived in the eighteenth century by Oliver Goldsmith and Richard Brinsley Sheridan, enjoyed a second revival in the late nineteenth century, and has endured into the twentieth century. Examples of comedies of manners include William Congreve's *The Way of the World* in the late seventeenth century, Oliver Goldsmith's *She Stoops to Conquer* and Richard Brinsley Sheridan's *The School for Scandal* in the eighteenth century, Oscar Wilde's *The Importance of Being Earnest* in the nineteenth century, and W. Somerset Maugham's *The Circle* in the twentieth century.

Comic Relief: The use of humor to lighten the mood of a serious or tragic story, especially in plays. The technique is very common in Elizabethan works, and can be an integral part of the plot or simply a brief event designed to break the tension of the scene. The Gravediggers' scene in William Shakespeare's *Hamlet* is a frequently cited example of comic relief.

Commedia dell'arte: An Italian term meaning "the comedy of guilds" or "the comedy of professional actors." This form of dramatic comedy was popular in Italy during the sixteenth century. Actors were assigned stock roles (such as Pulcinella, the stupid servant, or Pantalone, the old merchant) and given a basic plot to follow, but all dialogue was improvised. The roles were rigidly typed and the plots were formulaic, usually revolving around young lovers who thwarted their elders and attained wealth and happiness. A rigid convention of the *commedia dell'arte* is the periodic intrusion of Harlequin, who interrupts the play with low buffoonery. Peppino de Filippo's *Metamorphoses of a Wandering Minstrel* gave modern audiences an idea of what *commedia dell'arte* may have been like. Various scenarios for *commedia dell'arte* were compiled in Petraccone's *La commedia dell'arte, storia, technica, scenari,* published in 1927.

Complaint: A lyric poem, popular in the Renaissance, in which the speaker expresses sorrow about his or her condition. Typically, the speaker's sadness is caused by an unresponsive lover, but some complaints cite other sources of unhappiness, such as poverty or fate. A commonly cited example is "A Complaint by Night of the Lover Not Beloved" by Henry Howard, Earl of Surrey. Thomas Sackville's "Complaint of Henry, Duke of Buckingham" traces the duke's unhappiness to his ruthless ambition.

Conceit: A clever and fanciful metaphor, usually expressed through elaborate and extended comparison, that presents a striking parallel between two seemingly dissimilar things—for example, elaborately comparing a beautiful woman to an object like a garden or the sun. The conceit was a popular device throughout the Elizabethan Age and Baroque Age and was the principal technique of the seventeenth-century English metaphysical poets. This usage of the word conceit is unrelated to the best-known definition of conceit as an arrogant attitude or behavior. The conceit figures prominently in the works of John Donne, Emily Dickinson, and T. S. Eliot.

Concrete: Concrete is the opposite of abstract, and refers to a thing that actually exists or a description that allows the reader to experience an object or concept with the senses. Henry David Thoreau's *Walden* contains much concrete description of nature and wildlife.

Concrete Poetry: Poetry in which visual elements play a large part in the poetic effect. Punctuation marks, letters, or words are arranged on a page to form a visual design: a cross, for example, or a bumblebee. Max Bill and Eugene Gomringer were among the early practitioners of concrete poetry; Haroldo de Campos and Augusto de Campos are among contemporary authors of concrete poetry.

Confessional Poetry: A form of poetry in which the poet reveals very personal, intimate, sometimes shocking information about himself or herself. Anne Sexton, Sylvia Plath, Robert Lowell, and John Berryman wrote poetry in the confessional vein.

Conflict: The conflict in a work of fiction is the issue to be resolved in the story. It usually occurs between two characters, the protagonist and the antagonist, or between the protagonist and society or the protagonist and himself or herself. Conflict in Theodore Dreiser's novel *Sister Carrie* comes as a result of urban society, while Jack London's short story ''To Build a Fire'' concerns the protagonist's battle against the cold and himself.

Connotation: The impression that a word gives beyond its defined meaning. Connotations may be universally understood or may be significant only to a certain group. Both ''horse'' and ''steed'' denote the same animal, but ''steed'' has a different connotation, deriving from the chivalrous or romantic narratives in which the word was once often used.

Consonance: Consonance occurs in poetry when words appearing at the ends of two or more verses have similar final consonant sounds but have final vowel sounds that differ, as with ''stuff'' and ''off.'' Consonance is found in ''The curfew tolls the knells of parting day'' from Thomas Grey's ''An Elegy Written in a Country Church Yard.'' Also known as Half Rhyme or Slant Rhyme.

Convention: Any widely accepted literary device, style, or form. A soliloquy, in which a character reveals to the audience his or her private thoughts, is an example of a dramatic convention.

Corrido: A Mexican ballad. Examples of *corridos* include ''Muerte del afamado Bilito,'' ''La voz de mi conciencia,'' ''Lucio Perez,'' ''La juida,'' and ''Los presos.''

Couplet: Two lines of poetry with the same rhyme and meter, often expressing a complete and self-contained thought. The following couplet is from Alexander Pope's ''Elegy to the Memory of an Unfortunate Lady'': 'Tis Use alone that sanctifies Expense, And Splendour borrows all her rays from Sense.

Criticism: The systematic study and evaluation of literary works, usually based on a specific method or set of principles. An important part of literary studies since ancient times, the practice of criticism has given rise to numerous theories, methods, and ''schools,'' sometimes producing conflicting, even contradictory, interpretations of literature in general as well as of individual works. Even such basic issues as what constitutes a poem or a novel have been the subject of much criticism over the centuries. Seminal texts of literary criticism include Plato's *Republic,* Aristotle's *Poetics,* Sir Philip Sidney's *The Defence of Poesie,* John Dryden's *Of Dramatic Poesie,* and William Wordsworth's ''Preface'' to the second edition of his *Lyrical Ballads.* Contemporary schools of criticism include deconstruction, feminist, psychoanalytic, poststructuralist, new historicist, postcolonialist, and reader- response.

D

Dactyl: See *Foot*

Dadaism: A protest movement in art and literature founded by Tristan Tzara in 1916. Followers of the movement expressed their outrage at the destruction brought about by World War I by revolting against numerous forms of social convention. The Dadaists presented works marked by calculated madness and flamboyant nonsense. They stressed total freedom of expression, commonly through primitive displays of emotion and illogical, often senseless, poetry. The movement ended shortly after the war, when it was replaced by surrealism. Proponents of Dadaism include Andre Breton, Louis Aragon, Philippe Soupault, and Paul Eluard.

Decadent: See *Decadents*

Decadents: The followers of a nineteenth-century literary movement that had its beginnings in French aestheticism. Decadent literature displays a fascination with perverse and morbid states; a search for novelty and sensation—the "new thrill"; a preoccupation with mysticism; and a belief in the senselessness of human existence. The movement is closely associated with the doctrine Art for Art's Sake. The term "decadence" is sometimes used to denote a decline in the quality of art or literature following a period of greatness. Major French decadents are Charles Baudelaire and Arthur Rimbaud. English decadents include Oscar Wilde, Ernest Dowson, and Frank Harris.

Deconstruction: A method of literary criticism developed by Jacques Derrida and characterized by multiple conflicting interpretations of a given work. Deconstructionists consider the impact of the language of a work and suggest that the true meaning of the work is not necessarily the meaning that the author intended. Jacques Derrida's *De la grammatologie* is the seminal text on deconstructive strategies; among American practitioners of this method of criticism are Paul de Man and J. Hillis Miller.

Deduction: The process of reaching a conclusion through reasoning from general premises to a specific premise. An example of deduction is present in the following syllogism: Premise: All mammals are animals. Premise: All whales are mammals. Conclusion: Therefore, all whales are animals.

Denotation: The definition of a word, apart from the impressions or feelings it creates in the reader. The word "apartheid" denotes a political and economic policy of segregation by race, but its connotations— oppression, slavery, inequality—are numerous.

Denouement: A French word meaning "the unknotting." In literary criticism, it denotes the resolution of conflict in fiction or drama. The *denouement* follows the climax and provides an outcome to the primary plot situation as well as an explanation of secondary plot complications. The *denouement* often involves a character's recognition of his or her state of mind or moral condition. A well-known example of *denouement* is the last scene of the play *As You Like It* by William Shakespeare, in which couples are married, an evildoer repents, the identities of two disguised characters are revealed, and a ruler is restored to power. Also known as Falling Action.

Description: Descriptive writing is intended to allow a reader to picture the scene or setting in which the action of a story takes place. The form this description takes often evokes an intended emotional response—a dark, spooky graveyard will evoke fear, and a peaceful, sunny meadow will evoke calmness. An example of a descriptive story is Edgar Allan Poe's *Landor's Cottage,* which offers a detailed depiction of a New York country estate.

Detective Story: A narrative about the solution of a mystery or the identification of a criminal. The conventions of the detective story include the detective's scrupulous use of logic in solving the mystery; incompetent or ineffectual police; a suspect who appears guilty at first but is later proved innocent; and the detective's friend or confidant—often the narrator—whose slowness in interpreting clues emphasizes by contrast the detective's brilliance. Edgar Allan Poe's "Murders in the Rue Morgue" is commonly regarded as the earliest example of this type of story. With this work, Poe established many of the conventions of the detective story genre, which are still in practice. Other practitioners of this vast and extremely popular genre include Arthur Conan Doyle, Dashiell Hammett, and Agatha Christie.

Deus ex machina: A Latin term meaning "god out of a machine." In Greek drama, a god was often lowered onto the stage by a mechanism of some kind to rescue the hero or untangle the plot. By extension, the term refers to any artificial device or coincidence used to bring about a convenient and simple solution to a plot. This is a common device in melodramas and includes such fortunate circumstances as the sudden receipt of a legacy to save the family farm or a last-minute stay of execution. The *deus ex machina* invariably rewards the virtuous and punishes evildoers. Examples of *deus ex machina* include King Louis XIV in Jean-Baptiste Moliere's *Tartuffe* and Queen Victoria in *The Pirates of Penzance* by William Gilbert and Arthur Sullivan. Bertolt Brecht parodies the abuse of such devices in the conclusion of his *Threepenny Opera.*

Dialogue: In its widest sense, dialogue is simply conversation between people in a literary work; in its most restricted sense, it refers specifically to the speech of characters in a drama. As a specific literary genre, a "dialogue" is a composition in which characters debate an issue or idea. The Greek philosopher Plato frequently expounded his theories in the form of dialogues.

Diction: The selection and arrangement of words in a literary work. Either or both may vary depending on the desired effect. There are four general types of diction: "formal," used in scholarly or lofty writing; "informal," used in relaxed but educated conversation; "colloquial," used in everyday speech; and "slang," containing newly coined words and other terms not accepted in formal usage.

Didactic: A term used to describe works of literature that aim to teach some moral, religious, political, or practical lesson. Although didactic elements are often found in artistically pleasing works, the term "didactic" usually refers to literature in which the message is more important than the form. The term may also be used to criticize a work that the critic finds "overly didactic," that is, heavy-handed in its delivery of a lesson. Examples of didactic literature include John Bunyan's *Pilgrim's Progress,* Alexander Pope's *Essay on Criticism,* Jean-Jacques Rousseau's *Emile,* and Elizabeth Inchbald's *Simple Story.*

Dimeter: See *Meter*

Dionysian: See *Apollonian and Dionysian*

Discordia concours: A Latin phrase meaning "discord in harmony." The term was coined by the eighteenth-century English writer Samuel Johnson to describe "a combination of dissimilar images or discovery of occult resemblances in things apparently unlike." Johnson created the expression by reversing a phrase by the Latin poet Horace. The metaphysical poetry of John Donne, Richard Crashaw, Abraham Cowley, George Herbert, and Edward Taylor among others, contains many examples of *discordia concours.* In Donne's "A Valediction: Forbidding Mourning," the poet compares the union of himself with his lover to a draftsman's compass: If they be two, they are two so, As stiff twin compasses are two: Thy soul, the fixed foot, makes no show To move, but doth, if the other do; And though it in the center sit, Yet when the other far doth roam, It leans, and hearkens after it, And grows erect, as that comes home.

Dissonance: A combination of harsh or jarring sounds, especially in poetry. Although such combinations may be accidental, poets sometimes intentionally make them to achieve particular effects. Dissonance is also sometimes used to refer to close but not identical rhymes. When this is the case, the word functions as a synonym for consonance. Robert Browning, Gerard Manley Hopkins, and many other poets have made deliberate use of dissonance.

Doppelganger: A literary technique by which a character is duplicated (usually in the form of an alter ego, though sometimes as a ghostly counterpart) or divided into two distinct, usually opposite personalities. The use of this character device is widespread in nineteenth- and twentieth- century literature, and indicates a growing awareness among authors that the "self" is really a composite of many "selves." A well-known story containing a *doppelganger* character is Robert Louis Stevenson's *Dr. Jekyll and Mr. Hyde,* which dramatizes an internal struggle between good and evil. Also known as The Double.

Double Entendre: A corruption of a French phrase meaning "double meaning." The term is used to indicate a word or phrase that is deliberately ambiguous, especially when one of the meanings is risque or improper. An example of a *double entendre* is the Elizabethan usage of the verb "die," which refers both to death and to orgasm.

Double, The: See *Doppelganger*

Draft: Any preliminary version of a written work. An author may write dozens of drafts which are revised to form the final work, or he or she may write only one, with few or no revisions. Dorothy Parker's observation that "I can't write five words but that I change seven" humorously indicates the purpose of the draft.

Drama: In its widest sense, a drama is any work designed to be presented by actors on a stage. Similarly, "drama" denotes a broad literary genre that includes a variety of forms, from pageant and spectacle to tragedy and comedy, as well as countless types and subtypes. More commonly in modern usage, however, a drama is a work that treats serious subjects and themes but does not aim at the grandeur of tragedy. This use of the term originated with the eighteenth-century French writer Denis Diderot, who used the word *drame* to designate his plays about middle- class life; thus "drama" typically features characters of a less exalted stature than those of tragedy. Examples of classical dramas include Menander's comedy *Dyscolus* and Sophocles' tragedy *Oedipus Rex.* Contemporary dramas include Eugene O'Neill's *The Iceman Cometh,* Lillian Hellman's *Little Foxes,* and August Wilson's *Ma Rainey's Black Bottom.*

Dramatic Irony: Occurs when the audience of a play or the reader of a work of literature knows something that a character in the work itself does not know. The irony is in the contrast between the intended meaning of the statements or actions of a character and the additional information understood by the audience. A celebrated example of dramatic irony is in Act V of William Shakespeare's *Romeo and Juliet,* where two young lovers meet their end as a result of a tragic misunderstanding. Here, the audience has full knowledge that Juliet's apparent "death" is merely temporary; she will regain her senses when the mysterious "sleeping potion" she has taken wears off. But Romeo, mistaking Juliet's drug-induced trance for true death, kills himself in grief. Upon awakening, Juliet discovers Romeo's corpse and, in despair, slays herself.

Dramatic Monologue: See *Monologue*

Dramatic Poetry: Any lyric work that employs elements of drama such as dialogue, conflict, or characterization, but excluding works that are intended for stage presentation. A monologue is a form of dramatic poetry.

Dramatis Personae: The characters in a work of literature, particularly a drama. The list of characters printed before the main text of a play or in the program is the *dramatis personae.*

Dream Allegory: See *Dream Vision*

Dream Vision: A literary convention, chiefly of the Middle Ages. In a dream vision a story is presented as a literal dream of the narrator. This device was commonly used to teach moral and religious lessons. Important works of this type are *The Divine Comedy* by Dante Alighieri, *Piers Plowman* by William Langland, and *The Pilgrim's Progress* by John Bunyan. Also known as Dream Allegory.

Dystopia: An imaginary place in a work of fiction where the characters lead dehumanized, fearful lives. Jack London's *The Iron Heel,* Yevgeny Zamyatin's *My,* Aldous Huxley's *Brave New World,* George Orwell's *Nineteen Eighty-four,* and Margaret Atwood's *Handmaid's Tale* portray versions of dystopia.

E

Eclogue: In classical literature, a poem featuring rural themes and structured as a dialogue among shepherds. Eclogues often took specific poetic forms, such as elegies or love poems. Some were written as the soliloquy of a shepherd. In later centuries, "eclogue" came to refer to any poem that was in the pastoral tradition or that had a dialogue or monologue structure. A classical example of an eclogue is Virgil's *Eclogues,* also known as *Bucolics.* Giovanni Boccaccio, Edmund Spenser, Andrew Marvell, Jonathan Swift, and Louis MacNeice also wrote eclogues.

Edwardian: Describes cultural conventions identified with the period of the reign of Edward VII of England (1901-1910). Writers of the Edwardian Age typically displayed a strong reaction against the propriety and conservatism of the Victorian Age. Their work often exhibits distrust of authority in religion, politics, and art and expresses strong doubts about the soundness of conventional values. Writers of this era include George Bernard Shaw, H. G. Wells, and Joseph Conrad.

Edwardian Age: See *Edwardian*

Electra Complex: A daughter's amorous obsession with her father. The term Electra complex comes from the plays of Euripides and Sophocles entitled *Electra,* in which the character Electra drives her brother Orestes to kill their mother and her lover in revenge for the murder of their father.

Elegy: A lyric poem that laments the death of a person or the eventual death of all people. In a conventional elegy, set in a classical world, the poet and subject are spoken of as shepherds. In modern criticism, the word elegy is often used to refer to a poem that is melancholy or mournfully contemplative. John Milton's "Lycidas" and Percy Bysshe Shelley's "Adonais" are two examples of this form.

Elizabethan Age: A period of great economic growth, religious controversy, and nationalism closely associated with the reign of Elizabeth I of England (1558-1603). The Elizabethan Age is considered a part of the general renaissance—that is, the flowering of arts and literature—that took place in Europe during the fourteenth through sixteenth centuries. The era is considered the golden age of English literature. The most important dramas in English and a great deal of lyric poetry were produced during this period, and modern English criticism began around this time. The notable authors of the period—Philip Sidney, Edmund Spenser, Christopher Marlowe, William Shakespeare, Ben Jonson, Francis Bacon, and John Donne—are among the best in all of English literature.

Elizabethan Drama: English comic and tragic plays produced during the Renaissance, or more narrowly, those plays written during the last years of and few years after Queen Elizabeth's reign. William Shakespeare is considered an Elizabethan dramatist in the broader sense, although most of his work was produced during the reign of James I. Examples of Elizabethan comedies include John Lyly's *The Woman in the Moone,* Thomas Dekker's *The Roaring Girl, or, Moll Cut Purse,* and William Shakespeare's *Twelfth Night.* Examples of Elizabethan tragedies include William Shakespeare's *Antony and Cleopatra,* Thomas Kyd's *The Spanish Tragedy,* and John Webster's *The Tragedy of the Duchess of Malfi.*

Empathy: A sense of shared experience, including emotional and physical feelings, with someone or something other than oneself. Empathy is often used to describe the response of a reader to a literary character. An example of an empathic passage is William Shakespeare's description in his narrative poem *Venus and Adonis* of: the snail, whose tender horns being hit, Shrinks backward in his shelly cave with pain. Readers of Gerard Manley Hopkins's *The Windhover* may experience some of the physical sensations evoked in the description of the movement of the falcon.

English Sonnet: See *Sonnet*

Enjambment: The running over of the sense and structure of a line of verse or a couplet into the following verse or couplet. Andrew Marvell's ''To His Coy Mistress'' is structured as a series of enjambments, as in lines 11-12: ''My vegetable love should grow/Vaster than empires and more slow.''

Enlightenment, The: An eighteenth-century philosophical movement. It began in France but had a wide impact throughout Europe and America. Thinkers of the Enlightenment valued reason and believed that both the individual and society could achieve a state of perfection. Corresponding to this essentially humanist vision was a resistance to religious authority. Important figures of the Enlightenment were Denis Diderot and Voltaire in France, Edward Gibbon and David Hume in England, and Thomas Paine and Thomas Jefferson in the United States.

Epic: A long narrative poem about the adventures of a hero of great historic or legendary importance. The setting is vast and the action is often given cosmic significance through the intervention of supernatural forces such as gods, angels, or demons. Epics are typically written in a classical style of grand simplicity with elaborate metaphors and allusions that enhance the symbolic importance of a hero's adventures. Some well-known epics are Homer's *Iliad* and *Odyssey,* Virgil's *Aeneid,* and John Milton's *Paradise Lost.*

Epic Simile: See *Homeric Simile*

Epic Theater: A theory of theatrical presentation developed by twentieth-century German playwright Bertolt Brecht. Brecht created a type of drama that the audience could view with complete detachment. He used what he termed ''alienation effects'' to create an emotional distance between the audience and the action on stage. Among these effects are: short, self- contained scenes that keep the play from building to a cathartic climax; songs that comment on the action; and techniques of acting that prevent the actor from developing an emotional identity with his role. Besides the plays of Bertolt Brecht, other plays that utilize epic theater conventions include those of Georg Buchner, Frank Wedekind, Erwin Piscator, and Leopold Jessner.

Epigram: A saying that makes the speaker's point quickly and concisely. Samuel Taylor Coleridge wrote an epigram that neatly sums up the form: What is an Epigram? A Dwarfish whole, Its body brevity, and wit its soul.

Epilogue: A concluding statement or section of a literary work. In dramas, particularly those of the seventeenth and eighteenth centuries, the epilogue is a closing speech, often in verse, delivered by an actor at the end of a play and spoken directly to the audience. A famous epilogue is Puck's speech at the end of William Shakespeare's *A Midsummer Night's Dream.*

Epiphany: A sudden revelation of truth inspired by a seemingly trivial incident. The term was widely used by James Joyce in his critical writings, and the stories in Joyce's *Dubliners* are commonly called ''epiphanies.''

Episode: An incident that forms part of a story and is significantly related to it. Episodes may be either self- contained narratives or events that depend on a larger context for their sense and importance. Examples of episodes include the founding of Wilmington, Delaware in Charles Reade's *The Disinherited Heir* and the individual events comprising the picaresque novels and medieval romances.

Episodic Plot: See *Plot*

Epitaph: An inscription on a tomb or tombstone, or a verse written on the occasion of a person's death. Epitaphs may be serious or humorous. Dorothy Parker's epitaph reads, ''I told you I was sick.''

Epithalamion: A song or poem written to honor and commemorate a marriage ceremony. Famous examples include Edmund Spenser's

''Epithalamion'' and e. e. cummings's ''Epithalamion.'' Also spelled Epithalamium.

Epithalamium: See *Epithalamion*

Epithet: A word or phrase, often disparaging or abusive, that expresses a character trait of someone or something. ''The Napoleon of crime'' is an epithet applied to Professor Moriarty, arch-rival of Sherlock Holmes in Arthur Conan Doyle's series of detective stories.

Exempla: See *Exemplum*

Exemplum: A tale with a moral message. This form of literary sermonizing flourished during the Middle Ages, when *exempla* appeared in collections known as ''example-books.'' The works of Geoffrey Chaucer are full of *exempla.*

Existentialism: A predominantly twentieth-century philosophy concerned with the nature and perception of human existence. There are two major strains of existentialist thought: atheistic and Christian. Followers of atheistic existentialism believe that the individual is alone in a godless universe and that the basic human condition is one of suffering and loneliness. Nevertheless, because there are no fixed values, individuals can create their own characters—indeed, they can shape themselves—through the exercise of free will. The atheistic strain culminates in and is popularly associated with the works of Jean-Paul Sartre. The Christian existentialists, on the other hand, believe that only in God may people find freedom from life's anguish. The two strains hold certain beliefs in common: that existence cannot be fully understood or described through empirical effort; that anguish is a universal element of life; that individuals must bear responsibility for their actions; and that there is no common standard of behavior or perception for religious and ethical matters. Existentialist thought figures prominently in the works of such authors as Eugene Ionesco, Franz Kafka, Fyodor Dostoyevsky, Simone de Beauvoir, Samuel Beckett, and Albert Camus.

Expatriates: See *Expatriatism*

Expatriatism: The practice of leaving one's country to live for an extended period in another country. Literary expatriates include English poets Percy Bysshe Shelley and John Keats in Italy, Polish novelist Joseph Conrad in England, American writers Richard Wright, James Baldwin, Gertrude Stein, and Ernest Hemingway in France, and Trinidadian author Neil Bissondath in Canada.

Exposition: Writing intended to explain the nature of an idea, thing, or theme. Expository writing is often combined with description, narration, or argument. In dramatic writing, the exposition is the introductory material which presents the characters, setting, and tone of the play. An example of dramatic exposition occurs in many nineteenth-century drawing-room comedies in which the butler and the maid open the play with relevant talk about their master and mistress; in composition, exposition relays factual information, as in encyclopedia entries.

Expressionism: An indistinct literary term, originally used to describe an early twentieth-century school of German painting. The term applies to almost any mode of unconventional, highly subjective writing that distorts reality in some way. Advocates of Expressionism include dramatists George Kaiser, Ernst Toller, Luigi Pirandello, Federico Garcia Lorca, Eugene O'Neill, and Elmer Rice; poets George Heym, Ernst Stadler, August Stramm, Gottfried Benn, and Georg Trakl; and novelists Franz Kafka and James Joyce.

Extended Monologue: See *Monologue*

F

Fable: A prose or verse narrative intended to convey a moral. Animals or inanimate objects with human characteristics often serve as characters in fables. A famous fable is Aesop's ''The Tortoise and the Hare.''

Fairy Tales: Short narratives featuring mythical beings such as fairies, elves, and sprites. These tales originally belonged to the folklore of a particular nation or region, such as those collected in Germany by Jacob and Wilhelm Grimm. Two other celebrated writers of fairy tales are Hans Christian Andersen and Rudyard Kipling.

Falling Action: See *Denouement*

Fantasy: A literary form related to mythology and folklore. Fantasy literature is typically set in nonexistent realms and features supernatural beings. Notable examples of fantasy literature are *The Lord of the Rings* by J. R. R. Tolkien and the Gormenghast trilogy by Mervyn Peake.

Farce: A type of comedy characterized by broad humor, outlandish incidents, and often vulgar subject matter. Much of the ''comedy'' in film and television could more accurately be described as farce.

Feet: See *Foot*

Feminine Rhyme: See *Rhyme*

Femme fatale: A French phrase with the literal translation "fatal woman." A *femme fatale* is a sensuous, alluring woman who often leads men into danger or trouble. A classic example of the *femme fatale* is the nameless character in Billy Wilder's *The Seven Year Itch,* portrayed by Marilyn Monroe in the film adaptation.

Fiction: Any story that is the product of imagination rather than a documentation of fact. characters and events in such narratives may be based in real life but their ultimate form and configuration is a creation of the author. Geoffrey Chaucer's *The Canterbury Tales,* Laurence Sterne's *Tristram Shandy,* and Margaret Mitchell's *Gone with the Wind* are examples of fiction.

Figurative Language: A technique in writing in which the author temporarily interrupts the order, construction, or meaning of the writing for a particular effect. This interruption takes the form of one or more figures of speech such as hyperbole, irony, or simile. Figurative language is the opposite of literal language, in which every word is truthful, accurate, and free of exaggeration or embellishment. Examples of figurative language are tropes such as metaphor and rhetorical figures such as apostrophe.

Figures of Speech: Writing that differs from customary conventions for construction, meaning, order, or significance for the purpose of a special meaning or effect. There are two major types of figures of speech: rhetorical figures, which do not make changes in the meaning of the words, and tropes, which do. Types of figures of speech include simile, hyperbole, alliteration, and pun, among many others.

Fin de siecle: A French term meaning "end of the century." The term is used to denote the last decade of the nineteenth century, a transition period when writers and other artists abandoned old conventions and looked for new techniques and objectives. Two writers commonly associated with the *fin de siecle* mindset are Oscar Wilde and George Bernard Shaw.

First Person: See *Point of View*

Flashback: A device used in literature to present action that occurred before the beginning of the story. Flashbacks are often introduced as the dreams or recollections of one or more characters. Flashback techniques are often used in films, where they are typically set off by a gradual changing of one picture to another.

Foil: A character in a work of literature whose physical or psychological qualities contrast strongly with, and therefore highlight, the corresponding qualities of another character. In his Sherlock Holmes stories, Arthur Conan Doyle portrayed Dr. Watson as a man of normal habits and intelligence, making him a foil for the eccentric and wonderfully perceptive Sherlock Holmes.

Folk Ballad: See *Ballad*

Folklore: Traditions and myths preserved in a culture or group of people. Typically, these are passed on by word of mouth in various forms—such as legends, songs, and proverbs— or preserved in customs and ceremonies. This term was first used by W. J. Thoms in 1846. Sir James Frazer's *The Golden Bough* is the record of English folklore; myths about the frontier and the Old South exemplify American folklore.

Folktale: A story originating in oral tradition. Folktales fall into a variety of categories, including legends, ghost stories, fairy tales, fables, and anecdotes based on historical figures and events. Examples of folktales include Giambattista Basile's *The Pentamerone,* which contains the tales of Puss in Boots, Rapunzel, Cinderella, and Beauty and the Beast, and Joel Chandler Harris's Uncle Remus stories, which represent transplanted African folktales and American tales about the characters Mike Fink, Johnny Appleseed, Paul Bunyan, and Pecos Bill.

Foot: The smallest unit of rhythm in a line of poetry. In English-language poetry, a foot is typically one accented syllable combined with one or two unaccented syllables. There are many different types of feet. When the accent is on the second syllable of a two syllable word (con- *tort*), the foot is an "iamb"; the reverse accentual pattern (*tor* - ture) is a "trochee." Other feet that commonly occur in poetry in English are "anapest", two unaccented syllables followed by an accented syllable as in in-ter-*cept*, and "dactyl", an accented syllable followed by two unaccented syllables as in *su*-i- cide.

Foreshadowing: A device used in literature to create expectation or to set up an explanation of later developments. In Charles Dickens's *Great Expectations,* the graveyard encounter at the beginning of the novel between Pip and the escaped convict Magwitch foreshadows the baleful atmosphere and events that comprise much of the narrative.

Form: The pattern or construction of a work which identifies its genre and distinguishes it from other genres. Examples of forms include the different genres, such as the lyric form or the short story form, and various patterns for poetry, such as the verse form or the stanza form.

Formalism: In literary criticism, the belief that literature should follow prescribed rules of construction, such as those that govern the sonnet form. Examples of formalism are found in the work of the New Critics and structuralists.

Fourteener Meter: See *Meter*

Free Verse: Poetry that lacks regular metrical and rhyme patterns but that tries to capture the cadences of everyday speech. The form allows a poet to exploit a variety of rhythmical effects within a single poem. Free-verse techniques have been widely used in the twentieth century by such writers as Ezra Pound, T. S. Eliot, Carl Sandburg, and William Carlos Williams. Also known as *Vers libre.*

Futurism: A flamboyant literary and artistic movement that developed in France, Italy, and Russia from 1908 through the 1920s. Futurist theater and poetry abandoned traditional literary forms. In their place, followers of the movement attempted to achieve total freedom of expression through bizarre imagery and deformed or newly invented words. The Futurists were self-consciously modern artists who attempted to incorporate the appearances and sounds of modern life into their work. Futurist writers include Filippo Tommaso Marinetti, Wyndham Lewis, Guillaume Apollinaire, Velimir Khlebnikov, and Vladimir Mayakovsky.

G

Genre: A category of literary work. In critical theory, genre may refer to both the content of a given work—tragedy, comedy, pastoral—and to its form, such as poetry, novel, or drama. This term also refers to types of popular literature, as in the genres of science fiction or the detective story.

Genteel Tradition: A term coined by critic George Santayana to describe the literary practice of certain late nineteenth- century American writers, especially New Englanders. Followers of the Genteel Tradition emphasized conventionality in social, religious, moral, and literary standards. Some of the best-known writers of the Genteel Tradition are R. H. Stoddard and Bayard Taylor.

Gilded Age: A period in American history during the 1870s characterized by political corruption and materialism. A number of important novels of social and political criticism were written during this time. Examples of Gilded Age literature include Henry Adams's *Democracy* and F. Marion Crawford's *An American Politician.*

Gothic: See *Gothicism*

Gothicism: In literary criticism, works characterized by a taste for the medieval or morbidly attractive. A gothic novel prominently features elements of horror, the supernatural, gloom, and violence: clanking chains, terror, charnel houses, ghosts, medieval castles, and mysteriously slamming doors. The term ''gothic novel'' is also applied to novels that lack elements of the traditional Gothic setting but that create a similar atmosphere of terror or dread. Mary Shelley's *Frankenstein* is perhaps the best-known English work of this kind.

Gothic Novel: See *Gothicism*

Great Chain of Being: The belief that all things and creatures in nature are organized in a hierarchy from inanimate objects at the bottom to God at the top. This system of belief was popular in the seventeenth and eighteenth centuries. A summary of the concept of the great chain of being can be found in the first epistle of Alexander Pope's *An Essay on Man,* and more recently in Arthur O. Lovejoy's *The Great Chain of Being: A Study of the History of an Idea.*

Grotesque: In literary criticism, the subject matter of a work or a style of expression characterized by exaggeration, deformity, freakishness, and disorder. The grotesque often includes an element of comic absurdity. Early examples of literary grotesque include Francois Rabelais's *Pantagruel* and *Gargantua* and Thomas Nashe's *The Unfortunate Traveller,* while more recent examples can be found in the works of Edgar Allan Poe, Evelyn Waugh, Eudora Welty, Flannery O'Connor, Eugene Ionesco, Gunter Grass, Thomas Mann, Mervyn Peake, and Joseph Heller, among many others.

H

Haiku: The shortest form of Japanese poetry, constructed in three lines of five, seven, and five syllables respectively. The message of a *haiku* poem usually centers on some aspect of spirituality and provokes an emotional response in the reader. Early masters of *haiku* include Basho, Buson,

Kobayashi Issa, and Masaoka Shiki. English writers of *haiku* include the Imagists, notably Ezra Pound, H. D., Amy Lowell, Carl Sandburg, and William Carlos Williams. Also known as *Hokku.*

Half Rhyme: See *Consonance*

Hamartia: In tragedy, the event or act that leads to the hero's or heroine's downfall. This term is often incorrectly used as a synonym for tragic flaw. In Richard Wright's *Native Son,* the act that seals Bigger Thomas's fate is his first impulsive murder.

Harlem Renaissance: The Harlem Renaissance of the 1920s is generally considered the first significant movement of black writers and artists in the United States. During this period, new and established black writers published more fiction and poetry than ever before, the first influential black literary journals were established, and black authors and artists received their first widespread recognition and serious critical appraisal. Among the major writers associated with this period are Claude McKay, Jean Toomer, Countee Cullen, Langston Hughes, Arna Bontemps, Nella Larsen, and Zora Neale Hurston. Works representative of the Harlem Renaissance include Arna Bontemps's poems "The Return" and "Golgotha Is a Mountain," Claude McKay's novel *Home to Harlem,* Nella Larsen's novel *Passing,* Langston Hughes's poem "The Negro Speaks of Rivers," and the journals *Crisis* and *Opportunity,* both founded during this period. Also known as Negro Renaissance and New Negro Movement.

Harlequin: A stock character of the *commedia dell'arte* who occasionally interrupted the action with silly antics. Harlequin first appeared on the English stage in John Day's *The Travailes of the Three English Brothers.* The San Francisco Mime Troupe is one of the few modern groups to adapt Harlequin to the needs of contemporary satire.

Hellenism: Imitation of ancient Greek thought or styles. Also, an approach to life that focuses on the growth and development of the intellect. "Hellenism" is sometimes used to refer to the belief that reason can be applied to examine all human experience. A cogent discussion of Hellenism can be found in Matthew Arnold's *Culture and Anarchy.*

Heptameter: See *Meter*

Hero/Heroine: The principal sympathetic character (male or female) in a literary work. Heroes and heroines typically exhibit admirable traits: idealism, courage, and integrity, for example. Famous heroes and heroines include Pip in Charles Dickens's *Great Expectations,* the anonymous narrator in Ralph Ellison's *Invisible Man,* and Sethe in Toni Morrison's *Beloved.*

Heroic Couplet: A rhyming couplet written in iambic pentameter (a verse with five iambic feet). The following lines by Alexander Pope are an example: "Truth guards the Poet, sanctifies the line,/ And makes Immortal, Verse as mean as mine."

Heroic Line: The meter and length of a line of verse in epic or heroic poetry. This varies by language and time period. For example, in English poetry, the heroic line is iambic pentameter (a verse with five iambic feet); in French, the alexandrine (a verse with six iambic feet); in classical literature, dactylic hexameter (a verse with six dactylic feet).

Heroine: See *Hero/Heroine*

Hexameter: See *Meter*

Historical Criticism: The study of a work based on its impact on the world of the time period in which it was written. Examples of postmodern historical criticism can be found in the work of Michel Foucault, Hayden White, Stephen Greenblatt, and Jonathan Goldberg.

Hokku: See *Haiku*

Holocaust: See *Holocaust Literature*

Holocaust Literature: Literature influenced by or written about the Holocaust of World War II. Such literature includes true stories of survival in concentration camps, escape, and life after the war, as well as fictional works and poetry. Representative works of Holocaust literature include Saul Bellow's *Mr. Sammler's Planet,* Anne Frank's *The Diary of a Young Girl,* Jerzy Kosinski's *The Painted Bird,* Arthur Miller's *Incident at Vichy,* Czeslaw Milosz's *Collected Poems,* William Styron's *Sophie's Choice,* and Art Spiegelman's *Maus.*

Homeric Simile: An elaborate, detailed comparison written as a simile many lines in length. An example of an epic simile from John Milton's *Paradise Lost* follows: Angel Forms, who lay entranced Thick as autumnal leaves that strow the brooks In Vallombrosa, where the Etrurian shades High over-arched embower; or scattered sedge Afloat, when with fierce winds Orion armed Hath vexed the Red-Sea coast, whose waves o'erthrew Busiris and his Memphian chivalry, While with perfidious hatred they pursued The sojourners of Goshen, who beheld From the safe shore their floating carcasses And broken chariot-wheels. Also known as Epic Simile.

Horatian Satire: See *Satire*

Humanism: A philosophy that places faith in the dignity of humankind and rejects the medieval perception of the individual as a weak, fallen creature. ''Humanists'' typically believe in the perfectibility of human nature and view reason and education as the means to that end. Humanist thought is represented in the works of Marsilio Ficino, Ludovico Castelvetro, Edmund Spenser, John Milton, Dean John Colet, Desiderius Erasmus, John Dryden, Alexander Pope, Matthew Arnold, and Irving Babbitt.

Humors: Mentions of the humors refer to the ancient Greek theory that a person's health and personality were determined by the balance of four basic fluids in the body: blood, phlegm, yellow bile, and black bile. A dominance of any fluid would cause extremes in behavior. An excess of blood created a sanguine person who was joyful, aggressive, and passionate; a phlegmatic person was shy, fearful, and sluggish; too much yellow bile led to a choleric temperament characterized by impatience, anger, bitterness, and stubbornness; and excessive black bile created melancholy, a state of laziness, gluttony, and lack of motivation. Literary treatment of the humors is exemplified by several characters in Ben Jonson's plays *Every Man in His Humour* and *Every Man out of His Humour.* Also spelled Humours.

Humours: See *Humors*

Hyperbole: In literary criticism, deliberate exaggeration used to achieve an effect. In William Shakespeare's *Macbeth,* Lady Macbeth hyperbolizes when she says, ''All the perfumes of Arabia could not sweeten this little hand.''

I

Iamb: See *Foot*

Idiom: A word construction or verbal expression closely associated with a given language. For example, in colloquial English the construction ''how come'' can be used instead of ''why'' to introduce a question. Similarly, ''a piece of cake'' is sometimes used to describe a task that is easily done.

Image: A concrete representation of an object or sensory experience. Typically, such a representation helps evoke the feelings associated with the object or experience itself. Images are either ''literal'' or ''figurative.'' Literal images are especially concrete and involve little or no extension of the obvious meaning of the words used to express them. Figurative images do not follow the literal meaning of the words exactly. Images in literature are usually visual, but the term ''image'' can also refer to the representation of any sensory experience. In his poem ''The Shepherd's Hour,'' Paul Verlaine presents the following image: ''The Moon is red through horizon's fog;/ In a dancing mist the hazy meadow sleeps.'' The first line is broadly literal, while the second line involves turns of meaning associated with dancing and sleeping.

Imagery: The array of images in a literary work. Also, figurative language. William Butler Yeats's ''The Second Coming'' offers a powerful image of encroaching anarchy: Turning and turning in the widening gyre The falcon cannot hear the falconer; Things fall apart. . . .

Imagism: An English and American poetry movement that flourished between 1908 and 1917. The Imagists used precise, clearly presented images in their works. They also used common, everyday speech and aimed for conciseness, concrete imagery, and the creation of new rhythms. Participants in the Imagist movement included Ezra Pound, H. D. (Hilda Doolittle), and Amy Lowell, among others.

In medias res: A Latin term meaning ''in the middle of things.'' It refers to the technique of beginning a story at its midpoint and then using various flashback devices to reveal previous action. This technique originated in such epics as Virgil's *Aeneid.*

Induction: The process of reaching a conclusion by reasoning from specific premises to form a general premise. Also, an introductory portion of a work of literature, especially a play. Geoffrey Chaucer's ''Prologue'' to the *Canterbury Tales,* Thomas Sackville's ''Induction'' to *The Mirror of Magistrates,* and the opening scene in William Shakespeare's *The Taming of the Shrew* are examples of inductions to literary works.

Intentional Fallacy: The belief that judgments of a literary work based solely on an author's stated or implied intentions are false and misleading. Critics who believe in the concept of the intentional fallacy typically argue that the work itself is sufficient matter for interpretation, even though they may concede that an author's statement of purpose can be useful. Analysis of William Wordsworth's *Lyrical Ballads* based on the observations about poetry he makes in his "Preface" to the second edition of that work is an example of the intentional fallacy.

Interior Monologue: A narrative technique in which characters' thoughts are revealed in a way that appears to be uncontrolled by the author. The interior monologue typically aims to reveal the inner self of a character. It portrays emotional experiences as they occur at both a conscious and unconscious level. images are often used to represent sensations or emotions. One of the best-known interior monologues in English is the Molly Bloom section at the close of James Joyce's *Ulysses.* The interior monologue is also common in the works of Virginia Woolf.

Internal Rhyme: Rhyme that occurs within a single line of verse. An example is in the opening line of Edgar Allan Poe's "The Raven": "Once upon a midnight dreary, while I pondered weak and weary." Here, "dreary" and "weary" make an internal rhyme.

Irish Literary Renaissance: A late nineteenth- and early twentieth-century movement in Irish literature. Members of the movement aimed to reduce the influence of British culture in Ireland and create an Irish national literature. William Butler Yeats, George Moore, and Sean O'Casey are three of the best-known figures of the movement.

Irony: In literary criticism, the effect of language in which the intended meaning is the opposite of what is stated. The title of Jonathan Swift's "A Modest Proposal" is ironic because what Swift proposes in this essay is cannibalism—hardly "modest."

Italian Sonnet: See *Sonnet*

J

Jacobean Age: The period of the reign of James I of England (1603-1625). The early literature of this period reflected the worldview of the Elizabethan Age, but a darker, more cynical attitude steadily grew in the art and literature of the Jacobean Age. This was an important time for English drama and poetry. Milestones include William Shakespeare's tragedies, tragi-comedies, and sonnets; Ben Jonson's various dramas; and John Donne's metaphysical poetry.

Jargon: Language that is used or understood only by a select group of people. Jargon may refer to terminology used in a certain profession, such as computer jargon, or it may refer to any nonsensical language that is not understood by most people. Literary examples of jargon are Francois Villon's *Ballades en jargon,* which is composed in the secret language of the *coquillards,* and Anthony Burgess's *A Clockwork Orange,* narrated in the fictional characters' language of "Nadsat."

Juvenalian Satire: See *Satire*

K

Knickerbocker Group: A somewhat indistinct group of New York writers of the first half of the nineteenth century. Members of the group were linked only by location and a common theme: New York life. Two famous members of the Knickerbocker Group were Washington Irving and William Cullen Bryant. The group's name derives from Irving's *Knickerbocker's History of New York.*

L

Lais: See *Lay*

Lay: A song or simple narrative poem. The form originated in medieval France. Early French *lais* were often based on the Celtic legends and other tales sung by Breton minstrels—thus the name of the "Breton lay." In fourteenth-century England, the term "lay" was used to describe short narratives written in imitation of the Breton lays. The most notable of these is Geoffrey Chaucer's "The Minstrel's Tale."

Leitmotiv: See *Motif*

Literal Language: An author uses literal language when he or she writes without exaggerating or embellishing the subject matter and without any tools of figurative language. To say "He ran very quickly down the street" is to use literal language, whereas to say "He ran like a hare down the street" would be using figurative language.

Literary Ballad: See *Ballad*

Literature: Literature is broadly defined as any written or spoken material, but the term most often refers to creative works. Literature includes poetry, drama, fiction, and many kinds of nonfiction writing, as well as oral, dramatic, and broadcast compositions not necessarily preserved in a written format, such as films and television programs.

Lost Generation: A term first used by Gertrude Stein to describe the post-World War I generation of American writers: men and women haunted by a sense of betrayal and emptiness brought about by the destructiveness of the war. The term is commonly applied to Hart Crane, Ernest Hemingway, F. Scott Fitzgerald, and others.

Lyric Poetry: A poem expressing the subjective feelings and personal emotions of the poet. Such poetry is melodic, since it was originally accompanied by a lyre in recitals. Most Western poetry in the twentieth century may be classified as lyrical. Examples of lyric poetry include A. E. Housman's elegy ''To an Athlete Dying Young,'' the odes of Pindar and Horace, Thomas Gray and William Collins, the sonnets of Sir Thomas Wyatt and Sir Philip Sidney, Elizabeth Barrett Browning and Rainer Maria Rilke, and a host of other forms in the poetry of William Blake and Christina Rossetti, among many others.

M

Mannerism: Exaggerated, artificial adherence to a literary manner or style. Also, a popular style of the visual arts of late sixteenth-century Europe that was marked by elongation of the human form and by intentional spatial distortion. Literary works that are self-consciously high-toned and artistic are often said to be ''mannered.'' Authors of such works include Henry James and Gertrude Stein.

Masculine Rhyme: See *Rhyme*

Masque: A lavish and elaborate form of entertainment, often performed in royal courts, that emphasizes song, dance, and costumery. The Renaissance form of the masque grew out of the spectacles of masked figures common in medieval England and Europe. The masque reached its peak of popularity and development in seventeenth-century England, during the reigns of James I and, especially, of Charles I. Ben Jonson, the most significant masque writer, also created the ''antimasque,'' which incorporates elements of humor and the grotesque into the traditional masque and achieved greater dramatic quality. Masque-like interludes appear in Edmund Spenser's *The Faerie Queene* and in William Shakespeare's *The Tempest.* One of the best-known English masques is John Milton's *Comus.*

Measure: The foot, verse, or time sequence used in a literary work, especially a poem. Measure is often used somewhat incorrectly as a synonym for meter.

Melodrama: A play in which the typical plot is a conflict between characters who personify extreme good and evil. Melodramas usually end happily and emphasize sensationalism. Other literary forms that use the same techniques are often labeled ''melodramatic.'' The term was formerly used to describe a combination of drama and music; as such, it was synonymous with ''opera.'' Augustin Daly's *Under the Gaslight* and Dion Boucicault's *The Octoroon, The Colleen Bawn,* and *The Poor of New York* are examples of melodramas. The most popular media for twentieth-century melodramas are motion pictures and television.

Metaphor: A figure of speech that expresses an idea through the image of another object. Metaphors suggest the essence of the first object by identifying it with certain qualities of the second object. An example is ''But soft, what light through yonder window breaks?/ It is the east, and Juliet is the sun'' in William Shakespeare's *Romeo and Juliet.* Here, Juliet, the first object, is identified with qualities of the second object, the sun.

Metaphysical Conceit: See *Conceit*

Metaphysical Poetry: The body of poetry produced by a group of seventeenth-century English writers called the ''Metaphysical Poets.'' The group includes John Donne and Andrew Marvell. The Metaphysical Poets made use of everyday speech, intellectual analysis, and unique imagery. They aimed to portray the ordinary conflicts and contradictions of life. Their poems often took the form of an argument, and many of them emphasize physical and religious love as well as the fleeting nature of life. Elaborate conceits are typical in metaphysical poetry. Marvell's ''To His Coy Mistress'' is a well-known example of a metaphysical poem.

Metaphysical Poets: See *Metaphysical Poetry*

Meter: In literary criticism, the repetition of sound patterns that creates a rhythm in poetry. The patterns are based on the number of syllables and the presence and absence of accents. The unit of rhythm in a line is called a foot. Types of meter are classified according to the number of feet in a line. These are the standard English lines: Monometer, one foot; Dimeter, two feet; Trimeter, three feet; Tetrameter, four feet; Pentameter, five feet; Hexameter, six feet (also called the Alexandrine); Heptameter, seven feet (also called the ''Fourteener'' when the feet are iambic). The most common English meter is the iambic pentameter, in which each line contains ten syllables, or five iambic feet, which individually are composed of an unstressed syllable followed by an accented syllable. Both of the following lines from Alfred, Lord Tennyson's ''Ulysses'' are written in iambic pentameter: Made weak by time and fate, but strong in will To strive, to seek, to find, and not to yield.

Mise en scene: The costumes, scenery, and other properties of a drama. Herbert Beerbohm Tree was renowned for the elaborate *mises en scene* of his lavish Shakespearean productions at His Majesty's Theatre between 1897 and 1915.

Modernism: Modern literary practices. Also, the principles of a literary school that lasted from roughly the beginning of the twentieth century until the end of World War II. Modernism is defined by its rejection of the literary conventions of the nineteenth century and by its opposition to conventional morality, taste, traditions, and economic values. Many writers are associated with the concepts of Modernism, including Albert Camus, Marcel Proust, D. H. Lawrence, W. H. Auden, Ernest Hemingway, William Faulkner, William Butler Yeats, Thomas Mann, Tennessee Williams, Eugene O'Neill, and James Joyce.

Monologue: A composition, written or oral, by a single individual. More specifically, a speech given by a single individual in a drama or other public entertainment. It has no set length, although it is usually several or more lines long. An example of an ''extended monologue''—that is, a monologue of great length and seriousness—occurs in the one-act, one-character play *The Stronger* by August Strindberg.

Monometer: See *Meter*

Mood: The prevailing emotions of a work or of the author in his or her creation of the work. The mood of a work is not always what might be expected based on its subject matter. The poem ''Dover Beach'' by Matthew Arnold offers examples of two different moods originating from the same experience: watching the ocean at night. The mood of the first three lines— The sea is calm tonight The tide is full, the moon lies fair Upon the straights. . . . is in sharp contrast to the mood of the last three lines— And we are here as on a darkling plain Swept with confused alarms of struggle and flight, Where ignorant armies clash by night.

Motif: A theme, character type, image, metaphor, or other verbal element that recurs throughout a single work of literature or occurs in a number of different works over a period of time. For example, the various manifestations of the color white in Herman Melville's *Moby Dick* is a ''specific'' *motif,* while the trials of star-crossed lovers is a ''conventional'' *motif* from the literature of all periods. Also known as *Motiv* or *Leitmotiv.*

Motiv: See *Motif*

Muckrakers: An early twentieth-century group of American writers. Typically, their works exposed the wrongdoings of big business and government in the United States. Upton Sinclair's *The Jungle* exemplifies the muckraking novel.

Muses: Nine Greek mythological goddesses, the daughters of Zeus and Mnemosyne (Memory). Each muse patronized a specific area of the liberal arts and sciences. Calliope presided over epic poetry, Clio over history, Erato over love poetry, Euterpe over music or lyric poetry, Melpomene over tragedy, Polyhymnia over hymns to the gods, Terpsichore over dance, Thalia over comedy, and Urania over astronomy. Poets and writers traditionally made appeals to the Muses for inspiration in their work. John Milton invokes the aid of a muse at the beginning of the first book of his *Paradise Lost:* Of Man's First disobedience, and the Fruit of the Forbidden Tree, whose mortal taste Brought Death into the World, and all our woe, With loss of Eden, till one greater Man Restore us, and regain the blissful Seat, Sing Heav'nly Muse, that on the secret top of Oreb, or of Sinai, didst inspire That Shepherd, who first taught the chosen Seed, In the Beginning how the Heav'ns and Earth Rose out of Chaos. . . .

Mystery: See *Suspense*

Myth: An anonymous tale emerging from the traditional beliefs of a culture or social unit. Myths use supernatural explanations for natural phenomena. They may also explain cosmic issues like creation and death. Collections of myths, known as mythologies, are common to all cultures and nations, but the best-known myths belong to the Norse, Roman, and Greek mythologies. A famous myth is the story of Arachne, an arrogant young girl who challenged a goddess, Athena, to a weaving contest; when the girl won, Athena was enraged and turned Arachne into a spider, thus explaining the existence of spiders.

N

Narration: The telling of a series of events, real or invented. A narration may be either a simple narrative, in which the events are recounted chronologically, or a narrative with a plot, in which the account is given in a style reflecting the author's artistic concept of the story. Narration is sometimes used as a synonym for ''storyline.'' The recounting of scary stories around a campfire is a form of narration.

Narrative: A verse or prose accounting of an event or sequence of events, real or invented. The term is also used as an adjective in the sense ''method of narration.'' For example, in literary criticism, the expression ''narrative technique'' usually refers to the way the author structures and presents his or her story. Narratives range from the shortest accounts of events, as in Julius Caesar's remark, ''I came, I saw, I conquered,'' to the longest historical or biographical works, as in Edward Gibbon's *The Decline and Fall of the Roman Empire,* as well as diaries, travelogues, novels, ballads, epics, short stories, and other fictional forms.

Narrative Poetry: A nondramatic poem in which the author tells a story. Such poems may be of any length or level of complexity. Epics such as *Beowulf* and ballads are forms of narrative poetry.

Narrator: The teller of a story. The narrator may be the author or a character in the story through whom the author speaks. Huckleberry Finn is the narrator of Mark Twain's *The Adventures of Huckleberry Finn.*

Naturalism: A literary movement of the late nineteenth and early twentieth centuries. The movement's major theorist, French novelist Emile Zola, envisioned a type of fiction that would examine human life with the objectivity of scientific inquiry. The Naturalists typically viewed human beings as either the products of ''biological determinism,'' ruled by hereditary instincts and engaged in an endless struggle for survival, or as the products of ''socioeconomic determinism,'' ruled by social and economic forces beyond their control. In their works, the Naturalists generally ignored the highest levels of society and focused on degradation: poverty, alcoholism, prostitution, insanity, and disease. Naturalism influenced authors throughout the world, including Henrik Ibsen and Thomas Hardy. In the United States, in particular, Naturalism had a profound impact. Among the authors who embraced its principles are Theodore Dreiser, Eugene O'Neill, Stephen Crane, Jack London, and Frank Norris.

Negritude: A literary movement based on the concept of a shared cultural bond on the part of black Africans, wherever they may be in the world. It traces its origins to the former French colonies of Africa and the Caribbean. Negritude poets, novelists, and essayists generally stress four points in their writings: One, black alienation from traditional African culture can lead to feelings of inferiority. Two, European colonialism and Western education should be resisted. Three, black Africans should seek to affirm and define their own identity. Four, African culture can and should be reclaimed. Many Negritude writers also claim that blacks can make unique contributions to the world, based on a heightened appreciation of nature, rhythm, and human emotions—aspects of life they say are not so highly valued in the materialistic and rationalistic West. Examples of Negritude literature include the poetry of both Senegalese Leopold Senghor in *Hosties noires* and Martiniquais Aime-Fernand Cesaire in *Return to My Native Land.*

Negro Renaissance: See *Harlem Renaissance*

Neoclassical Period: See *Neoclassicism*

Neoclassicism: In literary criticism, this term refers to the revival of the attitudes and styles of expression of classical literature. It is generally used to describe a period in European history beginning in the late seventeenth century and lasting until about 1800. In its purest form, Neoclassicism marked a return to order, proportion, restraint, logic, accuracy, and decorum. In England, where Neoclassicism perhaps was most popular, it reflected the influence of seventeenth- century French writers, especially dramatists. Neoclassical writers typically reacted against the intensity and enthusiasm of the Renaissance period. They wrote works that appealed to the intellect, using elevated language and classical literary forms such as satire and the ode. Neoclassical works were often governed by the classical goal of instruction. English neoclassicists included Alexander Pope, Jonathan Swift, Joseph Addison, Sir Richard Steele, John Gay, and Matthew Prior; French neoclassicists included Pierre Corneille and Jean-Baptiste Moliere. Also known as Age of Reason.

Neoclassicists: See *Neoclassicism*

New Criticism: A movement in literary criticism, dating from the late 1920s, that stressed close textual analysis in the interpretation of works of literature. The New Critics saw little merit in historical and biographical analysis. Rather, they aimed to examine the text alone, free from the question of how external events—biographical or otherwise—may have helped shape it. This predominantly American school was named ''New Criticism'' by one of its practitioners, John Crowe Ransom. Other important New Critics included Allen Tate, R. P. Blackmur, Robert Penn Warren, and Cleanth Brooks.

New Negro Movement: See *Harlem Renaissance*

Noble Savage: The idea that primitive man is noble and good but becomes evil and corrupted as he becomes civilized. The concept of the noble savage originated in the Renaissance period but is more closely identified with such later writers as Jean-Jacques Rousseau and Aphra Behn. First described in John Dryden's play *The Conquest of Granada,* the noble savage is portrayed by the various Native Americans in James Fenimore Cooper's ''Leatherstocking Tales,'' by Queequeg, Daggoo, and Tashtego in Herman Melville's *Moby Dick,* and by John the Savage in Aldous Huxley's *Brave New World.*

O

Objective Correlative: An outward set of objects, a situation, or a chain of events corresponding to an inward experience and evoking this experience in the reader. The term frequently appears in modern criticism in discussions of authors' intended effects on the emotional responses of readers. This term was originally used by T. S. Eliot in his 1919 essay ''Hamlet.''

Objectivity: A quality in writing characterized by the absence of the author's opinion or feeling about the subject matter. Objectivity is an important factor in criticism. The novels of Henry James and, to a certain extent, the poems of John Larkin demonstrate objectivity, and it is central to John Keats's concept of ''negative capability.'' Critical and journalistic writing usually are or attempt to be objective.

Occasional Verse: poetry written on the occasion of a significant historical or personal event. *Vers de societe* is sometimes called occasional verse although it is of a less serious nature. Famous examples of occasional verse include Andrew Marvell's ''Horatian Ode upon Cromwell's Return from England,'' Walt Whitman's ''When Lilacs Last in the Dooryard Bloom'd''— written upon the death of Abraham Lincoln—and Edmund Spenser's commemoration of his wedding, ''Epithalamion.''

Octave: A poem or stanza composed of eight lines. The term octave most often represents the first eight lines of a Petrarchan sonnet. An example of an octave is taken from a translation of a Petrarchan sonnet by Sir Thomas Wyatt: The pillar perisht is whereto I leant, The strongest stay of mine unquiet mind; The like of it no man again can find, From East to West Still seeking though he went. To mind unhap! for hap away hath rent Of all my joy the very bark and rind; And I, alas, by chance am thus assigned Daily to mourn till death do it relent.

Ode: Name given to an extended lyric poem characterized by exalted emotion and dignified style. An ode usually concerns a single, serious theme. Most odes, but not all, are addressed to an object or individual. Odes are distinguished from other lyric poetic forms by their complex rhythmic and stanzaic patterns. An example of this form is John Keats's ''Ode to a Nightingale.''

Oedipus Complex: A son's amorous obsession with his mother. The phrase is derived from the story of the ancient Theban hero Oedipus, who unknowingly killed his father and married his mother. Literary occurrences of the Oedipus complex include Andre Gide's *Oedipe* and Jean Cocteau's *La Machine infernale,* as well as the most famous, Sophocles' *Oedipus Rex.*

Omniscience: See *Point of View*

Onomatopoeia: The use of words whose sounds express or suggest their meaning. In its simplest sense, onomatopoeia may be represented by words that mimic the sounds they denote such as ''hiss'' or ''meow.'' At a more subtle level, the pattern and rhythm of sounds and rhymes of a line or poem may be onomatopoeic. A celebrated example of onomatopoeia is the repetition of the word ''bells'' in Edgar Allan Poe's poem ''The Bells.''

Opera: A type of stage performance, usually a drama, in which the dialogue is sung. Classic examples of opera include Giuseppi Verdi's *La traviata,* Giacomo Puccini's *La Boheme,* and Richard Wagner's *Tristan und Isolde.* Major twentieth- century contributors to the form include Richard Strauss and Alban Berg.

Operetta: A usually romantic comic opera. John Gay's *The Beggar's Opera,* Richard Sheridan's *The Duenna,* and numerous works by William Gilbert and Arthur Sullivan are examples of operettas.

Oral Tradition: See *Oral Transmission*

Oral Transmission: A process by which songs, ballads, folklore, and other material are transmitted by word of mouth. The tradition of oral transmission predates the written record systems of literate society. Oral transmission preserves material sometimes over generations, although often with variations. Memory plays a large part in the recitation and preservation of orally transmitted material. Breton lays, French *fabliaux,* national epics (including the Anglo- Saxon *Beowulf,* the Spanish *El Cid,* and the Finnish *Kalevala*), Native American myths and legends, and African folktales told by plantation slaves are examples of orally transmitted literature.

Oration: Formal speaking intended to motivate the listeners to some action or feeling. Such public speaking was much more common before the development of timely printed communication such as newspapers. Famous examples of oration include Abraham Lincoln's ''Gettysburg Address'' and Dr. Martin Luther King Jr.'s ''I Have a Dream'' speech.

Ottava Rima: An eight-line stanza of poetry composed in iambic pentameter (a five-foot line in which each foot consists of an unaccented syllable followed by an accented syllable), following the abababcc rhyme scheme. This form has been prominently used by such important English writers as Lord Byron, Henry Wadsworth Longfellow, and W. B. Yeats.

Oxymoron: A phrase combining two contradictory terms. Oxymorons may be intentional or unintentional. The following speech from William Shakespeare's *Romeo and Juliet* uses several oxymorons: Why, then, O brawling love! O loving hate! O anything, of nothing first create! O heavy lightness! serious vanity! Mis-shapen chaos of well-seeming forms! Feather of lead, bright smoke, cold fire, sick health! This love feel I, that feel no love in this.

P

Pantheism: The idea that all things are both a manifestation or revelation of God and a part of God at the same time. Pantheism was a common attitude in the early societies of Egypt, India, and Greece—the term derives from the Greek *pan* meaning ''all'' and *theos* meaning ''deity.'' It later became a significant part of the Christian faith. William Wordsworth and Ralph Waldo Emerson are among the many writers who have expressed the pantheistic attitude in their works.

Parable: A story intended to teach a moral lesson or answer an ethical question. In the West, the best examples of parables are those of Jesus Christ in the New Testament, notably ''The Prodigal Son,'' but parables also are used in Sufism, rabbinic literature, Hasidism, and Zen Buddhism.

Paradox: A statement that appears illogical or contradictory at first, but may actually point to an underlying truth. ''Less is more'' is an example of a paradox. Literary examples include Francis Bacon's statement, ''The most corrected copies are commonly the least correct,'' and ''All animals are equal, but some animals are more equal than others'' from George Orwell's *Animal Farm.*

Parallelism: A method of comparison of two ideas in which each is developed in the same grammatical structure. Ralph Waldo Emerson's ''Civilization'' contains this example of parallelism: Raphael paints wisdom; Handel sings it, Phidias carves it, Shakespeare writes it, Wren builds it, Columbus sails it, Luther preaches it, Washington arms it, Watt mechanizes it.

Parnassianism: A mid nineteenth-century movement in French literature. Followers of the movement stressed adherence to well-defined artistic forms as a reaction against the often chaotic expression of the artist's ego that dominated the work of the Romantics. The Parnassians also rejected the moral, ethical, and social themes exhibited in the works of French Romantics such as Victor Hugo. The aesthetic doctrines of the Parnassians strongly influenced the later symbolist and decadent movements. Members of the Parnassian school include Leconte de Lisle, Sully Prudhomme, Albert Glatigny, Francois Coppee, and Theodore de Banville.

Parody: In literary criticism, this term refers to an imitation of a serious literary work or the signature style of a particular author in a ridiculous manner. A typical parody adopts the style of the original and applies it to an inappropriate subject for humorous effect. Parody is a form of satire and could be considered the literary equivalent of a caricature or cartoon. Henry Fielding's *Shamela* is a parody of Samuel Richardson's *Pamela.*

Pastoral: A term derived from the Latin word ''pastor,'' meaning shepherd. A pastoral is a literary composition on a rural theme. The conventions of the pastoral were originated by the third-century Greek poet Theocritus, who wrote about the experiences, love affairs, and pastimes of Sicilian shepherds. In a pastoral, characters and language of a courtly nature are often placed in a simple setting. The term pastoral is also used to classify dramas, elegies, and lyrics that exhibit the use of country settings and shepherd characters. Percy Bysshe Shelley's ''Adonais'' and John Milton's ''Lycidas'' are two famous examples of pastorals.

Pastorela: The Spanish name for the shepherds play, a folk drama reenacted during the Christmas season. Examples of *pastorelas* include Gomez Manrique's *Representacion del nacimiento* and the dramas of Lucas Fernandez and Juan del Encina.

Pathetic Fallacy: A term coined by English critic John Ruskin to identify writing that falsely endows nonhuman things with human intentions and feelings, such as ''angry clouds'' and ''sad trees.'' The pathetic fallacy is a required convention in the classical poetic form of the pastoral elegy, and it is used in the modern poetry of T. S. Eliot, Ezra Pound, and the Imagists. Also known as Poetic Fallacy.

Pelado: Literally the ''skinned one'' or shirtless one, he was the stock underdog, sharp-witted picaresque character of Mexican vaudeville and tent shows. The *pelado* is found in such works as Don Catarino's *Los effectos de la crisis* and *Regreso a mi tierra.*

Pen Name: See *Pseudonym*

Pentameter: See *Meter*

Persona: A Latin term meaning ''mask.'' *Personae* are the characters in a fictional work of literature. The *persona* generally functions as a mask through which the author tells a story in a voice other than his or her own. A *persona* is usually either a character in a story who acts as a narrator or an ''implied author,'' a voice created by the author to act as the narrator for himself or herself. *Personae* include the narrator of Geoffrey Chaucer's *Canterbury Tales* and Marlow in Joseph Conrad's *Heart of Darkness.*

Personae: See *Persona*

Personal Point of View: See *Point of View*

Personification: A figure of speech that gives human qualities to abstract ideas, animals, and inanimate objects. William Shakespeare used personification in *Romeo and Juliet* in the lines ''Arise, fair sun, and kill the envious moon,/ Who is already sick and pale with grief.'' Here, the moon is portrayed as being envious, sick, and pale with grief—all markedly human qualities. Also known as *Prosopopoeia.*

Petrarchan Sonnet: See *Sonnet*

Phenomenology: A method of literary criticism based on the belief that things have no existence outside of human consciousness or awareness. Proponents of this theory believe that art is a process that takes place in the mind of the observer as he or she contemplates an object rather than a quality of the object itself. Among phenomenological critics are Edmund Husserl, George Poulet, Marcel Raymond, and Roman Ingarden.

Picaresque Novel: Episodic fiction depicting the adventures of a roguish central character (''picaro'' is Spanish for ''rogue''). The picaresque hero is commonly a low-born but clever individual who wanders into and out of various affairs of love, danger, and farcical intrigue. These involvements may take place at all social levels and typically present a humorous and wide-ranging satire of a given society. Prominent examples of the picaresque novel are *Don Quixote* by Miguel de Cervantes, *Tom Jones* by Henry Fielding, and *Moll Flanders* by Daniel Defoe.

Plagiarism: Claiming another person's written material as one's own. Plagiarism can take the form of direct, word-for- word copying or the theft of the substance or idea of the work. A student who copies an encyclopedia entry and turns it in as a report for school is guilty of plagiarism.

Platonic Criticism: A form of criticism that stresses an artistic work's usefulness as an agent of social engineering rather than any quality or value of the work itself. Platonic criticism takes as its starting point the ancient Greek philosopher Plato's comments on art in his *Republic.*

Platonism: The embracing of the doctrines of the philosopher Plato, popular among the poets of the Renaissance and the Romantic period. Platonism is more flexible than Aristotelian Criticism and places more emphasis on the supernatural and unknown aspects of life. Platonism is expressed in the love poetry of the Renaissance, the fourth book of Baldassare Castiglione's *The Book of the Courtier,* and the poetry of William Blake, William Wordsworth, Percy Bysshe Shelley, Friedrich Holderlin, William Butler Yeats, and Wallace Stevens.

Play: See *Drama*

Plot: In literary criticism, this term refers to the pattern of events in a narrative or drama. In its simplest sense, the plot guides the author in composing the work and helps the reader follow the work. Typically, plots exhibit causality and unity and have a beginning, a middle, and an end. Sometimes, however, a plot may consist of a series of disconnected events, in which case it is known as an "episodic plot." In his *Aspects of the Novel,* E. M. Forster distinguishes between a story, defined as a "narrative of events arranged in their time- sequence," and plot, which organizes the events to a "sense of causality." This definition closely mirrors Aristotle's discussion of plot in his *Poetics.*

Poem: In its broadest sense, a composition utilizing rhyme, meter, concrete detail, and expressive language to create a literary experience with emotional and aesthetic appeal. Typical poems include sonnets, odes, elegies, *haiku,* ballads, and free verse.

Poet: An author who writes poetry or verse. The term is also used to refer to an artist or writer who has an exceptional gift for expression, imagination, and energy in the making of art in any form. Well-known poets include Horace, Basho, Sir Philip Sidney, Sir Edmund Spenser, John Donne, Andrew Marvell, Alexander Pope, Jonathan Swift, George Gordon, Lord Byron, John Keats, Christina Rossetti, W. H. Auden, Stevie Smith, and Sylvia Plath.

Poetic Fallacy: See *Pathetic Fallacy*

Poetic Justice: An outcome in a literary work, not necessarily a poem, in which the good are rewarded and the evil are punished, especially in ways that particularly fit their virtues or crimes. For example, a murderer may himself be murdered, or a thief will find himself penniless.

Poetic License: Distortions of fact and literary convention made by a writer—not always a poet—for the sake of the effect gained. Poetic license is closely related to the concept of "artistic freedom." An author exercises poetic license by saying that a pile of money "reaches as high as a mountain" when the pile is actually only a foot or two high.

Poetics: This term has two closely related meanings. It denotes (1) an aesthetic theory in literary criticism about the essence of poetry or (2) rules prescribing the proper methods, content, style, or diction of poetry. The term poetics may also refer to theories about literature in general, not just poetry.

Poetry: In its broadest sense, writing that aims to present ideas and evoke an emotional experience in the reader through the use of meter, imagery, connotative and concrete words, and a carefully constructed structure based on rhythmic patterns. Poetry typically relies on words and expressions that have several layers of meaning. It also makes use of the effects of regular rhythm on the ear and may make a strong appeal to the senses through the use of imagery. Edgar Allan Poe's "Annabel Lee" and Walt Whitman's *Leaves of Grass* are famous examples of poetry.

Point of View: The narrative perspective from which a literary work is presented to the reader. There are four traditional points of view. The "third person omniscient" gives the reader a "godlike" perspective, unrestricted by time or place, from which to see actions and look into the minds of characters. This allows the author to comment openly on characters and events in the work. The "third person" point of view presents the events of the story from outside of any single character's perception, much like the omniscient point of view, but the reader must understand the action as it takes place and without any special insight into characters' minds or motivations. The "first person" or "personal" point of view relates events as they are perceived by a single character. The main character "tells" the story and may offer opinions about the action and characters which differ from those of the author. Much less common than omniscient, third person, and first person is the "second person" point of view, wherein the author tells the story as if it is happening to the reader. James Thurber employs the omniscient point of view in his short story "The Secret Life of Walter Mitty." Ernest Hemingway's "A Clean, Well-Lighted Place" is a short story told from the third person point of view. Mark Twain's novel *Huck Finn* is presented from the first person viewpoint. Jay McInerney's *Bright Lights, Big City* is an example of a novel which uses the second person point of view.

Polemic: A work in which the author takes a stand on a controversial subject, such as abortion or religion. Such works are often extremely argumentative or provocative. Classic examples of polemics include John Milton's *Aeropagitica* and Thomas Paine's *The American Crisis.*

Pornography: Writing intended to provoke feelings of lust in the reader. Such works are often condemned by critics and teachers, but those which can be shown to have literary value are viewed less harshly. Literary works that have been described as pornographic include Ovid's *The Art of Love,* Margaret of Angouleme's *Heptameron,* John Cleland's *Memoirs of a Woman of Pleasure; or, the Life of Fanny Hill,* the anonymous *My Secret Life,* D. H. Lawrence's *Lady Chatterley's Lover,* and Vladimir Nabokov's *Lolita.*

Post-Aesthetic Movement: An artistic response made by African Americans to the black aesthetic movement of the 1960s and early '70s. Writers since that time have adopted a somewhat different tone in their work, with less emphasis placed on the disparity between black and white in the United States. In the words of post-aesthetic authors such as Toni Morrison, John Edgar Wideman, and Kristin Hunter, African Americans are portrayed as looking inward for answers to their own questions, rather than always looking to the outside world. Two well-known examples of works produced as part of the post-aesthetic movement are the Pulitzer Prize-winning novels *The Color Purple* by Alice Walker and *Beloved* by Toni Morrison.

Postmodernism: Writing from the 1960s forward characterized by experimentation and continuing to apply some of the fundamentals of modernism, which included existentialism and alienation. Postmodernists have gone a step further in the rejection of tradition begun with the modernists by also rejecting traditional forms, preferring the anti-novel over the novel and the anti-hero over the hero. Postmodern writers include Alain Robbe-Grillet, Thomas Pynchon, Margaret Drabble, John Fowles, Adolfo Bioy-Casares, and Gabriel Garcia Marquez.

Pre-Raphaelites: A circle of writers and artists in mid nineteenth-century England. Valuing the pre-Renaissance artistic qualities of religious symbolism, lavish pictorialism, and natural sensuousness, the Pre-Raphaelites cultivated a sense of mystery and melancholy that influenced later writers associated with the Symbolist and Decadent movements. The major members of the group include Dante Gabriel Rossetti, Christina Rossetti, Algernon Swinburne, and Walter Pater.

Primitivism: The belief that primitive peoples were nobler and less flawed than civilized peoples because they had not been subjected to the tainting influence of society. Examples of literature espousing primitivism include Aphra Behn's *Oroonoko: Or, The History of the Royal Slave,* Jean-Jacques Rousseau's *Julie ou la Nouvelle Heloise,* Oliver Goldsmith's *The Deserted Village,* the poems of Robert Burns, Herman Melville's stories *Typee, Omoo,* and *Mardi,* many poems of William Butler Yeats and Robert Frost, and William Golding's novel *Lord of the Flies.*

Projective Verse: A form of free verse in which the poet's breathing pattern determines the lines of the poem. Poets who advocate projective verse are against all formal structures in writing, including meter and form. Besides its creators, Robert Creeley, Robert Duncan, and Charles Olson, two other well-known projective verse poets are Denise Levertov and LeRoi Jones (Amiri Baraka). Also known as Breath Verse.

Prologue: An introductory section of a literary work. It often contains information establishing the situation of the characters or presents information about the setting, time period, or action. In drama, the prologue is spoken by a chorus or by one of the principal characters. In the "General Prologue" of *The Canterbury Tales,* Geoffrey Chaucer describes the main characters and establishes the setting and purpose of the work.

Prose: A literary medium that attempts to mirror the language of everyday speech. It is distinguished from poetry by its use of unmetered, unrhymed language consisting of logically related sentences. Prose is usually grouped into paragraphs that form a cohesive whole such as an essay or a novel. Recognized masters of English prose writing include Sir Thomas Malory, William Caxton, Raphael Holinshed, Joseph Addison, Mark Twain, and Ernest Hemingway.

Prosopopoeia: See *Personification*

Protagonist: The central character of a story who serves as a focus for its themes and incidents and as the principal rationale for its development. The protagonist is sometimes referred to in discussions of modern literature as the hero or anti-hero. Well-known protagonists are Hamlet in William Shakespeare's *Hamlet* and Jay Gatsby in F. Scott Fitzgerald's *The Great Gatsby.*

Protest Fiction: Protest fiction has as its primary purpose the protesting of some social injustice, such as racism or discrimination. One example of protest fiction is a series of five novels by Chester Himes, beginning in 1945 with *If He Hollers Let Him Go* and ending in 1955 with *The Primitive.* These works depict the destructive effects of race and gender stereotyping in the context of interracial relationships. Another African American author whose works often revolve around themes of social protest is John Oliver Killens. James Baldwin's essay "Everybody's Protest Novel" generated controversy by attacking the authors of protest fiction.

Proverb: A brief, sage saying that expresses a truth about life in a striking manner. "They are not all cooks who carry long knives" is an example of a proverb.

Pseudonym: A name assumed by a writer, most often intended to prevent his or her identification as the author of a work. Two or more authors may work together under one pseudonym, or an author may use a different name for each genre he or she publishes in. Some publishing companies maintain ''house pseudonyms,'' under which any number of authors may write installations in a series. Some authors also choose a pseudonym over their real names the way an actor may use a stage name. Examples of pseudonyms (with the author's real name in parentheses) include Voltaire (Francois-Marie Arouet), Novalis (Friedrich von Hardenberg), Currer Bell (Charlotte Bronte), Ellis Bell (Emily Bronte), George Eliot (Maryann Evans), Honorio Bustos Donmecq (Adolfo Bioy-Casares and Jorge Luis Borges), and Richard Bachman (Stephen King).

Pun: A play on words that have similar sounds but different meanings. A serious example of the pun is from John Donne's ''A Hymne to God the Father'': Sweare by thyself, that at my death thy sonne Shall shine as he shines now, and hereto fore; And, having done that, Thou haste done; I fear no more.

Pure Poetry: poetry written without instructional intent or moral purpose that aims only to please a reader by its imagery or musical flow. The term pure poetry is used as the antonym of the term ''didacticism.'' The poetry of Edgar Allan Poe, Stephane Mallarme, Paul Verlaine, Paul Valery, Juan Ramoz Jimenez, and Jorge Guillen offer examples of pure poetry.

Q

Quatrain: A four-line stanza of a poem or an entire poem consisting of four lines. The following quatrain is from Robert Herrick's ''To Live Merrily, and to Trust to Good Verses'': Round, round, the root do's run; And being ravisht thus, Come, I will drink a Tun To my *Propertius.*

R

Raisonneur: A character in a drama who functions as a spokesperson for the dramatist's views. The *raisonneur* typically observes the play without becoming central to its action. *Raisonneurs* were very common in plays of the nineteenth century.

Realism: A nineteenth-century European literary movement that sought to portray familiar characters, situations, and settings in a realistic manner. This was done primarily by using an objective narrative point of view and through the buildup of accurate detail. The standard for success of any realistic work depends on how faithfully it transfers common experience into fictional forms. The realistic method may be altered or extended, as in stream of consciousness writing, to record highly subjective experience. Seminal authors in the tradition of Realism include Honore de Balzac, Gustave Flaubert, and Henry James.

Refrain: A phrase repeated at intervals throughout a poem. A refrain may appear at the end of each stanza or at less regular intervals. It may be altered slightly at each appearance. Some refrains are nonsense expressions—as with ''Nevermore'' in Edgar Allan Poe's ''The Raven''—that seem to take on a different significance with each use.

Renaissance: The period in European history that marked the end of the Middle Ages. It began in Italy in the late fourteenth century. In broad terms, it is usually seen as spanning the fourteenth, fifteenth, and sixteenth centuries, although it did not reach Great Britain, for example, until the 1480s or so. The Renaissance saw an awakening in almost every sphere of human activity, especially science, philosophy, and the arts. The period is best defined by the emergence of a general philosophy that emphasized the importance of the intellect, the individual, and world affairs. It contrasts strongly with the medieval worldview, characterized by the dominant concerns of faith, the social collective, and spiritual salvation. Prominent writers during the Renaissance include Niccolo Machiavelli and Baldassare Castiglione in Italy, Miguel de Cervantes and Lope de Vega in Spain, Jean Froissart and Francois Rabelais in France, Sir Thomas More and Sir Philip Sidney in England, and Desiderius Erasmus in Holland.

Repartee: Conversation featuring snappy retorts and witticisms. Masters of *repartee* include Sydney Smith, Charles Lamb, and Oscar Wilde. An example is recorded in the meeting of ''Beau'' Nash and John Wesley: Nash said, ''I never make way for a fool,'' to which Wesley responded, ''Don't you? I always do,'' and stepped aside.

Resolution: The portion of a story following the climax, in which the conflict is resolved. The resolution of Jane Austen's *Northanger Abbey* is neatly summed up in the following sentence: ''Henry and Catherine were married, the bells rang and every body smiled.''

Restoration: See *Restoration Age*

Restoration Age: A period in English literature beginning with the crowning of Charles II in 1660 and running to about 1700. The era, which was characterized by a reaction against Puritanism, was the first great age of the comedy of manners. The finest literature of the era is typically witty and urbane, and often lewd. Prominent Restoration Age writers include William Congreve, Samuel Pepys, John Dryden, and John Milton.

Revenge Tragedy: A dramatic form popular during the Elizabethan Age, in which the protagonist, directed by the ghost of his murdered father or son, inflicts retaliation upon a powerful villain. Notable features of the revenge tragedy include violence, bizarre criminal acts, intrigue, insanity, a hesitant protagonist, and the use of soliloquy. Thomas Kyd's *Spanish Tragedy* is the first example of revenge tragedy in English, and William Shakespeare's *Hamlet* is perhaps the best. Extreme examples of revenge tragedy, such as John Webster's *The Duchess of Malfi,* are labeled "tragedies of blood." Also known as Tragedy of Blood.

Revista: The Spanish term for a vaudeville musical revue. Examples of *revistas* include Antonio Guzman Aguilera's *Mexico para los mexicanos,* Daniel Vanegas's *Maldito jazz,* and Don Catarino's *Whiskey, morfina y marihuana* and *El desterrado.*

Rhetoric: In literary criticism, this term denotes the art of ethical persuasion. In its strictest sense, rhetoric adheres to various principles developed since classical times for arranging facts and ideas in a clear, persuasive, appealing manner. The term is also used to refer to effective prose in general and theories of or methods for composing effective prose. Classical examples of rhetorics include *The Rhetoric of Aristotle,* Quintillian's *Institutio Oratoria,* and Cicero's *Ad Herennium.*

Rhetorical Question: A question intended to provoke thought, but not an expressed answer, in the reader. It is most commonly used in oratory and other persuasive genres. The following lines from Thomas Gray's "Elegy Written in a Country Churchyard" ask rhetorical questions: Can storied urn or animated bust Back to its mansion call the fleeting breath? Can Honour's voice provoke the silent dust, Or Flattery soothe the dull cold ear of Death?

Rhyme: When used as a noun in literary criticism, this term generally refers to a poem in which words sound identical or very similar and appear in parallel positions in two or more lines. Rhymes are classified into different types according to where they fall in a line or stanza or according to the degree of similarity they exhibit in their spellings and sounds. Some major types of rhyme are "masculine" rhyme, "feminine" rhyme, and "triple" rhyme. In a masculine rhyme, the rhyming sound falls in a single accented syllable, as with "heat" and "eat." Feminine rhyme is a rhyme of two syllables, one stressed and one unstressed, as with "merry" and "tarry." Triple rhyme matches the sound of the accented syllable and the two unaccented syllables that follow: "narrative" and "declarative." Robert Browning alternates feminine and masculine rhymes in his "Soliloquy of the Spanish Cloister": Gr-r-r—there go, my heart's abhorrence! Water your damned flower-pots, do! If hate killed men, Brother Lawrence, God's blood, would not mine kill you! What? Your myrtle-bush wants trimming? Oh, that rose has prior claims— Needs its leaden vase filled brimming? Hell dry you up with flames! Triple rhymes can be found in Thomas Hood's "Bridge of Sighs," George Gordon Byron's satirical verse, and Ogden Nash's comic poems.

Rhyme Royal: A stanza of seven lines composed in iambic pentameter and rhymed *ababbcc.* The name is said to be a tribute to King James I of Scotland, who made much use of the form in his poetry. Examples of rhyme royal include Geoffrey Chaucer's *The Parlement of Foules,* William Shakespeare's *The Rape of Lucrece,* William Morris's *The Early Paradise,* and John Masefield's *The Widow in the Bye Street.*

Rhyme Scheme: See *Rhyme*

Rhythm: A regular pattern of sound, time intervals, or events occurring in writing, most often and most discernably in poetry. Regular, reliable rhythm is known to be soothing to humans, while interrupted, unpredictable, or rapidly changing rhythm is disturbing. These effects are known to authors, who use them to produce a desired reaction in the reader. An example of a form of irregular rhythm is sprung rhythm poetry; quantitative verse, on the other hand, is very regular in its rhythm.

Rising Action: The part of a drama where the plot becomes increasingly complicated. Rising action leads up to the climax, or turning point, of a drama. The final "chase scene" of an action film is generally the rising action which culminates in the film's climax.

Rococo: A style of European architecture that flourished in the eighteenth century, especially in France. The most notable features of *rococo* are its extensive use of ornamentation and its themes of lightness, gaiety, and intimacy. In literary criticism, the term is often used disparagingly to refer to a decadent or over-ornamental style. Alexander Pope's "The Rape of the Lock" is an example of literary *rococo.*

Roman a clef: A French phrase meaning "novel with a key." It refers to a narrative in which real persons are portrayed under fictitious names. Jack Kerouac, for example, portrayed various real-life beat generation figures under fictitious names in his *On the Road.*

Romance: A broad term, usually denoting a narrative with exotic, exaggerated, often idealized characters, scenes, and themes. Nathaniel Hawthorne called his *The House of the Seven Gables* and *The Marble Faun* romances in order to distinguish them from clearly realistic works.

Romantic Age: See *Romanticism*

Romanticism: This term has two widely accepted meanings. In historical criticism, it refers to a European intellectual and artistic movement of the late eighteenth and early nineteenth centuries that sought greater freedom of personal expression than that allowed by the strict rules of literary form and logic of the eighteenth-century neoclassicists. The Romantics preferred emotional and imaginative expression to rational analysis. They considered the individual to be at the center of all experience and so placed him or her at the center of their art. The Romantics believed that the creative imagination reveals nobler truths—unique feelings and attitudes—than those that could be discovered by logic or by scientific examination. Both the natural world and the state of childhood were important sources for revelations of "eternal truths." "Romanticism" is also used as a general term to refer to a type of sensibility found in all periods of literary history and usually considered to be in opposition to the principles of classicism. In this sense, Romanticism signifies any work or philosophy in which the exotic or dreamlike figure strongly, or that is devoted to individualistic expression, self-analysis, or a pursuit of a higher realm of knowledge than can be discovered by human reason. Prominent Romantics include Jean-Jacques Rousseau, William Wordsworth, John Keats, Lord Byron, and Johann Wolfgang von Goethe.

Romantics: See *Romanticism*

Russian Symbolism: A Russian poetic movement, derived from French symbolism, that flourished between 1894 and 1910. While some Russian Symbolists continued in the French tradition, stressing aestheticism and the importance of suggestion above didactic intent, others saw their craft as a form of mystical worship, and themselves as mediators between the supernatural and the mundane. Russian symbolists include Aleksandr Blok, Vyacheslav Ivanovich Ivanov, Fyodor Sologub, Andrey Bely, Nikolay Gumilyov, and Vladimir Sergeyevich Solovyov.

S

Satire: A work that uses ridicule, humor, and wit to criticize and provoke change in human nature and institutions. There are two major types of satire: "formal" or "direct" satire speaks directly to the reader or to a character in the work; "indirect" satire relies upon the ridiculous behavior of its characters to make its point. Formal satire is further divided into two manners: the "Horatian," which ridicules gently, and the "Juvenalian," which derides its subjects harshly and bitterly. Voltaire's novella *Candide* is an indirect satire. Jonathan Swift's essay "A Modest Proposal" is a Juvenalian satire.

Scansion: The analysis or "scanning" of a poem to determine its meter and often its rhyme scheme. The most common system of scansion uses accents (slanted lines drawn above syllables) to show stressed syllables, breves (curved lines drawn above syllables) to show unstressed syllables, and vertical lines to separate each foot. In the first line of John Keats's *Endymion,* "A thing of beauty is a joy forever:" the word "thing," the first syllable of "beauty," the word "joy," and the second syllable of "forever" are stressed, while the words "A" and "of," the second syllable of "beauty," the word "a," and the first and third syllables of "forever" are unstressed. In the second line: "Its loveliness increases; it will never" a pair of vertical lines separate the foot ending with "increases" and the one beginning with "it."

Scene: A subdivision of an act of a drama, consisting of continuous action taking place at a single time and in a single location. The beginnings and endings of scenes may be indicated by clearing the stage of actors and props or by the entrances and exits of important characters. The first act of William Shakespeare's *Winter's Tale* is comprised of two scenes.

Science Fiction: A type of narrative about or based upon real or imagined scientific theories and technology. Science fiction is often peopled with alien creatures and set on other planets or in different dimensions. Karel Capek's *R.U.R.* is a major work of science fiction.

Second Person: See *Point of View*

Semiotics: The study of how literary forms and conventions affect the meaning of language. Semioticians include Ferdinand de Saussure, Charles Sanders Pierce, Claude Levi-Strauss, Jacques Lacan, Michel Foucault, Jacques Derrida, Roland Barthes, and Julia Kristeva.

Sestet: Any six-line poem or stanza. Examples of the sestet include the last six lines of the Petrarchan sonnet form, the stanza form of Robert Burns's ''A Poet's Welcome to his love-begotten Daughter,'' and the sestina form in W. H. Auden's ''Paysage Moralise.''

Setting: The time, place, and culture in which the action of a narrative takes place. The elements of setting may include geographic location, characters' physical and mental environments, prevailing cultural attitudes, or the historical time in which the action takes place. Examples of settings include the romanticized Scotland in Sir Walter Scott's ''Waverley'' novels, the French provincial setting in Gustave Flaubert's *Madame Bovary,* the fictional Wessex country of Thomas Hardy's novels, and the small towns of southern Ontario in Alice Munro's short stories.

Shakespearean Sonnet: See *Sonnet*

Signifying Monkey: A popular trickster figure in black folklore, with hundreds of tales about this character documented since the 19th century. Henry Louis Gates Jr. examines the history of the signifying monkey in *The Signifying Monkey: Towards a Theory of Afro-American Literary Criticism,* published in 1988.

Simile: A comparison, usually using ''like'' or ''as'', of two essentially dissimilar things, as in ''coffee as cold as ice'' or ''He sounded like a broken record.'' The title of Ernest Hemingway's ''Hills Like White Elephants'' contains a simile.

Slang: A type of informal verbal communication that is generally unacceptable for formal writing. Slang words and phrases are often colorful exaggerations used to emphasize the speaker's point; they may also be shortened versions of an often-used word or phrase. Examples of American slang from the 1990s include ''yuppie'' (an acronym for Young Urban Professional), ''awesome'' (for ''excellent''), wired (for ''nervous'' or ''excited''), and ''chill out'' (for relax).

Slant Rhyme: See *Consonance*

Slave Narrative: Autobiographical accounts of American slave life as told by escaped slaves. These works first appeared during the abolition movement of the 1830s through the 1850s. Olaudah Equiano's *The Interesting Narrative of Olaudah Equiano, or Gustavus Vassa, The African* and Harriet Ann Jacobs's *Incidents in the Life of a Slave Girl* are examples of the slave narrative.

Social Realism: See *Socialist Realism*

Socialist Realism: The Socialist Realism school of literary theory was proposed by Maxim Gorky and established as a dogma by the first Soviet Congress of Writers. It demanded adherence to a communist worldview in works of literature. Its doctrines required an objective viewpoint comprehensible to the working classes and themes of social struggle featuring strong proletarian heroes. A successful work of socialist realism is Nikolay Ostrovsky's *Kak zakalyalas stal* (*How the Steel Was Tempered*). Also known as Social Realism.

Soliloquy: A monologue in a drama used to give the audience information and to develop the speaker's character. It is typically a projection of the speaker's innermost thoughts. Usually delivered while the speaker is alone on stage, a soliloquy is intended to present an illusion of unspoken reflection. A celebrated soliloquy is Hamlet's ''To be or not to be'' speech in William Shakespeare's *Hamlet.*

Sonnet: A fourteen-line poem, usually composed in iambic pentameter, employing one of several rhyme schemes. There are three major types of sonnets, upon which all other variations of the form are based: the ''Petrarchan'' or ''Italian'' sonnet, the ''Shakespearean'' or ''English'' sonnet, and the ''Spenserian'' sonnet. A Petrarchan sonnet consists of an octave rhymed *abbaabba* and a ''sestet'' rhymed either *cdecde, cdccdc,* or *cdedce.* The octave poses a question or problem, relates a narrative, or puts forth a proposition; the sestet presents a solution to the problem, comments upon the narrative, or applies the proposition put forth in the octave. The Shakespearean sonnet is divided into three quatrains and a couplet rhymed *abab cdcd efef gg.* The couplet provides an epigrammatic comment on the narrative or problem put forth in the quatrains. The Spenserian sonnet uses three quatrains and a couplet like the Shakespearean, but links their three rhyme schemes in this way: *abab bcbc cdcd ee.* The Spenserian sonnet develops its theme in two parts like the Petrarchan, its final six lines resolving a problem, analyzing a narrative, or applying a proposition put forth in its first eight lines. Examples of sonnets can be found in Petrarch's *Canzoniere,* Edmund Spenser's *Amoretti,* Elizabeth Barrett Browning's *Sonnets from the Portuguese,* Rainer Maria Rilke's *Sonnets to Orpheus,* and Adrienne Rich's poem "The Insusceptibles."

Spenserian Sonnet: See *Sonnet*

Spenserian Stanza: A nine-line stanza having eight verses in iambic pentameter, its ninth verse in iambic hexameter, and the rhyme scheme ababbcbcc. This stanza form was first used by Edmund Spenser in his allegorical poem *The Faerie Queene.*

Spondee: In poetry meter, a foot consisting of two long or stressed syllables occurring together. This form is quite rare in English verse, and is usually composed of two monosyllabic words. The first foot in the following line from Robert Burns's "Green Grow the Rashes" is an example of a spondee: Green grow the rashes, O

Sprung Rhythm: Versification using a specific number of accented syllables per line but disregarding the number of unaccented syllables that fall in each line, producing an irregular rhythm in the poem. Gerard Manley Hopkins, who coined the term "sprung rhythm," is the most notable practitioner of this technique.

Stanza: A subdivision of a poem consisting of lines grouped together, often in recurring patterns of rhyme, line length, and meter. Stanzas may also serve as units of thought in a poem much like paragraphs in prose. Examples of stanza forms include the quatrain, *terza rima, ottava rima,* Spenserian, and the so-called *In Memoriam* stanza from Alfred, Lord Tennyson's poem by that title. The following is an example of the latter form: Love is and was my lord and king, And in his presence I attend To hear the tidings of my friend, Which every hour his couriers bring.

Stereotype: A stereotype was originally the name for a duplication made during the printing process; this led to its modern definition as a person or thing that is (or is assumed to be) the same as all others of its type. Common stereotypical characters include the absent- minded professor, the nagging wife, the troublemaking teenager, and the kindhearted grandmother.

Stream of Consciousness: A narrative technique for rendering the inward experience of a character. This technique is designed to give the impression of an ever-changing series of thoughts, emotions, images, and memories in the spontaneous and seemingly illogical order that they occur in life. The textbook example of stream of consciousness is the last section of James Joyce's *Ulysses.*

Structuralism: A twentieth-century movement in literary criticism that examines how literary texts arrive at their meanings, rather than the meanings themselves. There are two major types of structuralist analysis: one examines the way patterns of linguistic structures unify a specific text and emphasize certain elements of that text, and the other interprets the way literary forms and conventions affect the meaning of language itself. Prominent structuralists include Michel Foucault, Roman Jakobson, and Roland Barthes.

Structure: The form taken by a piece of literature. The structure may be made obvious for ease of understanding, as in nonfiction works, or may obscured for artistic purposes, as in some poetry or seemingly "unstructured" prose. Examples of common literary structures include the plot of a narrative, the acts and scenes of a drama, and such poetic forms as the Shakespearean sonnet and the Pindaric ode.

Sturm und Drang: A German term meaning "storm and stress." It refers to a German literary movement of the 1770s and 1780s that reacted against the order and rationalism of the enlightenment, focusing instead on the intense experience of extraordinary individuals. Highly romantic, works of this movement, such as Johann Wolfgang von Goethe's *Gotz von Berlichingen,* are typified by realism, rebelliousness, and intense emotionalism.

Style: A writer's distinctive manner of arranging words to suit his or her ideas and purpose in writing. The unique imprint of the author's personality upon his or her writing, style is the product of an author's way of arranging ideas and his or her use of diction, different sentence structures, rhythm, figures of speech, rhetorical principles, and other elements of composition. Styles may be classified according to period (Metaphysical, Augustan, Georgian), individual authors (Chaucerian, Miltonic, Jamesian), level (grand, middle, low, plain), or language (scientific, expository, poetic, journalistic).

Subject: The person, event, or theme at the center of a work of literature. A work may have one or more subjects of each type, with shorter works tending to have fewer and longer works tending to have more. The subjects of James Baldwin's novel *Go Tell It on the Mountain* include the themes of father-son relationships, religious conversion, black life, and sexuality. The subjects of Anne Frank's *Diary of a Young Girl* include Anne and her family members as well as World War II, the Holocaust, and the themes of war, isolation, injustice, and racism.

Subjectivity: Writing that expresses the author's personal feelings about his subject, and which may or may not include factual information about the subject. Subjectivity is demonstrated in James Joyce's *Portrait of the Artist as a Young Man,* Samuel Butler's *The Way of All Flesh,* and Thomas Wolfe's *Look Homeward, Angel.*

Subplot: A secondary story in a narrative. A subplot may serve as a motivating or complicating force for the main plot of the work, or it may provide emphasis for, or relief from, the main plot. The conflict between the Capulets and the Montagues in William Shakespeare's *Romeo and Juliet* is an example of a subplot.

Surrealism: A term introduced to criticism by Guillaume Apollinaire and later adopted by Andre Breton. It refers to a French literary and artistic movement founded in the 1920s. The Surrealists sought to express unconscious thoughts and feelings in their works. The best-known technique used for achieving this aim was automatic writing—transcriptions of spontaneous outpourings from the unconscious. The Surrealists proposed to unify the contrary levels of conscious and unconscious, dream and reality, objectivity and subjectivity into a new level of "super-realism." Surrealism can be found in the poetry of Paul Eluard, Pierre Reverdy, and Louis Aragon, among others.

Suspense: A literary device in which the author maintains the audience's attention through the buildup of events, the outcome of which will soon be revealed. Suspense in William Shakespeare's *Hamlet* is sustained throughout by the question of whether or not the Prince will achieve what he has been instructed to do and of what he intends to do.

Syllogism: A method of presenting a logical argument. In its most basic form, the syllogism consists of a major premise, a minor premise, and a conclusion. An example of a syllogism is: Major premise: When it snows, the streets get wet. Minor premise: It is snowing. Conclusion: The streets are wet.

Symbol: Something that suggests or stands for something else without losing its original identity. In literature, symbols combine their literal meaning with the suggestion of an abstract concept. Literary symbols are of two types: those that carry complex associations of meaning no matter what their contexts, and those that derive their suggestive meaning from their functions in specific literary works. Examples of symbols are sunshine suggesting happiness, rain suggesting sorrow, and storm clouds suggesting despair.

Symbolism: This term has two widely accepted meanings. In historical criticism, it denotes an early modernist literary movement initiated in France during the nineteenth century that reacted against the prevailing standards of realism. Writers in this movement aimed to evoke, indirectly and symbolically, an order of being beyond the material world of the five senses. Poetic expression of personal emotion figured strongly in the movement, typically by means of a private set of symbols uniquely identifiable with the individual poet. The principal aim of the Symbolists was to express in words the highly complex feelings that grew out of everyday contact with the world. In a broader sense, the term "symbolism" refers to the use of one object to represent another. Early members of the Symbolist movement included the French authors Charles Baudelaire and Arthur Rimbaud; William Butler Yeats, James Joyce, and T. S. Eliot were influenced as the movement moved to Ireland, England, and the United States. Examples of the concept of symbolism include a flag that stands for a nation or movement, or an empty cupboard used to suggest hopelessness, poverty, and despair.

Symbolist: See *Symbolism*

Symbolist Movement: See *Symbolism*

Sympathetic Fallacy: See *Affective Fallacy*

T

Tale: A story told by a narrator with a simple plot and little character development. Tales are usually relatively short and often carry a simple message. Examples of tales can be found in the work of Rudyard Kipling, Somerset Maugham, Saki, Anton Chekhov, Guy de Maupassant, and Armistead Maupin.

Tall Tale: A humorous tale told in a straightforward, credible tone but relating absolutely impossible events or feats of the characters. Such tales were commonly told of frontier adventures during the settlement of the west in the United States. Tall tales have been spun around such legendary heroes as Mike Fink, Paul Bunyan, Davy Crockett, Johnny Appleseed, and Captain Stormalong as well as the real-life William F. Cody and Annie Oakley. Literary use of tall tales can be found in Washington Irving's *History of New York,* Mark Twain's *Life on the Mississippi,* and in the German R. F. Raspe's *Baron Munchausen's Narratives of His Marvellous Travels and Campaigns in Russia.*

Tanka: A form of Japanese poetry similar to *haiku.* A *tanka* is five lines long, with the lines containing five, seven, five, seven, and seven syllables respectively. Skilled *tanka* authors include Ishikawa Takuboku, Masaoka Shiki, Amy Lowell, and Adelaide Crapsey.

Teatro Grottesco: See *Theater of the Grotesque*

Terza Rima: A three-line stanza form in poetry in which the rhymes are made on the last word of each line in the following manner: the first and third lines of the first stanza, then the second line of the first stanza and the first and third lines of the second stanza, and so on with the middle line of any stanza rhyming with the first and third lines of the following stanza. An example of *terza rima* is Percy Bysshe Shelley's ''The Triumph of Love'': As in that trance of wondrous thought I lay This was the tenour of my waking dream. Methought I sate beside a public way Thick strewn with summer dust, and a great stream Of people there was hurrying to and fro Numerous as gnats upon the evening gleam,. . .

Tetrameter: See *Meter*

Textual Criticism: A branch of literary criticism that seeks to establish the authoritative text of a literary work. Textual critics typically compare all known manuscripts or printings of a single work in order to assess the meanings of differences and revisions. This procedure allows them to arrive at a definitive version that (supposedly) corresponds to the author's original intention. Textual criticism was applied during the Renaissance to salvage the classical texts of Greece and Rome, and modern works have been studied, for instance, to undo deliberate correction or censorship, as in the case of novels by Stephen Crane and Theodore Dreiser.

Theater of Cruelty: Term used to denote a group of theatrical techniques designed to eliminate the psychological and emotional distance between actors and audience. This concept, introduced in the 1930s in France, was intended to inspire a more intense theatrical experience than conventional theater allowed. The ''cruelty'' of this dramatic theory signified not sadism but heightened actor/audience involvement in the dramatic event. The theater of cruelty was theorized by Antonin Artaud in his *Le Theatre et son double* (*The Theatre and Its Double*), and also appears in the work of Jerzy Grotowski, Jean Genet, Jean Vilar, and Arthur Adamov, among others.

Theater of the Absurd: A post-World War II dramatic trend characterized by radical theatrical innovations. In works influenced by the Theater of the absurd, nontraditional, sometimes grotesque characterizations, plots, and stage sets reveal a meaningless universe in which human values are irrelevant. Existentialist themes of estrangement, absurdity, and futility link many of the works of this movement. The principal writers of the Theater of the Absurd are Samuel Beckett, Eugene Ionesco, Jean Genet, and Harold Pinter.

Theater of the Grotesque: An Italian theatrical movement characterized by plays written around the ironic and macabre aspects of daily life in the World War I era. Theater of the Grotesque was named after the play *The Mask and the Face* by Luigi Chiarelli, which was described as ''a grotesque in three acts.'' The movement influenced the work of Italian dramatist Luigi Pirandello, author of *Right You Are, If You Think You Are.* Also known as *Teatro Grottesco.*

Theme: The main point of a work of literature. The term is used interchangeably with thesis. The theme of William Shakespeare's *Othello*—jealousy—is a common one.

Thesis: A thesis is both an essay and the point argued in the essay. Thesis novels and thesis plays share the quality of containing a thesis which is supported through the action of the story. A master's thesis and a doctoral dissertation are two theses required of graduate students.

Thesis Play: See *Thesis*

Three Unities: See *Unities*

Tone: The author's attitude toward his or her audience may be deduced from the tone of the work. A formal tone may create distance or convey politeness, while an informal tone may encourage a friendly, intimate, or intrusive feeling in the reader. The author's attitude toward his or her subject matter may also be deduced from the tone of the words he or she uses in discussing it. The tone of John F. Kennedy's speech which included the appeal to "ask not what your country can do for you" was intended to instill feelings of camaraderie and national pride in listeners.

Tragedy: A drama in prose or poetry about a noble, courageous hero of excellent character who, because of some tragic character flaw or *hamartia*, brings ruin upon him- or herself. Tragedy treats its subjects in a dignified and serious manner, using poetic language to help evoke pity and fear and bring about catharsis, a purging of these emotions. The tragic form was practiced extensively by the ancient Greeks. In the Middle Ages, when classical works were virtually unknown, tragedy came to denote any works about the fall of persons from exalted to low conditions due to any reason: fate, vice, weakness, etc. According to the classical definition of tragedy, such works present the "pathetic"—that which evokes pity—rather than the tragic. The classical form of tragedy was revived in the sixteenth century; it flourished especially on the Elizabethan stage. In modern times, dramatists have attempted to adapt the form to the needs of modern society by drawing their heroes from the ranks of ordinary men and women and defining the nobility of these heroes in terms of spirit rather than exalted social standing. The greatest classical example of tragedy is Sophocles' *Oedipus Rex.* The "pathetic" derivation is exemplified in "The Monk's Tale" in Geoffrey Chaucer's *Canterbury Tales.* Notable works produced during the sixteenth century revival include William Shakespeare's *Hamlet, Othello,* and *King Lear.* Modern dramatists working in the tragic tradition include Henrik Ibsen, Arthur Miller, and Eugene O'Neill.

Tragedy of Blood: See *Revenge Tragedy*

Tragic Flaw: In a tragedy, the quality within the hero or heroine which leads to his or her downfall. Examples of the tragic flaw include Othello's jealousy and Hamlet's indecisiveness, although most great tragedies defy such simple interpretation.

Transcendentalism: An American philosophical and religious movement, based in New England from around 1835 until the Civil War. Transcendentalism was a form of American romanticism that had its roots abroad in the works of Thomas Carlyle, Samuel Coleridge, and Johann Wolfgang von Goethe. The Transcendentalists stressed the importance of intuition and subjective experience in communication with God. They rejected religious dogma and texts in favor of mysticism and scientific naturalism. They pursued truths that lie beyond the "colorless" realms perceived by reason and the senses and were active social reformers in public education, women's rights, and the abolition of slavery. Prominent members of the group include Ralph Waldo Emerson and Henry David Thoreau.

Trickster: A character or figure common in Native American and African literature who uses his ingenuity to defeat enemies and escape difficult situations. Tricksters are most often animals, such as the spider, hare, or coyote, although they may take the form of humans as well. Examples of trickster tales include Thomas King's *A Coyote Columbus Story,* Ashley F. Bryan's *The Dancing Granny* and Ishmael Reed's *The Last Days of Louisiana Red.*

Trimeter: See *Meter*

Triple Rhyme: See *Rhyme*

Trochee: See *Foot*

U

Understatement: See *Irony*

Unities: Strict rules of dramatic structure, formulated by Italian and French critics of the Renaissance and based loosely on the principles of drama discussed by Aristotle in his *Poetics.* Foremost among these rules were the three unities of action, time, and place that compelled a dramatist to: (1) construct a single plot with a beginning, middle, and end that details the causal relationships of action and character; (2) restrict the action to the events of a single day; and (3) limit the scene to a single place or city. The unities were observed faithfully by continental European writers until the Romantic Age, but they were never regularly observed in English drama. Modern dramatists are typically more concerned with a unity of impression or emotional effect than with any of the classical unities. The unities are observed in Pierre Corneille's tragedy *Polyeuctes* and Jean-Baptiste Racine's *Phedre.* Also known as Three Unities.

Urban Realism: A branch of realist writing that attempts to accurately reflect the often harsh facts of modern urban existence. Some works by Stephen Crane, Theodore Dreiser, Charles Dickens, Fyodor Dostoyevsky, Emile Zola, Abraham Cahan, and Henry Fuller feature urban realism. Modern examples include Claude Brown's *Manchild in the Promised Land* and Ron Milner's *What the Wine Sellers Buy.*

Utopia: A fictional perfect place, such as ''paradise'' or ''heaven.'' Early literary utopias were included in Plato's *Republic* and Sir Thomas More's *Utopia,* while more modern utopias can be found in Samuel Butler's *Erewhon,* Theodor Herzka's *A Visit to Freeland,* and H. G. Wells' *A Modern Utopia.*

Utopian: See *Utopia*

Utopianism: See *Utopia*

V

Verisimilitude: Literally, the appearance of truth. In literary criticism, the term refers to aspects of a work of literature that seem true to the reader. Verisimilitude is achieved in the work of Honore de Balzac, Gustave Flaubert, and Henry James, among other late nineteenth-century realist writers.

Vers de societe: See *Occasional Verse*

Vers libre: See *Free Verse*

Verse: A line of metered language, a line of a poem, or any work written in verse. The following line of verse is from the epic poem *Don Juan* by Lord Byron: ''My way is to begin with the beginning.''

Versification: The writing of verse. Versification may also refer to the meter, rhyme, and other mechanical components of a poem. Composition of a ''Roses are red, violets are blue'' poem to suit an occasion is a common form of versification practiced by students.

Victorian: Refers broadly to the reign of Queen Victoria of England (1837-1901) and to anything with qualities typical of that era. For example, the qualities of smug narrowmindedness, bourgeois materialism, faith in social progress, and priggish morality are often considered Victorian. This stereotype is contradicted by such dramatic intellectual developments as the theories of Charles Darwin, Karl Marx, and Sigmund Freud (which stirred strong debates in England) and the critical attitudes of serious Victorian writers like Charles Dickens and George Eliot. In literature, the Victorian Period was the great age of the English novel, and the latter part of the era saw the rise of movements such as decadence and symbolism. Works of Victorian literature include the poetry of Robert Browning and Alfred, Lord Tennyson, the criticism of Matthew Arnold and John Ruskin, and the novels of Emily Bronte, William Makepeace Thackeray, and Thomas Hardy. Also known as Victorian Age and Victorian Period.

Victorian Age: See *Victorian*

Victorian Period: See *Victorian*

W

Weltanschauung: A German term referring to a person's worldview or philosophy. Examples of *weltanschauung* include Thomas Hardy's view of the human being as the victim of fate, destiny, or impersonal forces and circumstances, and the disillusioned and laconic cynicism expressed by such poets of the 1930s as W. H. Auden, Sir Stephen Spender, and Sir William Empson.

Weltschmerz: A German term meaning ''world pain.'' It describes a sense of anguish about the nature of existence, usually associated with a melancholy, pessimistic attitude. *Weltschmerz* was expressed in England by George Gordon, Lord Byron in his *Manfred* and *Childe Harold's Pilgrimage,* in France by Viscount de Chateaubriand, Alfred de Vigny, and Alfred de Musset, in Russia by Aleksandr Pushkin and Mikhail Lermontov, in Poland by Juliusz Slowacki, and in America by Nathaniel Hawthorne.

Z

Zarzuela: A type of Spanish operetta. Writers of *zarzuelas* include Lope de Vega and Pedro Calderon.

Zeitgeist: A German term meaning ''spirit of the time.'' It refers to the moral and intellectual trends of a given era. Examples of *zeitgeist* include the preoccupation with the more morbid aspects of dying and death in some Jacobean literature, especially in the works of dramatists Cyril Tourneur and John Webster, and the decadence of the French Symbolists.

Cumulative Author/Title Index

Y

Z

Nationality/Ethnicity Index

Subject/Theme Index

*Boldface terms appear as subheads in Themes section.

D

E

F

G